Sports Medicine
The School-Age Athlete

This book is dedicated with love and gratitude
to my wife, Trish
and my parents, Edward and Blanche Reider

CONTRIBUTORS

JOHN P. ALBRIGHT, M.D.
Professor, Department of Orthopaedic Surgery, University of Iowa College of Medicine, Iowa City; Director of Sports Medicine Services, University of Iowa Hospitals and Clinics, Iowa City, Iowa
Wrestling

ROBERT K. ALEJO, B.A.
Conditioning Coach, Department of Athletics, University of California at Los Angeles, Los Angeles, California
Endurance Training

DAVID W. ALTCHEK, M.D.
Assistant Professor, Department of Surgery (Orthopaedics), Cornell University Medical College, New York; Assistant Attending Orthopaedic Surgeon, The Hospital for Special Surgery, New York, New York
Shoulder Instability

ROBERT BELNIAK, M.D.
Clinical Associate, Department of Orthopaedic Surgery, University of Connecticut Health Sciences Center; Attending Orthopaedist, New Britain General Hospital, New Britain, Connecticut
Football

TURNER A. BLACKBURN, Jr.
Adjunct Assistant Professor, Department of Sports Medicine, Columbus College, Columbus; Director of Physical Therapy, Rehabilitation Services of Columbus, Inc., Columbus, Georgia
Physical Modalities in Rehabilitation

MICHAEL BRAGE, M.D.
Chief Resident, Section of Orthopaedic Surgery and Rehabilitation Medicine, Department of Surgery, University of Chicago Hospitals, Chicago, Illinois
Ankle Injuries

WILLIAM BRYAN, M.D.
Clinical Associate Professor, Division of Orthopedics, Baylor College of Medicine, Waco; Team Physician, Houston Astros, Houston; Fondren Orthopedic Group, Joe W. King Institute for Orthopedic Surgery, Houston; Attending Physician, The Methodist Hospital, Houston, Texas
Baseball

WILLIAM G. CLANCY, Jr., M.D.
Clinical Professor, Department of Orthopedic Surgery, University of Virginia School of Medicine, Charlottesville; Virginia; Staff Physician, Health South Medical Center, Birmingham, Alabama
Running

v

CONTRIBUTORS

KENNETH E. DeHAVEN, M.D.
Professor and Associate Chairman, Department of Orthopaedics, University of Rochester Medical Center, Rochester; Director of Athletic Medicine, Strong Memorial Hospital, Rochester, New York
Meniscus Tears

PETER J. FOWLER, M.D., F.R.C.S.(C)
Professor, Department of Orthopaedic Surgery, University of Western Ontario Medical School, London, Ontario; Orthopaedic Surgeon, University Hospital, London, Ontario, Canada
Swimming

JONATHAN L. FRANKLIN
Clinical Instructor, Department of Orthopaedics, University of Washington, Seattle; Active Staff, Ballard Community Hospital, Seattle; Active Staff, Swedish Medical Center, Seattle, Washington
Skiing

FREDDIE H. FU, M.D.
Blue Cross of Western Pennsylvania Professor, Department of Orthopaedic Surgery, Head Team Physician, Chief, Division of Sports Medicine, University of Pittsburgh, Pittsburgh; Center for Sports Medicine and Rehabilitation, Presbyterian-University Hospital, Pittsburgh, Pennsylvania
Injuries Involving the Clavicle; Elbow Dislocations

C. KEITH FUJISAKI, M.D.
Assistant Clinical Professor, Department of Orthopaedic Surgery, University of Colorado, Denver, Colorado
Disorders of the Patellar Tendon

WILLIAM E. GARRETT, Jr., M.D., Ph.D.
Assistant Professor, Division of Orthopaedic Surgery and Department of Cell Biology, Duke University Medical Center, Durham; Consultant and Attending Physician, Orthopaedic Surgery, Durham V. A. Hospital, Durham; Consultant, Orthopaedic Surgery, Person County Memorial Hospital, Roxboro, North Carolina
Muscle Strains and Contusions; Soccer

WAYNE GERSOFF, M.D.
Assistant Professor and Director, Division of Sports Medicine, Department of Orthopedic Surgery, Team Orthopedic Surgeon, University of Colorado, Denver, Colorado
Head and Neck Injuries

BEN K. GRAF, M.D.
Assistant Professor, Division of Orthopaedic Surgery, University of Wisconsin, Madison; University of Wisconsin Hospital, Madison, Wisconsin
Osteochondritis Dissecans; Disorders of the Patellar Tendon

MICHAEL L. GROSS, M.D.
Private Practice; Orthopedic and Sports Medicine Associates, Westwood, New Jersey
Spondylolysis and Spondylolisthesis

WILLIAM G. HAMILTON, M.D.
Assistant Clinical Professor, Department of Orthopedic Surgery, College of Physicians and Surgeons, Columbia University, New York; Senior Attending Orthopedic Surgeon, The Roosevelt Hospital, New York; Assistant Attending Orthopedic Surgeon, The Hospital for Special Surgery, New York; Assistant Attending Orthopedic Surgeon, The Presbyterian Hospital, New York; Orthopedic Surgeon for the New York City Ballet, the American Ballet Theatre, and the School of American Ballet, New York, New York
Ballet

SALLY S. HARRIS, M.D., M.P.H.
Clinical Instructor and Sports Medicine Fellow, Division of Family Medicine, University of California at Los Angeles, Los Angeles, California
The Preparticipation Exam

HERBERT A. HAUPT, M.D.
Missouri Baptist Medical Center; Attending Orthopaedic Surgeon, St. Luke's West Hospital; West County Surgery Center, St. Louis, Missouri
Strength Training; Ergogenic Aids

JOHN HEIL
Clinical Psychologist and Coordinator of Psychological Services, Pain Control Center, Lewis-Gale Clinic, Salem, Virginia
Psychological Aspects of Sports Medicine

JAMES T. HOEGH, A.T.C., L.P.T.
Assistant Trainer, University of Iowa, Iowa City, Iowa
Wrestling

ROBERT HUNTER
Clinical Associate Professor, Department of Orthopaedic Surgery, University of Colorado, Denver; Staff, Aspen Valley Hospitals, Aspen; Valley View Hospital, Glenwood Springs, Colorado
Hockey

PATRICIA A. KOLOWICH, M.D.
Center for Athletic Medicine, Henry Ford Hospital, Detroit, Michigan
Patellar Instability and Pain

RICHARD H. LANGE, M.D.
Assistant Professor, Division of Orthopaedic Surgery, University of Wisconsin, Madison; University of Wisconsin Hospital, Madison, Wisconsin
Osteochondritis Dissecans

JOHN LARKIN, M.D.
Assistant Professor, Section of Orthopaedic Surgery and Rehabilitation Medicine, Department of Surgery, The University of Chicago, Chicago; Attending Orthopaedic Surgeon, The University of Chicago Hospitals, Chicago, Illinois
Ankle Injuries

CONTRIBUTORS

B. CRAIG LEE, P.T., A.T.C.
Director of Rehabilitation Services, The Medical Center, Inc., Columbus, Georgia
Physical Modalities in Rehabilitation

JOHN LOHNES, P.A.-C., B.H.S.
Physician Assistant, Duke University Medical Center, Durham, North Carolina
Muscle Strain and Contusions; Soccer

DANIEL P. MASS, M.D.
Professor, Section of Orthopaedic Surgery and Rehabilitation Medicine Department of Surgery, The University of Chicago, Chicago; The University of Chicago Hospitals, Chicago, Illinois
Hand and Wrist Injuries

BERT R. MANDELBAUM, M.D.
Adjunct Assistant Professor, University of California at Los Angeles, Los Angeles; Attending Surgeon, St. Johns Hospital, Santa Monica; University of California at Los Angeles Hospital, Los Angeles; Santa Monica Hospital, Santa Monica, California
Spondylolysis and Spondylolisthesis; Gymnastics

ANGUS McBRYDE, Jr., M.D.
Clinical Assistant Professor, Department of Orthopaedics, Duke University Medical Center, Durham; Attending Physician, Carolinas Medical Center, Charlotte; Senior Attending Physician, Orthopaedic Hospital of Charlotte, Charlotte, North Carolina
Great Toe Metatarsophalangeal Joint Problems

WALTER McCOMBS, B.S., A.T., C
Head Basketball Trainer, University of Kentucky, Lexington, Kentucky
Basketball and Volleyball

DARRYL W. MILLER, M.S., Exer. Phys., A.T.C.
Program Director and Instructor, Health Sciences Center, University of Colorado, Denver, Colorado
Football

ROBERT P. NIRSCHL, M.D.
Founding Medical Director, Virginia Sports Medicine Institute, Arlington; Senior Attending Orthopedic Surgeon, Arlington Hospital, Arlington, Virginia; Assistant Clinical Professor, Department of Orthopedic Surgery, Georgetown University School of Medicine, Washington, D.C.
Tennis

PAUL A. NITZ, M.D.
Staff, St. Elizabeth Hospital, Dayton, Ohio
Anterior Cruciate Ligament Injuries; Posterior Cruciate Ligament Injuries

LONNIE E. PAULOS, M.D.
Associate Clinical Professor, Department of Orthopaedic Surgery, The University of Utah School of Medicine, Salt Lake City; Co-Director, Intermountain Orthopaedic Research Lab, Salt Lake City; Co-Director Salt Lake City Knee and Sports Medicine Research Foundation, Salt Lake City, Utah
Patellar Instability and Pain; Skiing

ROBERT M. POOLE, M.Ed., P.T., A.T.C.
Adjunct Associate Professor, Department of Sports Medicine, Columbus College, Columbus, Georgia
Physical Modalities in Rehabilitation

WILLIAM G. RAASCH, M.D.
Chief Resident, Section of Orthopaedic Surgery and Rehabilitation Medicine, Department of Surgery, The University of Chicago Hospitals, Chicago, Illinois
Hand and Wrist Injuries

JAMES MICHAEL RAY, M.D.
Associate Professor, Department of Orthopedic Surgery, Director of Sports Medicine Section, Division of Orthopedics, University of Kentucky Medical Center, Lexington, Kentucky
Basketball and Volleyball

BRUCE REIDER, M.D.
Associate Professor, Section of Orthopaedic Surgery and Rehabilitation Medicine, Department of Surgery, The University of Chicago, Chicago; Director of Sports Medicine, The University of Chicago Hospitals, Chicago, Illinois.
Collaterial Ligament Injuries; Disorders of the Patellar Tendon; Football

THOMAS D. ROSENBERG, M.D.
Associate Clinical Professor, Department of Orthopaedic Surgery, The University of Utah School of Medicine, Salt Lake City; Co-Director, Intermountain Orthopaedic Research Lab, Salt Lake City; Co-Director Salt Lake City Knee and Sports Medicine Research Foundation, Salt Lake City, Utah
Skiing

ROBERT J. ROTELLA, M.A., Ph.D.
Director, Sport Psychology, Department of Health and Physical Education, Curry School of Education, The University of Virginia, Charlottesville, Virginia
Psychosocial Aspects of Sports Medicine

DESMOND K. RUNYAN, M.D., Ph.D.
Associate Professor, Department of Social Medicine and Pediatrics, School of Medicine, The University of North Carolina at Chapel Hill, Chapel Hill; Attending Phsyician, The University of North Carolina Hospitals, Chapel Hill, North Carolina
The Preparticipation Exam

GEORGE J. SALEM, M.S.
Instructor, Department of Kinesiology, Conditioning Coach, Department of Athletics, The University of California at Los Angeles, Los Angeles, California
Endurance Training; Flexibility Training

STEVE SALYERS, M.D.
Sports Medicine Fellow, The University of Pittsburgh, Pittsburgh, Pennsylvania; Clarksville Memorial Hospital, Clarksville, Tennessee
Injuries Involving the Clavicle; Elbow Dislocation

CONTRIBUTORS

WAYNE J. SEBASTIANELLI, M.D.
Associate Professor, Department of Orthopaedics, University of Rochester Medical Center, Rochester; Assistant Director of Athletic Medicine, Strong Memorial Hospital, Rochester, New York
Meniscus Tears

K. DONALD SHELBOURNE, M.D.
Clinical Assistant Professor, Department of Orthopaedic Surgery, Indiana University School of Medicine, Indianapolis; Staff, Methodist Hospital, Indianapolis, Indiana
Anterior Cruciate Ligament Injuries; Posterior Cruciate Ligament Injuries

JANET SOBEL, R.P.T.
Director of Rehabilitation, Virginia Sports Medicine Institute, Arlington, Virginia
Tennis

ROY A. STERNES, B.S., M.S., A.T., C
Athletic Trainer, University of Kentucky, Lexington, Kentucky
Basketball and Volleyball

M. SUSAN WEBSTER-BOGAERT, B.Sc. (Kin), M.A.
Clinical Kinesiologist, University Hospital, London, Ontario, Canada
Swimming

RUSSELL F. WARREN, M.D.
Professor, Department of Orthopaedic Surgery, Cornell University Medical College, Ithaca; Attending Orthopaedic Surgeon and Chief, Sports Medicine and Shoulder Services, The Hospital for Special Surgery, New York; Attending Orthopaedic Surgeon, The New York Hospital, New York, New York
Shoulder Instability

RANDALL R. WROBLE, M.D.
Clinical Instructor, Department of Surgery, Wright State University School of Medicine, Dayton; Associate Director, Cincinnati Sports Medicine and Orthopaedic Center, Deaconess Hospital, Cincinnati, Ohio
Wrestling

RONALD F. ZERNICKE, Ph.D.
Professor and Chairman, Department of Kinesiology, The University of California at Los Angeles, Los Angeles, California
Endurance Training; Flexibility Training

ACKNOWLEDGMENTS

The editor would like to acknowledge the special contributions of Mrs. Lucy Beck. Her tireless work in the preparation of the manuscript and her skillful coordination of the contributors were instrumental to the completion of this text.

The following also are acknowledged for their important contributions.

Editorial Assistance:	Edward Wickland, Kitty McCollough, Elise Oranges
Content:	Todd Harburn, D.O. (Football History)
	Bruce Gantz, M.D. (Wrestling—Otolaryngology)
	John Strauss, M.D. (Wrestling—Dermatology)
	Dan Foster, M.S., A.T.C. (Wrestling)
	Diana Grey, R.P.T. (Electric Modalities)
Photography:	Bob Broxterman and Yvonne Ehrhart
Manuscript Preparation:	Mrs. Chris Grisson (Chapters 2 and 4)
	Mrs. Gwen West (Chapters 2 and 4)
	Carlene Gray (Chapters 18 and 19)
	Andre Smith (Chapter 22)
	Kathy Zettl (Chapter 23)
	Judy Koren
	Sandra Lewis

PREFACE

Before the development of the discipline of orthopaedic sports medicine, most orthopaedic surgeons were trained to treat athletic injuries but not necessarily to treat injured athletes. In recent years, many individual orthopaedists and sports medicine societies have strived to integrate the care of sports injuries into the overall context of the demands of the athlete's training and competition.

The goal of this text is to equip the orthopaedist or team physician with the knowledge he or she needs to provide complete care to injured school-age athletes and to function as part of a treatment team that includes coaches, athletic trainers, and therapists. Almost all of the clinical authors are team physicians on the college or professional level, practitioners who must make daily decisions in the treatment of competing athletes. The authors' aim is to apply criteria of scientific objectivity wherever possible, yet to provide the reader with the many bits of practical knowledge necessary to deal with the unique situations that occur in sports. As in other areas of medicine, many treatment regimes follow personal or collective experience that is yet unverified by objective studies. An effort has been made to point out major divergent opinions where appropriate. The general tone of the work reflects the editor's interest in the aggressive mobilization and rehabilitation techniques that dominate current trends in sports injury treatment.

The concept of sports medicine assumes a patient for whom participation in a sport carries special significance, a patient with specific achievement goals and for whom return to training and competition has considerable importance. Thus, sports medicine has not been a valid concept in children below a certain age. These are patients who play rather than train or compete, and their treatment appropriately deserves a more leisurely and less goal-oriented tone. Current social and athletic trends, however, have pushed the commencement of serious training to adolescent and even pre-pubescent levels in many sports. School-age athletes have become our largest group of competitors; their optimum care requires more than just a handful of elite sports specialists.

This text is aimed at the orthopaedic community, but it will be a valuable resource for any medical professional involved in the care of school-age athletes. It is divided into three parts. The first part reviews training and rehabilitation techniques applicable to all athletes. The second part discusses specific injuries that occur commonly in many sports. Each of these is the subject of considerable interest—and often controversy—in contemporary sports medicine. The third part is organized by individual sports. Each chapter begins with an overview of the training and performance demands of the specific sport, and then discusses injuries that are particularly relevant to that sport. The injuries have been selected for discussion in particular sections because they are characteristic of that sport or because they require special techniques of treatment within the context of that sport. Most of these injuries may occur in several other sports, so they are cross-indexed anatomically for easy reference. The purpose of this method of organization is to permit complete integration of the injury treatment into the athlete's sports participation.

BRUCE REIDER

CONTENTS

PART I
TRAINING AND REHABILITATION TECHNIQUES

1
ENDURANCE TRAINING 1
Ronald F. Zernicke, George J. Salem, and Robert K. Alejo

2
STRENGTH TRAINING 19
Herbert A. Haupt

3
FLEXIBILITY TRAINING 40
Ronald F. Zernicke and George J. Salem

4
ERGOGENIC AIDS 52
Herbert A. Haupt

5
PHYSICAL MODALITIES IN REHABILITATION 67
Robert M. Poole, B. Craig Lee, and Turner A. Blackburn, Jr.

6
THE PREPARTICIPATION EXAM 88
Sally S. Harris and Desmond K. Runyan

PART II
COMMON SPORTS INJURIES

7
PSYCHOSOCIAL ASPECTS OF SPORTS MEDICINE 105
Robert J. Rotella and John Heil

8
MUSCLE STRAINS AND CONTUSIONS 118
William E. Garrett, Jr., and John Lohnes

9
HEAD AND NECK INJURIES 130
Wayne Gersoff

10
SPONDYLOLYSIS AND SPONDYLOLISTHESIS 144
Bert R. Mandelbaum and Michael L. Gross

11
SHOULDER INSTABILITY 157
David W. Altchek and Russell F. Warren

12
INJURIES INVOLVING THE CLAVICLE 190
Freddie H. Fu and Steve Salyers

13
ELBOW DISLOCATIONS 207
Freddie H. Fu and Steve Salyers

14
HAND AND WRIST INJURIES 217
Daniel P. Mass and William G. Raasch

15
OSTEOCHONDRITIS DISSECANS 240
Ben K. Graf and Richard H. Lange

16
MENISCUS TEARS 255
Kenneth E. DeHaven and Wayne J. Sebastianelli

17
COLLATERAL LIGAMENT INJURIES 272
Bruce Reider

18
ANTERIOR CRUCIATE LIGAMENT INJURIES 284
K. Donald Shelbourne and Paul A. Nitz

19
POSTERIOR CRUCIATE LIGAMENT INJURIES 317
K. Donald Shelbourne and Paul A. Nitz

20
PATELLAR INSTABILITY AND PAIN 332
Lonnie E. Paulos and Patricia A. Kolowich

21
DISORDERS OF THE PATELLAR TENDON 355
Ben K. Graf, C. Keith Fujisaki, and Bruce Reider

22
ANKLE, HINDFOOT, AND MIDFOOT INJURIES 365
John Larkin and Michael Brage

23
GREAT TOE METATARSOPHALANGEAL JOINT PROBLEMS 406
Angus McBryde, Jr.

PART III
SPORT-SPECIFIC SPORTS MEDICINE

24
GYMNASTICS 415
Bert R. Mandelbaum

25
SWIMMING 429
Peter J. Fowler and M. Susan Webster-Bogaert

26
BASEBALL 447
William Bryan

27
BALLET 484
William G. Hamilton

28
WRESTLING 520
Randall R. Wroble, James T. Hoegh, and John P. Albright

29
FOOTBALL 559
Bruce Reider, Robert Belniak, and Darryl W. Miller

30
HOCKEY 590
Robert Hunter

31
BASKETBALL AND VOLLEYBALL 601
James Michael Ray, Walter McCombs, and Roy A. Sternes

32
RUNNING 632
William G. Clancy, Jr.

33
SOCCER 651
William E. Garrett, Jr., and John Lohnes

34
TENNIS 664
Robert Nirschl and Janet Sobel

35
SKIING 673
Thomas D. Rosenberg, Jonathan L. Franklin, and Lonnie E. Paulos

INDEX 689

Part I

TRAINING AND REHABILITATION TECHNIQUES

1

ENDURANCE TRAINING

RONALD F. ZERNICKE
GEORGE J. SALEM
ROBERT K. ALEJO

In recent years, children and adolescents have become increasingly involved in competitive sports that require intensive physical training. Currently, athletes less than 12 years old compete internationally in sports such as gymnastics and tennis. The once-rare participation of children in marathons and other endurance competitions has become common. Questions about the long-term implications of such participation are being answered, however, and only recently have sports medicine specialists and exercise scientists begun to focus on the child in sport. The increase in participation parallels the increase in risk of musculoskeletal injuries that result from repetitive microtrauma related to overuse.[71] The same methods for etiologically assessing overuse injuries in the adult athlete, to isolate injury-contributing factors[82] and to design training techniques to minimize injuries, have been applied to school-age athletes. Whether these same methods can be applied carte blanche to the young athlete, however, needs to be examined and validated carefully.

In this chapter, we discuss general principles of endurance conditioning, including parameters of aerobic fitness, factors affecting endurance training, and training techniques. Second, we apply these general principles to the school-age athlete, with emphasis on endurance training and its inherent risks.

PARAMETERS OF FITNESS

CARDIOVASCULAR, RESPIRATORY, AND BODY COMPOSITIONAL ADAPTATIONS TO ENDURANCE TRAINING

$\dot{V}O_2max$

Muscular contraction depends on the transfer of energy from high-energy phosphate bonds to muscle contractile elements (actin and myosin).[49] The energy stored in these bonds, however, is minute,[97] and sustained physical activity requires the energy to be replenished. Replenishment occurs when energy is released during the breakdown of stored foodstuffs in the presence of oxygen. Oxygen serves as an electron acceptor and combines with hydrogen generated during glycolytic, beta oxidation, or Krebs cycle reactions. During endurance or aerobic activities, therefore, performance depends indirectly on the maximum amount of oxygen the athlete can consume ($\dot{V}O_2max$). $\dot{V}O_2max$ can increase with endurance training, and $\dot{V}O_2max$ measurements are commonly used to assess aerobic fitness. $\dot{V}O_2max$ increases until postpuberty in boys,[27] whereas in females $\dot{V}O_2max$ increases until puberty and then stays constant until early adulthood.[86] Throughout growth, average $\dot{V}O_2max$ values are lower in girls than in boys.[48]

Cardiac Output

More than any other factor, cardiac output distinguishes elite endurance athletes from well-trained or untrained individuals. For example, the average maximum cardiac output of sedentary individuals is 10 to 22 liters of blood per minute, whereas an elite endurance athlete can have a cardiac output of 35 to 40 liters of blood per minute.[68] Changes in maximum cardiac outputs can be traced to the increased stroke volume that results with increased aerobic fitness. These exercise-related increases in cardiac output are proportional to increases in $\dot{V}O_2$max.[97]

Stroke Volume

Elite endurance athletes have significantly larger resting and maximum cardiac stroke volumes. In a classic study by Saltin,[89] the average stroke volume of well-trained endurance athletes was compared with the average stroke volume of sedentary college students, both before and after the students' participation in a 55-day aerobic training program (Fig. 1–1). The study results showed that the resting level stroke volume of the endurance athletes was greater than that of the untrained students; maximum stroke volumes were greater in the endurance athletes; the difference between maximum and resting level stroke volume was much greater in the endurance athletes; and the 55-day endurance-training program increased both the resting and maximum cardiac stroke volumes of the students.

Because increases in stroke volume can occur with endurance training, the remarkable differences between sedentary and trained individuals are probably due to endurance-conditioning programs and not simply differences in genetics. But the relative contributions of genetics versus training are difficult to parcel out. Further, because exercise-induced increases in stroke volume are limited in the untrained individual, increases in cardiac output in the untrained individual are due primarily to increases in heart rate. In contrast, the cardiac output increases in a trained athlete are due to increases in both heart rate and stroke volume.[68]

Heart Rate

Aerobic training decreases resting and submaximal heart rates for athletes and even sedentary individuals.[91] Resting and submaximal heart rate changes provide an index of endurance fitness, and submaximal heart rate is often used to predict $\dot{V}O_2$max[5, 24, 35, 68] (Fig. 1–2). Increases in maximum heart rate due to training are usually minimal, and decreases are more likely to occur.[69] Conse-

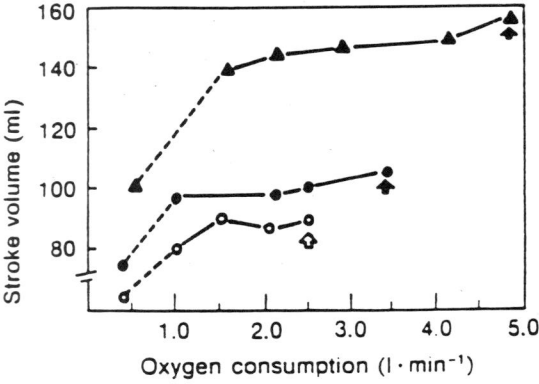

FIGURE 1–1. Stroke volume in relation to oxygen uptake during exercise in endurance athletes (▲) and sedentary college students before (○) and after (●) 55 days of aerobic training. Maximum values are indicated by *arrows*. (Adapted from SALTIN, B. Physiological effects of physical conditioning. *Med. Sci. Sports* 1: 50–56, 1969. Reprinted with permission.)

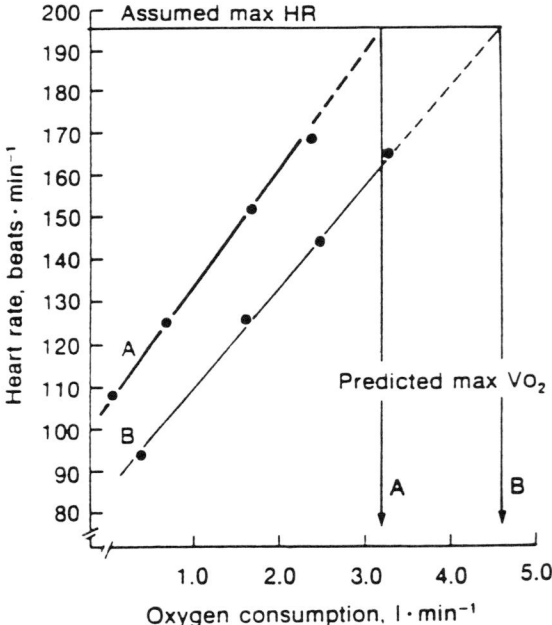

FIGURE 1–2. Application of the linear relationship between submaximal heart rate and oxygen consumption to predict max $\dot{V}O_2$ in two subjects. (Adapted from McARDLE, W. D., F. I. KATCH, and V. L. KATCH. *Exercise Physiology: Energy, Nutrition, and Human Performance.* Philadelphia: Lea and Febiger, 1986. Reprinted with permission.)

quently, maximum heart rate is not an effective criterion for predicting aerobic fitness. Maximum heart rate is unrelated to race or male-female differences for both adults and children and can be estimated, in beats per minute, as 220 minus a person's age.

Blood Volume

Hemoglobin and blood volume can increase with endurance training and decrease with inactivity.[59] These changes facilitate oxygen delivery by enhancing circulatory and thermoregulatory dynamics.[23, 68]

Blood Pressure

Endurance training can decrease both systolic and diastolic blood pressures of hypertensive[22] or normotensive[103] adults and hypertensive adolescents.[39] The mechanism by which endurance training decreases resting blood pressure is not fully known, but decreases in epinephrine and norepinephrine have been proposed as possible mechanisms. Although some researchers question the degree that exercise can benefit hypertensive individuals,[93] exercise is an integral component of most therapeutic hypertension programs.[68]

Heart Hypertrophy

Since 1628, when correlations between heart size and physical activity were first noted,[41] many studies have reported an increase in heart size in response to exercise training.[29] Using X-ray techniques, Åstrand[4] examined young female swimmers and found that their hearts were much larger than would be expected, based solely on body size. Increases in heart size may also be related to specificity of training. For example, Herxheimer found that long-distance runners and bicyclists had comparatively larger hearts than weight lifters or short-distance runners.[43] Changes in heart size may take longer than other exercise-related adaptations, such as $\dot{V}O_2$max increases and submaximal exercise heart rate decreases.[80]

Respiratory Changes

A common measure of ventilation efficiency is the ventilatory equivalent ($\dot{V}_E/\dot{V}O_2$). Measured in liters, this ratio is typically 25:1 in healthy young adults and persists to about 55 percent of $\dot{V}O_2$max.[114] This ratio may be considerably greater in children.[3] During exercise, the ratio may increase to 35 or 40 liters of air per $\dot{V}O_2$.[68, 97] This increase in ventilation is a necessary consequence of carbon dioxide accumulation, a byproduct of lactic acid buffering. During submaximal exercise, the endurance-trained athlete shows a lower, more efficient ventilatory equivalent,[2] resulting in greater oxygen extraction per breath; so the energy cost of breathing is reduced. During maximal exercise, however, the increase in $\dot{V}O_2$max (oxygen usage) must be met by a concurrent increase in ventilation.

Body Composition

Each athlete should focus on his or her body composition or lean body weight instead of simple scale weight. Body composition is most usefully reported as percent body fat. Recommended body fat percentages are 15 for average men and 26 for average women.[33] Although average body fat percentages for athletes are sport specific, the recommended range of body fat is 8 to 10 percent for male athletes and 12 to 14 percent for female athletes.[33] Generally, male endurance athletes have body fat percentages between 5 and 14 percent and females between 14 and 22 percent.[116]

Peripheral Circulatory Adaptations

Although increases in $\dot{V}O_2$max and improved submaximal adjustments to exercise have traditionally been attributed to central circulatory adaptations, evidence suggests that important peripheral adaptations also occur in response to endurance training.[45, 51, 81] Training has also been shown to increase oxygen extracted from circulating blood.[64, 83] For example, when Magel and colleagues[64] measured oxygen extraction [arteriovenous oxygen difference (a-v) O_2 diff] before and after 10 weeks of arm-interval training, they found significant increases in maximum (a-v) O_2 diff because of the endurance training. They attributed these changes either to increased peripheral blood flow or to increased cellular metabolic capacity, or both. Others[45, 81] have also reported increases in both peripheral blood flow and cellular metabolic capabilities due to endurance training.

During submaximal exercise, in the trained individual, blood flow to exercising muscles is apparently reduced.[111] Decreased oxygen delivery, which would accompany these changes, is limited by a parallel increase in (a-v) O_2 diff of the exercising muscles. Adequate oxygen transfer is maintained. In contrast, blood flow may be greater in trained

TABLE 1–1. Hypothetical Physiological and Body Composition Changes in a Sedentary Normal Individual Resulting from an Endurance Training Program,* Compared with Values of a World-Class Endurance Runner of the same age

Variables	Sedentary Normal		World-Class
	Pretraining	*Posttraining*	*Endurance Runner*
Cardiovascular			
HR rest, beats/min	71	59	36
HR max, beats/min	185	183	174
SV rest, ml†	65	80	125
SV max, ml†	120	140	200
$\dot{Q}$ rest, liters/m	4.6	4.7	4.5
$\dot{Q}$ max, liters/m	22.2	25.6	34.8
Heart volume, ml	750	820	1200
Blood volume, liters	4.7	5.1	6.0
Systolic BP rest mm Hg	135	130	120
Systolic BP max mm Hg	210	205	210
Diastolic BP rest mm Hg	78	76	65
Diastolic BP max mm Hg	82	80	65
Respiratory			
$\dot{V}_E$ rest, liters/min (BTPS)	7	6	6
$\dot{V}_E$ max, liters/min (BTPS)	110	135	195
Metabolic			
a-$\bar{v}$ O_2 diff rest, mil/100 ml	6.0	6.0	6.0
a-$\bar{v}$ O_2 diff max, mil/100 ml	14.5	15.0	16.0
$\dot{V}O_2$ rest ml/kg · min	3.5	3.7	4.0
$\dot{V}O_2$ max ml/kg · min	40.5	49.8	76.7
Body composition			
Weight, lb	175	170	150
Relative fat, %	16.0	12.5	7.5

* 6-month training program, jogging 3–4 times/wk, 30 min/d at 75% $\dot{V}O_2$ max.
† Upright position.
Source: From JENSEN, C. R., AND A. G. FISHER. *Scientific Basis of Athletic Conditioning*. 2nd ed. Philadelphia: Lea and Febiger, 1979.

muscles during maximal work load. The increases in (a-v) O_2 diff and blood flow in exercising muscles are consistent with $\dot{V}O_2$max increases.

To summarize these adaptive physiological factors, briefly described above, Jensen and Fisher[51] compared values of a world-class endurance runner with the hypothetical physiological and body compositional changes that could result from an endurance-training program in a sedentary normal person of the same age. Jensen and Fisher's comparisons are reproduced in Table 1–1.

SKELETAL MUSCLE ADAPTATIONS TO ENDURANCE TRAINING

Mitochondria

Endurance training significantly increases muscle cell oxidative capacity and mitochondrial enzymes. Early studies by Holloszy[44] and later studies[8] show that mitochondrial enzyme levels increase in response to endurance training, but controversy still persisted about these mitochondrial enzyme increases. Were the increases due to increases in the number or the size of the mitochondria? Electron microscopy studies by Gollnick and King,[38] Morgan et al.,[74] and Hoppler et al.[47] now show that both the number and size of the mitochondria increase with endurance training.

Endurance training also affects mitochondrial enzyme content. Increased levels of enzymes responsible for fatty acid,[7] ketone,[118] NADH (nicotinamide adenine dinucleotide, reduced), and succinate[44] oxidation occur after endurance training. Muscle homogenate and isolated mitochondrial studies document that endurance training increases a muscle's ability to oxidize fatty acids,[7] ketones,[118] and pyruvate.[7] Enzymes responsible for a muscle's glycolytic capacity decrease after chronic stimulation of a muscle.[42]

Myoglobin Content

With training, the myoglobin content of muscle can increase by as much as 80 percent.[77] As a result, oxygen in a muscle cell is increased, and mitochondrial diffusion is facilitated. The eased diffusion is consistent with a muscle cell's increased oxidative capabilities.

Muscle Fiber Types

Generally, humans have about 50 percent type I (slow-twitch) fibers and 50 percent type II (fast-twitch) skeletal muscle fibers. Although sprinters tend to have a higher percentage of type II fibers and endurance athletes a higher percentage of type I fibers, these differences are probably genetically determined and predispose an athlete to one or the other sporting conditions. Conversion of type II fibers to type I fibers due to exercise training has not been shown to occur[46] but conversion of IIb (fast-twitch white, glycolytic) to IIa (fast-twitch red, oxidative) can result with endurance training. Some forms of endurance training can produce complete conversion of type IIb fibers to type IIa fibers, and the adaptive increases in oxidative capacity appear greater in the type II fibers than in the type I fibers.[21] The species studied appears to have an influence on the amount and type of fibers that can convert with endurance training; although conversion of type IIb fibers to type IIa fibers can occur in humans, similar fiber conversions do not appear to occur in rats.[7, 98]

ENDURANCE-TRAINING EFFECTS ON CONNECTIVE TISSUES

Bone

Wolff's law indicates that bone will model and remodel in response to specific loading regimens. Physical activity is considered an important factor in skeletal growth and change. Immature bone appears especially sensitive to cyclic loading,[19] and it is proposed that sensitivity to exercise is at a maximum during periods of most rapid growth.[55] Comparisons of animal studies examining the effects of exercise on bone are often confounded by differences in animal species and strains, anatomical site of the bone, and exercise protocols. For example, Kiiskinen and Heikkinen[56] found a dose-response effect of exercise for mouse femur. Mice run for 80 minutes per day for 12 weeks had longer and heavier femurs than controls. Conversely, mice run for 120 minutes per day for 21 weeks had shorter and lighter femurs than controls. Matsuda et al.[65] studied the effects of treadmill running on a limb bone of growing roosters, run 5 days per week at 70 to 80 percent $\dot{V}O_2$max. They found that exercise significantly lowered bending stiffness, tensile yield stress, and mature collagen cross-links (pyridinoline) in the bone. Woo et al.[119] studied the training effects resulting from the running of immature swine for 12 months and found that the density and biochemical composition of the femoral diaphysis were comparable with controls but that total volume and dry, ash, and calcium weights, and maximum load and energy absorption were significantly increased in the exercised animals. McDonald et al.[70] reported age-related differences in bone mineralization patterns of rats following exercise. They noted that following training mineralization of weight-bearing bones appeared more pronounced, compared with the axial skeleton of immature animals. Other studies have reported either significant bone length increases[101] or decreases[104] and density increases[57] with training. In surveying studies, clearly the response of bone to physical training is exercise, species, and bone specific.

Cartilage

Endurance-training effects on both articular and fibrocartilage show that those structures are sensitive to exercise-related loading changes. Pedrini-Mille et al.[78] found that endurance-trained chickens had premature decreases in dermatan sulfate proteoglycans, increases in chondroitin sulfate containing molecule aggregation, and decreases in pyridinoline cross-links in the menisci. These biochemical changes may significantly affect the compressive stiffness, strength, and stability of the cartilage and increase the risk of tearing or related injuries. Kiviranta et al.[58] found that an endurance-training program of 10 weeks increased the thickness and the glycosaminoglycans and nonglycosaminoglycans oligosaccharides of articular cartilage in young dogs (15 weeks old). Here again, such biochemical changes probably affect the mechanical properties of the cartilage. Others have found that diminished weight bearing[76] and repetitive impact loads[79] lead to degeneration of the articular cartilage. It appears that sufficient loading is necessary for healthy articular cartilage but that excessive cyclic loading may cause cartilage maladaptation.

Ligaments and Tendons

It is generally accepted that exercise increases the ultimate strength of tendons and ligaments. But change in strength is intimately related to both the type and duration of exercise. Single exercise bouts[106] or sprint training[105] may not produce increases in ligament junction strength, although activity level and junction strength are positively correlated.[79]

Studies examining the effects of endurance training on tendons and ligaments of children and adolescents have not been done, but—consistent with bone and cartilage—it appears that activity and cyclic loading are important for maintaining the biochemical and structural integrity of tendons and ligaments.[75]

ADAPTATIONS TO CESSATION OF TRAINING

Detraining effects occur rapidly with the cessation of exercise. Significant reductions in the cardiovascular measures of $\dot{V}O_2max$, stroke volume, and cardiac output can occur after only 2 weeks of detraining.[90] Saltin et al. found decreases to 27 percent of physical working capacity in people confined to bedrest for 20 consecutive days.[90]

Reductions in muscle mitochondrial enzymes also result after exercise cessation. For example, rats treadmill run for 14 weeks had increases in mitochondrial marker enzymes to 100 percent in hindleg muscles. Stopping the training resulted in an exponential reduction of these enzymes to baseline levels within 35 days.[14] Studies using humans showed that increased enzyme levels resulting from 3 to 12 weeks of endurance training returned to normal within 6 to 8 weeks after cessation of exercise.[42, 60] Although mitochondrial enzyme decreases due to training cessation appear slower in subjects trained for longer durations (6 to 20 years), significant declines can occur within 12 weeks.[21] Training effects are transient, and their maintenance requires continued exercise.

MEASURING AEROBIC FITNESS

$\dot{V}O_2max$

The best test of aerobic fitness is the $\dot{V}O_2max$ test. Because this test measures the actual oxidative capacity of the individual, it should be used whenever a high level of accuracy is needed. Typically, these tests begin at a low level of work on a treadmill, bicycle ergometer, or rowing ergometer, and the work loads are increased until the individual reaches maximum oxygen consumption. Maximum oxygen consumption can be determined when further increases in work load do not elicit similar increases in oxygen consumption or when these consumption increases are less than 2 ml/kg/min (*American College of Sports Medicine Guidelines*). Other indications of near-maximum oxygen uptake include blood lactate levels greater than 80 mg/100 ml and respiratory exchange quotients (R) greater than 1. Maximum oxygen uptake comparisons for athletes of different sports are provided in Figure 1–3.[6]

Specificity of training principles may limit the validity of aerobic fitness appraisal, using these methods. For example, swimmers whose endurance training is very dependent on arm motion may not achieve high $\dot{V}O_2max$ scores using a bicycle ergometer. $\dot{V}O_2max$ measures are also influenced by gender,[51] body composition,[120] and age.[68]

$\dot{V}O_2max$ measures for children are more difficult to obtain than for adults. Bicycle ergometers frequently must be modified to fit the smaller dimensions of children,[62] and proper pedal cadences must be maintained to ensure commensurate work loads.[110] Bicycle ergometer measures can have the disadvantage of causing leg muscle fatigue before maximum cardiac output.[117] For example, $\dot{V}O_2max$ measures of children tested on a bicycle ergometer can be 7 to 19 percent lower than those obtained during treadmill locomotion.[13, 110] And the plateauing of oxygen uptake with increased work loads is less probable in children, as compared with adults.[3, 25] Even with these drawbacks, $\dot{V}O_2max$ measures are the most accurate measures of aerobic fitness in children, and the reliability and reproducibility of $\dot{V}O_2max$ measures in children are similar to those found in adults.[13, 25]

Indirect Measures of Aerobic Fitness

While direct measures of $\dot{V}O_2max$ are accurate and reproducible, these tests require

ENDURANCE TRAINING

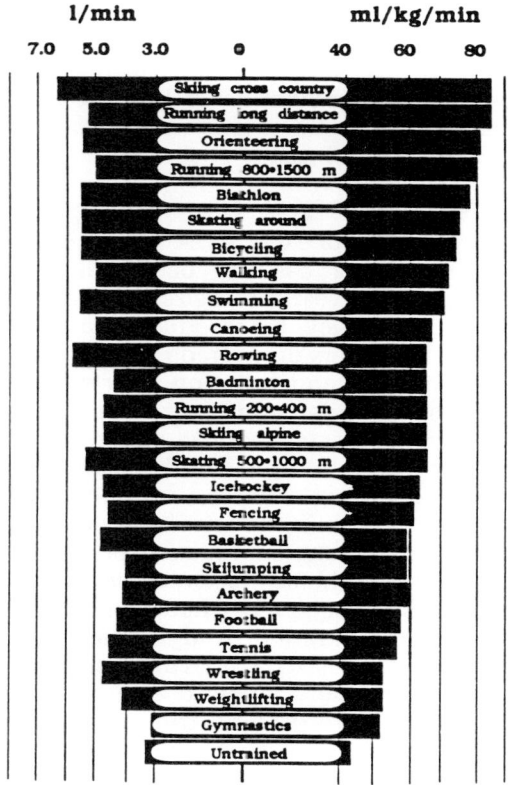

FIGURE 1–3. Comparison of maximum oxygen uptake for athletes of different sports. (Adapted from ÅSTRAND, P. O., and K. RODAHL. *Textbook of Work Physiology.* New York: McGraw-Hill Book Co., 1970. Reprinted with permission.)

use of costly, nonportable ergometers and spirometers and may not be suitable for the testing of many subjects. As a result, many tests of aerobic fitness have been developed and standardized that may be more practical for the testing of children and adolescents. Generally, these tests fall into two categories: *distance runs*, where performance is correlated with $\dot{V}O_2$max or compared with existing standards,[63] and *submaximal exercises*, where heart rates can be used to predict $\dot{V}O_2$ max[16] (see Fig. 1–2). Many studies have examined the validity and reliability of such indirect aerobic fitness tests,[18,53] but conclusions vary. Generally, it appears that the longer-distance runs have greater validity and reliability than shorter runs, although the long-distance runs can be influenced by the pacing pattern adopted by the person and the person's experience.[53] $\dot{V}O_2$max predictions from submaximal heart rates are typically only accurate to within 10 to 20 percent of directly measured values.[68] That level of error may be acceptable, however, for routine assessment of aerobic fitness of school-age athletes.

FACTORS AFFECTING ENDURANCE TRAINING

To improve aerobic fitness and performance for a particular sport, athletes must train using activities that stress the cardiovascular system by using proper muscle groups (i.e., those groups most commonly used in the sport). Further, the training exercises must reach minimum thresholds to stress or overload the targeted systems sufficiently for improvement to occur. The factors that influence the stress placed on a targeted system include fitness level, intensity of exercise, duration of exercise, and frequency of exercise.

Fitness Level

Generally, people who are least aerobically fit will show the greatest improvement with endurance training.[36,68,94,96] Conversely, those who already have a high level of aerobic power will manifest a small improvement—although even that small improvement could have practical significance. For instance, using Shephard's fitness response equation, a person with an early aerobic power of 41.8 ml/kg/min showed a 19.5 percent gain in aerobic power using a certain training prescription, whereas a person with an early aerobic power of 51.8 ml/kg/min showed only a 5.8 percent gain using the same prescription.[97] Other factors affecting endurance training, including intensity, duration, and frequency of exercise, can be manipulated, based on early fitness measures, to produce the desired adaptive responses while avoiding injury.

Exercise Intensity

The intensity of exercise prescription is usually based on a percentage of $\dot{V}O_2$max or maximum heart rate. Initial or current levels of fitness must be known, so that the intensity of exercise can be prescribed. Practically, however, oxygen consumption during an exercise is difficult to measure, and therefore heart rate (linearly correlated with oxygen consumption) is the most commonly used indicator of exercise intensity. A relationship between percent maximum $\dot{V}O_2$max and per-

TABLE 1–2. Relation Between Percent max $\dot{V}O_2$ and Percent max Heart Rate

Percent max/HR	Percent max/$\dot{V}O_2$
50	28
60	42
70	56
80	70
90	83
100	100

Source: From MCARDLE, W. D., F. I. KATCH, AND V. L. KATCH. *Exercise Physiology: Energy, Nutrition, and Human Performance.* Philadelphia: Lea and Febiger, 1986.

cent maximum heart rate is given in Table 1–2. Training intensity must exceed a minimum threshold to improve aerobic fitness. Karvonen[52] found this minimum level to be 60 percent of the difference between resting and maximal heart rate, whereas others report that 70 percent of maximum heart rate—50 to 55 percent $\dot{V}O_2$max—is enough to produce a response.[1] It also appears that the higher the intensity above threshold, the greater the training improvement.[95] Consistent with these findings, Shephard[96] reported that the ratio of intensity of effort to a person's initial anaerobic power is the main factor influencing training adaptations. An increase in exercise intensity necessitates increased muscle fiber recruitment, cell metabolism, and oxygen demand—a greater adaptational response—but excessive intensity will place greater demands on anaerobic systems or lead to rapid fatigue. An upper limit of aerobic exercise intensity undoubtedly exists, but specifying that limit is an elusive target.

Exercise Duration

Currently, exercise duration thresholds for endurance-training effects have not been quantified, but it is reasonable that high-intensity exercises may need shorter duration for aerobic fitness increases, and low-intensity exercises may need longer durations for aerobic fitness increases. Even at low intensity levels, exercises of long duration can produce fatigue of some muscle fibers and the recruitment of others. Both duration and intensity levels may be involved in aerobic fitness adaptations. Interestingly, studies claiming that the effects of training are directly related to the intensity of exercise often do not account for increase in total work done. When Sharkey[94] examined variations in intensity while stabilizing the amounts of work done by varying duration, significant intensity-related training differences could not be found. It appears that total work load, a combination of intensity and duration, may be the important variable for aerobic fitness training.

Exercise Frequency

The exact role of exercise frequency in endurance training has not been fully explained. Some investigators stress the importance of frequency for producing aerobic fitness,[37] but others downgrade its role in favor of intensity and duration effects.[96] To complicate matters, studies examining frequency effects have produced equivocal results. For example, some studies show that exercise bouts two or three times per week elicit the best training effects,[50] but other results recommend more frequent exposures.[96]

The recurrent theme of exercise specificity must also be considered when determining the intensity, duration, and frequency of training. Exercises of a high intensity and moderate frequency may need long recovery periods. This is especially true during the competition phase of training, where competitors perform at maximum levels of intensity and duration.

In summary, fitness levels and exercise intensity, duration, and frequency are interdependent variables that influence training prescription and adaptation for each individual athlete. Thus, a general recommendation for a training prescription for all young athletes, who have varying levels of exerience, is virtually impossible. Each athlete must be evaluated individually and prescribed a training program accordingly. Further, in training programs where periods or training cycles are included, these variables must be adjusted as well. Failure to recognize these relationships can lead to poor performance or injury.

TRAINING SPECIFICITY

Specificity of training separates the competitive school-age athlete from the recreational athlete. To raise athletic performance, principles of training specificity must be incorporated into an endurance-training program. Specificity and its placement within a program allow the athlete to optimize physical capacities for athletic success. Endurance training of athletes should be sport specific;

for example, if one wants to improve rowing capacity, the individual must row. As basic as that statement is, so is the concept of specificity. Take the example of a football player, just finishing a season of playing and training. Although football training can be of a high intensity, as this athlete begins participation in track and field, he may find it difficult to complete running workouts. The training of the neuromuscular system appears to be motor-skill specific,[30] and the primary movement patterns used in football are probably not those used in hurdling, for example. The football player may be in better physical condition than someone with no previous training, but he will lack the advantage of someone who has been training specifically for a track and field event. Training programs should contain activities related as closely as possible to the skill used in competition.

TRAINING PROGRAM DESIGN

Before describing the details of designing and implementing such a training program, the concept of training periods or cycling needs clarification. The effectiveness of training specificity is directly related to a well-planned training aim, implemented throughout the following three training periods.

Training Periods

A yearly training plan should be divided into discrete epochs (e.g., days, months) in which specific aspects are emphasized. Typically, there are three periods of training: preparatory, competitive, and transitional.[34, 40, 66] Each period must follow the other in the order they are discussed. Proceeding in this order will allow proper and sufficient entry into successive periods. The length of each period may vary from athlete to athlete. Fundamentally, the athlete must exhibit certain physical qualities that will clue the conditioning coach to move to the next period. For example, certain strength levels must be attained in the preparatory period before progressing to the competitive period. These levels will be determined by the coach, based on the individual athlete's previous performance levels or the performance levels of others involved in the same sport. As an athlete continues to train year-round, data can be evaluated and the lengths of each period can be determined. The more years an athlete trains, the more precise the training schedule becomes.

As a training objective becomes clear, the coach and the athlete may become impatient. It is important not to rush the training effect but to stick to rigid training periods as they apply. By defining each period and the requirements for progress, the athlete should be able to derive the greatest benefits from his or her training program.

Preparatory. The preparatory period—maybe the most important of the three—contains two phases (general and specific training) and has the highest volume and lowest intensity of work. Endurance athletes need up to 6 months of preparatory work to allow the athlete to hold a specific working capacity for 4 to 5 months.[112] If this training period is not properly executed, the more intense work later in the year may lead to poor performances and increased risk of injury.

Competitive. The competitive period includes the time following the specific training phase of the preparatory period up to and during competition. Here, the principal aim is maximal performance. All programming tries to simulate closely sporting movements and situations as competition draws near. This could mean running parts of marathons, controlled distance swims with starts and competitors, or executing training session goals of equaling competitive times or distances.

Transition. After intense training, a period of rest and transition is wise. In reality, this is active rest and has general low-intensity training and few competitive-specific movements. A renewal of mental and physical capacities and rehabilitation of any injuries are benefits of this phase of training.[107]

Training Program Details

To design a sport-specific endurance-training program, the athlete, coach, and trainer should (1) determine the major energy sources used in the sport, (2) determine the primary movements necessary for top performance, (3) evaluate which muscles are important for the major movements, and (4) implement exercises and training techniques to challenge those muscle groups. After these four program design points have been determined, it is necessary to develop the training parameters. Complete details of this concept are beyond the scope of this chapter, but the basic guidelines are straightforward.

Phase 1 of the preparatory period, general training, is composed of general strength skills. Strength is basic to all types of training, including power and endurance.[121] Phase 2, specific training, develops local muscular endurance.[112] Strength derived in the general preparatory training phase is put to the test by increasing muscular contractions at a given load.

The competitive period increases $\dot{V}O_2$max to delay the onset of oxygen debt and to build lactic acid tolerance while maintaining competitive form.[113] The effects of phases 1 and 2 in the preparatory period will be reduced because of the specificity of training in the competitive period, but those athletes who retain the best results from each period will have a distinct performance advantage. The durations of each training period will be different for each athlete, but each period is essential.

Overtraining. Training volume (e.g., mileage, yardage, minutes) appears related to endurance performance.[36] In this context, the trainer and endurance athlete must be alert for overtraining symptoms. If training volume is necessary for success, then specific practice sessions must also be emphasized. To ignore either volume or practice when establishing conditioning parameters may produce overtraining and potential injuries.[17] The premise that more is better is a major contributor to overtraining problems. Symptoms appear to be both mental and physical. Signs of mental overtraining stem from "burnout syndrome." Daily preparation for training at stressful levels can cause mental fatigue. Adrenaline flow that is necessary for hard training begins to take its toll after a number of bouts. Being able to "get up" for workouts and competition becomes difficult. Lethargy, low morale, and lack of enthusiasm are just a few signs of mental overtraining.

Symptoms of physical overtraining can be due to too much work or the same type of training without change for an extended period of time. The human body is a very adaptive mechanism but when overstimulated will break down. Physical signs of overtraining include chronic injuries, persistent postworkout joint and muscle soreness, and loss of strength and endurance. Rest, certain therapeutic measures, or restorative measures are most effective prescriptions for overtraining symptoms.

Interval Training. Besides continuous low-intensity exercise, interval training can significantly modify aerobic systems.[26, 30] Interval training is nothing more than a series of repeated bouts of exercise alternated with periods of relief or rest. Interval training can include all types of modulates for exercise, as long as there is a work-rest interval. Some distinct advantages of interval training include specific training of the energy systems involved in the sport and an accurate control of the stressor. Owing to the exactness of times and distances during interval prescription, the athlete can closely monitor the training process. A prescription might take the form of a 400-meter sprint followed by a 1:20 rest for three repetitions. A different but exact training response can be elicited by manipulating the distance or rest interval. Many work-rest ratios are possible, and work intervals can be expressed as either time or distance. Choosing the best combination of intervals depends on the athlete's fitness level, training period, and sport.

In theory, aerobic metabolism can be taxed by modifying frequency, intensity, or duration; related to these parameters, training time and heart rate or maximum $\dot{V}O_2$ are critical. But, in practice, it is an ill-designed training program that determines aerobic training by distances, time, or heart rate alone. A well-designed training program integrates and simultaneously monitors frequency, intensity, and duration.

The final step in a training program design is testing. Gains in strength and endurance are specific to the type of training, and to be valid, the tests should measure the proper parameters. If the training program and sport use dynamic movements, then the testing should be dynamically, instead of isometrically or concentrically, oriented. During the testing, the coach or trainer should always be alert for submaximal performances due to physical or mental fatigue. Typically, tests of strength, muscular endurance, aerobic fitness, and performance level should be done at the beginning of the preparatory and competition training periods.

Training Program Example

Designing a training program sounds more difficult than it is. To make clearer the process of program design, we take an adolescent swimmer from beginning to end.

Our swimmer is a distance (1650-meter) free-style athlete. Here, energy utilization will be primarily aerobic, and the muscles used in the primary propulsion of this athlete will include the pectoralis, deltoids, lattissimus dorsi, erectors, gluteals, biceps femoris, and hip flexors.

Phase 1 of the prepatory period, general strengthening, requires the athlete to execute strength exercises that are general to the sport. This would include weight training, elastic bands, paddles in the water, and kick only or pull only sets of swimming. Even the use of two swimsuits or shorts to create drag in the pool may be employed. Although absolute strength may seem to be unimportant for endurance or aerobic activities, there are positive effects of strength training on muscular endurance.

Phase 2 in the preparatory period will concentrate on local muscular endurance. During this time, an increase of work periods and shortened rest periods are used to gain endurance. The objective in phase 2 is to create a condition of high lactic acid levels through training. Weight training should follow this same philosophy, whereas, stroke-specific exercises in the pool are increased.

The competitive period will be specific to the sport. Increasing $\dot{V}O_2$max while maintaining competitive form is the main objective. Rest periods between work sets are now minimal and would present the right conditions for interval training. The training protocol in the pool would reflect racelike conditions in a controlled manner. Parts of races (starts, turns, wall touches) or the whole race would serve as repetitions during training. Training sessions should be tapered immediately prior to competitions so that the athlete is well rested and can exhibit his or her fastest times of the year.

Lastly, testing parameters are determined prior to the onset of training and might be modified by the coach when testing occurs. These parameters should be closely related to swimming distances in that some correlation should be made between test scores and swimming performance.

ENDURANCE TRAINING IN CHILDREN AND ADOLESCENTS

EVALUATION OF TRAINING RESPONSES IN CHILDREN

Tests of children's responses to training are limited by ethical considerations and by methodological and physiological restrictions. Ethical considerations obviate many standard evaluation procedures typically performed on adults, including muscle and fat biopsies.[9, 87] Examinations should expose a child to a minimum of discomfort. Any experimental procedures to study training responses in children must be scrutinized carefully.

Assessment of aerobic fitness using existing protocols and equipment designed for adults must be modified to fit the variety of body geometries of children. Short attention spans and limited motivational factors also limit the use of many protocols, including some $\dot{V}O_2$max measures.[23, 62] Even the examination of chronologically age-matched children may need instrument and protocol adaptations to match differences in maturation, intelligence, or growth.[87]

Many cardiovascular changes resulting from training can occur solely because of growth and maturation changes, and exercise studies researching children must account for such natural changes. To evaluate cardiorespiratory adaptations in children, cross-sectional studies can be made of active versus nonactive children, or various types of longitudinal studies may prove useful: (1) Cohort groups can be followed over time, as some children become active, whereas others remain inactive; (2) child athletes, who increase their training efforts over time, may be monitored; or (3) children may be randomly assigned to experimental or control groups.[87]

ENDURANCE-TRAINING ACTIVITIES IN CHILDREN

The results from studies examining the effects of endurance training for children do not always agree. Factors that confound the interpretation of many results include poorly quantified training protocols; variations in age, sex, and maturation; and differences in early fitness levels. Even with those limits in mind, the consensus is that endurance training positively influences the aerobic fitness of children.

Cross-sectional studies by Åstrand[4] and Vaccaro et al.[109] on experienced child swimmers found that the average $\dot{V}O_2$max of the swimmers was significantly greater than that of untrained children of similar ages. Consistent with these findings, others reported increased aerobic fitness in child runners,[67] swimmers,[99] hockey players,[28] and wrestlers.[88]

Many longitudinal studies in which children participated in endurance training also support the notion that children increase their aerobic fitness with proper training. For example, improvements were found in the cardiorespiratory capacity of children who trained via swimming[108] and running.[32]

Some investigators, however, did not find increases in aerobic fitness after exercise training. Stewart and Gutin[102] found no significant $\dot{V}O_2max$ changes in boys 10 to 12 years of age after 8 weeks of interval training. Bar-Or and Zirwin[10] found that an increase in the frequency of physical education classes over a 9-week period had no effect on the $\dot{V}O_2max$ of 9- and 10-year-old boys. Others report no significant increase in $\dot{V}O_2max$ or cardiovascular fitness after endurance training in children.[11] Some of these results, however, are open to question because the training program was not of sufficient intensity or duration.[110] Because prepubertal children are inherently active, they may have a higher threshold level for training effects. Training-induced increases in $\dot{V}O_2max$ may only happen when training intensity and duration are high.[15]

Another reason for these dissident results may be an apparent maturation-related sensitivity of training responses. Schmücker and Hollmann[92] examined well-trained juvenile male and female swimmers, cyclists, and field hockey players and found that an increase in endurance training did not affect the aerobic capacity in athletes less than 11 years of age. Male athletes older than 12 years, however, did show aerobic capacity increases, although the effect in females was less obvious. Several researchers have tried to standardize maturation levels by expressing data about an individual's age at peak height velocity (PHV), that age when the most rapid changes in growth occur.[61, 73] The age at PHV is approximately 12 years in girls and 14 years in boys.[103] Kobayashi et al.[61] found that increases in aerobic fitness were small in males before PHV but significant during and after PHV. Mechanisms proposed to explain these findings include increases in testosterone levels and muscle tissue.[73] While the measure appears to have utility, some reservations remain about the relationship.[115]

Comparisons between the effects of endurance training in adults and in children have shown few differences between the two groups. Eisenman and Golding,[31] for example, endurance-trained 12- to 13-year-old girls and 18- to 21-year-old women, using running and bench-stepping methods. After 14 weeks, significant and similar $\dot{V}O_2max$ increases were found in both the girls and the women.

It appears that endurance training of enough intensity and duration can increase the aerobic fitness of children and adolescents. And the training responses of adults and children appear similar when training programs are of adequate intensity, but in children, especially males, endurance-training adaptations may be sensitive to maturational changes.

POTENTIAL RISKS

Although there is some discussion about the frequency, necessary depth, and usefulness of preparticipatory physical exams,[84] most agree that physical exams given before initial sports participation (middle and high school), and again during high school, are advisable.[12, 85] Preparticipational physical exams should be given to all children starting an endurance-training program who have not been examined earlier and especially those who may be at high risk because of prior injury or disease. Information collected from these exams can be useful for excluding or modifying exercises that otherwise may be contraindicated. In this section, we discuss the potential risks of endurance training for school-age athletes who, through physical examination, were free of immediate risk of injury.

Because exercise can influence the modeling and remodeling of connective tissues, concern has developed about the effects of strenuous exercise on the growth and development of children and adolescents. To date, however, few studies have examined the effects of endurance-training influence on growth in the young athlete. In a recent report,[100] 39 boys, classified by physical activity, were assessed yearly between the ages of 11 and 18 years to determine height and weight changes, plus cardiovascular measures. Results showed that training did not modify growth acceleration, the age at PHV, or the peak of the growth rate. Similar findings were reported by Kemper et al.,[54] who found that increasing the number of activity classes did not influence growth. Drawing broad conclusions from these studies must be viewed with caution, because training stimuli were not well quantified and might have been at subthreshold levels.[15] Other studies have reported increased stature with physical training.[32,72] But close examination of these studies also shows that maturity status was not controlled and that accelerated growth could be explained by adolescent height spurts.[15] Currently, there are no compelling data that endurance training in child or school-age athletes will either limit or enhance growth. Animal studies, however, have shown that exercise can significantly influence the modeling and remodeling of connective tissues, such as bone, cartilage, ligaments, and tendon.

CONCLUDING COMMENTS

Unfortunately, endurance training of optimal intensity, duration, and frequency in child and adolescent athletes has yet to be defined. Sady[87] believes that guidelines established by the *American College of Sports Medicine* for adults may also be proper for the school-age athlete while acknowledging that these standards may not reflect the aerobic fitness of this younger population. Despite the standards used, however, periodical and systematical evaluations of the young athlete are needed during an endurance-training program to ensure improvement or maintenance of aerobic fitness without exacerbating the risk of injury.

References

1. American College of Sports Medicine: Guidelines for Graded Exercise Testing and Exercise Prescription. Philadelphia: Lea & Febiger, 1975.
2. Andrew, G. M. C. A. Guzman, and M. R. Becklake. Effect of athletic training on exercise cardiac output. J. Appl. Physiol. 21:603–608, 1966.
3. Åstrand, P. O. *Experimental Studies of Physical Working Capacity in Relation to Sex and Age.* Copenhagen: Munksgaar, 1952.
4. Åstrand, P. O., L. Engström, B. O. Eriksson, P. Karlberg, I. Nylander, B. Saltin, and C. Thorén. Girl swimmers with special references to respiratory and circulatory adaptation and gynaecological and psychiatric aspects. Acta Paediatr. Scand. 147(Suppl.):5–75, 1963.
5. Åstrand, P. O., and I. Rhyming. A nomogram for calculation of aerobic capacity (physical fitness) from pulse rate during submaximal work. J. Appl. Physiol. 7:218–221, 1954.
6. Åstrand, P. O., and K. Rodahl. Textbook of Work Physiology. New York: McGraw-Hill Book Co., 1970.
7. Baldwin, K. M., G. H. Klinkerfuss, R. L. Terjung, P. A. Molé, and J. O. Holloszy. Respiratory capacity of white, red, and intermediate muscle: Adaptive response to exercise. Am. J. Physiol. 222:373–378, 1972.
8. Barnard, R. J., V. R. Edgerton, and J. B. Peter. Effect of exercise on skeletal muscle. I. Biochemical and histochemical properties. J. Appl. Physiol. 28:762–766, 1970.
9. Bar-Or, O. Pediatric Sports Medicine for the Practitioner. New York: Springer-Verlag, New York, Inc., 1983.
10. Bar-Or, O., and L. D. Zirwin. Physiological effects of increased frequency of physical education classes and of endurance conditioning on 9- to 10-year-old girls and boys. In: Pediatric Work Physiology, Proceedings 4th International Symposium, Wingate Institute, Israel, pp. 183–198, 1973.
11. Benedict, G., P. Vaccaro, and B. D. Hatfield. Physiological effects of an eight-week precision jump rope program in children. Am. Correct. Ther. J. 5:108–111, 1985.
12. Blum, R. W. Preparticipation evaluation of the adolescent athlete. Postgrad. Med. 78:52–69, 1985.
13. Boileu, R. R., V. H. Heyward, and B. H. Massey. Maximal aerobic capacity on the treadmill and bicycle ergometer of boys 11–14 years of age. J. Sports Med. Phys. Fitness 17:153–162, 1977.
14. Booth, F. W., and J. O. Holloszy. Cytochrome C turnover in rat skeletal muscles. J. Biol. Chem. 252:416–419, 1977.
15. Borms, J. The child and exercise: An overview. J. Sports Sciences 4:3–20, 1986.
16. Brouha, L. The step test: A simple method of measuring physical fitness for muscular work in young men. Res. Quart. 14:31–36, 1943.
17. Brown, R. Training concepts for Mary Decker. Track and Field Quart. Rev. 85:25–26, 1985.
18. Burke, E. J. Validity of selected laboratory and field tests of physical working capacity. Res. Quart. 47:95–104, 1976.
19. Carter, D. R. Mechanical loading histories and cortical bone remodeling. Calcif. Tissue Int. 38:519–524, 1984.
20. Chausow, S. A., W. F. Riner, and R. A. Boileau. Metabolic and cardiovascular responses of children during prolonged physical activity. Res. Quart. Exerc. Sport 55:1–7, 1984.
21. Chi, M. M. -Y., C. S. Hintz, E. F. Coyle, W. H. Martin III, J. L. Ivy, P. M. Nemeth, J. O. Holloszy, and O. H. Lowry. Effects of detraining on enzymes of energy metabolism in individual human muscle fibers. Am. J. Physiol. 244(Cell Physiol. 13):C276–C287, 1983.
22. Choquette, G., and R. J. Ferguson. Blood pressure reduction in "borderline" hypertensives following physical training. Conn. Med. Assoc. J. 108:699–703, 1973.
23. Convertino, V. A. Heart rate and sweat rate responses associated with exercise-induced hypervolemia. Med. Sci. Sports Exerc. 15:77–82, 1983.

24. Cooper, K. Correlation between field and treadmill testing as a means for assessing maximal oxygen uptake. JAMA 203:201–204, 1968.
25. Cunningham, D. A. Reliability and reproducibility of maximal oxygen uptake measurement in children. Med. Sci. Sports 9:104–108, 1977.
26. Cunningham, D. A., D. McCrimmon, and L. F. Vlach. Cardiovascular response to interval training and continuous training in women. Europ. J. Appl. Physiol. 41:187–197, 1979.
27. Cunningham, D. A., D. H. Paterson, C. J. R. Blimkie, and A. P. Donner. Development of cardiorespiratory function in circumpubertal boys: A longitudinal study. J. Appl. Physiol. Respirat. Environ. Exercise Physiol. 56:302–307, 1984.
28. Cunningham, D. A., P. Telford, and G. T. Swart. The cardiopulmonary capacities of young hockey players: Age 10. Med. Sci. Sports 8:23–25, 1976.
29. De Maria, A. N., A. Neumann, G. Lee, W. Fowler, and D. T. Mason. Alterations in ventricular mass and performance induced by exercise training in man by echocardiography. Circulation 57:237–244, 1978.
30. Eddy, D. O., K. L. Sparks, and D. A. Adelizi. Effects of continuous and interval training in women and men. Europ. J. Appl. Physiol. 7:136–138, 1977.
31. Eisenman, P. A., and L. A. Golding. Comparison of effects of training $\dot{V}O_2$max in girls and young women. Med. Sci. Sports 7:136–138, 1975.
32. Ekblom, B. Effect of physical training in adolescent boys. J. Appl. Physiol. 27:350–355, 1969.
33. Ellison, A. E. Athletic Training and Sports Medicine, A. L. Boland, K. E. DeHaven, P. Grace, G. A. Snook, H. Calehuff (Eds.). Chicago, IL: American Academy of Orthopaedic Surgeons, 1984.
34. Fleck, S. J., and W. J. Kraemer. Designing Resistance Training Programs. Champaign, IL: Human Kinetics Books, 1987.
35. Fox, E. L. A simple accurate technique for predicting maximal aerobic power. J. Appl. Physiol. 35:914–916, 1973.
36. Fox, E. L. Sports Physiology. New York: CBS Educational & Professional Publishing, p. 205, 1984.
37. Gettman, L. R., M. L. Pollock, J. L. Durstine, A. Ward, J. Ayres, and A. C. Linnerod. Physiological responses of men to 1, 3, and 5-day per week programs. Res. Quart. 47:638–646, 1976.
38. Gollnick, P. D., and D. W. King. Effect of exercise and training on mitochondria of rat skeletal muscle. Am. J. Physiol. 216:1502–1509, 1969.
39. Hagberg, J. M., D. Golding, A. A. Ehasani, G. W. Heuth, A. Hernandez, M. K. Schecht, and J. O. Holloszy. Effects of exercise training on the blood pressure and hemodynamics of adolescent hypertensives. Am. J. Cardiol. 52:763–768, 1981.
40. Harre, D. Principles of Sports Training: Based on Experience and Scientific Research in Sports in the German Democratic Republic. Berlin: Sportverlag Publication, pp. 78–87, 1982.
41. Harvey, W. Exercitatio Anatomica de motu cordis et sanguinis in animali. Frankfurt: Fitzeri (Reprinted in: Founders of Experimental Physiology, W. Blasius, J. Boylan, K. Kramer [Eds.]). Munich: Lechmanns, 1971.
42. Henriksson, J., and J. S. Reitmann. Time course of changes in human skeletal muscle succinate dehydrogenase and cytochrome oxidase activities and maximal oxygen uptake with physical activity and inactivity. Acta Physiol. Scand. 99:91–97, 1977.
43. Herxheimer, H. Untersuchungen über die Änderung der Herzguösse unter dem Einfluss bestimmter sportarten. Z. Klin. Med. 3:376–393, 1929.
44. Holloszy, J. O. Biochemical adaptations in muscle: Effects of exercise on mitochondrial oxygen uptake and respiratory enzyme activity in skeletal muscle. J. Biol. Chem. 242:2278–2282, 1967.
45. Holloszy, J. O., and J. W. Booth. Biochemical adaptations to endurance exercise in muscle. Annu. Rev. Physiol. 38:273–291, 1976.
46. Holloszy, J. O., and E. F. Coyle. Adaptations of skeletal muscle to endurance exercise and their metabolic consequences. J. Appl. Physiol.: Respirat. Environ. Exercise Physiol. 56:831–838, 1984.
47. Hoppler, H., P. Lüthi, H. Claasen, E. R. Weibel, and H. Howald. The ultrastructure of normal human skeletal muscle: A morphometric analysis on untrained men, women, and well-trained orienters. Pfluegers Arch. 344:217–232, 1973.
48. Hughson, R. Children in competitive sports: A multidisciplinary approach. Can. J. Appl. Sport Sci.11:162–172, 1986.
49. Hultman, E., J. Bergström, and N. McLennan Anderson. Breakdown and resynthesis of phosphorylcreatine and adenosine-triphosphate in connection with muscular work in man. Scand. J. Lab. Invest. 19:56–66, 1967.
50. Jackson, J. H., B. J. Sharkey, and L. P. Jonston. Cardiorespiratory adaptations to training at specified frequencies. Res. Quart. 39:295–300, 1968.
51. Jensen, C. R., and A. G. Fisher. Scientific Basis of Athletic Conditioning. 2nd ed. Philadelphia: Lea and Febiger, 1979.
52. Karvonen, M. J. Effects of vigorous exercise on the heart. In: Work and the Heart, F. F. Rosenbau, E. L. Belnap (Eds.). New York: Paul B. Hoeber, Inc., 1959.
53. Katch, F. I., G. S. Pechar, W. D. McArdle, and A. L. Weltman. Relationship between individual differences in a steady pace endurance running performance and maximal oxygen intake. Res. Quart. 44:206–215, 1973.
54. Kemper, H. C. G., J. G. A. Ras, J. Snel, P. G. Splinter, L. W. C. Tavecchio, and R. Verschuur. Invloed van extra lichamelijke opvoeding (The influence of extra physical education). Haarlem: De Vrieseborch, 1974.
55. Kiiskinen, A. Physical training and connective tissue in young mice: Physical properties of Achilles tendon and long bone growth. Growth 41:123–127, 1977.
56. Kiiskinen, A., and E. Heikkinen. Effects of physical training on development and strength of tendons and bones in growing mice. Scand. J. Clin. Lab. Invest. 29: (Suppl. 123) 60, 1973.
57. King, D. W., and R. G. Pengelly. Effect of running exercise on the density of rat tibias. Med. Sci. Sports Exerc. 5:68–69, 1973.
58. Kiviranta, I., M. Tammi, J. Jurvelin, A-M Säämänen, and H. J. Helminen. Moderate running exercise augments glycosaminoglycans

and thickness of articular cartilage in the knee joint of young Beagle dogs. J. Orthop. Res. 6:188–195, 1988.
59. Kjellberg, S. R., U. Rudhe, and T. Sjostrance. Increase of the amount of hemoglobin and blood volume in connection with physical training. Acta Physiol. Scand. 19:146–151, 1949.
60. Klausen, K., L. B. Anderson, and I. Pelle. Adaptive changes in work capacity, skeletal muscle capillerization, and enzyme levels during training and detraining. Acta Physiol. Scand. 113:9–16, 1981.
61. Kobayashi, K., K. Kitamora, M. Miura, H. Sodeyama, Y. Murase, M. Miyshira, and H. Natsui. Aerobic power as related to body growth and training in Japanese boys: A longitudinal study. J. Appl. Physiol.: Respirat. Environ. Exerc. Physiol. 45:666–672, 1978.
62. Krahenbuhl, G. S., J. S. Skinner, and W. M. Kohrt. Developmental aspects of maximal aerobic power in children. Exerc. Sport Sci. Rev. 13:503–538, 1985.
63. Léger, L. A., and J. Lambert. A maximal multistage 20-meter shuttle run test to predict $\dot{V}O_2$max. Europ. J. Appl. Physiol. 49:1–12, 1982.
64. Magel, J. R., W. D. McArdle, M. Toner, and D. J. Delio. Metabolic and cardiovascular adjustments to arm training. J. Appl. Physiol. 45:75–79, 1978.
65. Matsuda, J. J., R. F. Zernicke, A. C. Vailas, V. A. Pedrini, A. Pedrini-Mille, and J. A. Maynard. Structural and mechanical adaptation of immature bone to strenuous exercise. J. Appl. Physiol.: Respirat. Environ. Exerc. Physiol. 60:2028–2034, 1986.
66. Matveyev, I. Fundamentals of Sports Training (English translation of revised Russian edition). Moscow: USSR Progress Publishers, 1981.
67. Mayer, N., and B. Gutin. Physiological characteristics of elite prepubertal cross-country runners. Med. Sci. Sports Exerc. 11:172–179, 1979.
68. McArdle, W. D., F. I. Katch, and V. L. Katch. Exercise Physiology: Energy, Nutrition, and Human Performance. Philadelphia: Lea & Febiger, 1986.
69. McArdle, W. D., et al. Specificity of run training on $\dot{V}O_2$max and heart rate changes during running and swimming. Med. Sci. Sports 10:1–20, 1978.
70. McDonald, R., J. Hegenaver, and P. Saltman. Age-related differences in the bone mineralization pattern of rats following exercise. J. Gerontol. 41:445–452, 1986.
71. Micheli, L. J. Pediatric and adolescent sport injuries: Recent trends. In: Exerc. Sport Sci. Rev. Vol. 14. New York: Macmillan Publishing Co., 1988.
72. Milicer, H., and L. Denisiuk. The physical development of youth. In: International Research in Sport and Physical Education, E. Jokl, E. Simon (Eds.). Springfield: Charles C. Thomas, Publisher, 1964.
73. Mirwald, R. L., D. A. Bailey, N. Cameron, and R. L. Rasmussen. Longitudinal comparison of aerobic power on active and inactive boys aged 7.0 to 17.0 years. Ann. Hum. Biol. 8:405–414, 1981.
74. Morgan, T. E., L. A. Cobb, F. A. Short, R. Ross, and D. R. Gunn. Effect of long-term exercise on human muscle mitochondria. In: Muscle Metabolism During Exercise, B. Perrow, B. Saltin (Eds.). New York: Plenum Publishing Corp., 1971.
75. Noyes, F. R., P. J. Torvik, W. B. Hyde, and J. L. De Lucas. Biomechanics of ligament failure. II. An analysis of immobilization, exercise, and reconditioning effects in primates. J. Bone Joint Surg. 56A:1406–1418, 1974.
76. Palmoski, M. J., and K. D. Brandt. Running inhibits the reversal of atrophic changes in canine knee cartilage after removal of a leg cast. Arthritis. Rheum. 24:1329–1337, 1981.
77. Pattengale, P. K., and J. O. Holloszy. Augmentation of skeletal muscle myoglobin by programs of treadmill running. Am. J. Physiol. 213:783–785, 1967.
78. Pedrini-Mille, A., V. A, Pedrinii, J. A. Maynard, and A. C. Vailas. Response of immature chicken meniscus to strenuous exercise: Biochemical studies of proteoglycan and collagen. J. Orthop. Res. 6:196–204, 1988.
79. Radin, E. L., R. B. Martin, D. B. Burr, B. Caterson, R. D. Boyd, and C. Goodwin. Effects of mechanical loading on the tissues of the rabbit knee. J. Orthop. Res. 2:221–234, 1984.
80. Ricci, G., D. Lajoie, R. Petitcle, F. Peronnet, R. J. Ferguson, M. Fournier, and A. W. Taylor. Left ventricular size following endurance, sprint, and strength training. Med. Sci. Sports Exerc. 14:344–347, 1982.
81. Rochelle, R. H., R. L. Stumpner, S. Robinson, D. B. Dill, and S. M. Horvath. Peripheral blood flow response to exercise consequent to physical training. Med. Sci. Sports 3:122–129, 1971.
82. Rooks, D. S., and L. J. Micheli. Musculoskeletal assessment and training: The young athlete. Clin. Sports Med. 7:641–677, 1988.
83. Rowell, L. Human cardiovascular adjustments to exercise and thermal stress. Physiol. Rev. 54:75–159, 1974.
84. Rowland, T. W. Preparticipation sports examination of the child and adolescent athlete: Changing views of an old ritual. Pediatrician 13:3–9, 1986.
85. Runyan, K. The preparticipation examination of the young athlete. Clin. Pediatr. 22:674–679, 1983.
86. Rutenfranz, J., K. L. Anderson, V. Seliger, F. Klimmer, I. Berndt, and M. Ruppel. Maximum aerobic power and body composition during the puberty growth period: Similarities and differences between children of two European countries. Europ. J. Pediatr. 136:123–133, 1981.
87. Sady, S. P. Cardiorespiratory exercise training in children. Clin. Sports Med. 5:493–514, 1986.
88. Sady, S. P., W. H. Thompson, K. Berg, and M. Savage. Physiological characteristics of high-ability prepubescent wrestlers. Med. Sci. Sports Exerc. 16:72–76, 1984.
89. Saltin, B. Physiological effects of physical conditioning. Med. Sci. Sports 1:50–56, 1969.
90. Saltin, B., G. Bloomquist, J. Mitchell, R. Johnson, K. Wildenthal, and C. Chapman. Response to exercise after bed-rest and after training. Circulation 38(Suppl. 7), 1968.
91. Scheuer, J., and C. M. Tipton. Cardiovascular adaptations to training. Annu. Rev. Physiol. 39:221–251, 1977.
92. Schmücker, B., and W. Hollmann. The aerobic capacity of trained athletes from 6 to 7 years of

age on. In: Children and Exercise, J. Borms, M. Hebbelinck (Eds.), Acta Paediatr. Belg. 28 (Suppl.) 92–101, 1974.
93. Seals, D. R., and J. M. Hagberg. The effect of exercise training on human hypertension. Med. Sci. Sports Exerc. 16:207–215, 1984.
94. Sharkey, B. J. Intensity and duration of training and the development of cardiorespiratory endurance. Med. Sci. Sports 2:197–202, 1970.
95. Sharkey, B. J., and J. P. Holleman. Cardiorespiratory adaptations to training at specified intensities. Res. Quart. 38:398–704, 1967.
96. Shephard, R. J. Intensity, duration, and frequency of exercise as determinants of the response to a training regime. Int. Z. Angew. Physiol. 26:272–278, 1968.
97. Shephard, R. J. Endurance Fitness. 2nd ed. Toronto and Buffalo: University of Toronto Press, 1977.
98. Sjodin, B. Lactate dehydrogenase in human skeletal muscle. Acta Physiol. Scand. 436 (Suppl.): 9–18, 1976.
99. Soto, K. I., C. W. Zauner, and A. B. Otis. Cardiac output in preadolescent competitive swimmers and in untrained normal children. J. Sports Med. Physiol. Fit. 23:291–299, 1983.
100. Spryharova, S. The influence of training on physical and functional growth before, during, and after puberty. Europ. J. Appl. Physiol. 56:719–724, 1987.
101. Steinberg, M. E., and J. Trueta. Effects of activity on bone growth and development in the rat. Clin. Orthop. Rel. Res. 156:52–60, 1981.
102. Stewart, K., and B. Gutin. Effects of physical training on cardiorespiratory fitness in children. Res. Quart. 47:110–120, 1976.
103. Terjung, R. I., K. M. Baldwin, J. Cooksey, B. Samson, and R. A. Sutter. Cardiovascular adaptation to twelve minutes of mild daily exercise in middle-aged sedentary men. J. Am. Geriatr. Soc. 21:164–168, 1973.
104. Tipton, C. M., R. D. Matthes, and J. A. Maynard. Influence of chronic exercise on rat bones. Med. Sci. Sports 4:55, 1972.
105. Tipton, C. M., R. D. Matthes, and D. S. Sandage. *In situ* measurements of junction strength and ligament elongation in rats. J. Appl. Physiol. 37:758–761, 1974.
106. Tipton, C. M., R. J. Schild, and R. J. Tomanek. Influence of physical activity on the strength of knee ligaments in rats. Am. J. Physiol. 212:783–787, 1967.
107. Tivrin, T. A report on the preparation of ULMASOVA-3000m champion of Europe. Track and Field Quart. Rev. 83:55, 1983.
108. Vaccaro, P., and D. H. Clarke. Cardiorespiratory alterations in 9- to 11-year-old children following a season of competitive swimming. Med. Sci. Sports 10:204–207, 1978.
109. Vaccaro, P., D. H. Clarke, and A. F. Morris. Physiological characteristics of young well-trained swimmers. Europ. J. Appl. Physiol. 44:61–66, 1980.
110. Vaccaro, P., and A. Mahon. Cardiorespiratory responses to endurance training in children. Sports Med. 4:352–363, 1987.
111. Varnauskas, E., P. Bjorntorp, M. Fahlen, I. Prerovsky, and J. Stenberg. Effects of physical training on blood flow and enzymatic activity in skeletal muscle. Cardiovasc. Res. 4:418–422, 1970.
112. Verkhoshansky, Y. V. Programming and Organization of Training. Moscow: Fizkultura I. Spovt Publishers.
113. Warhurst, R. Training for distance running and the steeplechase. Track and Field Quart. Rev. 85:13, 1985.
114. Wasserman, K., B. J. Whipp, S. N., Koyal, and W. L. Beaver. Anaerobic threshold and respiratory gas exchange during exercise. J. Appl. Physiol. 35:236–243, 1973.
115. Weber, G., W. Kartodihavdjo, and V. Klissouras. Growth and physical training with reference to heredity. J. Appl. Physiol. 40:211–215, 1976.
116. Wilmore, J. H. Body composition and athletic performance. In: Nutrition and Athletic Performance, W. Haskell, J. Skala, J. Whittan (Eds.). Palo Alto, CA: Bull Publishing Co., 1981.
117. Wilmore, J. H. Training for Sport and Activity: The Physiological Basis of the Conditioning Process. Boston: Allyn & Bacon, Inc., 1982.
118. Winder, W. W., K. M. Baldwin, and J. O. Holloszy. Enzymes involved in ketone utilization in different types of muscle: Adaptation to exercise. Europ. J. Biochem. 47:461–467, 1974.
119. Woo, S. L- Y., S. L. Kuei, D. Amiel, M. A. Gomez, W. C. Hayes, F. C. White, and W. H. Akeson. The effect of prolonged physical training on the properties of long bone: A study of Wolff's law. J. Bone Joint Surg. 63A:780–787, 1981.
120. Wyndnam, C. A., and A. J. A. Hegns. Determinants of oxygen consumption and maximum oxygen intake of Caucasians and Bantu males. Int. Z. Angew. Physiol. 27:51–75, 1969.
121. Zakharchenko, S. A. Development of strength endurance in young long-distance runners in the yearly cycle of training. Soviet Sports Rev. 21:34, 1986.

STRENGTH TRAINING

HERBERT A. HAUPT

For many years the use of weight lifting was condemned for producing musclebound athletes who had little, if any, flexibility, with significantly impaired sports performance. Only recently have the advantages of properly supervised and organized resistance training programs been realized. Resistance training, when integrated into an overall fitness program that emphasizes aerobic and flexibility conditioning, can serve to prevent injuries in allied sporting activities as well as improve the overall performance in these activities. Improperly organized resistance training programs, especially those that do not emphasize proper technique and nutrition, can be ineffective and result in injury.

It was once thought that prepubescents and females would achieve little benefit from resistance training owing to decreased testosterone levels. It is now known that females and participants as young as 7 years old may realize significant improvement in strength and sports performance through properly supervised resistance training.

In this chapter, I will review the known physiological effects of resistance training. I will discuss in detail the injury patterns associated with resistance training, with recommendations for preventative measures including proper training techniques and nutrition. Emphasis will also be placed on how a resistance training program can be organized and implemented.

This chapter should provide a working knowledge of the benefits and risks of resistance training and allow the reader to organize a program that emphasizes safety while maximizing results.

CONCEPTS AND DEFINITIONS

Strength training is best defined as the use of progressive resistance methods to increase one's ability to exert or resist force. The resistance methods may include the use of body weight, free weights, machines, or other such equipment.[1]

Resistance training employs one or more of the following training modalities: isometric, isotonic, isokinetic, and variable resistance. Competitive events include Olympic weight lifting, bodybuilding, and power lifting. There are specific strength training programs used by athletes in these competitive events to best prepare for the events. Weight training, circuit training, and plyometrics are training programs that are designed to achieve activity-specific or sports-specific training.

Strength development requires muscle to contract against an unyielding load. A *concentric* contraction involves shortening of the muscle against resistance. Pushing a weight off the chest, as in the bench press, and flexing the elbow with weight held in the hand, as in the arm curl, are examples of concentric muscle contraction. *Eccentric* contraction involves lengthening of the muscle against resistance such as lowering the weight to the chest during the bench press or slowly extending the arm after the arm curl. The most effective strength training programs employ both concentric and eccentric training modalities.

ISOMETRIC EXERCISES

Isometrics involve forceful muscle contractions against an unyielding load without the muscle changing length. Isometric exercises require a minimum of equipment, and since there is no joint motion, the exercises can be employed when joints must be immobilized because of trauma or surgery. Isometrics have the disadvantage of not allowing eccentric muscle contraction; in addition, the strength that is developed is specific for the angle at which the joint was positioned during the isometric exercise. It has also been demonstrated that isometric work leads more rapidly to fatigue, owing to reduced peripheral blood flow, compared with rhythmic exercise, which facilitates circulation.[2]

ISOTONIC EXERCISES

Isotonic resistance training employs a constant load to the muscles usually in the form of weights. Free weights are the most common isotonic equipment. Isotonic exercises employ both concentric and eccentric muscle contraction as the weight is both lifted and then slowly lowered to its starting point. Performing a lifting motion with free weights requires the use of assisting muscles beyond those that are the primary movers to help stabilize the weight during the lift. Isotonic resistance training has the disadvantage of not matching load to strength of a muscle at different joint angles. At different positions in the joint motion, the power that may be exerted by muscle changes as the length of that muscle changes. A constant load cannot accommodate this, and the amount lifted is therefore defined by the weakest point in the range of motion. Lifting weight greater than this minimum would not allow a full range of motion. Other disadvantages of free weights include acceleration at the end of an arc of motion that decreases muscle loading and danger of falling weights requiring spotters to protect against injury.[3]

VARIABLE-RESISTANCE EXERCISES

Machines have been developed to minimize the mismatch of strength and resistance during a joint's range of motion. These machines, for example, Nautilus, employ a cam to vary the amount of force presented to the muscle. The cam allows maximum load during the range of the motion where strength is greatest. *Variable-resistance* machines allow both concentric and eccentric training for the muscles. However, they suffer from the disadvantage of forcing the user into the defined arc of the machine through its radius of motion. As a consequence, users who have extremities that have a different radius of motion than the machine may be subject to decreased efficiency on the exercise equipment and possible injury. Additionally, there is less synergistic muscle action with the use of machines since the equipment does not require stabilization during the lift, as is required with free weights.

ISOKINETIC EXERCISES

Isokinetic exercises employ reciprocating resistance that is a function of the force applied to maintain a constant velocity through the range of motion. This minimizes the effect of acceleration as is found in variable-resistance or isotonic exercises. Isokinetic exercise programs are primarily concentric, but recently, some of the newer machines allow eccentric isokinetic training as well. Isokinetic machines, such as Cybex, have their greatest use in determining muscle strength at various velocities corresponding to power and endurance.

CIRCUIT TRAINING

Circuit weight training employs stations through which the participant moves rapidly performing a set of exercises at approximately 50 to 70 percent of the maximum weight. The training program uses machines that allow rapid migration through the stations with minimal rest between lifts. The program is oriented toward increased cardiovascular endurance as well as strength improvement. While strength does improve with this training program, the improvement in VO_2 max is significantly less than would be expected as the result of an aerobic training program.[4]

WEIGHT TRAINING

Weight training is the term given to strength training used to supplement or improve performance in other sports or activities. Weight training typically utilizes both machine and free weights and often incorporates circuit training techniques.

PLYOMETRICS

Plyometrics are exercises that force a rapid lengthening of a muscle prior to its contraction. Rapid prestretching of a muscle before a contraction facilitates the contraction and causes it to be more forceful.[5] One of the most popular plyometric exercises is the depth jump, which requires a participant to drop from controlled height and, on landing, to perform a maximum vertical jump immediately. There have been reported improvements in explosive events following plyometric training.[6] Plyometric training maximizes the coordination between neuromuscular skills and muscular strength.[6] Maximum benefit occurs when weight training is combined with plyometric training to improve sports performance that requires explosive yet powerful muscular contractions.[7,8] Plyometrics have the potential disadvantage of overloading tendons and ligaments and therefore should be restricted to the well-trained athlete after adequate warm-up.

OLYMPIC WEIGHT LIFTING

Olympic weight lifting is a competitive event restricted to two lifts. The "clean and jerk" brings weight to the chest in one movement and then above the head in the second movement. The "snatch" brings weight from the floor to above the head in one single movement. It is a potentially dangerous activity if the lifter's balance should be lost while performing a lift. Performance of the Olympic lift requires balance and speed in addition to tremendous strength.

POWER LIFTING

Power lifting is also a competitive event, but here the emphasis is on three lifts—the bench press; the dead lift, where weight is lifted from the floor to waist level; and the squat, where weight is placed on the shoulders and the participant lowers himself or herself until the knees are parallel to the floor and then rises again. The power lifter trains with very heavy weights where only one or two repetitions are performed, with prolonged rest periods between lifts. Injuries occur in this event owing to the extreme weights employed that can potentially overload bones, tendons, or muscles.

BODYBUILDING

In *bodybuilding*, the objective is to present the most muscular physique. The training program employs much higher repetitions per lift and a higher-intensity training program. Because of the higher intensity, bodybuilders are often in better aerobic condition compared with power lifters or Olympic lifters with lipid profiles that are similar to those found in runners.[9] They also have increased capillary density within a muscle and increased slow-twitch muscle fiber development compared with the Olympic lifter and power lifter.[10]

REPETITIONS/RM/SETS

Repetitions are the number of times that a resistance training motion is performed without rest. 1-RM is the maximum amount of weight that a participant can lift on a particular exercise for just one repetition. 6-RM is the maximum amount of weight that a participant can lift for six repetitions without stop. Authorities believe that loads that range from 2-RM to 10-RM performed at a maximum number of repetitions are the most effective for strength development[11] 6-RM appears to be the optimum load.[12] Repetitions beyond 20 have progressively less effect.[11] A weight training program is organized into "sets" of repetitions with brief periods of rest between each set for a given exercise. The optimum number of sets appears to be three when utilizing six repetitions per set with 6-RM loads.[12]

ORGANIZATION OF A RESISTANCE TRAINING PROGRAM

Optimizing strength increases from resistance training requires manipulation of the number of repetitions, sets, and frequency of the exercise program. General guidelines can be given, but customization of the program is highly individual.

DeLorme was the first to propose the concept of progressive resistance exercise (PRE).[13] The PRE technique creates an environment where the individual muscle exercises to full capacity against an ever-increasing resistance. The program consists of multiple sets of an exercise performed for 10 repetitions per set, with progressively increasing resistance up to the maximum of 10-RM. Weekly, the participant establishes a new 10-RM load for the following week's exercise program. Recently, the PRE technique has been modified by Knight to allow better determination of the daily strength increase of the athlete and to modify the load accordingly. This new technique is called the Daily Adjustable Progressive Resistance Exercise (DAPRE).[14] In this program, the participant performs four sets of an exercise. A working weight is established based on the previous day's efforts. The first set is one half of that working weight for 10 repetitions. The second set is three fourths of that working weight for six repetitions. The third set is the full working weight for a maximum number of repetitions. Based on the number of repetitions performed, the weight is adjusted for the fourth set and again is performed for a maximum number of repetitions. Based on the number of repetitions performed during the fourth set, the weight is again adjusted and becomes the new working weight for the following day's exercise (Tables 2–1 and 2–2). This program helps to ensure that a participant works near his or her optimal capacity during each training session. This is particularly helpful for patients undergoing rehabilitation following surgery or injury.[15]

There are many other combinations of sets and repetitions that may be used to maximize strength gains. As noted earlier, the optimum number of repetitions appears to be six with a 6-RM load. This is the ideal working weight in the DAPRE technique. However, effective training can occur with loads that range from 2-RM to 10-RM. Using progressively lighter loads below 10-RM results in decreasing improvements in strength.[11] An ideal resistance training program would emphasize maximum repetitions for three to five sets. The load may have to be adjusted in later sets to account for fatigue.

A successful program employing these techniques pyramids the resistance used. In this program, five sets of an exercise are performed with progressively increasing resistance for the first three sets. Maximum resistance is employed on the third set. The result is that the participant performs a higher number of repetitions on the first set, usually eight to ten repetitions; six to eight repetitions on the second set; and perhaps one to three repetitions on the third set. Between six and ten repetitions are performed on the fourth and fifth sets.

Another variation employs multiple exercises that train the same muscle group and are done consecutively. This allows training of the muscle at different angles and velocities. This "giant set" is usually composed of a total of three to eight sets for each muscle trained. It is sometimes advisable to give a muscle rest between sets by working antagonistic muscles on alternate sets. For instance, biceps and triceps may be trained together with one set of a bicep exercise, followed immediately by a "superset" of a tricep exercise. The remaining sets would continue to alternate between bicep and tricep exercises.

Giant sets, supersets, and PRE and DAPRE techniques all provide alternatives that the participant should explore to maximize strength gains.

Optimal strength gains occur when the resistance training program is performed between three and five times per week.[16] To avoid overtraining, a muscle should be given

TABLE 2–1. DAPRE Technique

Set	Weight	Repetitions
1	One-half working weight	10
2	Three-quarters working weight	6
3	Full working weight	Maximum[a]
4	Adjusted working weight[a]	Maximum[b]

[a] The number of repetitions performed during the third set is used to determine the adjusted working weight for the fourth set according to the guidelines in Table 2–2.
[b] The number of repetitions performed during the fourth set is used to determine the working weight for the next session according to the guidelines in Table 2–2.
Source: From Knight, K., Knee rehabilitation by the daily adjustable progressive resistive exercise technique. Am. J. Sports Med. 7:336–337, 1979. Reprinted with permission.

TABLE 2–2. General Guidelines for Adjustment of Working Weight

No. of Repetitions Performed During Set	Adjusted Working Weight	
	Fourth Set[a]	*Next Session*[b]
0–2	Decrease 5–10 lb	Decrease 5–10 lb
3–4	Decrease 0–5 lb	Keep the same
5–6	Keep the same	Increase 5–10 lb
7–10	Increase 5–10 lb	Increase 5–15 lb
11–	Increase 10–15 lb	Increase 10–20 lb

[a] The number of repetitions performed during the third set is used to determine the adjusted working weight for the fourth set (Table 2–1).
[b] The number of repetitions performed during the fourth set is used to determine the working weight for the next session (usually the next day) (Table 2–1).
Source: Knight, K., Knee rehabilitation by the daily adjustable progressive resistive exercise technique. Am. J. Sports Med. 7:336–337, 1979. Reprinted with permission.

between 24 and 36 hours of rest before it is trained again. To allow an adequate number of training sessions per week and yet minimize overtraining, alternate body parts can be trained on subsequent days. In this technique, a participant may train Monday, Tuesday, Thursday, and Friday with Wednesday, Saturday, and Sunday as rest days. Ideally, aerobic training would be performed on rest days. Monday and Thursday training sessions would train one set of body parts, whereas the alternate body parts would be trained on Tuesday and Friday. Typically, muscles that flex joints are trained on Monday and Thursday, and those that extend joints are trained on Tuesday and Friday. Other programs train all body parts 3 days a week, with a rest day between each training day. More sophisticated "split" programs train alternate body parts on the same day in two separate training sessions. Another two body parts are trained the following day, and so on. This technique is commonly employed by the competitive bodybuilder who will train one body part per training session. Maximum energy for each body part is ensured by splitting the training into morning and evening sessions on the same day.

Periodization is the technique of varying the number of sets and repetitions performed during training sessions. Changing the intensity and volume of exercise over a period of time optimizes physiological adaptation. Such a program may go through two or three cycles per year where volume and intensity are gradually increased and then decreased.[11]

There are a myriad of options available to customize a resistance training program. Integration of a resistance training program with an aerobic training program ensures maximum strength and cardiovascular development.

PHYSIOLOGICAL EFFECTS

NEURAL

Increased strength through resistance training involves not only muscle adaptations but neural adaptations as well. Trained participants are able to activate prime mover muscles more fully, producing more force. There is improved motor unit recruitment as a result of training, so that there is less electromyogram (EMG) activity required to produce a submaximal force. Additionally, there is improved synchronization of motor unit recruitment.[17] While the effect of synchronization on the amount of force output is not clear, it is known that synchronization does increase duration of maximal force output.[11]

There is evidence that, through training, the Golgi tendon organs may become desensitized, and therefore greater force production occurs because of disinhibition of the muscle.[11] Also, training induces an increase in the number of vesicles that store acetylcholine in a neuron terminal as well as an increase in the area of apposition at the neuromuscular junction. The result is improved neurochemical transmission of impulses.[11]

When naive subjects begin strength training, there is a rapid increase in strength without significant changes in the muscles themselves. These immediate strength increases are attributed to neural factors. Following short-term improvment in strength as a result of neural factors, further strength increases are a result of muscle adaptation.[18]

Neural effects are also at work when bilateral training effects are considered. Cross training is the noted increased strength in a contralateral limb when the other limb has performed strength training exercises. The muscles in the contralateral limb show no change associated with the strength increases. The mechanism for the strength improvement appears to be central neural adaptation.[17, 18] A similar central neural effect occurs during bilateral deficit, where the amount of force produced by a particular muscle group in one limb is less when the contralateral limb is concurrently performing a maximal activation. In other words, the total force produced when both limbs are performing an exercise is less than the sum of the forces that can be produced by each limb individually. Bilateral deficit can be decreased by training both limbs simultaneously.[17, 18]

There appears to be a neural component to specificity of training as well. Heavy resistance weight training is associated with increased EMG recordings late in the EMG pattern. Participants in plyometric strength training programs demonstrate increased EMG readings early in the EMG pattern consistent with the training that emphasizes explosive muscle contraction.[17] Additionally, participants who have been trained in plyometrics demonstrate facilitation of eccentric contraction in the muscles trained.

Patterns of motor unit recruitment are developed for each exercise performed, with improved coordination of synergistic and antagonistic muscle activity for the exercise. Antagonistic muscles, such as the triceps and the biceps, work against each other, whereas synergistic muscles, such as the biceps and the forearm flexor muscles, assist one another. The result is increased skill, coordination, and power.[17] To develop capabilities of motor units optimally, resistance training programs must employ numerous exercises that are performed at various velocities and angles.[11]

It is possible to excite muscle by applying electric current across the muscle or its peripheral nerve. Electrical stimulation employs these techniques. Strength gains associated with electromyostimulation are similar to those that occur through voluntary training but take place more quickly. It is unclear whether long-term electrical stimulation would result in strength increases that are superior to voluntary training.[18] Electrical stimulation appears to activate preferentially the largest motor units that are difficult to train under voluntary conditions. The strength increases associated with electrical stimulation appear to be mediated by neural adaptation.[18]

CARDIOVASCULAR

Strength training really has very little effect on the endurance capacity of the participant. $\dot{V}O_2$max is considered the best measurement of the aerobic capacity of an athlete. Strength training programs that emphasize high-intensity exercise with short rest periods between exercises are associated with only minimal improvements in $\dot{V}O_2$max.[19, 20] One paper demonstrated a 5 to 8 percent increase in $\dot{V}O_2$max following high-intensity resistance training, but this was relatively small compared with the average 20 percent improvement associated with endurance-based programs.[4] This same study demonstrated that a program that employs high-resistance loads with longer rest periods is associated with a 0.5 to 9 percent decrease in $\dot{V}O_2$max. $\dot{V}O_2$max appears to be unchanged with resistance training because the $\dot{V}O_2$ rarely exceeds 45 percent of the $\dot{V}O_2$max of the athlete during the training program. Aerobic training programs consistently drive $\dot{V}O_2$ in excess of 50 percent of $\dot{V}O_2$max, which is considered the threshold for aerobic improvement.[19] However, there is a significant increase in the heart rate during resistance training.[19, 21] Unlike aerobic training, maintaining heart rate above 60 percent of maximum heart rate is not associated with improvement in aerobic capacity during resistance training.[19] In aerobic events, heart rate increases to maximize cardiac output in the face of maximized stroke volume. In these conditions, increased heart rate reflects increased aerobic stress. In resistance training, the increased heart rate is the result of an increased release of catecholamines coupled with decreased venous return due to blood shunting not noted during aerobic training.[19, 21, 22] Therefore, in resistance training heart rate is uncoupled from aerobic performance.

During the performance of a resistance exercise, blood pressure may be markedly increased. The greatest increase in blood pressure occurs during concentric motions and is related to increased cardiac output combined with increased abdominal and thoracic pressure.[23] Long-term resistance training decreases the blood pressure and heart rate response to resistance training.[24] Resistance training is not associated with elevated resting blood pressure.[23]

Resistance training does cause increased absolute left ventricular wall thickness and left ventricular mass. However, these increases normalize when expressed relative to body surface area or lean body mass.[23]

Plasma volume decreases by as much as 14.3 percent during resistance training exercises.[25] This decrease is approximately the same as seen during cycling and running training programs.[25] The plasma volume returns to normal in approximately 30 minutes. Plasma volume appears to decrease secondary to muscular contraction, which increases filtration pressure, and increased osmotic effects secondary to the breakdown of lactate in the interstitial fluid.[25]

Bodybuilding is associated with favorable alterations in lipoprotein fractions.[20] Bodybuilders, whose training is considered high intensity, have an LDL/HDL (low-density lipoprotein/high-density lipoprotein) ratio of approximately 2.0, compared with 2.4 in runners. Power lifters, on the other hand, whose resistance training is considered low intensity, characterized by high resistance and long rest periods, have an LDL/HDL ratio of 3.7 as a result of decreased HDL and increased LDL fractions.[26] Participants who already have a low LDL/HDL ratio may not notice significant improvements during a bodybuilding training program.[27] As with other exercises, the most significant improvements in lipid profiles occur in individuals who enter the training program with relatively unfavorable profiles. The use of anabolic steroids by resistance training participants causes a significant increase in LDL and cholesterol and a decrease in HDL.[26,28] The LDL/HDL ratio may increase by as much as 280 percent during the use of anabolic steroids.[26]

Increased insulin sensitivity is associated with a decreased risk for coronary artery disease. Resistance training may be associated with increased insulin sensitivity.[9] This effect appears to be related to the intensity of the resistance training, as power lifters demonstrate decreased insulin sensitivity.[9]

Therefore, resistance training programs that are higher in intensity as used in bodybuilding and circuit training may be associated with decreased cardiovascular risk factors. This is not the case with lower-intensity, high-resistance programs as used by power lifters. Resistance training programs have little effect on aerobic capacity.

SKELETAL MUSCLE

Resistance training results in muscle hypertrophy. The hypertrophy is the result of an increase in both the total number of fibers and the size of the fibers. The size of the fibers increase as a result of the addition of actin and myosin filaments to the outside of the myofibril.[11] Hyperplasia of muscle fibers occurs as a unique result of resistance training.[29]

Resistance training increases the cross-sectional area of both type I, or slow-twitch, fibers and type II, or fast-twitch fibers. Hypertrophy of fast-twitch fibers is greater than that of slow-twitch fibers.[10] Interestingly, compared with other power-trained athletes, bodybuilders have a relatively higher percentage of slow-twitch fibers. Bodybuilders also demonstrate a relatively higher capillary density in muscle compared with Olympic weight lifters or power lifters.[10,11] Increased glycogen levels are also noted in muscles of bodybuilders. All these findings suggest that bodybuilder muscle development is more like that found in endurance athletes.[10]

All resistance-trained athletes, including bodybuilders, demonstrate a decrease in the enzymes associated with aerobic energy metabolism. Resistance training is also associated with a reduced mitochondrial volume density in muscle, the result of the relative increase in myofibril volume, whereas mitochondrial volume remains unchanged.[10,11] These findings support the incompatibility of resistance training and aerobic capacity development.

Therefore, resistance training can result in muscle hypertrophy through increased fiber size and number. Bodybuilders are unique among resistance-trained athletes in that they have muscle composition that is more like that of the endurance athlete.

STRENGTH

It is well established that resistance training does increase the strength of the participant. This occurs regardless of the age or sex of the participant. Prepubescents as well as women have all demonstrated significant increases in strength when employing resistance training techniques.[30,31,32] Novice weight trainers experience a more rapid rate of strength development compared with initially stronger and experienced weight trainers,[11] owing to neural adaptation. Intensity of muscle contractions is important for maximal strength development. Intensities at 50 percent or less of maximum yield little or no gains in strength.[33] Once strength has been developed, it can generally be maintained with a once-a-week resistance training program. Once all resistance training is terminated, strength is lost at approximately one third the rate at which it was gained.[16] Comparisons between isotonic free-weight exercises and isokinetic exercises demonstrate that both methods are equally effective in developing strength.[3] When evaluating the effects of plyometrics, the addition of weight training to the plyometrics program significantly improves strength performance, compared with the use of plyometrics alone.[8]

PSYCHOLOGICAL EFFECTS

Weight training can significantly improve the body concept of the participant. In the male, a more muscular physique is perceived as reflecting a more ideal body image, with significant increases in body satisfaction and feelings of personal pride.[34] Additionally, mesomorphic males are generally viewed by others as more skillful, capable, and psychologically sound than are less-developed males.[35] Males who enter a weight training program in comparatively weak condition gain significantly more body satisfaction than do males who begin a program with a relatively more mesomorphic appearance.[34] Even in prepubescence, weight training can serve to increase attentiveness to homework and other activities.[36] Therefore, weight training can have significantly positive physical and psychological effects on the participant.

BODY COMPOSITION

A resistance training program will increase lean body mass and decrease the percentage of body fat. The increase in lean body mass is the result of increased muscle tissue. Only slight changes in total body weight occur as a result of short-term resistance training. Increases in body weight require long periods of training. Resistance-trained male athletes have body fat percentages that range from 8.3 to 12.2 percent. Female bodybuilders measure approximately 13 percent. The average norm for body fat of college-age males and females is between 14 and 26 percent.[11] A change in the mesomorphic component may be slow to occur. Significant strength increases may occur much sooner than a change in physique.[37]

ENERGY REQUIREMENTS

The energy requirements of resistance training are met through hydrolysis of high-energy phosphate bonds in skeletal muscle. As increasing numbers of repetitions per set and decreasing rest intervals occur during the weight training program, glycolysis plays an increasingly important role in energy contribution.[38] There is evidence that lipolysis may also provide an energy source.[38,39] The performance of a severely intensive resistive training session causes a decline in the high-energy phosphate and glycogen stores in the muscle and the accumulation of glycogenolytic/glycolytic intermediates including lactate,[38] findings consistent with anaerobic metabolism. There are also data to support the importance of aerobic energy production in the later phases of continuous maximal glycolytic anaerobic work to meet the energy demands.[40]

As an adaptation, resistance training results in significant increases in the intramuscular high-energy phosphate pool between training sessions. The increased energy stores probably do not relate to improvements in maximum strength but may prolong maximum muscular contractions.[11]

BONE AND CONNECTIVE TISSUE

Bodybuilding results in an absclute increase in the collagen within muscle sheaths, resulting in increased strength of the sheath.[41] In addition, resistance training can bring about increases in the size and strength of ligaments and tendons as a result of elevated collagen content.[11, 42] Other effects include thickening of the hyaline cartilage on the articular surfaces of bones.[43] Studies of the lumbar spine during heavy weight lifting demonstrate loads on the L3 vertebral body between 18.8 and 36.4 kilonewtons. This is much higher than the ultimate compressive strength of normal human vertebral bodies, which is 10 to 12 kilonewtons. The vertebral bodies in intensively trained power lifters are able to tolerate these significantly increased compressive loads as a result of increased bone mineral content. The increases in bone mineral content are a function of the amount of training performed. Those participants who lift greater than 1000 tons annually have the highest levels of bone mineral content in their lumbar vertebra.[44]

Therefore, resistance-trained athletes adapt to the training programs by increasing the strength of tendons, ligaments, and bone. These adaptations would certainly be expected to decrease injury rates in other sports in which the athlete may participate.

HORMONAL EFFECTS

Intense resistance training is associated with increased postexercise serum testosterone levels in males.[45] There appears to be a threshold of intensity of training as measured by the percent of 1-RM, the volume of training as measured by the number of repetitions and sets, and finally, the muscle mass used in the exercise to produce increases in testosterone concentrations.[46] Increases in serum testosterone do not appear to occur in females following heavy resistance training.[45, 46] Higher resting baseline levels of total testosterone have also been observed in athletes who have been involved in resistance training compared with untrained subjects.[47]

Testosterone has both anticatabolic and anabolic effects. The anabolic effect is mediated by interaction with cytoplasmic receptors on muscle cells stimulating protein synthesis. The anticatabolic effect is the result of displacement of cortisol from its receptors. It has been demonstrated that the testosterone/cortisol ratio is a useful indicator of anabolic activity in the resistance-trained athlete.[48, 49] Elevations in the testosterone/cortisol ratio are associated with strength increases. A decrease in this ratio is associated with detraining strength decreases or strength decreases as a result of overtraining.[4, 49] Plateaus in strength increases during a resistance training program are often the result of overtraining. Overtraining can be defined as a decrease in the testosterone/cortisol ratio by more than 30 percent.[48] Therefore, the balance between the anabolic effects of testosterone and the catabolic effects of cortisol are quite important in developing and maintaining strength through resistance training.

Growth hormone levels are increased during intense resistance training. The high-resistance, low-repetition exercise program performed by power lifters is associated with greater increases in endogenous growth hormone release than is the lower-resistance, higher-repetition program performed by bodybuilders.[50] The growth hormone release is a delayed response. It begins approximately 16 minutes after the commencement of exercise and remains elevated for a short time after exercise cessation.[50]

Resistance training is also associated with the release of epinephrine and norepinephrine from the adrenal medulla and sympathetic neurons. Additionally, there are associated increases in dopamine levels, probably as a result of an inability to convert dopamine to norepinephrine owing to limits in enzymatic conversion.[51] The increased catecholamine concentrations are similar to those found in other intense anaerobic activities such as sprinting and cycling. These levels are all significantly greater than those associated with aerobic activities.[46]

RESISTANCE TRAINING INJURIES

As with any athletic endeavor, resistance training can result in injury. Awareness of the mechanism of injury and appropriate preventative measures can minimize these risks. Injuries will be reviewed by body part.

BACK AND NECK

During resistance training, the back sustains extremely high compressive loads. During a half-squat exercise with a barbell load between 0.8 and 1.6 times body weight, compressive loads at L3 and L4 vertebral bodies vary between 6 and 10 times body weight.[52] Through prolonged resistance training with high loads, the vertebral bodies will increase their bone mineral content, as noted earlier in this chapter.

Lumbosacral strains are not uncommon during resistance training. These strains are often associated with poor technique or lifting loads that are greater than the subject can handle.

In the more elite competitive weight lifters, *spondylolysis* is a relatively common finding. In one study, 21 of 47 competitive weight lifters demonstrated spondylolytic changes.[53] It is hypothesized that back hyperextension during heavy lifts is the etiology. Specifically, the clean and jerk and snatch in Olympic lifting and the squat and dead lift in power lifting are associated with this injury. *Spondylolisthesis* has also been demonstrated. This may be a preexisting condition that is exacerbated by weight lifting.[54] Herniated nucleus pulposus has also been documented.[54]

Cervical strain syndrome is not uncommon during resistance training[54] and is often the result of the participant's using paracervical muscles to help stabilize the head and torso on a weight-lifting bench. Only rarely are these injuries associated with significant cervical pathology.

CHEST

Avulsion of the pectoralis major tendon may occur while performing arm curls with dumbbells[55] or, more commonly, doing weighted dip exercises. The weighted dip exercise is performed with weights strapped to the waist while performing a dip between parallel bars (Fig. 2–1). Attempted surgical correction of a tear at the musculotendinous junction may not be successful. Repairs of pectoralis tendon avulsions from the humerus have been successful.[55] Weighted dip

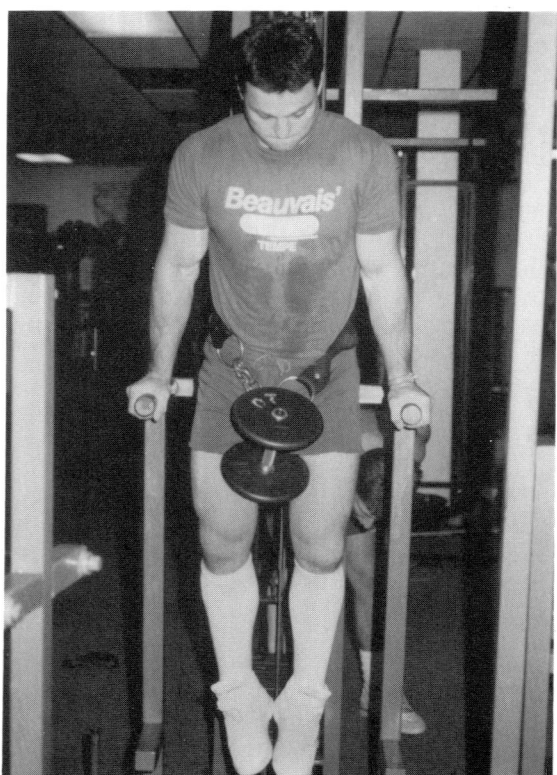 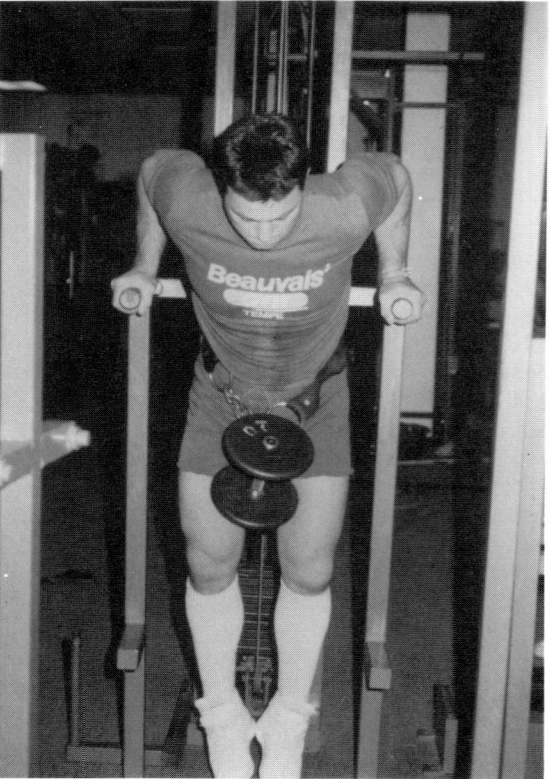

FIGURE 2–1. The weighted dip exercise places undue stress on the pectoralis major tendon insertion on the humerus and can result in tendon avulsions or tears in the pectoralis muscle.

exercises are a potentially dangerous activity and should be avoided.

PELVIS

Avulsion of the anterior superior iliac spine may occur in young athletes.[54] This injury has occurred during the dead lift exercise and during the back hyperextension exercise as the participant flexes his or her hyperextended upper torso while lying supine on an elevated bench.

KNEE AND LEG

Patellofemoral pain syndrome is frequently associated with poor technique while performing the leg extension exercise. Most leg extension equipment allows a full range of motion at the knee so that the participant extends the knee from a hyperflexed position to full extension against resistance. Only the last 30 to 45 degrees of extension are of real benefit to the participant. Extension against resistance with the knee hyperflexed can be associated with patellofemoral pain (Fig. 2–2A). A safer technique is to limit the range of motion in the exercise from 45 degrees of flexion to full extension (Fig. 2–2B and Fig. 2–2C) unless the patellofemoral joint is already crepitant, or painful, in a certain arc of motion. In this case it is better to restrict knee extension exercises to the non-crepitant or pain-free arc. Additionally, improper seat adjustment on a stationary bicycle can also be associated with patellofemoral pain. If the seat of the stationary bicycle is not high enough, the knee is again hyper-

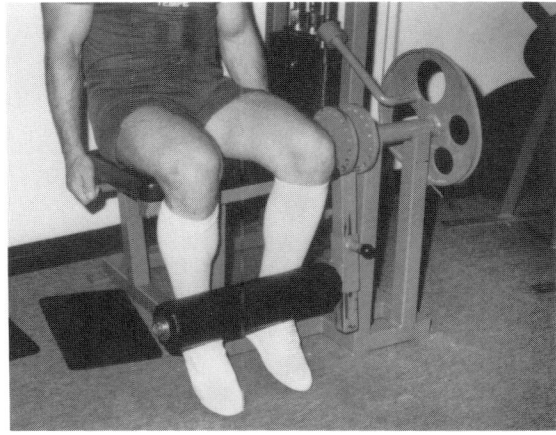
A

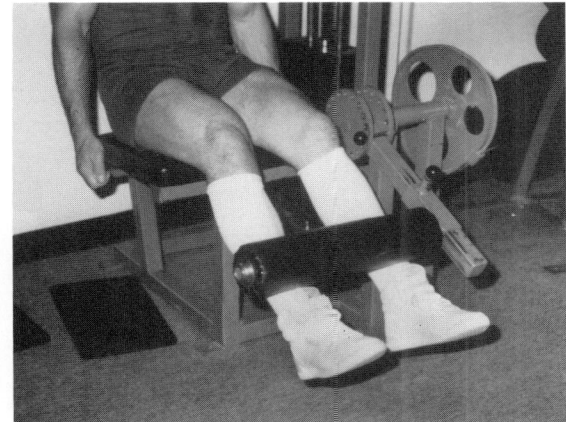
B

C

FIGURE 2–2. The leg extension exercise can be associated with patellofemoral pain if full flexion of the knee is allowed, as in A. A less painful variation of the exercise is a limited range of motion from 45 degrees of flexion to full extension, as in B and C. If the patellofemoral joint is already crepitant or painful during a certain arc of motion, this arc should be avoided.

flexed when the pedal (Fig. 2–3) is in the "up" position. This will result in patellofemoral pain as the participant forces the hyperflexed knee to extend against the resistance of the pedal. Proper seat adjustment is obtained by placing the heel of the foot on the "down" pedal and adjusting the height of the seat until the leg is fully extended (Fig. 2–4). Quadriceps and patellar tendinitis can occur with more intense training programs, including those associated with plyometrics. Higher repetition and lower-weight leg extension exercises, combined with massage and modalities including nonsteroidal anti-inflammatories, can usually resolve the tendinitis in time. Patellar and quadriceps tendon ruptures have been documented.[56, 57] These injuries have occurred during the use of very heavy weights in the squat or the Olympic lifts.

Meniscal tears have occurred during leg curls that emphasize the hamstring muscles and during dead lifting exercises.[54]

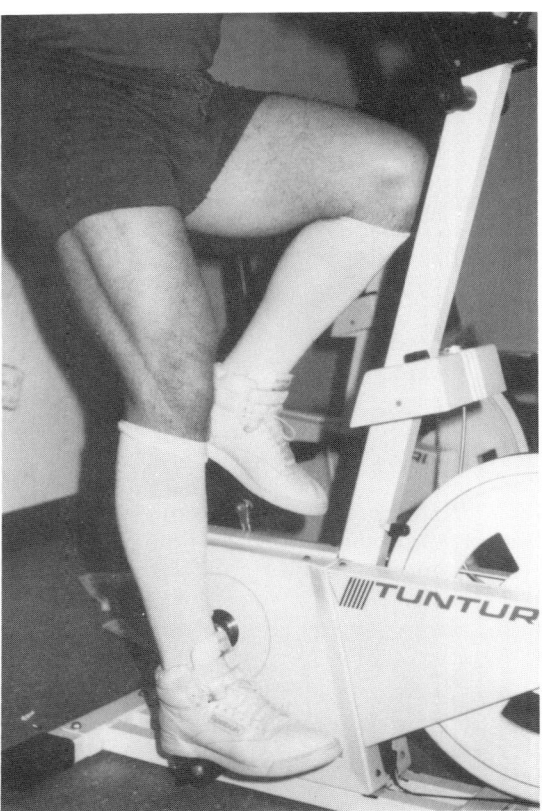

FIGURE 2–4. Proper stationary bicycle seat adjustment allows full extension of the leg when the heel is placed on the down pedal. As noted in this figure, this places less flexion on the knee in the up-pedal position and reduces the risk of patellofemoral pain.

SHOULDER

Dislocations of the shoulder during heavy bench pressing have been documented and have occurred bilaterally simultaneously.[58] Dislocation occurs as the weight is in the low position on the chest, causing the shoulder to be placed in the position of vulnerability.

Biceps tendinitis is often considered shoulder pain by the athlete and may be related to improper technique using arm curls. If the participant is not careful to prevent the shoulder from flexing as an arm curl is performed, added stress is placed on the long head biceps tendon as it passes through the intertubercular groove. This injury may be avoided by stabilizing the elbows at the torso so that all motion occurs at the elbow with elbow flexion.

Weight lifter's shoulder is a common complaint in heavy-resistance-trained athletes. In this condition, loss of subchondral bone

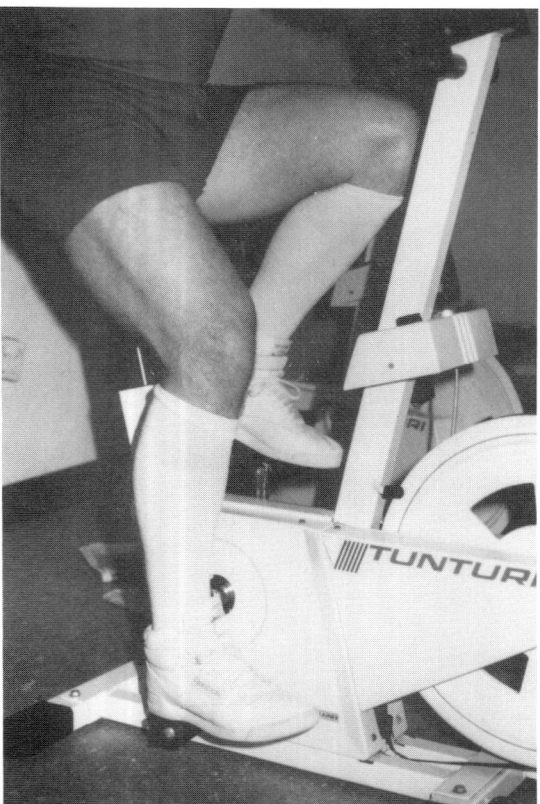

FIGURE 2–3. If the stationary bicycle seat height adjustment is not high enough, the knee will hyperflex in the up position on the pedal, which can be associated with patellofemoral pain.

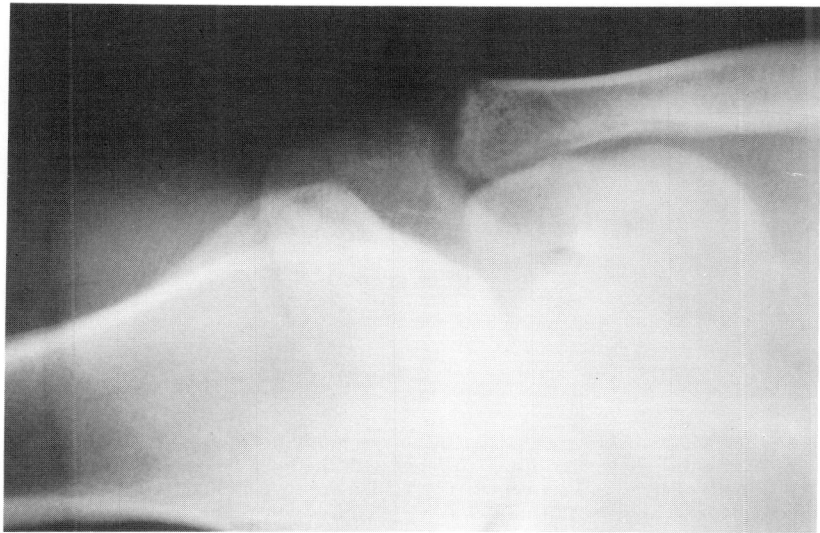

FIGURE 2–5. Osteolysis of the distal end of the clavicle is noted in this transaxillary view of a patient who was involved in heavy resistance training with the bench press. Acromioclavicular joint tenderness is associated with this finding.

and cystic changes at the distal end of the clavicle are present and are collectively referred to as *osteolysis of the distal end of the clavicle*[59] (Fig. 2–5). Bone scans demonstrate increased activity in this region. The pathognomonic clinical sign of weight lifter's shoulder is pain at the acromioclavicular joint associated with the bench press and the dip. The pain is usually more severe the night following a weight-lifting exercise program. Wide-grip bench pressing appears to be the etiology of this complaint. The wide grip is considered the grip of preference for increased power during the bench press, but it places the acromioclavicular joint as well as the anterior deltoid at risk when the weight is lowered to the chest (Fig. 2–6).

It has been recommended that excision of the distal clavicle be performed for relief of pain if osteolysis is present.[59] However, I have had great success in treating this condition conservatively. Conservative treatment includes abstinence from the bench press and the dip exercises. In place of these exercises, cable crossovers (Fig. 2–7), decline presses with dumbbells (Fig. 2–8), incline presses with a straight bar (Fig. 2–9), and dumbbell flies may be performed. Finally, all

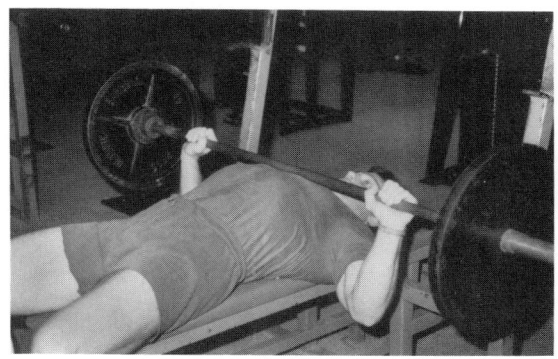
A

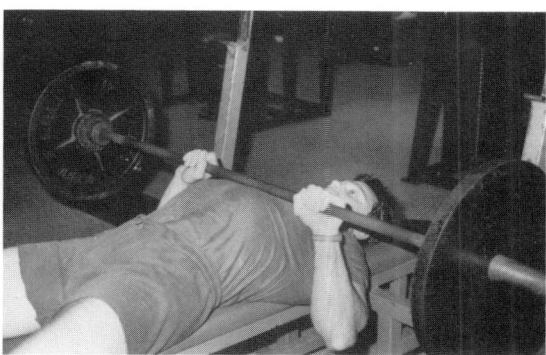
B

FIGURE 2–6. The wide-grip bench press is often associated with weight lifter's shoulder syndrome, as it places increased sheer stress across the acromioclavicular joint, as noted in *A*. Using a more narrow grip reduces the stress on the acromioclavicular joint, as shown in *B*.

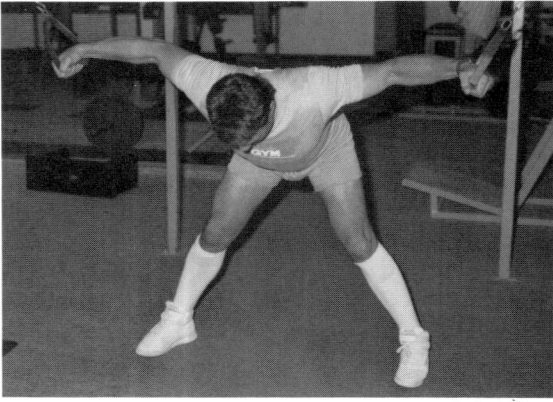 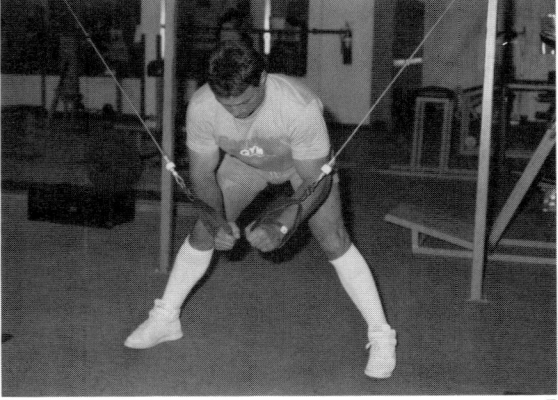

A B

FIGURE 2–7. Cable cross-overs are effective pectoralis major training exercises that minimize acromioclavicular joint pain. The exercise is performed with the torso flexed at 90 degrees, maintaining slight flexion of both elbows, as noted in A. The cables are then pulled down in front of the body, maintaining the elbow flexion as shown in B.

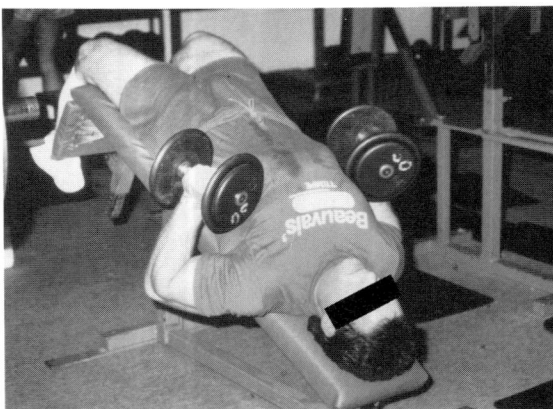 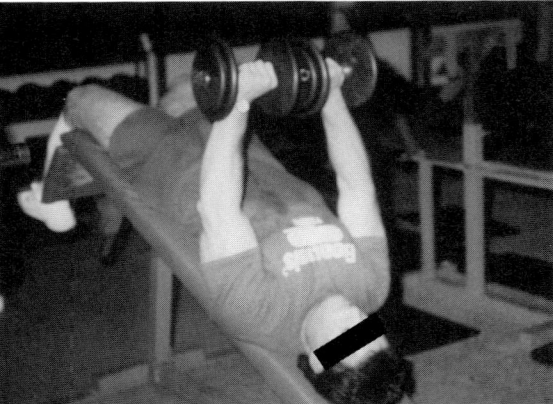

A B

FIGURE 2–8. The decline press with dumbbells is performed with the dumbbells held parallel to the body in the down position, and the arms are pronated in the up position. This exercise minimizes stress on the acromioclavicular joint.

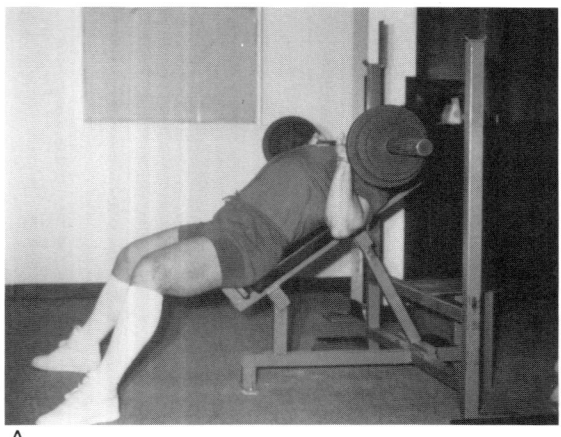 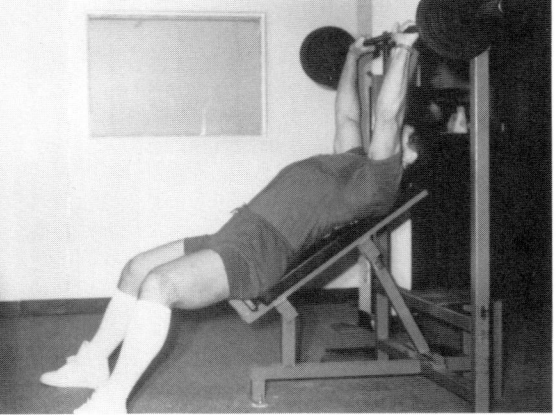

A B

FIGURE 2–9. The incline press allows pectoralis muscle development while minimizing stress on the acromioclavicular joint.

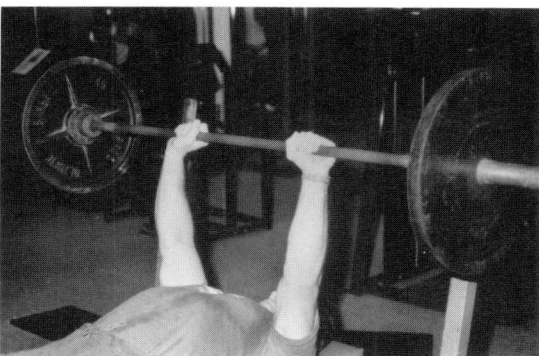

FIGURE 2–10. The narrow grip during bar presses minimizes shoulder injury. The hands should grasp the bar at shoulder width and no wider.

pressing exercises should be performed with a shoulder-width grip, which is considered narrow to most weight lifters (Fig. 2–10). With this program, including appropriate ice massage of the injured area and use of nonsteroidal antiinflammatories, the participants usually notice improvement within 6 to 8 weeks. In addition, most find that their chest development and strength improve with the program.

In my experience, the bench press carries with it significant risks while it fails to isolate properly the pectoralis muscle for maximal development. I recommend that the bench press be restricted to the competitive power lifter who competes with the exercise and avoided by all others.

I am not aware of any compelling indication for the use of the dip exercise and recommend that it be abandoned entirely. It is associated not only with painful shoulder syndromes but, as noted earlier, with tearing of the pectoralis major muscle and tendon.

ARM

Ruptures of the tricep tendon have occurred during heavy bench pressing[60] and during the snatch Olympic lift. It has also occurred as the result of striking the posterior aspect of the arm during a fall in a professional bodybuilder.[31] The condition may go unrecognized and present with symptoms that are similar to the cubital tunnel syndrome with paresthesias in the fourth and fifth finger.[60] Delayed surgical repair is successful.[60, 61, 62] An association with anabolic steroid use has been suggested.[60, 62]

WRIST AND FOREARM

Bilateral distal radius and ulna fractures have occurred in adolescent weight lifters doing overhead lifting exercises. The radius fractures were Salter II epiphyseal fractures.[63] The injury is the result of hyperextension of the wrist that is pronated during the military press or the clean and jerk. As excessive weight is raised overhead, control of the weight may be lost, causing the weight to roll off the back of the wrist and resulting in dorsal displacement of the wrist and a Salter II fracture. The importance of avoidance of competitive lifting by the adolescent and prepubescent is made apparent by this injury.

Ulnar forearm pain is a relatively common problem in weight lifters. It is often associated with arm curls using a straight bar that causes the wrists to be held in extreme supination (Fig. 2–11). This places stress on the flexor and extensor carpi ulnaris muscles, resulting in a mild periostitis of the ulna (Fig. 2–12). A stress fracture of the diaphysis of the ulna has occurred by the same mechanism.[64] It is my recommendation that arm curls be performed with either dumbbells or a curl bar that is shaped like a camshaft. By grasping the curl bar at the cam angulation, hypersupination of the wrists is avoided (Fig. 2–13A). Using dumbbells, the wrists can be positioned where they are most comfortable for the athlete, avoiding hypersupination of the wrist (Fig. 2–13B).

Compartment syndrome in the forearm following intense weight lifting has been documented.[65]

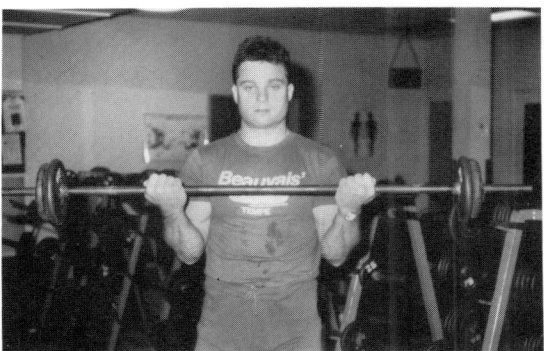

FIGURE 2–11. The use of a straight bar for bicep curls forces the wrist into maximum supination and can result in forearm pain.

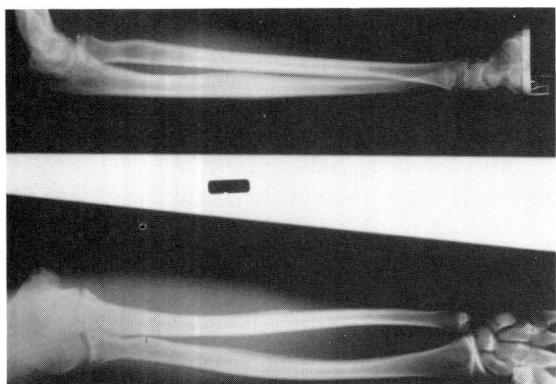

FIGURE 2–12. These X rays represent periostitis associated with ulnar forearm pain as a result of using the straight bar for bicep curls as in Figure 2–9B.

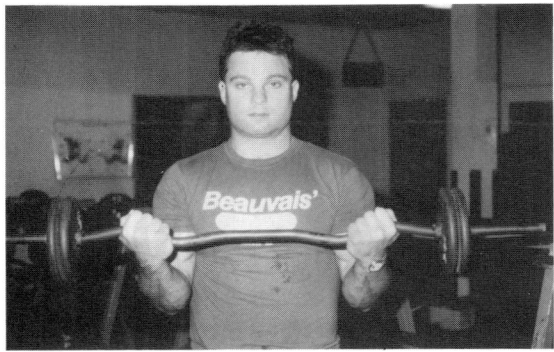

A

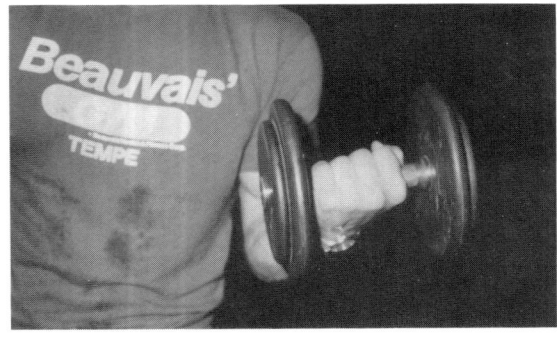

B

FIGURE 2–13. Using the cam-shaped curl bar as in *A*, or dumbbells as in *B*, avoids hypersupination of the forearm and minimizes ulnar forearm pain associated with bicep curls.

OTHER INJURIES

Esophageal varices has been reported in a heavy weight lifter, presumably as a result of increased venous pressure during Valsalva maneuvers.[66] Severe injuries, including death, may occur if heavy weights are dropped while performing exercises such as the bench press or the overhead press. For this reason, the use of spotters to stabilize the weight or to catch the weight if it is dropped is very important when free weights are used. The use of machines for resistance training minimizes the need for spotters.

CEPHALGIA

Exertional headache as a result of resistance training is usually abrupt and of brief duration and subsides with cessation of the exercise. It is usually a benign condition, but medical evaluation should be performed to rule out underlying dangerous conditions such as aneurysms, arteriovenous (AV) malformations, or tumors. Serious conditions are found in only 10 percent of the cases.[67, 68]

LOSS OF FLEXIBILITY

Resistance training not associated with a flexibility program may result in decreased range of motion.[69] By maintaining an adequate flexibility program in conjunction with the resistance training program, range of motion may actually increase.[32, 36, 69]

REHABILITATION AND IMPROVED SPORTS PERFORMANCE

Most physical therapy programs incorporate some form of resistance training. Isometric exercises for immobilized limbs, ankle weights and wrist weights for early resistive exercises through range of motion, isokinetic devices, and free weights and variable-resistance machines all play a role in effective rehabilitation for injured or postoperative patients. Resistance training may be the primary mode of rehabilitation following injury or may be combined with some of the modalities described in Chapter 5 into an integrated rehabilitation program.

Performance in sports-related activities can be improved through resistance training. The use of weight training alone or in combination with plyometric training has been demonstrated to improve significantly the 40-yard dash times, vertical jump height, shuttle run times, and number of pull-ups performed compared with either program alone.[7, 8] In addition, there appears to be a decreased risk of injury to muscles and tendons as a result of preparticipation resistance training.

Therefore, resistance training is fundamental to injury prevention and treatment for the athlete. Appropriately organized strength training can also enhance athletic performance.

NUTRITION

Resistance-training athletes have for years sought supplements that would increase their size and strength. Many have assumed that strength training requires increased protein intake. As a result, large markets for protein supplements have developed. However, recent research indicates that the nutritional needs of the resistance-trained athlete are no different than those of other athletes. Both need adequate carbohydrate intake to sustain intense training. The National Research Council recommended dietary allowance for protein for the average population is set at 0.8 grams protein/kg bodyweight. Strength-trained athletes probably require an amount greater than this. However, it is unlikely that even with intense resistance training that an athlete would require more than 1.0 to 1.5 grams/kg body weight to be in nitrogen balance.[70] The average American diet supplies between 12 and 15 percent of its calories as protein.[70] An athlete consuming 50 kilocalories/kg body weight of everyday foods will have a protein intake between 1.5 and 1.75 grams/kg body weight, which is more than adequate to sustain muscle development. Therefore, the average American diet supplies plenty of protein, even for resistance-trained athletes. Certainly, when athletes restrict their caloric intake to maintain body weight, as in wrestling, gymnastics, and boxing, protein supplementation may be required. In these cases, in order to maintain adequate protein intake, foods should be selected that are low in calories without sacrificing protein. If protein supplements are required, milk or milk powders are effective and inexpensive protein sources.[70]

More important than protein for the resistance-trained athlete is adequate carbohydrate intake. Resistance-trained athletes consuming 65 percent of their caloric intake in the form of carbohydrates demonstrated significantly increased lean body mass, compared with a similar group of resistance-trained athletes consuming 40 percent of their calories in the form of carbohydrates.[71] Additionally, when comparing a group of resistance-trained athletes using anabolic steroids and obtaining 37 percent of their calories in the form of carbohydrates to resistance-trained athletes who through liquid supplements obtained 47 percent of their calories in the form of carbohydrates and did not use steroids, the steroid and the supplement group gained equal amounts of lean body mass. The supplement group actually reduced body fat, whereas the steroid group increased body fat, resulting in overall increased body weight. The steroid group enjoyed only a statistically insignificant increase in strength over the supplement group.[72]

An athlete who consumes 5 grams carbohydrate/kg body weight will absorb 1.5 to 2.0 grams protein/kg. The resistance-trained athlete who maintains this daily intake of carbohydrates is ensured adequate energy and protein for strength development.[73]

Glycogen resynthesis is required following intense training whether the training is aerobic or anaerobic. Over a 24-hour period, the amount of glycogen resynthesis is the same whether simple or complex carbohydrates are consumed.[74] However, at 48 hours there is a significant improvement in glycogen resynthesis, using the complex carbohydrates. Obviously, athletes are not working on a 48-hour schedule, and therefore even simple carbohydrates can be of significant benefit to the resistance-trained athlete. While increased insulin levels may occur in response to a simple carbohydrate load compared with a complex carbohydrate load, only a very small percentage of athletes, 1 to 5 percent, will experience hypoglycemic episodes.[73] Therefore, simple carbohydrates may actually be as efficacious to the resistance-trained athlete as complex carbohydrates. Most dietary authorities, however, do recommend complex carbohydrates.

It has been recommended that athletes of all types spread their caloric intake over several meals a day. However, it has been demonstrated that glycogen resynthesis is the same with either two or seven meals per day, assuming that the same total amount of carbohydrate is being absorbed.[75]

Amino acid supplements are being heavily marketed to resistance-trained athletes. Whether amino acid supplements are effective is unclear at this point, although there is theoretical support for their use. Resistance training does increase amino acid uptake by the muscle cell. In addition, heavy resistance training may result in amino acid oxidation.[76] Supplementation with amino acids may help reverse a potential deficit. Well-formulated studies investigating this question are not available at this time.

Increased endogenous growth hormone levels have been noted in response to amino acid challenges. The combination of arginine and lysine taken orally in the amounts of 1200 mg each have stimulated the release of growth hormone.[77] Orally administered lysine or arginine alone do not have this effect.[76] Further study in this area is required before definitive statements can be made regarding the benefits of amino acid supplementation for the resistance-trained athlete.

In summary, the resistance-trained athlete would be well served to concentrate on a well-balanced diet that maintains adequate levels of carbohydrate. Ideally, the resistance-trained athlete would consume 5 grams carbohydrate/kg body weight. Protein supplements are not required unless the athlete is restricting caloric intake. In these cases, milk can be used as a supplement to achieve 1.0 to 1.5 grams protein/kg body weight. The benefits of amino acid supplementation are theoretical and probably small if they do exist.

STRENGTH TRAINING FOR THE PREPUBESCENT AND ADOLESCENT

There is confusion among athletes, coaches, and physicians regarding the benefits and risks of resistance training for the prepubescent. The American Academy of Pediatrics in 1983 concluded that "maximal benefits are obtained from appropriate weight training in the postpubertal athlete and minimal benefits are obtained from weight training in the prepubertal athlete. In contrast, weight lifting is a competitive sport with a high injury rate that should not be practiced by pre-adolescents."[11, 78] It was felt that insufficient circulating androgens would not allow prepubertal boys to improve strength or increase muscle mass as a result of a weight training program. Since then, there have been numerous reports of significant strength increases in both the prepubescent as well as the pubescent participant as a result of resistance training.[31, 32, 36, 37, 79] In fact, prepubescents developed as much strength as the pubescent and postpubescent participants.[31] Similar results were found comparing pubescent participants with young men; both groups increased strength equally. Minimal injuries were noted in the prepubescent and pubescent participants involved in strength training.[32, 36, 37] Bone scans performed in prepubescent participants following an intense training program with concentric resistance techniques were all negative.[32, 36] This finding would suggest that there was no damage to physis, bone, or muscle as a result of the training programs. Several studies investigated flexibility following resistance training; there were no findings of decreased flexibility, and in some cases, flexibility actually increased.[32, 36, 79] An interesting finding was an increase in the height of the participants, compared with controls.[32, 36, 37] There were no significant changes in mesomorphic appearances during the short-term resistance programs, and neural adaptation seemed to play a significant role in the strength development of these participants.[36, 37] The importance of proper supervision, avoidance of competitive weight-lifting techniques, and use of only concentric resistance training techniques are important in achieving these results.[32, 36]

Therefore, available studies contradict the position statement by the American Academy of Pediatrics. Under properly supervised conditions, both prepubescent and pubescent participants can significantly increase their strength with minimal injury and loss of flexibility as a result of resistance training.

The American Orthopedic Society for Sports Medicine sponsored a symposium to examine strength training in the prepubescent. The objective of this conference was to consider the relative risks and benefits of strength training for the prepubescent and establish guidelines for its use in this population.[1] The results of this conference were that strength training can be beneficial and safe for youngsters—that it can increase muscle strength, improve motor skills, protect against injury, increase muscle endurance, and have positive psychological benefits. The risks of strength training were considered controllable. Developing equipment that better fits the size of the prepubescent and that offers lighter weight would further improve safety. Flexibility was not considered at risk. It was also suggested that the number and severity of musculotendinous injuries in other sports could be decreased as a result of strength training. While the potential for epiphyseal injuries has to be considered, the risk was considered minimal. The conference condemned competitive weight-lifting programs for the prepubescent including Olympic and power lifting. Close supervision must be maintained to avoid competition among the participants during the training program. Because of lower thresholds of dangerous core temperature and the inability to lose heat efficiently through small skin surfaces, prepubescents may be at more risk for dehydration following intense programs in warm climates. The potential for sustained and transient hypertension was noted, but this was considered a small risk.

The conference proposed a program design for prepubescent resistance training that includes a thorough medical examination, adequate emotional maturity by the participants, proper supervision, dynamic concentric contractions as opposed to eccentric contractions, full-range-of-motion exercises, and integration of the strength training program with an overall conditioning program for fitness. Appropriate warm-up and cool-down periods were emphasized, and competition was strictly prohibited. It was recommended that two to three training sessions per week be performed, lasting 20 to 30 minutes per session. This would inlcude both the warm-up and cool-down periods. One to three sets per exercise was recommended with between 6 and 15 repetitions per set. To allow adaptation to the techniques, no resistance or weight should be used initially. The amount of weight used by the participant is established when the participant can barely perform six repetitions with that weight. The participant continues training with that amount of weight until 15 repetitions can be performed. At that point, resistance is increased in 1- to 3-pound increments to bring the resistance high enough so that only six repetitions can be performed. No maximum lifts are allowed. Following these guidelines, children as young as 7 years old can benefit from resistance training. Increased strength, improved self-image, and minimal risk can be expected within the guidelines proposed.

SUMMARY

Resistance training has specific physiological effects on the participant. Such training serves to stimulate both neural and muscular effects, which results in increased strength in the participant. While not considered activities that improve the cardiovascular status of the athlete as measured by VO_2max, appropriately designed programs can serve to diminish the risk factors associated with cardiovascular disease. The other positive effects of resistance training include improved mesomorphic appearance, positive psychological effect, and improvement in sports-related activities. Women and adolescents as well as prepubescents all benefit in a similar fashion from resistance training. In a properly supervised program employing concentric resistance techniques, prepubescents as young as 7 years old can safely participate in resistance training and expect significant improvements in strength.

As with any athletic activity, there are specific injury patterns associated with resistance training. Injuries generally are the result of either poor or improper technique, the use of resistance loads beyond the participant's limit, and of course, overuse. Most injury patterns can be treated in a conservative fashion, but there are some rare entities that require surgical intervention. Preventative measures include emphasis on proper technique and organization of the resistance training program to allow adequate rest periods and avoid excessive weight.

Resistance training can serve to improve the performance in other sporting activities. It can also serve to prevent injuries in these activites and provide the rehabilitation modality for existing injuries.

To be most effective for the athlete, resistance training should be integrated into an overall fitness program. Such a program would place equal emphasis on aerobic conditioning and flexiblity. The fitness program would also emphasize proper nutrition stressing the benefit of carbohydrate intake, preferably complex carbohydrates. With such an integrated program, the participant can expect improved health and longevity as well as improved strength and sports performance.

References

1. American Orthopedic Society for Sports Medicine. Proceedings of the conference on strength training and the prepubescent. 1988, pp 1–14. Bernard Cahill, MD, moderator and editor.
2. Lind A. R., McNicol G. W. Muscular factors which determine the cardiovascular responses to sustained and rhythmic exercise. Can Med Assoc J 96:706–713, 1967.
3. Lander J., Bates B., Sawhill J., Hamill J. A comparison between free-weight and isokinetic bench pressing. Med Sci Sports Exerc 17(3):344–353, 1985.
4. Gettman L. R., Pollack M. L. Circuit weight training: a critical review of its physiological benefits. Phys Sports Med 9:44–60, 1981.
5. Wilt F. Plyometrics: what it is—how it works. Athlet J, pp 76–90, 1975 (May).
6. Brown M., Mayhew J., Boleach L. Exercise physiology: effect of plyometric training on vertical jump performance in high school basketball players. J Bone Joint Surg 64A (7):1053, 1982.
7. Blakey J., Southard D. The combined effects of weight training and plyometrics on dynamic leg strength and leg power. J Appl Sports Sci Res 1(1):14–16, 1987.
8. Ford H. T., Puckett J. R., Drummond J. P., et al. Effects of three combinations of plyometric and weight training programs on selected physical fitness test items. Percept Mot Skills 56:919–922, 1983.
9. Hurley B., Kokkinos P. Effects of weight training on risk factors for coronary artery disease. Sports Med 4:231–238, 1987.
10. Tesch P. Skeletal muscle adaptations consequent to long term heavy resistance exercise (Supplement). Med Sci Sports Exerc 20(5):S132–S134, 1988.
11. Kraemer W., Deschenes M., Fleck S. Physiological adaptations to resistance exercise: implications for athletic conditioning. Sports Med 6:246–256, 1988.
12. Berger R. A. Optimum repetitions for the development of strength. Res Q Exerc Sport 33:334–338, 1962.
13. DeLorme T. Restoration of muscle power by heavy-resistance exercises. J Bone Joint Surg 27(4):645–667, 1945.
14. Knight K. Knee rehabilitation by the daily adjustable progressive resistive exercise technique. Am J Sports Med 7:336–337, 1979.
15. Knight K. Quadriceps strengthening with the DAPRE technique: case studies with neurological implications. Med Sci Sports Exerc 17(6):646–650, 1985.
16. Basford J. Literature review: weightlifting, weight training and injuries. Orthopedics 8(8): 1051–1056, 1985.
17. Sale D. Neural adaptation to resistance training (Supplement). Med Sci Sports Exerc 20(5):S135–S145, 1988.
18. Enoka R. Muscle strength and its development: new perspectives. Sports Med 6:146–168, 1988.
19. Hurley B. F., Seals D. R., Ehsani A. A., et al. Effects of high-intensity strength training on cardiovascular function. Med Sci Sports Exerc 16(5): 483–488, 1984.
20. Ullrich I., Reid C., Yeater R. Increased HDL-cholesterol levels with a weight lifting program. South Med J 80(3): 328–331, 1987.
21. Duda M. Elite lifters at risk for spondylolysis. Phys Sportsmed 15(10): 57–59, 1987.
22. Khalil T. M., Genaidy A. M., Asfour S. S., Vinciguerra T. Physiological limits in lifting. Am Ind Hyg Assoc J 46(4): 220–224, 1985.
23. Fleck S. Cardiovascular adaptations to resistance training (Supplement). Med Sci Sports Exerc 20(5): S146–S151, 1988.
24. Fleck S., Dean L. Resistance training experience and the pressor response during resistance exercise. J Appl Physiol 63(1): 116–120, 1987.
25. Collins M., Hill D., Cureton K., DeMello J. Plasma volume change during heavy resistance weight lifting. Eur J Appl Physiol 55:44–48, 1986.
26. Hurley B., Seals D., Hagberg J., et al. A high density lipoprotein cholesterol in bodybuilders vs powerlifters: negative effects of androgen use. JAMA 252:507–513, 1984.
27. Kokkinos P. F., Hurley B. F., Vaccaro P., et al. Effects of low and high repetition resistive training on lipoprotein lipid profiles. Med Sci Sports Exerc 20(1): 50–54, 1988.
28. McKillop G., Ballantyne D. Lipoprotein analysis in bodybuilders. Int J Cardiol 17:281–286, 1987.
29. Hurley B., Kokkinos P. Effects of weight training on risk factors for coronary artery disease. Sports Med 4:231–238, 1987.
30. Giddings C. J., Neaves W. B., Gonyea W. J. Muscle fiber necrosis and regeneration induced by prolonged weight-lifting exercise in the cat. Anat Rec 211:133–141, 1985.
31. Pardee S., Eisenman P. The influence of resistive exercise on somatotype and selected skin folds in college women. J Sports Med 28:93–98, 1988.
32. Pfeiffer R., Francis R. Effects of strength training on muscle development in prepubescent, pubescent, and the postpubescent males. Phys Sports Med 14(9): 134–143, 1986.
33. Rians C., Weltman A., Cahill B., Janney C., et al. Strength training for prepubescent males: is it safe? Am J Sports Med 15:483–489, 1987.
34. Tucker L. Effect of weight training on body attitudes: who benefits most? J Sports Med 27:70–78, 1987.
35. Berscheid E., Walster E. Beauty and the beast. Psychol Today 5(10): 42–46, 1972.
36. Weltman A., Janney C., Rians C., et al. The effects of hydraulic resistance strength training in prepubertal males. Med Sci Sports Exerc 18(6): 629–638, 1986.
37. Sailors M., Berg K. Comparison of responses to weight training in pubescent boys and men. J Sports Med 27:30–37, 1987.
38. Dudley G. Metabolic consequences of resistive-type exercise (Supplement). Med Sci Sports Exerc 20(5): S158–S161, 1988.
39. Guezennec Y., Leger L., Lhoste F., et al. Hormone and metabolite response to weight lifting training sessions. Int J Sports Med 7:100–105, 1986.
40. Hakkinen K., Kauhanen H., Komi P. Aerobic, anaerobic, assistant exercise and weightlifting performance capacities in elite weightlifters. J Sports Med 27:240–256, 1987.
41. Stone M. Implications for connective tissue and bone alterations resulting from resistance exercise training (Supplement). Med Sci Sports Exerc 29(5): S162–S168, 1988.

42. Fahey T. D., Akka L., Rolph R. Body composition and VO$_2$max of exceptional weight trained athletes. J Appl Physiol 39:559–561, 1975.
43. Ingelmark B. E., Elsholm R. A study on variations in the thickness of the articular cartilage in association with the rest and periodical load. Ups Lakaret Foxhandl 53:61–64, 1948.
44. Granhed H., Jonson R., Hansson T. The loads on the lumbar spine during extreme weight lifting. Spine 12(2): 146–149, 1987.
45. Fahey T. D., Rolph R., Moungmee P., et al. Serum testosterone, body composition, and strength of young adults. Med Sci Sports 8:31–34, 1976.
46. Kraemer W. Endocrine responses to resistance exercise (Supplement). Med Sci Sports Exerc 20(5): S152–S157, 1988.
47. Cumming D. C., Wall S. R., Galbraith M. A., Belcastro A. N. Reproductive hormone responses to resistance exercise. Med Sci Sports Exerc 19:234–238, 1987.
48. Adlercreutz H., Harkonen M., Kuoppasalmi K., et al. Effect of training on plasma anabolic and catabolic steroid hormones and their response during physical exercise (Supplement). Int J Sports Med 7:27–28, 1986.
49. Hakkinen K., Pakarinen A., Alen M., Komi P. Serum hormones during prolonged training of neuromuscular performance. Eur J Appl Physiol 53:287–293, 1985.
50. Vanhelder W. P., Radomski M. W., Goode R. C. Growth hormone responses during intermittent weight lifting exercise in men. Eur J Appl Physiol 53:31–34, 1984.
51. Kraemer W. J., Noble B. K., Clark M. J., Culver B. W. Physiologic responses to heavy resistance exercise with very short rest periods. Int J Sports Med 8:247–252, 1987.
52. Cappozzo A., Felici F., Figura F., Gazzani F. Lumbar spine loading during half-squat exercises. Med Sci Sports Exerc 17(5): 613–620, 1985.
53. Duda M. Elite lifters at risk for spondylolysis. Phys Sportsmed 15(10): 57–59, 1987.
54. Brady T. A., Cahill B. R., Bodnar L. M. Weight training related injuries in the high school athlete. Am J Sports Med 10(1): 1, 1982.
55. Egan T., Hall H. Avulsion of the pectoralis major tendon in a weight lifter: repair using a barbed staple. Can J Surg 30(6): 434–435, 1987.
56. Grenier R., Guimont A. Simultaneous bilateral rupture of the quadriceps tendon and leg fractures in a weightlifter: a case report. Am J Sports Med 11:451–453, 1983.
57. Kurland P. N. The injured athlete. Philadelphia, JB Lippincott Co, 1982, p 382.
58. Jones M. (Editorial) Br J Sports Med 21(3): 139, 1987.
59. Cahill B. R. Osteolysis of the distal part of the clavicle in male athletes. J Bone Joint Surg 64A(7): 1053, 1982.
60. Herrick R., Herrick S. Ruptured triceps in a powerlifter presenting as a cubital tunnel syndrome: a case report. Am J Sports Med 15(5): 514–516, 1987.
61. Sherman O. H., Snyder S. J., Fox J. M. Triceps tendon avulsion in a professional body builder: a case report. Am J Sports Med 12: 328–329, 1984.
62. Bach B., Warrenn R., Wickiewicz T. Triceps rupture: a case report and literature review. Am J Sports Med 15(3): 285–289, 1987.
63. Gumbs V. L., Segal D., Halligan J. B., et al. Bilateral distal radius and ulnar fractures in adolescent weight lifters. Am J Sports Med 10(6): 375, 1982.
64. Hamilton H. K. Stress fracture of the diaphysis of the ulna in a body builder. Am J Sports Med 12(5): 405–406, 1984.
65. Bird C., McCoy J. Weight lifting as a cause of compartment syndrome in the forearm: a case report. J Bone Joint Surg 63A(3): 406, 1983.
66. Feed S. S., Dagradi A. E. Esophageal varices in weightlifters. Endoscopy 25:981, 1979.
67. Powell B. Weight lifter's cephalgia: case report. Ann Emerg Med 11(8): 449–451, 1982.
68. Rooke E. D. Benign exertional headache. Med Clin North Am 52:801–808, 1968.
69. Chang D., Buschbacher L., Edlich R. Limited joint mobility in power lifters. Am J Sports Med 16(280–284, 1988.
70. Meredith C. Protein needs and protein supplements in strength trained men, in Garrett W. E. Jr., Malone T. R. (eds): Muscle development: nutritional alternatives to anabolic steroids, report of the Ross symposium. Columbus, Ohio, Ross Laboratories, 1988, pp 68–71.
71. Rinehardt K. Effects of diet on muscle and strength gains during resistive training, in Garrett W. E. Jr., Malone T. R. (eds): Muscle development: nutritional alternatives to anabolic steroids, report of the Ross symposium. Columbus, Ohio, Ross Laboratories, 1988, pp 78–83.
72. Harberson D. Weight gain and body composition of weightlifters: effects of high calorie supplementation vs anabolic steroids, in Garrett W. E. Jr., Malone T. R. (eds): Muscle development: nutritional alternatives to anabolic steroids, report of the Ross symposium. Columbus, Ohio, Ross Laboratories, 1988, pp 72–76.
73. Grandjean A. Current nutrition beliefs and practices in athletics for weight/strength gains, in Garrett W. E. Jr., Malone T. R. (eds): Muscle development: nutritional alternatives to anabolic steroids, report of the Ross symposium. Columbus, Ohio, Ross Laboratories, 1988, pp 56–61.
74. Costill D. L., Miller J. M. Nutrition for endurance sports: carbohydrate and fluid balance. Int J Sports Med 1:6, 1980.
75. Costill D. L., Sherman W. M., Fink W. J., et al. The role of dietary carbohydrate in muscle glycogen resynthesis after strenuous running. Am J Clin Nutr 34:1831, 1981.
76. Lemon P., Chaney M. Physiologic effects of amino-acid supplementation, in Garrett W. E. Jr., Malone T. R. (eds): Muscle development: nutritional alternatives to anabolic steroids, report of the Ross symposium. Columbus, Ohio, Ross Laboratories, 1988, pp 62–67.
77. Isidori A., LoMonaco A., Cappa M. A study of growth hormone release in man after oral administration of amino acids. Curr Med Res Opin 7:475, 1981.
78. American Academy of Pediatrics. Weight training and weight lifting: information for the pediatrician. Phys Sportsmed 11(3): 157–161, 1983.
79. Sewall L., Micheli L. Strength training for children. J Pediatr Orthop 6(2): 143–146, 1986.

3

FLEXIBILITY TRAINING

RONALD F. ZERNICKE
GEORGE J. SALEM

Specificity-of-training principles have dramatically influenced concepts of fitness training, and currently, individually tailored and highly specific training programs are the norm for athletes in preparation for competition. World-class athletes have strength, speed, power, and endurance programs planned months and sometimes years in advance of a competition. These highly specific programs aim to have the athlete peak at the time of competition. Although these relatively new training concepts are routinely being used to enhance strength, speed, power, and endurance, not infrequently, flexibility training is often only an afterthought.

Certainly, flexibility training has long been practiced by selected athletes (e.g., gymnasts, dancers, wrestlers); nevertheless, many athletes, coaches, and trainers have failed to recognize the importance of this essential component of fitness. Research findings correlating flexibility with athletic performance,[14, 20, 22, 27, 49] prevention of injury,[15, 33, 52] and increased range of motion[21, 27] emphasize to athletes, coaches, and trainers that flexibility training should be included with their programs of strength, speed, power, and endurance training. But improper technique and inadequate understanding of flexibility training could be disastrous to the athlete. Further, different stretch techniques and the myths surrounding them can exacerbate the problems of developing a proper stretching program. Therefore, we have provided information on the parameters, techniques, and development of flexibility.

PARAMETERS OF FLEXIBILITY

TYPES OF FLEXIBILITY

Although *flexibility* is defined in many ways, the definition provided by Corbin et al. 1981[9]—range of motion available in a joint or group of joints—will be used here. In addition, flexibility can be categorized as either static or dynamic. *Static flexibility* refers to the mobility of a joint without regard for the speed of the movement, whereas *dynamic flexibility* includes the speed at which full joint mobility can be attained.[24]

A person can have good static flexibility in a joint without good dynamic flexibility. Consequently, although the person may exhibit good range of motion in a joint, it may take a relatively long time to achieve the movement. Because most sports require highly specific and, frequently, quick movements, dynamic flexibility is particularly important. Measuring dynamic flexibility, however, is difficult and can be dangerous to an athlete. Thus, most flexibility measurements are static.

EVALUATING FLEXIBILITY

Numerous instruments can be used to measure flexibility. A manual goniometer is typically employed to evaluate flexibility in most joints. Numerous investigators have used this device to evaluate stretching techniques for improved joint flexibility.[21, 48, 53] For more sophisticated measurements, electrogoniometers, radiogoniometers, and photogoniometers are used. Flexometers, which measure degrees of bending, are also accepted,[13, 31, 37, 51, 62] but the simplest and most widely used flexibility measuring devices are tape measures and rulers. With tape measure techniques, the amount of flexibility is considered the distance a person can reach or move a body segment from or to a given reference point.[18, 25, 27, 38] Variations of these methods, using trigonometric functions to determine joint angles, have also been reported.[56]

TESTS OF FLEXIBILITY

Flexibility measurements are important tools for evaluating overall flexibility conditioning, injury, posttreatment recovery, and flexibility training techniques. Numerous methods have been used to evaluate joint flexibility in hip, shoulder, trunk, knee, or ankle joints.[14, 18, 31, 48, 51] Although not exhaustive, the methods outlined by Corbin[9] provide a straightforward procedure for evaluating general anatomical flexibility in the school-aged athlete. Additional testing procedures and flexibility standards can be found in several sources.[9, 10, 11, 16, 24, 31]

Hip

The compound flexibility test for the hip involves the hip, knee, and trunk, along with several muscle groups, and is a most important measure (Fig. 3–1). One method often used has the individual sitting on the floor or in a specially designed flexibility box with his or her feet against an immovable object. The athlete then reaches as far as possible without flexing at the knees, and flexibility is measured as the distance the athlete can reach.

Shoulder

Two methods are typically used to evaluate shoulder flexibility (Fig. 3–2). The first method requires the athlete to raise the right elbow and reach down between the shoulder blades with the right hand. The left hand is placed in the small of the back with the palm facing away from the back. As the athlete attempts to overlap hands, the distance between hands is measured (Fig. 3–2). The second method requires the athlete to lift a stick above his or her head, while lying prone, with chin on the floor and wrists held fixed. The height the stick can be raised above the ground is indicative of the shoulder flexibility.

Hamstrings

Although a hip flexion test indirectly measures hamstring flexibility along with other muscle groups, a specific evaluation of hamstring flexibility may be desirable (Fig. 3–3). The athlete needs to sit in a straight-backed chair, with his hip flexed 90 degrees, with one leg hanging off the chair also flexed at 90 degrees at the knee; he or she now extends the contralateral leg. Full extension indicates good hamstring flexibility, and lack of flexi-

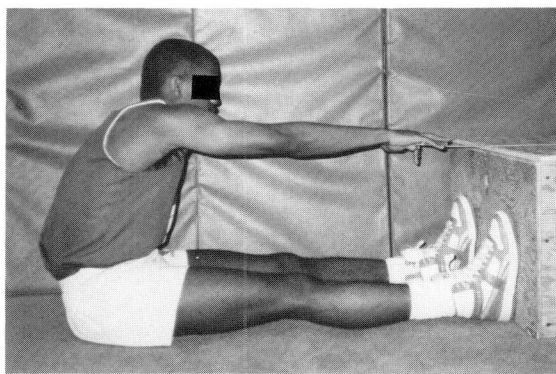

FIGURE 3–1. A standard test for hip, knee, and trunk flexibility.

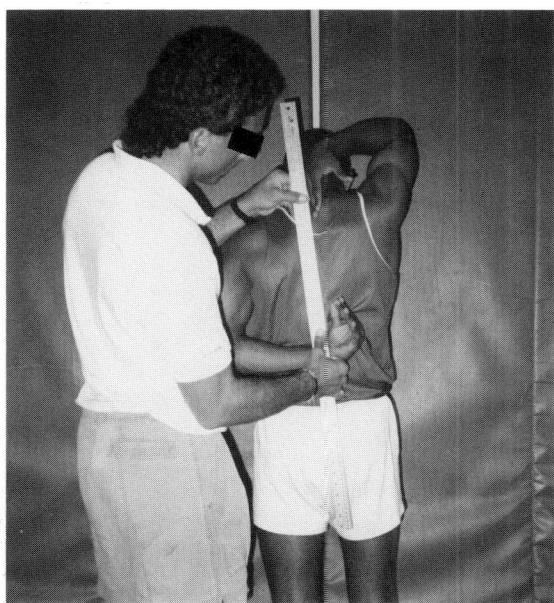

FIGURE 3–2. A standard test for shoulder flexibility.

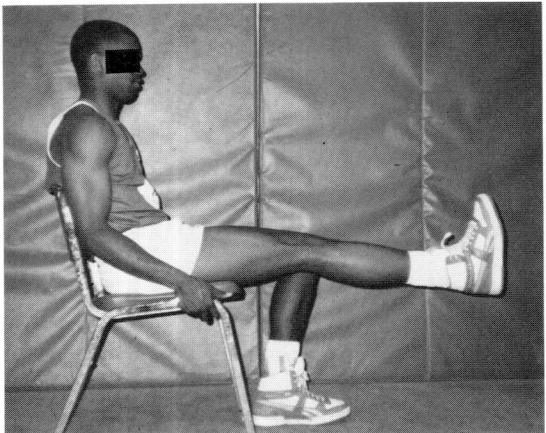

FIGURE 3-3. A standard test for hamstring flexibility.

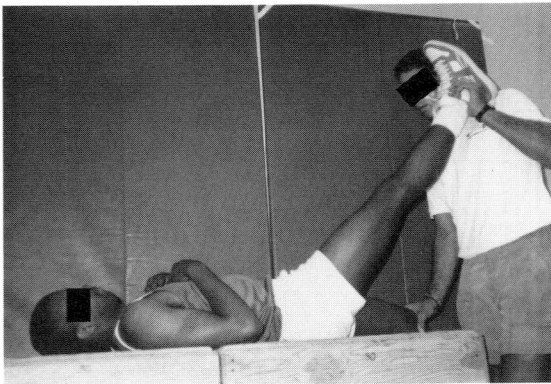

FIGURE 3-5. A standard test for hip flexor flexibility.

bility can be measured by the degree of knee flexion remaining at the end of the range of motion.

Quadriceps and Hip Flexors

The athlete lies prone on the floor or table while the trainer holds and stabilizes the ipsilateral buttocks, thus immobilizing the pelvis (Fig. 3-4). The knee, flexed to 90 degrees, is slowly lifted off the floor, and the distance from the floor to the knee is measured.

Hip Flexor Length

The athlete lies supine on a table with the knee of the measured limb flexed at 90 degrees and hanging off the end of the table (Fig. 3-5). The coach then slowly assists the athlete in lifting the contralateral limb off the table until hip flexor tightness is felt in the measured limb. The assisted leg should remain straight and the lower back kept flat on the table. The angle between limbs can be measured and used as an indication of flexibility.

Trunk Hyperextension

The athlete lies prone on the floor or testing table with hands locked behind the head while the trainer stabilizes the athlete's hips (Fig. 3-6). Next, the athlete lifts the trunk off the floor or table as high as possible with the assistance of the trainer. The distance from the clavicular notch to the floor or table is then measured. Additionally, trunk rotational flexibility can be evaluated by having the athlete elevate his or her shoulder off the floor or table during the hyperextension test. The distance from the shoulder to the floor or table can now be calculated.

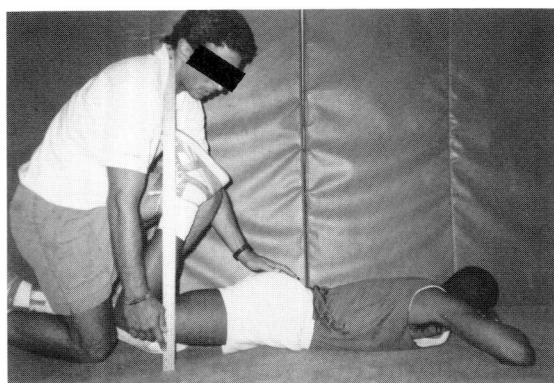

FIGURE 3-4. A standard test for quadriceps and hip flexibility.

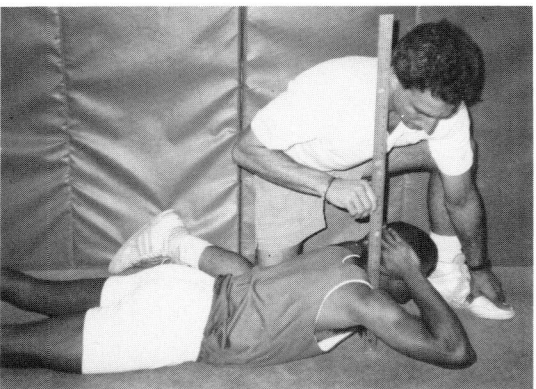

FIGURE 3-6. A standard test for trunk flexibility.

FLEXIBILITY TRAINING 43

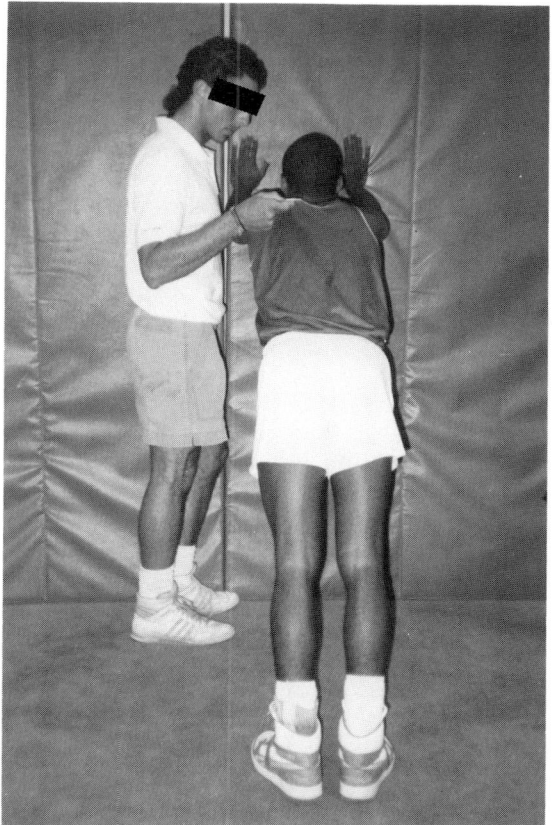

FIGURE 3–7. A standard test for calf and ankle flexibility.

Calf and Ankle

The subject stands facing a wall with his or her feet at shoulder width and 1 meter from the wall (Fig. 3–7). Hands are placed on the wall, and elbows are slowly flexed, allowing the torso and head to move toward the wall. With the athlete's back straight and heels on the floor, the distance from the clavicular notch to the wall can be measured as an indication of calf and ankle flexibility.

PHYSIOLOGICAL BASES OF FLEXIBILITY

The mobility of any joint is limited in varying degrees by periarticular connective tissues including bone, tendon, ligament, joint capsule, fascial sheath, and aponeurosis. In addition, joint mobility can be hindered substantially by the connective tissue framework of passive muscles.[2, 7, 47] Conversely, damage to one or more of these structures may result in abnormal joint flexibility or joint laxity. Thus, an understanding of connective tissue properties and the mechanisms underlying flexibility training is imperative.

CONNECTIVE TISSUE CONTRIBUTIONS

Typically, flexibility exercises increase joint mobility by decreasing the passive resistance of ligamentous joint capsules, tendons, and muscle. In a classic study by Johns and Wright,[30] these structures were found to be the principal sources of passive restraint to joint mobility. They recorded joint stiffness as the torque necessary to produce passive motion at the wrists of anesthetized cats. Structures including skin, tendons, and joint capsule were systematically removed between torque measurements, and they assumed that the reduction in torque, produced by severing a structure, represented the torque that structure contributed to total torque. The relative torque contributions of the various structures were 47 percent in the joint capsule, 41 percent in muscles, 10 percent in tendons, and 2 percent in skin. These results may be species related, however.

VISCOELASTIC PROPERTIES

Connective tissues are viscoelastic; that is, they exhibit both viscous and elastic properties in response to stretching. Their *viscous* properties are dependent on rate of deformation (velocity) and can result in *plastic*—that is, permanent—deformation. Their *elastic* properties are dependent on the amount of deformation and result in *elastic*—that is, recoverable—deformation. All connective tissues exhibit viscoelastic properties, undergoing elastic and plastic changes in length, and the relative contributions depend on factors such as the amount, duration, and speed of the stretch and the tissue temperature during the stretch.

Numerous rheological models have been proposed to explain connective tissue properties.[58, 60] While some models are quite elaborate and specific for a given connective tissue structure, the model proposed by Warren et al.[60] is sufficient to explain the general viscoelastic effects of connective tissue properties. This model predicts that low-force, long-duration stretching techniques result in greater plastic deformation and increased stretching. In contrast, high-force, short-duration stretching results in elastic deformations, and stretching gains are quickly lost. Thus, slow, passive stretching techniques are recommended over ballistic, rapid-stretch techniques.

Temperature can also significantly modify connective tissue mechanical properties. The stiffness of soft connective tissues is inversely proportional to temperature.[60] LaBan[35] and Lehmann et al.[36] found that in response to an initial stretch the elongation of a tendon unit could be increased when the temperature was raised above 103° F. Others suggest that at about 104° F a change in collagen microstructure occurs to produce a greater plastic deformation than occurs at lower temperatures.[50] Further, the increase in temperature decreases the stiffness of collagenous tissues. Within the rheological model,[60] presumably the increased temperature decreases the stiffness of the elastic element to produce greater deformations. Other studies suggest that the amount of structural weakening produced by stretching a tissue may be reduced by increasing the temperature within a "therapeutic range" (101° to 110° F).[60] Because warm-up exercises may elevate muscle and joint temperatures to within this range, they are recommended by most authors.[1, 3, 52] For example, during 10 minutes of moderate bicycle exercise, thigh muscle temperature increases to about 102° F.[40] Questions still persist regarding the value of warm-up exercises for improving flexibility.[62] However, because results indicate warm-up exercises may decrease the stiffness[54] and structural weakening[60] of connective tissues while increasing the load to failure of musculotendinous units,[52] we recommend approximately 10 minutes of moderate aerobic exercise prior to all flexibility training.

MYOTACTIC REFLEXES

The stretch reflex may be invoked whenever a muscle-tendon unit is stretched. During the stretch, sensory organs are deformed, generating a receptor potential and activating muscle spindle afferents. Spindle afferent excitation facilitates contraction of the stretched muscle, via the stretch-reflex loop. These spindle afferents code both static and dynamic stretch, and the amount and rate of firing depend on the amount and rate of stretch. Jerky ballistic stretching elicits a strong spindle afferent response and subsequently a strong contraction.

An inverse stretch reflex can be invoked whenever a muscle contracts. Here, the reflex loop facilitates relaxation of the contracted muscle. Discussion continues about Golgi tendon organ receptor sensitivity to muscle stretch,[28, 55] but nevertheless, the inverse stretch reflex appears to have a higher threshold than the stretch reflex.[19] Further, there is some question as to whether complete relaxation of a muscle can occur after forceful contractions that invoked the inverse stretch reflex.[45] In theory, however, the PNF stretching techniques described below take advantage of this relaxation phenomenon following muscular contraction.

STRETCHING TECHNIQUES

The three most common stretching techniques include: *dynamic*, *static*, and *proprioceptive neuromuscular facilitation (PNF)*. While each can increase flexibility, no single technique has emerged as the most effective, and some techniques may actually place the athlete at greater risk of injury.

Dynamic

Dynamic, or ballistic, stretching uses bounces or jerky motions to load and stretch a muscle group. It is difficult to control such ballistic movements, and overstretching may cause an injury. Because the stretch reflex is sensitive to rate of stretch, dynamic stretching involves a strong stretch reflex and contraction. Tension created in the muscle during dynamic stretching is more than double that created during slow, gentle stretching.[59] The elevated muscular tension may further increase the injury risk. Thus, this method of stretching is usually discouraged by most trainers.

Static

Static, passive, or slow stretching involves a slow, deliberate, sustained lengthening of the muscle. Each stretching position is held for approximately 20 seconds to facilitate connective tissue plastic elongation. Compared with other techniques, static stretching produces the least amount of muscle tension[45, 59] and is the stretching technique advocated by most experts and trainers.[1, 3, 15, 18]

PNF

The PNF technique, originally developed at the Kabat-Kaiser Institute for use with paralyzed individuals, maximally exploits myotactic reflexes. Although several variations of the PNF technique exist, two methods, the contract-relax (CR) method and contract-relax-antagonist-contract (CRAC) method, are most prevalent. The CR method incorporates three steps: (1) a static stretch, (2) followed by an isometric contraction and relaxation and finally (3) an additional static stretch. The CRAC method is similar to CR except that the anatomical agonist is contracted during the final stretch. Studies comparing the PNF methods with static stretching methods have frequently produced differing results, but essentially all data suggest that CR and CRAC are equal[25] or generally superior[25, 26, 45, 51, 56] to static stretching results. Further, the CRAC has been shown superior to the CR method in some cases.[21, 26, 45] These results emphasize the effectiveness of the PNF methods. While effective, PNF methods are more difficult and require more instruction and supervision than the simple static method. PNF methods, consequently, are advisable for the experienced and well-supervised athlete.

All three of these basic stretching methods can be varied, done in combination with other methods, or done with assistance of other individuals. Such variations in techniques, however, require additional experience by the athlete, coach, and trainer.

FLEXIBILITY AND PERFORMANCE

Is performance enhanced with flexibility training? Unfortunately, very little scientific data exist to answer that important question. Intuitively, however, some sports likely demand greater flexibility in athletes than other sports. For example, a gymnast or wrestler needs a flexibility level that exceeds the flexibility demands of sports such as archery or cycling. Further, specificity requires a swimmer to have greater shoulder flexibility than the long-distance runner. In sports requiring a generalized use of muscles—for example dancing, wrestling, or gymnastics—athletes must have good overall flexibility. Those sports requiring more restrictive movements—for example archery, hiking, or golf—may attract athletes with excellent flexibility at critical joints but who may be relatively inflexible otherwise.

While few studies exist to substantiate performance enhancement as a result of increased flexibility, correlational and observational studies of flexibility and performance are available. Interpretation of these studies requires caution, however, because it is impossible to conclude whether flexibility resulted from participation or was a prerequisite for participation.

Cureton, in the 1930s, examined flexibility requirements of swimmers and concluded that swimmers generally were more flexible than athletes of other sports and nonathletes.[14] Dittmer[20] and Felton[22] positively correlated running patterns and standing broad jump performance with flexibility, and Reser[49] found a significant relationship between range of motion and height of vertical jump. Reid and colleagues found that classical ballet dancers are significantly more flexible than nondancers, particularly in hip external rotation, hip flexion, hip abduction, and knee extension, but less flexible than nondancers in passive hip adduction and internal rotation.[48]

Existing data suggest that more flexible athletes have better performances. But those joints demanding flexibility are specific to a given sport, and therefore flexibility training should be prescribed accordingly. On the other hand, greater flexibility (not the same as joint laxity) does not appear to limit performance, nor have sports such as weight lifting been shown to decrease flexibility.[34, 39]

FLEXIBILITY AND INJURY

The most important benefit of proper stretching and flexibility training may be the prevention of injury. It is generally believed that a shortened, tight muscle is susceptible to injury (strains). (See Chapter 8.)

Proper flexibility training and preexercise stretching can reduce both joint stiffness and muscle tightness, and stretching leads to the prevention of injuries.[42, 46] For example, Safran et al.[52] and Taylor et al.[57] found that warm-up exercise and passive stretching can increase the load to failure of the musculotendinous unit and decrease resting muscle tension. Miller[42] found that the likelihood of reinjuring calf muscles could be reduced to less than 1 percent as a result of specific stretching exercises. Conversely, athletes lacking flexibility may have a greater risk of injury. For example, knee and hip injuries account for up to 40 percent of injuries in classical ballet dancers. Recently, Reid et al. found that dancers who experienced lateral hip and knee pain had significantly less flexibility in hip adduction than dancers not exhibiting symptoms.[48] The lack of flexibility and subsequent injury risks may be related to an unbalanced flexibility program stressing hip abduction and external rotation. Such findings emphasize the need for both specific stretching prescriptions and general flexibility training. In addition to injury prevention, stretching may also minimize and alleviate muscular distress.[17, 61] For example, muscle soreness was reportedly minimized during early season workouts of football players as a result of a carefully implemented stretching program.[61] Reportedly, flexibility exercises may produce some musculotendinous injuries,[4, 23] but almost without exception, such injuries are related to improper stretching techniques. Thus, careful prescription, supervision, and execution of the indicated exercises are essential elements of a well-coordinated flexibility training program.

AGE, SIZE, AND SEX DIFFERENCES IN FLEXIBILITY

AGE

Although reports are inconclusive, flexibility tends to decrease with age.[9, 31] The controversy centers on precisely what age flexibility begins its decline. Milne et al.[43] found significant decreases in flexibility between kindergarten and second-grade children; however, Clarke[8] reported flexibility decreases beginning at age 10 for males and age 12 for females, and others suggest that flexibility increases until adolescence and then levels off or declines through adulthood.[29] Generally, it is agreed that flexibility in adults is less than that for juveniles and that older adults have less flexibility than younger adults.[31] Because flexibility appears to reduce joint stiffness and muscle tightness,[42, 46] ligamentous injuries and musculotendinous strains common among adults may be reduced in children. Here again, though, other factors including increases in training intensity, body weight, collision forces, and tissue weakening may also contribute to age-related increases in ligamentous and musculotendinous injuries. Extracting those flexibility changes exclusively related to structural and physiological changes that occur with age from the influence of differing levels of physical activity is difficult, therefore, and these findings must be viewed with reasonable caution.

SIZE

Although body size appears to be unrelated to flexibility,[9, 31] anthropometric differences among people may give an advantage to some people during some tests used to assess flexibility. Broer and Galles[6] found that people with longer trunks and arms had an advantage with the standard hip flexion test. Those differences, however, could be eliminated with use of a correction procedure[41] that accounts for the differences of body size. Muscle size also does not influence flexibility,[32] and athletes who both strength and flexibility train typically have flexibility measures greater than or equal to most nonathletes.[9] The term *muscle bound*, implying decreased flexibility with muscle hypertrophy, is a *misnomer*. In general, body size and anthropometric differences have little practical effect on an athlete's flexibility.[9]

SEX

Females appear to be more flexible than males, and the differences may be greater in children.[9, 43] Nevertheless, anatomical and environmental differences may account for some of the reported differences in flexibility,[12] and more information is needed to determine the validity of sex differences in flexibility.

IMPROVING FLEXIBILITY

Although joint flexibility is determined in part by genetic factors, improvements in flexibility can be obtained through the implementation of appropriate flexibility training programs. For example, shoulder, trunk, hip, knee, and ankle flexibility have been increased with static, PNF, and even ballistic stretching methods.[18, 38, 51, 56] Unfortunately, the variation in experimental protocols is high, and research to determine the ideal training frequency, stretch duration, and program length has been minimal. Borms et al.[5] investigated the effect of static stretching duration (the preferred stretching method for adolescents) and divided subjects into three groups based on stretch duration. Subjects flexibility trained for 10 weeks, 2 days per week, holding each stretch for either 10 seconds, 20 seconds, or 30 seconds. Sessions lasted 50 minutes, and exercises were targeted at increasing hip flexibility. No differences were found among the three groups at 3, 7, or 10 weeks, but hip flexibility improved significantly for all groups by the seventh week. These results suggest two important conclusions: (1) Stretch durations as short as 10 seconds may elicit significant training adaptations, and (2) significant adaptations occur between 3 and 7 weeks.

Questions, however, still remain regarding the following issues: Would adaptations occur earlier if training frequency were increased? Or would 10-second stretch durations still elicit similar responses if training sessions were less than 50 minutes? De Vries,[18] in his comparison of static and ballistic stretching, found significant increases in flexibility using stretch durations of 30 to 60 seconds after 5 weeks. Others recommend stretch durations as short as 8 seconds.[44] Further, flexibility training frequency recommendations also show considerable variability. For example, suggested flexibility training frequencies range from daily programs[12] to 2 days per week programs.[18]

There is much debate and little consensus about recommendations of frequency and duration for flexibility training, and gains in flexibility have been made through a variety of flexibility programs. We recommend flexibility exercises before and after all athletic practices and competitions. We also recommend stretching durations of approximately 20 seconds and a training frequency of between 3 and 5 days per week. Significant gains in flexibility, although gradual, can occur within about 5 weeks. Improvements in flexibility, however, cannot be rushed. If significant gains have not occurred by 5 weeks, changes in the flexibility training program, including exercise selection and frequency, may be indicated. Lastly, stretching exercises are not recommended for injured joints and musculotendinous units until significant healing has begun to occur.

DEVELOPING A FLEXIBILITY PROGRAM

Specificity-of-exercise principles apply to flexibility training just as they apply to strength, endurance, and power training. Flexibility programs must be tailored to the individual athlete, and factors influencing the development of a program include the sport, flexibility desired, competition scheduled, and experience of the athlete. Because some or all of those factors may change throughout a year, flexibility tests to help evaluate both the athlete and the program should be done two to three times per year. In addition, periodic supervision of the athlete should occur throughout a given program, with more frequent evaluations made during the initiation and early phases of a new program.

To develop a sound flexibility training program, the sport-specific flexibility demands must be determined. Although a complete sport-specific profile of flexibility is not routinely available, repeated and systematic observations of practice and competition movements can help estimate an athlete's flexibility needs. For example, swimmers need sufficient flexibility in their shoulders, ankles, and trunk, whereas sprinters need flexibility in knee, hip, and ankle joints. Because many children and adolescent athletes compete in more than one sport, the total flexibility requirements for all sports in which the athlete will compete should be assessed.

Next, the athlete should be tested for flexibility to determine his or her strengths and weaknesses. The tests outlined by Corbin[9] and presented earlier may be performed on a school-age athlete to obtain a general flexibility profile. Other tests of flexibility involving sport-specific muscle groups and joints may be warranted to gain a descriptive and specific profile. The references provide several sources for additional testing procedures.[10, 11, 16, 24, 31] In addition to flexibility testing, a physical evaluation to determine existing or previous injuries should be performed, so that contraindicated flexibility exercises that may overstress a joint or muscle can be excluded.

The competitive schedule of the athlete must also be considered. While preparing for competition, training programs for strength, power, speed, and endurance should proceed from general exercises (multiple-joint and whole-body movements) to specific exercises using competition-specific movements. To facilitate performance and reduce injury risk throughout training and competition, flexibility training should also proceed in this general-to-specific manner. Thus, flexibility exercises prescribed during early phases of training should be simple, anatomically comprehensive, and designed to promote overall body flexibility. As the athlete nears a competitive phase, flexibility exercises should include more specific stretches, and the number of stretches per muscle group or joint should be increased. Consequently, the overall length of a flexibility routine will increase during a training cycle.

Finally, the experience of the athlete must be considered. More experienced athletes will be familiar with flexibility programs and the flexibility demands of his or her sport. Additionally, the experienced athlete will be able to appraise more accurately a flexibility program and judge better the effectiveness and risks of each exercise. The more experienced athlete can also be given a program that may include "risk" exercises. Such risk exercises, as described by Beaulieu,[3] may be too advanced for the novice athlete. Because they place considerable force on the muscles being stretched, such stretching should only be attempted by sufficiently experienced and flexible athletes. These exercises should never be performed on an injured joint or muscle. An example of a risk exercise is provided in the following section. Experienced athletes may also be prescribed PNF, partner exercises, or both, but the maturity and experience of the athlete should be carefully assessed prior to using one of these more advanced methods. Beginning or novice athletes should start with static stretching methods. Most preadolescent and school-age youths will fall into such a category.

Once these evaluation methods have been completed, the coach, physician, or trainer can design an appropriate program to be used before and after training or competition workouts. A full description of available flexibility exercises is beyond the scope of this chapter, but good sources are available, and some of those are listed in the References section (e.g., see Anderson[1] and Beaulieu[3]). We provide one example of a detailed flexibility program, however, to illustrate the use of the described concepts.

ATHLETE PROFILE

Our athlete is a male sprint swimmer, aged 16. Currently, he has no injuries; however, he did experience a mild quadriceps strain while playing basketball 6 months ago. He has been swimming competitively for 4 years and is approximately 5 months away from the first competition of the season. When his flexibility was tested recently, he showed average ranges of flexibility in the shoulders, hip, hamstrings, hip flexors, trunk, and ankles in comparison with other team members. Quadriceps flexibility was, however, significantly less than that of his cohorts. Consequently, the following flexibility program was prescribed.

Exercises 1, 3, 4, 8, 9, 12, 13, 14, 16, and 17, as described by Beaulieu, are initially recommended. (Fig. 3–8). These general flexibility exercises will increase range of motion in the lower leg, ankle, groin, abdomen, chest, hamstring, hip, and quadriceps, and particular emphasis is placed on shoulder (1, 13), trunk (8, 12), and quadriceps (3, 17) flexibility. The previous quadriceps injury and tightness exclude the use of a risk exercise (7) for ankle flexibility. As flexibility improves in the quadriceps, ankle exercise 7 may be included. As the athlete approaches the initial competition phase (2 months precompetition), exercises 2, 5, 6, and 15 may be added. Exercises 10 and 11 can be added if assistance is provided by a qualified coach, physician, or trainer. All exercises should be done in order, be held without pain for 20 seconds, and be preceded by a warm-up exercise of approximately 10 minutes. A warm-up exercise of jogging, bicycling, or gentle swimming will raise body temperature, decrease joint stiffness and promote stretching. Repeating these exercises after training sessions and competitions will reduce muscle distress. Flexibility tests to determine gains in flexibility and program effectiveness should be done after 3 to 4 months. By using the athlete's new flexibility measures and competition schedule, the coach, physician, or trainer can effectively make modifications to the existing program.

SWIMMING

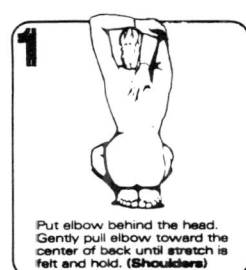
1. Put elbow behind the head. Gently pull elbow toward the center of back until stretch is felt and hold. **(Shoulders)**

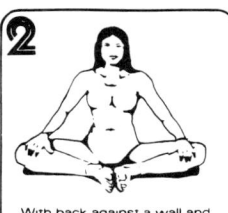
2. With back against a wall and feet together, push down on knees until stretch is felt and hold. **(Groin)**

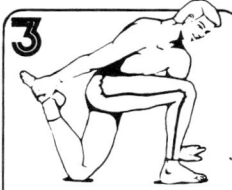
3. Assume the position shown by grabbing left foot with right hand. Pull the left foot towards the buttocks until stretch is felt and hold. **(Quadriceps)**

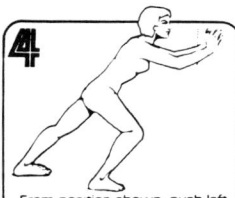
4. From position shown, push left knee forward with the chest until stretch is felt and hold. Keep toes of left foot even with knee of right leg. **(Lower Leg)**

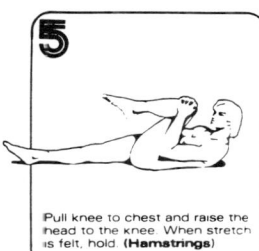
5. Pull knee to chest and raise the head to the knee. When stretch is felt, hold. **(Hamstrings)**

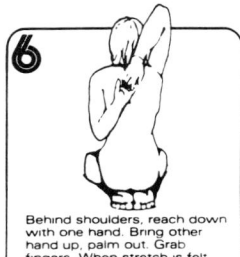
6. Behind shoulders, reach down with one hand. Bring other hand up, palm out. Grab fingers. When stretch is felt, hold. **(Shoulders)**

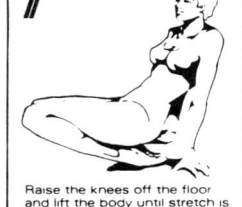
7. Raise the knees off the floor and lift the body until stretch is felt and hold. **(Ankles)**

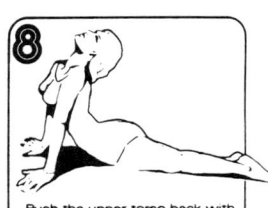
8. Push the upper torso back with the arms until stretch is felt and hold. Arch the back as far back as it will go. **(Abdomen and Chest)**

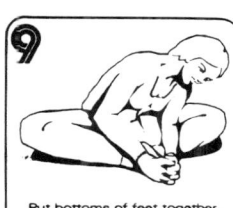
9. Put bottoms of feet together, pull heels toward groin and body forward until stretch is felt and hold. **(Groin)**

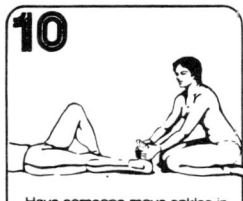
10. Have someone move ankles in each of four directions: forward, back, left, and right, until stretch is felt and hold. **(Ankles)**

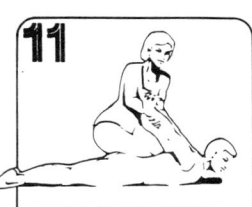
11. Interlock fingers behind back. Have partner raise arms slowly until stretch is felt and hold. **(Shoulders)**

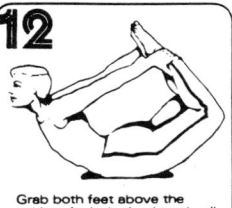
12. Grab both feet above the ankles. Arch the back and pull the feet toward the head until stretch is felt and hold. **(Abdomen and Chest)**

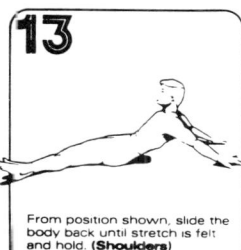
13. From position shown, slide the body back until stretch is felt and hold. **(Shoulders)**

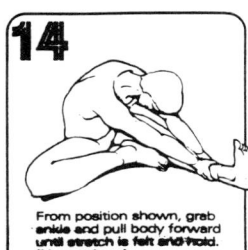
14. From position shown, grab ankle and pull body forward until stretch is felt and hold. **(Hamstrings)**

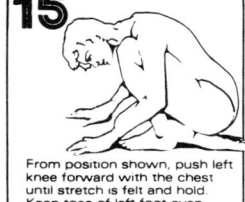
15. From position shown, push left knee forward with the chest until stretch is felt and hold. Keep toes of left foot even with knee of right leg. **(Lower Leg)**

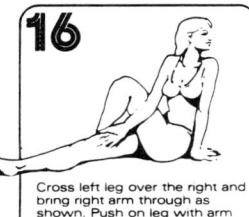
16. Cross left leg over the right and bring right arm through as shown. Push on leg with arm and twist body until stretch is felt and hold. Turn head to the rear. **(Hip and Oblique)**

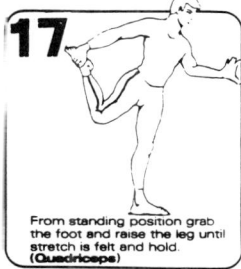
17. From standing position grab the foot and raise the leg until stretch is felt and hold. **(Quadriceps)**

FIGURE 3-8. Adapted from J. E. Beaulieu, Stretching Charts 'Swimming,' P. O. Box 3288, Dept. P, Eugene, OR 97403.

References

1. Anderson, B. Stretching. Bolinas, CA, Shelter Publishers, 1980.
2. Banus, M. G., and, A. M. Zetlin. The relation of isometric tension to length in skeletal muscle. J. Cell. Comp. Physiol. 12:403–420, 1938.
3. Beaulieu, J. E. Developing a stretching program. Physician Sports Med. 9:59–65, 1981.
4. Benjamin, B., and P. Roth. Warming up vs. stretching. Running Times 34:15–21, 1979.
5. Borms, J., P. Van Roy, J. P. Santens, and A. Haentjens. Optimal duration of static stretching exercises for improvement of coxo-femoral flexibility. J. Sports Sci. 5:39–47, 1987.
6. Broer, M., and N. Galles. Importance of relationship between various body measurements in performance of the toe-touch test. Res. Quart. 29:262, 1958.
7. Casealla, C. Tensile force in total striated muscle, isolated fibre, and sarcolemma. Acta Physiol. Scand. 21:380–401, 1950.
8. Clarke, H. H. Joint and body range of movement. Phys. Fitness Res. Dig. 5:16–18, 1975.
9. Corbin, C. B. Flexibility. Clin. Sports Med. 3:101–117, 1984
10. Corbin, C. B., L. J. Dowell, R. Lindsey, et al. Concepts in Physical Education, 4th ed. Dubuque, IA, William C. Brown Co., 1981.
11. Corbin, C. B., and R. Lindsey. Fitness for Life, 2nd ed. Glenview, IL, Scott, Foresman and Co., 1983.
12. Corbin, C. B., and L. Noble. Flexibility: A major component of physical fitness. JOPERD 51:23–24, 1980.
13. Cornelius, W. L., and M. M. Hinson. The relationship between isometric contractions of hip extensors and subsequent flexibility in males. J. Sports Med. 20:75–80, 1980.
14. Cureton, T. K., Jr. Observation and tests of swimmers at the 1932 Olympic Games. J. Physical Educ. 30:125–130, 1933.
15. Cureton, T. K. Flexibility as an aspect of physical fitness. Res. Quart. 12:381–390, 1941.
16. Cureton, T. K. Physical Fitness of Champion Athletes. Urbana, IL, University of Illinois Press, 1951.
17. De Vries, H. A. Prevention of muscular distress after exercise. Res. Quart. 32:177–185, 1961.
18. De Vries, H. A. Evaluation of static stretching procedures for improvement of flexibility. Res. Quart. 33:222–229, 1962.
19. De Vries, H. A. Physiology of Exercise for Physical Education and Athletics, 2nd ed. Dubuque, IA, William C. Brown Co., 1974.
20. Dittmer, J. A. A kinematic analysis of the running pattern of grade school girls and certain factors which distinguish good from poor performance at the observed ages (thesis), University of Wisconsin, Madison, 1962.
21. Ethyre, B. R., and L. D. Abraham. Gains in range of ankle dorsiflexion using three popular stretching techniques. Am. J. Phys. Med. 65:189–196, 1986.
22. Felton, E. A. A kinesiological comparison of good performers (and poor) in the standing broad jump (thesis), University of Wisconsin, Madison, 1960.
23. Fixx, J. Second Book of Running. New York, Random House, 1980.
24. Fleischman, F. A. The Structure and Measurement of Physical Fitness. Englewood Cliffs, NJ, Prentice-Hall, Inc., 1964.
25. Hartley-O'Brien, S. J. Six mobilization exercises for active range of hip flexion. Res. Quart. 51:625–635, 1980.
26. Holt, L. E., T. M. Travis, and T. Okita. Comparative study of three stretching techniques. Percept. Mot. Skills 31:611–616, 1970.
27. Hortobagyi, T., J. Faludi, J. Tihanyi, and B. Merkely. Effects of intense "stretching"-flexibility training on the mechanical profile of the knee extensors and on the range of motion of the hip joint. Int. J. Sport Med. 6:317–321, 1985.
28. Houk, J. C., J. J. Singer, and E. Henneman. Adequate stimulus for tendon organs with observation of the mechanics on the ankle joint. J. Neurophysiol. 34:1051–1065, 1971.
29. Hupprich, F. L., and P. Sigersth. The specificity of flexibility in girls. Res. Quart. 21:32, 1950.
30. Johns, R. J., and V. Wright. Relative importance of various tissues in joint stiffness. J. Appl. Physiol. 17:824–828, 1962.
31. Johnson, B. L., and J. K. Nelson. Practical Measurement for Evaluation in Physical Education, 4th ed. Edina, MN, Burgess Publishing Co., 1986.
32. Jones, A. Flexibility as a result of exercise. Athletic J. 57:32–40, 1977.
33. Krause, H., B. Prudden, and K. Hisrschaven. Role of inactivity in production of disease. J. Am. Geriatr. Soc. 4:463–471, 1956.
34. Kusinitz, J., and C. E. Keeney. Effects of progressive weight training on health and physical fitness of adolescent boys. Res. Quart. 29:294, 1958.
35. LaBan, M. M. Collagen tissue: Implications of its response to stress *in vitro*. Arch. Phys. Med. Rehabil. 43:265–283, 1962.
36. Lehmaan, J. F., A. J. Masock, C. G. Warren, et al. Effect of therapeutic temperatures on tendon extensibility. Arch. Phys. Med. Rehabil. 51:481–487, 1970.
37. Leighton, J. R. Instrument and technic for measurement of range of joint motion. Arch. Phys. Med. Rehabil. 36:571–578, 1955.
38. Lucas, R. C., and R. Koslow. Comparative study of static, dynamic, and proprioceptive neuromuscular facilitation stretching techniques on flexibility. Percept. Mot. Skills 58:615–618, 1984.
39. Massey, B. H., and N. L. Chaudet. Effects of systematic, heavy resistive exercise on range of joint movement in young male adults. Res. Quart. 27:50, 1956.
40. McArdle, W. D., F. I. Katch, and V. L. Katch. Exercise Physiology: Energy, Nutrition, and Human Performance. Philadelphia, PA, Lea & Febiger, 1986.
41. McCloy, C. H., and N. D. Young. Tests and Measurements in Health and Physical Education. New York, Appleton-Century-Crofts, 1954.
42. Miller, A. P. Strains of the posterior calf musculature (tennis leg). Am. J. Sports Med. 7:172–174, 1979.
43. Milne, C., V. Seefeldt, and P. Reuschlein. Relationship between grade, sex, race, and motor performance in young children. Res. Quart. 47:726–730, 1976.
44. Möller, M., J. Ekstrand, B. Oberg, and S. Gillquist. Duration of stretching effect on range of motion

45. Moore, M. A., and R. S. Hutton. Electromyographic investigation of muscle stretching techniques. Med. Sci. Sports Exerc. 12:322–329, 1980.
46. O'Neil, R. Prevention of hamstring and groin strain. Athletic Training 11:27–31, 1976.
47. Ramsey, R., and S. Street. The isometric length-tension diagram of isolated skeletal muscle fibers of the frog. J. Cell. Comp. Physiol. 15:11–34, 1940.
48. Reid, D. C., R. S. Burnham, L. A. Saboe, and S. F. Kushner. Lower extremity flexibility patterns in classical ballet dancers and their correlation to lateral hip and knee injuries. Am. J. Sports Med. 15:347–352, 1987.
49. Reser, J. M. The effects of increasing range of motion on vertical jump (thesis), UCLA, 1961.
50. Rigby, B. J. The effect of mechanical extension under the thermal stability of collagen. Biochem. Biophys. Acta 79:634–636, 1964.
51. Sady, S. P., M. Wortman, and D. Blande. Flexibility training: Ballistic, static, or proprioceptive neuromuscular facilitation. Arch. Phys. Med. Rehabil. 63:261–263, 1982.
52. Safran, M. R., W. E. Garrett, Jr., A. V. Seaber, R. R. Glisson, and B. M. Ribbeck. The role of warmup in muscular injury prevention. Am. J. Sports Med. 16:123–129, 1988.
53. Starring, D. T., M. R. Gossman, G. G. Nicholson, Jr., and J. Lemons. Comparison of cyclic and sustained passive stretching using a mechanical device to increase resting length of hamstring muscles. Phys. Ther. 68:314–320, 1988.
54. Stoller, D. W., K. L. Markoff, S. A. Zager, and S. C. Shoemaker. The effects of exercise, ice and ultrasonography on torsional laxity of the knee. Clin. Orthop. 174:172–180, 1983.
55. Stuart, P. G., G. E. Goslow, C. G. Mosher, and R. M. Reinking. Stretch responsiveness of Golgi tendon organs. Exp. Brain Res. 10:463–476, 1970.
56. Tanigawa, M. C. Comparison of the hold-relax procedure and passive mobilization on increasing muscle length. Phys. Ther. 52:725–735, 1972.
57. Taylor, D. C., A. V. Seaber, and W. E. Garrett, Jr. Response of muscle tendon units to cyclic repetitive stretching. Trans. Orthop. Res. Soc. 10:84, 1985.
58. Viidik, A. Rheological model for uncalcified parallel-fibred collagenous tissue. J. Biomech. 1:3–11, 1968.
59. Walker, S. M. Delay of twitch relaxation induced by stress and stress relaxation. J. Appl. Physiol. 16:801–806, 1961.
60. Warren, C. G., J. F. Lehman, and J. N. Koblanski. Heat and stretch procedures: An evaluation using rat tail tendon. Arch. Phys. Med. Rehabil. 57:122–126, 1976.
61. Wilkerson, G. B. Developing flexibility by overcoming the stretch reflex. Physician Sports Med. 9:189–191, 1981.
62. Williford, H. N., J. B. East, F. H. Smith, and L. A. Burrys. Evaluation of warm-up for improvement in flexibility. Am. J. Sports Med. 14:316–319, 1986.

4
ERGOGENIC AIDS

HERBERT A. HAUPT

As financial and social incentives continue to motivate athletes to win at all costs, more and more athletes are turning to ergogenic aids to supplement years of training. Ergogenic aids are physical, mechanical, nutritional, psychological, or pharmacological substances or treatments that either directly improve physiological variables associated with exercise performance or remove subjective restraints that may limit physiological capacity.[3] Great publicity surrounds the detected use of banned ergogenic aids by athletes. Dealing with athletes today demands a thorough knowledge of banned ergogenic aids so that effective counseling for the athletes can be provided. In this chapter I will discuss the more well known ergogenic aids that have been banned by the National Collegiate Athletic Association (NCAA) or the U.S. Olympic Committee (USOC). These are the anabolic compounds, which include anabolic steroids and growth hormone; the stimulants, which include cocaine, crack, amphetamines, phenylpropanolamine, and caffeine; beta blockers; and blood doping. Since most athletes will encounter drug testing at some point in their careers, drug testing techniques, including a detailed description of specimen collection, are reviewed.

I would like to extend special thanks to Mrs. Chris Grissom of Orthopedic Associates, Inc., for her invaluable help in the preparation of this manuscript.

ANABOLIC COMPOUNDS

ANABOLIC STEROIDS

While anabolic steroids have been used as ergogenic aids by athletes as early as 1954, it was not until the 1983 Pan American Games in Carracas, Venezuela, that they captured the attention of the general public. Several athletes tested positive for drugs during those games, and since then the use of anabolic steroids by athletes has certainly become one of the most controversial issues in sports today. As recently as the 1988 Summer Olympics anabolic steroids have dominated sporting events. The media coverage of the astounding world record set by the Canadian sprinter Ben Johnson, followed by his disqualification for abuse of anabolic steroids, became one of the major events of the 1988 Summer Olympics.

Educating athletes on anabolic steroids requires particular care. Athletes are aware that anabolic steroids can increase their size and strength. Athletes who use steroids are also amazingly well educated regarding their potential side effects, and they are also aware that these side effects are generally reversible following short-term use. Unfortunately, most athletes are not aware of the damaging psychological effects of anabolic steroids. Anabolic steroids can cause significant personality alterations that may force its user into violent behavior. These steroids can also become addictive. They may be the most destructive drugs that an athlete can encounter.

Anabolic steroids are synthetic derivatives of testosterone. These compounds were developed in an attempt to dissociate the androgenic and anabolic effects of testosterone to minimize the masculinizing androgenic side effects. Complete dissociation of these effects is impossible, and therefore, all anabolic steroids have associated with them some androgenic side effects.[32] There are both oral and injectable forms of anabolic steroids. Athletes who use anabolic steroids frequently use combinations of both the oral and the injectable forms simultaneously at dosages much higher than their recommended therapeutic dosage. This technique is called *stacking*.[16, 43] Table 4–1 lists the generic and trade names of the more commonly used anabolic steroids.

While the use of anabolic steroids as an ergogenic aid by competitive athletes has been well publicized by the media, in my experience the greatest abuse of anabolic steroids is in the noncompetitive athlete who takes the steroids for cosmetic reasons, simply to look bigger and stronger. Today's fashion stresses a more muscular physique, and peer-sensitive young adults are anxious to develop this appearance. Being impatient with the normally slow muscular growth pattern associated with weight lifting, many turn to anabolic steroids to achieve this appearance as quickly as possible. It has been reported that 6.6 percent of all high school male seniors have tried anabolic steroids by the age of 18. This represents between 250,000 and 500,000 adolescents.[10]

Anabolic steroids can increase both the size and strength of their user only under proper conditions. To achieve positive results, the athlete must have been previously trained in intense weight training prior to the use of the steroids, continue to train during the use of the steroids, and maintain a diet adequate in carbohydrates and protein. If these conditions are not met, the anabolic steroid will have little or no effect on the athlete's size and strength.[25]

Anabolic steroids have no effect on aerobic performance.[25] Therefore, endurance athletes would not benefit from use of anabolic steroids. However, sprinters and other participants in anaerobic events that require short bursts of power would certainly be expected to improve their performance through the

TABLE 4–1. Generic and Trade Names of Anabolic Steroids in Common Use

Oral			Intramuscular	
17-Alpha-methyl Derivatives of Testosterone	*17 Alpha-ethyl Derivatives of Testosterone*	*1-Methyl Derivatives*	*Esters of Testosterone*	*Esters of 19-Nortestosterone*
Methyltestosterone Android (Brown) Metandren (Ciba) Oreton (Schering) Vigorex (Marin) Virilon (Stor) Testred (ICN) Fluoxymesterone Android-F (Brown) Halotestin (Upjohn) Methandrostenolone Dianabol (Ciba) Oxandrolone Anavar (Searle) Oxymetholone Anadrol-50 (Syntex) Adroyd (Parke, Davis) Stanozolol Winstrol (Winthrop)	Ethylestrenol Maxibolin (Organon) Orabolin (Organon) Norethandrolone Nilevar (Searle)	Methenolone acetate Nibal (Squibb) Mesterolone Mestoranum (Schering)	Testosterone propionate Oreton Propionate (Shering) Testosterone enanthate Delatestryl (Squibb) Testosterone cypionate Depo-Testosterone (Upjohn)	Nandrolone decanoate Deca-Durabolin (Organon) Nandrolone phenpropionate Durabolin (Organon)

Haupt, HA, Rovere GD, Anabolic steroids: A review of the literature. Am J of Sports Med 12:469–484, 1984.

strength-enhancing characteristics of anabolic steroids.

The mechanism of action of anabolic steroids involves both anabolic and anticatabolic effects. The anticatabolic effects of anabolic steroids include their ability to reverse the catabolic effects of endogenous glucocorticosteroids that are released during periods of stress, including intense training. Anabolic steroids can also cause a shift from a negative nitrogen balance to a positive nitrogen balance through improved utilization of ingested protein.[25, 32] The anabolic effects of anabolic steroids are at the cellular level, where they can induce protein synthesis in skeletal muscle cells. They attach to cytoplasmic receptors found on muscle cells and activate the synthesis of protein within the cells.[25, 32] Another anabolic effect is their ability to stimulate the release of endogenous growth hormone.[2] Finally, there is a motivational effect associated with anabolic steroid use. Athletes taking anabolic steroids experience a state of euphoria, diminished fatigue, and increased aggression, all of which can be focused into intense training sessions.[25] A profound placebo effect has also been associated with the use of steroids.[6]

While anabolic steroids can increase both size and strength, this effect is maintained only as long as the use of anabolic steroids is continued. Following discontinuance of the steroid, a significant percentage of the increased size and strength disappears, which seems to be related to the seriously depressed levels of testosterone in the athlete who uses anabolic steroids. Without the exogenous steroid supplementation, the athlete's depleted testosterone levels cannot maintain the muscularity. In addition, the motivational efects of the steroid are eliminated, and the intense training sessions cannot be maintained. The result is a rapid decrease in size and strength. It is for this reason that athletes who wish to maintain their competitive edge or their appearance must continue the anabolic steroids indefinitely.

A variety of side effects may be noted by athletes taking anabolic steroids. These include increased acne about face and torso, male-pattern baldness, changes in sex drive, testicular atrophy, irritability, aggression, and gynecomastia. Most of these changes are reversible when the steroids are discontinued.[25] Females taking anabolic steroids take on many male characteristics including increased muscularity, male-pattern baldness, hirsutism, deepening of the voice, and clitoral enlargement. Some of these effects may be permanent.[50] Adolescents taking anabolic steroids prior to epiphyseal closure may accelerate the epiphyseal closure, resulting in short stature.[25, 33]

Anabolic steroids can adversely affect the reproductive system of the athlete. While taking anabolic steroids, the male athlete's endogenous testosterone levels are markedly decreased. The result is abnormal spermatogenesis and resultant transient infertility. These changes appear to be reversible when the steroids are discontinued.[25, 26]

The orally active anabolic steroids can have a profound effect on the liver while the injectable forms of anabolic steroids appear to have little effect on the liver. With the use of the orally active anabolic steroid liver function tests often become elevated. Intense weight lifting alone may also cause changes in liver function tests, including serum glutamic-oxaloacetic transaminase (SGOT), serum glutamic-pyruvic transaminase (SGPT), and lactic dehydrogenase (LDH). It is therefore recommended that more specific liver function tests be used to monitor liver function in weight training athletes. These include the alkaline phosphatase liver isoenzyme and the LDH liver isoenzyme. The altered liver function tests usually return to normal following discontinuance of the steroids.[25, 33]

Peliosis hepatis is a rare entity historically associated with tuberculosis. It is characterized by hemorrhagic cystic degeneration of the liver. Of the 23 cases of peliosis hepatis that have been reported in the literature, all patients but 1 were taking orally active anabolic steroids for periods between 6 and 24 months continuously, and all were being treated with anabolic steroids for medical illnesses.[25] There have been at least 36 reported cases of liver tumors associated with the use of anabolic steroids. All but one of these were reported in patients taking anabolic steroids for medical treatment. The majority of the tumors were malignant, associated with the orally active anabolic steroids, and the patients were treated for longer than 24 months continuously with the anabolic steroids.[25] There has been at least one report of a liver tumor in an athlete using anabolic steroids for bodybuilding purposes.[40]

Epidemiological studies have demonstrated that the risk of coronary heart disease is directly related to plasma levels of low-density lipoprotein (LDL) cholesterol concentration and inversely related to high-density lipoprotein (HDL) cholesterol concentrations. While intense exercise can serve to lower the LDL/HDL ratio, the use of anabolic steroids, even with short-term use and despite exercise, can cause a significant increase in the LDL/HDL ratio. In one study, the ratio increased by 280 percent.[27] These altered ratios return to normal following discontinuance of the steroids. The question of how detrimental short-term elevations in the LDL/HDL ratio are to coronary health is unanswered at this time. However, recently there have been two separate reports of strokes in athletes taking anabolic steroids for bodybuilding purposes.[17, 38] As athletes take anabolic steroids for more prolonged periods, we are likely to see more severe cardiovascular disturbances.

The most disturbing adverse effects of anabolic steroids may be their psychological effects. A high percentage of athletes who take anabolic steroids will suffer some degree of personality change that may range from increased irritability to a toxic psychosis that may require hospitalization.[42, 43] Athletes taking anabolic steroids often become extremely intense, aggressive, and sometimes violent individuals. These characteristics allow the athlete to train in a much more strenuous and focused manner. However, these aggressive side effects carry over into everyday life as well. The athletes assume a Jekyll and Hyde personality where even a slight provocation can cause them to react in a violent and sometimes uncontrolled manner. They can become virtual sociopaths who can no longer maintain effective relationships with friends, family, or loved ones. Their only release is in the weight room or on the playing field where violent behavior may be more acceptable. These individuals not uncommonly lose girlfriends, suffer divorces, move away from family, and frequently find themselves in trouble with the law. Recently, there have been reports of psychotic episodes in a small percentage of anabolic steroid users. Hospitalizations were required in some instances, and the psychoses reversed following discontinuance of the steroids.[43] Ultimately, personality alterations return to normal following discontinuance of the steroids. Unfortunately, scars on relationships between friends, family, and loved ones and any arrest records will remain with the athlete for the rest of his or her life.

An equally disturbing and potentially more devastating effect of anabolic steroids is addiction. There is both a psychological and a physiological component to this addiction.[52] Athletes who take anabolic steroids usually do so out of insecurity. It may be the insecurity of a professional football player who feels that he cannot maintain his position without the aid of the steroid, or just the insecurity of a young athlete feeling that he is smaller than his peers in a local health club. It may be the insecurity of a world-class sprinter and current world-record holder as he approaches the most important race of his life. In all these cases, the athletes use the steroids to supplement their perceived deficiencies. Under the proper conditions, anabolic steroids will in fact stimulate increased size and strength. An athlete whose competitive success is contingent on this increased size and strength may find it quite difficult to discontinue the steroids for fear of losing this competitive edge. Even more disturbing is the use of anabolic steroids for cosmetic purposes. I am aware of more and more young teenage weight lifters who take anabolic steroids simply to look bigger and stronger as quickly as possible. These young men are extremely impatient with the normal slow muscular growth patterns that occur with weight lifting alone. They constantly review themselves in the mirror and critically perceive themselves as being smaller than their peers. They become obsessed with their appearance. This obsession with body image motivates them to seek to gain size and strength at any cost. They often turn to anabolic steroids. When these young athletes take steroids, assuming that they are adequately trained and maintain adequate diet, they do in fact realize an increase in size and strength. While taking the steroids, the athletes enjoy more intense training sessions, a euphoria well documented with any steroid use, and a markedly increased sexual drive. They thrive on the attention and admiration of their peer group as a result of their increased size and strength. However, as the young male athlete discontinues the steroid, his body's seriously depressed levels of testosterone cannot support the intense training sessions, and the size and strength improvements quickly disappear, as does the sexual drive, the steroid euphoria, and the peer admiration. The athlete becomes obsessed with his decreasing size and appearance, and this already-insecure athlete falls victim to a very real and serious depression. Most of the athletes cannot tolerate this withdrawal complex and quickly return to using the steroids to maintain their distorted body image. Back on the steroids, the athlete once again regains his size and strength, his sexual drive, and his self-esteem. The thought of long-term medical consequences rarely enters his mind. He has become psychologically addicted to the anabolic steroid. Recent evidence has also demonstrated a physiological component to the dependency on anabolic steroids that resembles that of opioid dependence.[52]

Compulsive behavior to maintain a distorted body image has been well known to specialists dealing with eating disorders such as anorexia nervosa. The same psychological disorder that affects the anorexia nervosa sufferer may be operating in young bodybuilders who become so obsessed with their body image that they must continue anabolic steroid use indefinitely to maintain their distorted body image.

Counseling the athlete who is entertaining the use of anabolic steroids is most effective when alternatives to steroids can be discussed with the athlete. Emphasizing the benefits of proper nutrition and stressing proper weight-lifting techniques are important considerations. It must be emphasized to the athlete that while the effects of anabolic steroids may be quite impressive, these effects remain only as long as the steroids are continued. Similar results can occur, more slowly, but permanently, through proper training techniques and proper nutrition. It is often most effective to find role models for these athletes who have developed their physiques through years of training without the use of steroids. In my experience, when the athlete is properly educated regarding the physiological and psychological effects of the steroids and is educated regarding effective alternatives to steroids, their interest in these drugs can be curbed.

Unfortunately, many still turn to steroids, initially as an experiment and ultimately as a long-term supplement. Counseling these individuals is quite difficult. Usually, education regarding physiological and psychological effects have little impact. These athletes are not interested in alternatives, as they feel they are maximizing their development already through the use of steroids. These athletes require professional counseling through appropriate psychiatric referrals. In the near future, I anticipate the development of rehabilitation programs dedicated to the treatment of anabolic steroid abuse.

I have found that many of the athletes who have used steroids in the past, or are currently using steroids, are concerned about any adverse effects they may have sustained. I have developed a blood study for these athletes investigating potential adverse liver and blood cholesterol effects. This testing program has been made available through a local hospital on an anonymous and inexpensive basis. The results are returned to the athlete with suggestions to seek medical evaluation if any of the parameters are out of normal limits. The study includes the routine iver enzymes SGOT and SGPT. It also includes the liver-specific isoenzymes of LDH and alkaline phosphatase as well as the liver-specific enzyme gamma-glutamic transaminase (GGT). These more specific enzymes are often within normal limits despite abnormal levels of SGOT and SGPT, which are elevated owing to skeletal muscle breakdown. In addition, LDL and HDL concentrations are included in this study. The athlete is warned that a normal profile does not ensure his or her health with steroid use, as other adverse effects may be occurring that are not studied in the profile.

Athletes are generally well educated regarding substances that they may use as ergogenic aids. This includes anabolic steroids. Unfortunately, the psychological consequences of steroids and their potential for addiction are not well known to the athlete. While the athletes may correctly perceive their risks for significant physiological side effects to be small if they use steroids for brief periods of time, many are unaware of the potential difficulties in discontinuing their use. The result may be incessant use of the steroids by an athlete who previously contemplated only short-term use. As we see athletes taking anabolic steroids for more prolonged periods, we are likely to see more severe physiological effects. Those who eventually do discontinue the steroids are dismayed to find that the improvements made with the steroids generally disappear, and they have little to show for hours and even years of intense training beyond

GROWTH HORMONE

Growth hormone (hGH) is the most abundant principle of the anterior pituitary in the human. In the human gland, 10 percent of the dry weight is growth hormone.[2, 35] Proper human growth from infancy is contingent on growth hormone, and growth hormone appears to affect the growth of just about every organ and tissue in the body.[24] Growth hormone release is cyclical, with the largest release occurring 60 to 90 minutes after sleep onset at the beginning of slow-wave sleep.[37] It also increases during exercise, with peak levels and duration being a function of the intensity of the exercise, duration of the exercise, and the training status of the athlete, with more hormone release occurring in the untrained than the trained individual during exercise.[13, 37] The mechanism by which growth hormone stimulates somatic growth is related to the production of somatomedins, which are synthesized in the liver and circulate in the blood following exposure to growth hormone. It appears that somatomedins may mediate the effects of growth hormone. The interaction of growth hormone and somatomedin effects are difficult to separate and are still under study.[13, 24, 37]

Athletes are turning to growth hormone because they believe that hGH can provide many of the benefits of anabolic/androgenic steroids, and as yet, no effective testing for the hormone exists.[13] In several species, growth hormone has been shown to cause a retention of nitrogen and an overall anabolic affect. It also increases the transport of amino acids in the tissues and accelerates their incorporation into protein.[24] In experimental conditions, growth hormone–treated muscles increased in size relative to untreated muscles. The effect here is in synergy with the amount of work that the muscles performed. It appears that the protein synthesis in the muscles is increased by both the growth hormone and the muscular work.[37] Additionally, growth hormone stimulates the mobilization of lipids from adipose tissue and increases their oxidation as a source of energy.[24, 37] Therefore, an athlete may realize an improvement in strength and perhaps overall performance with the use of hGH.

There are many factors that either stimulate or inhibit the release of growth hormone. It has been demonstrated that the amino acids arginine, ornithine, and lysine, either alone or in combination, can stimulate the endogenous release of growth hormone.[34] Many athletes are using these amino acid supplements in an attempt to stimulate their own production of growth hormone. Other athletes turn to growth hormone injections instead. Prior to recombinant DNA (deoxyribonucleic acid) technology, the only sources for growth hormone were those derived from the pituitary glands of human cadavers.[9, 44] Several cases of Creutzfeldt-Jakob disease were attributed to the use of cadaver pituitary glands that were infected with the Creutzfeldt-Jakob virus.[44] Recently, recombinant DNA research has produced biosynthetic growth hormone. The original synthetic hormone produced by Genentech differed from endogenous growth hormone by the presence of an extra methionine group not found on the natural growth hormone. In about 30 percent of the patients treated with this synthetic growth hormone, serum antibodies to growth hormone were formed.[9] Speculation regarding the possible interference with endogenous growth hormone by these antibodies has prompted concern regarding the use of this biosynthetic hormone.[9, 37] Recently, Lilly has formulated a synthetic growth hormone that has the same amino acid sequence as the endogenous hormone. This appears to be less likely to produce serum antibodies to naturally occurring growth hormone.[28] All forms of growth hormone are injectable.

The interest by athletes in growth hormone is limited by its cost and the need for syringes and needles. It has been estimated that the amount of growth hormone needed for an ergogenic effect would cost between $1000 and $1500 for an 8-week supply.[13] Despite the cost factor, there is still an interest in the hormone by some athletes.

Low levels, or absence, of growth hormone results in pituitary dwarfism. This is the only currently approved indication for growth hormone treatment.[28] Growth hormone excess in prepubertal subjects leads to gigantism and in postpubertal subjects to acromegaly. Acromegaly is a clinical syndrome characterized by an increase in the size of the skull, with prominent cheekbones, protruding jaw, and frontal bossing. The fingers and hands become broad and spadelike, with sausage-appearing fingers. Facial features become coarse as a result of increased growth of subcutaneous tissues. The protrusion of the jaw is secondary to increased growth of the mandible and maxilla. Generally, there is no increase in height because the bony growth centers have already fused in the adult. While the acromegalic appears muscular, the muscles are actually quite weak, owing to myopathy. Osteoporosis also becomes a problem with time.[45] Mortality is high and most patients ultimately die of cardiac failure—50 percent by the age of 50 and 89 percent by the age of 60.[37] Growth hormone excess can lead to diabetes.[37, 45] Approximately one third of the males with acromegaly develop impotence, and almost all women develop amenorrhea or at least menstrual irregularities.[45] Prepubertal growth hormone excesses result in gigantism. These individuals also suffer from osteoporosis and muscle weakness just like the acromegalics, and like the acromegalics, many ultimately die of cardiac failure.[49]

Athletes using growth hormone either to increase their size and strength or to increase their ultimate height, depending on the age of the user, will certainly be prone to the clinical syndromes described above. What effects short-term usage has on the athlete are difficult to predict at this point. Since it is an injectable drug, there are the added risks of hepatitis and acquired immune deficiency syndrome (AIDS) as a result of potentially shared needles and syringes. Growth hormone is banned by both the NCAA and the USOC.[39, 49]

STIMULANTS

COCAINE

Cocaine has been part of our society for many years. It occurs naturally in the leaf of the *Erythroxylon coca* plant. Its history of use includes use by Sigmund Freud for a variety of maladies, as an ingredient in the original formula of Coca-Cola until it was removed in 1903, and as a local anesthetic, for which it is still used as its only true therapeutic indication.[36] Recent studies estimate that 28 percent of adults between the ages of 20 and 40 and 16 percent of high school seniors have tried cocaine at least once.[36, 51] The untimely deaths of basketball star Len Bias and pro football player Don Rogers heralded public awareness of cocaine abuse by athletes. Their deaths also demonstrated the potential danger in the use of this drug.

The active drug is cocaine hydrochloride. Cocaine hydrochloride decomposes with heating, and for that reason, its major mode of absorption is by snorting, or sniffing the crystals. Cocaine limits its own absorption by this route by causing vasoconstriction of the nasal mucosal membranes.[14]

Cocaine is a potent stimulant and as such may be abused by athletes as an ergogenic aid. Once absorbed, it causes the release of norepinephrine from neurons while simultaneously blocking its reuptake, thus making more of the neurotransmitter available to receptor sites.[51] The result of this potentiation of the effects of norepinephrine are feelings of euphoria, decreased fatigue, and grandiosity of thought. In addition, the speed of peripheral reflexes is increased, but in an unsynchronized and uncoordinated fashion. As a result of these effects, the athlete may feel that he or she is performing at a higher level, both stronger and faster, but, in fact, this is a result of the individual's distorted perception of his or her performance. The athlete is in fact not stronger, and, while reflexes are quicker, actions are uncoordinated and often ineffective.[51]

Regardless of whether an athlete takes cocaine in an attempt to improve athletic performance or simply uses for recreation, dependence or addiction may certainly occur. It has been estimated that an individual consuming cocaine at the rate of 120 milligrams a day for 10 consecutive days will become dependent on the drug. A "line of coke" is approximately 25 milligrams.[51] Dependency may force an athlete to use cocaine anywhere from 4 to 20 times a day. Tolerance may develop so that an athlete can be addicted and continue to participate in sports before this abuse interferes significantly with his or her activities.[51]

The other side effects of cocaine abuse include potential ulceration and perforations of the nasal septum with chronic use. Rhinitis, sinusitis, and bronchitis are common with recurrent use. Hyperthermia is a potentially serious complication and is the result of peripheral vasoconstriction causing core temperature to elevate. This could be extremely hazardous to an athlete exercising in hot, humid climates.[36, 51] The use of cocaine can result in agitation, restlessness, insomnia, anxiety, and in some cases, toxic psychosis where the individual may hallucinate, become paranoid, and suffer from delusions. Time distortion also occurs.[36] As a result, the user may miss team buses and other appointments. Missed appointments, antisocial activity, restlessness, and disciplinary problems in a previously well adjusted individual may be the first signs of cocaine abuse.

The most disastrous side effects of cocaine use are cardiovascular and may result in death. Cocaine-induced release of norepinephrine can trigger serious ventricular arrhythmias or coronary artery vasospasms. The spasms can cause coronary thrombus formation even in the presence of a normal artery.[11] The result of these effects can be acute myocardial infarction or sudden death. In addition, cerebrovascular accidents can occur within minutes of cocaine use if there is cerebral aneurysm or other predisposing conditions.[8] Finally, seizure activity may occur as a result of central nervous system stimulation. Some experts feel that most deaths caused by cocaine are due to seizures leading to anoxia.[14]

CRACK

Crack is essentially pure cocaine produced by removing the hydrochloride from cocaine hydrochloride to produce a precipitate of pure cocaine. The final precipitate appears as a white rock. Its name comes from the popping sound made by the crystals as they are heated. Unlike cocaine hydrochloride, this material is not decomposed by heating. It vaporizes at higher temperatures, making it suitable for smoking. Smoking crack delivers large quantities of cocaine to the vascular bed of the lung, where it is quickly absorbed.[14] Absorption by this route is not limited as it is by nasal absorption. The result is an intense, short-lived but accelerated cocaine effect. Within minutes of the initial rush of euphoria, the user suffers a crushing "crash," forcing rapid repeat doses, which quickly leads to addiction. Also more intense are the potentially disastrous side effects, including cardiac arrhythmias, myocardial infarction, and seizure activity.[14] Overdosing with crack is an unfortunate and frequent occurrence. Crack is currently becoming widely available, as it is relatively inexpensive to produce, compared with cocaine. The unfortunate result is near-epidemic use, especially among adolescents.[14]

Athletes may feel that cocaine has a positive effect on their performance through enhanced reflexes, feelings of euphoria, and decreased fatigue. However, it carries with its use potential life-threatening cardiovascular effects, risks of addiction, and significant behavioral alterations. Cocaine's presence in an athlete's urine is detectable 18 to 36 hours after use. Cocaine is banned by both the NCAA and the USOC.[39, 49]

AMPHETAMINES

Amphetamines are potent stimulants that have been used as ergogenic aids by athletes for many years. Their use seems to be diminishing slightly in the athletic ranks, being replaced by cocaine. Amphetamines are indirect-acting sympathomimetic amines. As such, they indirectly stimulate the adrenergic nervous system through the release of endogenous catecholamines. Amphetamines are one of the most potent sympathomimetic amines with respect to stimulation of the central nervous system (CNS).[22] As a result of the CNS stimulation, the athlete becomes more alert and has a decreased sense of fatigue. Amphetamines seem to have their most profound effect when performance has been reduced by fatigue or lack of sleep. In these conditions, the amphetamine improves concentration and overall alertness despite the fatigued condition.[22, 29] Athletic performance in activities of strength, speed, and endurance have all been shown to improve with the use of amphetamines.[29, 48]

Amphetamines are also potent appetite suppressants. As such, they may be abused by athletes who must maintain their weight, as in gymnastics, wrestling, or ballet.[22, 35]

Tolerance and addiction to amphetamines can occur. The abrupt withdrawal of amphetamines may produce chronic fatigue and depression. Adverse effects on the CNS include anxiety, insomnia, nervousness, and agitation and even the possibility of a toxic pscyhosis with vivid hallucinations and paranoid characteristics.[22] Hyperthermia is a potentially serious problem in athletes performing in hot environments because of the peripheral vasoconstriction caused by the drug.[29, 35] Deaths have been associated with amphetamine use as a result of cerebrovascular hemorrhage, acute cardiac failure, and hyperthermia. Amphetamines are banned by both the NCAA and the USOC.[39, 49]

PHENYLPROPANOLAMINE

Phenylpropanolamine (PPA) is a sympathomimetic amine that is an active ingredient in many over-the-counter appetite suppressants, nasal decongestants, and cold remedies. It is becoming a frequently used ergogenic aid by athletes because of its stimulant characteristics. PPA is an amphetamine lookalike that differs from amphetamine by the presence of a single hydroxl group that decreases its central stimulatory effect compared with amphetamine.[21] PPA primarily stimulates alpha-adrenergic receptors and is therefore a potent nasal decongestant.[32] In the over-the-counter formulations, it is often combined with other drugs such as antihistamines or caffeine. The clinical effect of PPA occurs within 30 minutes of use and can last up to 3 hours.[5]

PPA can induce significant increases in blood pressure even at therapeutic dosages, especially when combined with caffeine, as found in many over-the-counter medications.[5, 41] Life-threatening hypertension can occur following ovedosage. Overdosage with PPA is not infrequent in adolescents who attempt to increase weight loss or in athletes who attempt to maximize the stimulant effect. In addition, seizures have occurred with PPA, again when taken in combination with caffeine.[41] Psychotic episodes, paranoia, homicidal behavior, hallucinations, and attempted suicide have all been reported after taking phenylpropanolamine. Acute renal failure has occurred in association with rhabdomyolysis. Cardiac arrhythmias and myocardial infarction have been documented with its use.[41] As athletes turn more and more to ergogenic aids, phenylpropanolamine, because of its availability, is subject to abuse. It is banned by both the NCAA and the USOC.[39, 49]

CAFFEINE

Caffeine is a member of the group of methylated xanthines that includes theophylline and theobromine. Theobromine is found in cocoa and theophylline in tea.[19] Coffee is a major source of caffeine in the American diet. However, it is also possible to obtain caffeine tablets, which are usually taken to combat drowsiness. Caffeine is frequently used by athletes as an ergogenic aid. Dosages of caffeine of 250 mg to 350 mg have been demonstrated to enhance performance in endurance athletic events.[30, 47] The effect on endurance performance appears to be mediated by central nervous system stimulation by caffeine; enhanced fatty acid utilization during activities, thereby sparing muscle glycogen; and increased skeletal muscle contractility.[12, 20, 30, 35]

The CNS effect of caffeine relates to its ability to block the adenosine receptors in the central nervous system. The result is a reduction in the adenosine inhibition of the release of neurotransmitters and its overall depressive effect.[15] The resultant stimulation decreases the athlete's perception of fatigue and increases his or her vigilance and intensity. Peak blood levels of caffeine are reached within 30 minutes.[47] Therefore, shortly after intake, either as tablets or from coffee, the athlete will experience the stimulatory effect. While the other methylxanthines have similar CNS effects, caffeine is the most active.[20]

Caffeine is lipolytic, thereby increasing the plasma levels of free fatty acids. Elevation of plasma free fatty acids results in an increased rate of lipid metabolism and decreased dependence on muscle glycogen during exercise. The longer muscle glycogen is spared, the lower the rate of exhaustion.[12] Therefore, caffeine does have a positive physiological effect on the performance of endurance activities. This effect would not improve performance in maximal short-term, high-intensity athletic activities.

Caffeine serves to strengthen the contraction of skeletal muscle and render it less susceptible to fatigue.[20, 35] Caffeine is the most active of all the methylxanthines in this effect.[20]

The adverse effects of caffeine on the athlete include a mild diuretic effect.[20] This could be potentially bothersome in long-distance running. Additionally, while there is a stimulant effect of caffeine and this may be ergogenic, fine-motor coordination can be affected. Occasional arrhythmias have been associated with the use of caffeine, including premature ventricular contractions and tachycardia. Discontinuance of the caffeine eliminates the arrhythmia. Caffeine also has sleep-altering effects, especially when coffee or caffeine is taken just prior to sleep. Finally, there is a withdrawal syndrome associated with discontinuance of caffeine in individuals who have taken significant amounts daily. This syndrome includes headache, drowsiness, lethargy, and, in some cases, irri-

TABLE 4–2. Caffeine Urine Concentrations

Product	Amt/Dose	Equivalent in Urine Within 2–3 Hours
Decaffeinated coffee	2–3 mg	0.03–0.04 mcg/ml
One cup coffee	100.0 mg	1.50 mcg/ml
1 Coca-Cola, Diet Coke	45.6 mg	0.68 mcg/ml
1 Tab	46.8 mg	0.70 mcg/ml
1 Dr Pepper	39.6 mg	0.59 mcg/ml
1 Diet Pepsi, Pepsi Light	36.0 mg	0.54 mcg/ml
1 No Doz	100.0 mg	1.50 mcg/ml
1 Vivarin	200.0 mg	3.00 mcg/ml
1 APC, Empirin, or Anacin	32.0 mg	0.48 mcg/ml
1 Excedrin	65.0 mg	0.97 mcg/ml
1 Midol	32.4 mg	0.48 mcg/ml

Source: Reprinted with permission of the U.S. Olympic Committee from Sportsmediscope—USOC Sports Med Sci Div Newslett 7(7):2, 1988.

tability and nervousness.[35] Some degree of tolerance develops to the diuretic and sleep disturbance effects. Little or no tolerance seems to develop to central nervous system stimulation.[20]

Currently, the NCAA bans caffeine only if its concentration in the urine exceeds 15 mcg/ml.[39] The USOC bans caffeine in amounts greater than 12 mcg/ml.[49] To achieve these levels would require the consumption of approximately 6 to 10 cups of coffee in one sitting and testing within 2 to 3 hours after this dose.[49] Table 4–2 demonstrates the effects of consuming various caffeine-containing products on urine caffeine concentration 2 to 3 hours after use.

BETA BLOCKERS

Beta blockers are used by a select group of athletes who require the ability to control tremor during periods of stress and exercise in such sports as the biathalon, riflery, and archery. Beta blockers antagonize epinephrine-induced tremor in humans and laboratory animals. The antitremor effect appears to be peripheral and is most profound when the tremor is accentuated by emotional or physical stress causing epinephrine release.[53] Propanolol—trade name, Inderal—is the most well known and frequently used beta blocker by athletes. It is a nonselective beta blocker and as such blocks both the beta-1 and beta-2 receptors. Specific beta blockers are beta-1 selective such as Metoprolol. While beta blockers are effective in decreasing tremor especially during exercise, they can have an adverse effect on the athletic performance of the athlete.

A highly trained athlete's $\dot{V}O_2$max is reduced by 15 percent or more during the use of beta blockers.[53]

The use of Propanolol and other beta blockers can adversely affect the respiratory system. They cause an increase in airway resistance, which may cause potentially life-threatening reactions in asthmatics. In addition, nausea, vomiting, mild diarrhea, and even constipation have been reported with use of Propanolol. Hallucinations, nightmares, insomnia, and depression have also been reported.[23] Beta blockers have been banned by both the NCAA and the USOC.

BLOOD DOPING

Blood doping as an ergogenic aid for endurance events was first publicized during the 1976 Olympic Games in Montreal.[3] Since then, there has been considerable interest on the part of athletes regarding this technique. This interest is fueled not only because blood doping appears to be an effective ergogenic aid but also because blood doping cannot be detected even though it is banned by the NCAA and the USOC.[7] The technique involves transfusion of an athlete 24 to 48 hours prior to a competition in an attempt to increase the red cell volume in the athlete's blood. The normovolemic erythrocythemia induced by the transfusion causes a small but significant increase in the endurance capacity of the athlete.[3, 7, 18, 31] Blood doping has been given other names including blood boosting, blood packing, and induced erythrocythemia.[3]

The capacity of a muscle to perform continuous activity depends on the ability of blood to transport enough oxygen to the contracting muscle cell. By increasing the red cell mass, oxygen delivery to the exercising muscle is increased with resultant improvements in $\dot{V}O_2$max and performance.[3, 18, 31]

Blood transfusion can be either a heterologous transfusion from a matching donor or an autologous transfusion with the subject's own blood. The use of heterologous blood carries significant risk. Immunologic reactions complicate approximately 3 percent of all heterologous transfusions, resulting in mild allergic reactions including fever, urticaria, and very infrequently, hemolytic transfusion reactions that could be potentially fatal.[31] Athletes given heterologous transfusions are also at risk for contracting AIDS or blood-borne hepatitis. For these reasons, autologous transfusions are used exclusively by athletes for blood doping. The collection of the athletes' blood, however, complicates the technique, because following phlebotomy the athletes' hematocrit requires at least 3 to 6 weeks to return to normal.[18] Therefore, in order to allow full normalization of the hemoglobin in the athlete following phlebotomy, extended storage periods are needed. This is achieved by storing the blood as frozen cells using a high glycerol freezing technique.[18] With this technique, unlike the refrigeration technique, the aging process of the red cells is interrupted, and storage can be maintained for up to several years. When this blood is reinfused, regardless of how long it is stored, nearly 85 percent of the original red cells remain viable.[18]

If the athlete has returned to a normal cythemic level following phlebotomy by waiting a period of at least 3 to 6 weeks, and if the red cells are stored with the technique previously described, a transfusion of 2 units of packed cells will increase the hemoglobin by approximately 10 percent.[7] Twenty-four hours after infusion, the $\dot{V}O_2$max has been demonstrated to increase by 3.9 percent to 12.8 percent and endurance capacity by 2.5 percent to 35 percent.[3] The athlete's hemoglobin remains elevated following tranfusion for approximately 7 days and then gradually decreases over a 15-week period. Presumably, the increase in $\dot{V}O_2$max and endurance capacity will remain increased for at least several weeks following transfusion.[18]

Even using the autologous technique of blood transfusion the athlete does encounter certain risks with the procedure. Transfusing more than 2 units of packed cells would risk raising the hematocrit over 60 percent, which could subject the individual to a hyperviscosity syndrome, including intravascular clotting and the potential for heart failure and even death.[3] Additionally, blood transfusion procedures not performed with accepted medical technique could result in infection and air or clot emboli.

Blood doping does appear to be an effective ergogenic aid in endurance activities. It would presumably have little or no effect on anaerobic performance. The complicated process of phlebotomy and autologous transfusion results in increased hemoglobin and a small but significant increase in aerobic capacity. For these reasons, blood doping is banned by both the NCAA and the USOC. While there are currently no available testing techniques for blood doping, research is ongoing in this area.[7]

DRUG TESTING

Drug testing is a fact of life today. It is becoming more prevalent in the workplace and in the athletic arena. Athletes may become subject to drug testing as a result of an educational institution policy or when they participate in events where the sanctioning organization requires testing, such as the NCAA or the USOC. Athletes should be made aware of the protocols of specimen collection and testing techniques and be well versed in what drugs are banned by the sanctioning organizations under which they compete.

It is often not practical to test all athletes in a given event or institution. For that reason, there are selection processes that might be either random, based on player position or player sport, or based on reasonable cause or suspicion. Once a participant is selected for drug testing, there is a fairly uniform process of specimen collection and chain of custody control of the specimen as it is tested. While athletes are at first somewhat insecure about providing a specimen under constant scrutiny, most athletes feel that it is an effective safeguard against the possibility of an unfair advantage by the competitor who may use an ergogenic aid.

Testing techniques typically consist of a screening test followed by a confirmation test. The screening test may be either an immunoassay or a chromatography technique. Confirmation requires a gas chromatography/mass spectrometry study (GC/MS). GC/MS is the only legally admissible test.[1, 39, 46] For anabolic steroids, initial screening requires the use of GC/MS because of difficulty testing for steroids using routine screening techniques. Positives for anabolic steroids are then confirmed with more specific GC/MS techniques.[1] The testing techniques for the various drugs are becoming more sophisticated, but there are still no effective techniques to test for growth hormone or blood doping.

Athletes have attempted to avoid positive urine tests through techniques of urine manipulation. The athletes may catheterize themselves prior to testing and fill their bladders with "clean" urine. They have also used the drug Probenecid to block the excretion of banned substances. Lasix has been used to dilute the urine and therefore the concentration of banned substances. Both Probenecid and Lasix can be tested in the urine and are considered banned substances for these reasons. In addition, the more refined drug testing techniques are able to detect very low levels of drug urine concentrations of previously difficult-to-detect drugs.

Drugs remain in the urine for different lengths of time. Table 4–3 shows the length of time that drugs may be detected in the urine following use. Notice that marijuana may test positive for between 10 and 30 days, where other substances may only be positive for 24 to 48 hours after use. In the NCAA, the categories of banned substances include psychomotor and central nervous system stimulants, sympathomimetic amines, anabolic steroids, substances banned for specific sports, such as beta blockers in rifle sports, and street drugs including heroin and marijuana. Table 4–4 lists the NCAA-banned drugs. In addition, the NCAA prohibits the practice of blood doping. The NCAA does allow the use of local anesthetics, but the NCAA testing coordinator must be advised by the team physician prior to competition. The use of certain asthma medications is approved by the NCAA if the team doctor notifies the NCAA crew chief of the need for the medication. The use of corticosteroids must be declared by the team physicians prior to testing. The use of banned sympathomimetic amines, which are present in over-the-counter cold and diet medications, must be declared by the student athlete. A decision for eligibility after the use of these over-the-counter medications will be made by the NCAA, based on declaration consistent with concentration levels determined by laboratory analysis and other data.

USOC-banned substances include stimulants, narcotic analgesics, anabolic steroids, beta blockers, diuretics, blood doping, and human growth hormone. In addition, International Olympic Committee (IOC) bans the use of substances and methods that may alter the integrity and validity of urine samples. Examples of these include catheterization, urine substitution, and use of substances such as Probenecid or related compounds.[49] Like the NCAA, the USOC does allow the use of certain asthmatic medications.

Drug testing when coupled with adequate drug education serves to deter the use of drugs by athletes. Drug education by itself is seldom adequate. However, as we enter into a world of drug testing, observance of individual rights, reliability of results, and equitable implementation of sanctions must be given the highest priority.

TABLE 4–3. Duration of Drug Urinary Excretion

Drug	Approximate Elimination Time
Stimulants	
amphetamines and derivatives	1–7 days
Cocaine	
Occasional use	6–12 hours
Repeated use, within 48 hours (Caution! possibly longer)	3–5 days
Codeine and narcotics in cough medicines	24–48 hours
Tranquilizers	4–8 days
Marijuana (tetrahydrocannabinol)	3–5 weeks
Anabolic steroids	
Fat, soluble injectable types	6–8 months
Oral or water-soluble types	3–6 weeks
Over-the-counter cold medications containing ephedrine derivatives as decongestants	48–72 hours

Source: Reprinted with permission of the U.S. Olympic Committee from USOC Drug Education Program—Questions and Answers, 1988 handbook, p 9.

TABLE 4–4. NCAA-Banned Drug Classes, 1988–89

Psychomotor and Central Nervous System Stimulants

Amiphenazole	Meclofenoxate
Amphetamine	Methamphetamine
Bemigride	Methylphenidate
Benzphetamine	Nikethamide
Caffeine[1]	Norpseudoephedrine
Chlorphentermine	Pemoline
Cocaine	Pentetrazol
Cropropamide	Phendimetrazine
Crothetamide	Phenmetrazine
Diethylpropion	Phentermine
Dimethylamphetamine	Picrotoxine
Doxapram	Pipradol
Ethamivan	Prolintane
Ethylamphetamine	Strychnine
Fencamfamine	AND RELATED COMPOUNDS

Sympathomimetic Amines[2]

Clorprenaline	Methoxyphenamine
Ephedrine	Methylephedrine
Etafedrine	Phenylpropanolamine
Isoetharine	Pseudoephedrine
Isoprenaline	AND RELATED COMPOUNDS

Anabolic Steroids

Boldenone	Nandrolone
Clostebol	Norethandrolone
Dehydrochlormethyl-testosterone	Oxandrolone
	Oxymesterone
Fluoxymesterone	Oxymetholone
Mesterolone	Stanozolol
Methonolone	Testosterone[3]
Methandienone	AND RELATED COMPOUNDS

Substances Banned for Specific Sports

Rifle

Alcohol	Pindolol
Atenolol	Propranolol
Metoprolol	Timolol
Nadolol	AND RELATED COMPOUNDS

Diuretics

Acetazolamide	Hydroflumethiazide
Bendroflumethiazide	Methyclothiazide
Benzthiazide	Metolazone
Bumetanide	Polythiazide
Chlorothiazide	Quinethazone
Chlorthalidone	Spironolactone
Ethacrynic acid	Triamterene
Flumethiazide	Trichlormethiazide
Furosemide	AND RELATED COMPOUNDS
Hydrochlorothiazide	

Street Drugs

Heroin	THC (tetrahydrocannabinol)[4]
Marijuana[4]	

Definition of *positive* depends on the following:

[1] For caffeine—if the concentration in urine exceeds 15 mcg/ml.

[2] Refer to Section no. 3.5 of the drug testing protocol or Executive Regulation 1–7–(c)–(5).

[3] For testosterone—if the ratio of the total concentration of testosterone to that of epitestosterone in the urine exceeds 6.

[4] For Marijuana and THC—if the concentration in the urine of THC metabolite exceeds 25 ngm/ml.

Source: Reprinted with permission of the National Collegiate Athletic Association from the 1988–89 NCAA Drug-Testing Program, pp 8–9.

CONCLUSION

Growth hormone and anabolic steroids may significantly increase the size and strength of their user. These positive effects, however, are just one of their many side effects. Just as real are the various adverse effects that these drugs have on the athlete. As stimulants, cocaine, crack, amphetamines, phenylpropanolamine, and caffeine may all have an ergogenic effect for the athlete. For this reason, all are banned by the NCAA and the USOC, including caffeine in higher dosages. Similarly banned are the use of beta blockers and blood doping. Effective testing techniques for growth hormone and blood doping do not exist at this point.

While athletes are just as susceptible to drug abuse with recreational drugs as are nonathletes, they are certainly more likely to abuse ergogenic aids. School-age athletes, often infused with a sense of invulnerability and immortality, may be particularly susceptible to the lure of these drugs. Drug education combined with aggressive drug testing appears to be an effective means to control the use of drugs and illegal ergogenic aids by the athlete. Only by maintaining high standards of education and testing can we hope to be successful in significantly curtailing the abuse of these substances by athletes.

References

1. A Round Table: Drug testing in sports. Physician Sportsmed 12:69–82, 1985.
2. Alen M., Rahkila P., Reinila M., et al; Androgenic-anabolic steroid effects on serum thyroid, pituitary, and steroid hormones in athletes. Am J Sports Med 15:357–361, 1987.
3. American College of Sports Medicine: Position and stand on blood doping as an ergogenic aid. Med Sci Sports 19(5):540–543, 1987.
4. American College of Sports Medicine: Position statement on the use of alcohol in sports. Med Sci Sports 14:ix–xi, 1982.
5. Ando K., Johanson C.: Sensitivity changes to dopaminergic agents in fine motor control of rhesus monkeys after repeated methamphetamine administration. Pharmacol Biochem Behav 22:737–743, 1985.
6. Ariel G., Saville W : Anabolic steroids: The physiological effects of placebos. Med Sci Sports 4:124–126, 1972.
7. Berglund B.: Development of techniques for the detection of blood doping in sports. Sports Med 5:127–135, 1988.
8. Bergman R. T.: Substance abuse in the very young athlete. Sports Med Dig 7(3):1–3, 1985.
9. Biosynthetic growth hormone. Med Lett Drugs Ther 27:101–104, 1985.
10. Buckley W., Yesalis C., Friedl K., et al: Estimated prevalence of anabolic steroid use among male high school seniors. JAMA 260:3441–3445, 1988.
11. Cantwill J. D., Rose F. D.: Cocaine and cardiovascular events. Physician Sportsmed 11: 77–82, 1986.
12. Costill D. L., Dalsky G. P., Fink W. J.: Effects of caffeine ingestion on metabolism and exercise performance. Med Sci Sports 10(3) 155–158, 1978.
13. Cowart V. S.: Human growth hormone: The latest ergogenic aid? Physician Sportsmed 3:175–185, 1988.
14. Crack. Med Lett Drugs Ther 28:69–72, 1986.
15. Eichner E. R.: The caffeine controversy: Effects on endurance and cholesterol. Physician Sportsmed 12:124–130, 1986.
16. Frankle M. A., Cicero G. J., Payne J.: Use of androgenic anabolic steroids by athletes. JAMA 252:482, 1984.
17. Frankle M. A., Eichberg R., Zachariah S. B.: Anabolic androgenic steroids and a stroke in an athlete: Case report. Arch Phys Med Rehabil 69:632–633, 1988.
18. Gledhill N.: Blood doping and related issues: A brief review. Med Sci Sports Exerc 14:183–189, 1982.
19. Goodman L. S., Gilman A.: The Pharmacologic Basis of Therapeutics, Fifth Edition. New York, Macmillan Publishing Co, pp 306–309, 1975.
20. Goodman L. S., Gilman A.: The Pharmacologic Basis of Therapeutics, Fifth Edition. New York, Macmillan Publishing Co, pp 367–378, 1975.
21. Goodman L. S., Gilman A.: The Pharmacologic Basis of Therapeutics, Fifth Edition. New York, Macmillan Publishing Co, pp 481, 505, 1975.
22. Goodman L. S., Gilman A.: The Pharmacologic Basis of Therapeutics, Fifth Edition. New York, Macmillan Publishing Co, pp 496–500, 1975.
23. Goodman L. S., Gilman A.: The Pharmacologic Basis of Therapeutics, Fifth Edition. New York, Macmillan Publishing Co, pp 547–552, 1975.
24. Goodman L. S., Gilman A.: The Pharmacologic Basis of Therapeutics, Fifth Edition. New York, Macmillan Publishing Co, pp 1376–1382, 1975.
25. Haupt H. A., Rovere G. D.: Anabolic steroids: A review of the literature. Am J Sports Med 12: 469–484, 1984.
26. Holma P. K.: Effects of an anabolic steroid (metandienone) on spermatogenesis. Contraception 15:151–162, 1977.
27. Hurley B. F., Seals D. R., Hagberg J. M., et al: High-density-lipoprotein cholesterol in bodybuilders vs powerlifters: Negative effects of androgen use. JAMA 252:507–513, 1982.
28. Ipratropium: Med Lett Drugs Ther 29:71–74, 1987.
29. Ivy J. L.: Amphetamines in sports: Are they worth the risk? Sports Med Dig 6(3):1–3, 1984.
30. Ivy J. L., Costill D. L., Fink W. J., et al: Influence of caffeine and carbohydrate feedings on endurance performance. Med Sci Sports 11:6–11, 1979.
31. Klein H. G.: Blood transfusions and athletics—games people play. New Engl J Med 312–854–856, 1985.
32. Kochakian C. D. (ed): Anabolic-Androgenic Steroids. Handbook of Experimental Pharmacology, New Series. Berlin, Springer-Verlag, 43:37–39, 49–52, 58–63, 67, 366–367, 388–401, 1976.
33. Lamb D. R.: Anabolic steroids in athletics: How

well do they work and how dangerous are they? Am J Sports Med 12:31–38, 1984.
34. Lemon P., Chaney M.: Physiologic effects of amino acid supplementation, in Garrett W. E. Jr., Malone T. R. (eds): Muscle Development: Nutritional Alternatives to Anabolic Steroids, Report of the Ross Symposium. Columbus, Ohio, Ross Laboratories, 1988 pp 62–65.
35. Lombardo J. A.: Stimulants and athletic performance (Part 1 of 2): Amphetamines and caffeine. Physician Sportsmed 11:128–142, 1986.
36. Lombardo J. A.: Stimulants and athletic performance (Part 2): Cocaine and nicotine. Physician Sportsmed 12:85–89, 1986.
37. Macintyre J. G.: Growth hormone and athletes. Sports Med 4:129–142, 1987.
38. Mochizuki R. M., Richter K. J.: Cardiomyopathy and cerebrovascular accident associated with anabolic-androgenic steroid use. Physician Sportsmed 16:108–114, 1988.
39. National Collegiate Athletic Association. The 1988–89 NCAA Drug-TEsting Program. Sept 1988.
40. Overly W. L., Dankoff J. A., Wang B. K., et al: Androgens and hepatocellular carcinoma in an athlete [editorial]. Ann Intern Med 100:158, 1984.
41. Phenylpropanolamine for weight reduction. Med Lett Drugs Ther 26:55–58, 1984.
42. Pope H. G. Jr., Katz D. L.: Bodybuilder's psychosis. Lancet 1:863, 1987.
43. Pope H. G. Jr., Katz D. L.: Affective and psychotic symptoms associatd with anabolic steroid use. Am J Psychiatry 145:487–490, 1988.
44. Problems with growth hormone. Med Lett Drugs Ther 27:57–60, 1985.
45. Robbins S. L.: Pathologic basis of disease. Philadelphia, WB Saunders Co, pp 1364–1365, 1974.
46. Rovere G. D., Haupt H. A., Yates C. S.: Drug testing in a university athletic program: Protocol and implementation. Physician Sportsmed 14:69–76, 1986.
47. Slavin J. L., Joensen D. J.: Caffeine and sports performance. Physician Sportsmed 13:191–193, 1985.
48. Smith G. M., Beecher H. K.: Amphetamine sulfate and athletic performance. I. Objective effects. JAMA 170:542–557, 1959.
49. Sportsmediscope. Guide to banned medications. 7:1–5, 1988.
50. Strauss R. H., Liggett M. T., Lanese R. R.: Anabolic steroid use and perceived effects in ten weight trained women athletes. JAMA 253:2871–2874, 1985.
51. Tennant F. S. Jr.: Dealing with cocaine use by athletes. Sports Med Dig 6(11):1–3, 1984.
51. Tennant F. S. Jr., Black D. L., Voy R. O.: Anabolic steroid dependence with opioid type features. N Engl J Med, pp 578, Sept 1988.
52. Wilmore J.: Exercise testing, training, and beta-adrenergic blockade. Physician Sportsmed 12:45–52, 1988.

PHYSICAL MODALITIES IN REHABILITATION

ROBERT M. POOLE
B. CRAIG LEE
TURNER A. BLACKBURN, JR.

This chapter discusses the use of therapeutic modalities in the care of athletic injuries in school-age athletes. The purpose of modality use is to reduce the inflammatory response that follows injury. Pain, crepitation, loss of motion, muscle atrophy, and joint dysfunction are possible results of inflammation. Therapeutic modalities reduce these debilitating effects and therefore facilitate the athlete's return to his or her sport or activity.[20]

CRYOTHERAPY

The use of ice as a therapeutic modality is one of the oldest known forms of treatment. Hippocrates (400 B.C.) suggested that an application of cold be used for acute trauma to reduce swelling and pain.[55] Cold compresses, ice packs, ice towels, cooling sprays, and ice baths are some currently used agents of tissue temperature reduction. New techniques continue to be tested to obtain more effective management of athletic injuries.

Special thanks go to the following for providing information and tables for use in this book: Diana Gray, P.T., University of Chicago, 5841 South Maryland Avenue, Chicago, IL; Kurt Jepson, P.T., Saco Bay Orthopaedic & Sports Physical Therapy, P.A., Saco, ME, Table 5–5; David Walsh, P.T., A.T.C., Rehabilitation Services of Columbus, Inc., Columbus, GA, Table 5–4; and to Judy Koren for her research expertise and tireless assistance.

PHYSICAL PRINCIPLES

Conduction and *evaporation* are two methods used for therapeutic cooling. Conduction is the more common method, causing a loss of heat from the tissues through direct contact with a cold agent. The amount of temperature change is dependent on the following:

1. The difference in temperature between the cold agent and the tissue
2. Application time
3. Conductivity of the area being cooled
4. Type of cooling agent
5. Mode of application

The greater the difference between the tissue temperature and the cold agent, the greater the resulting tissue temperature change. Exposure time is also important. Changes in skin temperature occur within the first minutes of application; however, reduction of the temperature of subcutaneous tissues and muscle requires 20 to 30 minutes of exposure.[44]

Thermoconductivity is the measure of a tissue's efficiency of heat conduction. Tissues with a high water content have greater thermoconductivity. Adipose tissue acts as an insulator resisting heat flow; therefore, the amount of fat may influence the degree and rate of cooling of muscle tissue.[44]

The mode of application of cold may also influence the degree of cooling. A greater difference is expected when using ice packs as compared with cold water compresses or gel packs. The difference may be in the amount of internal heat energy required to melt the ice. Internal energy must be used to change the ice to water before raising its temperature.

Evaporation is a cooling method that transfers energy through the use of vapocoolant sprays. These sprays are volatile liquids that begin to evaporate on contact with the skin, thereby removing heat. The spray is applied in sweeps across the skin. A few seconds of application have been found to decrease skin temperature to about 15° C but bring about negligible changes in subcutaneous tissue or muscle temperature.[44]

PHYSIOLOGICAL EFFECTS

Cold is a particularly good form of treatment in acute trauma because of physiological effects that include the following:

1. Arteriolar vasoconstriction
2. Reduction of inflammation
3. Reduction of muscle spasms
4. Decrease in pain

When cold is applied to the skin immediately after injury, the first response is vasoconstriction of cutaneous blood vessels, resulting in reduced blood flow. In acute injuries, the restriction of blood flow to the area reduces swelling and extravasation of blood into the skin and surrounding tissues. This in turn reduces inflammation.[40, 55]

Application of cold during the initial 24 to 48 hours following injury has been shown to reduce cellular metabolism, effectively decreasing swelling and oxygen consumption of surrounding uninjured tissues. This may allow marginally viable cells to survive, thus reducing the amount of necrotic tissue that the body must repair or remove following injury.

Muscle spasm may also be relieved by an application of cold. It is believed that a decrease in muscle activity may be brought about by reduction of muscle spindle firing or by reflex response of sensory nerves overlying the muscles.[40]

Nerve conduction velocity of gamma motor neurons and sensory neurons has been seen to decrease with therapeutic application of cold.[20, 35] Kowal[35] proposed that pain fibers were inhibited by cold faster than other fiber types. Following acute trauma, cold can be seen to produce initial vasoconstriction, control edema, promote absorption of exudate, and prevent further bleeding and exudate formation. In these ways, cold can be seen to break up the vicious cycle of pain, metabolites, muscle spasm, and pain.[55]

INDICATIONS AND CONTRAINDICATIONS

Therapeutic applications of cold are indicated in the following acute and chronic sports medicine situations:

1. Sprains
2. Strains
3. Contusions
4. Fractures
5. Heat illness
6. Acute phase of inflammatory bursitis, tendinitis, and tenosynovitis.

Cold may also be helpful during the rehabilitation phase of injury by providing relief of muscle spasm and pain, thus allowing therapeutic exercise to begin earlier.[40]

Most athletes are otherwise healthy individuals. The problems of swelling due to cardiac disease or renal and pulmonary disorders can usually be discounted. However, these, along with Raynaud's phenomenon, cold hypersensitivity, or compromised local circulation, should be kept in mind when treating athletic injuries. Another precaution for therapeutic cold application is use of cold directly over a superficial motor nerve, such as the peroneal nerve. Cryotherapy should not be continuously applied to skin for more than 30 minutes. Frostbite does not occur from a short-term application of cold directly to the skin; however, several cases of cold skin "burn" have been reported when using gel packs cooled below 32° F for more than 20 minutes.

Athletes should be advised against returning to participation following a 20-minute application of ice. Ice may compromise the protective pain mechanism, precipitating further injury.

APPLICATION TECHNIQUES

Ice Packs

The most inexpensive, efficient, and convenient method of therapeutic cold application is the placement of a plastic bag or towel filled with chipped, flaked, cubed, or crushed ice directly on the skin. The size of the pack can be varied according to the area treated. Treatment time varies, but 15 to 30 minutes should be sufficient to lower tissue temperatures to desired levels.[55] (See Figure 5–1 and Tables 5–1, 5–2, and 5–3.)

Gel Packs

Commercially available gel packs usually consist of a silica gel mixture in a heavy vinyl case. These are stored in a special refrigeration unit in most training rooms or clinic settings but can be kept in the freezer at home. Gel packs can be used repeatedly. They are applied over a wet towel for about 20 minutes. Some reports of cold injury have been made when gel packs were applied directly to the skin for more than 20 minutes (Fig. 5–2; refer to Tables 5–1 and 5–2).

Ice Towels

A terry cloth towel is placed in a bucket of crushed ice and water. When removed, ice particles stick to the towel. The towel can be wrapped over the area to be treated but must be changed often (every 4 to 5 minutes), since it warms rapidly.

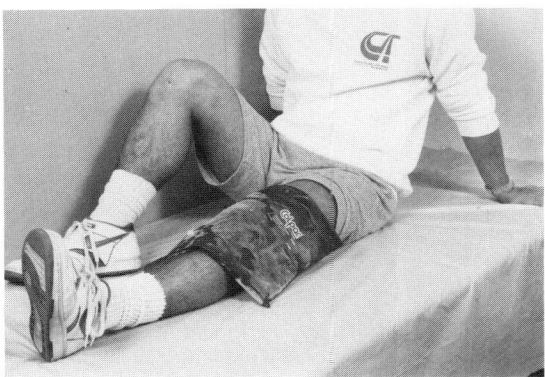

FIGURE 5–2. Application of commercially available gel-type cold pack. Gel packs are reusable many times.

Ice Massage

Massage of the affected area with ice in a styrofoam cup or frozen on a stick is an effective method of cold application. Water is frozen in a styrofoam cup, and the sides of the cup are peeled away to make a holder for the ice. A wooden tongue depressor may also be frozen in the cup with the water, making an ice pop. The affected area is massaged in small overlapping circles for a period of 10 to 15 minutes. The athlete may feel cold burning, aching, and then analgesia. The first stages pass rapidly. Skin temperature does not usually drop below 14° C; therefore, risk of tissue damage is minimal. This easy method may be taught to reliable patients for continued use at home (Fig. 5–3 and Table 5–4).

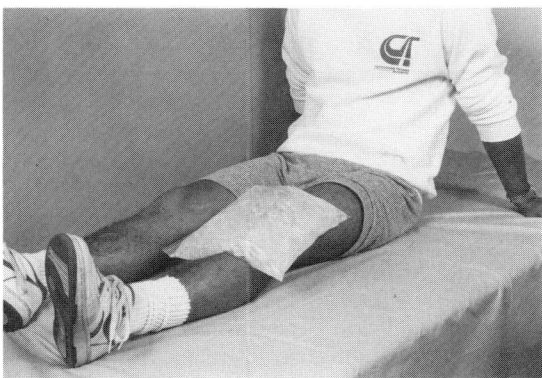

FIGURE 5–1. Ice pack applied to swollen left knee.

Economical, Reusable Ice Pack:

Fill a self-sealing plastic bag with ice, water, and isopropyl alcohol in a 2 : 1 : 1 ratio. This bag may be kept in a freezer. It will not freeze solid and may be used many times.

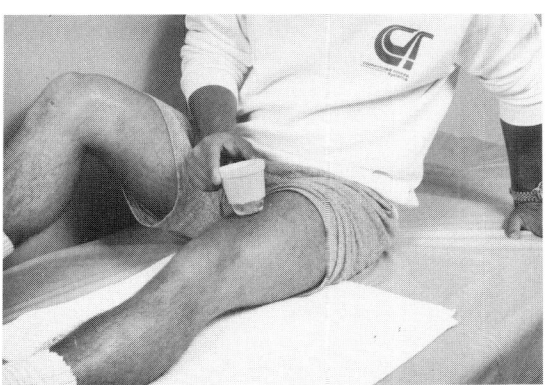

FIGURE 5–3. An ice pop is used to massage a contused left thigh.

TABLE 5–1. Physical Modalities in the Treatment of Hamstring Strains (Grade II or III)
by Turner A. Blackburn, Jr.

Acute, Day 1–3	Cryotherapy:	Ice packs, gel packs, 20–30 minutes, several times a day
	Compression:	½ inch foam or felt over injury with compression bandage
	Gait:	Assistive device if gait is with limp
	Modalities:	High-volt or MENS and/or phonophoresis at 1.5 watts/cm² × 10 minutes continuous output
Late Acute, Day 3–5	[Active bleeding stopped (3–5 days)]	
	Gait:	Progressive walking to tolerance Discontinue assistive device
	Modalities:	Contrast treatments, 15 minutes heat/15 minutes cold Electric stimulation, 15–18 milliamps × 15 minutes
	Exercise:	Active hamstring stretch, supine Gravity-assisted strengthening Biking Ice-walk—ice, 15 minutes; walk until anesthesia goes away; repeat × 3 Light massage Compression dressing
Subacute, 1 Week Postinjury	Gait:	Progressing walk to run as tolerated
	Modalities:	Moist heat Ultrasound and/or phonophoresis, 1.5 W/cm² × 10 minutes, continuous output Electric stimulation, 15–20 milliamps × 15 minutes
	Exercise:	Hamstring curls; sissy squats Hamstring stretch; step-ups (passive) Massage Compression dressing
Return to Activity, 4–6 Weeks	Criteria for return:	Full range of motion for involved joints Full flexibility Normal hamstring stretch Run/cut/accelerate to normal Progressive running—jog to sprint to agilities Progressive strengthening and flexibility Heavier weight training Compression support

MENS = Microcurrent electrical neuromuscular stimulation

Ice Immersion

An ice bucket containing a combination of crushed ice and water (mostly ice) is one of the more uncomfortable methods of cryotherapy. This technique ensures circumferential contact of the extremity with the cooling agent. Temperatures vary from about 13° to 18° C, with treatment times of 5 to 15 minutes. Once analgesia is obtained, range of motion is possible with decreased pain. This method is particularly suitable for feet, ankles, hands, wrists, arms, and elbows (Fig. 5–4). Cold whirlpools may be used for immersion of larger body parts.

Cold Compression Units

A commercially available cold compression unit, such as the Jobst Corporation's Cryotemp (Jobst Institute, Inc., Toledo, OH), can be adjusted and maintained at selected temperatures, usually 10° to 25° C. Cooled water is circulated through a sleeve applied over the elevated extremity. Intermittent pressure and cold provide a pumping action to reduce edema from the extremity (Figs. 5–5 and 5–6; Tables 5–2 and 5–3).

Vapocoolant Sprays

Fluoromethane spray has been used in sports for many years to reduce muscle spasm and swelling in acute injuries.[32] The affected area is sprayed unidirectionally from a distance of about 2 feet. The area is covered twice. Caution should be taken since repeated applications can lower skin temperature to 4° C, causing skin tissue damage.

TABLE 5–2. The Use of Modalities in Rehabilitation Following Arthroscopic Meniscectomy

by Turner A. Blackburn, Jr.

POD 1–2	Compression dressing
	Immobilizer (optional)
	Crutches PWB to tolerance
	TENS unit for pain
	Cryotherapy: ice packs, gel packs, or cold compression unit, 20–30 minutes, several times a day
	Exercises:
	    Quad sets
	    Hamstring stretches
	    Ankle pumps
	    Terminal knee extensions
	    Straight leg raises with terminal knee extensions
	    Active/active-assisted range of motion

POD 3	Dressing change: light compression wrap, Band-Aids over portals
	Progress toward full-weight bearing
	TENS discontinued
	Cryotherapy: ice packs, gel packs, or cold compression unit, 20–30 minutes, several times a day
	Electric stimulation for quad reeducation at 15–20 milliamps × 15 minutes, 5 to 7 days
	Continue above exercises with the addition of the following:
	    Hip flexion
	    Hamstring curls
	    Hip abduction
	    Biking, when range of motion permits

POD 10	Light compression dressing, as needed
	Walking program up to 2 miles
	Cryotherapy as necessary after exercise, 20 minutes
	Continue exercise program
	Functional activities:
	    Step-ups
	    Sissy squats
	    Swimming

POD 21–28	Criteria for return:
	    Full range of motion
	    Full flexibility
	    Run/cut/accelerate to normal
	    Progressive running: jog to sprint to agilities
	    Progressive strengthening and flexibility
	    Heavier weight training
	    Cryotherapy when necessary after activity

POD = Postoperative day
PWB = Progressive weight bearing
TENS = Transcutaneous nerve stimulation

Spray may be combined with gentle stretching to relieve painful muscle spasms (Fig. 5–7).

SUMMARY

The use of cold in treating acute athletic injuries is simple, inexpensive, and effective. It is beneficial in reducing blood flow in tissue metabolism and therefore reduces swelling and acute inflammation. Muscle spasms and pain are also decreased, allowing earlier range of motion and exercise to begin more comfortably.

THERMOTHERAPY

Thermotherapy, or the application of heat, has been used for several centuries as an analgesic, antispasmodic, and sedative. Primitive societies discovered that heat not only afforded analgesic effects but possessed healing qualities as well.[32] In modern society, heating agents are used to relieve pain, to

TABLE 5–3. The Use of Modalities in the Treatment of Acute Ankle Sprains (Grade I and II)
by R. M. Poole

Acute, Day 1–3	Tubular compression stocking applied to extremity from toes to just above the knee
	Cryotemp (Jobst Institute, Inc., Toledo, OH) × 20 minutes at 80 psi and 40° F, with elevation of the limb during treatment
	Remove extremity from Cryotemp sleeve
	Apply ½ inch felt horseshoe around malleoli bilaterally
	Place ankle in an open basketweave, taping over the felt horseshoes using 1½ inch white athletic tape
	Tubular compression stocking is reapplied to the extremity to cover an area from the toes to just below the knee; the athlete is allowed to weight-bear with crutches as tolerated
	Exercise program includes:
	Ankle pumps and elevation
	Isometrics for anterior tibialis, posterior tibialis, and peroneals, 20 repetitions every hour during the day
	Ice packs and elevation continued at home, 20 minutes, every other hour
Subacute, Day 4–6	Warm whirlpool (97° F) × 15 minutes with active range of motion
	Active exercises to follow whirlpool:
	Continue exercise program above and add the following exercises:
	Heel cord stretching using a heel cord box
	Heel raises
	Toe raises
	Strengthening (progressive resistive exercises) for anterior tibialis, posterior tibialis, and peroneals, 5 sets of 10 repetitions, with 1–5 pounds
	Proprioceptive exercises using balance board
	Cryotemp and tape after exercise as above
	Progress to gait without crutches, walking as tolerated
	Progress to straight-line jogging
	Progress to specific sport activities
	Running, cutting, and agility drills
	Ice after exercise × 20 minutes, as needed for swelling
Day 7 Onward	Progressive weight training
	Progressive running; progress to 2 miles jogging
	Progressive activities—sprints, then cutting activities
	Sport-specific activity
	Return to sport
	Cryotherapy when necessary after activity, 20 minutes

increase blood flow, to facilitate tissue healing, and to get stiff joints and tight muscles ready for exercise.[38, 44] Consequently, thermotherapy is one of the most common modalities in the treatment of athletic injuries. The most frequently used agents in tissue heating include superficial, deep, wet, dry, and chemical agents.

PHYSICAL PRINCIPLES

The transmission of heat energy is provided through either conduction, convection, radiation, or conversion. Superficial heat is conveyed through conduction, convection, or radiation, and deep heat is conveyed through conversion.[41] *Conduction* occurs when heat is transferred from a warm object to a cooler one by direct contact, as in the application of moist hot packs, electric heating pads, or paraffin baths. The use of these types of superficial heat can affect skin temperature directly and muscle temperature indirectly through reflex circulation increases and conduction. *Convection* refers to the transference of heat through the movement of fluids or gases, as in the whirlpool bath. *Radiation* is the process whereby heat energy is transmitted through empty space by electromagnetic waves, as in infrared or ultraviolet light.

Conversion refers to the generation of heat from another source such as sound, electrical

TABLE 5–4. Treatment of Acromioclavicular Sprains and Shoulder Pointers
by David Walsh

When an athlete sustains a grade I acromioclavicular (A-C) separation in which stability is not compromised and excessive motion is not evident, the most limiting factor is pain. By using ice immediately and following with iontophoresis, the healing process is aided and pain is decreased. Early motion may then be started.

Acute Phase: Ice with compression for approximately 15 minutes. After the area has warmed from the ice, follow with iontophoresis with Marcaine and Decadron directly over the area of pain. Treatment time is 20 minutes.

24–36 Hours: Treatment same as above. Start range of motion within pain-free limits: abduction, flexion, and horizontal abduction/adduction not over 90 degrees. Avoid shoulder shrugs, as this may irritate the area treated. Ice massage with ice pop after exercise for 15 minutes.

48–72 Hours: If no swelling is present and pain has not increased, use ice and iontophoresis, then follow with pulsed ultrasound at 1.0 W/cm^2 to drive the medication further into the joint. Try to increase active range of motion within pain-free limits. Ice massage with ice pop after exercise for 15 minutes.

Since iontophoresis is used to decrease pain, the athlete should refrain from contact drills until dissipation of the anesthetic properties in order to prevent further injury.

agents, or chemical agents.[32] In ultrasound, the mechanical energy produced by high-frequency sound waves changes to heat energy at tissue interfaces. Chemical agents in the form of liniments and balms create counterirritation of sensory nerve endings,

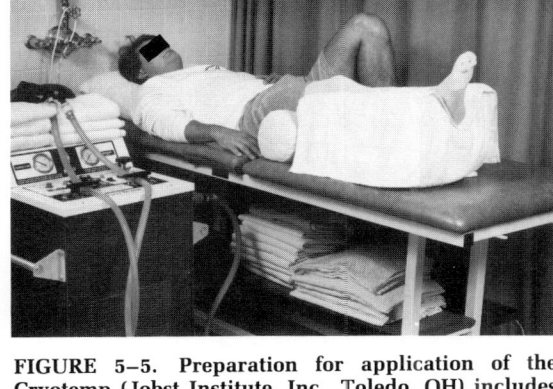

FIGURE 5–5. Preparation for application of the Cryotemp (Jobst Institute, Inc., Toledo, OH) includes elevation of the limb and application of compression stocking.

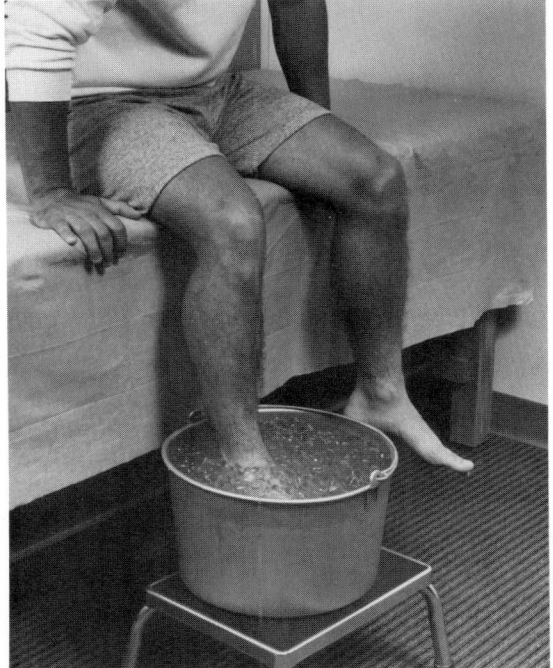

FIGURE 5–4. Ice immersion. Immersion of a swollen ankle in a bucket of ice and water.

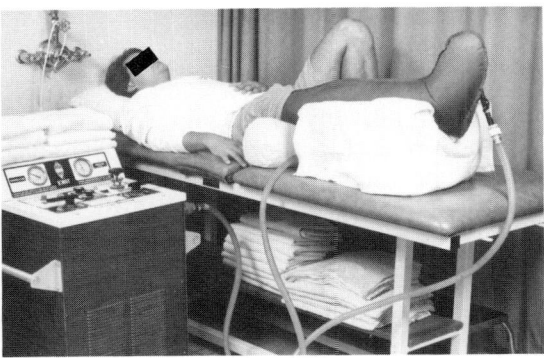

FIGURE 5–6. Cryotemp sleeve in place, showing compression and cold applied to lower extremity.

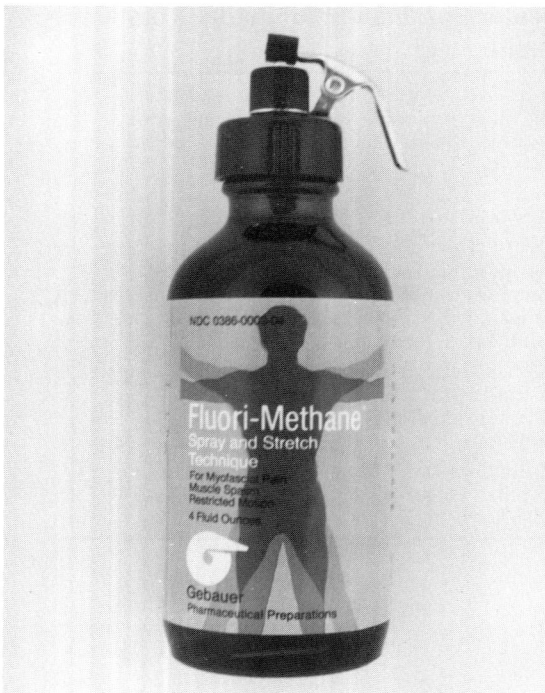

FIGURE 5–7. Commercially available Fluori-Methane spray for quick surface cooling.

producing an increase in tissue temperature by increasing capillary blood flow.

PHYSIOLOGICAL EFFECTS

Many physiological effects can occur as a result of the body's response to an increase in tissue temperature. The extent and significance of these physiological changes depend on a number of factors:[44]

1. Type of heat energy applied
2. Intensity of heat energy
3. Duration of application
4. Unique tissue response to heat

In order for a physiological response to occur, heat must be absorbed into the tissues, causing an increase in molecular activity.[32] The temperature of the tissue must be elevated to between 40° and 45° C in order to meet therapeutic levels of heating.[38, 57]

When considering a heat agent for therapeutic intervention, it is important to understand the metabolic, vascular, neuromuscular, and connective tissue effects of temperature elevation. Chemical activity in cells and metabolic rate increase two- to threefold for each 10° C that the temperature rises.[18, 26] If the temperature rises past 45° C, the tissues burn because the metabolic activity required to repair tissue is not capable of keeping up with thermally induced protein denaturation. Chemical reaction rate increases can cause an increase in oxygen uptake by tissues, resulting in the availability of more nutrients for tissue healing.[2]

An increase in tissue temperature is associated with vasodilation and an increase in blood flow to the tissues.[26, 57] Heat is often used as a modality prior to exercise to enhance the effects of the vasodilation. Greenberg[22] compared hot packs alone, exercise alone, and hot packs plus exercise. He reported that the increase in blood flow from exercise was greater than that from heat alone. The vasodilation effects of the combined use of hot packs and exercise were additive and greater than with either modality used alone.

Thermotherapy is used to assist in the resolution of muscle spasms and to provide analgesia. Although the mechanism of action for these neuromuscular effects is not totally understood, the underlying basis for their use may be related to the ability of heat to elevate the pain threshold,[37] alter nerve conduction velocity,[3] and change muscle spindle firing rates.[43] Temperature elevation in skeletal muscle can also change temporarily the ability to build tension and sustain prolonged activity.[11, 15] The heating of connective tissues in combination with a stretch can alter the viscoelastic properties of the connective tissues.[36] The viscous properties permit a residual elongation of the connective tissue after the stretch is applied, and the elastic properties are responsible for the tissue's recoverable deformation.[53]

INDICATIONS AND CONTRAINDICATIONS

Therapeutic applications of heat or thermotherapy are indicated in the following sports medicine situations:

1. Musculoskeletal pain
2. Muscle spasm
3. Joint stiffness
4. After acute phase:
    a. Contusions
    b. Strains

c. Bursitis
   d. Tendinitis
   e. Tenosynovitis
   f. Capsulitis

Contraindications for clinical use of superficial heat modalities include the following:

1. Loss of sensation
2. Immediately following injury (first 48 to 72 hours)
3. Decreased arterial circulation
4. Directly over eyes or genitals
5. Over abdomen during pregnancy

APPLICATION TECHNIQUES

Moist Hot Pack

Commercial moist hot packs or hydrocollator packs heat by conduction and should remain immersed in thermostatically controlled hot water at a temperature of 71° to 79° C until time to be used. Cover the pack with six layers of dry towels or commercial cover. Treat the area for 15 to 20 minutes and remove the layers of towels as the pack cools (Figs. 5–8 and 5–9).

Whirlpool

The whirlpool provides both conduction and convection heating of tissues. Set the water temperature according to injury: 33° to 35° C, neutral; 35° to 37° C, warm; 37° to 45° C, hot. Increase the temperature and the duration of treatment (5 to 20 minutes) according to the healing phase. The use of water as a treatment agent is discussed later in the chapter.

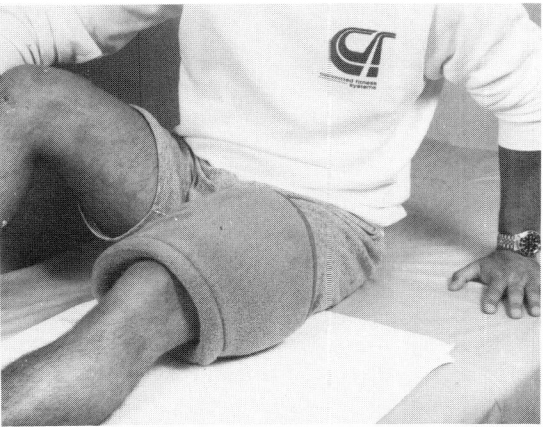

FIGURE 5–9. Application of moist hot pack to a subacute thigh contusion.

Ultrasound

Ultrasound may be considered a deep heating modality. It is covered in detail later in the chapter.

SUMMARY

The use of deep heat is an important portion of the therapeutic program in treating athletic injuries. The beneficial effects of temperature elevation include elevation of pain threshold, decrease in muscle spasm, decrease in joint stiffness, increase in blood flow, and increase in collagen tissue extensibility.

HYDROTHERAPY

Hydrotherapy, or water therapy, is one of the oldest therapeutic methods for managing athletic injuries.[29] The therapeutic use of water at various temperatures has been advocated for the treatment of joint stiffness, painful scars, adhesions, and arthritis, and as a warm-up to assist with exercises.[59] Hydrotherapy is mainly used for its effects in heating,[6] cooling, debridement,[1, 34] pain relief, and relaxation of muscles. The most commonly used forms of hydrotherapy include leg and arm whirlpool (extremity tank), low boy, hubbard tank, and therapeutic pool.[44]

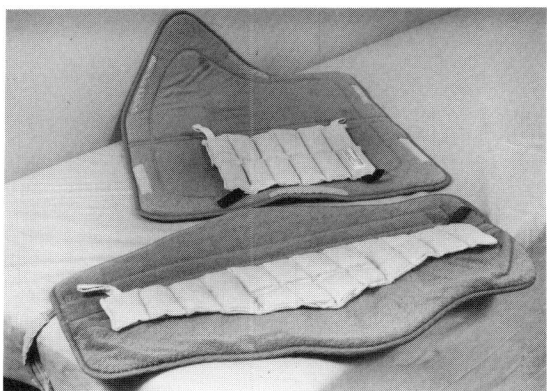

FIGURE 5–8. Two types of moist hot packs available for use in the clinic with appropriately sized covers.

PHYSICAL PROPERTIES

Whirlpools provide the most effective means of applying circumferential heat or cold while stimulating movement of the affected part. The combination of temperature, agitation, and water's buoyant properties provides pain relief and muscle relaxation and enables active assistive movement. The cleansing ability of the water is especially important after cast removal or for the treatment of abrasions, blisters, and other associated skin lesions.[41]

Hydrotherapy is performed in water tanks of various sizes and shapes. Whirlpools are tanks used for partial body immersion; hubbard tanks or low boys are tanks used for full body immersion. Heat or cold is exchanged between the tissues and the water by two methods: conduction and convection.[44]

PHYSIOLOGICAL EFFECTS

One of the main reasons for using hydrotherapy is to gain the therapeutic value of heat or cold. The physiological effects are the same as for other thermal agents, except a larger body surface area is immersed in water. Consequently, exposure of the body to varying temperatures will have not only a local effect but also systemic effects on the cardiovascular and other organ systems.[44]

Water temperature must vary according to each patient's tolerance and specific injury. For the treatment of acute injuries, 55° to 65° F (13° to 18° C) water temperature is used for 10 minutes. For chronic injuries, 100° to 110° F (38° to 43° C) water is employed for 20 minutes. At temperatures above 116.7° F (47° C), most individuals experience a burning sensation. When total body immersion is used, significantly less surface area for evaporative cooling is available; therefore, water temperatures must be lowered 5° to 10° F. As the water temperature increases above 110° F (43° C), the body temperature increases 1° or 2° F.[41] The selection of temperature must be influenced by the indication for treatment, duration since injury, and the inflammatory reaction state.[52]

Physiologically, the whirlpool acts as an analgesic agent, relaxing muscle spasm, relieving joint pain, improving mechanical debridement,[47] and facilitating exercise.[48] Whirlpool agitation provides mechanical stimulation to skin receptors, which may explain its pain-relieving effects. The agitation may also act as a stimulus to large sensory afferent nerve fibers, closing the gate to pain.[44]

INDICATIONS AND CONTRAINDICATIONS

Hydrotherapy is extremely useful in treating chronic traumatic injuries, inflammatory conditions, stiffness, pain, adhesions, arthritis, tenosynovitis, open wounds, sprains, and strains and permits early facilitation of active assistive or active movement.

In addition to contraindications similar to those for respective superficial heat or cold, (1) complete immersion bath should be avoided for cardiac patients, (2) extremes in temperatures should be avoided for patients with peripheral vascular disease of the lower extremities, and (3) whirlpools are relatively contraindicated for patients with multiple sclerosis. Warm whirlpools after exercise, especially in hot environments, should be avoided unless the body is allowed to cool down; 20 to 30 minutes of rest should precede any generalized superficial heat application following strenuous activity. Dehydration after exercise and vasodilation from whirlpools may cause fainting.

APPLICATION TECHNIQUES

Whirlpool (Refer to Table 5–3)

1. Select the proper whirlpool size.
2. Select the proper water temperature

Acute (0 to 48 hours) = Cold 55° to 65° F (12.8° to 18.3° C)

Subacute (48 to 72 hours) = Warm 93° to 98° F (33.9° to 36.7° C)

Chronic = Hot 98° to 104° F (36.5° to 40° C)

3. Properly position agitator so that the flow is not aimed directly at an acute lesion.
4. Treatment time is usually 20 to 30 minutes.

Contrast Bath

1. Limb is placed in hot water at 105° to 110° F (40.6° to 43° C) for 4 minutes,[32] followed by 2 minutes ice/water.
2. The athlete alternates 4 minutes hot water with 2 minutes cold water for a period

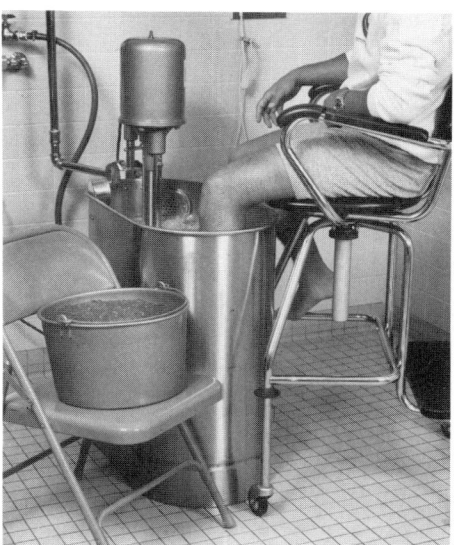

FIGURE 5–10. An extremity tank is used for active range-of-motion activities prior to ice immersion, as in contrast baths.

of 24 minutes, or four cycles (Figs. 5–10 and 5–11).

Therapeutic Pools

Therapeutic pools are standard swimming pools heated to approximately 95° F. The athlete can work through active range-of-motion and strengthening activities in the pool, surrounding the affected joints with warm wa-

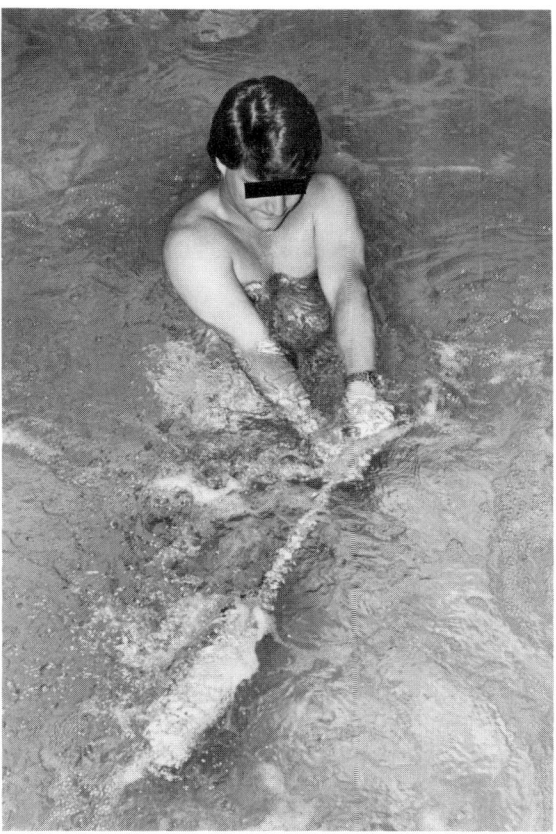

FIGURE 5–12. Active range-of-motion/strengthening activity in the therapeutic pool, using a baseball bat to simulate hitting.

ter. Working against the resistance of the water can also help to increase strength and endurance (Fig. 5–12). Flotation vests can be used to allow the injured athlete to continue training in the supportive aquatic environment (Fig. 5–13).

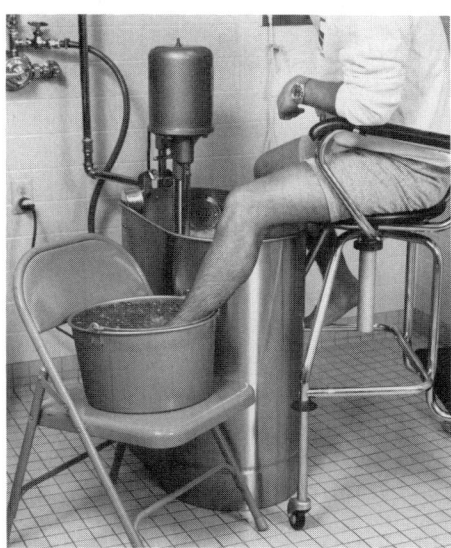

FIGURE 5–11. Ice immersion phase of contrast bath.

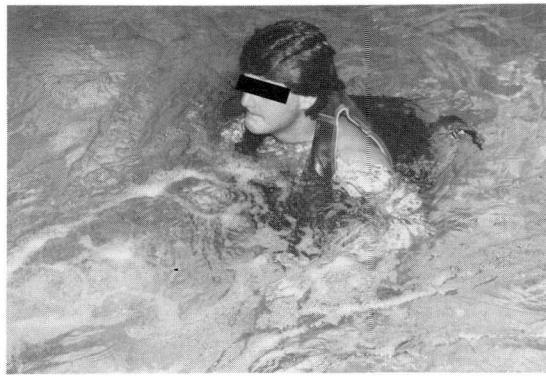

FIGURE 5–13. Active range-of-motion/strengthening activity in the therapeutic pool, using a flotation vest to assist in running exercise.

SUMMARY

A thorough knowledge and understanding of (1) the physical properties of water and the method of thermal energy transfer, (2) normal physiology, (3) indications and contraindications, and (4) appropriate application techniques are needed in order to determine the proper use of hydrotherapy for the treatment of athletic injuries.

ULTRASOUND

Ultrasound, in use for more than 40 years,[44] is a form of high-frequency sound energy that can produce changes in tissue temperature as deep as 5 centimeters. The therapeutic benefits of ultrasound include pain relief and reduction of muscle spasm.

PHYSICAL PRINCIPLES

The range of high-frequency sound beyond the normal human audible range of 20,000 hertz is known as ultrasound. Therapeutic ultrasound uses these high-frequency sound waves to produce mechanical and thermal effects in tissues. Clinical ultrasound has a frequency of 1,000,000 to 3,000,000 hertz, or 1 to 3 megahertz. The three parts of an ultrasound generator are: the power supply, normally 120 volts; an oscillating circuit, which applies power from the power supply to a crystal, producing sound energy; and a transducer, which transmits the sound energy through a metal diaphragm to the tissue surface to be treated.

When high-frequency alternating current is applied to a crystal, a mechanical distortion of the crystal is created, producing vibrations. The electromechanical distortion of the crystal structure is called the piezoelectric effect. This is the principle on which clinical ultrasound is based.[20]

PHYSIOLOGICAL EFFECTS

Applications of therapeutic ultrasound have been shown to produce thermal, mechanical, and chemical effects on human tissues.

The thermal effects of ultrasound have been demonstrated to warm tissue to a depth of 5 centimeters or greater.[23, 44] The acoustic transmission properties of skin, muscle, and fat are similar, although not identical; the percentages of sound that they attenuate are 39 percent, 24 percent, and 13 percent, respectively.[44] In these tissues, the thermal effects diminish with tissue depth. A 1.8° to 3.6° F temperature rise has been demonstrated in these tissue types to a depth of 5 cm.

The acoustic properties of muscle and bone are very different. At the muscle/bone interface, sound waves are reflected, and shear stress waves are produced, releasing greater heat energy.[55] Temperatures of 106.7° F have been recorded at the muscle/bone interface and 117.5° F at joint capsules.[23]

The mechanical effects of ultrasound include micromassage, the result of the alternating positive and negative pressures of the sound waves passing through the tissues at the ultrasound frequency. Some of the biological effects of micromassage include increase in tissue temperature, acceleration of diffusion across cell membranes, and increase in circulation.[55]

The chemical effects of ultrasound application on adenosine triphosphate (ATP) activity have been described as an increase in ATP in skeletal muscle with ultrasound, as well as increased cell membrane permeability and accelerated enzyme activity.[5]

INDICATIONS AND CONTRAINDICATIONS

Therapeutic ultrasound is generally used in the treatment of many types of sports-related problems such as sprains, muscular strains, tendinitis, bursitis, and tenosynovitis. It has also been indicated in the reduction of pain and muscle spasm, scar tissue, and joint contracture management and as a noninvasive technique to introduce medication through the skin (phonophoresis) (refer to Table 5–4).

Contraindications for clinical use of ultrasound in school-age athletes are few. Burns may occur if the transducer head is moved too slowly and/or if there is insufficient coupling agent on the skin. A burn may also occur if the intensity is too great or the ultrasound is applied directly over a bony prominence. Application directly over bone may cause local decalcification. Ultrasound should not be used in cases of circulatory problems such as thrombus or hemorrhage. It should not be used around the eyes or over a pregnant uterus, tumor, or the epiphyseal plates in young children.[44, 55]

APPLICATION TECHNIQUES

Unlike other forms of energy, ultrasound does not travel well through air. A coupling agent must be used to transmit ultrasound energy from the transducer to the tissue surface. There are several commercially available ultrasound gels that are very effective in providing transmission of sound waves. Other coupling agents that may be used are water, mineral oil, and glycerol. None of these are as effective as the gels, although they may have applications in special situations.

Two treatment methods are used in applying ultrasound: the stationary transducer and the moving transducer. With the stationary technique, lower intensities are necessary to prevent tissue damage, owing to uneven energy distribution. With the moving technique, the transducer is slowly moved over the tissue surface using firm, overlapping, longitudinal or circular strokes. This distributes the energy as evenly as possible throughout an area that is usually two to three times as large as the transducer head (Fig. 5–14).

The intensity of the ultrasound is recorded in watts per square centimeter (W/cm^2). Intensities of 0.5 to 2.0 W/cm^2 may be considered the effective range of therapeutic ultrasound.

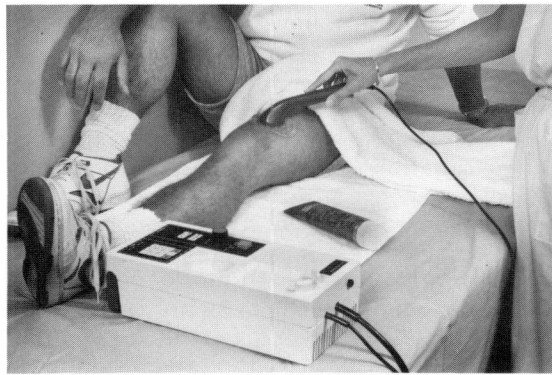

FIGURE 5–14. Ultrasound treatment to the left thigh in a subacute thigh contusion (Mettler Ultrasound Unit, Mettler Corporation, Anaheim, CA).

There are two modes available with modern clinical ultrasound. These are continuous output and pulsed output. Continuous output ultrasound is a constant output of energy during treatment. With pulsed output, the energy is delivered in periodic bursts, with the power on for a fixed duration and off for a fixed duration. On and off times are measured in milliseconds. Since the efficacy of pulsed ultrasound is still undergoing clinical debate, the continuous ultrasound mode is the recommended choice for athletic applications.[44]

Ultrasound can be applied using an underwater technique. For this application, the affected part is placed in a basin or bucket of water. The transducer is submerged and held approximately 10 to 30 millimeters from the surface to be treated and parallel to that surface. Care should be taken to be sure that there are no air bubbles on the patient's skin or the transducer head during treatment. Treatment time is approximately 10 minutes at 1.5 W/cm^2 if tissue temperature rise is needed. The sound head may be moved during treatment or left stationary. This is an especially effective technique with the extremities.

If an irregular surface such as a bony prominence is to be treated, a rubber balloon may be filled with water and used as a coupling agent. A layer of coupling gel is used between the balloon and the skin, and between the transducer and the balloon. The balloon can also be attached to the transducer head and the sound energy delivered through the water and into the irregular area of skin.

Phonophoresis, as previously mentioned, is the delivery of medication through the skin into the tissues. This technique is used in inflammatory processes where an antiinflammatory agent is driven into the area to help decrease inflammatory response.

In 1967, Griffin et al.[24] treated 66 patients with clinical diagnoses of bicipital tendinitis, knee and shoulder osteoarthritis, shoulder bursitis, and bicipital tendinitis with ultrasound and hydrocortisone. Of these patients, 68 percent were able to demonstrate pain-free, normal functional range of motion after treatment. Of the 36 patients treated with ultrasound and a placebo, only 45 percent were improved in range of motion or pain after treatment.

When hydrocortisone cream is used, it is rubbed into the skin. A layer of coupling gel is spread over the area, and ultrasound is delivered. A 10 percent hydrocortisone cream has been shown to produce the best results.[33] (Refer to Table 5-1.)

Some clinicians prefer to use hydrocortisone mixed by a pharmacist with commercially available ultrasound gel (12.5 grams hydrocortisone powder mixed with 8.45 fluid ounces of ultrasound transmission gel). This is used with normal ultrasound procedures to deliver molecules of antiinflammatory drug throughout the treatment time.

SUMMARY

Ultrasound is a versatile deep-heating modality that can be used in a variety of situations in sports medicine. It has been shown to be effective in treating muscle sprains and strains and in reducing pain associated with inflammation.

ELECTRICAL STIMULATION

Many types of electrical stimulation can be used during the acute care and rehabilitation of athletes. Included in this group are high-volt pulsed galvanic stimulation (HVPGS), Russian stimulation, microcurrent electrical neuromuscular stimulation (MENS), transcutaneous nerve stimulation (TENS), and diathermy. The reported effects of different forms of electrical stimulation are often similar. Reduction of pain, increased strength, reduction of atrophy, acceleration of healing, reduction of edema, and muscle relaxation are all common effects attributed to electrical stimulation. Because the reported benefits of different forms of electrical stimulation are often very similar, it can be difficult to choose the most appropriate type.

Electrical stimulators can be classified several ways. A common differentiation is between direct or alternating current. Stimulators utilizing an alternating current (AC) will not create a polar effect in the tissues. It is also not possible to drive ions or stimulate denervated muscle with alternating current. AC stimulators are generally more comfortable; consequently, a higher net current can be tolerated. AC stimulators include Russian stimulators, diathermy, and TENS.

Direct current (DC) will create a polar effect in the tissues being treated. Ion flow will be unidirectional. At the anode, the result is production of acids and free oxygen. At the cathode, free hydrogen is formed. If the current is of sufficient intensity, cauterization of underlying tissue can result.[25] Direct current can be pulsed or continuous. High-volt pulsed galvanic stimulators produce interrupted or pulsed direct current. HVPGSs deliver very short pulses (less than 100 microseconds) of current, allowing much higher peak current (up to 500 volts) to be tolerated. Because of the short duration of pulses, the above-mentioned chemical effects do not occur with HVPGS.[25] Uninterrupted direct current is used for iontophoresis. Denervated muscle requires either uninterrupted current or pulses longer than 50 microseconds.[57] Uninterrupted current requires lower intensities to avoid acid or alkaline burns. Uninterrupted DC is also much less comfortable, again dictating lower intensities.

Another classification that is used to help understand the differences among electrical stimulators is high or low voltage. This relates to the intensity of the peak current. An example of high-voltage stimulation is the HVPGS. Low-voltage units have voltage under 150 volts and milliamperage of less than 80. Examples of low-voltage stimulation include TENS, MENS, and iontophoresis.

Tissues respond differently to electrical stimulation. For example, large-diameter nerve fibers have a lower threshold for depolarization than small fibers. Muscle fibers do not respond to alternating currents. Denervated muscle requires a stimulus with a frequency of less than 40 hertz. By adjusting characteristics of the electrical stimulation, the desired tissue response can be biased. TENS units are most effective in stimulating nerve. However, if a sufficient intensity is used, a motor response can be elicited. Russian muscle stimulators have a current that allows significant muscle responses with relative comfort, when compared with other stimulators.

The parameters of current can be adjusted to change the bias of an electrical stimulator. Pulse duration or width, rate or frequency of pulse and waveform can all be manipulated to elicit more selective responses. As an example, Delitto and Rose[13] compared the relative comfort of three different waveforms. The quadriceps muscle of 20 normal subjects was stimulated three times with current that was identical except for the waveform. Intensity of current was increased to provide 60 percent of maximum voluntary contraction (MVC). Results showed that different waveforms significantly altered the perception of comfort, although no one waveform consistently provided the most comfortable contraction.

With similar results from many types of stimulators being reported, it is important to understand how tissues respond to variations in electrical current. It is equally important to understand the specific nature of current that a stimulator delivers in order to make appropriate choices in the selection of electrical stimulation. Several electrical stimulators commonly used in rehabilitation of athletes are discussed in more detail below.

HIGH-VOLTAGE PULSED GALVANIC STIMULATION

In recent years, the use of high-voltage pulsed galvanic or direct current stimulation in the treatment of athletic injuries has become increasingly popular. The HVPGS, by definition, is a transcutaneous electric nerve stimulator[20] that delivers more than 100 volts, has a microsecond pulse duration, a low average current (up to 1.5 ampere), and a twin peak waveform.[46] The new DC waveform characteristics allow nonirritating stimulation of the muscles and nerves directly.[41] The therapeutic purposes of HVPGS are to reduce acute pain and postoperative pain, diminish swelling,[51] retard muscle atrophy,[16, 54] reduce muscle spasm,[52] and increase joint mobility.[30]

PHYSICAL PROPERTIES

The name high-voltage pulsed galvanic stimulator incorrectly implies that a galvanic current is being used. Similar to galvanic or direct current, the waveform is monophasic, but the short pulse width prevents the current from being classified as galvanic. Although the HVPGS lacks the ability to stimulate denervated muscles or perform iontophoresis because it is pulsed, the unit has the capability of providing 300 to 500 volts, which exceeds the 100- to 150-volt requirement for a "high-voltage" classification. The low average current generated by the unit eliminates its use as an iontophoretic device. These units do allow a high peak current to be generated, providing better penetration into the tissues.

High-voltage pulsed galvanic stimulators have three major pulse characteristics: pulse duration, peak current, and pulse rate or frequency. The major influence of pulse duration is on the perception of comfort of stimulation. The shorter the pulse duration, the less pain is perceived. The pulse duration of HVPGS ranges between 5 and 100 microseconds and permits selective stimulation of predominantly sensory and motor axons with much less stimulation of pain-conducting nerve fibers.

The magnitude of the peak current is associated with the depth of penetration of the current into the tissue. Although some HVPGS units can provide a maximum peak current of approximately 300 to 400 milliamperes, they are very safe since the average current is very low. The pulse rate or number of pulses per second determines the type of muscle contraction (twitch or tetanic) and the fatigability of the contracting muscle.

PHYSIOLOGICAL EFFECTS

HVPGS has been used to reduce pain, diminish edema, retard muscle atrophy, reduce muscle spasm, and increase joint mobility. The following is a short summary of the mechanism by which HVPGS achieves its results.

Reduction of Pain

The current physiological hypothesis is that pain can be reduced through electric stimulation (the gate theory) that causes the release of opiate substances, endorphins and enkephalins, from several sites within the central nervous system. These substances act to suppress pain.[42]

Edema Reduction

The electrical field concept and the muscle-pumping mechanism are believed to be involved in the physiological mechanism of this effect (refer to Table 5–5).

Reduction of Muscle-Disuse Atrophy

The HVPGS unit has the capability to stimulate muscle fibers. A 1 : 3 ratio of contraction to relaxation time is necessary to maintain muscular activity without fatigue. The proposed mechanism involved in reducing disuse atrophy via electric stimulation is the superimposition of voluntary and ergogeneously stimulated exercise.[20]

TABLE 5–5. High-Volt Pulsed Galvanic Stimulation (HVPGS) for Edema Reduction
by Kurt Jepson

Acute Stage 0–48 Hours	Identify medial and lateral electrode locations Thoroughly clean skin before application Place limb in an elevated position Use a large proximal dispersive ground monopolar technique Sandwich joint with two active electrodes Set active electropolarity to positive Continuous mode Pulse rate at 120 pulses per second Intensity based on patient tolerance, usually between 150–250 milliamps Combine with cold packs and compression Treatment time 20–30 minutes, twice daily Treatment daily up to 48 hours
Subacute Stage 48–72 Hours	Appropriately classify posttraumatic physiological stage Place limb in elevated position Skin preparation: as above Use a large proximal dispersive ground monopolar technique Sandwich joint with two active electrodes Set polarity to positive Surge mode: 2 seconds on, 2 seconds off Pulse rate at 120 pulses per second Intensity set to patient tolerance, maximal after tolerance Combine with cold packs and compression Treatment time 15–20 minutes Treatment daily up to 72 hours
Chronic Edema	Place limb in elevated position Use a large proximal dispersive ground monopolar technique Identify hamstrings and quad motor points Prepare skin for active electrode placement Assign active electrode channel to each muscle Polarity to negative reciprocal mode Pulse rate at 60 pulses per second On time to 2.5 seconds Intensity to induce tetany Treatment time 15–20 minutes Follow with cold packs and compression Treat daily until significant reduction is noted

Reduction of Muscle Spasm

In theory, HVPGS reduces muscle spasm by stimulating a stronger contraction than the athlete can produce volitionally (owing to increased pain), resulting in muscle fatigue and greater relaxation.[31] Another possible mechanism is the previously discussed gate pain relief theory, in which the pain-spasm-pain cycle is broken.

Increased Joint Mobility

The physiological response to electrical stimulation that causes the observed change in range of motion is unclear. If range-of-motion limitation is associated with pain, then reduction of such pain by use of electrical stimulation should improve joint mobility. Other mechanisms may include a direct electrical effect on blood vessels that increases circulation or other unknown electrical effects on connective tissues surrounding the joint.

INDICATIONS AND CONTRAINDICATIONS

Therapeutic applications of HVPGS are indicated in the following sports medicine situations:

1. Acute pain
2. Postsurgical pain
3. Posttraumatic edema
4. Muscle spasm
5. Joint contracture
6. Disuse atrophy

Contraindications for clinical use of HVPGS are as follows:

1. Patients with pacemakers
2. Patients with cancer
3. During pregnancy

We rarely see these patients in a sports medicine setting; therefore, the contraindications are few.

APPLICATION TECHNIQUES

The following instructions may be used as guidelines to provide a typical treatment using HVPGS[28] (Fig. 5–15; refer to Table 5–5 in addition to Tables 5–1 and 5–2).

1. Explain to the athlete what will be felt during the treatment.
2. Expose the surface area and check the skin for abrasions and good conductance.
3. Place the dispersive pad on the body surface some distance away from the treatment site.
4. Prepare the treatment electrodes by properly saturating the sponges with water. Alternative treatments may include the hand-held spot electrode or placement of the electrode leads into a pail of water. The submersion technique enables the circumferential and simultaneous application of cryotherapy.
5. Select the treatment parameters: frequency, mode, and duration. A frequency between 30 and 40 pulses per second will produce a tetanus period that should be relieved by a time of relaxation. A ratio of 1 : 3 is desirable, with 10 seconds of contraction to be followed by 30 seconds of relaxation. Treatment time usually ranges from 15 to 30 minutes.
6. Turn on the unit to elicit the desired motor or sensory response.
7. Instruct the athlete to adjust the intensity to maintain the predetermined response with emphasis on a gradual increase of intensity to maintain comfort.

SUMMARY

The use of high-voltage pulsed galvanic stimulation units has significantly increased in recent years in the treatment of athletic injuries. It is becoming the treatment of choice for acute pain, postoperative pain, and reduction of muscle spasms.

RUSSIAN STIMULATION

Russian stimulation is a modality used by some therapists to stimulate muscle contraction. During the late 1970s, claims from Russia of 30 to 50 percent increases in strength from use of muscle stimulation were reported. Attempts at reproducing these results outside Russia have not been successful.[12, 14, 16] However, increases in muscle torque production in healthy and postoperative patients have been shown. Delitto et al. compared two groups of patients after anterior cruciate ligament (ACL) reconstruction.[14] One group received electrically elicited cocontractions of the quadriceps and hamstrings five times a week for 3 weeks. The other group performed equal numbers of voluntary maximal cocontractions. A statistically higher torque production was reported in the electrical stimulation group than in the voluntary exercise group after 3 weeks of treatment.

Russian stimulation utilizes higher frequencies, delivered in bursts (typically 2500 hertz in 50 bursts per second). Because higher frequencies are used, higher peak intensities can be tolerated. Within several sessions, 50 to 70 percent of MVC can usually be elicited.

A treatment with Russian stimulation involves 10 to 15 contractions of a muscle. Optimum intensity elicits greater than 50 percent of MVC. Rest times between contractions should be two to three times longer than the actual contraction time, to avoid fatigue. Most clinicians instruct the athlete to use voluntary contractions during electrical stimulation to facilitate greater strength gains

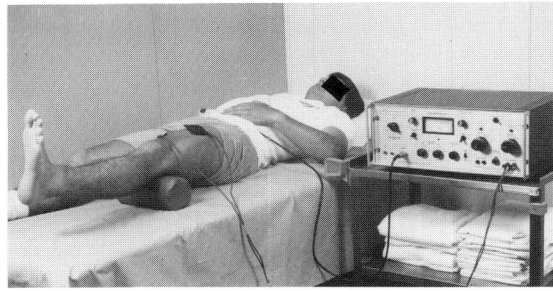

FIGURE 5–15. Electrical stimulation of the left quadriceps, using the Electrostim 180 HVPGS unit (Micromed Instruments, Canada).

and improve motor control. Russian stimulators can be used to reeducate muscles after surgery or to enhance muscle contraction in the treatment of conditions such as patellofemoral pain.[59]

TENS

Transcutaneous nerve stimulation (TENS) is the introduction of electrical stimulation across the skin with the purpose of relieving pain. The analgesia produced by TENS is attributed to two mechanisms: the gate control theory and stimulation of release of endorphins and enkephalins. It is likely that both of these mechanisms play a role in the success of TENS.

The use of TENS gained considerable popularity during the late 1960s when the battery-powered portable unit was designed. The current delivered from TENS is a pulsed current without a net polar effect. Most units commercially available today have several parameters that can be adjusted. These include pulse width, pulse rate, and pulse amplitude. TENS can be used with two to eight electrodes and can be used as a 20- to 30-minute treatment or can be worn continuously throughout the day.

The obvious indication for TENS is pain that is appropriate to mask. TENS is frequently used to control postoperative pain by placing long electrodes along an incision immediately after surgery. Postoperative use usually continues for 3 to 4 days. TENS has also been shown to be effective in decreasing pain from fractures, acute tendinitis, and patellofemoral pain.[17, 50] It is important to remember that TENS is not effective in all cases, and clear-cut guidelines on patient selection have not been established. TENS should not be used to allow athletes to work through acute trauma because of the possibility of increasing injury. The contraindications are similar to other forms of electrical stimulation. TENS can be used with pacemakers.[49] The most frequent complication from TENS is skin irritation from prolonged tape or electrode use.

MENS

Microcurrent electrical neuromuscular stimulation (MENS) has recently been attributed with dramatic clinical results in pain relief, restoration of function, and wound healing. MENS is treatment with low-intensity (200 to 300 microamperes),[19] long-pulse-duration current used for point stimulation. Because intensity is usually below or slightly above sensory level, true muscular depolarization does not occur. Consequently, many clinicians are using the term "low-volt" microcurrent to describe the treatment.[19]

Promotion of wound healing by low-intensity current has been well documented in controlled studies.[10, 58] It is suggested that tissue injuries disturb the normal flow of electrical current in the body. This disturbance may be responsible for triggering the healing process. The introduction of an external electrical current may also be helpful in triggering this process.[7] The acceleration of wound healing using low-intensity currents supports the clinical observation of early restoration of function after acute athletic injuries.

Relief of pain is not as well supported with controlled studies. Despite this, a wealth of unpublished and uncontrolled data exist regarding the ability of MENS to decrease or relieve pain. One study done by Lerner and Kirsch[39] compared low-volt microcurrent stimulation with placebo stimulation on 201 patients with chronic neuromuscular pain. Results showed that the patients who received actual treatment reported longer and more significant pain relief.

Treatment with MENS utilizes point stimulation over areas of low skin impedance. Stimulation to each point typically lasts 6 seconds and is repeated several times per week. Intensity is adjusted at or just below sensory perception.

Low-volt microcurrent treatment shows considerable promise for treatment of athletes. In addition to the pain relief effects that are provided by TENS, MENS may prove to be effective in promoting the healing of soft tissue injuries. As research continues, MENS may take an accepted and important role in the treatment of athletic injuries.

IONTOPHORESIS

Early in the twentieth century, the feasibility of using electricity to deliver drugs across the skin was demonstrated by Leduc in a study using rabbits.[4] Since that time, the treatment has been refined and is rapidly becoming a popular conservative treatment for musculoskeletal inflammatory conditions.

Iontophoresis is the technique of introducing ions into the tissues by means of low-voltage electric current for the purpose of producing a therapeutic effect.[8] Glass et al.[21] used radiolabeled dexamethasone sodium phosphate (Decadron) delivered iontophoretically into the tissues of rhesus monkeys. The study demonstrated delivery of the drug into all tissue layers underlying the electrode, including tendon and cartilage tissue.[21]

In 1982, Bertolucci[8] completed a double-blind study in which he iontophoretically administered test drugs of lidocaine hydrochloride and dexamethasone sodium phosphate or a placebo to 53 patients. The patients receiving the test drugs were significantly improved after treatment, and the group receiving the placebo received no benefit from treatment.

PHYSICAL PRINCIPLES

Iontophoresis treatment must be administered using a low-voltage generator capable of delivering continuous direct current. The manner in which the specific compound ionizes must be known, as well as whether the compound is to be driven into the skin by the positive or negative electrode.[25] Iontophoresis is based on the principle that like charges repel and unlike charges attract. By applying an electric current of specific polarity, ions of medication of similar charge are repelled from the source electrode and driven into the skin.

PHYSIOLOGICAL EFFECTS

The injection of antiinflammatory drugs into inflamed tissue has been demonstrated to reduce an inflammatory response significantly. Iontophoresis, however, has several advantages over local injection. Iontophoresis is noninvasive, delivers a low systemic dose of medication, is less painful, and does not cause the tissue damage that may be seen with injection as a result of needle penetration or subcutaneous injection of fluid.[8]

INDICATIONS AND CONTRAINDICATIONS

Iontophoresis has been indicated in the treatment of tendinitis, bursitis, epicondylitis, trigger point tenderness, and fasciitis.[20] The contraindication for school-age athletes is placement of electrodes over abraded skin or recent scars. Drug sensitivity varies with individuals, so this should also be taken into account.[27]

APPLICATION METHODS

There are currently on the market two models of iontophoretic devices that have widespread sports applications. They are the Iontophor-PM, Model 6110 (Life Tech, Inc., Tampa, FL) and the Phoresor-PM 700 (Iomed, Inc., Salt Lake City, UT). Both are transistorized galvanic DC generators that produce up to 4 milliamperes of current. They have built-in sensors for determining the level of skin resistance (Fig. 5–16).

There are a number of different drug combinations for specific situations. However, the one most often used for sports-related injury is a combination of 4 percent lidocaine hydrochloride noninjectable solution and dexamethasone sodium phosphate (4 mg/ml). The drugs are used in a 2:1 ratio in the electrode. Treatment time varies according to the electrode size and averages 16 to 20 minutes.

The active electrode (the positive electrode in the case of lidocaine and dexamethasone) is placed directly over the painful area and

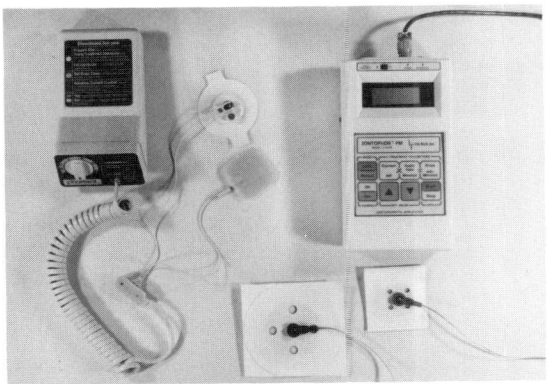

FIGURE 5–16. Two types of iontophoresis: current generators and electrodes. The Phoresor (Iomed, Inc., Salt Lake City, UT) on the *left* and Iontophor-PM (Life Tech, Inc., Tampa, FL) on the *right*.

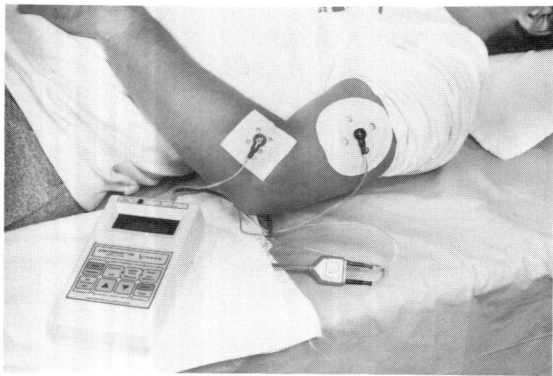

FIGURE 5–17. Treatment of lateral epicondylitis, using the Iontophor-PM (Life Tech, Inc., Tampa, FL).

the dispersive pad approximately 2 inches away. The electrodes are filled and the galvanic generator is turned on slowly. The current should be adjusted to a comfortable setting (Fig. 5–17; refer to Table 5–4).

SUMMARY

Physical modalities vary in sophistication from a bag of ice to complex electric devices. They have a role in reducing pain, edema, stiffness, and other effects of soft tissue trauma and are useful in facilitating rehabilitation. Much remains to be learned about their effects on human tissues, and many traditional clinical uses have not yet been investigated with controlled studies. Their use is most appropriate when combined with therapeutic exercise into an integrated rehabilitation program such as the ones described in Tables 5–1 through 5–5.

References

1. Abraham, E. A., McMaster, W. E., Krijger, M., Waugh, T. R. Whirlpool therapy for the treatment of soft tissue wounds complicating extremity fractures. J Trauma 14:222–267, 1974.
2. Abramson, D. L. Changes in blood flow, oxygen uptake and tissue temperatures produced by the topical application of wet heat. Arch Phys Med Rehabil 42:305, 1961.
3. Abramson, D. L., Chu, L. S. W., Tuck, S. Jr., Lee, S. W., Richardson, G, Levin, M. Effects of tissue temperatures and blood flow on motor nerve conduction velocity. JAMA 198:1082–1088, 1966.
4. Banga, A. K., Chien, Y. W. Iontophoretic delivery of drugs: Fundamentals, developments, and biomedical applications. J Contr Release 7:1–24, 1988.
5. Barany, M., Barany, K., Oppenheimer, H. Effects of ultrsonic energy on adenosine triphosphate. Nature 199:694, 1963.
6. Beasley, R. W., Kester, N. C. Principles of medical-surgical rehabilitation of the hand. Med Clin North Am 53:645–659, 1969.
7. Becker, R. O., Selden, G. Method for producing cellular dedifferentiation by means of very small electrical current. Trans NY Acad Sci 29:606–615, 1967.
8. Bertolucci, L. E., Introduction of anti-inflammatory drugs by iontophoresis: Double blind study. J Orthop Sports Phys Ther 4 (No 2):103–108, 1982.
9. Bourbon, B. Use of the low watt laser in treatment of lymphedema: A single case study. Phys Ther 68:813, 1988.
10. Carley, L. C., Wainapel, S. F. Electrotherapy for acceleration of wound healing: Low intensity direct current. Arch Phys Med Rehabil 66:443–445, 1985.
11. Chastain, P. B. The effect of deep heat on isometric strength. Phys Ther 58:543–546, 1978.
12. Currier, D. E. P., Mann, R. Muscular strength development by electrical stimulation in healthy individuals. Phys Ther 63:915, 1985.
13. Delitto, A., Rose, R. J. Comparative comfort of three waveforms used in electrically eliciting quadriceps femoris muscle contractions. Phys Ther 66:1704, 1986.
14. Delitto, A., Rose, R. J., McKowen, J. M., Lehman, R. C., Thomas, J. A., Shively, R. A. Electrical stimulation versus voluntary exercise in strengthening thigh musculature after anterior cruciate ligament surgery. Phys Ther 68:660–663, 1988.
15. Edwards, H. T. Effects of temperature on muscle energy metabolism and endurance during successive isometric contraction, sustained to fatigue of the quadriceps muscle in man, J Physiol 220:335, 1972.
16. Eriksson, E., Haggmark, T. Comparison of isometric muscle training and electrical stimulation supplementing isometric muscle training in the recovery after major knee ligament surgery. Am J Sports Med 7:169–171, 1979.
17. Ersek, R. A. Relief of acute musculoskeletal pain using transcutaneous electrical neurostimulation. J Am Coll Emerg Phys 6:300, 1977.
18. Fischer, E., Soloman, S. Physiologic response to heat and cold. In Licht, S (ed), Therapeutic Heat and Cold (ed 2). Baltimore: Waverly Press, 1965.
19. Gersh, M. R. Microcurrent electrical stimulation: Putting it in perspective. Clin Mgmt Phys Ther 9:51–54, 1989.
20. Gieck, J. H., Saliba, E. N. Application of modalities in overuse syndromes. Clin Sports Med 6 (No 2): 427–466, 1987.
21. Glass, J. M., Stephen, R. L., Jacobson, S. C. The quantity and distribution of radiolabelled dexamethasone delivered to tissue by iontophoresis. Int J Dermatol 19:519–525, 1980.
22. Greenberg, R. S. The effects of hot packs and exercise on local blood flow. Phys Ther 52:273–278, 1972.
23. Griffin, J. E. Physiological effects of ultrasound as it is used clinically. J Am Phys Ther Assoc 46:18, 1966.
24. Griffin, J. E., Enternach, J. L., Price, R. E., Touch-

stone, J. C. Patients treated with ultrasonic driven hydrocortisone and with ultrasound alone. Phys Ther 47:594–601, 1967.
25. Griffin, J., Karselis, T. Physical Agents for Physical Therapists (ed 3). Springfield: Charles C. Thomas, Publisher, 1988.
26. Hardy, J. D., Bard, P. Body temperature regulation. In Mount-Castle, VD (ed), Medical Physiology 2 (ed 13). St. Louis: CV Mosby Co, 1974.
27. Harris, P. R. Iontophoresis: Clinical research in musculoskeletal inflammatory conditions. J Orthop Sports Phys Ther 4 (No 2): 109–122, 1982.
28. Hayes, K. M. Manual for Physical Agents. Chicago: Northwestern University, 1984.
29. Holmes, G. Hydrotherapy as a means for rehabilitation. Br J Sports Med 5:93, 1942.
30. Kahn, J. Low Volt Technique. Syossett, NY: John Kahn (author–publisher), 1976.
31. Killian, C., Malone, I. High Frequency and High Voltage Protocols. Minneapolis: Metronic, 1984.
32. Klafs, C. E., Arnheim, D. D. Modern Principles of Athletic Training. St. Louis: CV Mosby Co, 1989.
33. Kleinkort, J. A., Wood, F. Phonophoresis with 1 percent versus 10 percent hydrocortisone. Phys Ther 55 (No 12): 1320–1324, 1975.
34. Koepke, G. H. The role of physical medicine in the treatment of burns. Surg Clin North Am 50: 1385–1399, 1970.
35. Kowal, M. A. Review of physiologic effects of cryotherapy. J Orthop Sports Phys Ther 5:66–73, 1983.
36. LeBan, M. M. Collagen tissue: Implications of its response to stress in vitro. Arch Phys Med Rehabil 43:461, 1962.
37. Lehmann, J. D., Brunner, G. D., Stow, R. W. Pain threshold measurements after therapeutic application of ultrasound, microwave and infrared. Arch Phys Med Rehabil 39:560, 1958.
38. Lehmann, J. F., de Lateur, B. J. Therapeutic heat. In Lehmann, J. F. (ed), Therapeutic Heat and Cold (ed 3). Baltimore: Williams & Wilkins, 1982.
39. Lerner, F. N., Kirsch, D. L. Micro-stimulation and placebo effect in short term treatment of the chronic back pain patient. ACA J Chiropr 15:101–106, 1981.
40. Loane, S. R. Cryotherapy—using cold to treat injuries. In Appenzeller, O (ed), Sports Medicine: Fitness, Training, Injuries. Baltimore: Urban & Schwarzenberg, 447–452, 1988.
41. Marino, M. Principles of therapeutic modalities: Implications for sports injuries. In Nicholas, JA, Hershman, EB (eds), The Lower Extremity and Spine in Sports Medicine. St. Louis: CV Mosby Company, 1986.
42. Mellzack, R., Wall, P. D. Pain mechanisms: A new theory. Science 150:971, 1965.
43. Mense, S. Effects of temperature on the discharge of muscle spindles and tendon organs. Arch Eur J Physiol 374:159, 1978.
44. Michlovitz, S. L. Thermal Agents in Rehabilitation. Philadelphia: FA Davis Co, 1986.
45. Mueller, F., Blyth, C. Epidemiology and sports injuries in children. Clin Sports Med 1 (No 3): 343–352, 1982.
46. Newton, R. A., Karselis, T. C. Skin pH following high voltage pulsed galvanic stimulation. Phys Ther 63 (No 10): 1593–1596, 1983.
47. Nylin, J. The use of water in therapeutics. Arch Phys Med Rehabil 13:261, 1932.
48. Pope, C. Physiologic action and therapeutic valve of general and local whirlpool baths. Arch Phys Med Rehabil 10:498, 1929.
49. Rasmussen, M. J., Hayes, D., Vlietstra, R., Thorsteinsson, G. Can transcutaneous electrical nerve stimulation be safely used in patients with permanent cardiac pacemakers? Mayo Clin Proc 63:443–445, 1988.
50. Roeser, W., Meeks, L., Venis, R., Strickland, G. The use of transcutaneous nerve stimulation for pain control in athletic medicine. A preliminary report. Am J Sports Med 4 (No 5):210, 1976.
51. Ross, C. R., Segal, D. High voltage galvanic stimulation—an aid to post-operative healing. Curr Podiatry 34:19, 1981.
52. Roy, S., Irvin, R. Sports Medicine Prevention, Evaluation, Management, and Rehabilitation. Englewood Cliffs: Prentice-Hall, Inc, 1983.
53. Sapega, A. A., Quedenfeld, T. C., Moyer, R. A., Butler, R. A. Biophysical factors in range-of-motion exercise. Physician Sportsmed 9:57–65, 1981.
54. Stamford, B. The myth of electrical exercise. Physician Sportsmed 11:144, 1983.
55. Wadsworth, H., Chanmugam, A. P. P. Electrophysical Agents in Physiotherapy. Australia: Science Press, 1983.
56. Ward, A. R., Electricity Fields and Waves in Therapy. Marrickville, NSW: Science Press, 1983.
57. Warren, C. G. The use of heat and cold in the treatment of common musculoskeletal disorders. In Kessler, R. M., Hertling, D (Eds), Management of Common Musculoskeletal Disorders. Philadelphia: Harper & Row Publishers, Inc, 1983.
58. Wolcott, L. E., Wheeler, P. C., Hardwicke, H. M., et al. Accelerated healing of skin ulcers by electrotherapy: Preliminary clinical results. South Med J, 795–801, 1969.
59. Zisles, J. Hydrotherapy. In Krusen, F (ed), Handbook of Physical Medicine and Rehabilitation (ed 2). Philadelphia: WB Saunders Co, 1971.

6

THE PREPARTICIPATION EXAM

SALLY S. HARRIS
DESMOND K. RUNYAN

Although a large body of literature addresses the subject of preparticipation exams, there exists no clear consensus regarding the objectives, format, and content of the ideal examination. Current recommendations are based largely on clinical experience and conventional wisdom, rather than formal scientific evidence. However, there exists a growing body of epidemiological evidence from observational studies by which to evaluate objectively specific components of the preparticipation exam. This chapter will examine current recommendations and present a rational, focused approach to performing preparticipation exams, with specific emphasis on those recommendations that have the strongest empirical support.

OBJECTIVES

Most experts in sports medicine advocate a focused, limited approach to performing preparticipation exams, directed at identifying conditions that could put the athlete at risk for adverse effects (injury, illness, or death) owing to participation in sports. Others argue that the preparticipation exam is frequently an athlete's only contact with the health care system and therefore advocate a more comprehensive evaluation of general health status and physical fitness. Indeed, several studies of adolescent athletes have found that between 80 and 90 percent seek routine health care only for clearance for sports participation.[1,2] Two studies have found that in 8 percent and 21.6 percent, respectively, of adolescent athletes screened during a preparticipation exam, medical problems unrelated to athletic participation were identified.[3,1] However, there is no evidence that a comprehensive exam is more effective in detecting conditions that would limit athletic participation. Attempts to perform a more extensive evaluation in the context of the preparticipation exam may detract from the effectiveness of screening for sports participation; consume unnecessary time, money, and manpower; and give the misleading impression that the preparticipation exam can serve as a substitute for routine health care. It is important that the purpose and limitations of the preparticipation exam be made clear to athletes and their parents. Ideally, the preparticipation exam form should include a written statement explaining that the exam is not a substitute for a comprehensive medical evaluation. However, physicians should use the opportunity to encourage the athlete to seek routine health care.

An increasingly common objective of the preparticipation exam is to fulfill legal or insurance requirements. A 1985 survey of 45 states found that 35 states required yearly examination of high school athletes.[4] Thirty-six states had an official state form; however, 11 of these did not include medical history questions, and only 28 specified physical exam guidelines. In 38 states, a physician was required to perform the exam; however, in the remainder, the exam could be performed by other health care providers, such as nurse practitioners or physician assistants.

Only three states provided a list of specific contraindications for participation, and only one state form included a statement of the purpose or limitations of the exam. In general, state requirements vary greatly and often lack specific guidelines necessary for a directed and complete preparticipation exam. State, local, or institutional requirements may need to be supplemented by additional information derived from the examining physician's own expertise or from guidelines issued by appropriate medical organizations, such as those of the American Academy of Pediatrics.[5]

FORMAT

The preparticipation exam can be performed in one of several formats: personal physician office-based exam, multiple-examiner station exam, or single-file lineup exam.

Traditionally, most preparticipation exams have been carried out in the primary-care physician's private office. This format has the advantages of an established patient-physician relationship, access to medical records, a comfortable private setting, and the opportunity for personal follow-up.

The multiple-examiner station exam is a format in which a team of individuals evaluates a group of athletes in a station-by-station fashion. The team is usually composed of a variety of individuals, such as nurses, coaches, teachers, parents, and one or more physicians, who are each responsible for one examination station. Typical stations would include registration, medical history, vital signs, height and weight measurements, and one or more physical examination stations focusing on specific organ systems. Optional additional stations could include vision, hearing, and laboratory testing and administration of immunizations, if necessary. The exam can be done in a variety of settings, such as in a group of classrooms, an all-purpose room, or gymnasium, as long as care is taken to partition the area to ensure privacy within the examination stations. This station exam format has the advantage of being able to handle a large group of athletes in a single setting at one point in time and therefore tends to be more time efficient and less costly than the office-based exam. In addition, the exam tends to be sports oriented and performed by physicians with a special interest in sports medicine. Often it is possible to incorporate relevant specialists, such as orthopedists and cardiologists, who would otherwise not be directly involved and thus facilitate consultation. However, this format requires a great deal of prior planning, organization, and cooperation and has the disadvantage of lack of continuity of care.

One study has compared the effectiveness of the office-based exam with the multiple-examiner station exam in a group of 922 high school students.[6] The multiple-examiner station format identified a higher percentage of athletes with physical abnormalities (predominantly musculoskeletal), more athletes requiring further evaluation prior to participation, and more conditions indicating disqualification. In addition, single physicians in the officed-based setting were less likely to recommend additional evaluation or conditioning for athletes with previous injury. It is not surprising that when a physician focuses on only a portion of the examination that he or she is more likely to detect abnormalities than a single physician performing the entire exam. However, the clinical importance and predictive value of abnormalities detected during preparticipation exams are unknown.

The single-file lineup examination in which one physician examines a team of athletes in a group setting, such as in a locker room, is not recommended. This format does not provide adequate conditions for either accurate physical diagnosis or appropriate patient privacy and has been denounced by the American Academy of Pediatrics and most experts in sports medicine.

FREQUENCY AND TIMING

There are no published data on which to base recommendations regarding the frequency at which preparticipation exams should be done. Most experts agree that an annual exam for all athletes is not necessary and has a poor cost-benefit ratio.[1] The American Academy of Pediatrics recommends a complete preparticipation exam every 3 to 4 years or prior to beginning any new level of competition.[5] For most athletes, a complete preparticipation exam would be indicated prior to the onset of junior high, high school, and college participation or when beginning any new sport. Athletes returning to sports in which they have participated in the previous year need only undergo an interim medical history to address complaints, illnesses, or injuries that have occurred in the intervening period. If there has been a change in health status, the need for further evaluation is then determined by the physician on an individual basis. This policy has been adopted by the National Collegiate Athletic Association (NCAA) and an increasing number of high school athletic associations.[7]

The timing of the preparticipation exam should take into account two factors: (1) the need to assess health status as close as possible to the onset of athletic participation, so that relevant problems arising in the interval are not missed, and (2) the need to allow sufficient time to respond to conditions detected during the exam that require further evaluation or treatment, such as injury rehabilitation, cardiology referral, or orthopedic consultation. Approximately 1 month before the onset of athletic participation seems to be an appropriate time to perform the preparticipation exam.

MEDICAL HISTORY

The medical history is perhaps the most important component of the preparticipation exam. Two studies of high school athletes have shown that at least 74 percent of conditions limiting clearance for sports, whether temporarily or permanently, can be detected on the basis of medical history alone.[1,2] The most frequent conditions relevant to sports clearance that were identified on the medical history were history of joint problems (such as knee injury, subluxing patella, ankle injury, and chondromalacia patella) and history of cardiac problems (such as undiagnosed heart murmur, congenital heart disease, or arrhythmia). Other less frequently reported conditions affecting sports clearance were history of multiple concussions, history of syncope with activity, severe scoliosis, poorly controlled asthma, and presence of a single testicle. Those few conditions affecting sports clearance that were not evident from the medical history but that were only detected by the physical exam included hypertension, moderate or severe knee instability, and scoliosis. These findings suggest that a focused medical history, in conjunction with an orthopedic exam and measurement of blood pressure, is probably adequate to detect the majority of conditions limiting athletic participation. An appropriate medical history directed at identifying conditions that limit athletic participation would include:

1. Assessment of general health status
2. History of past injuries and hospitalizations
3. Limitations of function
4. Cardiac, pulmonary, and musculoskeletal review of systems

The review of other systems, family, and social histories have not been shown to be useful. A sample medical history for the preparticipation exam is shown in Figure 6–1.

PHYSICAL EXAM

The preparticipation physical exam should be limited in scope and concentrate on those parts likely to influence a decision regarding clearance for athletic participation. In addition, the exam should be sports specific, addressing those problems of relevance to the athlete's particular sport. The purpose of the exam may also vary according to the age and experience of the athlete. Significant medical problems are most likely to be discovered in younger or less experienced athletes. In contrast, the older, experienced athletes have undergone a sort of selection process in which significant medical problems would have been identified in previous exams and in some cases precluded athletic participation. Therefore, the exam in the older athlete should focus primarily on evaluation of previous injury and rehabilitation status.

In general, the physical exam appears to be of low yield in identifying conditions affecting sports clearance, largely owing to the low prevalence of disqualifying conditions among young athletes.[8] Our review of six recent studies identified a disqualification rate between 0 and 1.3 percent.[1,2,3,6,9,10] Conditions leading to disqualification in these studies were mitral insufficiency, hypertrophic cardiomyopathy, congenital heart disease, missing testicle, unilateral asymptomatic hydronephrosis, meniscal tear, subluxing patella, history of multiple concussions, ventricular arrhythmia with syncope during exercise, severe scoliosis, severe knee instability, and recent fracture.

Many conditions identified on the basis of physical exam lead to referrals for further medical evaluation prior to sports clearance.

PREPARTICIPATION EXAM HISTORY

This exam is not a substitute for a complete physical but is solely for the purpose of sports clearance.

Name _____
   Address _____
   Phone _____
Birthdate _____
Family Physician _____
   Address _____
   Phone _____
Person to contact in case of emergency _____
   Phone _____
School/Grade _____
Sport/Position _____

	No	Yes	Explain
Have you ever had surgery?	___	___	___
Have you ever been hospitalized for a reason other than surgery?	___	___	___
Have you ever broken, dislocated, or injured a bone or joint?	___	___	___
Have you had any serious illness in the past?	___	___	___
Do you have any ongoing medical problems (such as anemia, asthma, bleeding disorders, diabetes, eating disorder, heart disease, hernia, kidney disease, liver disease, mononucleosis, seizures, skin problems, or other conditions)?	___	___	___
Do you have any known deformities (such as curvature of the spine, one kidney, one testicle, blindness in one eye?	___	___	___
Have you ever been told you have a heart murmur, high blood pressure, extra heartbeats, or a heart abnormality?	___	___	___
Are you taking any medications?	___	___	___
Do you have any allergies (hay fever, hives, asthma, or to medicines)?	___	___	___
Have you ever "passed out" or been "knocked out" (concussion)?	___	___	___
Have any members of your family had a "heart attack" or "heart problem" or died sucdenly before the age of 50?	___	___	___
Do you ever have difficulty breathing after you have *stopped* exercising, such as shortness of breath, coughing, wheezing, chest pain, or chest tightness?	___	___	___
Have you ever had a problem that caused you to miss a game or practice? *more than 2 days of work.*	___	___	___
Do you wear glasses or contact lenses?	___	___	___
Do you have any chipped teeth, braces, or bridges?	___	___	___
Have you ever missed menstrual periods for 6 months or more? (females only)	___	___	___

When was your last tetanus shot? Date _____

FIGURE 6–1.

Preparticipation exam studies report referral rates between 1.2 and 13.6 percent.[1,2,3,6,9,10] The most common conditions triggering referral were musculoskeletal problems in need of rehabilitation and heart murmurs, most of which are subsequently found to be benign. The majority of these conditions turn out to be false positives, and the athletes are subsequently cleared for participation. Since the majority of these conditions could be identified on the basis of history alone, the physical exam is a relatively noncontributory component of the preparticipation exam.

Despite the lack of evidence regarding the

PREPARTICIPATION PHYSICAL EXAM

Name _____   Date _____

Ht _____   Wt _____   BP _____   Pulse _____
Vision (if not recently checked): L 20/ ____   R 20/ ____   Visual fields _____
Eyes: pupil size _____
Skin: _____
Mouth: _____
Lymph nodes: _____
Heart: PMI _____
       Pulses _____
       Rhythm _____
       Murmurs _____
Lungs: _____
Abdomen: Liver _____   Spleen _____
Orthopedic: Cervical spine/back   _____
               Shoulders   _____
               Arm/elbow   _____
               Wrist/hand   _____
               Knees   _____
               Ankles/feet   _____

Other (from positive history): _____

Participation status:
___ Cleared
___ Cleared with limitations   Limitations: _____
___ Clearance deferred pending further evaluation Reason _____
___ Disqualification   Reason _____

Physician's signature: _____

FIGURE 6–2.

overall effectiveness of the physical exam, it seems prudent that a focused physical exam be done at appropriate stages in each athlete's career. Those parts of the exam that appear to have the greatest utility are the cardiovascular exam and musculoskeletal exam; these will be discussed in more detail below. A sample physical exam form for preparticipation exams is shown in Figure 6–2.

CARDIOVASCULAR EXAM

The cardiovascular portion of the exam should include blood pressure measurement, palpation of peripheral pulses, and auscultation of the heart.

Hypertension

Hypertension is a relatively common occult condition found during preparticipation exams[2] but is rarely grounds for disqualification from most sports. Care should be taken to use an appropriate cuff size and to evaluate blood pressure measurements against age-specific norms. Blood pressure measurements exceeding 130/75 for children 11 years of age and younger, and 140/85 for children 12 and older, require further evaluation.[5] Suspected hypertension should be confirmed by several subsequent measurements, as anxiety in young athletes can often lead to transient elevations. Some experts recommend that individuals with hypertension should be discouraged from weight lifting, because it can cause acute elevations in blood pressure.[11]

Arrhythmias

Athletes have a higher prevalence of bradycardia and some irregular rhythms than the general population.[12] These include first- and second-degree heart block, Wenckebach phenomenon, and junctional rhythms. In most cases, the irregular rhythm disappears with the usual tachycardic response to exercise and does not require further evaluation. Similarly, isolated premature ventricular contractions are common in young people in general and are rarely of clinical consequence.

Heart Murmurs

Heart murmurs are extremely common findings in young athletes. The vast majority are benign pulmonic ejection murmurs and have been reported to be present in up to 85 percent of young athletes.[13] Other benign murmurs include Stills murmur, venous hums, and carotid bruits.

It is important to distinguish benign functional murmurs from pathological murmurs associated with conditions that put one at risk for sudden death. Hypertrophic cardiomyopathy may be the most common cause of sudden death in athletes.[14] The murmur in this condition, when present, is characterized by an apical systolic murmur that increases with valsalva manuever and when going from a sitting to supine position. Prolapsed mitral valve is the most common cardiac abnormality found in athletes but does not constitute a contraindication to sports participation unless associated with arrhythmias. The murmur is characterized by a midsystolic click, followed by a late systolic murmur heard in the apex, and best heard with the patient in a sitting or standing position. This condition is more common in females and has been associated with nonspecific chest pain, arrhythmias, pectus excavatum, scoliosis, and Marfan syndrome. Marfan syndrome itself can present a risk for sudden death owing to the possibility of aortic rupture secondary to cystic medial necrosis. It is generally not possible to detect this cardiac abnormality on the basis of auscultation, chest X ray, or electrocardiogram (ECG). However, individuals with Marfan syndrome can be identified by the presence of other features such as a positive family history of Marfan syndrome, kyphoscoliosis, anterior thoracic deformity, tall stature, arm span greater than height, upper-to-lower-body ratio greater than one standard deviation below the mean, myopia, lenticular dislocation, arachnodactyly, and joint laxity. Individuals suspected of having Marfan syndrome should be evaluated by echocardiography, since 84 percent will have evidence of aortic roof dilatation.[15] Marked valvular aortic stenosis would represent a contraindication to strenuous sports participation. This murmur is typically characterized by a crescendo-decrescendo systolic ejection murmur often preceded by a systolic ejection click, heard at either the right or left sternal border, with radiation to the carotid arteries. Since most cases of marked aortic stenosis would be associated with a prominent murmur, this condition is usually detected early in childhood.

In general, screening athletes for significant cardiovascular disorders has been found to be of low yield. In one study, 90 (17.9 percent) of 501 intercollegiate athletes screened for cardiovascular disease were found to have findings suggestive of heart disease on either history, physical exam, or ECG.[16] However, on further evaluation, 84 percent of these had no evidence of cardiovascular disease, and 15 percent had mild mitral valve prolapse that did not preclude sports participation. Three other athletes had mild ventricular septal hypertrophy and were also cleared for participation. In no case was a cardiovascular condition identified that was a contraindication to sports participation. It is unclear whether failure to detect important cardiovascular disorders is due to the low prevalence of such conditions in ostensibly healthy athletes or poor sensitivity of the screening methods.

Sudden Death

Of particular interest has been the question of whether athletes with the potential for sudden death may be identified in advance on the basis of the preparticipation exam. A recent review of 29 athletes with sudden death suggests that in young athletes (less than 35 years old) sudden death is due to congenital cardiovascular disease.[17] Over half the cases were associated with hypertrophic cardiomyopathy, whereas the remainder were associated with congenital coronary artery anomalies, ruptured aorta secondary to cystic medial necrosis (Marfan syndrome), idiopathic left ventricular hypertrophy, and coronary artery atherosclerosis. Myocarditis, mitral valve prolapse, aortic valve stenosis, and sarcoidosis were relatively uncommon causes of sudden death. In only 25 percent of these cases was underlying cardiovascular disease suspected on the basis of prior histories or physical exams, and in most cases, sudden death was the first manifestation of disease. Although a history of syncope during exercise or a family history of sudden death is often associated with hypertrophic cardiomyopathy, these findings lack sensitivity to detect the majority of cases. Similarly, the physical exam also frequently fails to detect those with hypertrophic cardiomyopathy, because the majority with the disease have a nonobstructive form and therefore a soft or absent murmur.[18]

One study has addressed the question of whether a history of syncope is associated with increased risk of sudden death.[19] Although this study did not pertain exclusively to risk of sudden death during exercise, it suggests that risk is increased only in those individuals for whom a cardiac etiology can be determined. Risk does not appear to be increased in those with syncope due to noncardiovascular or unknown causes in the absence of severe underlying illnesses. In most cases for which a cardiac etiology could be determined, it was done on the basis of the history and physical exam. From the standpoint of risk of sudden death, these findings would suggest that in the absence of cardiovascular disease detectable by history or physical exam, further evaluation for cause of syncope is not necessary for sports clearance.

The use of chest X rays, ECG, or echocardiography as screening procedures in the preparticipation exam is not recommended, owing to economic limitations and the low incidence of sudden death. Although the exact incidence of sudden death during sports participation is unknown, it has been estimated that 200,000 athletes would need to be screened in order to identify 1 athlete who may die suddenly during athletic participation.[20] One study found that ECG evaluation of all athletes during a preparticipation exam did not significantly improve the ability of the screening process to detect important cardiovascular disease, beyond that which could be detected on the basis of the history and physical exam alone.[16] Echocardiography, however, is a relatively sensitive and specific diagnostic test for cardiovascular disease but impractical to use for screening purposes. Chest X ray, ECG, and echocardiography should be used discriminately on an individualized basis for purposes of further evaluation of suspected disease. Table 6–1 summarizes the value of the medical history, physical exam, chest X ray, ECG, and echocardiography in the diagnosis of those cardiovascular disorders associated with sudden death during exercise.

ORTHOPEDIC EXAM

The orthopedic exam appears to be the component of the physical exam with the greatest sensitivity and specificity in detecting conditions relevant to sports clearance.[2] Since a history of previous injury appears to be a risk factor for future injury,[21, 22, 23, 24] a main goal of the orthopedic exam should be to evaluate residual deficits due to past injuries. This should include an evaluation of strength, flexibility, and range of motion of the affected joint and referral for rehabilitation when indicated. Several studies support the effectiveness of preseason conditioning programs in the prevention of knee injuries in particular.[24, 25] In the absence of weight-lifting apparatus, bilateral comparison of midthigh girth and clinical muscle strength testing appear to be a practical way to evaluate knee strength and detect weakness due to previous injury in the office setting; the diagnostic accuracy of this approach has not been established.

There appears to be no correlation between measurements of flexibility or ligamentous laxity and risk of sports injuries. Although one early study found such a correlation in regard to ligamentous injuries of the knee in professional football players,[26] these findings have not been found to hold true in subsequent studies involving varying age groups and several different sports.[27, 28, 29, 30, 31, 32]

The orthopedic exam should focus on those joints most relevant to the athlete's specific sport, particularly when there is a history of previous injury or when the athlete is experiencing joint-specific symptoms. In the absence of specific problems, the 90-second orthopedic screening exam (shown in Table

TABLE 6–1. Major Causes of Sudden Death in Athletes and Potential Efficacy of Screening Studies

Causes	Screening Procedures	Sensitivity	Predictive Value
Hypertrophic cardiomyopathy	History*	Poor	Poor
	Chest X-ray film	Fair	Poor
	Auscultation	Fair	Excellent
	Echocardiogram	Excellent	Excellent‖
	12-lead ECG	Good†	Poor
Cystic medial necrosis	History	Poor	Poor
	Chest X-ray film	Fair	Excellent
	Auscultation	Poor	Fair
	Echocardiogram	Excellent	Excellent
	12-lead ECG	—	—
CAD/congenital coronary abnormalities	History	Poor	Poor
	Chest X-ray film	Poor	Fair**
	Auscultation	—	—
	12-lead ECG	Poor	Poor
	Exercise ECG	Fair-good	Poor‡
	Radionuclide studies	Excellent	Poor‡
Aortic valve stenosis	History	—	—
	Chest X-ray film	Poor	Poor
	Auscultation	Excellent	Good§
	12-lead ECG	Fair	Poor
	Echocardiogram	Poor	Poor

CAD = Coronary artery disease
ECG = Electrocardiogram
* Specifically, a history of syncope or sudden premature death in a close family member.
† Both in making the diagnosis of hypertrophic cardiomyopathy and identifying patients at risk of sudden death.
‡ Of increasing value in subjects older than 40 years of age when the prevalence of coronary artery disease increases; however, most abnormal responses will still be falsely positive.
§ The predictive value of auscultation depends on intensity of murmur; the high prevalence of softer innocent murmurs will necessitate a more sophisticated and expensive evaluation in many individuals.
‖ Predictive value is critically dependent on the magnitude of ventricular septal thickness (septal thickness > 20 mm would be highly indicative of hypertrophic cardiomyopathy; septal thickness of 13 to 14 mm, as an isolated clinical finding, would provide only suggestive evidence of disease).
** Only if coronary calcifications are detected by fluoroscopy; poor if fluoroscopy is not carried out.
Note: The rating system is based on the following sequence: excellent > good > fair > poor.
Source: Maron BJ, Epstein SE, Roberts WC: Causes of sudden death in competitive athletes. J Am Coll Cardiol 7:204–214, 1986.

6–2) has been recommended to screen for unrecognized problems that might adversely affect athletic participation.[5] Positive findings would require a more extensive evaluation of the target area. Although this is a very practical screening test, the sensitivity of this test with regard to detecting orthopedic abnormalities has not been tested.

ADDITIONAL CONCERNS

The physician should be aware of other components of the physical exam that may be applicable in specific situations. For instance, athletes involved in sports with direct skin-to-skin contact, such as wrestling, should be evaluated for the presence of contagious skin infections, such as impetigo, herpes gladiatorum, or lice. Organomegaly should be assessed in individuals participating in contact sports, owing to risk of rupture. A baseline neurological examination is recommended in athletes with a history of head trauma and documentation of anisocoria in any athlete at risk for head trauma. A menstrual history may be important in female athletes participating in endurance sports, because they are prone to amenorrhea and associated decreases in bone density. A history of amenorrhea is not a contraindication to athletic participation, but such individuals should be referred for further evaluation and counseling. Auscultation of the lung fields is unlikely to yield positive findings in the absence of a history of acute or chronic

TABLE 6–2. The 90-Second Orthopedic Screening Exam

Instructions to Athlete	Observation
Stand facing examiner	Acromioclavicular joints; general habitus
Look at ceiling, floor, over both shoulders; touch ears to shoulders	Cervical spine motion
Shrug shoulders (examiner resists)	Trapezius strength
Abduct shoulders 90° (examiner resists at 90°)	Deltoid strength
Full external rotation of arms	Shoulder motion
Flex and extend elbows	Elbow motion
Arms at sides, elbows 90°flexed; pronate and supinate wrists	Elbow and wrist motion
Spread fingers; make fist	Hand or finger motion and deformities
Tighten (contract) quadriceps; relax quadriceps	Symmetry and knee effusion; ankle effusion
"Duck walk" four steps (away from examiner with buttocks on heels)	Hip, knee, and ankle motion
Back to examiner	Shoulder symmetry; scoliosis
Knees straight, touch toes	Scoliosis, hip motion, hamstring tightness
Raise up on toes, raise heels	Calf symmetry, leg strength

Source: American Academy of Pediatrics, Committee on Sports Medicine: Sports Medicine: Health Care for Young Athletes. Evanston, IL: American Academy of Pediatrics, 1983.

respiratory symptoms. Otoscopy, ophthalmoscopy, and scoliosis screening have not been found to be useful in the absence of a relevant history[2] but may be prudent if no recent evaluation has been done. Similarly, the traditional hernia examination is not relevant to the decision of sports clearance, as the presence of a reducible hernia would not constitute a contraindication to participation, and surgical repair can safely be deferred until after the end of the athletic season. However, examination of the genitalia may serve important non–sports-related purposes, such as screening for testicular cancer, cryptorchidism, sexually transmitted diseases, and maturational staging. General measurements of physical fitness such as body composition, strength, flexibility, and endurance are important for training, performance, and rehabilitation but have not been proven useful in the context of the preparticipation exam as predictors of injury or other adverse outcomes.

LABORATORY TESTS

There is no evidence that routine blood testing or urinalysis is worthwhile as part of the preparticipation exam. In none of six studies of preparticipation exams were any athletes excluded because of an abnormal laboratory test.[1, 2, 3, 6, 9, 10] In one study, 40 of 701 athletes had evidence of proteinuria on urine screening, but none was found to have any urinary tract abnormality upon further evaluation.[2] Similarly, determination of hemoglobin or hematocrit has not proven to be productive because of the low prevalence of iron deficiency serious enough to affect performance adversely. The American Academy of Pediatrics supports the position that routine blood or urine testing is not recommended as part of the preparticipation exam.[5] Specific laboratory tests are indicated only on an individual basis, when suggested by relevant medical history or physical exam findings. Drug screening for ergogenic or recreational drugs should not be part of the preparticipation exam at the high school level. Such screening is currently done on an institutional basis at the collegiate and elite levels. The American Academy of Pediatrics states in a recent policy statement that "student athletes should not be singled out for involuntary screening for drugs of abuse. Except for health-related purposes, such testing should not be a condition for participation in sports or any school function."[33]

EXERCISE-INDUCED BRONCHOSPASM

Exercise-induced bronchospasm (EIB) is a relatively common condition estimated to occur in 3 to 10 percent of athletes.[34] The condition is prevalent even among elite athletes, as shown by the finding that 11.2 percent of the 1984 Olympic Team had a history of EIB and/or asthma.[35] EIB is typically characterized by the onset of bronchospasm 5 to 10 minutes after cessation of 5 to 8 minutes of strenuous exercise. Symptoms usually last 5 to 15 minutes and may be followed by a 30- to 90-minute refractory period in about 50 percent of individuals.[36] A late bronchospastic response may occur 3 to 6 hours after exercise in 30 to 40 percent of subjects who have recovered from an earlier response.[37] Symptoms may be manifested as frank wheezing or only as shortness of breath, chest tightness, or coughing.

The medical history is a relatively sensitive way to identify athletes with EIB. A history of asthma or allergic rhinitis should trigger specific questioning, since at least 80 percent of individuals with asthma and approximately 40 percent of individuals with allergic rhinitis have been found to have EIB.[35] The prevalence of EIB in nonallergic individuals is thought to be low, on the order of 3 to 4 percent,[35] although some authorities believe that it does not exist as an independent disorder in the absence of at least mild asthma.[38] Among athletes on the 1984 U.S. Olympic Team, 90 percent of those with EIB could be identified on the basis of medical history, although many were previously unaware of their diagnosis.[35] Similarly, Rice et al. found in their study of 983 intercollegiate athletes that EIB was previously undiagnosed in 19 of 28 athletes, despite the presence of a suggestive medical history.[39]

The physical exam is a relatively poor screening tool for detecting EIB. The occurrence and severity of EIB cannot be predicted from auscultation or pulmonary function studies performed with the subject at rest.[35,36] Response to an exercise challenge can confirm the diagnosis of EIB when illicited, but lack of a response does not rule out EIB, as the response can be highly variable and inconsistent.[36] Other diagnostic tests for asthma, such as methacholine or histamine challenge, correlate poorly with the presence of EIB.[40]

Neither asthma nor EIB is usually a contraindication to sports participation. In most cases, the condition can be controlled by pharmacological agents and may even be improved by physical conditioning. The treatment of choice for EIB is beta-adrenergic aerosols administered 30 minutes prior to exercise. These agents have been found to be effective in reducing or preventing EIB in 90 percent of cases.[36] Cromolyn sodium is effective in 60 to 70 percent of patients with EIB,[36] whereas antihistamines, anticholinergics, theophylline, and steroids are generally not effective in the prevention of EIB.[36,41]

PHYSICAL MATURATION

Some authorities advocate examination of the genitalia of peripubertal athletes for the purpose of maturational staging, in order to identify less physically mature athletes who may be at increased risk of injury while competing in contact sports against more physically mature peers. Although common sense suggests that marked physical mismatching in contact sports may be inadvisable, there is currently no strong evidence to suggest that less physically mature individuals are at increased risk of injury. In fact, risk of injury in contact sports increases with age and weight of the participants;[42] injury rates are significantly higher among high school and college athletes than among younger adolescents in whom the greatest variation in maturational status exists.[42] One study suggesting an increased risk of injury in physically immature athletes[43] suffers from significant methodological shortcomings. A recent prospective study of soccer injuries found that physical immaturity was not a risk factor for injury, since the highest rate of injury was found in older, taller, more physically mature boys.[44] However, this study suggests that among the high-risk group of physically mature boys, weak muscular strength may be a risk factor for injury. In absence of compelling evidence showing an association, we cannot recommend physical maturation assessment for purposes of injury prevention. In addition, one must consider the psychological sequelae of excluding physically immature individuals from participation in contact sports as well as the logistical difficulty of matching athletes by maturational age rather than chronological age. Whereas assessment of physical maturation is not relevant to the decision of clearance for athletic participation, it may be useful on an individual basis for counseling purposes. The physician may be more accurate in estimation of eventual adult height or judging the potential benefits of weight lifting in peripubertal athletes. None of 36 official state forms for preparti-

TABLE 6–3. Recommendations for Participation in Competitive Sports

	Contact/ Collision	Limited Contact/Impact	Noncontact		
			Strenuous	*Moderately Strenuous*	*Nonstrenuous*
Atlantoaxial instability	No	No	Yes	Yes	Yes
*Swimming: no butterfly, breast stroke, or diving starts					
Acute illnesses	*	*	*	*	*
*Needs individual assessment, e.g., contagiousness to others, risk of worsening illness					
Cardiovascular					
Carditis	No	No	No	No	No
Hypertension					
Mild	Yes	Yes	Yes	Yes	Yes
Moderate	*	*	*	*	*
Severe	*	*	*	*	*
Congenital heart disease	†	†	†	†	†
*Needs individual assessment					
†Patients with mild forms can be allowed a full range of physical activities; patients with moderate or severe forms, or who are postoperative, should be evaluated by a cardiologist before athletic participation					
Eyes					
Absence or loss of function of one eye	*	*	*	*	*
Detached retina	†	†	†	†	†
*Availability of American Society for Testing and Materials (ASTM)-approved eye guards may allow competitor to participate in most sports, but this must be judged on an individual basis					
†Consult ophthalmologist					
Inguinal hernia	Yes	Yes	Yes	Yes	Yes
Kidney: absence of one	No	Yes	Yes	Yes	Yes
Liver: enlarged	No	No	Yes	Yes	Yes
Musculoskeletal disorders	*	*	*	*	*
*Needs individual assessment					
Neurologic					
History of serious head or spine trauma, repeated concussions, or craniotomy	*	*	Yes	Yes	Yes
Convulsive disorder					
Well controlled	Yes	Yes	Yes	Yes	Yes
Poorly controlled	No	No	Yes†	Yes	Yes‡
*Needs individual assessment					
†No swimming or weight lifting					
‡No archery or riflery					
Ovary: absence of one	Yes	Yes	Yes	Yes	Yes
Respiratory					
Pulmonary insufficiency	*	*	*	*	Yes
Asthma	Yes	Yes	Yes	Yes	Yes
*May be allowed to compete if oxygenation remains satisfactory during a graded stress test					
Sickle cell trait	Yes	Yes	Yes	Yes	Yes
Skin: boils, herpes, impetigo, scabies	*	*	Yes	Yes	Yes
*No gymnastics with mats, martial arts, wrestling, or contact sports until not contagious					
Spleen: enlarged	No	No	No	Yes	Yes
Testicle: absence or undescended	Yes*	Yes*	Yes	Yes	Yes
*Certain sports may require protective cup					

Source: American Academy of Pediatrics, Committee on Sports Medicine: Recommendations for participation in competitive sports. Pediatrics 81:737–738, 1988.

cipation exams requires evaluation of physical maturation.[4]

DOWN SYNDROME

Physicians are increasingly called on to perform preparticipation exams for individuals with Down syndrome, owing to widespread participation of these individuals in Special Olympics sports programs. Of special concern is the issue of atlantoaxial instability. This condition is associated with Down syndrome in 10 to 20 percent of individuals, is usually asymptomatic, and is believed to be gradually progressive with advancing age.[45] It is not known whether those with atlantoaxial instability are at increased risk of subluxation.[45] Both the American Academy of Pediatrics[46] and regulations of the Special Olympics[47] recommend obtaining cervical spine X rays on all individuals with Down syndrome participating in sports with risk of trauma to the head or neck and excluding from participation those with atlantoaxial instability. However, evidence of atlantoaxial instability on cervical spine X rays (atlantoaxial interval equal to or greater than 5 mm) has not been found to be predictive of subluxation.[45] In addition, there are no reported spinal cord injuries in over 500,000 athletes with Down syndrome participating in the Special Olympics during the last 17 years.[45] A review of 31 cases in which subluxation occurred in individuals with Down syndrome found that all but 3 had a history of preceding neurological signs and symptoms for several months.[45] Since the predictive value of cervical spine X rays is poor and the incidence of subluxation seemingly low, these findings suggest that a careful neurological history and physical exam are likely to be more worthwhile than routine cervical spine X rays in evaluating the potential for atlantoaxial subluxation in athletes with Down syndrome.

DISQUALIFYING CONDITIONS

The most recent guidelines for disqualification from sports participation are the 1988 recommendations of the American Academy of Pediatrics (AAP),[48] shown in Table 6–3. The AAP guidelines classify their recommendations by categories of sports, divided on the basis of degree of strenuousness and probability for collision (Table 6–4). These guidelines were formulated in order to update the existing 1976 recommendations of the American Medical Association,[49] which were considered to be overly restrictive in

TABLE 6–4. Classification of Sports

		Noncontact		
Contact/Collision	Limited Contact/Impact	Strenuous	Moderately Strenuous	Nonstrenuous
Boxing	Baseball	Aerobic dancing	Badminton	Archery
Field hockey	Basketball	Crew	Curling	Golf
Football	Bicycling	Fencing	Table tennis	Riflery
Ice hockey	Diving	Field		
Lacrosse	Field	Discus		
Martial arts	High jump	Javelin		
Rodeo	Pole vault	Shot put		
Soccer	Gymnastics	Running		
Wrestling	Horseback riding	Swimming		
	Skating	Tennis		
	Ice	Track		
	Roller	Weight lifting		
	Skiing			
	Cross-country			
	Downhill			
	Water			
	Softball			
	Squash, handball			
	Volleyball			

Source: American Academy of Pediatrics, Committee on Sports Medicine: Recommendations for participation in competitive sports. Pediatrics 81:737–738, 1988.

some cases in light of changes in societal attitudes and improvements in protective equipment. For instance, hemophilia is no longer a contraindication for participation in noncontact sports, and presence of inguinal hernia is no longer a contraindication for participation in contact sports. The new guidelines also reflect an increased sensitivity to the civil rights of athletes, recognizing that sports participation can be allowed in risky situations if the patient has a full understanding and acceptance of inherent risk associated with sports participation in the presence of preexisting medical conditions. In general, the courts have upheld the right of the individual to participate in sports despite the presence of disqualifying conditions, such as loss of vision in one eye, undescended testicle, and single kidney.

According to the AAP guidelines, disqualification from nonstrenuous noncontact sports is rarely necessary, but disqualification from strenuous or contact sports may be necessary either during an acute illness or because of chronic disease. Owing to the availability of many different types of sports, complete disqualification is rarely necessary. Since there is little scientific evidence on which to base recommendations for sports disqualification, the AAP recommendations should serve only as guidelines. The final decision should be based on the physician's clinical judgment and the individual circumstances of the athlete, after weighing the risks and benefits of participation in each case.

References

1. Risser W. L., Hoffman H. M., Bellah G. G., Jr, et al: A cost benefit analysis of preparticipation sports examinations of adolescent athletes. J School Health 55:270–273, 1985.
2. Goldberg B., Saraniti A., Witman P., et al: Preparticipation sports assessment—an objective evaluation. Pediatrics 66:736–745, 1980.
3. Tennant F. S., Sorenson K., Day C.: Benefits of preparticipation sports examinations. J Fam Pract 13:287–288, 1981.
4. Feinstein R. A., Soileau E. J., Daniel W. A., Jr: A national survey of preparticipation physical examination requirements. Phys Sportsmed 16:51–59, 1988.
5. American Academy of Pediatrics, Committee on Sports Medicine: Sports Medicine: Health Care for Young Athletes. Evanston, IL: American Academy of Pediatrics, 1983.
6. DuRant R. H., Seymore C., Linder C. W., et al: The preparticipation examination of athletes: comparison of single and multiple examiners. Am J Dis Child 139:657–661, 1985.
7. Samples P: Preparticipation exams: are they worth the time and trouble? Phys Sportsmed 14:180–187, 1986.
8. Runyan D. K.: The preparticipation examination of the young athlete. Clin Pediatr 22:674–679, 1983.
9. Thompson T. R., Andrish J. T., Bergfeld J. A.: A prospective study of preparticipation screening examinations of 2670 young athletes: methods and results. Cleve Clin Q 49:225–233, 1982.
10. Linder C. W., DuRant R. H., Seklecki R. M., et al: Preparticipation health screening of young athletes: results of 1268 examinations. Am J Sports Med 9:187–193, 1981.
11. McKeag D. B.: Preparticipation screening of the potential athlete. Clin Sports Med 8:373–396, 1989.
12. Salem D., Isner J.: Cardiac screening for athletes. Orthop Clin North Am 11:687–695, 1980.
13. Shaffer T. E., Rose K. D.: Cardiac evaluation for participation in school sports. JAMA 228:398, 1974.
14. Maron B. J., Epstein S. E., Roberts W. C.: Causes of sudden death in competitive athletes. J Am Coll Cardiol 7:204–214, 1986.
15. Missri J. C., Swett D. D.: Marfan syndrome: a review. Cardiovasc Rev Rep 3:1645–1654, 1982.
16. Maron B. J., Bodison S. A., Wesley Y. E., et al: Results of screening a large group of intercollegiate competitive athletes for cardiovascular disease. J Am Coll Cardiol 10:1214–1221, 1987.
17. Maron B. J., Roberts W. C., McAllister H. A., et al: Sudden death in young athletes. Circulation 62:218–229, 1980.
18. Epstein S. E., Henry W. L., Clark C. E., et al: Asymmetric septal hypertrophy. Ann Intern Med 81:650–680, 1974.
19. Kapoor W. N., Karpf M., Wieand S., et al: A prospective evaluation and follow-up of patients with syncope. N Engl J Med 309:197–204, 1983.
20. Epstein S. E., Maron B. J.: Sudden death and the competitive athlete: perspectives in preparticipation screening studies. J Am Coll Cardiol l7:220–230, 1986.
21. Ekstrand J., Gillquist J.: Soccer injuries and their mechanisms: a prospective study. Med Sci Sports Exerc 15:267–270, 1983.
22. Goldberg B., Witman P. A., Gleim G. W., et al: Children's sports injuries: are they avoidable? Phys Sportsmed 7:93–101, 1979.
23. Lysens R., Steverlynck A., Van Den Auweele Y., et al: The predictability of sports injuries. Sports Med 1:6–10, 1984.
24. Abbott H., Kress J.: Preconditioning in the prevention of knee injuries. Arch Phys Med Rehabil 50:326–333, 1969.
25. Cahill B., Griffith E.: Effect of preseasoning conditioning on the incidence and severity of high school football knee injuries. Am J Sports Med 6:180–184, 1978.
26. Nicholas J. A.: Injuries to knee ligaments: relationship to looseness and tightness in football players. JAMA 212:2236–2239, 1970.
27. Moretz J. A., Walters R., Smith L.: Flexibility as a predictor of knee injuries in college football players. Phys Sportsmed 10:93–97, 1982.
28. Kalenak A., Morehouse C. A.: Knee stability and knee ligament injuries. JAMA 234:1143–1145, 1975.

29. Grana W. A., Moretz J. A.: Ligamentous laxity in secondary school athletes. JAMA 240:1975–1976, 1978.
30. Godshall R. W.: The predictability of athletic injuries: an eight-year study. Sports Med 3:50–54, 1975.
31. Glick J. M.: A study of ligamentous looseness in football players and its relation to injury. Abbott Proc 1:34–39, 1971.
32. Marshall W. A.: A longitudinal study of the injury potential of the collateral ligaments of college football players, thesis. University of Wisconsin, Madison, 1970.
33. American Academy of Pediatrics, Committee on Adolecence, Committee on Bioethics, and Provisional Committee on Substance Abuse: Screening for drugs of abuse. Pediatrics 84:396–398, 1989.
34. Pierson W. E.: Exercise-induced bronchospasm in children and adolescents. Pediatr Clin North Am 35:1031–1040, 1988.
35. Voy R. O.: The U.S. Olympic Committee experience with exercise-induced bronchospasm, 1984. Med Sci Sports Exerc 18:328–330, 1986.
36. Anderson S. D.: Exercise-induced asthma. In: Middleton E Jr, Reed CE, Ellis ET, et al, eds. Allergy—Principles and Practice. 3rd ed. St. Louis, MO: CV Mosby Co, 1988, 1156–1175.
37. Sly R. M.: History of exercise-induced asthma. Med Sci Sports Exer 18:314–317, 1986.
38. Godfrey S.: Exercise-induced asthma. In: Bierman CW, Pearlman DS, eds. Allergic Diseases from Infancy to Adulthood. 2nd ed. Philadelphia, PA: WB Saunders Co, 1988, 597–606.
39. Rice S. G., Bierman C. W., Shapiro G. G., et al: Indentification of exercise-induced asthma among intercollegiate athletes. Ann Allergy 55:790–793, 1985.
40. Chatam M., Bleecker E. R., Smith P. L., et al: A comparison of histamine, methacholine, and exercise airway reactivity in normal and asthmatic subjects. Am Rev Respir Dis 126:235–240, 1982.
41. Katz R. M.: Prevention with and without the use of medications for exercise-induced asthma. Med Sci Sports Exerc 18:331–333, 1986.
42. Goldberg B., Rosenthal P. P., Robertson L. S., et al: Injuries in youth football. Pediatrics 81:255–261, 1988.
43. Hafner J. K., Scott S. E., Veras C., et al: Interscholastic athletics: method for selection and classification of athletes. NY State J Med 82:1449–1459, 1982.
44. Backous D. D., Friedl K. E., Smith N. J., et al: Soccer injuries and their relation to physical maturity. Am J Dis Child 142:839–842, 1988.
45. Davidson R. G.: Atlantoaxial instability in individuals with Down syndrome: a fresh look at the evidence. Pediatrics 81:857–865, 1988.
46. American Academy of Pediatrics, Committee on Sports Medicine: Atlantoaxial instability in Down syndrome. Pediatrics 74:152–154, 1984.
47. Special Olympics Bulletin: Participation by individuals with Down syndrome who suffer from the atlantoaxial dislocation condition. Washington, DC, Special Olympics Inc, March 31, 1983.
48. American Academy of Pediatrics, Committee on Sports Medicine: Recommendations for participation in competitive sports. Pediatrics 81:737–738, 1988.
49. American Medical Association: Medical Evaluation of the Athlete: A Guide. rev ed. Chicago, IL: American Medical Association, 1976.

Part II

COMMON SPORTS INJURIES

7

PSYCHOSOCIAL ASPECTS OF SPORTS MEDICINE

ROBERT J. ROTELLA
JOHN HEIL

Team physicians and orthopedic surgeons have long realized the necessity of a wholistic approach to their patients. There is no getting around the basic fact that the mind and body work together and thus influence each other.

In recent years, it has become increasingly evident that psychosocial factors also play an important part in sports medicine. This chapter will discuss psychosocial issues considered important to physicians working with school-age athletes. These will include (1) stress and adolescent athletes, (2) burnout, (3) overuse injuries, (4) malingering athletes, (5) postoperative and postinjury adjustment, (6) drug use, (7) eating disorders, and (8) psycho-social-emotional issues related to injury, pain, and sport performance.

Work with school-age athletes presents a special challenge to physicians because of the extent to which consent for treatment rests with parents. The scope and intensity of parental involvement should generally decrease with increasing age of the athletes. However, it is easy to envision situations where there is a difficult balance to be struck between recognizing the confidentiality of patient communication, on one hand, and respecting the rights of parents as care taker of their children, on the other. It can be useful at times to think of parents as part of the treatment team. In contrast, parental behavior—in particular, from a psychological point of view—can be problematic to the extent that it may need to be a focus of treatment as well.

In work with athletes of any age, it is also important to consider the role of the coach. Because he or she is a great resource and a potential ally in the management of the athlete, it can be quite helpful to have the coach play an active role. However, in this situation as well as that with parents, similar concerns regarding confidentiality and benevolent disclosure can sometimes arise.

STRESS AND ADOLESCENT ATHLETES

In the world of sport the demand to perform is often the basic cause of stress. Stress typically occurs when a young athlete feels compelled or forced to perform to a standard or against a competitor that is perceived to exceed his or her capacity to perform. The stress that young athletes experience may lead to increased motivation and high-level performance. But it may also lead to burnout, overuse injuries, malingering, and/or drug and substance abuse. Whether the response is positive or negative often depends on the athletes' perceptions, their abilities to cope, and their physical and psychological abilities to meet demands and expectations.

Stress is probably far more prevalent in American society than most would care to admit. Desires to be successful and to achieve status, recognition, and acceptance can place a tremendous burden on parents and children alike. Children are less prepared for handling these demands effectively. In today's American society, even toddlers are not immune to the pervasive emphasis on striving for success and the impact of the associated values on how we perceive ourselves, our friends, and our performances. Children are commonly being overloaded by parents, coaches, teachers, and peers. They are being rushed into roles and responsibilities that many are not ready mentally and physically to handle. In many cases, young athletes are pushed to succeed before learning to enjoy the activity. It is only natural for athletes facing such experiences regularly to learn that winning is far more important than enjoying the game.

Clearly, the stress of competition alone can create an imbalance in the emotional well-being of young athletes, but the demands to win compound this emotional imbalance even further. It is easier for young athletes to accept competitive demands when the results are positive. Few adolescent athletes are prepared for losing on a regular basis. But even with regular success, there are often underlying stressors associated with performance expectations and demands to continue winning and improving. It is no longer enough to "try to win"; at this point, the athlete "has" to win or is expected to win. When repeated successes occur, others respond calmly as if it is no big deal—it is expected. But losses are responded to with "What's wrong?" As the pressure to win mounts, many times adolescent athletes cannot cope when unexplained losses occur. Such athletes often perceive themselves as not as good as people expected them to be, and soon they become afraid of losing. The problem is further exaggerated by the public scrutiny and evaluation that is a part of sport.

The inevitability of fatigue and injury creates additional stressors for young athletes. When athletes are fatigued or injured, exhortation by adults for that "extra effort" rarely brings about the desired result of improved performance. They simply cannot do more. Even greater problems occur when they try to do so in order to win approval from respected adults. The child's inability to distinguish between serious injuries and simple body fatigue at times will have youngsters competing despite pain and injuries. The inability simply to "shake off" the body's signal of pain is puzzling to the coach or parent who wants the youngster to do *better*. Such individuals often view the young athlete as a miniature professional who must be tough and play through pain and injury.

Some young athletes will leave their sport after experiencing regular pain. Others will simply lose interest or decrease motivation for their sport. Some will reject the values of their coaches or parents. Still others will push themselves twice as hard through pain, wishing to earn the respect and admiration of adults.

It is not unusual for young athletes to use fatigue or injury as a reason for poor performance. But most quickly learn that adults do not like excuses, and it is safer not to complain or mention it to them. For many highly motivated athletes, the fear of getting out of shape and losing ground to competitors drives them to refuse to rest or take time off from intense training to allow their bodies to heal. This response is usually reinforced by coaches and parents. All the problems just discussed are usually exaggerated when athletes choose to specialize in one sport in order to have an increased chance to excel.

BURNOUT

Burnout can be defined as a reaction to the stresses of athletic competition that can be characterized by feelings of emotional exhaustion or an impersonal attitude toward those the athlete associates with and decreased athletic performance. Simply put, such athletes are fed up with what they are doing and feel fatigued and frustrated as a result of persistent devotion to a cause that failed to produce an expected reward.

Burnout usually occurs in young athletes when an imbalance between environmental demands and response capabilities is experienced. Athletes cognitively assess the demands of their sport and the resources available. When athletes make a negative appraisal, they decide the costs outweigh the rewards. A typical response is that sport simply is not fun anymore.

Because he or she encounters the athlete in the acute injury situation, the team physician or orthopedic surgeon is often in the best position to detect the early signs of burnout in young athletes. Although one of the primary goals of sports medicine is restoring the athlete to competition, the physician must

TABLE 7–1. Burnout Avoidance

1. Keep sport fun.
2. Keep winning and losing in perspective.
3. Play at least one lifetime sport just for fun and recreation.
4. Take periodic breaks from practice and competition.
5. Remember it is productive to take time off from practice for even minor injuries.
6. When pain is experienced, be smart—rest, relax, rehabilitate, and wait before returning to competition.

avoid becoming one of the stressors placing demands on the young patient. The physician should be sensitive to the athlete who needs more time to recover psychologically and should adjust the pace of rehabilitation accordingly. Sometimes it will be necessary to reassure the burned-out athlete that "it's okay to be hurt." Table 7–1 lists many bits of advice the physician may give the overstressed athlete to avoid burnout.

Many athletes quit sports because they practice and play in constant pain and do not wish to live in pain or go through the daily rehabilitation procedures necessary in order to compete pain free. This may be a very wise and mature decision.

OVERUSE INJURIES

In today's highly competitive world of sport, it is common for youngsters to suffer from overuse injuries by the time the teenage years are reached. It is quite likely that overuse injuries will gradually appear at a younger age over the next 20 years as parents feel pressured to push their children into sport at increasingly younger ages.

Most overuse injuries appear in adolescent athletes who have focused their time, energy, and efforts into one particular sport. It is a common misperception that athletes must be single-minded in order to be highly successful. But this viewpoint persists and will likely continue to be a widely accepted view in a culture in love with the "work ethic," "self-sacrifice," and "paying the painful price of success."

Physicians play a most important role in helping athletes with overuse injuries. The physician as a highly respected professional has the ability to get adolescent athletes to back off, take a rest, engage in exercises utilizing typically unused body parts, or try a new sport.

Physicians should in particular be alert to danger signs likely to predispose young athletes to overuse injuries. These include the following:

- Extremely high levels of commitment
- Very dedicated
- Never misses practice
- Always sacrificing and paying the price of success
- Often try too hard in competition
- Perfectionistic
- Believe hard work is always the answer to success
- Self-worth is closely attached to their sport performance
- Brag about always being tough and pushing through pain
- Have a no-pain-no-gain attitude
- Always giving 110 percent effort
- Love and need approval constantly from coaches

When a physician realizes that an adolescent is suffering from overuse syndrome, the following should be done:

1. Take the time to discuss the problem with the coach, the athlete, and the parents.
2. Attempt to figure out why the problem is occurring:
   a. Is the athlete being worked too hard in practice? Too frequently?
   b. Is the athlete not physically ready?
   c. Is the athlete working too hard outside practice time?
   d. Has the athlete given up all other sports and thus overused certain body parts or muscle groups?
3. Make a specific plan that limits the number of hours per week the athlete is allowed to practice.
4. Decide if specific exercises must be done and do not allow the athlete to practice if these are not done.
5. Make a rest and relaxation plan that is just as important as the practice plan.
6. Emphasize the importance of reading early pain signals and responding to them appropriately.
7. Teach the athlete that success in sport requires knowing when to take time off, to take it easy, and to rest and allow the body to recover.

8. Make it clear that if changes are not made, the athlete may be forced to quit the sport.
9. Encourage the athlete to take up a recreational lifetime sport engaged in regularly just for fun.
10. Let the athlete choose the lifetime sport.
11. Meet alone with the athlete to find out if the athlete is in pain and wishes to quit but parents or coaches are pressuring him or her to continue.

THE MALINGERING ATHLETE

Athletes who malinger are typically quite challenging to orthopedic surgeons and team physicians. Such athletes present a dilemma. It is a challenge to determine whether the athlete is a malingerer or is truly hurt. "It is easy to think you are 90 percent sure one way or the other, but there is always the possibility that you are wrong, and it is a mistake you do not want to make. But like it or not, there is no way to ever know for sure."

The malingerer in sport—the athlete who intentionally lies about an injury in order to avoid practice or competition—has been a topic of interest to specialists in sports medicine for years.

While there are little empirical data available, case histories and personal experience provide helpful insight to understanding malingering athletes.

A HEALTHY PERSPECTIVE

Specialists in sports medicine should always begin with a viewpoint that trusts that athletes are telling them the truth about how their bodies feel. Snap judgments leading to a malingering label are a serious mistake. Develop a philosophy of considering an athlete to be a malingerer only as a last resort. No one should pretend they can identify a malingerer when they see one. There is no foolproof way of knowing for sure, but caring and concerned orthopedic surgeons and team physicians can learn from observing the repeated behavior of athletes that would logically lead them to suggest malingering to be a problem. When such a conclusion is reached *for the purpose of helping such athletes*, it can be appropriate and useful to do so.

THE WHY OF MALINGERING

The habit of malingering typically is a result of (1) a need for attention or (2) fears. For an array of reasons, the need for attention becomes a higher priority than the need to play. The malingerer seeks treatment with the goal of getting out of practice and/or competition and still receiving the desired attention, perhaps in the form of sympathy.

The true malingerer is a master at faking it. Pain and suffering can be displayed whenever necessary. Oftentimes the degree to which these presentations are overdone is the giveaway to the physician. Malingerers do not typically wish to wait in the wings. They want everyone to know they are hurt and if possible wish to stay the center of attention. It is often the unnatural and exaggerated response that allows malingering athletes to be identified and differentiated from athletes who have low pain thresholds or who have developed psychological sequelae to injury that complicate rehabilitation.

It must be clearly understood that, like other behaviors, malingering is simply a *learned* behavior. Experience has taught such athletes that malingering behaviors are acceptable. In the past, they have been rewarded for their behaviors, and now they malinger either willfully and intentionally or as a result of habit for clear gain. Either at home or in their sport environment, most malingerers were allowed to get away with lying and deceit. When caught they were typically given a second chance. Some malingerers are gifted athletes who have realized that most adults will let them get away with normally unacceptable behaviors because of their exquisite talents.

HELPFUL ADVICE

Strategies for helping malingerers vary as greatly as the causes, but it is always crucial to view each athlete on an individual basis. The following are basic suggestions for helping malingerers.

1. Take time to get to know and understand athletes.
2. Strive to develop a trusting relationship with athletes, particularly those who are initially most difficult to like, respect, and admire.

3. Do not take lies and manipulations by athletes personally—these are simply well-learned habits used on adults who show care and concern.

4. Attempt to reward such athletes with more attention when they are honest rather than dishonest—catch them being honest.

5. Avoid attacking or accusing the athlete of lying, but sit down with the athlete and confront this issue honestly and directly. Be sure to display empathy for the possibility of an undetected injury. Make it clear that the best interests of the athlete and team are the primary concerns. Let the athlete present his or her perspective and listen carefully. Encourage truth, honesty, and openness and call the athlete on obvious inconsistencies in behavior.

6. Remember that the better the relationship between athlete and physician in the adolescent years, the less likelihood of an athlete becoming a malingerer later in life.

7. Empathy promotes growth and positive development, whereas pity breeds weakness.

8. Malingering is done only if there is something to be gained from the behavior.

9. Honestly admit to the athlete that you are frustrated and confused in trying to understand the athlete's behavior and that you are receptive to any suggestions. Make it clear you are trying to determine if the athlete is afraid of playing and needs help managing stress and fear or if the athlete is seeking attention.

10. At some point, a malingering athlete must be given strictly defined boundaries for behavior and detailed consequences of stepping outside those boundaries. Make it clear that these steps are being taken for the best interests of the athlete and team. Reward desired behavior and withdraw rewards for malingering.

CONCLUDING THOUGHTS

Helping malingerers requires tremendous patience and understanding. But the long-term benefits of helping such athletes during the adolescent years are enormous. Orthopedic surgeons and team physicians must remember that some injuries have unusual or subtle signs and symptoms that even the best eye, hands, or modern equipment may not detect. Thus, while malingering may be suspected, the potential always exists that the athlete is in fact injured.

POSTOPERATIVE AND POSTINJURY ADJUSTMENT

ROUTINE MANAGEMENT

Injury is obviously disruptive both physically and emotionally. A dysphoric or "disorganized" emotional response to immediate loss and the threat of an uncertain future commonly occurs. Depression, anger, confusion, contradictory emotional response, and even denial may occur and can undermine the speed and thoroughness of recovery. It is recommended that the physician assess each patient on a "denial-distress-determination" continuum. *Denial* implies failure to recognize the severity of a given problem. *Distress* is the magnitude of emotional response that may be either appropriate to the severity of an injury or illness situation or relatively more exaggerated. *Determination* refers to determined purposeful motivation to return to optimal level of functioning.

The basis of any therapeutic relationship is careful listening and response to questions, both asked and implied. In particular, in working with athletes a strong goal orientation is an important aspect of treatment. Clearly stated goals help the athlete see the way back to recovery and help direct his or her determination in a purposeful and directive way (Danish, 1984). A rehabilitation program that contains clearly defined functional goals is not only medically sound but psychologically appropriate for the goal-oriented athlete. (See Table 17–2.) When the athlete is given specific functional criteria as requirements for returning to competition, the physician is removed from the adversarial role of the opponent who is keeping the athlete away from the activities he or she loves. Having intermediate goals as steps in the rehabilitation process also gives the athlete the reinforcement of accomplishment along the difficult path to complete recovery.

One additional consideration merits mention: As athletes develop their skills, they gain greater and greater mastery over themselves and their environment, cultivating a sense of control and even invulnerability. Injury renders the athlete vulnerable, especially where hospitalization occurs. The hospital environment is in many respects the antithesis of "personal control." Here management of such basic functions as sleep, voiding, and physical activity are often routinely taken over by treatment providers. Tim Kerr of the Philadelphia Flyers, who played through chronic injury and had to rehabilitate eventually through a series of protracted surgeries, in retrospect identified fear of anesthesia as one of his most difficult challenges related to injury (Cataldi, 1987).

LASTING DEFICITS

An injury that permanently limits the performance capabilities of the athlete is a tremendous challenge in psychological management. The prospect of unrealized athletic potential is frustrating not only for the athlete but for parents and friends as well as treatment providers. This situation presents the greatest risk of difficulties in emotional adjustment. Reliance on denial as a coping mechanism can be a management problem. As a general consideration, denial can be helpful when it allows the athlete to adjust gradually to loss. However, it becomes problematic when it interferes with recovery and adaptation to injury. In such situations, careful clinical judgment should prevail. It may be useful to delay presenting this difficult information to the athlete until it is ready to be "heard." Depending on the age of the athlete, it is helpful to consult the parents regarding the timing of the delivery of this message. In addition, it is important to realize that this can be a significant loss for the parents as well. Candid acknowledgment of one's own frustration with not being able to provide a better alternative to the athlete can often validate the athlete's feelings of frustration and help him or her work through their denial.

A strong goal orientation plays an important role here as well. Once athletes are made aware of lasting deficits, it becomes important to let them know as clearly as possible what they can do eventually in regard to sport and physical activity. It is also necessary to inform them in relatively specific details about the demands of rehabilitation. Where injury involves undergoing particularly complex, painful, or frightening procedures, some special measures may be taken. Providing careful description of procedures, allowing the athlete where possible to exercise some control over the situation (even when this is minimal), and encouraging utilization of existing coping mechanisms all can be quite helpful (Chapman and Turner, 1986). This process may be facilitated by formal involvement by a psychologist.

PROBLEMATIC ADJUSTMENT

Despite everyone's best efforts, problems in psychological adjustment to injury may occur, and ultimately, referral may be necessary. The best predictor before the fact is the existence of concurrent or chronic problems in psychological adjustment. The role of preexisting overtraining syndrome (marked by decreased performance, rapid onset of fatigue, emotional discord, and psychophysiological signs) in precipitating injury and complicating recovery should be considered (Ryan et al., 1983).

During the recovery process, pain problems that fail to respond to routine management acutely and pain that persists beyond natural healing are leading signs in the early identification of problems in rehabilitation. This is of greater concern where pain problems are accompanied by any of the following: poor compliance (including overdoing prescribed activity), inability to identify realistic goals for recovery, and evident difficulties in psychological adjustment.

While a "controversial" topic, it is important to note that pain is a complexly determined "sensory and emotional" response (as defined by the International Association for the Study of Pain, 1986). It is influenced by peripheral and central physiological factors as well as environmental ones. When pain problems occur, an initial important measure is reassurance of the athlete regarding the benign status of pain. At the same time, a particularly thorough goal orientation to all aspects of treatment (including medication use) should be instituted. This involves specification of rehabilitation measures on a "time contingent" versus "pain contingent" basis (Fordyce et al., 1986). For example, medications or modalities should be prescribed for use at specified times in accord with a prearranged schedule, as opposed to "for pain." The physician should, of course, thoroughly reevaluate the patient to detect any physical problem that is not being optimally treated.

Where initial efforts are not effective, prompt referral is indicated. This is particularly important because of the well-recognized role that early identification of difficulties in adjustment plays in eventual successful outcome. The longer the pain and related symptoms persist, the more likely they are to become enmeshed with psychological symptoms such as decreased confidence, fear of reinjury, sleep disturbance, and depression.

The management of pain presents challenges as well to the maintenance of a good patient-doctor relationship. As pain persists in apparent disproportion to injury, there is a tendency for the physician to question the athlete's sincerity or motivation. In contrast, the athlete may question both the clinical judgment and the personal concern of the treatment provider. As problematic as these reactions can be, they tend to arise quite naturally from the different points of view held by the physician and the athlete. The physician, of course, focuses on objective physical signs of medical stability. In contrast, pain colors the world of the athlete and evokes concerns regarding functional limitations.

As a final caution, it is important in prolonged pain to rule out persistent pain syndromes such as myofascial pain (which has been identified in children) (Fine, 1987) and reflex sympathetic dystrophy.

DRUG USE

Drug use is a national concern. There is ample evidence as well that it is seen in school-age athlete populations (College of Human Medicine, 1985). The use of performance-enhancement drugs in sport presents an added dimension to the more widely recognized "recreational" drug use problem. There is an additional aspect of problematic drug use to be noted. This occurs where narcotics and other psychoactive substances are utilized in the long-term management of benign pain states, usually with eventual significant deleterious effect.

Awareness of increasing anabolic-androgenic steroid use has prompted a position paper by the American College of Sportsmedicine (1984). While the effects of these and other ergogenic substances have been recognized, their use has been widely denounced as unethical by key bodies governing amateur sport (National Collegiate Athletic Association [NCAA] and International Olympic Committee [IOC]/U.S. Olympic Committee [USOC]). Growing concern has been directed to the health risks associated with steroid use (Lubell, 1989). Because patterns of athlete use (e.g., "stacking" or use of multiple steroid preparations) deviate from typical medical use, long-term risks may be greater than present knowledge indicates. The effects of anabolic steroids and other ergogenic aids are discussed in Chapter 4. Psychological dysfunction is being increasingly recognized as a side effect. Symptoms can include aggressiveness, mood inflation, poor judgment, and imperturbability. Psychosis may also be seen in steroid use. It appears that a significant percentage of heavy users suffer also from a withdrawal syndrome, although this needs further investigation.

In approaching athletes regarding evidence of steroid use, it is important to appreciate the demands of their particular world. As one moves up the ladder of achievement, the pressure to push limits and to take risks increases. Steroid use can often be perceived as a necessary element in athletic success. To be judgmental or moralizing in this situation could be detrimental to the athlete, although ethically it is clearly the responsibility of the physician or other treatment provider to discourage use.

The dilemma that a physician may face is that the patient who is using steroids is at a critical point in his or her career and is determined to continue use despite any side effects. To report the athlete to the authorities would undermine the patient-physician relationship and put the athlete's career and reputation in jeopardy. Even if this occurs, there is no guarantee that use may not be continued. The added irony is that others who are continuing to use may be spared the same exposure because they chose not to disclose this information and not to trust their physicians. In contrast, it is probably accurate to assume that the athlete could proceed toward his or her goal more safely if under medical supervision. Faced with these two alternatives, a sympathetic physician could choose to supervise the athlete, reasoning that steroids will be used anyway. In our opinion, this would be a mistake because to do so is to serve as an "enabler," that is, to assist the athlete in participating in an unethical drug behavior. While one can rationalize that a lot of athletes are doing it, to support the athlete in this way makes it easier to continue to use drugs and gives him or her an advantage (i.e., medical consultation and advice) over other athletes. At the same time, it essentially perpetuates the problem. At what point additional steroid-assisted strength gains provide diminishing returns with effort better directed toward technical skill or other elements of training remains unclear. Even if steroid use were safe and legal, at a given point in time it may not necessarily be in the best competitive interest of an athlete.

Steroid and other drug use, especially where there may be medical or psychological effects involved, presents a complex treatment situation that must be approached on an individual basis. While it is given that the physician and other health care providers must work in the best interest of the patient athlete, this does not necessarily imply disclosure of the problem situation to others. However, it is difficult to envision a situation where sharing of information regarding drug use with the parent of a "minor" child should not be part of the overall treatment plan. For more information on drug use, see Chapter 4.

EATING DISORDERS

Rising evidence over the frequency of eating disorders (anorexia nervosa and bulimia) has prompted concerns in the worlds of medicine (American College of Physicians, 1986) and sport (United States Olympic Committee, 1987) and been met with special publications designed to provide information about symptoms, etiology, and referral. Female athletes appear to be an "at risk" population for two reasons (Thompson, 1987). The first of these has to do with the strong "body" consciousness that arises owing to the demands of sport. While this may be of issue in any sport, it is most likely to be problematic where sport success relies on subjective evaluation of physical form (e.g., gymnastics and dance). In addition, the pressures of athletic performance may exacerbate eating disorders where there is already a tendency toward this behavior (Thompson, 1987). When injury and eating disorders exist simultaneously, the situation is further complicated.

The etiology and clinical management both from a medical and psychological point of view of this set of disorders is quite complicated. Anorexia is marked by low weight and disturbed body image, with the perception that one is obese held persistently in contrast to other evidence. It eventually shows a wide variety of metabolic changes including amenorrhea. While bulimics may be virtually of any weight, their behavior is characterized by a binge-purge cycle, the latter of which may include both self-induced vomiting and laxative abuse. While problematic, it is generally less severe than anorexia nervosa. However, metabolic problems and menstrual irregularities frequently are noted. As a consequence of the eventual health risks involved in eating disorders, it is likely that those suffering from this particular problem will be found more frequently in clinical settings. Of particular note is the increasing evidence of a link between musculoskeletal injuries and amenorrhea (Lloyd et al., 1986).

When eating disorders are discovered, it is suggested that psychological referral be arranged in the most personal and least threatening of ways while a supportive relationship is maintained. In general, confrontation and deprivation from athletic performance should be utilized with the greatest of caution because of their potential detrimental effects on treatment relationships as well as motivation for treatment.

PSYCHO-SOCIAL-EMOTIONAL ISSUES

As sport performance for adolescent athletes has become increasingly popular and success has become desirable, thinking effectively has become a difficult challenge. Team physicians and orthopedic surgeons can help athletes understand how to maintain a healthy perspective, to manage disappointment, and to deal with feelings of quitting that are likely to occur when faced with recurring injuries and the related pain.

KEEPING PERSPECTIVE

Athletes who are committed to their goals want what they want badly. As a result, emotions will be elicited when setbacks and disappointments occur. Certain emotions tend to overrule the intellect and logic. Events and perceptions are quickly blown out of perspective and self-motivation deteriorates.

When perspective is lost, athletes see the world as if they had blinders on, limiting their vision. Frequently, events are misperceived, and important and obvious realities are not noticed. Selective attention narrows in counterproductive and often self-protective ways. Events and behaviors of coaches, teammates, and team physicians are misinterpreted.

At this point, athletes increasingly lose perspective. They become more sensitive. Instead of thinking logically, athletes just react, as if ruled by emotion rather than reason. Soon even a slightly unpleasant encounter is exaggerated. Problems in sport rapidly spill over into life outside of sport. Concentration toward schoolwork is destroyed. Relationships with others deteriorate. Gradually, problems from sport are carried into all areas of life.

Some athletes turn inward and get lost inside themselves, feeling sorry for themselves or criticizing themselves. Others focus externally, blaming their problems entirely on others. Whatever the case, there is a tremendous energy drain and a mental distraction from previous goals. Personal and emotional survival becomes the dominant goal. A perceived loss of control over life or sport success is pervasive.

Athletes often comment: "I can't switch gears. It's as if someone else is flipping my switch and I can't focus on anything when I'm supposed to do so. It's as though my projector is running so fast I could never catch up. My head can't catch up to my emotions."

At some point, if perspective deteriorates too fully, instead of fighting to survive through a renewed commitment, survival is attained by escaping. Athletes feeling this way start not to care. Instead of trying harder or trying to do it all alone, athletes give up the fight and their attitude deteriorates rapidly.

Team physicians and orthopedic surgeons must be ready and willing to recognize these signs. They are the danger signs of lost perspective. Events and reactions to them will be blown out of proportion. However, the good news is that these behaviors primarily occur when people really care about something, be it sport or love of another person. Team physicians and orthopedic surgeons must react intelligently and help athletes once again develop a healthy perspective. Table 7–2 lists 10 suggestions the physician may offer the troubled athlete for help in maintaining perspective.

TABLE 7–2. Helpful Thoughts for Maintaining Perspective

1. *Accept that it is human to have problems.*
2. *Avoid overstating or understating the severity of the problem.* When problems are overstated, athletes tend to get frozen in their tracks. As a result, they procrastinate and fail ever to get started. If eventually they do get started, it is too late, and then there is reason for fearing failure, which makes it more difficult to take the crucial first step. Understating operates differently. It primarily leads to a carefree attitude that leads to a lack of preparation. It is easiest to manage problems effectively when athletes and coaches are able to honestly and accurately appraise problems.
3. *Accept personal responsibility.* When facing problems, it is easy to blame others, which is a first step to certain defeat. To avoid inappropriate excuse making, negative emotions such as anger, self-pity, or threat must be controlled.
4. *Keep an open mind.* There are numerous effective solutions to any problem as long as an open mind is available.
5. *Alter perceptions.* Throughout a career, it is necessary to turn problems into opportunities, stumbling blocks into stepping stones to success.
6. *Provide inspiration.* Overcoming problems can be inspirational if a problem is allowed to be a challenge or measure of the size of one's heart. This can make athletes feel special when they surpass the test of character.
7. *Renew commitment.* Problems are great opportunities to determine how badly athletes want success. A decision will have to be made. Will the problem be accepted to the point of giving in and giving up the fight? Or will confronting the problem head on lead to added enthusiasm and dedication?
8. *Maintain optimism.* It is when athletes are faced with problems that it is most crucial to stay positive in their belief that they will succeed. When problems appear, the wolves will come out and remind athletes that success is impossible. Others will provide the sympathy that weakens.
9. *Look to friends.* It is important to remind athletes to look to true friends for advice. Do not let pride get in the way. A friend will be honest and helpful.
10. *Turn to trained professionals.* When a problem cannot be worked out alone or with friends, it is best to turn to a coach, physician, or a sport psychologist for help, depending on the nature of the problem.

COMMITMENT AND DISAPPOINTMENT

Committed athletes are quite ambitious. Usually, the more ambitious they are, the more difficulties, discouragements, and disappointments they experience during their sport careers. But, in general, to ambitious athletes these disappointments are sources of strength, growth, and success, once they learn how to deal with them. It is only when ambition deteriorates to "blind ambition" and athletes react to impulse that serious problems occur. Rather than trying to work at what they are doing and trying to get better at it, athletes in such a state waste excessive energy. At this point, their blind ambition leads to constant impatience. There is little room for tolerant waiting. These athletes become increasingly torn and restless. This attitude destroys composure and eventually hinders confidence and motivation. Ambition must be modified and controlled if disappointments are to be useful.

Disappointments can be separated into two major categories ranging from global disappointments to everyday disappointments. Global disappointments have a tendency to become pathological. When people get depressed following a severe disappointment, they often are unable to reexamine the conflicts and issues that have preceded the disappointment. Athletes in this serious a mindset are unable to look clearly at anything. When this condition persists over several days or weeks, professional help from psychiatrists, psychologists, or mental health centers is necessary.

However, most disappointments experienced by committed athletes are of the everyday kind: an injury at a most inopportune time of year, a bad first half, not coming through in the clutch, losing in the last seconds. At least in team sports, athletes have teammates, coaches, athletic trainers, team physicians, friends, and fans to share in their disappointments.

This is one time where it is beneficial that sport is a public endeavor. Disappointed athletes never need to be lonely, even though some choose to be so. Some who do so make the choice for healthy soul searching, which involves honest self-evaluation, reexamination, and growth and strength for the future. Others who choose to be alone do so in order to sit alone and feel sorry for themselves. This can be an extremely seductive and momentarily pleasant feeling but is counterproductive in the long run.

Committed athletes want something. When they do not get it, the result is disappointment. But there is more to disappointment than not getting what is wanted. Why does it hurt so? An athlete's wants often have enormous unconscious value, and consequently, failure to get what is wanted takes on greater significance. The exaggerated significance given to the event commonly leads to self-reflection and evaluation that can result in emotionally based interpretations suggesting worthlessness and meaninglessness. Committed athletes frequently place so much importance on success and dream attainment that personal meaning and self-worth become dependent on successful results.

However, it is most intriguing that getting what is wanted can also lead to disappointment. Great disappointment and disillusionment commonly occur when athletes attain their dreams and realize that in fact the world does not suddenly stand still or come together and the unconscious dreams are not realized.

HOW TO MANAGE DISAPPOINTMENT

There is something about disappointment that causes most people to see disappointment as bad. It tends to be viewed as a negative, equal to failure. But disappointment is usually an essential to success. So it is the management of disappointment that determines whether disappointment will be positive or negative. Once athletes are able to see disappointment in positive terms, they can learn a great deal from the experience.

The second common misconception is that disappointment is never to be shown. In American society in general and especially in sport, individuals are taught to hide or deny disappointment, particularly in public. Success is the dominant theme, and nobody loves a loser. So most competitors are taught always to show a winning smile and an upbeat look even in the toughest of times. The cultural pressure encourages the "winner's mask."

Certainly athletes must realize that with few exceptions others will not provide a lot of sympathy or empathy. Most who do not have the same degree of wanting will not be able to identify with the level of disappointment. Teammates will often be too concerned with their own disappointment, whereas competitors will usually be too excited with their own joy or their personal struggles.

There are several specific ideas for effectively helping athletes to manage disappointment. A place to begin is to realize that directing rage at one's self or feeling excessive shame or humiliation for failing to measure up to expected standards are counterproductive. When athletes are disappointed, they are likely to be emotionally hyperactive, make poor decisions, and say or do things they later wished they had not. Because athletes do not usually know how to manage disappointment, they are likely to be confused because they do not know what to do.

In general, there are two ways in which people respond to disappointments: (1) withdraw from others to be alone to think or (2) interact with others. Athletes who respond by withdrawing become introspective and self-reflective. This can be a most effective response for those who use the time to work through their disappointments and find out something new about themselves (perhaps a flawed training regimen, strategy, or conditioning program or lost composure, concentration, or confidence) that can lead to improvement. Initially, most athletes are not very good at this response.

While treating physicians can help athletes through role modeling and honest, open discussions on how to respond in this manner to disappointments, they can perhaps do even more good by encouraging athletes to show their feelings in the privacy of the locker room or physician's office. Here disappointments can be shared and expressed without negative ramifications. This approach provides for mental and emotional health, brings a team closer together, prevents false images of invulnerability, and provides a healthy acceptance of the true human condition for tough-minded athletes. It also helps athletes clear their minds and emotions. This process helps keep disappointments in perspective and prepares athletes to face their family, friends, and the media.

As all effective athletes eventually discover when facing disappointments, it takes courage to look at life as it is and to see athletes as they really are. It is from coming to terms with these realities that athletes grow stronger and reconfirm their commitments.

Some additional words of advice for helping athletes with disappointments include the following:

- Congratulate yourself for feeling disappointed; it means you are growing.
- Disappointments make the joys feel more pleasing.
- Do not run away from disappointments. Take time to think about them and review your experience.
- Check to be sure disappointments are not a result of constant unrealistic expectations.
- Assign probabilities to your expectations so you can be prepared for what to expect and why.
- Do not confuse success and failure with being loved and not loved.
- Keep eyes open to dreams but desire to know your abilities and possible limits while continuing to reach higher.
- Do not let all self-respect and personal identity be dependent on sport success.
- Learn to accept other people's negative feelings.
- Like and value yourself regardless of performance.
- Accept human vulnerability.
- Build close relationships.
- Maintain conscious control over personal drives.
- Learn from disappointments.
- Remember that cynicism is the scar tissue of unresolved disappointment.
- Renew your commitments and enthusiastically start anew.

FEELING LIKE QUITTING

Probably one of the most often repeated clichés in the world of sport is: "Quitters never win, and winners never quit." Dogged, unrelenting tenacity is a necessary aspect of commitment, but it must be realized that quitting is not the opposite of winning—it is part of winning. All committed people have moments when they feel like quitting.

A wise person long ago once said that it is easier to start a love affair than to end one. Similarly, in sport sometimes athletes have to quit, and sometimes it is the hardest but most important thing to do. Thankfully, because of the difficulty and the attachment to sport, committed athletes do not quit easily or readily.

Even the most highly committed of athletes at times let repeated injuries and the demands of rehabilitation take control over them. When this happens, athletes question their commitment, wonder about the meaning or value of sport, and ponder whether the time invested in sport and the other interests sacrificed, opportunities passed up, and social activities missed were worth it. Feeling like quitting is a normal human reaction to these thoughts. Those who maintain their commitment are the athletes who recognize the desire everyone has to quit when faced with adversity and develop ways for dealing with it.

For many athletes, the first impulse when things are not going well is to think: "There is no sense in continuing." "I quit." "It's not worth it." "I'll never get it right." The pressures to succeed from outside sometimes get to athletes. This is precisely when athletes must learn to control their *own* attitude rather than letting fan or social pressures control their attitudes. Occasionally, the athlete's best answer is to quit; other times, it is not.

Usually when in this state athletes are confused and unable to look at all the important issues. Team physicians must calmly and objectively help athletes decide what it is they want and how to get it. Too many adults respond to athletes who mention quitting (especially talented athletes) by getting angry, challenging their courage, and calling them names, hoping to shame them into returning. What athletes need from mature minds at such times is sensitivity, caring, understanding, and clear-thinking common sense. They do not need to hear they have a "bad" attitude. They need to consider what the results of quitting will be. How will they feel? What will they do with themselves? What are the advantages and disadvantages of quitting and continuing? No one else can answer these questions for individual athletes. At times, the answer is a few days or a week off. Other times, simply talking it out with an admired friend is all that is needed.

Whatever the case, most committed athletes feel like quitting every so often. A few actually quit and soon become committed to another endeavor. But the majority respond by quickly renewing their commitment with a fresh perspective on themselves and their sport. They usually continue with twice as much enthusiasm, feeling like real winners. These athletes realize that the closer they are to attaining their dreams, the more frustrated they will get and the stronger will be the urge to quit.

References

1. American College of Physicians (1986). Eating disorders: Anorexia nervosa and bulimia. Philadelphia, PA: American College of Physicians.
2. American College of Sportsmedicine (1984). Physicians stand on the use of anabolic-androgenic steroids in sports. Medicine and Science in Sports and Exercise, 19(5), 534–539.
3. Bandura, A. (1977). Self-efficacy: Toward a unifying theory of behavioral change. Psychological Review, 84, 191– 215.
4. Chapman, C. R. & Turner, J. A. (1986). Psychological control of acute pain in medical settings. Journal of Pain and Symptom Management, 1(1), 9–20.
5. College of Human Medicine (June 1985). The substance use and abuse habits of college student-athletes: Research paper #2: General findings. Michigan State University, East Lansing, MI.
6. Cook, D. & Tricker, R. (Eds.) (1989). Athletes at risk: Drugs in sport. Dubuque, IA: W. C. Brown.
7. Danish, S. (1984). Psychological aspects in the care and treatment of athletic injuries. In P. E. Vinger & E. Hoerner (Eds.), Sports injuries—the unthwarted epidemic (2nd ed.). Littleton, MA: PSG Publishing Co., Inc.
8. Dishman, R. K. (1982). Compliance/adherence in health-related exercise. Health Psychology, 1, 237–267.
9. Feigley, D. A. (1984). Psychological burnout in high-level athletes. Physician and Sportsmedicine, 12(10), 109–119.
10. Fender, L. K. (1989). Athlete burnout: Potential for research and intervention strategies. Sport Psychologist, 3, 63–71.
11. Fine, P. G. (1987). Myofascial trigger point pain in children. Journal of Pediatrics, 111, 547–548.
12. Fordyce, W. E., Brockway, J. A., Bergman, J. A., & Spangler, D. (1986). Acute back pain: A control-group comparison of behavioral versus traditional management methods. Journal of Behavioral Medicine, 9(2), 127–140.
13. Freudenberger, H. J. & Richelson, G. (1981). Burnout: How to beat the high cost of success. New York: Bantam Books.
14. Gould, D. (1987). Understanding attrition in children's sport. Advances in Pediatric Sport Sciences, 2, (4), 61–85.
15. International Association for the Study of Pain (ISAP) Subcommittee on Taxonomy (1986). Classification of chronic pain: Descriptions of chronic pain syndromes and definitions of pain terms. In H. Merskey (Ed.), Pain (Suppl. 3), S28–S30.
16. Kareszty, A. (1971). Overtraining. In L. Larson (Ed.), Encyclopedia of sport sciences and medicine (pp. 218–222). New York: Macmillan Publishing Co.
17. Lloyd, T., Trianthafyllou, S. T., Baker, E. R., Houts, P. S., Whiteside, J. A., Kalenak, A., & Stumpf, P. G. (1986). Women athletes with menstrual irregularity have increased musculoskeletal inju-

ries. Medicine and Science in Sports and Exercise, 18(4), 374–379.
18. Locke, E. A., Shaw, K. N., Saari, Z. M., & Latham, G. P. (1981). Goal setting and task performance: 1969–1980. Psychological Bulletin, 90, 125–152.
19. Lubell, A. (1989). Does steroid abuse cause—or excuse—violence? Physician and Sportsmedicine, 17(2), 176–185.
20. Maslach, C. & Pines, A. (1977). The burnout syndrome. Child Care Quarterly, 6, 100–114.
21. Morgan, W. P. & Brown, D. R. (September 1983). Diagnosis, prevention, and treatment of athletic staleness. Paper presented at the USOC Sports Medicine Councils' Workshop, Long Beach, CA.
22. Ogilvie, B. & Tutko, T. (1966). Problem athletes and how to handle them. London: Pelham Books.
23. Rotella, R. (1988). Psychological care of the injured athlete. In D. N. Kuland (Ed.), The injured athlete (pp. 213–224). Philadelphia: J. P. Lippincott Co.
24. Rotella, R. J. & Bunker, L. K. (1987). Parenting your superstar. Champaign, IL: Leisure Press.
25. Rotella, R. J. & Heyman, S. R. (1986). Stress, injury, and the psychological rehabilitation of athletes. In J. Williams (Ed.), Applied sport psychology. Mountain View, CA: Mayfield Publishing Co.
26. Ryan, A. J., Brown, R. L., Frederick, E. C., Falsetti, H. L., & Burke, E. R. (1983). Overtraining of athletes. A round table. Physician and Sportsmedicine, 11(6), 93–100.
27. Shank, R. H. (1988). Academic and athletic factors related to predicting compliance by athletes to treatments. Unpublished doctoral dissertation. University of Virginia, VA.
28. Smith, N., Smith, R., & Snroll, F. (1983). Kidsport: A survival guide for parents. Reading, MA: Addison-Wesley Publishing Co.
29. Smith, R . E. (1986). Toward a cognitive-affective model of athletic burnout. Journal of Sport Psychology, 8, 36–50.
30. Stuart, R. B. (1982). Adherence, compliance, and generalization in behavioral medicine. New York: Brunner/Mazel, Inc..
31. Thompson, R. A. (1987). Management of the athlete with an eating disorder: Implication for the sport management team. Sport Psychologist, 1, 114–126.
32. United States Olympic Committee (1987). Sports nutrition: Eating disorders. Colorado Springs, CO: United States Olympic Committee.
33. Cataldi, A. "Tim Kerr turns to family in a season that never was," Philadelphia Inquirer, December 24, 1987, D1–D3.

8
MUSCLE STRAINS AND CONTUSIONS

WILLIAM E. GARRETT, JR.
JOHN LOHNES

Muscle strains and contusions are among the most frequent sports injuries treated by medical personnel. However, there are a relatively small number of basic science and clinical studies to guide the treatment of muscle injuries, particularly in the growing child. This contrasts sharply with the much larger knowledge base for treating bone, articular cartilage, and ligament injuries. This chapter will first review the basic anatomy of muscles and muscle injuries, with particular reference to the growing child. The evaluation and treatment of muscle strains and contusions will then be discussed, with emphasis on the prevention of these injuries.

ANATOMY OF THE MUSCLE-TENDON UNIT

An accurate understanding of the anatomy of muscles and muscle injuries is essential for accurate diagnosis and treatment. Muscle generally originates from bone through a tendon or dense connective tissue and passes distally via tendon into a bony insertion. This musculotendinous unit can pass across one, two, or more joints, and it may have several shapes. Muscles that span two or more joints are typically less effective in producing tension throughout a range of motion than are single-joint muscles. In the lower extremity, two-joint muscles are situated more superficially, thus enhancing their phasic activities. An example is the gastrocnemius. Postural muscles are situated more deeply and are typically broad and flat, facilitating their function. This structural arrangement is illustrated by the soleus.

In children the tendon insertions on long bones may be near the relatively weaker epiphyseal plates, so that injuries normally resulting in musculotendinous strain in an adult will cause bone and growth plate damage in a child. During the adolescent growth spurt, the elongation of muscles tends to lag sightly behind the growth of long bones, presumably resulting in less flexibility during this period. Micheli and Smith[13] have suggested this may be an important predisposing factor for injury.

Individual muscles are frequently described by their fiber orientation, for example, pennate or fusiform (Fig. 8–1). The structure is closely related to its functional requirements. The amount of force a muscle can generate is proportional to the cross-sectional area of the fibers. The amount of shortening possible in a muscle is proportional to the length of the muscle fibers. The architectural arrangement of a muscle will therefore determine its biomechanical abilities. For example, the same muscle mass can be arranged in long parallel fibers or in shorter fibers of an increased number. The muscle with long parallel fibers will have more ability to shorten, and the muscle with more and shorter fibers will have the capacity for more force production and less shortening ability.

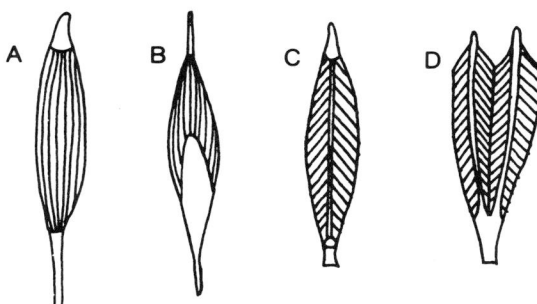

FIGURE 8–1. Fusiform (*A*), unipennate (*B*), bipennate (*C*), and multipennate (*D*) muscle architecture.

Individual fibers are grouped into small bundles known as *fascicles*. Usually, fascicles are not aligned parallel to the muscle axis but run obliquely from origin to insertion. It is important to recognize that frequently there may be tendons of origin and insertion running a considerable portion of the total length of the musculotendinous unit, thus providing musculotendinous junction throughout the length of the muscle belly.

In children, muscular strength increases gradually throughout the growing period as body size and long bone length increases. Growth of skeletal muscle results primarily from fiber hypertrophy rather than fiber hyperplasia. The amount of growth of skeletal muscle is determined by genetic factors, nutrition, and activity. Exercise appears to have a stimulating effect on growth of local muscle tissue in children after age 7.[12] In adults and postpubescent males, there is a marked ability of muscle fibers to hypertrophy in response to strength training. However, in prepubescent children, there is far less ability to hypertrophy even though the strength can increase considerably in response to training.[18]

Muscle fibers are divided into two types, based on structural, physiological, and metabolic differences. Type I fibers, also called *slow-twitch fibers*, respond more slowly to a motor nerve stimulus and are more resistant to fatigue. Type II fibers, or *fast-twitch fibers*, generate a peak tension more quickly than type I but are more subject to fatigue. Type II fibers are subdivided into type IIa and type IIb. Type IIa is somewhat intermediate between type I and type IIb, being fast contracting but also more resistant to fatigue than type IIb. Human muscles are made up of mixtures of these fiber types. In general, muscles with similar functions have similar fiber types. The deep tonic or postural muscles have more type I fibers. In contrast, the phasic, faster-contracting muscles have a higher proportion of type II fibers. Muscles at risk for strain injury often contain a higher percentage of type II fibers.

The composition of muscle fibers varies greatly from person to person. In a population of people, it would not be unusual to see proportions ranging from 90 percent type I fibers to 10 percent type I fibers in a vastus lateralis muscle biopsy. It is generally felt that persons with a higher proportion of type I fibers are intrinsically at an advantage in endurance sports, whereas a higher proportion of type II fibers might be advantageous in speed sports. Training can produce type I or type II fiber–type conversions in laboratory experiments or in extreme training programs. However, type IIa and type IIb conversions seem to occur more readily in response to more usual training regimens.

The growth and differentiation of muscle fibers are directed by utilization as the central and peripheral nervous system matures. The percentage of type I fibers appears to increase in children after infancy and may be the basis for the increasing muscular endurance observed with increasing age in young children.[23]

PATHOPHYSIOLOGY OF MUSCLE STRAIN

MECHANISM

Muscle strain is an indirect injury to muscle related to excessive stretch caused by antagonistic muscles, gravity, or external objects or by tension produced by active muscular contraction. These injuries are quite common in athletes and are sometimes called *muscle pulls, muscle tears,* or *muscle ruptures*. Most of these injuries have been found to occur in biarticular muscles, with a high percentage occurring in type II muscle fibers. The injuries frequently involve an eccentric contraction, thus stretching the active and passive components of the muscle-tendon unit. Although these injuries are common, few clinical or research studies have been conducted addressing the pathology and rehabilitation of these injuries, particularly in the pediatric and adolescent population.

An important distinction must be made between the muscle strain and tendinous lesion. Muscle injury is typically the result of macrotrauma. This type of injury is the result of a single event, the magnitude of which causes immediate clinical signs and symptoms. This is in contrast to the tendinous lesion, which is more frequently caused by microtrauma. Microtrauma is related to submaximal loading that eventually produces clinical signs and symptoms. Clinically, the majority of strains are partial and do not involve a complete disruption of the musculotendinous unit. Although this is the most common clinical injury, it is difficult to simulate in the animal model. Therefore, there are a limited number of studies on this topic.

Experimental studies of muscle strain injuries have been done in recent years, and these studies have increased our understanding of muscle strain injury.[15] Rabbit and rat models have been used most commonly. Hindlimb muscles have been mounted on biomechanical testing devices. Injury can be produced by stretching the muscle. Enough stretch will cause disruption of the muscle-tendon unit, with the tear occurring near the muscle-tendon junction.[15] The muscle can be activated by motor nerve stimulation, and stretch can be applied to simulate eccentric contractions. The length change and force developed before muscle failure do not change greatly with muscle activation. However, a contracting muscle can absorb much more energy prior to failure than a passively stretched muscle.[5] These data reinforce the concept that muscles act as energy absorbers in protecting themselves as well as bone and joint structures. Stronger muscles can absorb more energy than weak muscles. Similarly, fatigued muscles with their concomitant strength decrement are unable to absorb as much energy as nonfatigued muscles.

BODY RESPONSE TO MUSCLE STRAIN

The immediate response to the injury is an inflammatory sequence, characterized more by edema than bleeding. Bleeding occurs with many severe muscle strains. Ecchymosis and subcutaneous bleeding are sometimes present. However, studies using computed tomography have shown that the predominant response to muscle tissue in acute strains is a pattern of edema or inflammation.[5] The bleeding often escapes from the muscle and into the confined fascial compartment or actually into the subcutaneous space.

Experimental studies in rabbits have demonstrated the response of muscle to injury. The histology of healing muscle strains follows a characteristic sequence. The fibers have been observed to disrupt near the muscle-tendon junction (Fig. 8–2). In the study by Nikolaou et al.,[15] histological changes were not seen further away at the middle of the fiber even though the distal fiber was disrupted. The syncytial nature of muscle fibers is thought to ensure fiber viability even though the terminal portions of the fibers are disrupted. Hemorrhage is evident in the acute phase, surrounding the ruptured ends of the fibers. However, no large collection of blood or hematoma was seen experimentally, although the hemorrhage can escape from between the muscle fibers to elevate and collect under the epimysium.

Over the subsequent days, a typical cellular response to injury occurs. The disrupted fibers show changes of necrosis near the muscle-tendon junction. Macrophages can be seen within the disrupted fibers (Fig. 8–3). Inflammatory cells are prominent by the first day after injury and even more so by the second day (Fig. 8–4). The inflammatory reac-

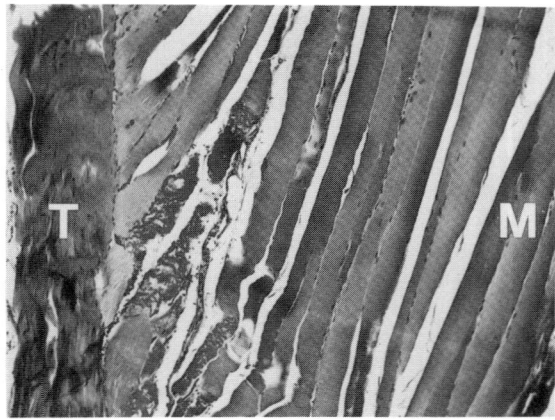

FIGURE 8–2. Histological appearance of rabbit tibialis anterior muscle immediately following strain injury. Limited rupture of distal fibers is seen along with hemorrhage. *T*, tendon; *M*, intact muscle fiber. (From Nikolaou, P. K., McDonald, B. L., Glisson, R. R., et al.: Biomechanical and histological evaluation of muscle after controlled strain injury. *Am. J. Sports Med.* 15:9–14, 1987.)

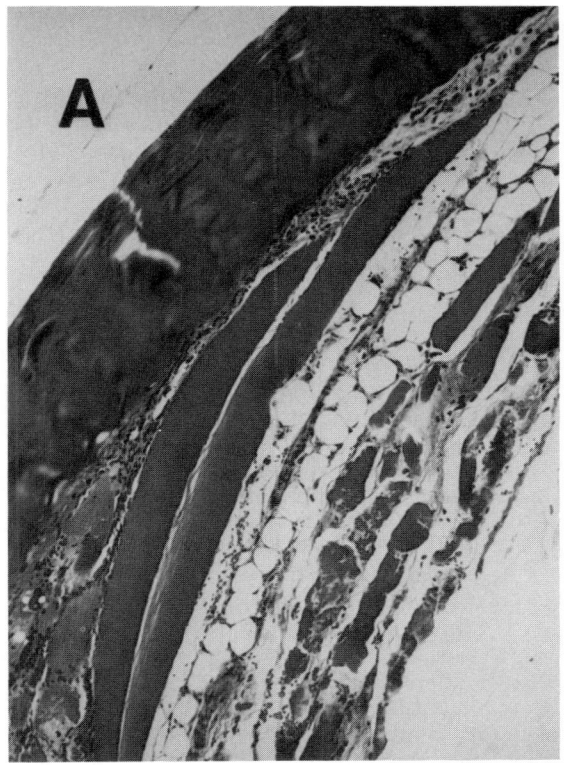

FIGURE 8–3. Histological appearance of rabbit tibialis anterior muscle (A) 24 hours after controlled strain. Image demonstrates muscle fiber necrosis with inflammation and hemorrhage. (From Nikolaou, P. K., McDonald, B. L., Glisson, R. R., et al.: Biomechanical and histological evaluation of muscle after controlled strain injury. *Am. J. Sports Med.* 15:9–14, 1987.)

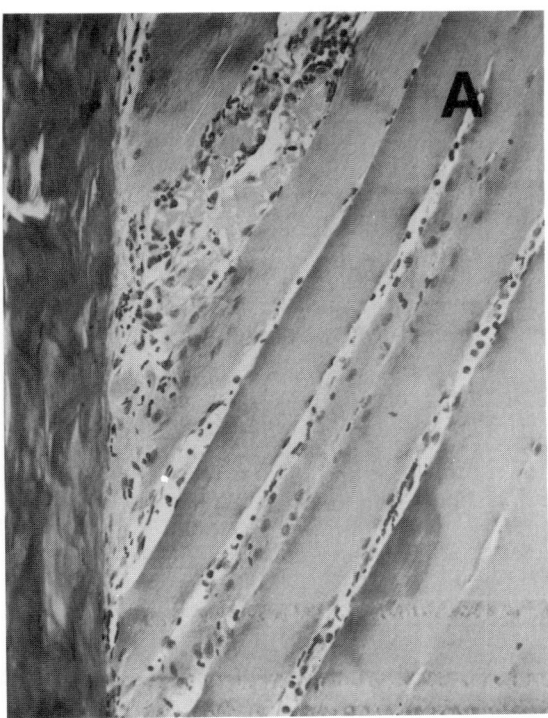

FIGURE 8–4. Histological appearance of rabbit tibialis anterior muscle (A) 48 hours after controlled strain injury, showing complete breakdown of muscle fibers and proliferation of inflammatory cells and fibroblastic activity at the myotendinous junction. (From Nikolaou, P. K., McDonald, B. L., Glisson, R. R., et al.: Biomechanical and histological evaluation of muscle after controlled strain injury. *Am. J. Sports Med.* 15:9–14, 1987.)

tion is most intense near the region of muscle fiber disruption, although the edema spreads further.

After the initial inflammatory changes, the cellular processes show a clearing of the necrotic muscle fibers and a proliferation of granulation tissue with fibroblasts, capillaries, and residual inflammatory cells (Fig. 8–5). Muscle regeneration processes are evident with myotube formation and fibrosis. An increase in fibrosis becomes more prominent between the fourth and eleventh day, with an increase in the connective tissue between the fibers and near the muscle-tendon junction.

AVULSION FRACTURES

In skeletally immature children, the epiphyseal plate is often less resistant to tensile forces than the muscle-tendon unit, resulting

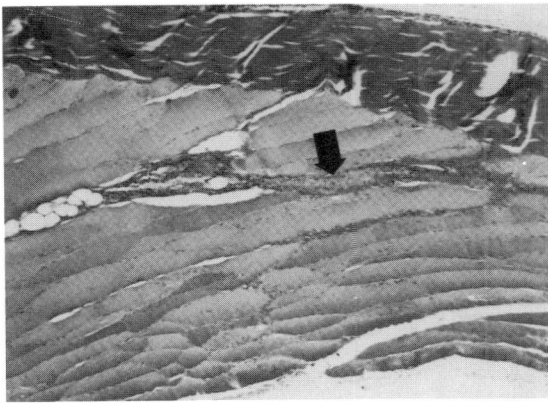

FIGURE 8–5. Histology of rabbit tibialis anterior muscle 7 days after controlled strain injury. Resolution of edema, hemorrhage, and inflammation with striking fibrotic changes localized to the site of injury (*arrow*) can be seen. (From Nikolaou, P. K., McDonald, B. L., Glisson, R. R., et al.: Biomechanical and histological evaluation of muscle after controlled strain injury. *Am. J. Sports Med.* 15:9–14, 1987.)

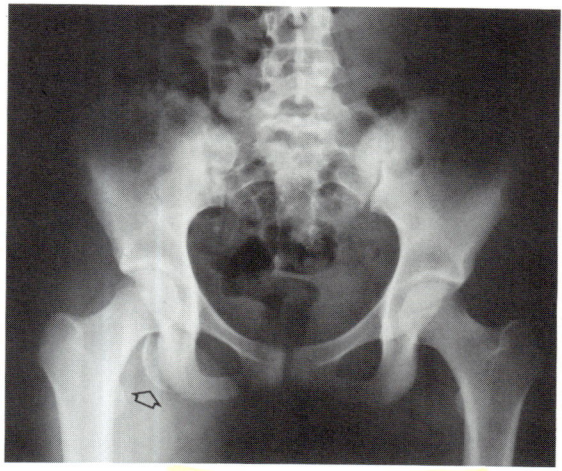

FIGURE 8–6. Avulsion of ischial apophysis in 14-year-old girl. (From Permanent Teaching File, Department of Radiology, Duke University Medical Center, Durham, NC.)

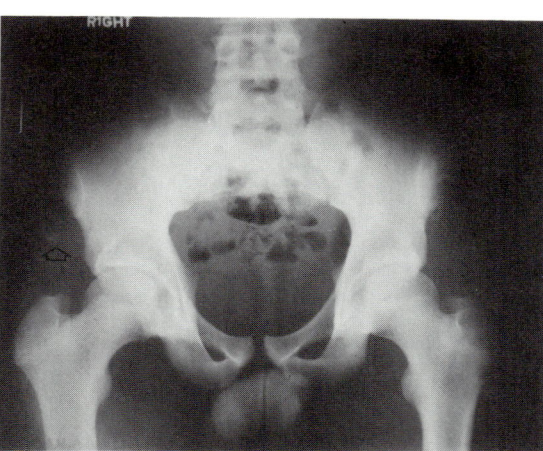

FIGURE 8–8. Bilateral avulsions of anterior superior iliac spines in a 15-year-old sprinter. (From Permanent Teaching File, Department of Radiology, Duke University Medical Center, Durham, NC.)

in avulsion fractures rather than muscle strain. These may occur before the appearance of secondary ossification centers. Avulsion fractures are particularly common in muscles originating on the pelvis and proximal femur and typically include injuries to the sartorius, rectus femoris, gluteus, iliopsoas, adductor longus, and hamstrings (Figs. 8–6 through 8–9). However, any tendinous origin or insertion may be involved.

The diagnosis should be confirmed by follow-up radiographs as callus forms. Significant displacement is unusual, but in rare cases, surgical reattachment of the avulsed bone and tendinous insertion or origin may be indicated if the fragment is large or there is instability or loss of function. Examples in which reattachment is appropriate include avulsion of the medial epicondyle of the elbow and avulsion of the tibial tubercle.

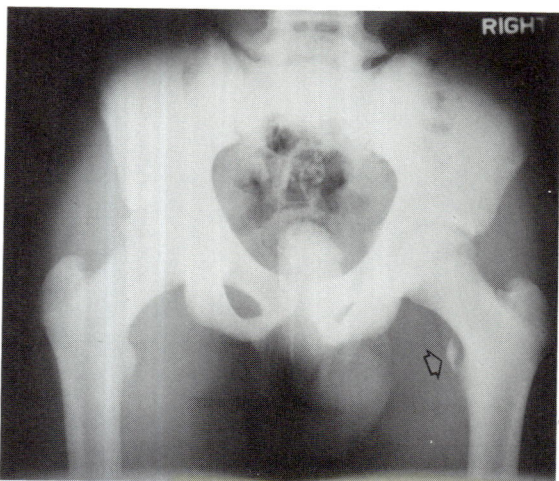

FIGURE 8–7. Avulsion of iliopsoas insertion on femur. (From Permanent Teaching File, Department of Radiology, Duke University Medical Center, Durham, NC.)

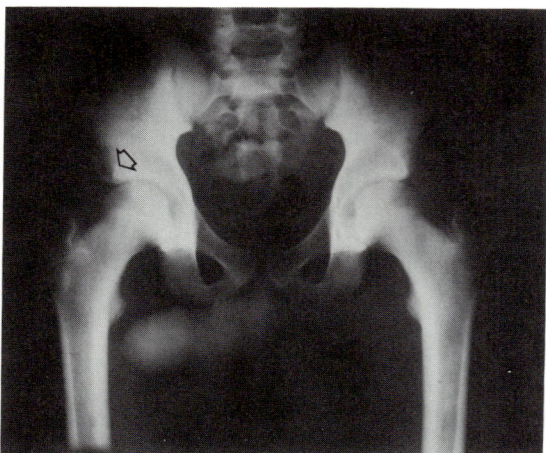

FIGURE 8–9. Avulsion of anterior inferior iliac spine in a 13-year-old. (From Permanent Teaching File, Department of Radiology, Duke University Medical Center, Durham, NC.)

GRADING OF MUSCLE STRAINS

Muscle strains are generally graded from I to III. In grade I strains, a small number of muscle fibers are crushed or torn, with the surrounding fascia remaining intact. The disruption of fibers is usually microscopic. There is pain with isolated resistance testing of the specific muscle and point tenderness at the site of strain. Some swelling or ecchymosis may be detectable during the first 24 hours.

Grade II muscle strains involve a large number of torn fibers. The fascia may also be torn. There is partial tearing or rupture of the musculotendinous junction. The athlete may feel a "pop" or tearing sensation, and a slight defect in the muscle is often palpable.

Grade III injuries involve complete rupture of the muscle. There is severe pain at the time of injury, and a defect is palpable. Muscle function is lost.

TREATMENT OF MUSCLE STRAINS

Treatment of muscle strains should be administered with an understanding of the anatomy of the particular muscle injured, the severity of injury, and the sequence of healing following partial (grade I and II) muscle tears described earlier.

Ice and a compression wrap are indicated during the first few hours following injury to control bleeding and edema. Nonsteroidal antiinflammatory medications have been shown to be effective in controlling the inflammatory response and associated pain during the first few days.[16] Although oral corticosteroids are effective in controlling inflammation, the side effects of their use in children for short doses has not been investigated thoroughly, and they should not routinely be the first line of antiinflammatory medication.

Immobilization may be indicated for comfort and protection during the first day or two following injury. However, prolonged immobilization is not necessary or desirable for successful healing to occur. Immobilization results in muscle atrophy and diminished ability to produce force. Long-term immobilization of a muscle in a flexed or extended position results in a deletion or addition of sarcomeres at the muscle-tendon junction to adapt to the new length. (A similar mechanism is responsible for the increased length of the developing muscle as it is stretched by growing bones.) One biomechanical study investigating the passive properties of immobilized rabbit muscle found that muscle immobilized in a shortened position developed less force and stretched to a shorter length before tearing than did the nonimmobilized contralateral control muscle.[10] Muscle immobilized in a lengthened position required more force and change in length before a tear occurred. Therefore, if immobilization is indicated for severe strains owing to pain, the position should be such that the muscle is lengthened. Generally, however, gentle passive range of motion should be started soon after muscle injury, followed by controlled active motion and stretching.

For grade I injuries, ice and compression should be applied for 30 minutes to 1 hour following injury. An oral nonsteroidal antiinflammatory medication should be given and continued for 5 to 7 days. A protective wrap may be appropriate. Active stretching should be begun the next day with controlled range of motion, passively at first within a pain-free range, then each day progressing to more active exercise including pool walking and stationary bike riding.

After muscle contraction is no longer painful, the athlete should begin a strengthening program before returning to functional activities. A common error in rehabilitation is to allow return to sport as soon as pain resolves. However, during the healing phase, muscle atrophies and weakens significantly during just a few days. Therefore, strength training using isokinetic equipment to isolate the involved muscle group should be an important part of rehabilitation to avoid reinjury. An appropriate muscle strengthening program for children will be discussed below. Although muscle reinjury is common, it is actually rare for reinjury to occur in a controlled rehabilitation program. Most reinjuries seem to occur following a premature return to sport or competition.

Grade II injuries require ice and compression for at least 1 hour. An oral corticosteroid taper can be given for severe injuries. From the beginning, motion and stretching should be performed within tolerable ranges. Gentle active exercise may be started when active contraction is painless, again followed by a strength program before resumption of sport.

Some grade III complete tears may be repaired if the muscle avulses from bone or if there is sufficient tendon left on the proximal and distal segments. This situation can exist in pectoralis ruptures. Again, avulsion fracture should be strongly suspected in children. Certain muscle ruptures do not require surgical repair, as the remaining muscles in the group will hypertrophy to compensate without noticeable loss of function.

EVALUATION AND TREATMENT OF SPECIFIC MUSCLE STRAINS

QUADRICEPS

Strains of the quadriceps generally involve the rectus femoris, which is the only two-joint muscle in this group. The injury is usually caused by a sudden, eccentric contraction while jumping or kicking. The athlete may feel a tearing sensation in the anterior thigh and experience subsequent swelling and tenderness. The grade of injury should be assessed to distinguish partial from complete disruption. A complete rupture usually occurs at the distal muscle-tendon junction. Clinically, a quadriceps contraction will cause a bulge in the proximal thigh. With complete disruption, early range of motion can be encouraged as soon as possible using antiinflammatory medicines to control pain and inflammation. Surgical repair is rarely indicated, as the other quadriceps muscles develop to compensate for the deficit.

With partial tears, the major concern is preventing reinjury and complete disruption due to the decreased tensile strength that occurs following injury. Rehabilitation should be progressive and sport specific. Passive and active range of motion and stretching should be started early, progressing to walking, pool running, and jogging. Isokinetic strength training is a helpful adjunct, beginning at higher functional velocities (300 degrees per second) and progressing to lower velocities requiring greater torque (60 degrees per second).

HAMSTRINGS

The hamstring muscles also span two joints and are prone to eccentric strain as decelerators of the lower leg during sprinting and kicking. The athletes most at risk are sprinters, kickers, and "tight-jointed" individuals. Any of the three hamstrings may be injured, but the long head of the biceps femoris is most commonly affected.[5] Occasionally, the tear may be complete. The healing of hamstring strains can be slow, and the treatment program is a delicate balance between measures designed to allow quick return and those necessary to avoid reinjury. It is probably best carried out with the close supervision of a therapist or trainer. Initial treatment involves ice, compression, and antiinflammatories, with weight bearing as tolerated, usually avoiding immobilization. Range of motion can be restored by static stretching and electrical stimulation, if available. Early functional exercises include jogging, pool running, and stationary biking. Strengthening includes resistive isokinetics, prone leg curls and hip extension with the knee flexed and extended, and backward running. Eccentric training rehabilitation may be helpful (Fig. 8–10).

GASTROCNEMIUS

Usually the medial head of the gastrocnemius is strained or ruptured. The athlete may feel a pop or feel as if he or she has been struck in the calf. Rupture of the Achilles' tendon should be ruled out, although this is rare in children. A gastrocnemius strain usually occurs much more proximally. Following acute treatment with ice and antiinflammatories, range of motion and strengthening should be carried out as with other strains. A heel wedge in the shoe is sometimes helpful for the first day or two to allow comfortable ambulation. This injury is not common in precollegiate athletes.

ADDUCTORS

A study of injuries in Swedish professional soccer players demonstrated that 54 percent of all groin injuries involved the adductor longus.[17] However, the adductor brevis, gracilis, pectineus, and iliopsoas may also be injured by forceful adduction of the thigh. Total rupture is uncommon but does occur and often presents as a tumorlike swelling in the upper medial thigh. More typically, an adductor strain is grade I or II and is characterized by groin pain with running and kicking. It is particularly aggravated by the inside kick of soccer.

A variety of other conditions may cause groin pain and should be ruled out before

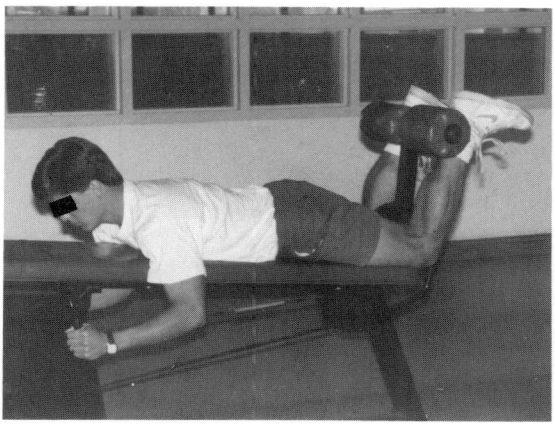 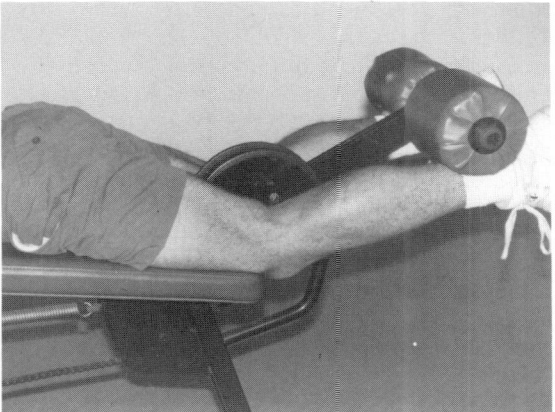

FIGURE 8–10. Eccentric muscle strength training of the hamstring group. Note the muscles are lengthening while simultaneously contracting as the weight is lowered.

assuming the problem is a muscular strain. These include osteitis pubis and spine abnormalities with radicular pain, hip pathology, hernia, and genitourinary infection. The treatment is rest, ice, and antiinflammatory medicines followed by adductor stretching and strengthening.

ROTATOR CUFF

Acute injuries to the rotator cuff in the young athlete are uncommon and are generally the result of shoulder dislocation. Where there is persistent pain referable to the rotator cuff, the presence of chronic shoulder laxity or instability should be evaluated.

In young throwing athletes, however, a pattern of recurrent strains of the rotator cuff, especially the supraspinatus muscle, can develop. This is an overuse problem seen particularly in young pitchers.[7] At the release of the throwing motion, the external rotators are stressed as they are eccentrically contracting to decelerate the arm. This results in a traction strain at the distal tendon or the muscle-tendon junction. Clinically, the symptoms resemble subacromial impingement problem or bursitis, which is unusual in children. Isolation of the supraspinatus by forward flexion and internal rotation against resistance will elicit pain, and usually there will be significant weakness with external rotation of the forearm with the elbow held at the side. Often the athlete will alter the overhead throw to a sidearm throw to alleviate stress on the rotator cuff.

Treatment consists of rest from throwing and nonsteroidal antiinflammatory medication until pain resolves, followed by a program designed to strengthen the rotator cuff. This consists of progressive external rotation resistance exercises using hand-held weights, pulleys with free weights, and elastic tubing.

LUMBAR PARASPINALS

Although back strains are extremely common in the adult population, they are less common in children. The young athlete complaining of back pain should always be evaluated for spinal abnormalities, including spondylolysis, spondylolisthesis, disk herniation, congenital deformity, or vertebral fracture. Hyperlordotic mechanical low back pain does occur in some adolescents during the growth spurt. This may be associated with tightness of the hip flexors. The treatment of back pain due to strains or postural causes is primarily rest, abdominal strengthening, hamstring stretching, and hip flexor stretching when indicated.

EXERCISE-INDUCED MUSCLE SORENESS

In addition to acute muscle strains with significant disruption of fibers near the muscle-tendon junction, there is another common injury to muscle occurring in the acute and subacute periods following intense exercise. The athletes suffering from this condition have not usually experienced a single acute injury but instead a more extended period of unaccustomed heavy exercise. Very often this exercise is eccentric in nature; that is, the muscles are being forcibly lengthened while they are contracting. Young athletes with exercise-induced muscle soreness often complain of an aching pain in several muscle groups after a period of exercise that has been more strenuous than usual. High-intensity exercises cause this type of discomfort. The onset is usually 12 to 24 hours after the exercise. The sore muscles are those contracting primarily eccentrically. For example, a baseball pitcher may note pain in the biceps and supraspinatus muscles; these muscles are the decelerators of the arm and forearm in the throwing motion.

In early studies, Hough[6] concluded that delayed muscle soreness was associated more with the amount of tension developed in the muscle than in its fatigue. He proposed that the diminution of the muscle's ability to produce tension and the increased soreness could be explained by small ruptures within the muscle. More recent studies have supported this theory and have shown that the weakness is transient, returning to normal in a few days. Eccentric contractions are more likely than concentric contractions to produce muscle soreness.[1]

Serology studies have demonstrated an elevation of intramuscular enzymes (notably hydroxyproline) during the period of muscle soreness, indicating the degradation of collagen.[4] In contrast, it has been shown that serum lactic acid concentration is not related to delayed onset muscle soreness.[3]

Clinical and animal studies support the involvement of an acute inflammatory response in the presence of exercise-induced muscle soreness. Treatment with nonsteroidal antiinflammatory medicines has been found to be effective in animal studies.[22] Stretching has also been recommended to assist the treatment of exercise-induced muscle soreness.[5] It is important to note that this condition of muscle soreness is very common, and it is not associated with any lasting deleterious effects in muscle. Many people involved with strength training consider that it may be a valuable or at least a necessary adjunct to successful training. This is known to athletes by the adage "no pain, no gain." A firm scientific basis for this common assumption is lacking, but it seems likely that delayed soreness is at least not harmful and perhaps may be associated with some benefits to training muscle.

PREVENTION OF MUSCLE STRAINS

Prevention of muscle injury is clinically important. There have been studies in groups of adult athletes showing the effectiveness of an overall conditioning program on the prevention of injuries to muscle. However, the various components of the conditioning programs have not been evaluated individually to determine which components are effective. The effect of conditioning programs in children remains controversial.

WARM-UP AND STRETCHING

Laboratory studies have shown that a warm-up period of muscle activation may indeed be beneficial in preventing strain injury. It has been found that preconditioned rabbit muscle is more elastic than a muscle that is "cold."[20] This study demonstrated that contracted muscle is capable of storing far more energy prior to failure than noncontracted muscle and that a single isometric contraction of rabbit muscle lasting 10 to 15 seconds was effective in changing several of the biomechanical parameters of the muscle. We recommend a warm-up routine for most athletic activities consisting of a 15-minute period of easy jogging, swimming, biking, and so on, and slow, controlled drills for the specific sport, for example, ball passing for soccer.

Stretching of muscle prior to stress has also been investigated experimentally. Passive stretching has been found to result in decreased stress on a muscle at a given length, owing to the viscoelastic nature of the muscle-tendon unit. It appears that no more than three or four repetitions of a stretch are required to provide adequate increases in tissue elasticity. Theoretically, stretching prior to activity should therefore also lead to fewer muscle injuries.

Stretching of all major muscle groups is recommended prior to practice or competition. There are various ways to stretch muscle. The three most common methods are ballistic stretching, static stretching, and modified proprioceptive neuromuscular facilitation (PNF). Ballistic (or bouncing) stretching has generally fallen into disfavor since it facilitates the stretch reflex and may actually make the muscle tighter. Static stretching—which places the muscle in an extended position, then sustains a slow, passive stretch—is now the most commonly used method. PNF is a method developed in the 1950s and involves alternately contracting and relaxing the agonist and antagonist muscle groups. (See Chapter 3.)

It should be noted that there are large individual variations in flexibility and that prepubescent children are generally more flexible than skeletally mature individuals. This range of motion and flexibility can be increased in both girls and boys in activities such as gymnastics and ballet. However, most of this increased joint laxity results from the repetitive stretching of ligamentous structures and has not been shown to result in fewer muscle strains.

Flexibility is affected by a number of different factors. Repetitive exercise can lead to flexibility in some muscle groups, but it may also lead to decreased flexibility in other groups.

MUSCLE CONTUSION

The most common injury seen in children in contact sports, particularly football and soccer, is the muscle contusion. This injury normally causes considerable pain and temporary disability in some cases; it also requires prolonged rehabilitation. Contusions typically occur in the lower extremities and are most common in the quadriceps ("charley horse") and anterior tibial muscles.

The pathology of a muscle contusion is different than a muscle strain. This injury has been investigated using several animal models. The rat calf muscle was used by Jarvinen and Sorvari.[9] Early healing following controlled contusion demonstrated histological patterns of hematoma formation and inflammatory process. A dense connective tissue scar replaced the hematoma. This dense connective tissue scar possessed large areas without muscle regeneration; this pattern is similar to the healing seen with muscle laceration. It is interesting to note that mobilization following injury led to less scar tissue and a more rapid recovery of tensile strength. It is also interesting to note in the context of this discussion that younger rats demonstrated stronger healing responses than older rats, although the implications of this finding for humans are speculative.

In sheep experiments conducted by Rothwell and Walton,[19] blunt trauma to the thigh caused rupture of the deep (postural) muscles near the bone and did not significantly injure the superficial musculature. A significant number of these controlled injuries resulted in periosteal hyperplasia within a week and eventual production of subperiosteal bone.

The clinical studies of contusions in animals as well as humans point to several considerations for their treatment. First, strict immobilization does not appear to be necessary or appropriate. Early mobilization should be encouraged within the pain-free tolerance of the individual. Second, acute reaction to muscle contusion involves hematoma formation and an inflammatory response. Therefore, acute treatment of muscle contusions should be directed toward controlling bleeding and minimizing secondary insult. Ice should be applied during the first 24 hours. Antiinflammatory agents may be useful, particularly during the acute phase. Massage is definitely contraindicated and in fact may cause further damage.[2] Finally, rapid protein synthesis occurs with these injuries, particularly when there is early mobilization, and complete recovery can be expected. However, painless full range of motion of the limb and normal muscle strength should be achieved before returning the athlete to sport. The recovery time may be anywhere from 2 days to 6 months, depending on the severity of injury and the development of complications such as myositis ossificans.

Human studies by Ryan[20] and Jackson and Feagin[8] stress the importance of grading the severity of quadriceps muscle contusions initially. The grade correlates well with the amount and length of the disability. A "mild" injury (grade I) is characterized by localized tenderness, knee range of motion greater than 90 degrees, and no alteration of gait. A "moderate" injury (grade II) shows greater tenderness and swelling, with less than 90 degrees of knee motion; the athlete walks with a limp and cannot do a deep knee bend. With a "severe" quadriceps contusion (grade III), there is marked swelling and tenderness, knee motion is less than 45 degrees, and the athlete may be unable to walk unassisted (see Fig. 8–11).

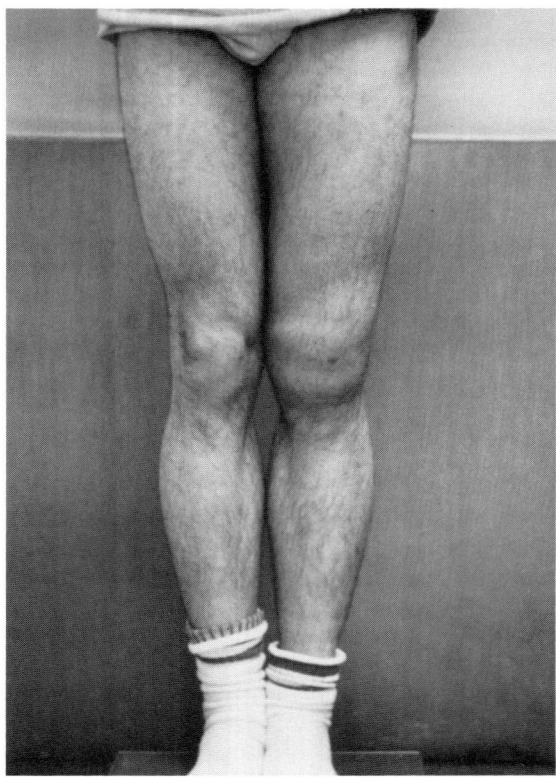

FIGURE 8–11. A severe quadriceps contusion, such as this one, may be accompanied by a knee effusion with no apparent intraarticular injury to the joint itself.

MYOSITIS OSSIFICANS

Ossification within the muscle at the site of the consolidated hematoma can occur following grade II or grade III contusions, particularly in the thigh. This ossification is called myositis ossificans, or heteroptic ossification. In Jackson and Feagin's series, myositis ossificans occurred in 13 of 18 athletes with moderate or severe injuries. It is most common during the second decade of life but can occur in much younger children.[24] Myositis ossificans can be detected radiographically between 2 and 4 weeks following injury and may increase until 6 months, after which further enlargement usually does not occur. The radiographic appearance may be either a calcific density connected to underlying bone by a stalklike structure, or it may be of the parosteal broad-based type. It may have no connection to underlying bone at all, but this is rare.

Localized pain and stiffness are the usual symptoms of myositis ossificans. Occasionally, there is a neurological deficit if the lesion is adjacent to peripheral nerves. A history of injury should always be confirmed, and the possibility of osteosarcoma or other cortical tumor ruled out if there is a questionable history. Because myositis ossificans is associated with more severe muscle contusions, its presence usually signifies that recovery will be relatively prolonged. However, the myositis ossificans itself does not require any specific treatment, and surgical excision is rarely indicated unless pain and limited motion persist beyond 1 year.[11]

PREVENTION OF MUSCLE CONTUSIONS

Attempts to reduce the risk of muscle contusions should be aimed at two areas: (1) use of protective equipment and (2) promotion of controlled, properly supervised and officiated play. In football, hockey, and lacrosse, protective padding is standard, yet even in these sports not all major muscle groups are protected, most notably the calf area. In baseball, basketball, and wrestling, there is generally little or no protective padding worn on the extremities (with the exception of the baseball catcher). In soccer, shin guards are the only protective gear worn by the field players; the goalkeeper may wear hip and thigh pads. Of course, it is unreasonable to expect that any contact sport can be made completely safe from contusions; there is simply a certain risk of injury inherent in certain sports that must be accepted by the participants. However, where protective equipment is allowed, it is the responsibility of the players, coaches, parents, and physicians to see that it is properly fitted and worn.

The provision of properly supervised and educated play is more easily achieved but commonly overlooked. Reckless, uncontrolled, or violent play predisposes players to injury of any kind but particularly so to direct blows and the resultant fractures and contusions. The practice of sportsmanlike conduct and a clear understanding of the rules of the game are essential for athletes of all ages and are best learned at the beginning stages of athletic development.

References

1. Abraham, W. M.: Factors in delayed muscle soreness. Med. Sci. Sports 9:11–20, 1977.
2. Antao, N. A.: Myositis of the hip in a professional soccer player. A case report. Am J Sports Med 16(1):82–83, 1988.
3. Armstrong, R. B., Garsnek, V., Schwane, J. A.: Muscle inflammation response eccentric exercise. Med. Sci Sports Exerc 12(2):94–95, 1980.
4. Besson, C., Rochcongar, P., Beauverger, Y., Dassonville, J., Auibree, M., Catheline, M.: Study of the valuations of serum muscular enzymes and myoglobin after maximal exercise test and during the next 24 hours. Eur J. Applied Physiol 47:47, 1981.
5. Garrett, W. E., Jr., Rich, F. R., Nikalaou, P. K., Vogler, J. B.: Computed tomography of hamstring muscle strain. Med Sci Sports Exerc 21(5):506–514, 1989.
6. Hough, T.: Ergographic studies in muscle soreness. Am J Physiol 7:76–92, 1902.
7. Ireland, M. L., Andrews, J. R.: Shoulder and elbow injuries in the young athlete. Clinics Sports Med 7(3):473–494, 1988.
8. Jackson, D., Feagin, J.: Quadriceps contusions in young athletes. JBJS 55–A:95–105, 1973.
9. Jarvinen, M., Sorvari, T.: Healing of crush injury in rat striated muscle: A histological study of the effect of early mobilization on the repair process. Acta Pathol Microbiol Scand 83:269–282, 1975.
10. Jones, V. T., Garett, W. E., Seaber, A. V.: Biomechanical changes in muscle after immobilization at different lengths. Trans Orthop Res Soc 10:6, 1985.
11. Lipscomb, A. B., Thomas, E. D., Johnston, R. K.: Treatment of myositis ossificans traumatica in athletes. Am J Sports Med 4(3):111–120, 1976.
12. Malina, R. M.: Exercise as an influence upon growth. Clin Pediatr 8(1):16–26, 1969.
13. Micheli, L. J., Smith, A. D.: Sports injuries in children. Curr Probl Ped 12(9):1–54, 1982.
14. Motajova, J.: Effect of special stress over a four-year period on certain morphological parameters and bone age in growing children. Folia Morphol 22(4):358–361, 1974.
15. Nikolaou, P. K., McDonald, B. L., Glisson, R. R., et al.: Biomechanical and histological evaluation of muscle after controlled strain injury. Am J Sports Med 15:9–14, 1987.
16. Obremskey, W. T., Seaber, A. V., Garrett, W. E., Jr.: Biomechanical and histological assessment of a controlled muscle strain injury treated with piroxicam. Trans Ortho Res Soc 13:338, 1988.
17. Renstrom, P., Peterson, L.: Groin injuries in athletes. Br J Sports Med 14:30–36, 1980.
18. Rians, C. B., Weltman, A., Cahill, B. R., Janney, C. A., Tippett, S. R., Katch, F. I.: Strength training for prepubescent males: Is it safe? Am J Sports Med 15(5):483, 489, 1987.
19. Rothwell, A. G., Walton, M.: The quadriceps hematoma: A clinical and experimental study. JBJS 62–B:270–271, 1980.
20. Ryan, A. J.: Quadriceps strain, rupture and charlie horse. Med Sci Sports 1(2):106–111, 1969.
21. Safran, M., Garrett, W. E., Jr., Seaber, A. V., Glisson, R. R., Ribbeck, B. M.: The role of warm-up in muscular injury prevention. Am J Sports Med 16(2):123–129, 1988.
22. Salminen, A., Kihlstrom, M.: Protective effect of indomethacin against exercise-induced injuries in mouse skeletal muscle fibers. Int J Sports Med 8:46–69, 1987.
23. Volger, C., Bove, K. E.: Morphology of skeletal muscle in children. Arch Pathol Lab Med 109(3):238–242, 1985.
24. Wilkes, L.: Myositis ossificans traumatica in a young child. Clin Orthop 118:151–152, 1976.

9
HEAD AND NECK INJURIES

WAYNE GERSOFF

When the potential injuries that can be sustained by athletic participation are considered, there are probably none more serious than injuries to the head and neck. There is no margin for poor evaluation or poor management of these injuries. The possible result is too catastrophic.

There are several sports that have been shown to have a higher incidence of head and neck injuries. The more common sports that can be classified as "collision" sports include tackle football, rugby, ice hockey, and lacrosse. There is also another group of sports that has been termed "self-destruct" sports by Bodnar.[5] The sports included in this category are automobile racing, motorcycle racing, skydiving, hang gliding, parachuting, and mountain climbing. In addition, certain individual sports such as diving, gymnastics, and wrestling are also associated with a high incidence of head and neck injuries (Table 9–1).

Unfortunately, the actual incidence of head and neck injuries is difficult to determine. Many injuries are often self-limited and are never reported to the physician or athletic trainer. This is most frequently seen with mild head injuries or minor brachial plexus injuries. It has also been shown by Albright et al. that athletes are reluctant to report previous minor injuries of the neck.[1] It was shown that although only 4 percent of the incoming freshmen football class at the University of Iowa reported previous significant cervical trauma, 35 percent demonstrated radiographic evidence of prior cervical spine injury. An additional factor that interferes with the development of an accurate epidemiological study is that most injuries tend to occur in practice situations. At least at the high school level, this is a time where appropriate medical personnel are usually not present.

It has been estimated that the incidence of all spinal injuries in athletic participation is approximately 10 percent. Those injuries associated with long-term neurological compromise occur in approximately 0.6 to 1.0 percent of athletic injuries.[27] The most accurate records of head and neck injuries are to be found in the sport of football. The greatest contribution to the study of head and neck injuries and the development of improved rules and equipment has been made by Torg. The creation of the National Football Head and Neck Injury Registry has tracked these injuries since 1971.[44] This registry was the major force behind the elimination of "spearing" tactics from tackle football in 1976 with the subsequent decrease in cervical spine injuries associated with quadriplegia in this sport.

As in all sports, there will be a certain percentage of injuries that are secondary to "bad luck." Fortunately, the overall incidence of head and neck injuries is relatively small. Unfortunately, these injuries are frequently the most catastrophic. While some injuries may be unavoidable, there are certain measures that can be implemented to prevent serious injuries. Modifications of equipment, rules, and playing techniques can contribute to the reduction of injuries to the head and cervical spine. In addition, the education of athletes, coaches, athletic trainers, and physicians can also make a significant contribu-

TABLE 9–1. Sports Associated with a High Incidence of Head and Neck Injuries

Collision Sports
Football
Rugby
Ice hockey
Lacrosse

"Self-Destruct" Sports
Automobile racing
Motorcycle racing
Hang gliding
Skydiving
Parachuting
Mountain climbing
Snowmobiling

Individual Sports
Diving
Gymnastics
Horseback riding

---

tion to the reduction of head and neck injuries. The role of accurate record keeping and a complete preseason physical examination is also significant in injury prevention.

This chapter will review the various types of injuries that can be sustained by the athlete to the head and cervical spine. Guidelines for the management and return to the participation of these injured athletes will also be presented. All physicians or athletic trainers involved with the coverage of athletic events must be familiar with the management of the unconscious athlete. Finally, an understanding of injury patterns can assist in the development of plans for the prevention of head and neck injuries.

MANAGEMENT OF THE UNCONSCIOUS ATHLETE

The unconscious athlete represents a true emergency situation. An organized, systematic approach to evaluating and managing this individual provides the safest mechanism for preventing potential catastrophe.[7,12,35]

Any physician or athletic trainer involved with athletic events where there is an increased risk of head injury must be familiar with the management of the unconscious athlete. In addition, owing to the high rate of injuries in practice, coaches must also be educated about this management plan. It is also highly recommended that all coaches, trainers, and physicians know how to perform cardiopulmonary resuscitation. There is no substitute for proper training. "On the job" training at the time of a catastrophe is not acceptable.

A disaster plan must be formulated in advance. All individuals involved in the care of athletes must know this plan and their individual assignments. Rehearsal of this plan is mandatory. The disaster plan should include (1) an equipment checklist, (2) telephone access, (3) emergency transportation, (4) properly trained personnel, and (5) an individual designated to be in charge. Proper equipment is essential and can often be a key factor in managing the unconscious athlete (Table 9–2).

When the unconscious athlete is approached on the field, the leader must be certain that no movements are initiated that could result in additional damage to the patient.[47] The prevention of further injury must be a primary objective in management. The unconscious athlete cannot communicate with you. Therefore, it must be assumed that in addition to a head injury there is also a cervical spine injury.[4] The head and neck should be initially immobilized in a neutral position simply by manual stabilization (Fig. 9–1).

An algorithm for field decision making is presented in Figure 9–2.[45] Initially, the athlete needs to be evaluated for breathing, pulse, and level of consciousness. In those sports involving the use of helmets, the chin strap and helmet should be left in place. Face masks can be easily removed from the helmet if it is necessary to initiate resuscitation. The helmet should not be removed until the athlete is at an appropriate medical facility and the head and neck area is either securely immobilized or cleared by radiographic studies.

Proper technique in moving the patient is extremely important. In general, the injured athlete should not be moved unless cardiopulmonary resuscitation (CPR) becomes necessary or transportation is available. Movement of the athlete should be done in a coordinated logrolling fashion that is con-

TABLE 9–2. Required Emergency Equipment for Athletic Events

Spine board
Bolt cutters
Sharp knife/scalpel
Telephone
Cervical collars

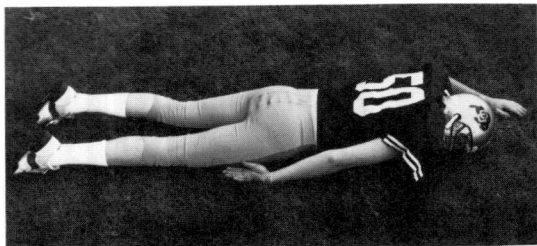 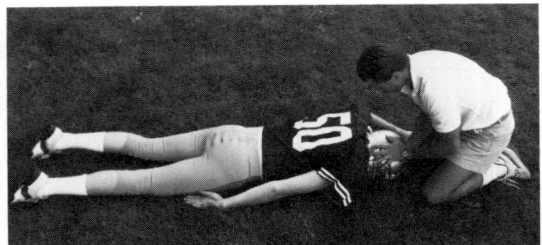

FIGURE 9–1. The head and neck of the unconscious athlete should be manually stabilized until it can be verified that there is no associated neck injury.

trolled by the leader (Fig. 9–3). A spine board should be used for lifting and carrying of the athlete. Again, this should be done in a careful, coordinated effort controlled by the team leader. At no time during the evaluation and management of the unconscious athlete should the physician or athletic trainer compromise care secondary to encouragement by coaches, officials, or fans to remove the athlete from the field. The care of the athlete takes complete precedence in this regard (Fig. 9–4).

HEAD INJURIES

Injuries to the head can be classified as either focal or diffuse brain injuries[7] or as severe or minor head injuries.[50] Diffuse brain injuries include concussions and diffuse axonal injury. Concussions are characterized by a transient alteration of consciousness and varying degrees of temporary neurological dysfunction, whereas diffuse axonal injuries are characterized by loss of consciousness for longer than 6 hours with associated neurological, psychological, and personality deficiencies. This type of injury is secondary to an event that causes inertial or acceleration changes of the brain in the skull—the so-called rattling of the brain.

Focal brain injuries are associated with an intracranial hematoma. This includes cerebral contusions, intracerebral hematomas, epidural hematomas, and acute subdural hematomas. This type of injury is more serious in nature and demands prompt recognition and treatment (Table 9–3).

Alternatively, head injuries can be described as severe or minor. Severe head injuries include cerebral contusion, intracranial hemorrhage, epidural hematoma, subdural hematoma, intracerebral hematoma, and diffuse axonal injury. Mild head injury includes all forms of concussion and is the most common head injury in sports (Table 9–3).[16,19,24,50]

CONCUSSION

Concussion is the typical example of a mild head injury or diffuse brain injury. It has been defined as an "immediate and transient impairment of neurofunction such as alteration of consciousness, disturbance of vision, equilibrium, and other similar systems."[16] Despite the fact that concussions are the most common head injury in sports, they are often overlooked or downplayed owing to their mild degree.[6,12,28]

Any athlete sustaining a direct blow to the head or forceful hit to the body that causes a sudden acceleration-deceleration injury to the head must be fully evaluated. Even if the athlete is conscious and ambulatory, an evaluation is required to determine the extent of injury. The initial screening examination should include the testing of (1) orientation

TABLE 9–3. Alternative Classification of Head Injuries

Severe	Mild
Cerebral contusion	Concussion (grades I–VI)
Intracranial hemorrhage	
Epidural hematoma	
Subdural hematoma	
Intracerebral hematoma	
Diffuse axonal injury	

Diffuse	Focal
Concussions	Cerebral contusions
Diffuse axonal injury	Intracerebral hematoma
	Epidural hematoma
	Acute subdural hematoma

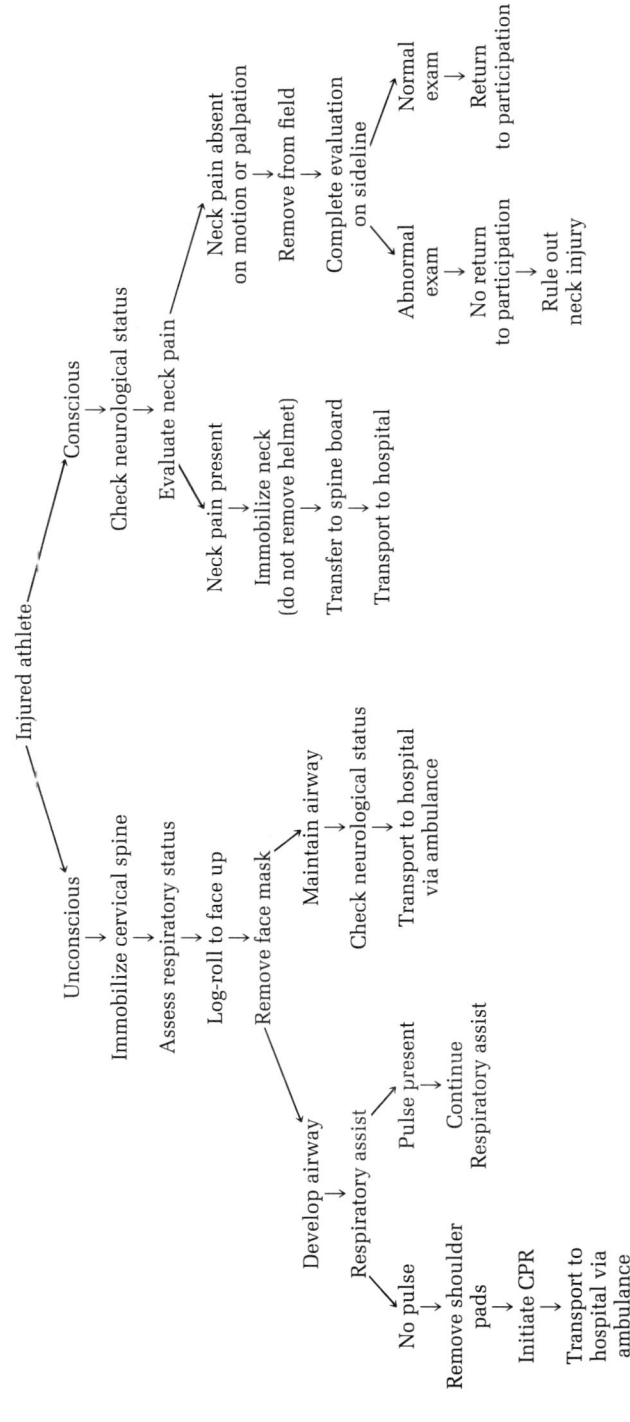

FIGURE 9–2. An algorithm for field decision making in head and neck injuries.

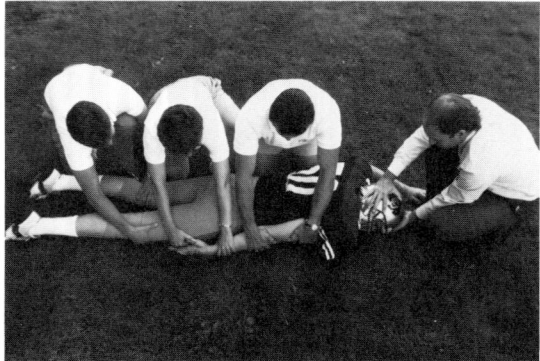 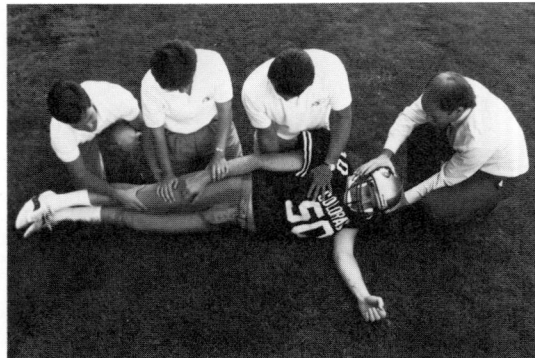

FIGURE 9–3. Turning of the athlete is coordinated by the leader, who maintains the relationship of the head to the body during the procedure.

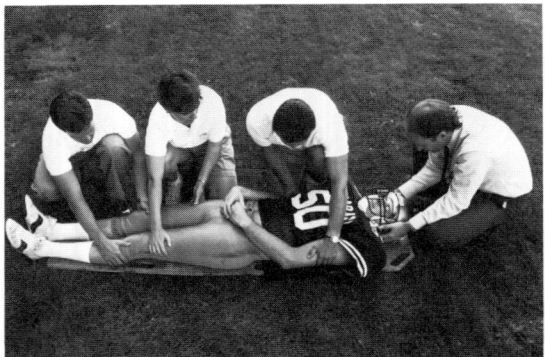 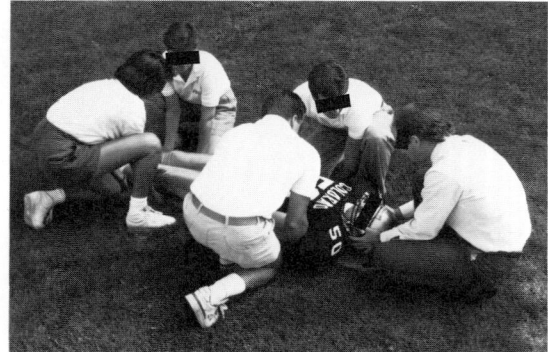

FIGURE 9–4. The athlete should be logrolled onto a spine board and securely immobilized for transport.

to person, place, and time; (2) facial expression; (3) posttraumatic amnesia; (4) retrograde amnesia; and (5) balance and gait. If there is any question in the initial screening examination, then the athlete should not be returned to participation and further observation or evaluation initiated.

Concussions can be defined as either mild, moderate, and severe or on a grading scale of I to VI (Table 9–4). The grade I concussion is typified by the athlete who gets his or her "bell rung" or sustains a "ding."[7,53] These individuals will not have posttraumatic or retrograde amnesia. Initially, this athlete will be mentally confused and project an equally confused facial expression. There may also be a mild alteration in balance, coordination, and gait. The period of confusion usually is short, lasting from 5 to 15 minutes before the athlete returns to his or her baseline mental status. When all symptoms and signs fully resolve, the athlete may return to participation. It is imperative that either the trainer or physician carefully observe the athlete for the remainder of the event. If the athlete develops any symptoms of dizziness, headache,

TABLE 9–4. Classification of Concussion

	I	II	III	IV	V	VI
Confusion	+	+	+	+	n.a.	n.a.
Loss of consciousness	–	–	–	+	n.a.	n.a.
Posttraumatic amnesia	–	+	+	+	n.a.	n.a.
Retrograde amnesia	–	–	+	+	n.a.	n.a.
Paralytic coma	–	–	–	+	n.a.	n.a.
Coma	–	–	–	–	+	+
Cardiorespiratory collapse	–	–	–	–	+/–	+
Death	–	–	–	–	+/–	+

n.a. = Not applicable

photophobia, or nausea, he or she should be held back from returning to competition. Any athlete who has sustained a minor head injury is at approximately a fourfold increased risk for sustaining a second minor head injury. It has also been shown that a second minor head injury that occurs while an athlete is still symptomatic from a previous minor head injury can result in fatal brain swelling.

Posttraumatic amnesia is described as the loss of memory of events that took place after the injury. The grade II concussion may include the symptoms of a grade I concussion but is characterized not only by confusion but also by posttraumatic amnesia. Even though there is no loss of consciousness, this athlete should not be allowed to return to participation on that day. In addition, it is recommended that these athletes receive continued observation and postinjury evaluation. It is not uncommon for the athlete who has sustained a grade II concussion to develop persistent headache, irritability, fatigue, double vision, dizziness, behavioral problems, and an inability to concentrate. This has been termed the *postconcussion syndrome*. Individuals who develop a postconcussion syndrome may have these symptoms for several weeks after the injury. The athlete should not be allowed to return to participation until all symptoms have resolved.

Grade III concussions are distinguished by the presence of all the previously described symptoms plus the inability to remember events prior to the injury or retrograde amnesia. There is no loss of consciousness. These athletes must be carefully examined and observed and the appropriate follow-up care initiated. Return to participation on that day is not permitted.

Loss of consciousness characterizes the grade IV concussion. There is a gradual return to consciousness after several seconds or minutes. This individual passes through various stages before becoming fully alert. These include stupor, confusion with or without delirium, and a lucid state. Both retrograde and posttraumatic amnesia are usually present in these individuals. Any athlete who demonstrates signs or symptoms of deteriorating neurological status or who remains unconscious for more than 3 to 5 minutes should be transported by ambulance to a hospital facility. In general, it is recommended that the athlete who sustains a grade IV concussion be observed at least overnight in a hospital facility.

The principals of management of the unconscious athlete must be applied. It must be determined if the athlete is breathing and if there is a pulse. The level of consciousness must also be determined. Owing to the high frequency of cervical spine injuries with head injuries, care must be taken not to unnecessarily move or manipulate the athlete. Once the athlete has regained consciousness, if he or she cannot walk from the playing field unassisted, then they should be removed on a spine board. If there is any suspicion of a cervical spine injury, then the athlete should be taken from the field of play on a spine board with the neck properly immobilized.

The classification of concussions as a minor head injury may seem inappropriate when grade V and grade VI concussions are considered. Grade V concussions are associated with impact injuries that are severe enough to produce paralytic comas lasting greater than 5 minutes, with possible cardiorespiratory collapse. If cardiorespiratory collapse does occur, CPR must be initiated immediately. Any athlete sustaining a grade V concussion must be immediately transported to a hospital by ambulance. The athlete should be transported to a facility that can provide both neurosurgical evaluation and computerized tomography (CT) scan evaluation. The grade VI concussion is of such great severity that it can result in death of the injured athlete. Fortunately, severe head injuries of this nature in athletic competition are rare.

Severe head injuries, although infrequent in sporting events, must be recognized because of the possible catastrophic potential of the injuries.[6,7,19,25] There are certain signs and symptoms that must be recognized by the physician, trainer, or coach that require emergency treatment. Following head injury, any athlete that develops increasing headaches, nausea and vomiting, inequality of pupils, disorientation, progressive or sudden impairment of consciousness, a gradual rise in blood pressure, or a decreasing pulse rate requires rapid emergency treatment and transportation to a hospital facility. The previously described signs and symptoms are indicative of increasing intracranial pressure. Increased intracranial pressure is associated with both epidural hematomas and subdural hematomas. Increased intracranial pressure, secondary to hemorrhage, represents the leading cause of death from head injury in sports. For example, in 1986, 9 of 12 reported fatalities in football were secondary to intracranial hemorrhage.[12]

Epidural hematomas result from the tearing of a meningeal artery as it crosses a bony groove in the skull secondary to a skull fracture. The middle meningeal artery is most frequently involved. These individuals may initially be unconscious at the time of injury. However, there is a recovery of consciousness, which is followed by a lucid period of time. Following this lucid state, there is a gradual appearance of the previously described emergency signs and symptoms. Unfortunately, this classic description of an epidural hematoma will not occur in all individuals. There will be some individuals who will not become unconscious until later in their course and others who will never regain consciousness during the course of their injury. The best diagnostic test for evaluating a patient suspected of having an epidural hematoma is the CT scan.

Subdural hemorrhage results from a contrecoup or rotational acceleration-deceleration injury to the head. The force of the injury causes the tearing of bridging veins between the brain and cavernous sinus. In general, more head injuries in athletic competition result from a lower inertial loading than do head injuries from high-speed vehicular accidents. Therefore, subdural hemorrhages occur more frequently than epidural hematomas in athletics. Subdural hematomas usually develop slowly owing to the low-pressure venous bleeding. Therefore, the signs and symptoms of increasing intracranial pressure may not be present for hours or even days after the time of injury.

RETURN TO COMPETITION

Head injuries that are mismanaged can have catastrophic consequences. A complete and accurate examination at the time of injury is essential. However, management must not stop there. Repeat examinations and careful observations are mandatory. If there is any uncertainty regarding any aspect of the examination, then it is better to be safe and protect the athlete.

The question of when an athlete can return to participation can be difficult to answer. Boxing is the only sport for which definite regulations concerning the return of participation of a head-injured athlete have been established.[33] There have been various guidelines suggested by several authors.[11,20,34,35] The majority of these guidelines are based on clinical observations and studies on performance. While these guidelines provide a framework from which to work, each injury must be individualized. Consideration must also be given to the type of sport in which the athlete is going to participate (Table 9–5).

In general, those individuals sustaining a grade I concussion can return to participation as soon as the confusion or other mild symptoms have cleared. Once participation is resumed, the athlete's performance should be carefully monitored. Any abnormal behavior, performance, or symptoms should result in the removal of the athlete from competition.

Grade II concussions in an athlete require that the athlete not be allowed to return to competition that day. This group of athletes requires postinjury evaluation. Observation and examination should continue for at least 1 week. At the end of 1 week, if the athlete is completely asymptomatic, then return to participation is permitted. If symptoms persist after 1 week, then return is not permitted until all symptoms are resolved.

Any athlete sustaining a grade III concussion should not be returned to competition that day. The management of these individuals is similar to that of the grade II concussion. It may take slightly longer for these individuals to become asymptomatic. However, it is imperative that these individuals not return to competition before they are completely asymptomatic.

It is generally recommended for an athlete to wait a minimum time of 1 month before

TABLE 9–5. Guidelines for Return to Competition After Concussion

Grade	Conditions for Return
I	After resolution of symptoms; may return to competition that day
II	No return to competition for 1 week; resolution of symptoms required
III	No return to competition for at least 1 week; resolution of symptoms required
IV	No return to competition for at least 1 month; resolution of symptoms required
V	No return to competition for season; recommend alternative sports

returning to participation when a grade IV concussion is sustained. Careful evaluation by a neurosurgeon at the time of injury, during recovery, and prior to return to competition is highly recommended. Any athlete sustaining a grade V concussion should not return to participation that season, and strong consideration should be given to changing to a mostly minimal or no-contact sport and certainly not returning to full-contact sports.

Special consideration must be given to an athlete who sustains multiple concussions while participating in a particular sport. When the type of concussion is of a mild nature, grade I or II, then a longer period of observation and evaluation is required before allowing the athlete to return to participation. An athlete sustaining a secondary concussion after a grade III concussion in the same season should be withheld from participation for the remainder of the season. Such an athlete may return to participation the following season if he or she is asymptomatic at both rest and exertion. A second concussion occurring after a grade IV injury should result in the athlete's being carefully evaluated, withheld from participation for the remainder of the season, and advised to change to at most a minimal contact sport.

The increased participation of children and adolescents in contact sports provides the potential for head injuries in a potentially vulnerable group.[6,12,23,32] Fortunately, data thus far indicate a lower incidence of serious head injuries in this population. This is most likely attributable in part to the inability of this younger age group to generate the impact force required to cause such an injury. It should be remembered that participation in sports is meant to contribute to athletes' mental and physical health. Therefore, the pressure to continue participation in an athletic event after sustaining a significant injury should not exist. Coaches, parents, and athletes must be educated about injury recognition and prevention. The tendency is usually for the athlete to minimize his or her injury and attempt to return to participation quickly. However, in the injured athlete, the risks of attempting to gain immediate goals must be overruled by the benefits of lifetime rewards. In adolescent athletes who sustain a grade IV concussion with loss of consciousness lasting greater than 5 minutes or multiple grade II or III concussions (with amnesia) in any season, it should be recommended that the athlete become involved in another sport where high-impact contact is not a factor. Athletes should also be encouraged to report their injuries. These reports should be carefully evaluated by the athletic trainer and team physician and not be automatically minimized.

CERVICAL SPINE FRACTURES

Injuries to C1 and C2 are unique vertebral fractures owing to their unique anatomical structure. Fractures of C3 through C7 can be grouped together because of their similar anatomical structures. Water sports, football, and trampoline have most often been associated with cervical spine injuries. Injuries to C3 through C7 are frequently encountered in football, whereas other accidents frequently involve C1 and C2.

The Special Olympics has provided the handicapped athlete with the ability to participate more fully in sports competition. These athletes require special consideration concerning their participation with regard to the stability of their cervical spine. The group that is of most concern is those athletes with Down syndrome. It has been reported that up to 40 percent of children with this condition can have cervical spine abnormalities.

The greatest amount of concern has been expressed over the association of Down syndrome with atlantoaxial instability, which was noted by Pueschel and Scola[31] in 15 percent of persons with this syndrome. In 1984, the American Academy of Pediatrics recommended that all children with Down syndrome who participate in high-risk sports such as gymnastics, swimming, or diving be screened with lateral radiographs in neutral, flexion, and extension. If they demonstrate an abnormal odontoid or greater than 4.5 mm between the odontoid and the anterior arch of the atlas, they are advised to avoid stressful sports. Burke and colleagues[9] evaluated 32 persons with Down syndrome in 1970 and 1985. They found that some children who demonstrated abnormal laxity in 1970 subsequently stabilized, whereas others who were normal in 1970 met criteria for instability in 1985. They concluded that atlantoaxial stability in Down syndrome is a chronic, potentially progressive lesion. They therefore advised that all persons with Down syndrome be excluded from high-risk activities. Although this recommendation has not been universally adopted, it would appear prudent to screen all athletes with Down syndrome for radiographic signs of atlantoaxial abnormalities, to preclude those with abnormalities from contact or other high-risk sports, and follow those with normal radiographs with periodic neurological evaluations and radiographic screenings.

The Jefferson fracture is the most common fracture of the C1 ring.[22] This is a burst type fracture of the ring of C1. The Jefferson fracture is a result of direct compression force in the cervical spine. Frequently, the mechanism of injury has a flexion, sheer, or rotatory component in addition to the direct compressive force. This type of fracture is rarely associated with neurological injury. It is usually treated with a halo or tongs, followed by 8 weeks in a halo vest.

Odontoid fractures are the most common injuries of the second cervical vertebrae. These fractures have been classified into three different types based on the area of the odontoid injured.[18] Type I odontoid fractures involve an avulsion of the tip of the odontoid where the alar ligament attaches. The type II fracture occurs through the base either at or slightly below the level of the superior articular surface. A type III odontoid fracture involves a fracture of the body of C2. Most injuries of the odontoid are either type II or type III. While type II fractures require surgical intervention, type III fractures can be treated by immobilization and a halo vest.

The os odontoidium represents a congenital failure of union of the odontoid process with the body of the C2 vertebrae. It may present as an unexpected finding on routine cervical spine radiographs. Evaluation by tomography may be required to distinguish this entity from a type II odontoid fracture. While the treatment of an asymptomatic os odontoidium may be controversial, it is generally agreed that an athlete presenting with an os odontoidium should not participate in a contact sport. This recommendation should be followed even if the os odontoidium is incidentally found.[18]

In addition to the odontoid, the pedicles of C2 can also be fractured.[22] This has been termed the *hangman's fracture*. This fracture received its name because of its association with the sudden hyperextension caused by the "hangman's noose." Spinal cord injuries secondary to this fracture vary from minimal to complete cord injury. If there is a complete cord injury, this will usually result in death.

Fractures of the C3 through C7 vertebrae result from a combination of compression and flexion forces. These fractures have been classified into four types. This classification system, developed by Cloward, is based on the comminution of the fracture.[27] Compression fractures without comminution are secondary to flexion injuries. Comminuted compression fractures of the cervical vertebrae are caused by axial loading, often with some degree of flexion. This type of injury has been termed the *tear-drop fracture*. It is most often associated with a diving accident when the head hits an immobile solid object, such as the bottom of the swimming pool.

The comminuted cervical vertebral fracture was frequently associated with the technique of spearing in American football. The landmark work of Torg,[10,42,43,44] analyzing the biomechanics of cervical spine injuries in football, cleared some common misconceptions surrounding this topic. Based on laboratory study, game films, and direct observation, several important conclusions were developed. Before Torg's work, many clinicians believed that hyperextension was the cause of many catastrophic cervical spine injuries in football. It was felt that the impact of the posterior rim of the helmet on the back of the neck during hyperextension caused a "guillotine" injury to the cervical spine. Others thought that hyperflexion was also an important cause of injury. Torg's game film analysis showed that most of the catastrophic cervical spine fractures in football were due to axial compression. This most commonly occurred during tackling when the tackler contacted his opponent with the crown of his head with the neck slightly flexed, a technique known as spearing. Fortunately, because of the work of Torg and others, this technique was made illegal in 1976. This resulted in a decrease in the number of cervical spine injuries resulting in quadriplegia in subsequent years.[26]

Fractures of the spinous process of the cervical vertebrae can be common in athletics. This type of injury is due to a severe flexion force resulting in avulsion of the spinous process of the vertebrae by the spine extensor and scapular elevator muscles. The term *clay shoveler's fracture* has been applied to spinous process avulsions. This is not a serious structural injury and can be treated symptomatically (Fig. 9–5).

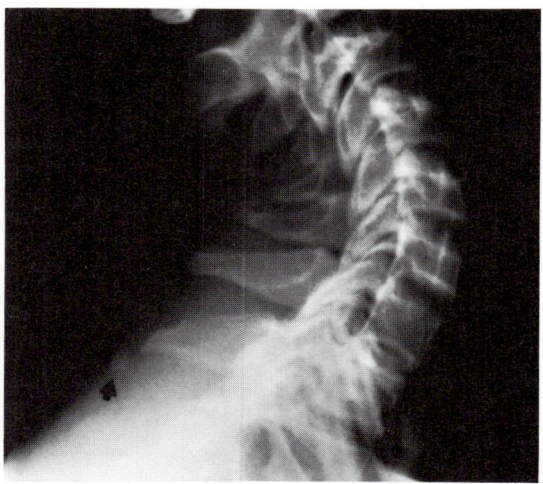

FIGURE 9–5. Avulsion of the tip of the spinous process—"clay shoveler's fracture"—is not a serious structural injury (*arrow*).

SOFT TISSUE INJURIES

Three types of soft tissue injuries are associated with athletic participation. These are injuries to the cervical disks, strains of the cervical musculature, and sprains of the cervical ligamentous structures.

Cervical musculature strains can be considered the most common injury to the neck in athletes. The injury is frequently caused by a "whiplash" type force. However, the athlete usually will not recall the specific incident causing the injury. The symptoms of injury to the cervical musculature are similar to other muscle injuries in the body. The athlete with an acute cervical strain will present with limited cervical spine motion and pain confined to the cervical spine area. This pain is usually greatest over the neck muscles. There is no radiation of the pain, paresthesias, or any neurological deficits. When the symptoms of pain and spasm have resolved and there is a painless full range of motion, the athlete may return to participation. Often the greatest discomfort and limitation of motion will not be realized until hours after the injury is sustained. The immediate application of ice to the muscles at the time of injury will help reduce the local bleeding of the torn muscle fibers. This is beneficial since it is the bleeding that greatly contributes to the pain and limitation of motion.

Cervical sprains involve some degree of injury to the ligamentous structures. While the sprain can be an isolated injury, there is often an associated muscular strain. Clinically, the two are often difficult to distinguish. The presentations of sprains and strains are extremely similar. If there is any question of ligamentous injury resulting in cervical instability, an appropriate radiographic evaluation is required. The decision to obtain complete radiographs is often difficult. However, it is always best to follow the more conservative approach. Any athlete sustaining a cervical spine injury with secondary pain and abnormal cervical motion should receive complete radiographic evaluation. If routine views of the cervical spine are normal, they are followed by flexion-extension views to detect occult instability. Flexion-extension views should be done by the patient moving his or her own neck rather than by the physician or radiologist moving the neck. The physician evaluating this patient should be familiar with the radiographic signs of instability outlined by White et al.[48] and White and Panjabi.[49]

Cervical disk injuries are caused either by acute herniation of the disk or by the presence of a degenerative disk. Acute disk herniations with associated neurological symptoms are more likely to occur in younger athletes. Fortunately, they are not that common. Cervical disk injuries in older athletes are usually associated with some degree of narrowing of the disk space and degeneration of the disk. In addition to localized cervical pain, the athlete sustaining an acute disk herniation will present with neurological findings appropriate to the level of disk injury. The athlete with a suspected disk herniation requires a careful and complete neurological examination. Evaluation by either CT myelogram or magnetic resonance imaging (MRI) is indicated if symptoms persist after conservative therapy and immobilization are attempted.

CERVICAL CORD NEUROPRAXIA

The occurrence of neuropraxia to the cervical spine cord in athletes has been excellently described by Torg and Pavlov[40] and Torg et al.[41] This neuropraxia can result from forceful hyperextension, hyperflexion, or axial loading. The athlete will present with sensory findings such as numbness, tingling, burning pain, or complete loss of sensation. This can be associated with motor changes, which can be either partial or complete. Surprisingly, these athletes do not complain of neck pain. Fortunately, the episode of symptoms usually lasts only 10 to 15 minutes. After this time period, there is complete recovery of function.

After sustaining an episode of neuropraxia with transient quadriplegia, the athlete needs to be evaluated thoroughly by both physical examination and radiographic analysis. Complete cervical spine films are needed to rule out the possibility of fractures or dislocations. Flexion and extension views of the lateral cervical spine can be utilized to determine the presence of cervical instability.

The lateral cervical spine roentgenogram is very important in determining the presence of cervical stenosis. Two methods of determination can be utilized. The first is frequently described as the standard method. In this method, the sagittal diameter of the spinal canal is determined by measuring the distance from the midpoint of the posterior aspect of the vertebral body to the nearest point on the corresponding spinolaminar line. An alternate method of determining cervical spinal stenosis has been developed by Torg and Pavlov (Fig. 9–6).[41] This is called the ratio method. One advantage of this method is that it compensates for variation in X-ray technique. To assess cervical spinal stenosis by the ratio method, the sagittal diameter, as measured by the standard method, is compared with the anteroposterior width of the vertebral body. Based on the findings of Torg and Pavlov, a ratio of less than 0.80 is diagnostic of cervical spinal stenosis.

Further radiographic studies, such as an MRI or CT scan, can also be utilized to obtain further information concerning the possible etiology of the neuropraxia. CT scans provide better information regarding the bony architecture of the cervical spine, whereas the MRI will provide information concerning a possible soft tissue etiology, such as cervical disk disease.

Cervical cord neuropraxia is associated with four different conditions: spinal stenosis, congenital fusion (Fig. 9–7), cervical instability, and disk disease. The underlying etiology associated with these conditions is a decrease in the anteroposterior diameter of the spinal canal. In athletes with decreased

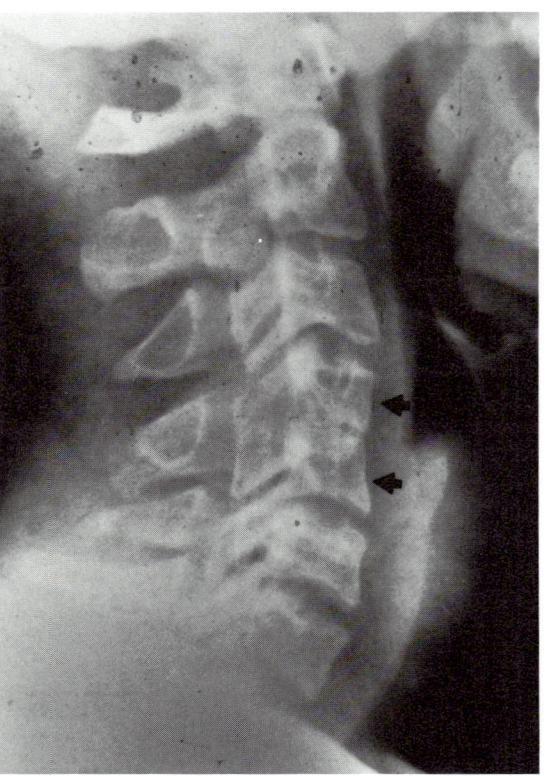

FIGURE 9–7. This 18-year-old football player had an episode of transient paresthesias. The radiograph reveals a congenital C4–C5 fusion.

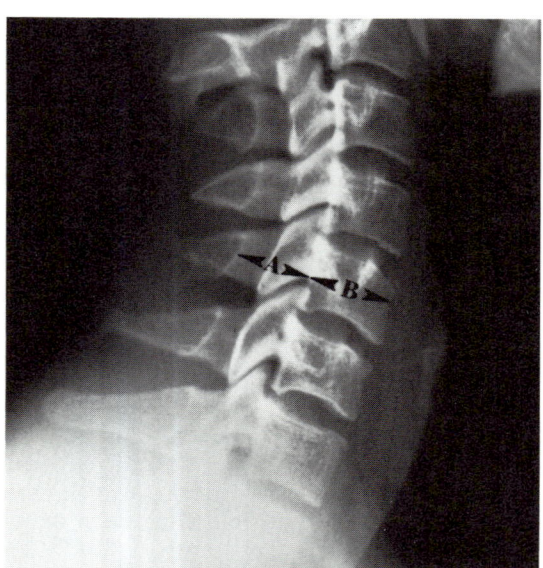

FIGURE 9–6. Torg's criteria for radiographic assessment of cervical spine stenosis compare the width of the vertebral body at the midpoint of its posterior aspect (B) to the distance from the body to the spinolaminar line at the same point (A). An A/B ratio of less than 0.80 is considered diagnostic of stenosis.

cervical canal diameter, if the neck is subjected to forced hyperflexion and hyperextension, the spinal cord can be compressed. This can subsequently result in transient sensory or motor changes. Torg has not found any evidence that an episode of cervical spinal cord neuropraxia predisposes the athlete to permanent neurological injury. He does recommend that those with cervical spine instability or degenerative change be precluded from further contact sports.[39] While it thus appears that there is no absolute medical indication that athletes without instability or degenerative changes should be disqualified from all further participation in contact sports after an episode of cervical cord neuropraxia, each treating physician should personally decide whether he or she wishes to assume the potential liability of returning such an athlete to competition.

BRACHIAL PLEXUS INJURIES

Injuries to the brachial plexus, while less potentially catastrophic than head or neck injuries, are more common in contact sports. Often referred to as *burners* or *stingers*, these injuries are frequently downplayed and not fully appreciated by coaches, trainers, and physicians.[29]

The most common mechanism of brachial plexus injury is to sustain a forceful impact to the shoulder girdle of the involved side while the head and neck are laterally flexed away from the site of injury. Less frequently, the injury can be sustained with the head laterally flexed toward the same side of injury or from forced hyperextension of the head and neck.

The underlying pathomechanics in brachial plexus injury are most likely due to traction on the nerves with varying degrees of damage to the nerve tissue. Clancy[14] and Clancy et al.[15] have classified these injuries into three grades that correlate with Seddon's classification of nerve injuries.[37]

Grade I injuries are secondary to a neuropraxia of the brachial plexus. They represent the most common neck injury in contact sports and are a classical type of burner or stinger. The athlete will initially experience a burning pain that starts in the shoulder area and then radiates distally down the extremity into the hand. There is a simultaneous development of numbness or tingling in the extremity and a feeling of the arm being "asleep." In most circumstances, there is spontaneous recovery shortly after the injury. The athlete may return to competition when there are no complaints or findings of pain or weakness on examination. However, the athlete should be reexamined after the event and the following day to make certain there has been no alteration in neurological function. Cervical spine radiographs are recommended for athletes who have sustained their first burner. It has been estimated that at least 50 percent of college football players have sustained at least one grade I brachial plexus injury during their careers.

Grade II brachial plexus injuries result from an axonotmesis of the nerve fibers. Electromyogram (EMG) studies have shown that the upper trunk of the brachial plexus is usually involved. Because the deltoid is the muscle most commonly affected, weakness of shoulder abduction should be routinely checked in all athletes with burners. Milder biceps weakness may also be present. These athletes initially experience a burning sensation in the extremity with an inability to use the arm. While the strength in the extremity may gradually return, as in a grade I injury, there is not a full return of strength. This weakness can persist for at least 3 to 4 weeks, with near full recovery of strength frequently by 6 weeks. Often, 6 months is required for the athlete to regain normal strength and endurance completely. These athletes do not routinely require EMG studies immediately after their injuries. However, if performed, EMG studies will usually demonstrate involvement of the upper trunk of the brachial plexus and its associated musculature. After 3 weeks, EMG can be performed if there is no improvement in strength testing. No athlete should be allowed to return to participation until all pain or any muscular weakness has resolved.

Grade III brachial plexus injuries involve neurotmesis of the nerve fibers. This type of injury is less common in contact sports. An athlete sustaining a grade III injury will have motor and sensory deficits that persist for at least 1 year. The athlete should be closely monitored for recovery of motion and sensory function. Owing to the severity of this type of injury, it is probably best to advise the athlete against returning to contact sports even in the event of full recovery.

The prevention and rehabilitation of brachial plexus injuries are closely interrelated. The use of various protective devices for the neck, such as neck rolls or collars, are discussed in the chapter on football injuries. In addition to these devices, the athlete should be placed on a specific program for upper body and neck strengthening and stretching. In the athlete sustaining a grade II injury, this is initiated after 2 to 3 weeks. Any athlete with a history of frequent grade I injuries needs to be started on the same stretching and strengthening program. If the burners continue to occur despite preventive measures, the only additional tool is to modify the tackling technique of the player. As long as the burners continue to be of the grade I category, there is no evidence that there is any danger in the athlete's continuing to participate. There are also no data to support resting the athlete for several weeks.

References

1. Albright, J. P., McAuley, E., Martin, R. K., et al.: Head and neck injuries in college football: An eight-year analysis. Am. J. Sports Med. 13:147, 1985.
2. Albright, J. P., Moses, J. M., Feldick, H. G., et al.: Nonfatal cervical spine injuries in interscholastic football. J.A.M.A. 236:1243, 1976.
3. Alves, W. M., Rimel, R. W. and Nelson, W. E.: University of Virginia prospective study of football-induced minor head injury: Status report. Clin. Sports Med. 6(1):211–218, 1987.
4. Bailes, J. E. and Maroon, J. C.: Management of cervical spine injuries in athletes. Clin. Sports Med. 8(1):43–58, 1989.
5. Bodnar, L. M.: Sports medicine with reference to back and neck injuries. Curr. Pract. Orthop. Surg. 7:116, 1977.
6. Bruce, D. A., Schut, L. and Sutton, L. N.: Brain and cervical spine injuries occurring during organized sports activities in children and adolescents. Clin. Sports Med. 1(3):495–514, 1982.
7. Bruno, L. A., Gennarelli, T. A. and Tory, J. S.: Management guidelines for head injuries in athletics. Clin. Sports Med. 6(1):17–30, 1987.
8. Buckley, W. E.: Concussions in college football. A multivariate analysis. Am. J. Sports Med. 16(1):51–56, 1988.
9. Burke, S. W., French, H. N. G., Roberts, J. M., et al.: Chronic atlanto-axial instability in Down syndrome. J. Bone Joint Surg. 67(9):1356–1360, 1985.
10. Burstein, A. H., Otis, J. C. and Torg, J. S.: Mechanisms and pathomechanics of athletic injuries to the cervical spine. In Torg, J. S. (ed.): Athletic injuries to the head, neck, and face. Philadelphia, Lea & Febiger, 1982.
11. Cantu, R. C.: Guidelines for return to contact sports after a cerebral concussion. Phys. Sports Med. 14:76–79, 1986.
12. Cantu, R. C.: Head and spine injuries in the young athlete. Clin. Sports Med. 7(3):459–472, 1988.
13. Carter, D. R. and Frankel, V. H.: Biomechanics of hyperextension injuries to the cervical spine in football. Am. J. Sports Med. 8(5):302–309, 1980.
14. Clancy, W. G.: Brachial plexus and upper extremity peripheral nerve injuries. In Torg, J. S. (ed.): Athletic injuries to the head, neck, and face. Philadelphia, Lea & Febiger, 1982.
15. Clancy, W. G., Brand, R. L. and Bergfield, J. A.: Upper trunk brachial plexus injuries in contact sports. Am. J. Sports Med. 5:209, 1977.
16. Committee on Head Injury Nomenclature of the Congress of Neurological Surgeons: Glossary of head injury including some definitions of injury to the cervical spine. Clin. Neurosurg. 12:386, 1966.
17. Davies, J. E.: The spine in sport-injuries, prevention, and treatment. Br. J. Sports Med. 14(1):18–21, 1980.
18. Fielding, J. W.: Athletic injuries to the atlanto-axial articulation. Am. J. Sports Med. 6:226, 1978.
19. Gennarelli, T. A.: Cerebral concussion and diffuse brain injuries. In Torg, J. S. (ed.): Athletic injuries to the head, neck, and face. Philadelphia, Lea & Febiger, 1982.
20. Hugenholtz, H. and Richard, M. T.: Return to athletic competition following concussion. Can. Med. Assoc. J. 127:827, 1982.
21. Hughston, J. C.: Whose neck next? (editorial) Am. J. Sports Med. 8(5):301, 1980.
22. Jackson, D. W. and Lohr, F. T.: Cervical spine injuries. Clin. Sports Med. 5(2):373–386, 1986.
23. Lehman, L. B.: Sports-related CNS injuries in children and adolescents. Postgrad. Med. 82(4):141–142, 1987.
24. Lehman, L. B.: Preventing and anticipating neurologic injuries in sports. Am. Fam. Physician 38(4):181–184, 1988.
25. Maroon, J. C., Steele, P. B. and Berline, A.: Football head and neck injuries—an update. Clin. Neurosurg. 27:414–428, 1980.
26. Mueller, F. O. and Blyth, C. S.: Football fatalities from head and cervical spine injuries occurring in tackle football: 40 years' experience. Clin. Sports Med. 6(1):185–196, 1987.
27. O'Leary, P. and Boiardo, R.: The diagnosis and treatment of injuries of the spine in athletes. In Nicholas, J. A. and Hershman, E. B. (eds.): The lower extremity and spine in sports medicine. St. Louis, C. V. Mosby Co., 1986.
28. Ommaya, A. K. and Gennarelli, T. A.: Cerebral concussion and traumatic unconsciousness correlation of experimental and clinical observations on blunt head injuries. Brain 97:633, 1974.
29. Patterson, D.: Legal aspects of athletic injuries to the head and cervical spine. Clin. Sports Med. 6(1):197–210, 1987.
30. Poindexter, D. P. and Johnson, E. W.: Football shoulder and neck injury: A study of the stinger. Arch. Phys. Med. Rehabil. 65(10):601–602, 1984.
31. Pueschel, S. M. and Scola, P. H.: Atlanto axial instability in individuals with Down syndrome. Pediatrics 80(4):555–560, 1987.
32. Rachesky, I., Boyce, W. T., Duncan, B., et al.: Clinical prediction of cervical spine injuries in children. Am. J. Dis. Child. 141(2):199–201, 1987.
33. Ryan, A. J.: Intracranial injuries resulting from boxing: A review (1918–1985). Clin. Sports Med. 6(1):31–40, 1987.

34. Saunders, R. L. and Harbaugh, R. E.: The second impact in catastrophic contact sports head trauma. J.A.M.A. 252:538–539, 1984.
35. Schneider, R. C.: Head and neck injuries in football. Baltimore, Williams & Wilkins, 1983.
36. Schneider, R. C.: Football head and neck injury. (editorial) Surg. Neurol. 27(5):507–508, 1987.
37. Seddon, H.: Surgical disorders of the peripheral nerves. Edinburgh, Churchhill Livingstone, Inc., 1972.
38. Tator, C. H.: Neck injuries in ice hockey: A recent, unsolved problem with many contributing factors. Clin. Sports Med. 6(1):101–114, 1987.
39. Torg, J. S.: Management guidelines for athletic injuries to the cervical spine. Clin. Sports Med. 6(1):53–60, 1987.
40. Torg, J. S. and Pavlov, H.: Cervical spinal stenosis with cord neuropraxia and transient quadriplegia. Clin. Sports Med. 6(1):115–134, 1987.
41. Torg, J. S., Pavlov, H., Genuario, S. E., et al.: Neuropraxia of the cervical spinal cord with transient quadriplegia. J. Bone Joint Surg. 68-A(9):1354, 1986.
42. Torg, J. S., Sennett, B. and Vegso, J. J.: Spinal injury at the level of the third and fourth cervical vertebrae resulting from the axial loading mechanism: An analysis and classification. Clin. Sports Med. 6(1):159–184, 1987.
43. Torg, J. S., Truex, R. C., Marshall, J., et al.: Spinal injury at the level of the third and fourth cervical vertebrae from football. J. Bone Joint Surg. 59A:1015, 1977.
44. Torg, J. S., Vegso, J. J., Sennett, B. S. and Das, M.: The National Football Head and Neck Registry: 14-year report on cervical quadriplegia (1971–1984). J.A.M.A. 254:3439–3443, 1985.
45. Torg, J. S., Wiesel, S. and Rothman, R.: Diagnosis and management of cervical spine injuries. In Torg, J. S. (ed.): Athletic injuries to the head, neck, and face. Philadelphia, Lea & Febiger, 1982.
46. Vegso, J. J. and Lehman, R. C.: Field evaluation and management of head and neck injuries. Clin. Sports Med. 6(1):16, 1987.
47. Watkins, R. G.: Neck injuries in football players. Clin. Sports Med. 5(2):215–246, 1986.
48. White, A. A., III, Johnson, R. M., Panjabi, M. M., et al.: Biomechanical analysis of clinical stability in the cervical spine. Clin. Orthop. 109:85–96, 1975.
49. White, A. A., III and Panjabi, M. M.: Clinical biomechanics of the spine. Philadelphia, J. B. Lippincott, Co., 1978.
50. Wilberger, J. E. and Maroon, J C.: Head injuries in athletes. Clin. Sports Med. 8(1):1–10, 1989.
51. Williams, P. and McKibbin, B.: Unstable cervical spine injuries in rugby—a 20 year review. Injury 18(5):329–332, 1987.
52. Wroble, R. R. and Albright, J. F.: Neck and low back injuries in wrestling. Clin. Sports Med. 5(2):295–326, 1986.
53. Yarnell, P. R. and Lynch, S.: The "ding" amnestic states in football trauma. Neurology 23:196, 1983.

10
SPONDYLOLYSIS AND SPONDYLOLISTHESIS

BERT R. MANDELBAUM
MICHAEL L. GROSS

As the number of young athletes participating in highly competitive sports programs has increased in recent years, the number of young athletes complaining of low back pain has increased as well. Although most low back pain in young athletes is related to trauma, these youngsters are, of course, not immune from the developmental, infectious, neoplastic, or visceral conditions that may cause back pain in any child. When treating school-aged athletes with low back pain, common conditions to consider include sprains and strains that can be relatively simple to diagnose and treat. More significant are apophyseal fractures, discogenic pain, infections, and neoplasms. Of great concern is one of the most common conditions that gives rise to low back pain in adolescent athletes: spondylolytic lesions of the pars interarticularis. Jackson reported that of young athletes seen with lumbar pain of greater than 3 months duration, 40 percent were eventually diagnosed as having symptomatic pathology related to the pars interarticularis at the lumbosacral junction.[36] Numerous authors have found a relationship between athletic participation and an increased incidence of spondylolysis and spondylolisthesis. Athletes in sports as varied as gymnastics, dance, football, martial arts, tennis, weight lifting, and rowing have all shown an increased incidence of symptomatic and asymptomatic defects in the posterior elements of the lumbar spine.[1,2,3,4]

The goals of the physician caring for young athletes should include (1) injury prevention, (2) early diagnosis and treatment, (3) minimization of morbidity, and (4) increased performance. These goals can only be achieved through efforts directed in several areas. Effective screening for potential problems combined with proper conditioning and training may reduce the overall incidence of symptomatic injuries. Education of athletes and coaches in safe training techniques will serve to decrease the rate of injury further. Early recognition of injuries and appropriate treatment will result in an early and safe return to competition, with decreased risks of either reinjury or exacerbation. Although the long-term significance of spondylolytic defects is unknown, a program that seeks to incorporate these principles will, in the least, serve to decrease any long-term sequelae such as chronic low back pain, disability, and degeneration of the lumbar spine.

This chapter will (1) outline the historical progression of important concepts in the understanding of spondylolysis and spondylolisthesis; (2) present the definitions of key terms and elements; (3) discuss the etiology and pathogenesis of the pars interarticularis defect with regard to heredity, embryology, and biomechanics (particular attention will be paid to how these factors affect, and are affected by, participation in athletic activities); (4) suggest a logical plan for clinical evaluation and treatment of young athletes with spondylolytic pain; and (5) present ideas for preventive measures.

HISTORY AND TERMS

In the simplest sense, *spondylolysis* refers to a defect in the pars interarticularis. The defect is either a break in its continuity or an elongation. Most often the lesion occurs at the L5–S1 articulation. *Spondylolisthesis* is the slipping of one vertebra forward over another owing to instability in the posterior elements. This instability, particularly in adolescent athletes, most frequently arises from a spondylolytic defect in the pars interarticularis.

Herbiniaux, a Belgian obstetrician, was the first to report on a patient with gross anterior displacement of the fifth lumbar vertebra on the first sacral vertebra in 1782.[5] In 1854, Kilian coined the term *spondylolisthesis* by combining the Greek *spondylo*, meaning "vertebra," and *olisthesis*, meaning "to slip forward."[6] In cadaveric studies the following year, 1855, Robert removed all the soft tissue attachments about the lumbosacral junction.[7] He established that anterior translation of the L5 vertebral body could take place only when a defect was created in the bony elements of the posterior neural arch. Also in 1855, Lambl concluded that the lesion responsible for anterior subluxation was located in the pars interarticularis.[8] During this same period, investigators began to identify spondylolisthesis at postmortem examination, but they were confused when a defect in the posterior neural arch could not be identified in every case. In 1881, Naugebauer resolved this conflict when he concluded that there were two distinct but related pathological entities that could result in spondylolisthesis: (1) elongation of the pars interarticularis or (2) spondylolysis, a frank disruption in the pars interarticularis.[9] Since then, authors have speculated that elongation may simply represent healing of a lytic defect in an elongated position.[49]

Through the years, classification systems have reflected the current thinking with regard to etiology of pars interarticularis defects. Wiltse, Newman, and Macnab have developed a system based on the different modes of pathogenesis of spondylolysis and spondylolisthesis. This comprehensive classification of spondylolysis and spondylolisthesis is in common usage today.[10,11] (See Table 10–1.)

Degenerative spondylolisthesis is a problem related to disk degeneration in older adults and is therefore not relevant to this dicussion. *Traumatic spondylolisthesis* deals with the acute situation of fracture dislocation, and *pathologic spondylolisthesis* refers to those situations where conditions such as tumors or metabolic bone disease lead to weakening of the bone; neither of these groups is relevant to the discussion of adolescent athletic injuries.

The lesion commonly encountered in young athletes is *isthmic spondylolisthesis*. The defect is located in the pars interarticularis and can be a stress fracture, an acute fracture, or an elongation of the bone. As noted, elongation may represent a secondary change after fracture. In either case, the important feature is that a defect in the pars interarticularis creates an instability pattern. This in turn leads to pain, forward displacement, or both. It remains unclear whether the pain arises from the fracture or the instability. However, it would appear that instability is the offending agent, since these defects can go undetected for many years until stress, such as the increased demands of athletic participation, brings them to light.

TABLE 10–1. Classification of Spondylolysis and Spondylolisthesis

Dysplastic
Congenital deficiency of the facet joint, leading to a gradual slipping forward of one vertebra over another

Isthmic
Spondylolysis defect in the pars interarticularis permitting forward slipping of one vertebral body over another, this group has three subdivisions:
Lytic fracture of the pars interarticularis
Elongated or attenuated, but intact, pars interarticularis
Acute fracture

Degenerative
Degeneration of the L5–S1 disk and facet joints, allowing forward displacement

Traumatic
Acute fracture in areas other than the pars interarticularis, such as the pedicle, lamina, or facet joint, that allows forward displacement (note that acute fractures of the pars interarticularis are placed in group II)

Pathological
Attenuation of the posterior neural arch secondary to structural weakness in the bone, such as in metabolic bone disease

There appears to be some confusion both in the literature and on the part of clinicians as to the terms *hereditary, congenital,* and *dysplasia. Hereditary* refers to a genetic condition. *Congenital* refers to a condition that occurs in utero. Congenital defects may be hereditary but are not necessarily so. *Dysplasia* refers to a developmental malformation that is the physical manifestation of either a congenital and/or a hereditary defect. It has been suggested that the term *congenital spondylolisthesis* be reserved for those newborn infants who demonstrate dysplastic elements at birth.[40,44] A thorough understanding of the differences and their implications for classification has important clinical significance. Children with a dysplastic spondylolisthesis have a worse prognosis for difficulties with progression of their slips.[12,48,49]

Once a spondylolisthesis occurs, slips are graded according to the classification developed by Meyerding.[45] The superior border of the inferior vertebra is divided into four equal quadrants; slips in the first quadrant are grade I, slips in the second quadrant are grade II, and so on. This same idea can also be expressed in terms of percentages.[46] In terms of prognosis, the angle of inclination of the lumbar spine on the sacrum is more important than the degree of slipping. This angle, known as the *slip angle,* is measured by the method described by Boxall et al.[47] The slip angle is formed by the intersection of a line drawn parallel to the inferior aspect of the fifth lumbar vertebra and a line drawn perpendicular to the posterior aspect of the first sacral vertebra.

ETIOLOGY

The etiology of spondylolysis and spondylolisthesis is multifactorial. Factors such as genetic predisposition, developmental defects, and trauma all come to bear in the pathogenesis of lesions in the pars interarticularis. Unique demands are placed on the musculoskeletal system by participation in sports. Often this involves repetitive stresses focused on the lower back beginning at a young age. The additional factors associated with athletic participation form the basis for controversy in the discussion of the etiology of pars interarticularis lesions in adolescent athletes.

Defects in the pars interarticularis appear only rarely in patients under the age of 5 years.[12,13,14,15,44] Cadaveric dissections of stillborn infants have failed to demonstrate any example of the defect.[12,15,20,28,50] However, Baker and McHollick[51] reported an incidence of pars defects in first-grade children between 5 and 6 percent. Although this precipitous rise in incidence is difficult to explain, it does appear to coincide with the increase in physical activity and organized physical education experienced by children as they enter school. The incidence reported in young schoolchildren does not differ widely from the reported incidence found in adults by Wiltse et al.[15] or from the occurrence rate found in the dissection of cadaveric specimens reported by Roche and Rowe.[16] Apparently, the majority of lesions appear early in life and become symptomatic later.

Historically, many investigators held the belief that the spondylolytic defect is a congenital one.[8,20,21,26] They theorized that the lesion developed either as a result of the failure of fusion between two centers of ossification that form the lateral portion of the neural arch[8] or from anomalous centers of ossification.[32,52] However, Hitchcock was unable to verify these findings in the dissections of 90 fetal specimens.[28] As previously noted, no investigators have been able to demonstrate a spondylolytic defect in fetal tissue or in newborns.[15,25,50] In view of these findings, the likelihood of a congenital defect seems low.

There does appear to be an important genetic component in the development of abnormalities in the pars interarticularis. In the cadaver study reported by Roche and Rowe, both racial and sex differences were identified. The incidence in white males was 6.4 percent; in black males, 2.8 percent; in white females, 2.3 percent; and black females, 1.1 percent.[16] Incidences of between 27 and 69 percent have been reported in the near relatives of patients with defects in the pars interarticularis.[13,18,20,21,22,25] In Eskimo tribes, an incidence as high as 50 percent has been reported.[18,23] Japanese studies have also demonstrated interracial differences.[19] The genetic role in the development of spondylolisthesis in the athlete appears to be in terms of a hereditary predisposition toward the development of the defect.

There is little doubt that a hereditary predisposition for spondylolysis exists and that it may play a role in the development of pars interarticularis defects. However, most investigators agree that in isthmic spondylolysis the defect is the pathological end result of repeated stresses that have produced a mechanical overload to the pars interarticularis. In other words, the spondylolytic defect is a stress fracture in the pars interarticularis, and this fracture has developed secondary to repeated trauma over a prolonged period.

The appearance of a spondylolytic defect can also be explained on a developmental basis. In early childhood, the normal lumbar lordosis is accentuated by the hip flexion contractures.[26] In humans, this is combined with an upright posture that focuses the strains of weight bearing on the pars interarticularis and leads to eventual disruption. Spondylolysis does not appear in primates other than man. In addition, Rosenberg et al. studied a group of patients with neurological impairments who had never walked and were unable to identify spondylolysis in any of them.[27] In the susceptible population, the stresses applied through the activities of daily living, particularly walking upright, can apply enough fatigue stress over time to create a spondylolysis.

Roche and Rowe were unable to produce the typical pars defects with vigorous attempts at both flexion and extension.[16,50] Hitchcock was only able to reproduce the defect with forced hyperflexion.[28] Other laboratory studies have demonstrated that a high degree of force is needed to produce an acute pars interarticularis lesion. This helps to verify the clinical assumption that most pars interarticularis fractures occur by way of a stress fracture mechanism rather than as an acute event.

Experimental studies have produced fractures of the pars interarticularis when cortical fatigue stresses were applied to the region.[30,31] Anatomical studies suggest that with continuous shear and compression the inferior facet is subject to alternating loads and forces that will produce fatigue failure.[29,30,31] In both flexion and extension, axial loading, shear stress, and torsional stress are produced in the lumbar spine. These forces are particularly increased in positions of hyperextension[30,31,32,33] and hyperflexion.[34,35] Biomechanically, it appears that the forces responsible for creating the spondylolytic lesion are a combination of flexion and extension torsional moments applied over time.

Controversy exists over whether it is flexion or extension that produces a lesion in the pars interarticularis. Arguments in favor of combined flexion and extension forces make particular sense when one considers that most flexible structures fail when alternating compression and tension stresses are applied. The pars interarticularis of the last lumbar vertebra is particularly at risk from these factors, since it is the link between the flexible lumbar spine and the rigid sacrum.

The effects of these factors are enhanced by participation in athletic activities. In athletes, the potentially damaging effect of continuous mechanical stresses, particularly torsional stress, is multiplied by the additional factor of a greater number of more forceful repetitions. What additive effect is produced in immature spines as rigorous participation begins at ever decreasing ages is not known.

Ciullo and Jackson have shown that the same high forces that create a pars interarticularis fracture in the laboratory are reproduced several times during a gymnastics practice session.[29] Jackson and colleagues noted that these forces are particularly accentuated by maneuvers such as back walkovers (hyperextension) and front walkovers (hyperflexion).[3,29] Hyperflexion is also noted in rowing. Hyperextension of the lumbar spine is achieved in baseball while pitching and in tennis while serving.[3,29] In football, Ferguson et al. found the players most often affected by pars interarticularis difficulties were interior linemen. They felt the reason for the higher incidence at this position was the stress placed on the lumbar spine by a three- or four-point stance.[1] This flexed position results in a loss of lumbar lordosis, with compression and narrowing of the disk spaces anteriorly. In turn, this puts great stress on the pars interarticularis of the fifth lumbar vertebra. Furthermore, the repetitive stresses resulting from driving forward and upward, combined with extension of the lumbar spine, such as in blocking or tackling, create shear at the apophyseal joints and may cause a stress fracture through the pars interarticularis as well. McCarrol et al. agreed that this was a possible explanation for the mechanism of injury in linemen but implicated other sources of stress such as weight lifting or improper training techniques as additional causes of spondylolysis and spondylolisthesis in players at other positions.[17]

Certain sports have been noted to have far greater incidence rates for pars interarticularis defects than those encountered in the general population. Classically, gymnastics is cited as the example of a sport with increased incidence of spondylosis among competitors. Jackson et al. reported an incidence of 11 percent among a group of female gymnasts studied.[3] Studies in college football players have found incidences as high as 15.2 percent.[17] Increased incidence has also been reported among divers, wrestlers, rowers, and tennis players.[2,3,36] Hoshina obtained roentgenographs of 677 Japanese male high school and college athletes; spondylolisthetic posterior elements were found in 21 percent, an incidence three times greater than that in the general population.[4]

As noted, spondylolysis is relatively nonexistent in children under the age of 5 years and seems to achieve its adult incidence by age 7 to 8 years. However, most reported series agree that the lesion does not become clinically obvious until the ages of 13 to 16 years.[3,15,17,37,49] In Lafond's series of 415 patients with low back pain, only 9 percent sought medical attention before adolescence.[38] In some series, the onset of symptoms coincides with adolescent growth spurt.[37,49,53] For adolescent athletes, this is also a time of increasing duration and intensity of athletic participation. One can conclude that there is a significant number of young athletes who begin their athletic careers with a preexisting, albeit undiagnosed, pars interarticularis defect. In this group, participation in sports, particularly during adolescence, may exacerbate symptoms secondary to their defect.

However, the incidence of both symptomatic and asymptomatic lesions is much higher in athletic participants. Therefore, it is likely that in some athletes participation in sports does more than simply exacerbate the symptoms of a preexisting abnormality or bring a genetic tendency to the surface. Athletic participation accentuates the torsional forces placed on the lumbar spine. It increases the number of repetitions with which the forces are applied. Finally, it increases the duration of time over which these forces are applied. Therefore, it seems probable that a second group of athletes with spondylolytic defects exists. In this group, fatigue loading of the pars interarticularis secondary to the unique and rigorous demands of participation in sports plays a pivotal role in the pathogenesis of the fresh defects.

There are, then, two sets of athletes with spondylolytic defects: those with long-standing defects made worse by participation and those who may or may not have genetic predisposition who acquire an acute stress fracture secondary to their athletic activities. This creates a two-part challenge: (1) to identify the first group in preparticipation physical examinations and prevent further injury through reconditioning and stretching programs and (2) to diagnose the second group early in their course and treat them appropriately. In this way, it may be possible to modify the natural history of the process. If so, the more overt manifestations of the disease process—stress fracture of the pars interarticularis or progression of slips—can hopefully be avoided. Ultimately, a thorough understanding of the pathological process will allow coaches, trainers, and physicians to implement training regimens that reduce the risk of injury in both groups.

CLINICAL FINDINGS

HISTORY

The usual presentation for a young athlete with a spondylolytic injury is one of chronic low back pain, frequently unilateral, that is increased by motions of hyperextension or twisting. While a cosmetic deformity secondary to a high-grade slip is often the presenting complaint in nonathletes, the young athlete usually presents earlier in the course and presents with pain. Pain often accompanies the activities of daily living and is exacerbated during practice or competition. In gymnasts, common aggravating maneuvers are walkovers, especially dismounts and vaults. Football players will complain that blocking drills are particularly troublesome. Tennis players will frequently complain of pain while serving. In general, the athletes will complain of any activities that are either jarring or require positions of extreme lumbar flexion or extension.

When localized, the pain is usually in the low back, particularly in the paraspinous area, and to some degree in the buttocks and posterior thighs. It is exceedingly rare for an athlete to present with radicular symptoms that are secondary to a pars lesion. Occasionally, athletes will remark that their discomfort is relieved by supine positioning. In taking a history, there are several other important items that should be included: previous back injury or back pain, duration since onset of symptoms, and family history of back problems.

PHYSICAL EXAMINATION

Physical findings can be variable, depending on the severity of the problem; however, there are several consistent findings that should alert the examiner to the possibility of a spondylolytic lesion. Patients will often demonstrate a hyperlordotic posture and weak abdominal musculature. Maximal tenderness is usually at the belt line. Extension of the spine will increase or reproduce the pain (Fig. 10-1). A useful, although perhaps overrated, diagnostic test is the unilateral hyperextension maneuver. The patient stands on one leg and hyperextends the low back. The maneuver is then repeated on the opposite leg. In cases of a unilateral lesion, pain is usually greatest while standing on the ipsilateral leg. Hamstring tightness is a common finding among symptomatic patients. It is important to realize that if a gymnast is experiencing pain with 90 degrees of straight leg raising, this may represent a substantial decrease in flexibility. We, therefore, employ the term *relative* hamstring tightness and take care to question the patients about previous levels of flexibility and whether they have noticed any changes. The exact etiology of hamstring tightness remains unclear. Historically, this was considered to be a sign of nerve root irritation.[53,54] Present thinking is that this phenomenon represents an attempt to stabilize the L5–S1 articulation.[12,40,49] This concept is borne out by the finding that many patients with hamstring tightness will have a resolution of their problem after an in situ fusion with no nerve root decompression. Hamstring tightness is responsible for the peculiar gait seen in some patients with spondylolytic defects known as the *pelvic waddle*. Neurological examination is usually normal in athletes with pain secondary to a pars interarticularis lesion, and although straight leg raising may demonstrate hamstring tightness, it will not reveal nerve root irritation.

Higher grade (III and IV) slips are unusual among highly competitive athletes, but they do occur. Earlier recognition and treatment may even further decrease the incidence of high-grade slips in the athletic population. More commonly, these patients can often be found on the high school level, particularly in preparticipation physical examinations. Therefore, the typical physical findings and characteristic posture in these patients should be recognized. Examination from each side will reveal something to the informed examiner. When viewed from the side, the patient has a severe lordosis. When viewed from the front, the lower abdomen is thrust forward, and a marked transverse crease is formed across the abdomen at the level of the umbilicus. When viewed from the back, the ilia are flared and the buttocks are flattened, or "heart-shaped." Occasionally, a step-off can be palpated between the spinous processes of L4 and L5. Patients with high degrees of slipping may show signs of nerve root compression; therefore, examination must include a careful neurological evaluation of the lower extremities.

Thorough examination of the spine in all athletes presenting with back pain should include inspection for structural abnormalities such as scoliosis and kyphosis. Organic

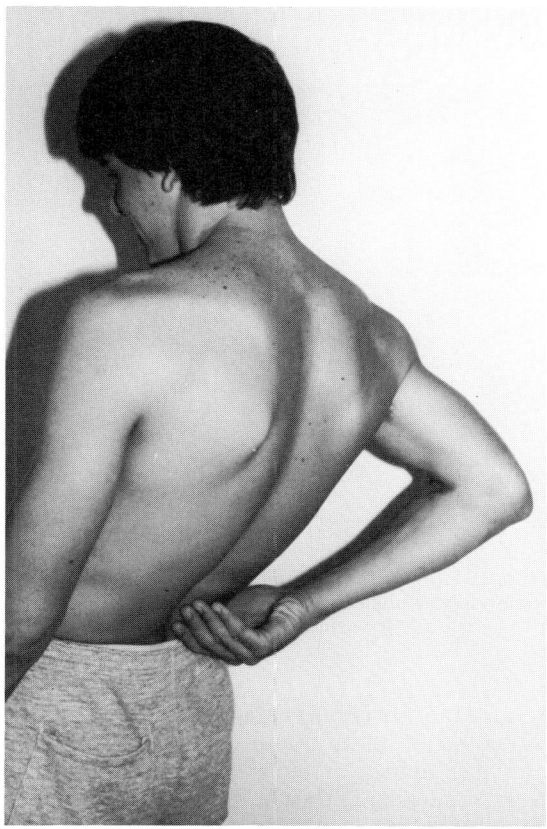

FIGURE 10–1. Active or passive extension of the spine will usually increase the pain in spondylolysis.

causes of low back pain, such as renal problems, must also be ruled out.

RADIOGRAPHIC FINDINGS

Routine radiographs of the lumbar spine should include anteroposterior, standing lateral, and both oblique views in all athletes with a suspected injury to the pars interarticularis. Although high-grade slips are easily identified on lateral views, young athletes do not often present for the first time with slips greater than grade I (Fig. 10–2). Lateral views may also expose other sources of low back pain such as osteoid osteoma, infection, or disk space degeneration. Oblique views will allow easy visualization of the pars interarticularis and readily expose a defect in spondylolysis. The "scotty dog" of Lachapele, with a collar on its neck, is a visual aid well known to all orthopedists (Fig. 10–3). Hensinger et al. have described the "greyhound" to represent the radiographic appearance of an elongated pars interarticularis.[49] Both oblique views are necessary since the defect may be unilateral or a second asymptomatic defect may appear on the contralateral side.

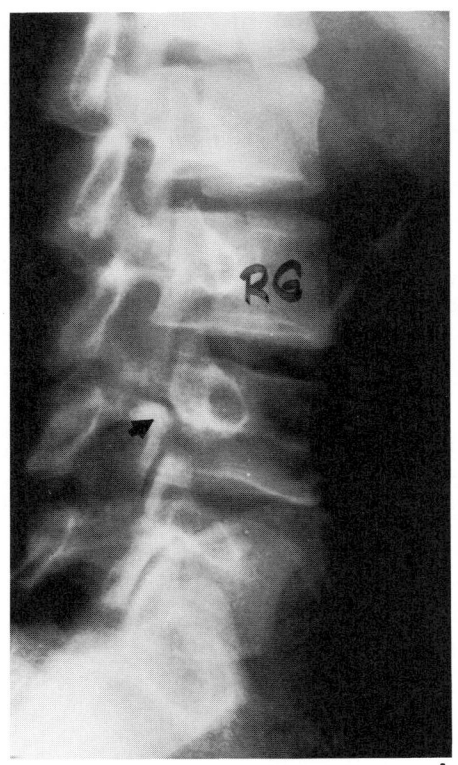

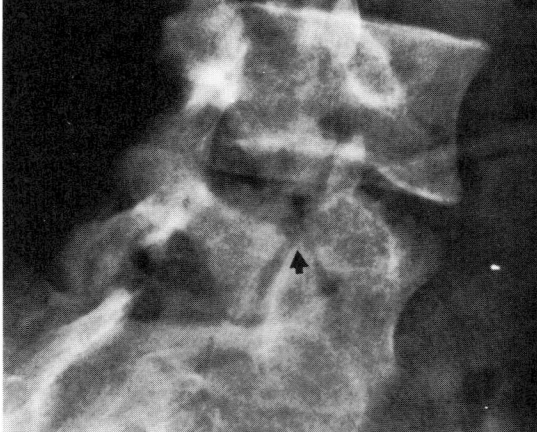

FIGURE 10–3. These oblique radiographs show spondylolysis of L4 in a 16-year-old football player (A) and L5 in an 18-year-old wrestler (B).

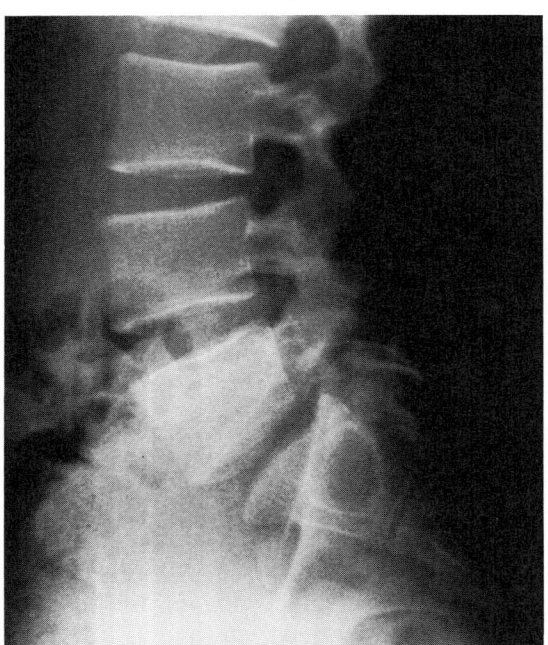

FIGURE 10–2. Radiograph of this 16-year-old linebacker shows spondylolysis of L5 with a grade I spondylolisthesis. He began having back pain a few months before this was taken.

If plain radiographs are normal, and a high index of suspicion remains for a pars interarticularis defect, a technetium 99 radionuclear bone scan of the lumbar spine should be obtained (Fig. 10–4). Increased uptake of the isotope in the region of the pars interarticularis confirms the diagnosis. Jackson et al.

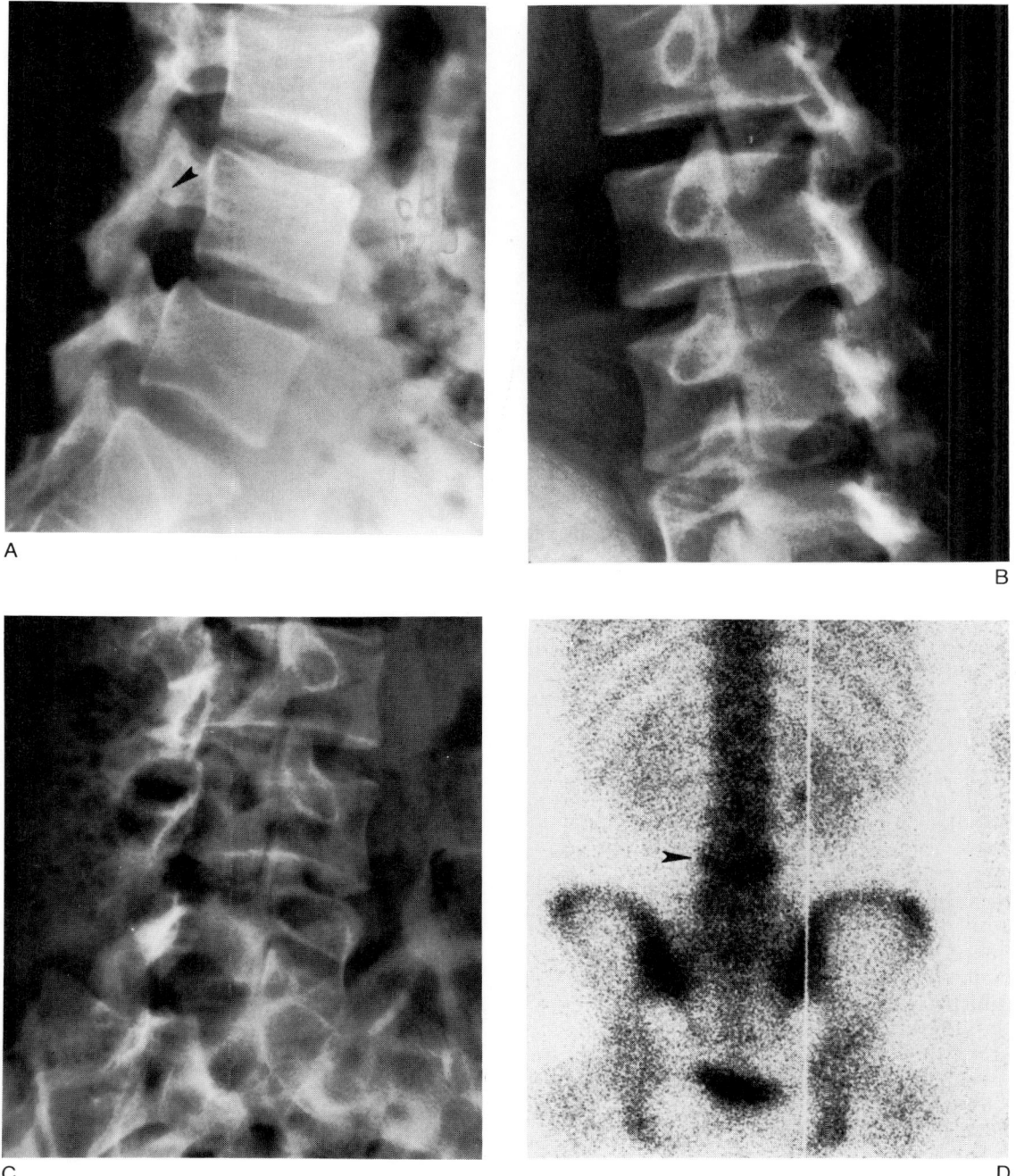

FIGURE 10–4. Spondylolysis of L4 is suggested on the lateral view in this 13-year-old female gymnast but not visible on the oblique views (B,C). A bone scan (D) shows increased uptake at L4.

have termed this subroentgenographic stage, with negative X rays and a positive bone scan, the "pars stress reaction."[29,36,39] This stage appears to coincide with the early phase of a stress fracture. Their studies have demonstrated both patients who have gone on to resolution from this stage and patients who have developed roentgenographic evidence of a pars interarticularis fracture. Early intervention at this point may avert the progression to radiographic changes. Micheli has stated that when clinical suspicion is great enough, a negative bone scan and negative roentgenograph should not be grounds to avoid treatment.[42]

If a pars interarticularis defect does appear on initial radiographs, then the physician must determine whether this reflects an acute or chronic condition. As stated, some athletes may have had an undiagnosed, asymptomatic lesion since the age of 5 years; others may have a fresh (6 months to 1 year) injury. In the acute condition, the gap is narrow, with irregular edges; in the chronic condition, the edges are rounded and smooth, showing signs of resorption. Bone scan can be useful in determining the age of a lesion. A positive bone scan will usually reflect a lesion of short standing, whereas a negative bone scan indicates a lesion that is usually 6 months to 1 year old. In treating a symptomatic lesion, the resolution of pain will often coincide with a change from hot to cold on the bone scan. Determining the age of a lesion may have important implications regarding treatment and prognosis. Although both lesions have the potential to heal, the odds are greater for the recent injury with a "hot" bone scan. Treatment for chronic lesions is often aimed simply at relieving symptoms.

In the absence of neurological findings, there is no indication for myelography in the work-up of these patients. Since the athletic population rarely presents with evidence of nerve root impingement, the myelogram is rarely used. Discography is usually recommended in the preoperative evaluation in adult patients with spondylolisthesis but is not of value in adolescents.[40] Magnetic resonance imaging (MRI) has not been used in the routine evaluation and treatment of school-age athletes with pars interarticularis defects. The role for MRI in the future may be in making an even earlier diagnosis of the subroentgenographic lesion. The fact that MRI is a nonionizing diagnostic modality makes it particularly attractive for use in the adolescent age group.

When the athlete fails to respond to treatment, the physician must always suspect other causes of adolescent low back pain (Fig. 10–5). Myelography, computerized tomography (CT) scanning, and MRI can be particularly useful in this situation or when neurological signs develop. If a tumor of the posterior elements is suspected, bone scan, CT scan, or MRI scan will help localize the lesion. Complete blood counts, sedimenta-

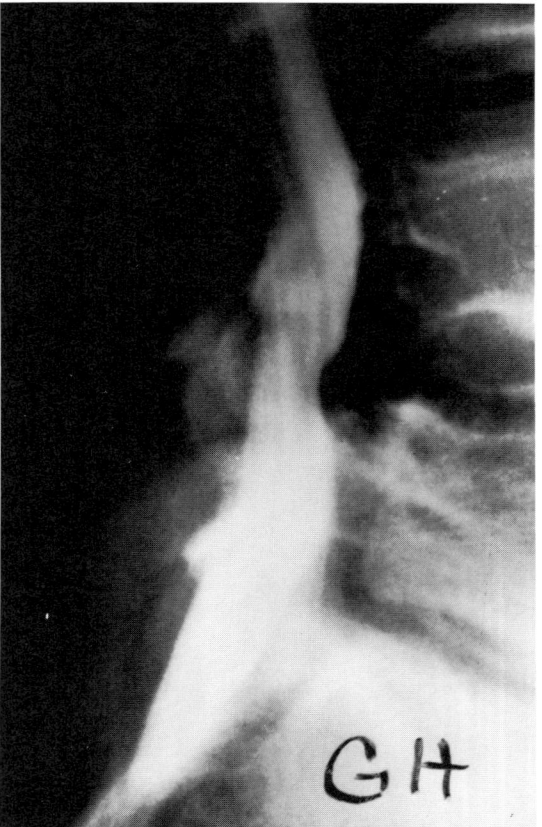

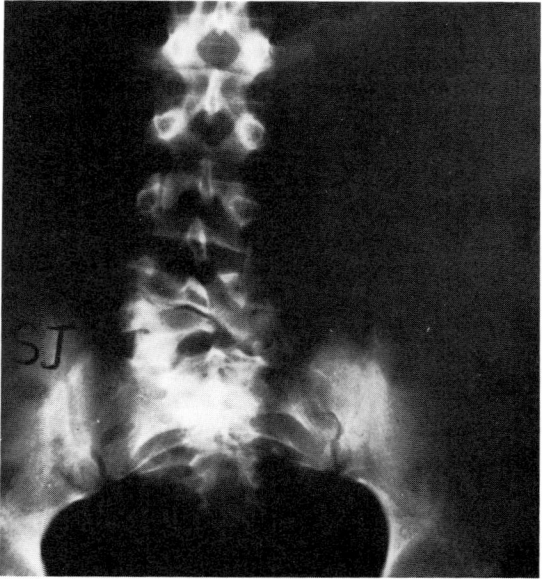

FIGURE 10–5. Not all adolescent back pain is caused by spondylolysis. A shows a central disk protrusion in a 200-pound 14-year-old football player; B, an anomalous L5–S1 in a 16-year-old female gymnast.

tion rates, and urinalysis can help in detection of neoplasm or infection.

TREATMENT

Treatment of the athlete with an injury to the pars interarticularis remains controversial, particularly in the earlier stages. Whatever course is chosen, the goals remain clear: pain relief, healing of the defect, and prevention of further slip. In terms of athletic participation, this can be translated into one phrase: "Safe return to participation." Furthermore, in treating the adolescent athlete, an important consideration are his or her goals for the future. These must be considered both in terms of sport and vocation.

In athletes with spondylolytic low back pain who have negative radiographs and a positive bone scan, Jackson et al. have recommended a program of restricted activity. In this subroentgenographic group, the cornerstone of the treatment regimen recommended by Jackson et al. is elimination of the aggravating activity. Athletes participate in a generalized fitness maintenance program that consists of swimming, cycling, and moderate weight lifting. Short periods of bedrest are utilized as necessary to reduce pain. This regimen evolved after treatment with plaster casts was found to be not well accepted in the adolescent population. Further impetus was given by the fact that they were able to document examples of pars defects that healed with continued athletic participation. In patients treated with a restricted activities regimen, a minimum of 3 months and sometimes considerably longer has been needed before a return to full activities is allowed. Resolution of pain has corresponded to reduction of activity on radioisotope bone scan.[3,15,29,36,39]

Micheli[43] has emphasized the use of a rigid polypropylene lumbosacral brace (Fig. 10–6). The brace is constructed with zero degrees of lumbar flexion to maximize the potential for healing. Immobilization is used for both the subroentgenographic and roentgenograph positive lesions. This more aggressive treatment is based on the belief that both lesions represent a fracture of the pars interarticularis and should be treated as such.[24,41,42,43] The brace is worn for 23 hours per day and utilized in conjunction with an exercise program. Exercises are designed to stretch the lumbodorsal fascia and hamstrings and to strengthen the abdominal muscles. When the athletes become asymptomatic, they are allowed to resume their sports while wearing the brace. Most patients were asymptomatic by 3 weeks.[24,41,43] Brace treatment is continued until there is radiographic evidence of healing or the bone scan changes from hot to cold. The average duration of treatment with the brace was 6 months.

Jackson has used a similar program in symptomatic athletes with documented lesions on radiographs.[29] In these patients, bone scan is used to differentiate fresh defects from older lesions. While treatment is the same, the prognosis for healing is greater in the fresh lesion. Both Hall[40] and Hensinger[12,40] prescribe an initial program of limited activity and exercises. The program is supplemented with immobilization when the patients do not experience a degree of relief within the first few weeks.

Our current program for treatment in athletes with symptomatic pars interarticularis defects that do not have a visible lesion on radiographs, but do show positive bone scans, begins with restricted activity and functional rehabilitation. Particular attention is paid to abdominal strengthening and lumbar stretching. Another important aspect of our regimen includes working with both the player and coach in a retraining program. Techniques that may exacerbate symptoms are corrected, and a modified training schedule with alternating hard and even days, particularly as pertaining to activities that can affect the low back, is adopted wherever possible. In athletes who do not show improvement within 4 weeks, immobilization is added. This usually consists of some form of molded polypropylene brace.

The same program is utilized when the athlete has a documented spondylolysis on radiographs. Patients with positive bone scans—that is, those with recent injuries—are more likely to heal with a period of immobilization. Therefore, treatment for these athletes is designed with eventual healing as a goal. Healing may be demonstrated on conventional radiographs or by conversion of bone scan from hot to cold. When patients are asymptomatic, they are allowed to return to their sports, provided they can do so in a brace. Brace wear is discontinued when healing is documented. Athletes with positive radiographs and cold scans, chronic lesions, are less likely to heal, and treatment for them is directed toward relief of symptoms. These athletes are braced as necessary for pain re-

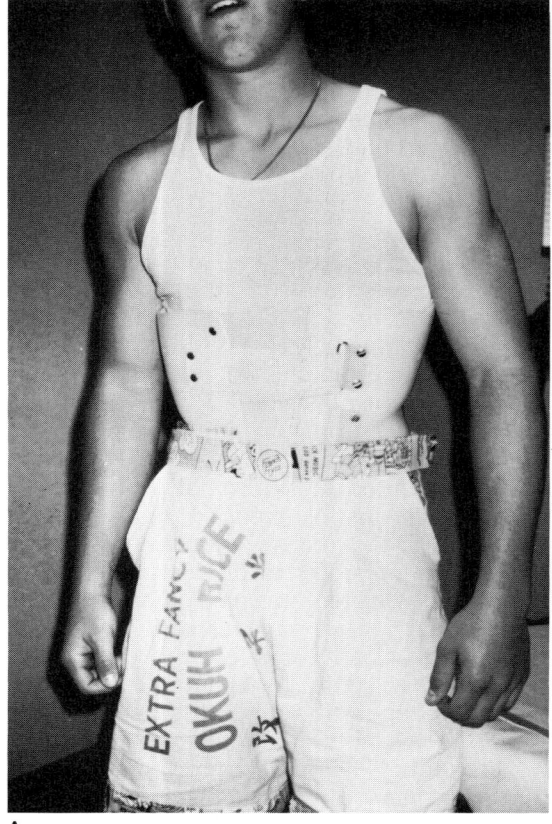 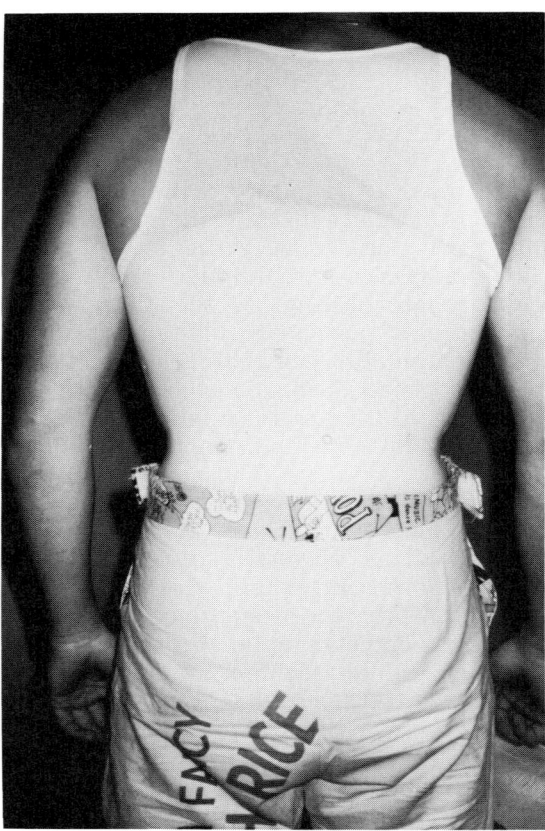

FIGURE 10–6. Immobilization in a rigid polypropylene brace may allow healing of some early lesions (*A,B*).

lief. Occasionally, an athlete will have recurrent episodes of pain. In this case, a decision is reached on an individual basis whether surgical intervention is warranted or whether to discontinue participation.

The question arises as to what to advise the young athlete with a known spondylolysis that is asymptomatic. There are no statistics available as to the number of low-grade slips that progress to a higher grade. The athletes are cautioned that the possibility does exist for increased slipping as well as for exacerbation of symptoms, and the highest risk is between the ages of 7 and 15 years. These athletes are followed very closely for progression of their defects. Serial radiographs are taken at 6-month intervals until skeletal maturity is reached to assess their status. The long-term significance of a pars defect is also unknown. If participation is continued after skeletal maturity is attained, X rays are repeated yearly. However, athletes are advised that they do run a risk of increased back problems in the future. In these cases, decisions again must be made on an individual basis as to what is the best course of treatment. The athlete and his or her family, physician, and coach should all participate in the decision as to whether continued participation in the chosen sport is warranted.

Higher degrees of spondylolisthesis (grade II or more) usually do not present for the first time in the athletically active population, particularly in the elite athlete. Occasionally, an athlete with a high degree of spondylolisthesis may be encountered on a high school or club level. These patients usually do not present with pain; rather, they are detected as part of a preparticipation physical examination or they are seeking attention for a cosmetic deformity. Athletes with slips of less than 50 percent are allowed full participation but are carefully advised of the risks of increased slipping and of the potential for future problems. In addition, they are reexamined periodically, either every 6 months or yearly, for increases in the slip. When an athlete with a low-grade spondylolisthesis has repeated exacerbations or prolonged pain (greater than 3 months) unresponsive to a nonoperative regimen or shows radiographic evidence of increased slipping, we recommend surgical treatment. If students present with spondylolisthesis greater than 50 percent, even if asymptomatic, we do not allow participation in a full athletic program. In addition, we implement a program of restricted activities. In these patients, strong consideration is given to surgical treatment to prevent further progression of the slip. The choice of operation is a complex one and varies with the preference of the operating surgeon.

Once successful surgery is completed, an athlete may be allowed to continue participation after an appropriate period of rehabilitation. We have seen athletes in a variety of sports, including gymnastics and football, continue at a highly competitive level after fusions for spondylolisthesis. This decision is made on an individual basis by the athlete, family, and operating surgeon.

SUMMARY

Spondylolysis and spondylolisthesis arise from defects in the pars interarticularis. Factors implicated in the pathogenesis of these defects include heredity, development, and biomechanical loading. Controversy exists as to the exact role that each of these factors plays in production of a lesion.

Treatment of the school-aged athlete with spondylolytic defects is a complex problem. A thorough understanding of the etiology and pathomechanics is necessary to devise a logical treatment program. Two groups of athletes with pars interarticularis defects exist. First, there is a group with preexisting defects or genetic predispositions that suffers exacerbations secondary to their athletic participation. Second, there is a group that sustains new injuries to the pars interarticularis; the injuries are produced by the unique demands of participation in certain sports, particularly those that require repeated positions of hyperflexion and extension. Athletes may be placed at further risk by increased forces, increased repetitions, and greater duration of the risk-producing activities.

The goals of treatment in athletes should be decreased risk of injury, early diagnosis and treatment, and safe return to participation. To achieve these goals, the efforts of a physician treating adolescent athletes must be directed toward both groups of injuries. Preparticipation physicals and screening will identify the first group. Recognition of the early manifestations of the entity, combined with rapid treatment in the second group, may modify the natural history of the disorder and prevent progression.

In the early phases, treatment includes restricted activity and rest, which is supplemented by immobilization in a molded polypropylene brace when necessary. When a patient fails to respond to treatment, care must be taken to rule out other causes of adolescent low back pain. Operative treatment is reserved for those with high-grade spondylolisthesis or for athletes unresponsive to conservative management.

Perhaps the most important role for the physician is in advising the coach on designing training techniques and practice schedules that will reduce the risk of injury.

References

1. Ferguson P. J., McMasters M. C., Stanitski C. L.: Low back pain in college football linemen. J Bone Joint Surg 56A:1300, 1974.
2. Semon R. L., Spengler D.: Significance of lumbar spondylolysis in college football players. Spine 6:172, 1981.
3. Jackson D. W., Wiltse L. L., Cirincione R. J.: Spondylolysis in the female gymnast. Clin Orthop 117:68, 1976.
4. Hoshina H: Spondylolysis athletes. Physician Sportsmed 3:75, 1980.
5. Herbiniaux G: Traité sur divers accouchements laborieux, et sur les polypes de la matrice. Brussels, 1782, JL DeBoubers.
6. Kilian H. F.: Schilderungen neuer Beckenformen und ihres Verhaltens im Leben. Manheim, 1854, Verlag von Basserman and Mahey.
7. Robert: Monatsschr. Gerburtskunde Frauenkran 5:81, 1855.
8. Lambl D. Z.: Zehn theses über Spondylolisthesis. Zbl Gynal Urol 9:250, 1855.
9. Naugebauer E.: Die Entschung der Spondylolisthesis. Centrlab f Gynak 5:260, 1881.
10. Wiltse L. L.: Spondylolisthesis: classification and etiology. In AAOS Symposium on the Spine. St. Louis, 1969, CV Mosby Co.
11. Wiltse L. L., Newman P. H , Macnab I.: Classification of spondylolysis and spondylolisthesis. Clin Orthop 117:23, 1976.
12. Hensinger R. N.: Spondylolysis and spondylolisthesis. In AAOS Instructional Course Lectures. St. Louis, 1983, CV Mosby Co.
13. Wiltse L. L.: Spondylolisthesis in children. Clin Orthop 21:156, 1961.

14. Borkow S. E., Klieger B.: Spondylolisthesis in the newborn, a case report. Clin Orthop 81:73, 1971.
15. Wiltse L. L., Widell E. H., Jackson D. W.: Fatigue fracture, the basic lesion in isthmic spondylolisthesis. J Bone Joint Surg 57A:17, 1975.
16. Roche M. B., Rowe G. G.: The incidence of separate neural arch and coincident bone variations: a survey. J Bone Joint Surg 34A:491, 1952.
17. McCarrol J. R., Miller J. M., Ritter M. A.: Lumbar spondylolysis and spondylolisthesis in college football players. Am J Sports Med 14:404, 1986.
18. Kettelkamp D. B., Wright D. G.: Spondylolisthesis in the Alaskan Eskimo. J Bone Joint Surg 53A:563, 1975.
19. Ota H.: Spondylolysis: familial occurrence and its genetic implications. J Jpn Orthop Assoc 41:931, 1967.
20. Friberg S.: Studies on spondylolisthesis. Acta Chir Scand 82 (Suppl 55):1, 1939.
21. Laurent L. E.: Spondylolisthesis. Acta Orthop Scand Suppl 35:1, 1958.
22. Wynne-Davies R., Scott J. H. S.: Inheritance and spondylolisthesis: a radiographic family survey. J Bone Joint Surg 61B:301, 1977.
23. Stewart T. D.: The age of neural arch defects in Alaskan natives considered from the standpoint of etiology. J Bone Joint Surg 35A:937, 1953.
24. Steiner M. E., Micheli L. J.: Treatment of symptomatic spondylolysis and spondylolisthesis with the modified Boston brace. Spine 10:937, 1985.
25. Wiltse L. L.: The etiology of spondylolisthesis. J Bone Joint Surg 44A:539, 1962.
26. Newman P. H.: The etiology of spondylolisthesis. J Bone Joint Surg 45B:39, 1963.
27. Rosenberg N. J., Bargar W. L., Friedman B.: The incidence of spondylolysis and spondylolisthesis in non-ambulatory patients. Spine 6:35, 1981.
28. Hitchcock H. H.: Spondylolisthesis, observations on its development, progression and genesis. J Bone Joint Surg 22:1, 1940.
29. Cuillo J. V., Jackson D. W.: Pars interarticularis stress reaction, spondylolysis and spondylolisthesis in gymnasts. Clin Sports Med 4:95, 1985.
30. Cyron B. M., Hutton W. C., Troup J. D.: Spondylolytic fractures. J Bone Joint Surg 58B:462, 1976.
31. Cyron B. M., Hutton W. C.: The fatigue strength of the lumbar neural arch in spondylolysis. J Bone Joint Surg 60B:234, 1978.
32. Munster J. K., Troup J. D.: The structure of the pars interarticularis of the lower lumbar vertebra and its relation to the etiology of spondylolysis. J Bone Joint Surg 55B:735, 1973.
33. Troup J. D.: Mechanical factors in spondylolisthesis and spondylolysis. Clin Orthop 117:59, 1976.
34. Farfan H. F., Osteria V., Lamy C.: The mechanical etiology of spondylolysis and spondylolisthesis. Clin Orthop 117:40, 1976.
35. Hutton W. C., Stott J. R. R., Cyron B. M.: Is spondylolysis a stress fracture? Spine 2:202, 1977.
36. Jackson D. W.: Low back pain in young athletes: evaluation of stress reaction and discogenic problems. Am J Sports Med 7:364, 1979.
37. Turner H., Bianco A. J.: Spondylolysis and spondylolisthesis in children and teenagers. J Bone Joint Surg 53A: 1298, 1971.
38. Lafond G.: Surgical treatment of spondylolisthesis. Clin Orthop 22:175, 1962.
39. Jackson D. W., Wiltse L. L., Dingeman R. D., Hayes M.: Stress reactions involving the pars interarticularis in young athletes. Am J Sports Med 9:304, 1981.
40. Wiltse L. L., et al. Symposium: current concepts in the management of spondylolisthesis. Contemp Orthop 18:231, 1989.
41. Micheli L. J.: Back injuries in gymnastics. Clin Sports Med 4:85, 1985.
42. Micheli L. J.: Low back pain in the adolescent: differential diagnosis. Am J Sports Med 7:362, 1979.
43. Micheli L. J., Steiner E. M.: The use of a modified Boston brace for back injuries in athletes. Am J Sports Med 8:351, 1980.
44. Zembo M. M., Roberts J. M., Burke S. W., et al.: Congenital spondyloptosis. Orthop Trans 11:111, 1987.
45. Meyerding H. W.: Spondylolisthesis. Surg Gynecol Obstet 54:371, 1932.
46. Taillard W.: Le spondylolisthesis chez l'enfant et l'adolecent. Acta Orthop Scand 14:115, 1955.
47. Boxall D., Bradford D. S., Winter R. B., Moe J. H.: Management of severe spondylolisthesis in children and adolescents. J Bone Joint Surg 61A:479, 1979.
48. Dandy Shannon M. J.: Lumbosacral subluxation (group I spondylolisthesis). J Bone Joint Surg 53B: 578, 1971.
49. Hensinger R. N., Lang J. R., MacEwen G. D.: Surgical management of spondylolisthesis in children and adolescents. Spine 1:207, 1976.
50. Roche M. B., Rowe G. G.: The etiology of separate neural arch. J Bone Joint Surg 35A:102, 1953.
51. Baker D. R., McHollick W.: Spondyloschisis and spondylolisthesis in children. In Proceedings of the AAOS. J Bone Joint Surg 38A:933, 1956.
52. Willis T. A.: The separate neural arch. J Bone Joint Surg 13:709, 1931.
53. Barash H. L., Galante J. O., Lambert R. D.: Spondylolysis and tight hamstrings. J Bone Joint Surg 52A: 1319, 1970.
54. Phalen G. S., Dickson J. A.: Spondylolisthesis and tight hamstrings. J Bone Joint Surg 43A:505, 1961.

SHOULDER INSTABILITY

DAVID W. ALTCHEK
RUSSELL F. WARREN

Shoulder instability is a common and sometimes complex problem in the school-age athlete. Although the anatomical factors remain the same as in older individuals, certain social and psychological factors make this group of patients a particular challenge to the clinician. The orthopedist often must communicate with the athletes, teachers, and coaches as well as parents to ensure that the planned treatment is being carried out. When a voluntary component to the instability exists, this in-depth knowledge of the patient becomes even more crucial.

Arthroscopy of the shoulder has attracted considerable interest and controversy. The role of the arthroscope in the management of the unstable shoulder is still in an evolutionary phase. We do not believe the arthroscope will ever replace a meticulous history and physical examination in the diagnosis of shoulder instability, but clearly, arthroscopic observation of such lesions as labral damage or a Hill Sachs deformity can help to classify more precisely the type of instability present. Final statements regarding the value of arthroscopic stabilization procedures must await studies with long-term follow-up and large numbers of patients.

ANATOMICAL CONSIDERATIONS IN THE UNSTABLE SHOULDER

As in any joint in the body, there are three factors that contribute to shoulder stability: the bony configuration, the capsular/ligamentous system, and the surrounding muscle-tendon units.

BONY STRUCTURES

In the glenohumeral joint, there are minimal bony constraints present. The elliptical glenoid, which averages 15 × 25 mm in size, has a radius of curvature less than that of the humeral head. The relatively flat glenoid is deepened by addition of the labrum, allowing for a more concentric glenohumeral articulation. Dysplasia or, more commonly, glenoid fracture can decrease the concentricity of the joint and permit instability to occur. Studies by Saha and at our institution have looked at the relationship between glenoid version and patients with clinical instability of the shoulder. In neither study did individual differences in glenoid version correlate with shoulder instability.[44]

The humeral head is normally retroverted 35 degrees in relation to the humeral condyles at the elbow. This amount of retroversion has been shown to increase in patients with Erb palsy, but apart from this situation, there has been no documentation of glenohumeral instability related to abnormalities in humeral head version. The Hill-Sachs or posterolateral indentation fracture of the humeral head that results from anterior dislocation has been implicated by several authors as a causative factor in recurrent dislocation. On this basis, authors such as Weber et al. have recommended humeral osteotomy to increase the retroversion of the humeral head, thereby preventing engagement of the defect on the anterior glenoid during external rotation.[54] We feel that the Hill-Sachs lesion is a secondary phenomenon. Once the primary capsular lesion is corrected, the bony defect alone will not permit recurrent instability. A humeral head defect can occur on the anteromedial aspect in patients with posterior instability of the shoulder. Unlike the Hill-Sachs lesion, which occurs with great frequency in patients with recurrent anterior dislocation, these anterior defects occur only rarely in patients with posterior instability. It is only in the chronic fixed posterior dislocation that these lesions are of a significant size. Discussion of this problem is not relevant to the adolescent athlete.

CAPSULE AND LIGAMENTS

The glenohumeral joint capsule arises anteriorly, posteriorly, and inferiorly about the anatomical neck of the humerus and inserts via the labrum in a circumferential fashion at the glenoid articular margin. Capsular redundancy is necessary for shoulder motion and demonstrates great individual variation. In most cases, capsular redundancy is greatest inferiorly (the axillary pouch) and posteriorly. Schlemm in 1860 first noted that three portions of the capsule are thickened and named them the superior, middle, and inferior glenohumeral ligaments.[45] These structures are not evident on the exterior surface of the joint capsule and become indistinct when the capsule is dissected free of its attachments. Arthroscopic examination has greatly increased our understanding of these structures and their variability. Anteriorly, the superior glenohumeral ligament is only variably present. Arising from the superior portion of the glenoid near the biceps tendon, it inserts alongside the lesser tuberosity of the humerus. The middle glenohumeral ligament is a distinct structure in the majority of individuals, arising from the superior one third of the anterior labrum and draping over the subscapularis tendon to insert below the superior ligament on the anterior portion of the humeral neck. The inferior glenohumeral ligament (IGHL), the most robust of the three, arises from the entire inferior one half of the labrum both anteriorly and posteriorly and acts as a sling to support the humeral head as it courses to its insertion around the bottom half of the anatomical neck of the humerus.

A study of the role of the glenohumeral ligaments and subscapularis tendon in anterior instability was carried out by Turkel et al.[51] They demonstrated that the subscapularis only played a role in preventing anterior dislocation when the arm was abducted less than 45 degrees. The primary restraint to anterior instability was the anterior portion of the inferior glenohumeral ligament, in particular the superior band of the ligament. A similar study was carried out at our institution.[47] We looked at the ligamentous restraints to both anterior and posterior instability of the shoulder. Using cadaveric shoulders, arthroscopy was performed to define the anatomy; then instrumented testing was performed to determine instability. Arthroscopic examination revealed the presence of a distinct superior band of the posterior portion of the inferior glenohumeral ligament, analogous to its anterior counterpart. Mechanical testing revealed that both the anterior and posterior limbs of the inferior glenohumeral complex act in concert to limit humeral head translation on the glenoid in both anterior and posterior directions. In addition, the posterior portion of the inferior glenohumeral ligament acts as the primary restraint to increased posterior translation and the secondary restraint to increased anterior translation. Similarly, the anterior portion of the glenohumeral ligament acts as a primary restraint for anterior limitation and a secondary restraint for posterior translation. Warren referred to this as the *circle concept* of the shoulder.[53]

This concept is important to the clinician in dealing with shoulder instability, particularly in the patient with underlying ligamentous laxity. These patients normally demonstrate large excursions of the humeral head. When damage occurs on one side of the joint, excursion will increase in both directions. Examination under anesthesia in these patients can be confusing, as the examiner will be able to demonstrate instability in more than one direction. A clear knowledge of the patient's history and documentation of the clinical direction of instability should dictate the direction of repair (i.e., either anterior or posterior). Capsular shift procedures that allow tension to be placed in both sides of the joint are ideal in this setting.

MUSCLE-TENDON UNIT

Mechanical cutting studies such as those cited above have demonstrated that division of the rotator cuff tendons will not, in the presence of an intact capsular unit, allow dislocation of the glenohumeral joint. When analyzed in a dynamic sense, it has been clearly demonstrated both by Poppen and Walker[34] and by our own study[46] that an intact rotator cuff is necessary to limit superior migration of the humeral head in relation to the glenoid during arm elevation. No study to this date has documented the dynamic role of the rotator cuff musculature in limiting anterior and posterior translation. Theoretically, the rotator cuff should function to share the load with the labral-ligamentous complex in restricting translation during activities such as throwing. If fatigue occurs, abnormal stresses will be generated, and labral or ligamentous injury can occur, leading to instability.

CLASSIFICATION OF SHOULDER INSTABILITY

The Hospital for Special Surgery utilizes the classification of shoulder instability shown in Table 11–1. The central components of the classification system include frequency of occurrence, etiology, direction, and degree of instability. Classification systems allow specific categorization for all types of shoulder instability. A classification system improves diagnostic forethought, streamlines treatment protocols, and facilitates comparative follow-up studies.

TABLE 11–1. Shoulder Instability Classification

Frequency
Acute
Recurrent
Fixed (chronic)
Etiology
Traumatic (macrotrauma)
Atraumatic
   Voluntary
   Involuntary
Microtrauma (repetitive use)
Congenital
Neuromuscular (Erb palsy, CP, seizures)
Direction
Anterior
Posterior
Inferior
Multidirectional
Degree
Dislocation
Subluxation
Micro (transient)

FREQUENCY

The initial event, either subluxation or dislocation, is termed *acute*, whereas those with repeated episodes are called *recurrent*. The term *fixed dislocation* refers to a missed episode of dislocation that leaves the humeral head in a chronically dislocated position.

ETIOLOGY

Etiology describes the degree of trauma occurring at the initiation of instability. Three possible categories are considered: traumatic, atraumatic, and repetitive microtrauma.

When the etiology is *traumatic*, the patient can describe a discrete episode in which an external force was applied to the arm, causing the shoulder to dislocate. The classical model for the traumatic etiology is the football player who attempts a tackle with the outstretched arm, which is forced into hyperextension, external rotation, and abduction, causing an anterior dislocation.

Patients who fall into the *atraumatic* category may describe a discrete episode initiating the instability but without the application of external force. An example would be the tennis player who suffers an acute dislocation while cocking the arm to serve. These patients often demonstrate generalized ligamentous laxity and frequently have instability in more than one direction. Patients in the traumatic group with recurrent instability may frequently develop an atraumatic pattern to their recurrences as progressive laxity and capsular stretching recur.

Repetitive microtrauma refers to a group of athletes often with subluxation who are never able to localize a discrete onset to the disability. These patients often present to their physicians with a complaint of pain or a "dead arm" rather than instability. It is only on careful examination by the physician, often with radiographic or arthroscopic documentation of ligament or labral damage, that instability is noted.

DIRECTION

A shoulder may be unstable in three primary directions: anterior, posterior, and inferior. Among these, anterior instability clearly predominates. Posterior instability, long considered to be present only after major trauma, after seizures, or on a voluntary basis, is now being increasingly recognized in the athletic population. Unlike anterior instability, which often presents as a dislocation rather than subluxation, posterior instability of the recurrent type is nearly always a subluxation, with dislocation being generally an isolated event.

For instability to occur in the inferior direction, generalized capsular laxity must be present. This defines multidirectional instability. Multidirectional instability occurs in one of three patterns: anterior and inferior dislocation with posterior subluxation, posterior and inferior dislocation with anterior subluxation, or dislocation in all three directions.

DEGREE

The categories of subluxation and dislocation attempt to quantify the amount of translation of the humeral head relative to the glenoid during the episodes of instability. *Dislocation* implies complete loss of articular contact between the humerus and glenoid that is not dynamic. Introduction of a new force is required to achieve reduction of the joint. Subluxation represents increased humeral head translation relative to the glenoid such that symptoms occur. It implies that the degree of laxity in the capsulolabral complex is greater than normal. The range of disorders that fall under this heading is enormous. At one end of the spectrum are symptomatic individuals in whom the examiner can translate the humeral head beyond the glenoid margin, and yet no clinical dislocation has ever occurred. The other end of the extreme are those patients, often throwing athletes, who complain only of pain and in whom no excessive translation can be demonstrated but who demonstrate obvious labral damage at arthroscopy. In these individuals, repetitive translation of the humeral head on the glenoid has damaged the labrum but not to the degree that macroscopic increases in translation are present. With repeated injury, this may progress to clinical subluxation if the labral injury affects the inferior glenohumeral ligament.

RADIOGRAPHIC EVALUATION OF SHOULDER INSTABILITY

The radiographic evaluation of suspected acute shoulder instability should include three views of the glenohumeral joint at right angles to each other. These are (1) the true anterior-posterior view (AP) taken perpendicular to the axis of the scapula (which lies at 30 to 40 degrees anterior to the coronal plane of the body), (2) a transcapular Y-view, and (3) an axillary view. These views are useful screening studies for fractures, glenohumeral dislocations, and acromioclavicular pathology. It is often important for the physician to be available to facilitate correct positioning of the patient's arm for the X-ray series.

The radiographic evaluation of recurrent shoulder instability was reviewed at our institution.[33] The pathology about the glenohumeral joint is most completely evaluated with an instability series. This consists

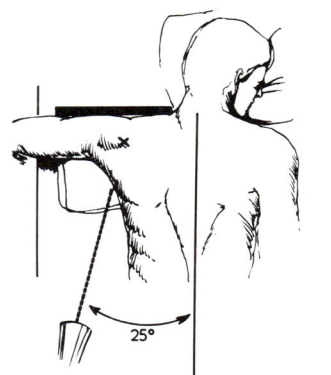
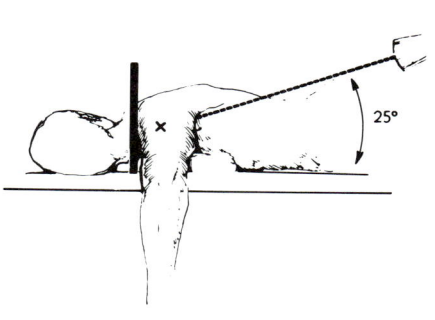

FIGURE 11–1. Illustration depicting the technique of the West Point axillary radiograph.

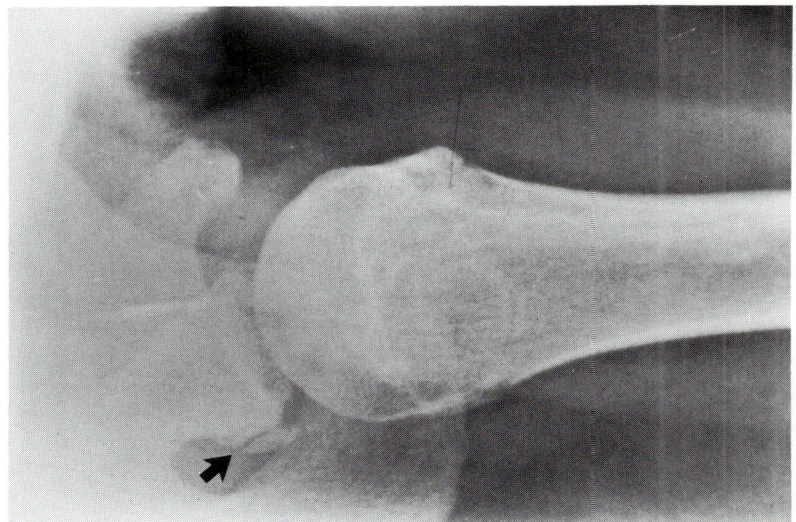

FIGURE 11-2. West Point axillary radiograph performed on a patient with recurrent posterior subluxation. Avulsion fracture (*arrow*) is seen on posterior glenoid margin.

of three radiographic views: an AP in internal rotation, a Stryker notch, and a West Point modified axillary view.[37] (See Fig. 11–1.) Bony lesions of the glenoid margin are best documented on the West Point view (Fig. 11–2). A combination of Stryker notch (Fig. 11–3) and AP internal rotation views (Fig. 11–4) will identify most Hill Sachs lesions in the posterolateral aspect of the humeral head. These two bony lesions are pathognomonic for glenohumeral instability.

Secondary studies such as arthrography, computerized tomography (CT) arthrography, and magnetic resonance imaging (MRI) can provide useful adjunctive information. In those individuals in whom a component of rotator cuff pathology is suspected, an arthrogram will identify any full thickness lesions. If glenoid fracture is suspected from the initial films, axial images from the CT will further define the location of the lesion (Fig. 11–5). The addition of intraarticular contrast to CT will allow evaluation of the anterior and posterior labrum (Fig. 11–6). Large labral detachments should be visible with this method. Recent development of a specific shoulder surface coil has improved the usefulness of the MRI in the evaluation of the unstable shoulder. Coronal images identify any evidence of rotator cuff pathology, and axillary images visualize the labrum, allowing assessment of its integrity. We found the MRI particularly useful in the evaluation of the painful shoulder in the throwing athlete in whom coexistence of labral lesions and rotator cuff pathology may occur.

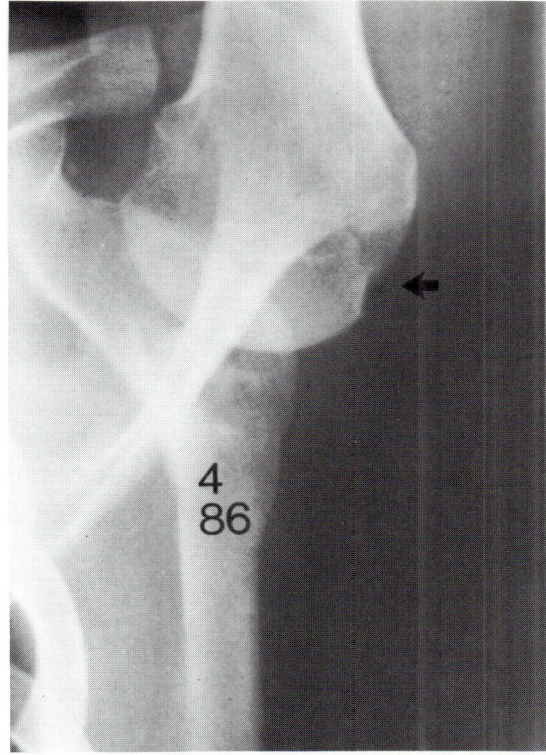

FIGURE 11-3. Stryker notch radiograph. Posterolateral portion of the humeral head has a (*arrow*) Hill-Sachs deformity.

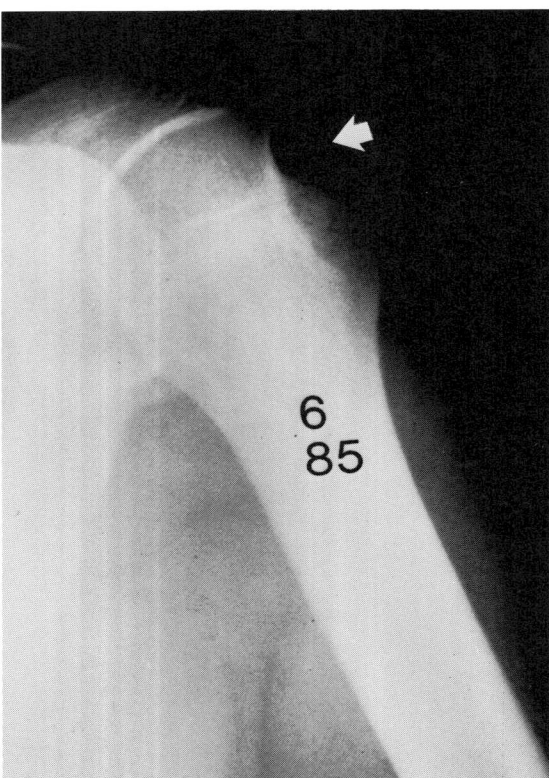

FIGURE 11–4. AP radiograph in internal rotation demonstrating (*arrow*) Hill-Sachs deformity.

ANTERIOR SHOULDER INSTABILITY

ACUTE TRAUMATIC ANTERIOR DISLOCATION

Dislocation of the glenohumeral joint as previously defined may occur secondary to direct or indirect forces. A direct force, such as a blow to the posterior aspect of the humeral head, is uncommon.[36] Indirect force is the most frequent etiology of anterior glenohumeral dislocation. The arm is usually forced in excessive abduction, external rotation, and extension. These forces cause disruption of the static and dynamic stabilizers of the joint. The humeral head most commonly dislocates into a subcoracoid position. The dislocated shoulder is usually very painful and associated with muscle spasm, causing the patient to become extremely apprehensive. Unless the traumatic incident is witnessed by the treating physician, a thorough history of the injury mechanism must be obtained. Specific questions about neurological involvement at the time of injury must be asked. Physical examination must include a detailed neurological examination of the upper extremity, paying particular attention to the axillary and musculcutaneous nerves.[9]

Ideally, radiographs should be obtained prior to attempted reduction of a suspected shoulder dislocation. However, when a

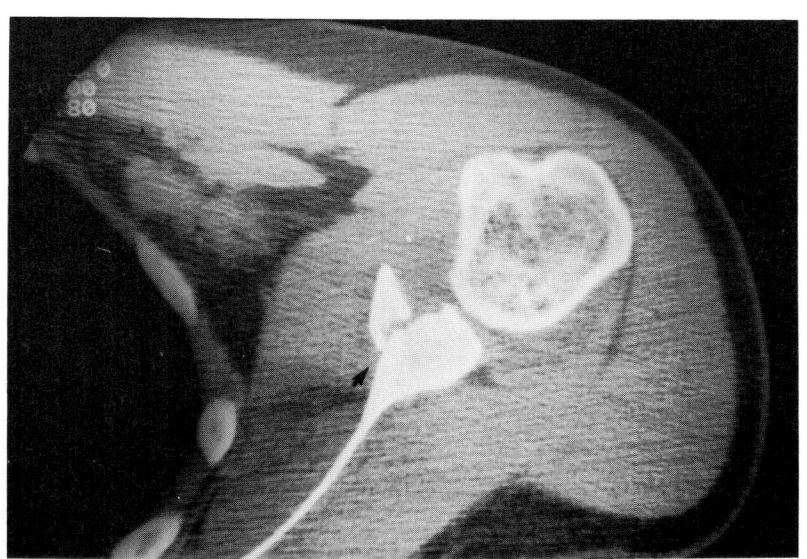

FIGURE 11–5. CT scan demonstrating displaced fracture (*arrow*) of the anterior glenoid in a patient with traumatic anterior dislocation.

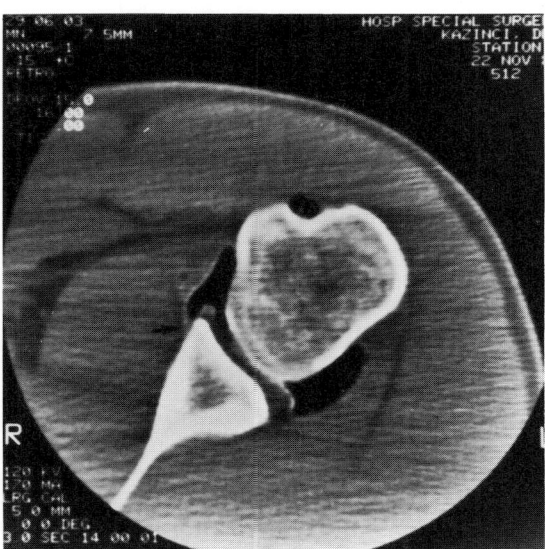

FIGURE 11–6. Normal CT arthrogram demonstrating normal anterior and posterior pouches. *Arrow* points to normal site of anterior capsule attachment.

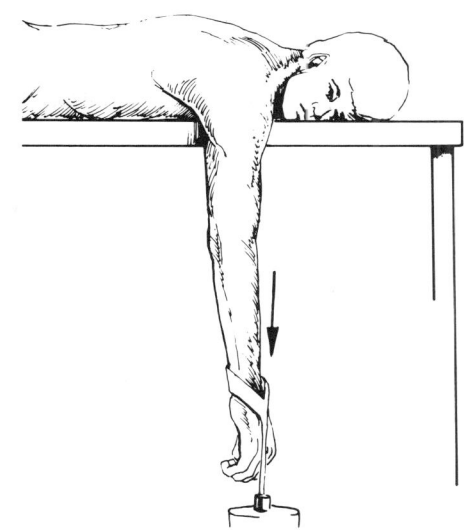

FIGURE 11–7. Illustration depicting prone reduction of the shoulder with weighted distraction.

young athlete sustains an acute witnessed dislocation on the field, immediate relocation should be attempted. Initially, simple elevation and gentle rotation of the humerus will often unlock the humeral head and effect a reduction. If this is unsuccessful, the patient should be transported to the locker room and placed prone on the training table. The scapular rotation maneuver is then performed.[3] The injured arm is allowed to hang in a dependent fashion off the edge of the table. The scapula is then rotated to unlock the humeral head, allowing the joint to be relocated spontaneously. If this is not successful, an intravenous line is started for the administration of muscle relaxants and pain medications as needed. At this point, radiographs should be obtained to assess the injury more completely. The next relocation maneuver we would try is Stimson's:[50] With the affected shoulder hanging free off the edge of the table, weights are used to apply traction to the arm; 5 pounds is usually sufficient, although the amount of weight will vary with the size of the patient (Fig. 11–7). After satisfactory relaxation has been achieved, traction is applied to the arm in a straight anterior direction with simultaneous posteriorly directed pressure applied directly to the humeral head. An alternative reduction technique is the double sheet method (Fig. 11–8). The patient is placed in a supine position with the arm and shoulder off the edge of the table. One sheet is placed around the patient's chest and held by an assistant. A second sheet is placed around the patient's upper arm for gentle lateral traction. The physician applies gradual gentle traction to the arm, grasping at the wrist and pulling in an axial direction. With the arm positioned in a comfortable amount of abduction, traction is applied in line with the arm and slowly increased until reduction occurs. Often gentle traction over a period of up

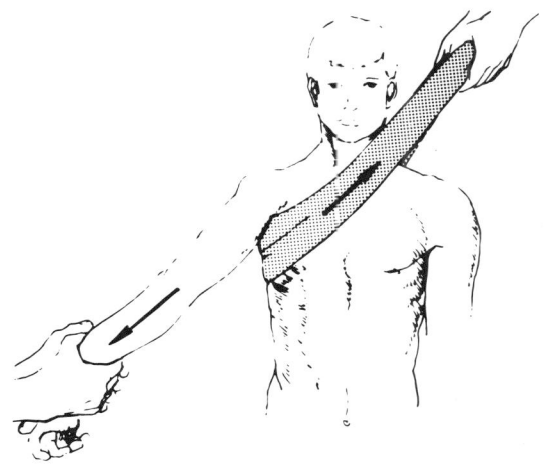

FIGURE 11–8. Illustration depicting double sheet method of shoulder reduction.

to 5 minutes is required to overcome muscle spasm. With this maneuver, the physician must be fully aware that undue traction forces may result in damage to the neurovascular structures about the shoulder. Iatrogenic fractures as well as displacement of existing fractures may also occur as a result of excessive traction. If this method fails, reduction under anesthesia should be performed. At present, we most often use scalene block anesthesia, which provides complete muscle relaxation as well as anesthesia, allowing easy reduction in all cases.

Radiographic confirmation using at least two views at right angles to each other is mandatory following reduction. The young athlete is immediately immobilized in a sling. Although controversy exists regarding the effect of immobilization on recurrence, our current philosophy in the young athlete is to recommend 6 weeks of immobilization after the index dislocation. Both Simonet and Cofield and Yoneda et al. in separate series have reported a reduction in recurrence rate using this period of immobilization.[49,55] The 6-week period is based on studies demonstrating the length of time required to achieve initial ligament and capsular healing.[11,27] After completion of the initial immobilization period, abduction is further limited to 80 degrees for 2 weeks to prevent capsular stretching and a rehabilitation program is begun. Exercises to strengthen the deltoid, rotator cuff, and scapular musculature emphasizing internal rotation are initiated and continued for 3 months postinjury. At the U.S. Naval Academy, Cox had demonstrated that the use of a prescribed exercise program will additionally lower the potential recurrence rate.[12]

Return to sport, particularly those involving contact, ideally should be delayed for a minimum of 3 months, provided a full range of motion has returned and no strength deficit persists. Strength, particularly internal rotation strength, should be quantitated using a Cybex dynamometer prior to return to play. Specific details of the rehabilitative program will be outlined in a later section of this chapter. These guidelines for return to play often must be tailored to fit individual circumstances. One common example is the high school athlete who may have a scholarship riding on his ability to complete a season. In this instance, we would counsel the parents that early return may increase the possibility of recurrence and allow the individual to resume participation if the patient and family are willing to accept this risk.

Recently, some investigators have proposed immediate arthroscopy of the acutely dislocated shoulder to define the pathology involved further, perhaps allowing individualization of initial treatment. If dislocation occurred without labral detachment or ligament tearing, as can occur in the ligamentously lax individual, theoretically the time of initial immobilization could be reduced, as no significant soft tissue healing would be expected. If, however, a labral detachment was noted and was reducible with simple internal rotation, immobilization in a sling for 6 weeks would be justified. If the labral lesion was not reduced to the glenoid margin by internal rotation alone, immediate arthroscopic reattachment of the labrum would be performed. A well-controlled perspective randomized study is now being performed at our institution to provide more information in this regard.

The risk of recurrent dislocation at present is most related to the patient's age at the time of index dislocation. In Rowe and Sakellarides's classic study of 324 anterior dislocations, the redislocation rate for patients under 20 was greater than 90 percent, whereas the rate for patients over 40 was below 25 percent.[41] In other studies, secondary factors such as generalized ligamentous laxity and the degree of associated trauma correlated positively with an increased recurrence rate.[23] Authors have theorized that the high recurrence rate in the young occurs because of the greater tissue elasticity present. This implies that a degree of irreversible capsular stretch occurs. Conservative treatment can influence the recurrence rate by allowing any capsular tearing or detachment to heal. It appears that there are multiple factors that influence the age effect on the recurrence rate. Clearly, the increase in sports activity in the younger age group plays a role. In the older individual, dislocation can cause midsubstance or lateral capsular tearing rather than glenoid detachment. Perhaps these lesions have a greater potential for healing than does the classic Bankart labral detachment, which is the most common lesion in traumatic anterior dislocation in the young athlete. In addition, the greater tissue elasticity of younger individuals may allow a greater amount of permanent plastic deformation of the capsule to occur, further predisposing the individual to laxity and subsequent instability.

RECURRENT ANTERIOR INSTABILITY

Recurrent anterior shoulder instability can be classified into the following subgroups: traumatic or atraumatic, voluntary and involuntary, and subluxation or dislocation. Factors that dictate placement within the recurrent subgroups include the magnitude of force the joint is experiencing, the extent of previous injuries, and the magnitude of ligamentous laxity.

RECURRENT ANTERIOR DISLOCATION

The extent of disability from recurrent anterior dislocation varies considerably among individuals. The majority experience no pain between episodes. The spectrum of instability ranges from rare traumatic dislocations to dislocations that occur while performing activities of daily living. As the individual experiences more frequent dislocations, attempts will usually be made to avoid those arm positions—abduction, extension, external rotation—that precipitate instability. Atraumatic shoulder dislocation can be either voluntary or involuntary. Voluntary dislocators generally have a long history of experiencing dislocations of the shoulder with minimal apprehension or discomfort. Although commonly associated with generalized ligamentous laxity (Fig. 11–9) or connective tissue disorders, this syndrome can also occur in patients with normal muscular development and no apparent increase in joint laxity.[40] Unfortunately, some patients use this as a trick to manipulate their social environment. It is important to detect these patients when considering treatment options. Voluntary dislocators may develop an involuntary component to their instability pattern. When this occurs, these individuals are often totally disabled from sports participation, owing to frequent instability.

Surgical stabilization can be considered for the voluntary dislocator after a supervised program of rotator cuff strengthening exercises fails to ameliorate the symptoms and complete psychiatric evaluation has been obtained. Psychiatric evaluation in these patients may demonstrate a character disorder. It is these patients who will most likely use the shoulder instability for secondary gain. Rowe has already reported that operative treatment of these often uncooperative patients results in a high percentage of failures.[40] Prior to consideration of surgery, the psychiatrist should evaluate the patient to rule out any such manipulative or destructive tendencies.

RECURRENT ANTERIOR SUBLUXATION

Subluxation is defined as increased humeral head translation on the glenoid without frank dislocation. Abnormally increased

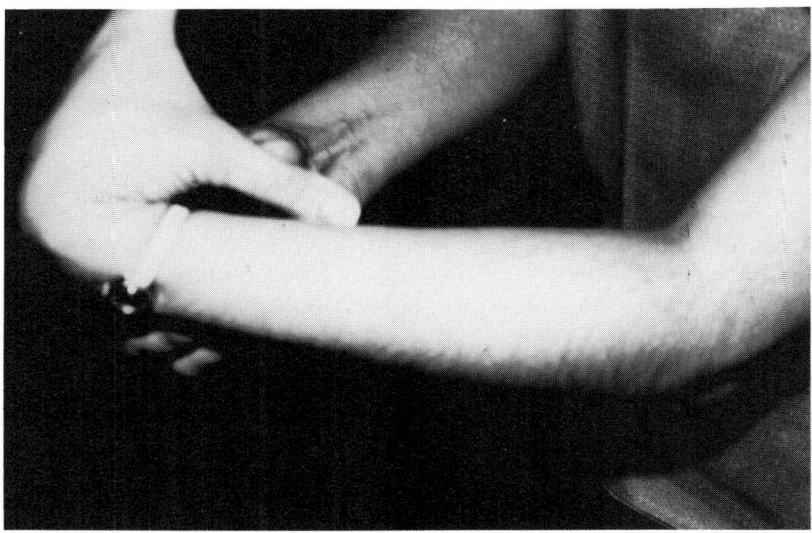

FIGURE 11–9. Photograph of a patient with generalized ligamentous laxity with positive thumb to forearm sign.

translation has been quantitated by our anatomical studies to be humeral head translation greater than one half the width of the glenoid. Dislocation is considered to occur when translation is greater than the sums of one half of the glenoid width and humeral head diameter.[47] It has been recognized that athletes involved in sports such as throwing or swimming exhibit a greater range of motion of the shoulder than the normal population. When asymptomatic athletes of this type are examined by a physician, translation equivalent to subluxation is frequently present. Undoubtedly, the capsule ligament complex as well as the rotator cuff musculature undergo repeated stresses in attempting to restrain this excess motion. This can lead to labral and rotator cuff damage accounting for the not-infrequent coexistence of instability and impingement in this group of athletes.

In marked contrast to the patient with recurrent anterior dislocation, the primary complaint of athletes with subluxation is often pain. If a thrower complains of painful anterior clicking or the so-called dead arm syndrome,[42] the diagnosis may not be difficult. However, the pain is often posterior and may mimic that of impingement. The dead arm syndrome describes a feeling of whole arm numbness and weakness that can occur accompanying an episode of subluxation. This has been reported to occur most frequently in throwing athletes with anterior subluxation.

Evaluation of patients with painful anterior subluxation must be carried out with a thorough understanding of the mechanism that produced the patient's complaints. When dealing with a throwing athlete, the clinician must have a working knowledge of the throwing sequence. Jobe et al. have divided the throwing mechanism into four phases.[22] Phase I, or windup, involves primary weight transfer to the back leg and minimal shoulder motion. Phase II, or the cocking phase, involves the arm achieving a position of 90 degrees of abduction coupled with humeral extension and maximal external rotation; in this phase of throwing, the tightly wound anterior capsular ligaments and subscapularis restrain excessive anterior translation of the humeral head. Phase III, or the acceleration phase, involves rapid unwinding of the capsule as the arm is forcibly internally rotated. In phase IV, or follow-through, the rotator cuff musculature and the tension in the capsular ligaments act to deaccelerate the arm. This analysis of throwing motion is described in greater detail in Chapter 29.

When analyzing the symptomatic throwing athlete, the clinician must attempt to localize his or her complaints to a portion of the throw. Pain in phase II of throwing often indicates anterior instability as the head is driven against the anterior structures. Howell et al.[19] looked at axillary radiographs of patients with both normal shoulders and known recurrent anterior dislocations. For both groups, radiographs were taken with the arm placed in a position of abduction and maximal external rotation analogous to the cocking position of throwing.[19] In the control group, the humeral head was found to move posterior to the center point of the glenoid. In the anterior instability group, the humeral head stayed centered or moved anterior to the midportion of the glenoid. This indicates that the competent anterior capsular labral complex tightens in the cocking phase and drives the head posteriorly, whereas the injured complex cannot properly position the head during this phase of throwing.

Pain in phase IV, follow-through, may be due to posterior subluxation but also occurs in conjunction with anterior instability due to traction on the anterior capsule.

Physical examination of the patient with suspected subluxation begins with inspection. The examiner is looking for signs of atrophy, particularly of the supraspinatus and infraspinatus. Atrophy can be a clue to the diagnosis of suprascapular nerve palsy, which does occur in the overhead athlete because of repetitive traction on the nerve. In these patients, weakness, particularly in external rotation, is profound. Pain occurs uniformly posteriorly. Electromyogram (EMG) should be obtained for documentation (Fig. 11–10).

Both passive and active range of motion are next assessed. Internal and external rotation should be checked both with the arms at the side and abducted to the 90-degree position. Frequently, patients with anterior instability will have some loss of external rotation in the abducted position, presumably secondary to apprehension. In throwing athletes, the dominant shoulder will normally exhibit 10 to 20 degrees of increased external rotation in the abducted position when compared with the nondominant arm. With the arm at the side, where apprehension will not play a role,

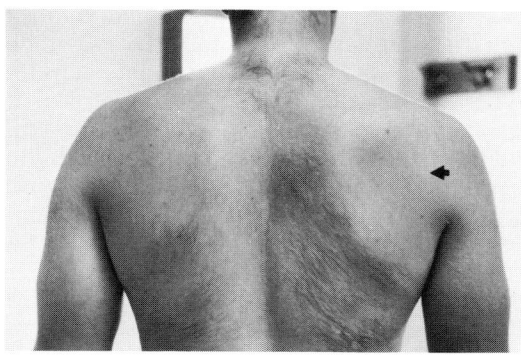

FIGURE 11-10. Photograph of a patient with suprascapular nerve palsy. *Arrow* points to area of muscle atrophy.

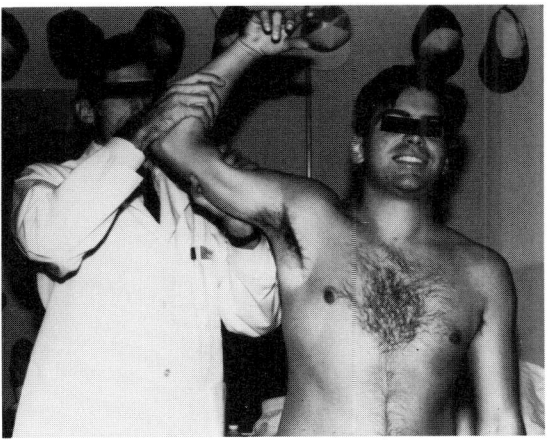

FIGURE 11-11. The anterior apprehension maneuver.

losses of 15 to 20 degrees of external rotation with respect to the opposite or normal arm are common. The reasons for this have not been well established.

Strength testing is then performed focusing on the deltoid, subscapularis, supra- and infraspinatus, and serratus anterior. As noted above, any gross weakness of external rotation strength should make the examiner suspicious for suprascapular nerve palsy. However, moderate weakness is also not an infrequent finding in patients with recurrent posterior subluxation. Weakness of the rotator cuff can also occur if there is simultaneous rotator cuff tendinitis.

The impingement sign should be assessed and compared with discomfort produced by the anterior apprehension maneuver.[30] In the apprehension maneuver, the arm is placed in the overhead abducted externally rotated position. The examiner gradually extends the humerus while applying an anterior stress to the humeral head (Fig. 11-11). Patients with gross anterior instability will react with apprehension, whereas those with subtle forms of subluxation will usually complain only of pain. However, patients with impingement may complain of pain as well on this maneuver. It is often helpful to perform an impingement test, injecting the subacromial bursa with lidocaine.[30] The examination is then repeated. If the pain is relieved on the impingement maneuver but remains present during the apprehension test, further confirmation of possible instability is obtained.

Stress testing in the supine position is then performed. The examiner must support the humerus in neutral rotation to prevent capsular windup, which would selectively limit translation. With the patient relaxed, the humeral head is translated anteriorly, posteriorly, and inferiorly, noting both the amounts of translation and discomfort produced (Fig. 11-12). Clicks or crepitus, particularly if associated with pain, are often a sign of labral damage. A typical patient with subtle anterior subluxation will demonstrate on awake examination only small increases in anterior translation, which are however, associated with marked discomfort. With the patient standing, an assessment of overall capsular laxity is performed by eliciting the sulcus sign. A sulcus sign occurs when distal traction on the adducted humerus causes inferior subluxation of the humeral head (Fig. 11-13). This results in a "sulcus" appearing between the acromion and humeral head.[31]

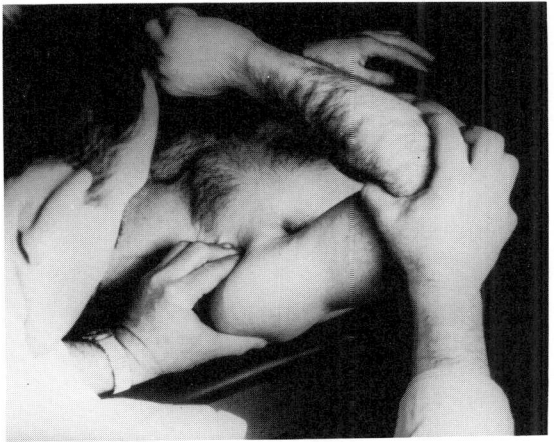

FIGURE 11-12. The supine stress test for shoulder instability. The examiner is kneeling or seated behind the patient.

168 PART II—COMMON SPORTS INJURIES

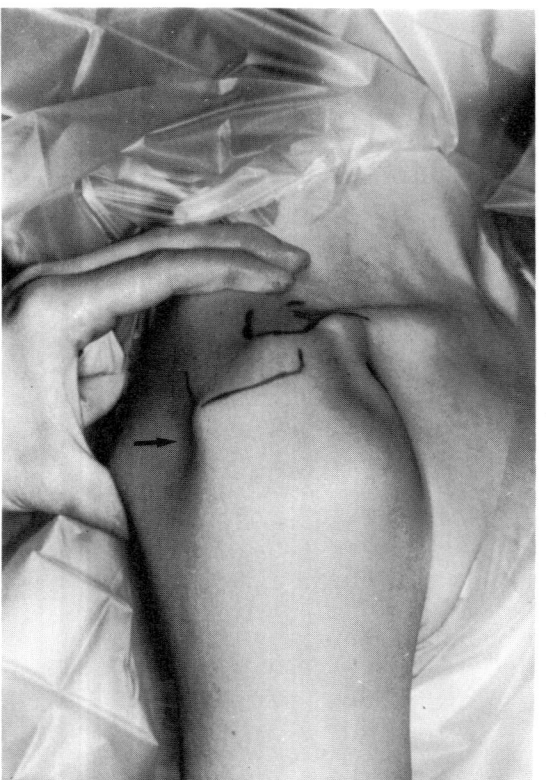

FIGURE 11–13. The sulcus sign. The examiner applies distal traction to the adducted arm. A gap (*arrow*) appears between the acromion and inferiorly subluxed humeral head.

gressive rehabilitation program. Rehabilitation first emphasizes restoration of motion by the use of passive and active assisted stretching exercises, avoiding the position of dislocation—abduction, extension, and external rotation (Figs. 11–14 and 11–15). Following restoration of motion, gentle strengthening exercises are begun, initially using light hand weights or surgical tubing. The scapular, trunk, and shoulder muscles are exercised in an arc restricted to the midranges of motion (Figs. 11–16, 11–17, 11–18). As strength improves, the arc and the resistance are increased. In the throwing athlete, emphasis is placed on eccentric training to better reproduce functional demands (see Table 11–2 and Fig. 11–19).

Return to sport is allowed at 3 to 4 months after acute dislocation, provided that the rehabilitation criteria of a full range of motion and adequate strength are met. Throwers are placed initially in an interval program, gradually increasing both the length and velocity of the throws. Rehabilitation continues during the first 2 to 3 months after return to sport.

The sulcus sign is graded 1+, 2+, or 3+, depending on the distance of the gap. A 1+ sulcus is 1 to 2 cm, a 2+ sulcus is 2 to 3 cm, and a 3+ sulcus is greater than 3 cm. Throwing athletes will commonly have enough inherent laxity to exhibit a 1+ sulcus in the normal dominant shoulder. A large 2+ or 3+ sulcus, when associated with instability, indicates that multidirectional instability is most likely present. The patient must be relaxed during the examination, as firing the deltoid can prevent inferior subluxation of the humeral head.

TREATMENT OF ANTERIOR SHOULDER INSTABILITY

ACUTE ANTERIOR DISLOCATION

As we have stated, acute anterior dislocation will be treated with internal rotation sling for a 6-week period, followed by a pro-

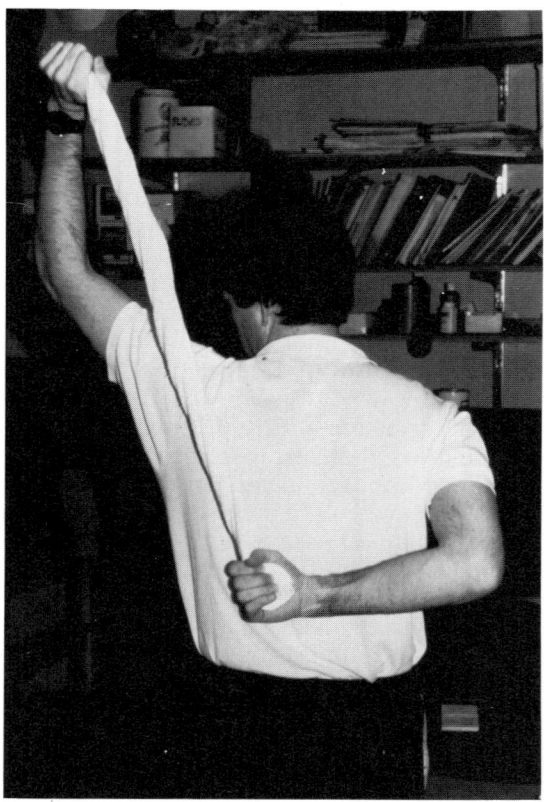

FIGURE 11–14. Stretching exercise using a towel to achieve maximal internal rotation.

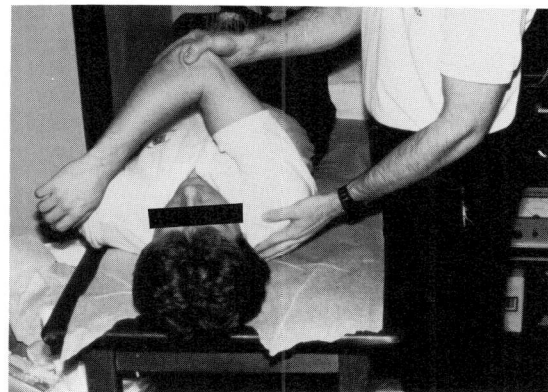

FIGURE 11-15. Posterior capsule stretching by passive arm adduction.

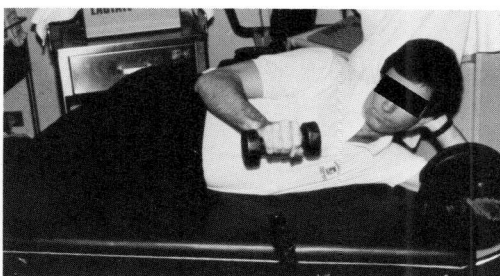

FIGURE 11-17. External rotation strengthening. Concentric strengthening is achieved by lifting the weight; eccentric strengthening, by slowly lowering the weight.

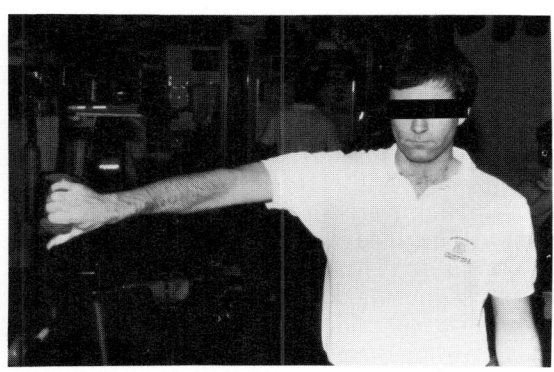

FIGURE 11-16. Selective supraspinatus strengthening with the humerus horizontally adducted 30 degrees and at maximal internal rotation.

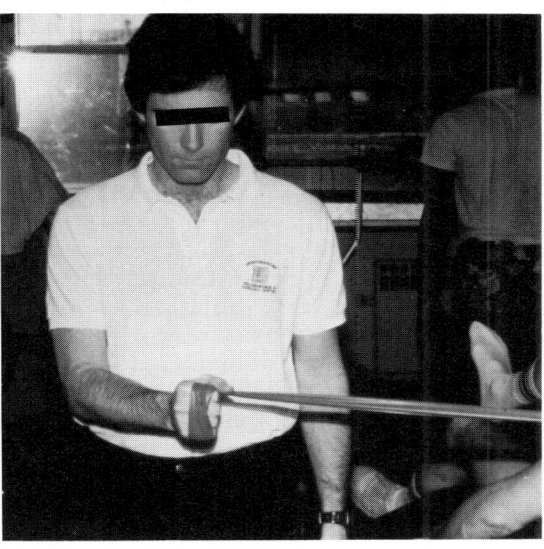

FIGURE 11-18. Internal and external rotation strengthening using the Theraband.

TABLE 11-2. Rehabilitation Following Acute or Recurrent Anterior Dislocation

Restoration of Motion
Passive and active assisted range-of-motion exercises (avoiding end range in the direction of instability)

Strengthening
Surgical tubing—restricted to painless arc initially
Progress to light hand weights—increase arc of motion, greater emphasis on eccentric work
Gradual initiation of instrumented isokinetic work—first, in concentric mode, progressing gradually to eccentric

Initial Return to Sport
Continue rehabilitation
Long warm-up periods
Interval participation initially with gradually decreasing rest periods

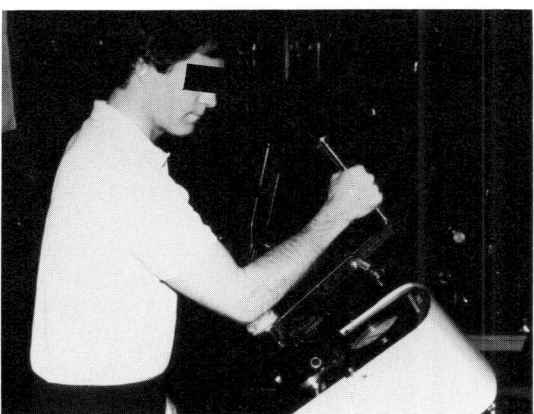

FIGURE 11-19. Isokinetic strengthening using a Cybex dynomometer.

RECURRENT ANTERIOR DISLOCATION

The patient with the recurrent involuntary anterior dislocation is treated with a sling only if pain and loss of range of motion are present following reduction. If there have been numerous recurrences, minimal trauma is often required to produce dislocation, and the athlete can reduce the shoulder himself or herself. In these patients, we avoid immobilization and immediately initiate rehabilitation in a fashion identical to that described above for the acute dislocation. Return to play is allowed often immediately.

It is in this group that surgical treatment should be considered. Once recurrent instability is established in a youthful athlete, it will most likely continue unless there is a major change in sports participation. If the instability is disabling, the parents and the athletes should be advised to consider surgical correction. Palliative treatment with a waist-arm strap is occasionally indicated to enable an athlete to complete a season. This device, worn around the waist with a strap connected to the affected arm, prevents the athlete with recurrent anterior instability from achieving the position of dislocation, that is, extreme abduction and external rotation. Obviously, this device is only useful in athletes who can limit their arm usage, such as football linemen and soccer players (Fig. 29–3).

TREATMENT OF ANTERIOR SUBLUXATION

Patients who have had an episode of acute traumatic shoulder subluxation should initially be placed at rest. The arm is immobilized in a sling for 5 weeks to allow potentially for capsular healing and decrease the recurrence rate. In those patients with insidious onset of instability, who are frequently throwing and swimming athletes, there is often the coexistent inflammation of the rotator cuff owing to instability-induced traction. In those patients with a more gradual onset, a shorter period of rest to decrease local inflammation may be allowed. In both cases, however, a flexibility and strengthening program is mandatory, and any gross loss of external rotation must be regained prior to returning to overhead sporting activities. Loss of motion can cause abnormal glenohumeral stresses as a result of asynchronous muscle

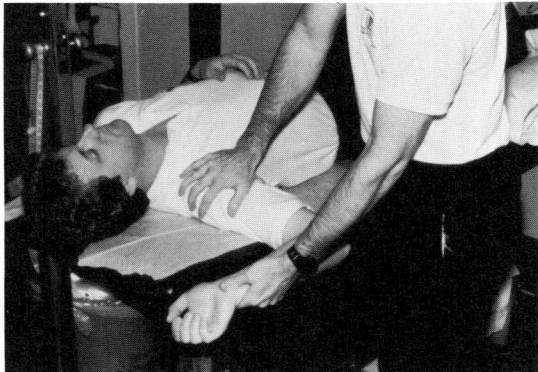

FIGURE 11–20. Passive stretching is performed in the abducted, externally rotated position.

activity. The flexibility program specifically aims at restoring any external rotation losses that may be present. Gradual stretching in the abducted, externally rotated position is performed both by the trainer and the athlete (Fig. 11–20).

Rehabilitation is carried out in a fashion similar to that outlined above for patients with anterior dislocation. Since many of these patients are throwers, greater emphasis should be placed on the eccentric phase of the program. This must be performed under careful supervision, as eccentric work tends to create greater amounts of muscle soreness. In addition, throwers require particular attention to the periscapular musculature: the rhomboids, lattismus dorsi, and serratus anterior. These muscles aid the scapula in acting as a moving platform from which the arm functions. As strength and flexibility return, the patient may gradually increase activity. The athlete usually requires 6 weeks to regain strength and motion and 6 more weeks to graduate to full activity. Rehabilitation is successful in the majority of patients with atraumatic onset and generalized ligamentous laxity. In patients with traumatic onset of instability, the results have been less successful. We generally consider 6 months an adequate time in which to judge whether therapy is effective.

DECISION MAKING IN ANTERIOR INSTABILITY

In patients who remain symptomatic either with persistent pain or instability despite maximal rehabilitative attempts, operative treatment should be considered. In the school-age athlete, timing of the procedure is critical to minimize time loss from both school and athletic participation. An important example is the high school quarterback with symptomatic anterior subluxation in whom the symptoms persist during the season despite a preseason course of rehabilitation. In this individual, surgery should be contemplated immediately following the playing season. This allows completion of convalescence and rehabilitation in time for participation in the next season.

The choice of arthroscopic versus open surgical treatment is discussed in detail in the section on technique. This decision is of particular importance when dealing with a throwing athlete. In our series as well as others, open stabilization has not frequently allowed the thrower to return to his or her preinjury status.[2,39] For this reason, we prefer to use an arthroscopic procedure for treatment of instability in the throwing athlete when feasible.

SURGICAL TREATMENT OF ANTERIOR SHOULDER INSTABILITY

RECURRENT ANTERIOR DISLOCATION

Specific clinical and pathological classification of the dislocation pattern are critical in choosing the correct method for eliminating instability. The physician must be able to reproduce the instability by examination and confirm that the instability is indeed unidirectional. Specifically, any element of inferior laxity must be noted. In most cases, history and physical examination in the office will provide the correct diagnosis. In some patients, apprehension may preclude any adequate examination of the shoulder; however, the maneuver producing the apprehension is helpful diagnostically. Examination under anesthesia is performed in a similar fashion to that in the office, noting especially the directions and magnitude of the instability. Experience is useful when performing an examination under anesthesia. The degree of nonpathological humeral head translation is often larger than expected, particularly posteriorly. Norris (personal communication) has observed that approximately 50 percent of the humeral head may be uncovered posteriorly during a normal examination. Our studies have demonstrated that the head will translate equidistant anteriorly and posteriorly if the arm is placed in the plane of the scapula and neutral rotation. If the arm is horizontally forward flexed, posterior excursion will decrease, whereas if the arm is horizontally extended, the anterior excursion will decrease.[36]

To stress the right shoulder, the examiner, while kneeling next to the patient, holds the patient's elbow with his or her right hand and gently applies an axial load. The left hand palpates the humeral head and acts as a fulcrum to lever the humeral head anteriorly or posteriorly. The degree of humeral head translation is noted with the arm abducted to 90 degrees and maintained in neutral rotation and neutral position relative to the scapular axis. Increasing external rotation will tighten the anterior capsule and prevent anterior translation. Similarly, internal rotation will tighten the posterior capsule and decrease perceived posterior laxity. By altering the degree of rotation and applied load, the optimal arm position provoking maximal glenohumeral instability can be found. At the Hospital for Special Surgery, shoulder instability is graded. Grade I implies greater than 50 percent humeral head translation on the glenoid without dislocation. Grade II implies that the examiner can dislocate the humeral head over the glenoid rim but that the reduction is spontaneous upon the release of examiner pressure. In grade III dislocation, the humeral head locks over the glenoid rim, requiring manipulation of the arm to achieve reduction. Translation is assessed in all three directions: anteriorly, posteriorly, and inferiorly. The sulcus is checked, applying distal traction of the adducted arm. The examiner should note the amount of generalized ligamentous laxity—thumb to forearm distance, the presence of elbow and knee recurvatum. The contralateral shoulder should be examined as well to quantitate translational increases.

If after the examination under anesthesia the diagnosis is in doubt, diagnostic arthroscopy of the glenohumeral joint should be performed. This will be discussed in detail in the section below on the patient with recurrent subluxation. This is rarely indicated in patients with documented recurrent dislocations. The role of arthroscopy in treating the unstable shoulder holds great potential. However, at present the gold standard for the treatment of recurrent anterior dislocation is the open stabilization. Arthroscopic stabilization will be outlined in a later section.

For the patient with recurrent anterior dislocation without a significant inferior component, we favor the open Bankart procedure. This procedure effectively treats the capsular lesion, whether it be labral detachment or capsular laxity, with a documented low recurrence rate in many series including our own. In addition, we believe that precise tensioning of the capsule allows proper restoration of motion, which is imperative in the athlete. Procedures such as the Putti Platt or Magnuson Stack that limit instability by limiting external rotation have no place in treating the athlete. Although many authors have reported excellent results, including a low recurrence rate and good preservation of motion, using the Bristow procedure, we have found only limited use for this procedure.[6] In rare instances of severe bony deficiency of greater than 30 percent of the anterior glenoid, we have supplemented our capsular repair with a transfer of the coracoid to the anterior glenoid. In our series, Hill Sachs lesions are present in over 80 percent of recurrent anterior dislocations.[3] Several authors have suggested that the bony defect plays a role in initiating instability by engaging the anterior lip of the glenoid. Recommended procedures to address this problem are of two types: filling the defect with bone graft or with the infraspinatus tendon or rotational osteotomy of the humerus.[54] We feel that these procedures are not necessary if the anterior capsular repair is performed correctly.

SURGICAL TECHNIQUES FOR RECURRING ANTERIOR DISLOCATION

Our procedure is a modification of that described by Bankart.[8] If the anterior glenoid labrum is detached, as occurs in the majority of patients, the lateral capsule is directly reattached under the correct tension to the bony glenoid margin. In a small percentage of patients, particularly those who are loose jointed, dislocation will occur without labral detachment. In those patients, the lateral capsule is sewn directly to the labrum. If inferior capsular laxity is present, a shift of the capsule is performed. This will be described in the section on multidirectional instability. In the presence of an intact glenoid labrum, sutures are set in the fibrocartilaginous labral base at 1, 3, and 5 o'clock. These sutures are utilized in an identical fashion to the bony sutures to repair the capsule.

After the induction of anesthesia and completion of the examination, the patient is positioned in the beach chair position. The affected arm is abducted in 45 degrees on an arm board. A folded sheet is placed in the midline between the scapulae, lifting the chest forward and allowing the scapula to fall backward. If the pad is placed under the medial border of the scapula, the scapula will be further rotated anteriorly, making access to the scapular neck difficult.

The skin incision is placed in the anterior skin fold to help minimize postoperative scar widening. If desired, it may be placed low in the axilla, as Leslie and Ryan described.[26] The Leslie incision provides for improved cosmesis but requires considerable subcutaneous dissection to create a normal pathway to the deltopectoral interval. In those patients with multidirectional instability, the Leslie incision is not recommended. The cephalic vein is identified and retracted laterally with the deltoid, as there are fewer branches entering medially. The coracoid is a good landmark for identification of the deltopectoral interval. Once the interval has been separated, the clavipectoral fascia will be encountered. The fascia is incised just lateral to the muscle belly of the short head of the biceps. As this layer is dissected proximally, it blends with the coracoacromial ligament, which is routinely transected. Prior to dividing the coracoacromial liagment, the interval beween the ligament and the underlying rotator cuff should be completely dissected. The conjoined tendon is partially incised in an oblique fashion, beginning at the midpoint of the tendon insertion on the coracoid exiting laterally and approximately 1.5 cm distally. This leaves a free lip of tendon proximally for reattachment. We have not found it necessary to osteotomize the coracoid, as simple partial tenotomy will allow adequate exposure. It is important to incise the tendon close to the coracoid because of the musculocutaneous nerve. Anatomical studies have shown that the nerve pierces the tendon an average of 50 mm from the coracoid tip, but variability does exist. Five percent of specimens had a branch entering only 1 to 2.5 cm distal to the coracoid tip.[4]

Attention is then directed to the inferior portion of the wound, where the surgeon should identify the circumflex humeral vessels. On occasion, a high insertion of the pectoralis major tendon may be present, necessitating a partial tenotomy to facilitate exposure. With the arm externally rotated, the vessels are isolated and ligated at a point approximately 2 cm medial to the lesser tuberosity. Using a small elevator, the lower border of the subscapularis is identified at this site. The underlying capsule is then identified using blunt dissection. A curved Kelly clamp is passed underneath the subscapularis to complete the dissection of the subscapularis from the capsule. By continuing medially, the dissection is easy and inadvertent entering of the capsule is avoided. Some manipulation of the clamp is usually necessary to allow dissection of the superior tendon of the subscapularis. With the clamp exiting in the subscapularis-supraspinatus interval, tagging sutures are placed along the medial border of the clamp. The tendon is then incised obliquely, beginning lateral to the clamp and exiting slightly lateral to the sutures. This oblique tenotomy leaves a long medial tendon flap, allowing secure subscapularis repair without shortening. Using blunt dissection, the capsule is dissected from the overlying subscapularis. Medial capsular exposure should extend 2 cm out on the scapular neck and inferior exposure to the 6 o'clock position on the glenoid. Because of the proximity of the axillary nerve, inferior dissection should be performed with great care, and blind attempts at hemostasis with the electrocautery must be avoided in this region.

If present, a rotator interval should be closed at this time. The term *rotator interval* refers to an area of capsular deficiency, usually 1 to 2 cm in size, that exists in the superior aspect of the capsule at the superior border of the subscapularis. As we will describe in the section on multidirectional instability, if a T-plasty procedure is planned, the rotator interval is incorporated in the horizontal capsular incision. To limit anterior subluxation of the humeral head, the elbow is lifted forward, thus directing the humeral head posteriorly. With the arm externally rotated to maintain tension on the capsule, a vertical incision is performed at the glenoid margin. Care must be exercised to avoid deviating laterally in the inferior portion of the capsule. A ring retractor is placed, and the labrum is inspected. In greater than 85 percent of our athletic patients, some degree of labral detachment is noted. However, this is significantly less common in the atraumatic type of instability. If present, the area of capsular detachment from the glenoid is extended medially and proximally to allow placement of a spiked retractor along the glenoid neck (Fig. 11–21). The joint is then irrigated to remove loose bodies, which are present in 20 percent of patients with recurrent instability. The glenoid rim is then roughened with an osteotome to create a bleeding bony surface for enhanced capsular healing. If possible, the surgeon should attempt to create a right angle between the glenoid face and scapular neck to facilitate suture passage. Using a dental drill, three to four drill holes are made in the edge of the glenoid from 1 to 6 o'clock. Nonabsorbable sutures are then passed through the drill holes. The ring retractor is removed and the joint reduced. With the arm held in 30 to 40 degrees of external rotation, the lateral capsule is reduced to the glenoid margin. If inferior laxity remains or redundancy of the capsule occurs, a T-plasty should be performed (see multidirectional instability section). The sutures are then passed through the reduced lateral capsule.

Following the repair, external rotation should be at least 30 degrees, or the repair is redone. The remaining medial capsule is

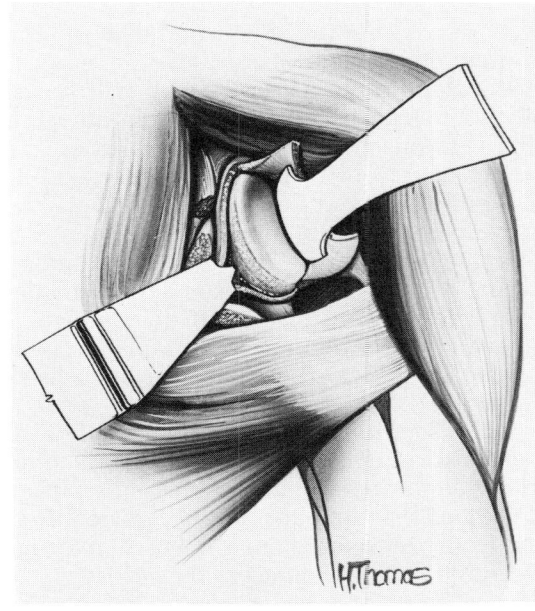

FIGURE 11–21. Illustration depicting exposure of the glenoid neck during the Bankart procedure.

then sutured on top of the lateral flap, providing a supplementary tissue buttress. The subscapularis is reattached to the tendon stump with nonabsorbable sutures, taking great care not to shorten the tendon. External rotation should be at least 30 degrees after the subscapularis repair without undue tension. The conjoined tendon is repaired anatomically and final hemostasis achieved. The wound is closed over a suction drain.

SURGICAL TREATMENT OF ANTERIOR SUBLUXATION

This group of patients becomes more clearly defined by the examination under anesthesia (EUA). If EUA reveals 3+ instability with any tendency toward inferior laxity, we proceed directly with open stabilization as described above. If only 2+ instability exists and there is no inferior laxity as judged by the absence of a sulcus, we perform an arthroscopic examination. The labrum, rotator cuff, and biceps tendon are carefully examined. Like Jobe, we have noted that the concurrence of rotator cuff and labral lesions in the throwing athlete is not infrequent.[21] Unlike the degenerative rotator cuff lesions that occur at the tendon insertion, we have found these to be articular side partial thickness tears occurring at both the musculotendinous junction and the insertion site. We believe that these are traction lesions that are secondary to the instability and thus require no treatment. Labral tears above the equator of the glenoid are not associated with instability and can be treated with simple excision. Lesions below the equator should be probed carefully to define whether tearing and/or detachment exists (Fig. 11-22). In the presence of a firmly attached labrum and a competent-appearing inferior glenohumeral ligament, inferior labral tears should be debrided to a stable margin. If detachment is present in this region, repair must be performed by either arthroscopic or open techniques.

Arthroscopic stabilization is a method of reestablishing continuity of the labral inferior glenohumeral ligament complex back to the glenoid rim. In principle, it is no different from the open Bankart, yet it requires the surgeon to have mastered arthroscopy of the shoulder and be comfortable with the arthroscopic anatomy. As of yet, no long-term data exist for the success rate of arthroscopic stabilization of the shoulder, regardless of technique. Thus, the patient and his or her family must be counseled of possible increased risk of failure of arthroscopic stabilization compared with open techniques. The potential advantage of arthroscopic stabilization is decreased morbidity and perhaps more rapid return to full activity, which is of critical importance in the athletic patient. At the Hospital for Special Surgery, we have utilized two methods for arthroscopic stabilization. The first is labral reattachment via transglenoid sutures. The second involves using an absorbable tack to reattach the soft tissue to the anterior glenoid[53] (Fig. 11-23). We have avoided the use of metallic implants for open or arthroscopic shoulder stabilization because inappropriate positioning, loosening, and subsequent articular injury have occurred all too frequently.[56]

We perform all shoulder arthroscopy in the modified beach chair position. The patient is placed on a bean bag and the table manipulated so that the torso is at a 70-degree angle from the horizontal. The bean bag is molded under the medial scapular border and around the patient's body, then inflated. The firm bean bag is then lateralized, allowing access to the entire scapula, and the arm is supported by an arm board (Fig. 11-24). Complete diagnostic arthroscopy of the glenohumeral joint is then performed, including examination of the labrum both anteriorly

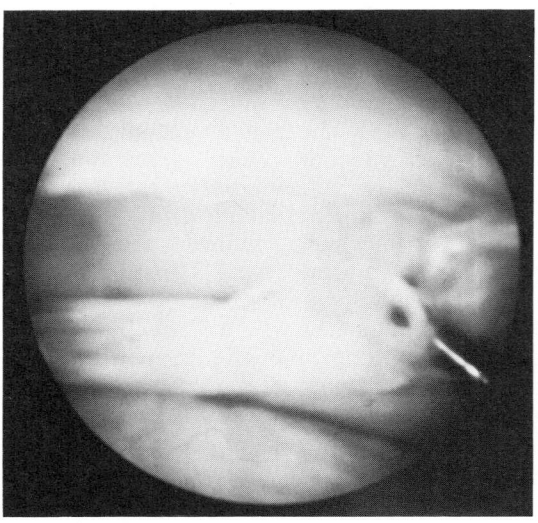

FIGURE 11-22. Arthroscopic photograph of a bucket handle tear of the anterior glenoid labrum. The probe (*center*) displaced the fragment (*left*) from the labral rim (*right*). The humeral head is in the *far left*.

SHOULDER INSTABILITY 175

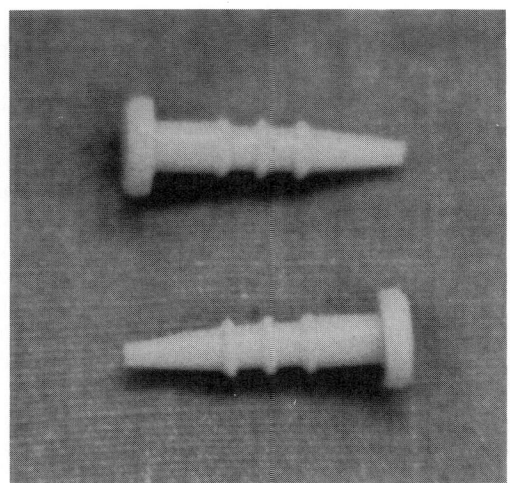

FIGURE 11–23. Absorbable cannulated tacks for arthroscopic stabilization procedure.

and posteriorly, the biceps tendon, the rotator cuff, and the posterolateral humeral head (the site of possible Hill Sachs lesion). Instruments are passed through a cannula system that allows exchange of inflow and instruments. Labral debridement, if indicated (see above), is performed using a motorized suction shaver. If arthroscopic stabilization is to be attempted using either the suture or tack technique, the tissue to be reattached should be carefully evaluated. The labrum must be of good quality and in continuity with the inferior glenohumeral ligament. If not, the labrum should be ignored and the inferior glenohumeral ligament directly reattached. Prior to reattachment, any nonfunctional labral tissue should be debrided and the scapula neck freshened to facilitate soft tissue healing to bone.

For the suture technique, absorbable sutures are placed in the tissue to be attached using a suture passer (Concepts). A Beath pin is then passed through an anterior cannula and placed on the glenoid margin 2 mm medial to the articular surface at a position that will require slight superior advancement of the reattached tissue. The pin is then drilled across the glenoid, beginning at the glenoid margin and aiming 30 degrees medially and 15 degrees inferiorly to avoid the suprascapular nerve coursing along the posterior glenoid neck. Half of the sutures are then passed through the glenoid, and a second pin is drilled superior and parallel to the first to allow passage of the remaining sutures (Fig. 11–25). With the arm held in neutral rota-

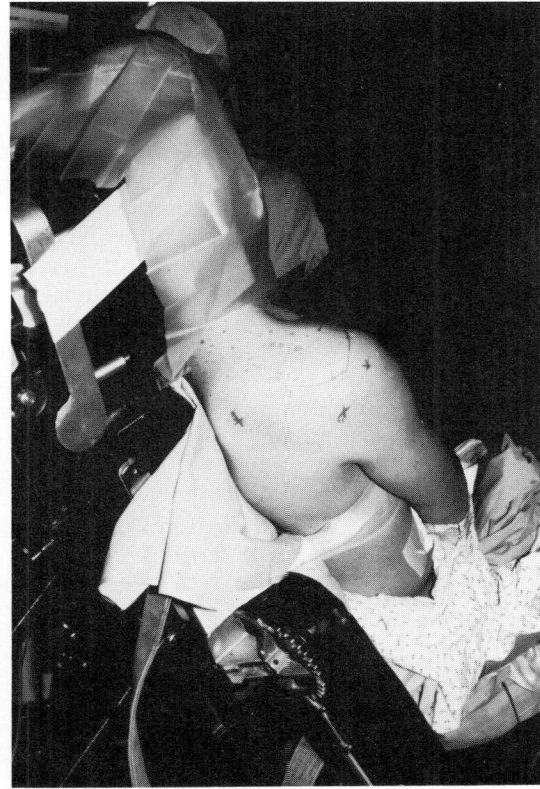

FIGURE 11–24. A posterior view of patient positioned for shoulder arthroscopy in the beach chair position. The scapula is free over the margin over the table.

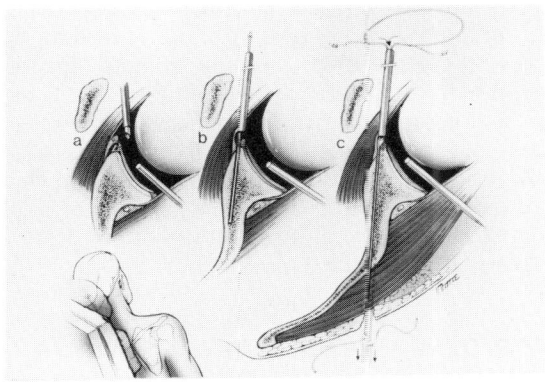

FIGURE 11–25. Illustration depicting technique of arthroscopic suture stabilization. (a) The burr entering anteriorly is used to debride the anterior glenoid neck while the arthroscope is posterior. (b) The Beath pin is drilled across the glenoid from anterior to posterior at an angle of 30 degrees medial to the plane of the glenoid. (c)

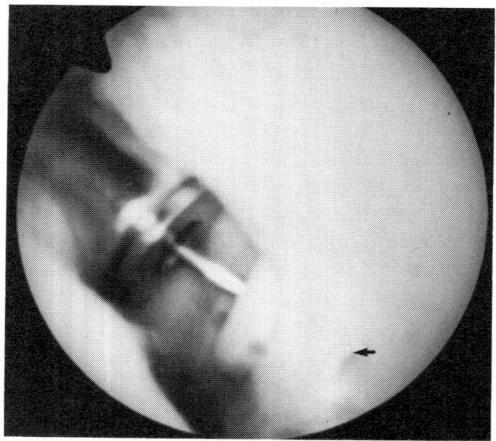

FIGURE 11–26. Arthroscopic photograph of absorbable tack impacting the labrum (*arrow*) to glenoid margin.

tion, posterior tension on the sutures should reduce the tissue to the glenoid margin. The sutures are then tied over the fascia posteriorly, taking care not to pucker the skin.

The tack avoids transglenoid drilling. After preparation identical to that of the suture technique, the soft tissue to be reattached is pierced by a guide wire and advanced superiorly. The guide wire is placed approximately 2 mm medial to the glenoid margin again at a position that will require slight superior advancement of the tissue. A cannulated drill is then passed over the guide wire and is used to penetrate the anterior glenoid to a depth of approximately 1 cm. The drill is then removed with the wire left in place and the tack impacted over the wire, fixing the tissue to the glenoid margin (Fig. 11–26). If an extensive area of labral detachment is present, a second tack is placed either superiorly or inferiorly to the first.

At present, inferior laxity (a 2+ to 3+ sulcus) is a contraindication to arthroscopic stabilization. Although it is conceivable in the future that capsular shifts may be performed arthroscopically, at present an open procedure is mandatory.

POSTOPERATIVE REHABILITATION

When only labral debridement has been performed, we use a sling only until the initial pain has resolved and begin immediate rehabilitation. After restoration of range of motion, strengthening is performed as detailed in the previous section. Return to sport is allowed when a full painless range of motion is present and strength is adequately restored.

After stabilization, whether arthroscopic or open, rehabilitation is tailored to the individual patient's needs. In the throwing athlete, we are aggressive with early restoration of motion. However, in the nondominant arm or the person with generalized ligamentous laxity, range-of-motion exercises are delayed. Immediately following surgery, the patient's arm is held in a universal shoulder immobilizer, which prevents external rotation. Pendulum exercises are begun at 2 weeks. Active exercises are added in the third week, with progressive increases in external rotation and elevation. The immobilization is discontinued at about 4 or 5 weeks. The degree of external rotation obtained on the operating table should be factored into the rehabilitation, so that the capsular repair will not be stretched or avulsed early in the postoperative period. In throwing athletes, the pendulum exercises are commenced during the first week, with the rehabilitation course following accordingly. The rehabilitation is less aggressive for a nondominant arm than for a dominant arm. As will be outlined later, in the patient with multidirectional instability the initiation of rehabilitation is delayed for 6 weeks (Table 11–3).

Our results have indicated that greater than 90 percent of nonthrowers demonstrate full return to sport. Although a similar percentage of throwing athletes are able to return to sport, the participation level they achieve is less predictable. In our series, approximately 50 percent of the throwers felt that they were able to participate at only a moderate level, owing to loss of throwing velocity. The reason for this is unclear. This limitation has

TABLE 11–3. Rehabilitation Following Anterior Stabilization

Begin pendulum exercises at 2 weeks
Active assisted forward flexion and external rotation to neutral at 3 weeks
Isometric deltoid exercises at 4 weeks
Discontinue immobilization at 4 weeks
Passive stretching to increase forward flexion and external rotation at 6 weeks
Concentric and eccentric exercises for the rotator cuff using surgical tubing at 8 weeks
Avoid greater than 10-pound hand-held weights for 3 months postoperatively
Return to noncontact or slow-pitch throwing at 4 months, contact or hard throwing at 6 months

been noted by other authors, most notably Rowe in his large series.[39] Jobe has described doing the capsular repair without dividing the subscapularis, suggesting that postoperative reduction in subscapularis function is the reason for throwing dysfunction.[21]

At 6 weeks, aggressive therapy to increase range of motion is undertaken. At 8 weeks, strengthening exercises using surgical tubing are initiated. Patients are prevented from carrying any heavy loads with the arm in a dependent position for 6 months to permit proper collagen maturation.

If the athlete is a thrower, 6 months should elapse prior to resumption of throwing activities to help prevent capsular stretching and possible reccurrence. Noncontact sports are recommenced at 4 months and contact sports at 6 months.

POSTERIOR SHOULDER INSTABILITY

Posterior instability of the shoulder is less common than anterior instability and often presents more of a diagnostic and therapeutic dilemma. Posterior shoulder instability has been reported to be present in approximately 2 to 4 percent of patients with an unstable shoulder.[10,14,38] The exact incidence is difficult to determine with precision, as the literature tends to discuss subluxation and dislocation interchangeably. In general, posterior subluxation is clearly more common than posterior dislocation, particularly in an athletic population.[52] As in cases of subtle anterior subluxation, the clinical picture is often vague, with the athlete complaining of shoulder pain rather than instability.

ANATOMICAL CONSIDERATIONS IN POSTERIOR SHOULDER INSTABILITY

The anatomical structures responsible for posterior shoulder instability and their relative contributions are not well defined in the literature at this time. At the Hospital for Special Surgery we have completed a series of cadaver studies to evaluate the static constraints to posterior translation of the humeral head.[24]

Incising the extrascapular posterior cuff musculature (the infraspinatus and teres minor) resulted in no increase in posterior instability. Cutting only the superior half of the posterior capsule also resulted in no increase in posterior instability. Posterior subluxation did occur when the posterior capsular incision was extended inferiorly to the 6 o'clock position on the glenoid. Translation further increased when the superior half of the anterior capsule, excluding the anterior portion of the inferior glenohumeral ligament, was also sectioned. Posterior instability also occurred when the inferior glenohumeral ligament was divided from its posterior superior margin to its anterior superior margin. When the intact specimens were placed through a range of motion, the capsular ligamentous function could be demonstrated. As the humerus was brought into a position that would reproduce posterior instability (i.e., arm flexion), adduction, and internal rotation, the posterior capsule expanded like a sling, supporting the humeral head. At the same time, the anterior capsule wound up, providing a tether to restrict posterior translation further.

It appears that, as in anterior instability, the intact inferior glenohumeral ligament is the essential structure primarily responsible for resisting posterior instability. However, anterior capsular integrity also plays a significant role in resisting posterior instability. This supports the circle concept of the shoulder, in which the capsule functions as a whole to limit instability.

Other rare anatomical factors that may contribute to posterior shoulder instability include glenoid retroversion greater than 10 degrees, retroversion of the head beyond 40 degrees, a hypoplastic glenoid, muscle imbalance, and generalized ligamentous laxity.[44]

ACUTE TRAUMATIC POSTERIOR DISLOCATION

Although available statistics are meager, approximately 98 percent of all posterior dislocation of the shoulder are subacromial. Subglenoid and subspinus posterior dislocations have been reported to occur on rare occasions.[36]

The mechanism of injury for posterior dislocation is either a direct blow to the anterior shoulder or, more commonly, an indirect force such as a fall on the outstretched arm. The arm is in a position of flexion, adduction, and internal rotation, which forces the humeral head directly posteriorly. This is a rare occurrence in sporting activities, as the forces required to produce the dislocation are high, such as those seen in a motor vehicle accident. Other causes are accidental electric shock and convulsive seizures, in which the stronger internal rotators, including the latissimus dorsi, pectoralis major, and subscapularis, overpower the external rotators.

Clinical signs and symptoms of posterior dislocation are often overlooked. The reported incidence of missed diagnosis at first examination is between 60 and 80 percent.[36] The most likely reason for this is reliance on AP X rays alone without the addition of lateral axillary views.

The patient usually presents with the arm adducted and internally rotated. The coracoid process appears prominent, and a corresponding posterior bulge is present. Any attempt at adduction or external rotation causes pain. Some examiners have noted that the patient cannot fully supinate the forearm with the arm forward flexed.[17]

Initial management includes a careful neurovascular examination, with specific attention to axillary nerve function. Since confusion may exist concerning the exact diagnosis, X-ray evaluation should be carried out prior to any attempt at reduction.

The standard trauma series should be obtained, including a true AP view of the shoulder (35 to 40 degrees oblique to the body); a transscapular view at right angles to the true AP film; and a physician-assisted axillary view. Classic roentgenographic findings to be aware of are the vacant glenoid sign, the 6-mm rim sign,[3] and the cystic sign.[5] Unlike the typical anterior dislocation where there is obvious inferior displacement of the humeral head, in the posterior dislocation there is often straight posterior translation. Consequently, the radiographic findings in a single plane are subtle, leading to possible diagnostic error. The vacant glenoid sign describes the appearance of an AP X ray of a posterior dislocation. The glenoid fossa is not fully filled with the humeral head and appears "vacant." In addition, there is a greater amount of overlap between the subcondral surfaces of the glenoid and humerus. The 6-mm rim sign is similar to the vacant glenoid sign and refers to the space between the anterior glenoid rim and the humeral head. If this space is greater than 6 mm, this is suggestive of a posterior dislocation. When a true AP of the glenoid is taken at 40 degrees to the central axis, neither of these two signs is present. The cystic sign refers to a lucency seen in the normal humeral head viewed in extreme internal rotation. This is seen in patients with posterior dislocation when the humerus is locked in the internally rotated position.

The axillary view is crucial to assess accurately the true position of the humeral head as well as any notch or depression fracture that occurred in the region of the lesser tuberosity. The presence of a large notch will preclude attempts at closed reduction without anesthesia. If the plain X-rays are not adequate, a CT scan can be valuable to define the anatomy more precisely (Figs. 11–27, 11–28, 11–29).

Reduction of the posterior dislocation is effected by first obtaining satisfactory patient relaxation through the use of medication. With the patient in the supine position, lateral traction is applied with internal rotation to dislodge the humeral head from behind the glenoid, followed by external rotation to relax the capsule. Anteriorly directed pressure is then placed on the humeral head to facilitate reduction. As reduction is achieved, the arm is gently adducted in slight external rotation and placed at the side. The

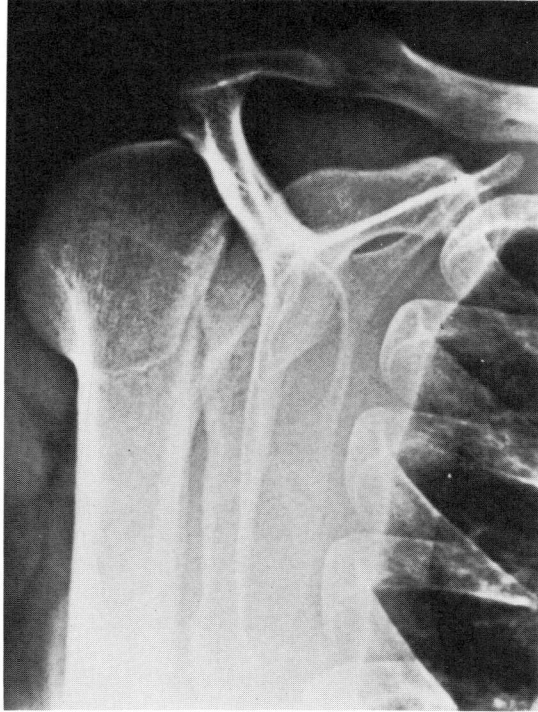

FIGURE 11–27. Transscapular radiograph demonstrating posterior dislocation of the humeral head.

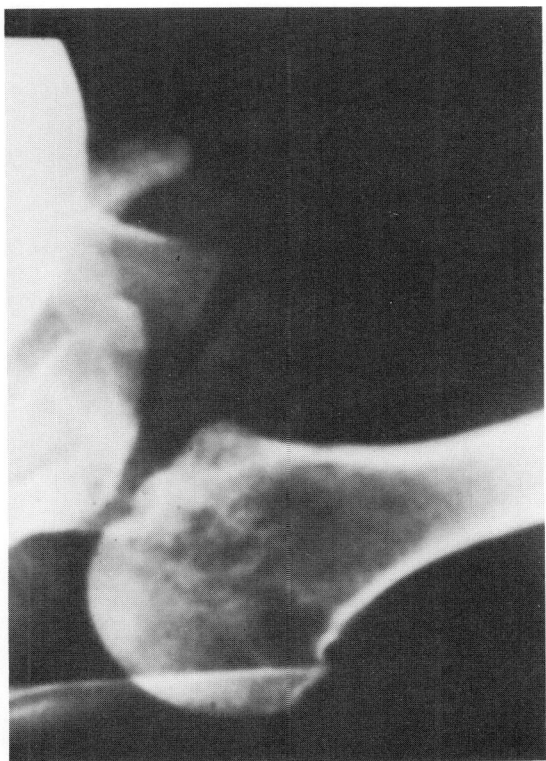

FIGURE 11-28. Axillary radiograph demonstrating posterior dislocation of the humeral head.

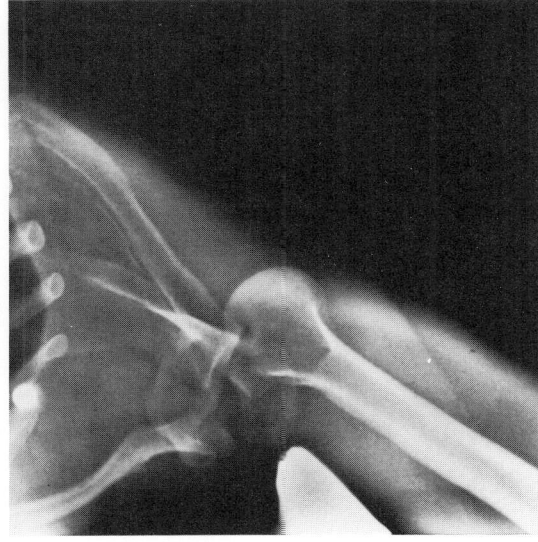

FIGURE 11-29. Axillary radiograph demonstrating posterior dislocation of the humeral head with large anterior humeral notch.

arm is then immobilized in a position of neutral rotation and slight humeral extension.[43] If a large anterior notch is present or the shoulder is grossly unstable, the arm is immobilized in a position of external rotation. Immobilization should be continued for 4 to 6 weeks, followed by an aggressive physical therapy program emphasizing strengthening of the external rotators of the shoulder.

Recurrence rates are not firmly established in the literature, but recurrences are clearly less frequent than those in anterior dislocations. One series reported by Roberts and Wickstein had recurrences in 30 percent of 24 patients.[35] Age is the most significant factor. As in anterior dislocation, the young athlete has the highest risk of recurrence.

RECURRENT POSTERIOR SUBLUXATION

Recurrent posterior subluxation is the most common form of recurrent posterior instability, particularly in the athletic patient. Unlike recurrent anterior dislocation, this condition does not occur secondary to posterior dislocation. Conversely, a patient with posterior subluxation does not progress to recurrent posterior dislocation. The etiology in the majority of cases is repetitive microtrauma as occurs owing to repetitive edge loading at the extremes of motion.

The majority of patients with posterior subluxation present with shoulder pain. Pain is usually posterior but may at times be anterior as well. In the throwing athlete, the pain will occur in the follow-through phase. With the humerus adducted, flexed, and internally rotated, stress is placed on the posterior capsular structures.[15] In football players, particularly offensive linemen, the act of blocking with a repetitive pushing maneuver also stresses the posterior structures, possibly leading to subluxation. If anterior pain is present, it is often due to traction occurring on the anterior ligamentous structures and/or stress-related impingement occurring to the tendon of the rotator cuff. More commonly than in anterior subluxation, the resulting impingement syndrome may be more disabling than the subluxation itself.

The patient with posterior instability will often describe a sensation of crepitation and/or clicking in the involved shoulder, and only rarely does the patient experience a frank sensation of instability. In a recent review of posterior instability at our institution,[15] crepitation or clicking was noted in 90 percent of the patients with symptomatic posterior subluxation. A voluntary component is present with greater frequency in patients with posterior subluxation than in patients with anterior subluxation. Two types of voluntary subluxation have been observed. Some patients induce subluxation by appropriate positioning of their arm into flexion adduction and internal rotation. Others use selective muscle group activation and suppression to create displacement of the humeral head. The latter group will frequently have a significant increase in generalized ligamentous laxity. In both groups, the subluxation appears to be a learned maneuver, a result of the patient's awareness of the specific action contributing to the subluxation. Some patients may use this as a trick to control their environment. These patients may require psychiatric evaluation, particularly those who produce subluxation by contracting their internal rotators. However, the majority of patients with voluntary posterior subluxation are not psychologically abnormal.

On physical examination, patients with grossly symptomatic recurrent posterior subluxation often have no posterior apprehension. This is in marked contrast to patients with anterior subluxation, in whom anterior apprehension is a common finding. Range of motion should be carefully documented. These patients frequently have loss of internal rotation, particularly with the arm at 90 degrees of abduction. Stability testing is performed with the patient supine as previously described. In addition, the arm is horizontally adducted, which in some patients will reproduce subluxation. As with anterior instability, we again assign a grade to the amount of posterior humeral head translation on physical exam. Instability is graded as 1+ if there is increased motion without a clunking sensation of the humeral head as it drops off the posterior glenoid; 2+ if a jump is noted without locking in the subluxated position; and 3+ if there is actual locking in a dislocated position. Careful assessment of inferior and anterior instability is necessary, as is examination of the contralateral shoulder (Figs. 11–30 and 11–31). In our population of patients with posterior subluxation, there is greater than a 70 percent incidence of generalized ligamentous laxity. We use four parameters to assess this: (1) the degree of

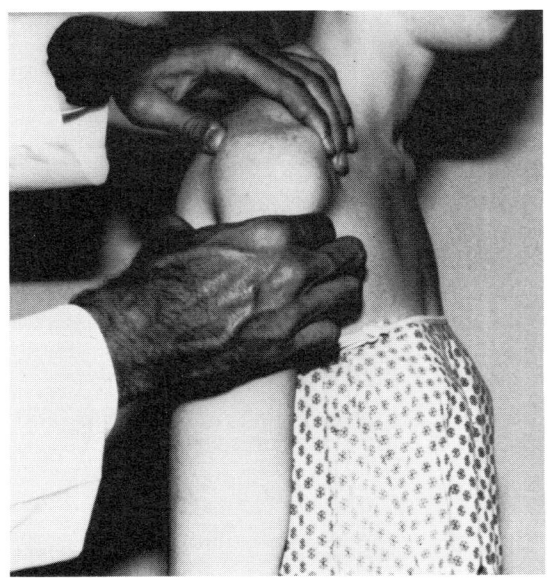

FIGURE 11–30. Examiner palpates clavicle anteriorly and acromion posteriorly with left hand while grasping the humeral head with the right hand.

thumb hyperabduction during wrist palmar flexion, (2) the degree of index finger metacarpal phalangeal joint hyperextension, and the degree of (3) elbow and (4) knee hyperextension.[25]

Radiographic evaluation of posterior instability includes the previously described[33] in-

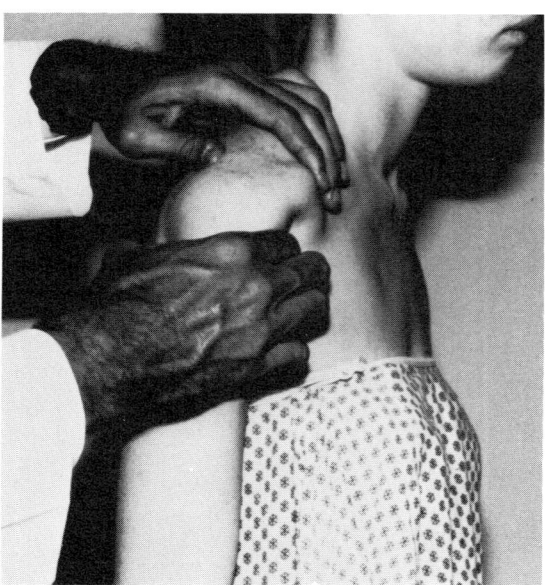

FIGURE 11–31. With right hand the examiner subluxes the humeral head posteriorly in a patient with posterior instability.

stability series: an AP in internal rotation, a Stryker notch view, and a West Point axillary view. In addition, an AP view in external rotation will identify any anterior notch fracture on the humeral head. We have found a much higher incidence of bony glenoid changes in patients with posterior instability than with anterior instability. In our series, 20 percent demonstrated posterior calcification along the capsule and labrum, and an additional 20 percent were noted to have 2 to 4 mm of frank bony erosion of the posterior glenoid rim.[15] On this basis, we have found the CT scan to be of particular value in the diagnostic work-up of these patients (Fig. 11–32). Owing to the significant overlap with impingement symptoms, diagnostic confusion frequently exists. A finding of posterior damage is an extremely important factor in deciding that subtle posterior instability is indeed present. Arthrography and arthrotomography have not been of great value in diagnosing posterior labral lesions. With the emergence of a high-quality surface coil for the shoulder, the MRI is becoming an increasingly useful tool in the diagnosis of posterior labral pathology. The diagnosis is in the majority of cases established on history and physical examination and routine radiographs. The arthroscope is rarely used as a primary diagnostic modality. If impingement is present, this will be immediately evident upon entering the subacromial space. The bursa will be thickened, with multiple adhesions obscuring visualization. In these cases, we debride the bursa and carefully examine the rotator cuff surface. If scarring or partial thickness tearing indicative of repetitive damage to the cuff is present, we proceed with division of the coracoacromial ligament and debridement of the undersurface of the acromion, removing any thickened scar tissue that has developed (Fig. 11–33). We generally avoid formal bony acromioplasty in these patients.

Treatment of recurrent posterior subluxation of the shoulder follows principles similar to those outlined for recurrent anterior subluxation. The goals for conservative management include (1) avoiding any voluntary episodes of instability or position that are likely to result in subluxation, (2) restoring normal shoulder motion, and (3) strengthen-

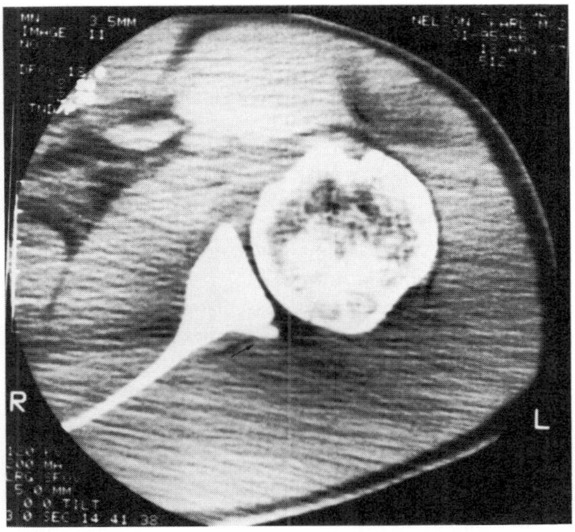

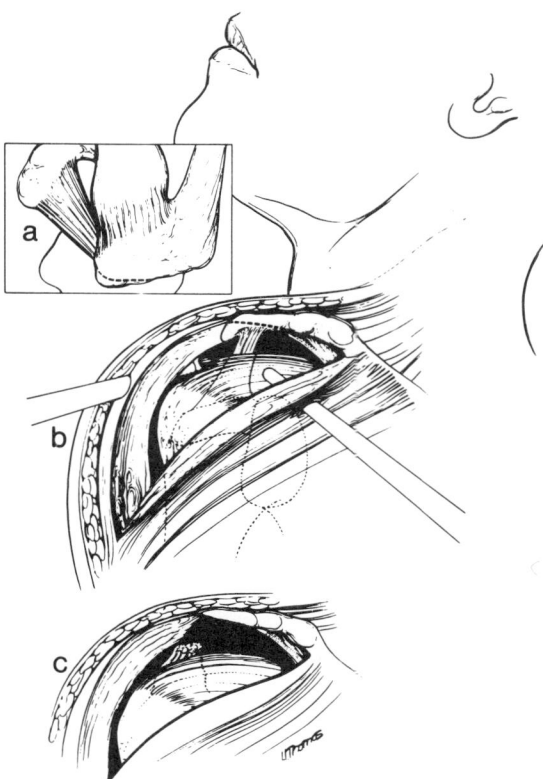

FIGURE 11–33. (a) Superior view of the coracoacromial arch. *Dotted line* represents area of proposed acromial resection. (b) Posterolateral view of the subacromial space (deltoid muscle partially removed). The arthroscope enters posteriorly; the burr enters anterolaterally. The *dotted line* represents the proposed area of acromial resection. (c) The acromioplasty has been completed; the coracoacromial ligament has been detached.

FIGURE 11–32. CT scan of a football lineman with recurrent posterior instability. Small osteophyte (*arrow*) of the posterior glenoid margin is seen.

ing the rotator cuff with emphasis on the external rotators. This must be performed in a careful, graduated fashion, avoiding positions that aggravate any preexisting tendinitis. We begin using isometric exercises and progress to the use of elastic tubing.

As strength increases, we emphasize the eccentric component of the exercise. The rationale for this has been derived from our own studies on the strength of shoulder rotators in tennis players. Previous studies that have analyzed the strength characteristics of the throwing arm have found that while the internal rotators are clearly stronger on the dominant side, the external rotators are in fact weaker when compared with the nondominant arm.[20] The shortcoming of these studies was that they measured concentric strength only. Since the external rotators are only firing concentrically to position the arm during the cock-up phase of the throw, it makes sense that they are not particularly strong when concentrically tested. It is during the follow-through phase when the external rotators fire eccentrically to decelerate the arm that great amounts of torque are generated.

We have conducted a study using tournament tennis players comparing both eccentric and concentric rotation strength in the dominant and nondominant shoulder. Although the external rotators are not significantly stronger in the dominant arm when measured concentrically, they are 50 to 75 percent stronger when measured eccentrically. Another study compared the effect of eccentric and concentric training of internal and external rotators in tennis players.[13] Torque and velocity of service were measured before and after training. The greatest strength and functional gains (as measured by increase in service velocity) were seen in the group that trained eccentrically. This indicates the importance of including eccentric training when conditioning the arm of a throwing athlete.

Surgical tubing provides a safe, effective means to begin eccentric training. We progress our athletes to isokinetic training only in the latter phases of the program. Eccentric training clearly increases muscle soreness and can itself induce rotator cuff inflammation. When the athlete with posterior instability has a profound amount of impingement pain, we initially manage the shoulder with immobilization in a sling and a nonsteroidal antiinflammatory agent. We generally avoid subacromial corticosteroid injections in the young athlete.

In our experience approximately 60 percent of patients with posterior instability will respond to a graduated exercise program.[15] Those patients with generalized ligamentous laxity and instability that occurs secondary to repetitive microtrauma are particularly apt to respond. Patients whose onset was associated with macrotrauma, such as football linemen, are less likely to be aided by an exercise program (Table 11–4).

Operative treatment is considered in patients who fail a minimum of 6 months of trial of conservative therapy and whose pain or instability prevents adequate function of the involved shoulder. A thorough examination under anesthesia is mandatory to confirm or refute preoperative findings. This should include an examination of the opposite shoulder.

Arthroscopy is a frequent first step in the operative procedure. Thorough arthroscopic examination of the glenohumeral joint is performed. If a rotator cuff lesion is discovered or impingement symptoms are profound, arthroscopy of the subacromial space is performed as well. Labral lesions may be present anteriorly as well as posteriorly in the patient with posterior subluxation. Arthroscopy may be of considerable value in treating posterior shoulder subluxation as well as diagnosing it. This is particularly true in the throwing athlete. Arthroscopic debridement of labral lesions will not diminish the instability but may relieve the mechanical limitation and diminish symptoms enough to allow a return to throwing. Subsequent stabilization proce-

TABLE 11–4. Rehabilitation for Posterior Instability

Decrease Inflammation
Nonsteriodal antiinflammatory agent and/or modalities
Restore Range of Motion
Active assisted and gentle passive stretching
Strengthen Rotator Cuff with Emphasis on the External Rotators
Isometric concentric/eccentric with surgical tubing
Strengthen the Scapular Musculature
Latissimus dorsi
Rhomoids
Trapezius
Avoid Aggravating Exercises
Avoid exercises that might aggravate tendinitis or stress posterior capsule such as resisted abduction above 90 degrees, bench pressing, or push-ups

dures may be required. However, some of these patients will become asymptomatic when they are no longer placing the shoulder under such high loads. Open posterior stabilization may prevent full return to high-level throwing. For this reason, we are more inclined to persist with exercises and possibly labral debridement in the athlete who wishes to return to competitive throwing. Contraindications to labral debridement are 3+ instability, findings of significant articular cartilage damage due to translation or voluntary instability. Arthroscopic debridement even when performed in well-selected patients tends to provide only temporary relief. Symptoms often reoccur in 2 to 3 years if activity is resumed.[1]

SURGICAL PROCEDURES FOR POSTERIOR SHOULDER INSTABILITY

Open posterior stabilization is indicated in those patients who are refractory to conservative care or labral debridement. Preoperative evaluation includes either an excellent-quality axillary view or a CT scan to assess the bony structure of the glenoid. In the majority of cases, capsular repair is sufficient. However, if the capsule is of poor quality or the glenoid is deficient, we do supplement with a posterior bone block.[29]

The patient is positioned in the lateral decubitis position with the affected side up. The arm is draped free to allow intraoperative manipulation. Our incision is placed longitudinally, directly over the glenoid margin and in line with the axillary crease, extending from just below the spine of the scapula distally for approximately 8 cm (Fig. 11–34). Circumferential skin flaps are created to allow identification of the posterior deltoid raphe, which courses obliquely across the wound. This raphe is split bluntly in line with the fibers of the deltoid. Inferior lateral dissection is limited by the axillary nerve as it exits below the teres minor. We have not found it necessary to detach the deltoid proximally to expand the exposure, but this can be done if needed. The interval between the teres minor and infraspinatus is identified and developed. The underlying capsule is located and dissected free from the infraspinatus. The tendon is split obliquely, leaving the deep portion long to potentially reinforce the capsular repair.

The capsule is then exposed by blunt dis-

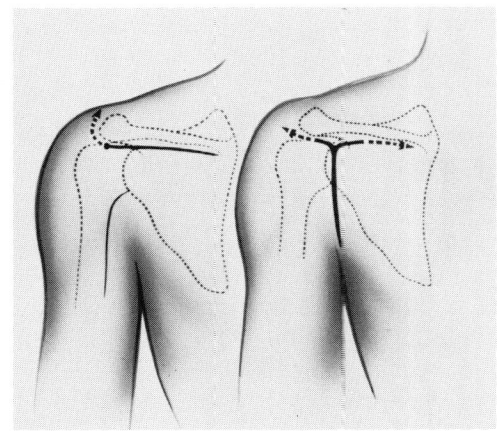

FIGURE 11–34. Illustration depicting the two options for posterior skin incision. On the *left*, horizontal with potential lateral extension. On the *right*, vertical with horizontal Chevron-type extension.

secting medially onto the scapular neck and inferiorly to the 6 o'clock position on the glenoid. Once exposed, the capsule is incised: Beginning with a transverse incision in the midportion, the glenoid margin is identified. A longitudinal incision is then performed just lateral to the glenoid labrum. The labrum and joint are inspected. The labrum often has vertical clefts from subluxation and may be partially detached, but an extensive posterior Bankart lesion is rarely present. In the majority of cases, the labrum is preserved. If the labrum is substantial, it may be used as the site for capsular reattachment. When the labrum is detached or of poor quality, the capsule is stripped from the scapula neck and a bony bed and glenoid drill holes are prepared for capsular reattachment in a manner identical to the method used in the anterior Bankart procedure. Posterior capsular repair always involves some degree of superior capsular advancement. By using the T-shaped capsular incision as described, the lower capsular flap can be advanced superiorly and the upper flap advanced inferiorly to create a buttress effect (Fig. 11–35). If marked inferior laxity is present, a second vertical incision can be created laterally, making the T into an H. Separate advancement of the lateral portion of the capsule allows for greater tension to be placed in the inferior portion of the recess. During suturing of the capsule, the arm should be held in slight extension and neutral rotation.

In the presence of an insufficient capsule, a posterior bone block is utilized (Fig. 11–36).

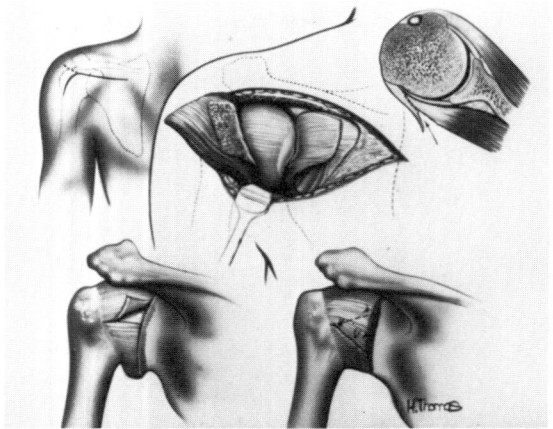

FIGURE 11–35. Illustration depicting the steps of posterior capsular shift for recurrent posterior instability.

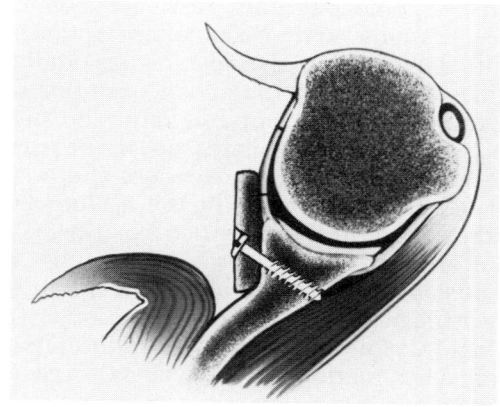

Figure 11–37. Illustration depicting the correct bone block position for posterior instability.

Despite the name "bone block," the primary goal is not for the graft to act as a mechanical block but rather to increase the size and depth of the glenoid fossa. Graft placement must be carefully done to prevent bony impingement on the humeral head. The graft is obtained from the spine of the scapula and is 3 cm long and about 15 mm wide. After the capsular repair has been completed, the graft is fixed by a bicortical screw to the inferior quadrant of the glenoid as close as possible to the joint margin. The graft should parallel the posterior scapular neck so that it functions to extend the joint (Fig. 11–37). Intraoperative X rays should be taken to confirm both the position of the bone block and the screw position.

In the case of the capsular repair alone, the infraspinatus tendon can be sewn into the capsule to buttress the repair.

Postoperatively, the patient is placed in a custom-made orthosis that supports the arm in neutral rotation and slight extension (Fig. 11–38). The splint is removed daily for hygiene and elbow extension exercises but is otherwise used at all times for 4 weeks. At 4 weeks, we begin Codman's exercises and gradual weaning out of the brace until at 6 weeks the brace is discontinued. At 6 weeks, a rehabilitation program is begun that first

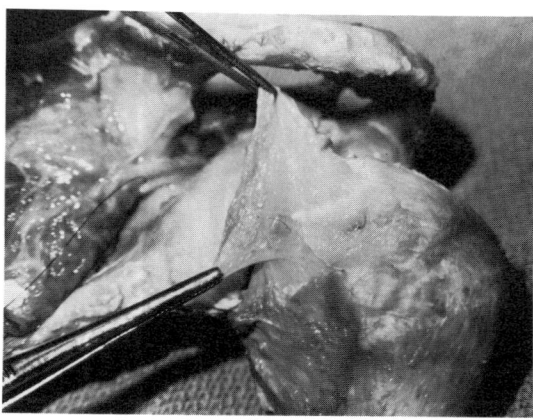

FIGURE 11–36. Photograph of thin posterior capsule (held between forceps).

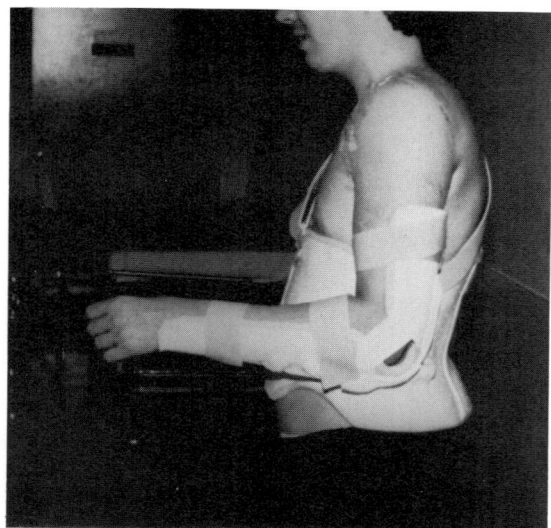

Figure 11–38. Orthroplast arm spica splint used for the patients after posterior stabilization and for those with multidirectional instability.

restores normal range of motion and then emphasizes strengthening of the external rotators. The patient gradually achieves range of motion by 8 weeks after beginning rehabilitation. The strengthening process is slow, and return to sports activities is usually delayed 9 to 12 months postoperatively.

In summary, the assessment of patients with suspected posterior subluxation of the shoulder should include evaluation of generalized ligamentous laxity, degree of trauma occurring during episodes, and presence of a voluntary component. Patients who experience repetitive microtrauma resulting in posterior subluxation often have generalized ligamentous laxity and are good candidates for the physical therapy program. However, only a portion of the macrotraumatic patients may benefit significantly from this program. When evaluated arthroscopically, these patients will show more evidence of posterior damage to both the articular and the labral cartilage than the microtraumatic group. The majority of the macrotraumatic patients will present with severe disability and are candidates for a posterior capsulorrhaphy. If the posterior capsule and infraspinatus tendon appear incompetent, augmentation of the reconstruction with a bone block is recommended. Arthroscopic debridement of labral tears may provide temporary symptomatic relief and is recommended for the competitive thrower.

MULTIDIRECTIONAL INSTABILITY OF THE SHOULDER

Multidirectional instability (MDI) is defined as instability occurring in more than one plane. As described by Neer and Foster,[31] three instability patterns occur most frequently: anterior dislocation with posterior and inferior subluxation, posterior dislocation with anterior and inferior subluxation, and dislocation occurring in all three directions. The common denominator among these patterns is the presence of inferior capsular laxity. As with other forms of instability, the etiology may be atraumatic, microtraumatic, or macrotraumatic. There is clearly a greater proportion of patients with generalized ligamentous laxity among patients with MDI than with unidirectional anterior or posterior instability.

In the athletic patient, there is usually an interplay between inherent tissue laxity and superimposed trauma that results in a multidirectional instability pattern. Multidirectional instability is merely a continuum within the instability spectrum and is not an entity entirely separate from unidirectional instability. Acutely, most, if not all, anterior and posterior dislocations are associated with some mild inferior laxity. The quality of soft tissue healing during the conservative treatment period as well as the degree of inferior laxity present prior to injury may determine the subsequent development of a multidirectional pattern of recurrent instability.

In patients without generalized ligamentous laxity, a history of multiple violent injuries to the shoulder is usually obtained. Athletes with increased laxity will generally relate repetitive activities such as throwing, swimming, or weight lifting as the cause of instability. This repetitive microtrauma has a cumulative effect, increasing the magnitude of MDI.

Of the three types of multidirectional instability, anterior inferior is the most common in the athletic population. On review of historical points, these patients may have little to differentiate them from those with unidirectional anterior instability. Some will complain of unusual fatigue or pain when attempting to carry a heavy object in the hand. Unlike patients with typical recurring anterior dislocation in whom pain is rarely present, these patients will more often exhibit impingementlike symptoms.

The most important and consistent finding on physical examination is the presence of a sulcus sign. Weighted X-ray views can provide supportive evidence, but false-negative results do occur, owing to inadequate relaxation.

The initial treatment for all types of multidirectional instability is conservative. Patients with atraumatic instability are more likely to respond to rehabilitation than those of traumatic origin. Approximately 50 to 70 percent of patients with multidirectional instability and ligamentous laxity will have a favorable response to rehabilitation, especially if they are willing to modify their activities. Patients with involuntary instability and a traumatic or microtraumatic origin to their instability are more likely to fail conservative care and be considered for surgical correction.

Confusion may exist regarding the primary direction of instability. This should be decided preoperatively based on historical data regarding the direction of instability, direction of apprehension, and awake stability examination. Examination under anesthesia on these patients can be misleading. There will often be a significant magnitude of instability in all directions when under anesthesia. For example, patients with anterior and inferior multidirectional instability will at times under anesthesia demonstrate posterior laxity equivalent to anterior laxity. The direction of surgical approach is dictated by the primary clinical direction of instability.

The details of the program for conservative treatment of multidirectional instability are identical to those for posterior instability.

Surgical procedures that successfully treat MDI must address the inferior capsular laxity. If a medial capsular detachment (Bankart lesion) is present, this must be corrected as well. Capsular shift procedures to eliminate the inferior redundancy have been described by several authors. Neer and Foster[31] have described a shift procedure performed on the extreme lateral margin of the capsule at the humeral neck. If a Bankart lesion is present, it must be repaired as a separate step. Others have utilized midlateral portions of the capsule for their shift procedures. These techniques also require separate repairs of medial detachments. Our modification of the Bankart procedure, the T-plasty, simplifies the performance of the capsular shift in conjunction with a Bankart repair. In our group of patients with anterior inferior multidirectional instability, the majority had anterior labral detachments as well as capsular laxity.[2] By incising the capsule as far medially as possible, a long lateral flap is created. Redundancy in the capsule is eliminated by superior advancement of the inferior lateral flap. This allows the surgeon to eliminate inferior laxity and repair the Bankart lesion in a single step. By doing so, there is a greater ability to preserve normal external rotation, which is a very important factor in the athletic patient. In our series of patients with multidirectional instability, the average postoperative loss of external rotation in the abducted position was 5 degrees. The lateral capsular incision, because of the ability to rotate externally the humerus intraoperatively, allows greater access to the posterior portion of the capsule and may be preferable if no Bankart lesion is present.

The T-plasty is performed by exposing the shoulder either anteriorly or posteriorly as described above. The capsule is exposed with greater attention paid to clear dissection of the inferior portion. This must be performed prior to any capsular incisions. The axillary nerve is dangerously close to the inferior capsule during this dissection, and the surgeon must be constantly aware of its position to avoid transsection or excessive traction.

A transverse incision in the capsule is performed first. We choose the midglenoid level, attempting to stay slightly superior to the inferior glenohumeral ligament. If a rotator interval is revealed during the anterior approach, this may be incorporated into the transverse incision. The joint is then inspected carefully, examining the labrum to define the presence or absence of a Bankart lesion. If the labrum is well attached to the glenoid, then the labral complex is not dissected off the glenoid neck, but instead a vertical capsular incision is made just lateral to the labrum. This is more often the case in posterior than in anterior instability. Should labral detachment be present, the vertical incision is carried out directly at the glenoid rim, and the medial capsule and labrum are stripped off the scapular neck. The glenoid rim is prepared using an osteotome to create a bleeding surface. Holes in the glenoid margin are created at 1, 3, and 5 o'clock using a dental burr, through which nonabsorbable sutures are passed. If no labral detachment is present, sutures are passed through the base of the labrum at these positions. The shoulder is then reduced and the arm held in the desired position of rotation, neutral for posterior instability and 30 degrees of external rotation for anterior instability. The inferior capsule is then drawn superiorly to decrease the infracapsular redundancy (Fig. 11–39). If after reattachment and maximal advancement there remains inferior redundancy and laxity, a second vertical capsular incision is made parallel to the first in the lateral portion of the capsule, creating an H configuration. The inferior limb is then advanced superiorly as needed to eliminate the inferior capsular redundancy further. The superior limb of the capsular T- or H-plasty is then advanced inferiorly and sutured over the inferior limb (Fig. 11–40). This places further tension in the capsular system and buttresses the repair. The goal is not to limit rotation of the arm but to restore a normal volume and tension to the glenohumeral capsule.

Postoperatively, the patient is immobilized in a thermoplastic splint, which sup-

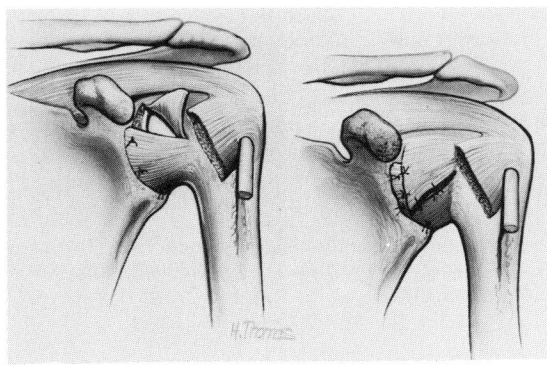

Figure 11-39. Illustration depicting the T-plasty capsular shift. On the *left*, the inferior flap is shifted superiorly. On the *right*, the superior flap is shifted inferiorly.

ports the arm from below and holds the arm in neutral rotation. The shoulder is kept immobilized for a full 6 weeks prior to starting any motion. Passive and active assisted motion is performed from 6 to 12 weeks postoperatively. Progressive resistance exercises are then added slowly. Full sporting activities are not allowed for 9 to 12 months until muscle strength and range of motion are symmetrical. When we reviewed the results for our anterior inferior group, we found overall excellent results.[2] Recurrent anterior instability was experienced only in 1 of 42 shoulders, and an additional three patients had episodic posterior instability postoperatively. However, only one had instability to the degree that he needed operative correction. As previously mentioned, there was minimal restriction of motion: The mean loss of external rotation with the arm abducted at 90 degrees was 5 degrees.

COMPLICATIONS OF SURGICAL TREATMENT FOR SHOULDER INSTABILITY

Several complications can occur with surgical repair for shoulder instability. Postoperative infection and hematoma can occur, as in all operations. Meticulous surgical technique, achieving hemostasis, use of suction drains, and prophylactic antibiotics can decrease the incidence of these problems. If an extensive hematoma occurs, early evacuation to prevent scarring and restricted range of motion is suggested.

Neurovascular injuries secondary to surgery are the next group of complications. The musculocutaneous nerve is susceptible to traction neuropraxia as it enters the coracobrachialis. The axillary nerve is at risk with inferior capsular dissection and repair. If a nerve injury occurs, initial conduction studies may be utilized to determine if conduction is still present before wallerian degeneration sets in at 48 hours. If conduction in the early period suggests that axonal continuity is present, then potential for recovery exists. In such a case, EMGs are obtained at 3-week intervals and the patient followed. However, if no conduction is present and no voluntary potential present on EMGs, then early exploration is indicated. It is important to avoid waiting too long in these patients, vainly hoping that recovery will occur. Urbaniak has noted that these lesions are frequently complete and require operative repair.

Failure of the surgical procedure is also a potential complication. This can vary from persistent instability in the shoulder to severe limitation of motion. The reported incidence of recurrent dislocation for surgical repair of anterior instability ranges from 0 to 11 percent.[18,28,36,39] Provided that pathological capsular abnormalities have been corrected at surgery, recurrent instability has been very uncommon at our institution. Range-of-motion losses are a function of surgical technique, tissue contracture, and rehabilitation programs. The capsular tension should be set at the proper degree of rotation and the subscapularis or infraspinatus muscle repaired anatomically. Potential serious complication concerns the use of hardware about the

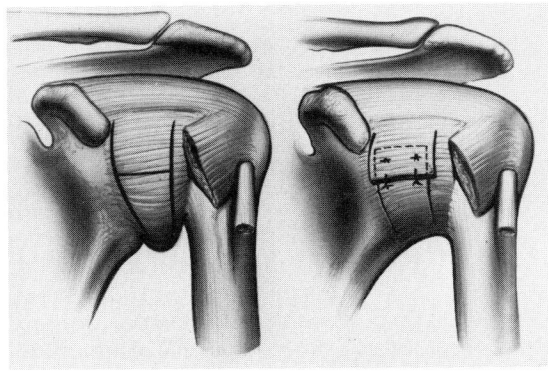

Figure 11-40. The H-plasty. An additional vertical incision is placed in the lateral capsule. The inferior and superior flaps are advanced accordingly.

shoulder. We have taken a position against the use of any metal implants in or about the shoulder joint in treating instability. Inappropriate placement or loosening may occur and cause damage to the glenohumeral joint.

References

1. Altchek, D. W., and Warren, R. F.: Arthroscopic labral debridement. A three year follow-up study. Orthop. Trans. (In press)
2. Altchek, D. W., and Warren, R. F.: T-plasty anterior repair for multidirectional instability of the shoulder. Orthop. Trans. (In press)
3. Anderson, D., Zvirbulis, R., and Ciullo, J.: Scapular manipulation for reduction of anterior shoulder dislocation. Clin. Orthop. 164:181–183, 1982.
4. Andrews, J. R., and Carson, W. G.: The arthroscopic treatment of glenoid labrum tears in the throwing athlete. Orthop. Trans. 8:44, 1984.
5. Arndt, J. H., and Sears, A. D.: Posterior dislocation of the shoulder. A.J.R. 94:639–645, 1965.
6. Bach, B. R., O'Brien, S. J., Warren, R. F., and Leighton, M.: An unusual neurological complication of the Bristow procedure. A case report. J. Bone Joint Surg. 70A(3): 458–460, 1988.
7. Bach, B. R., Warren, R. F., and Fronek, J.: Disruption of the lateral capsule of the shoulder. A cause of recurrent dislocation. J. Bone Joint Surg. 70B(2):274–276, 1988.
8. Bankart, A.S.B.: The pathology and treatment of recurrent dislocations of the shoulder joint. Br. J. Surg. 26:23, 1938.
9. Blom, S., and Dahlback, L.: Nerve injuries in dislocations of the shoulder joint and fractures of the neck of the humerus. Acta Chir. Scand. 136:461–466, 1970.
10. Boyd, H. B., and Sisk, T. D.: Recurrent posterior dislocation of the shoulder. J. Bone Joint Surg. 54A(4):779–786, 1972.
11. Clayton, M. L., and Weir, G. J., Jr.: Experimental investigations of ligamentous healing. Am. J. Surg. 98:373–378, 1959.
12. Cox, J. S.: Personal communication.
13. Ellenbecker, T. S., Davies, G. J., and Rowinski, M. J.: Concentric versus eccentric isokinetic strengthening of the rotator cuff. Objective data versus functional test. Am. J. Sports Med. 16(1):64–69, 1988.
14. English, E., and MacNab, I.: Recurrent posterior dislocation of the shoulder. Can. J. Surg. 17:147–151, 1974.
15. Fronek, J., Warren, R. F., and Bowen, M.: Posterior subluxation of the glenohumeral joint. J. Bone Joint Surg. 71A(2):205–216, 1989.
16. Galinat, B. J., Howell, S. M., and Kraft, T. A.: The glenoid-posterior acromion angle: an accurate method of evaluating glenoid version. Orthop. Trans. 12(3):727, 1988.
17. Hawkins, R. J., and Angelo, R. L.: Osteoarthritis following an excessively tight Putti-Platt repair. Orthop. Trans. 12(3):728, 1988.
18. Hovelius, L., Thorling, J., and Fredin, H.: Recurrent anterior dislocation of the shoulder: results after the Bankart and Putti-Platt operations. J. Bone Joint Surg. 61A(4): 566–569, 1979.
19. Howell, S. M., Galinat, B. J., and Renge, A. J.: Normal and abnormal mechanics of the glenohumeral joint in the horizontal plane. J. Bone Joint Surg. 70A(2):227–237, 1988.
20. Ivey, F. M., Calhoun, J. H., Rusche, K., and Bierschenk, J.: Normal values for isokinetic testing of shoulder strength. Med. Sci. Sports Exerc. 16(2):127, 1984.
21. Jobe, F. W.: Personal communication.
22. Jobe, F. W., Moynes, D. R., Tibone, J. E., and Perry, J.: An EMG analysis of the shoulder in pitching. A second report. Am. J. Sports Med. 12(3):218–220, 1984.
23. Kinnet, J. G., Warren, R. F., and Jacobs, B.: Recurrent dislocation of the shoulder after age fifty. Clin. Orthop. 149:164–168, 1980.
24. Kornblatt, I., Warren, R. F., and Marchand, R.: An analysis of the effects of capsular and tendon releases on posterior glenohumeral translation. Orthop. Trans. 8:89, 1984.
25. Koslin, B. L., Zeno, S., and Meyers, A.: Joint looseness: a function of the person and the joint. Med. Sci. Sports Exerc. 12:189–194, 1980.
26. Leslie, J. T., and Ryan, T. J.: The anterior axillary incision to approach the shoulder joint. J. Bone Joint Surg. 44A(6):1193–1196, 1962.
27. Mason, M. L., and Allen, H. S.: The rate of healing of tendinitis: an experimental study of the tensile strength. Am. J. Surg. 113:424–456, 1941.
28. Morrey, B. F., and Janes, J. M.: Recurrent anterior dislocation of the shoulder: long-term follow-up of the Putti-Platt and Bankart procedures. J. Bone Joint Surg. 58A(2): 252–257, 1976.
29. Mowery, C. A., Garfin, S. R., Booth, R. E., and Rothman, R. H.: Recurrent posterior dislocation of the shoulder: treatment using a bone block. J. Bone Joint Surg. 67A(5): 777–781, 1985.
30. Neer, C. S.: Anterior acromioplasty for the chronic impingement syndrome in the shoulder. A preliminary report. J. Bone Joint Surg. 54A(1):41–50, 1972.
31. Neer, C. S., and Foster, C. R.: Inferior capsular shift for involuntary inferior and multidirectional instability of the shoulder. J. Bone Joint Surg. 62A(6):897–908, 1980.
32. Nobuhara, K., and Hitoshi, I.: Rotator interval lesion. Clin. Orthop. 223:44–50, 1987.
33. Pavlov, H., Warren, R. F., Weiss, C., and Dines, D.: The roentgenographic evaluation of anterior shoulder instability. Clin. Orthop. 184:153–158, 1985.
34. Poppen, N. K., and Walker, P. S.: Normal and abnormal motion of the shoulder. J. Bone Joint Surg. 58A(2):195–201, 1976.
35. Robert, A., and Wickstrom, J.: Prognosis of posterior dislocations of the shoulder. Acta Orthop. Scand. 42:328–337, 1971.
36. Rockwood, C. A.: Subluxations and dislocations about the shoulder. In: Rockwood, C. A., and Green, D. P. (eds.): Fractures in adults, Vol. 1 Philadelphia: J. B. Lippincott Co., 1984, 2nd ed., pp 722–860.
37. Rokous, J. R., Faegin, J. A., and Abbott, H. G.: Modified axillary roentgenograms, a useful adjunct in the diagnosis of recurrent instability of the shoulder. Clin. Orthop. 82:84, 1972.
38. Rowe, C. R.: Prognosis in dislocations of the shoulder. J. Bone Joint Surg. 38A(5):957–977, 1956.
39. Rowe, C. R., Patel, D., and Southmayd, W. W.: The

40. Rowe, C. R., Pierce, D. S., and Clark, J. G.: Voluntary dislocation of the shoulder. A preliminary report on a clinical electromyographic and psychiatric study of twenty-six patients. J. Bone Joint Surg. 55A(3):445–460, 1973.
41. Rowe, C. R., and Sakellarides, H. T.: Factors related to recurrences of anterior dislocation of the shoulder. Clin. Orthop. 20:40–47, 1961.
42. Rowe, C. R., and Zarins, B.: Recurrent transient subluxation of the shoulder. J. Bone Joint Surg. 63A(6):863–872, 1981.
43. Rowe, C. R., and Zarins, B.: Chronic unreduced dislocations of the shoulder. J. Bone Joint Surg. 64A(4):494–505, 1982.
44. Saha, A. K.: Recurrent dislocations of the shoulder. New York: Thieme-Stratton, Inc., 1981, 2nd ed., p. 55.
45. Schlemm, F.: Über die Verstarklingsbander am Schultergelenk. Arch. Anat., 1860, pp 45–48.
46. Schwartz, E., Warren, R. F., and Otis, J.: Radiologic measurement of superior migration of the humeral head in impingement. Presented: American Shoulder and Elbow Society, New Orleans, LA, February 1990.
47. Schwartz, R. E., O'Brien, S. J., Warren, R. F., and Torzilli, P. A.: Capsular restraints to anterior-posterior motion of the shoulder. Orthop. Trans. 12(3):727, 1988.

Bankart procedure. A long-term end-result study. J. Bone Joint Surg. 60A(1):1–16, 1978.

48. Scott, D. J., Jr.: Treatment of recurrent posterior dislocations of the shoulder by glenoplasty. J. Bone Joint Surg. 49A(3):471–476, 1967.
49. Simonet, W. T., and Cofield, R. H.: Prognosis in anterior shoulder dislocation. Am. J. Sports Med. 12(1):19–24, 1984.
50. Stimson, L. A.: An easy method of reducing dislocation of the shoulder and hip. Med. Rec. 57: 356–357, 1900.
51. Turkel, S. J., Panio, M. W., Marshall, J. L., and Girgis, F. G.: Stabilizing mechanisms preventing anterior dislocation of the glenohumeral joint. J. Bone Joint Surg. 63A(8):1208–1217, 1981.
52. Warren, R. F.: Subluxation of the shoulder in athletes. Clin. Sports Med. 2(2):339–354, 1983.
53. Warren, R. F.: Personal communication.
54. Weber, B. G., Simpson, A., and Hardegger, F.: Rotational humeral osteotomy for recurrent anterior dislocation of the shoulder associated with a large Hill-Sachs lesion. J. Bone Joint Surg. 66A(9): 1443–1450, 1984.
55. Yoneda, B., Welsh, R. P., and MacIntosh, D. L.: Conservative treatment of shoulder dislocation in young males. J. Bone Joint Surg. 64B(2): 254–255, 1982.
56. Zuckerman, J. D., and Matsen, F. A.: Complications about the glenohumeral joint related to the use of screws and staples. J. Bone Joint Surg. 66A(2): 175–180, 1984.

12

INJURIES INVOLVING THE CLAVICLE

FREDDIE H. FU
STEVE SALYERS

Injuries to the clavicle and the acromioclavicular (AC) joint are quite common in sports. Somewhat suprisingly, treatment of these injuries continues to generate controversy. Good results are the norm, but complications can occur. At this time, there is a clear need for further study of these injuries in order to refine our treatment.

ANATOMY AND FUNCTION OF THE CLAVICLE

The clavicle is the only osseous attachment of the shoulder girdle to the trunk.[22] The clavicle is a unique bone, being the only long bone to ossify by an intramembranous process. This bone is S-shaped, with a convexity facing forward in the medial portion of the bone and a concavity facing forward in the lateral portion. The clavicle has numerous muscle and ligamentous attachments. The muscles attached to the clavicle include the deltoid, trapezius, pectoralis major, subclavius, and sternocleidomastoid (Fig. 12–1). The ligamentous attachments are the acromioclavicular ligaments, the coracoclavicular ligaments (conoid and trapezoid), the infraclavicular ligament, the rhomboid ligament, the sternoclavicular (SC) ligament, and the costoclavicular ligament. Usually, a fibrocartilaginous disk or meniscus is present at both the AC and the SC joints. The middle third of the clavicle is separated from the subcavian vessels and brachial plexus by the subclavius muscle and the clavipectoral fascia.[45]

The AC ligament is a thin capsule with superior and inferior thickenings that are somewhat stronger than the remainder of the capsule. There are also anterior and posterior thickenings, but these do not possess any great strength. The superior AC ligament blends with fibers from the deltoid and trapezius insertions and is thereby reinforced.[31] The coracoclavicular ligament is very strong and runs from the lateral and inferior portion of the clavicle to the base of the coracoid. This ligament has two parts: the conoid and the trapezoid.[31] The conoid is posterior and medial to the trapezoid ligament (Fig. 12–2).

Usually, only one epiphysis (at the sternal end) appears radiographically in adolescence, and it generally fuses by the third decade. An acromial epiphysis occasionally appears radiographically but fuses quickly in adolescence. The acromial epiphysis rarely ossifies and therefore is typically not seen radiographically. The acromial end makes a minimal contribution to the longitudinal growth of the clavicle.[18,48]

The clavicle has many functions. It acts as an anchor for the many muscle attachments mentioned above, and it also acts as a bony strut that holds the glenohumeral joint in space. The clavicle acts as a protector for the great vessels and the brachial plexus.

Urist[49] has shown that the coracoclavicular ligaments stabilize upward displacement of the clavicle relative to the acromion and

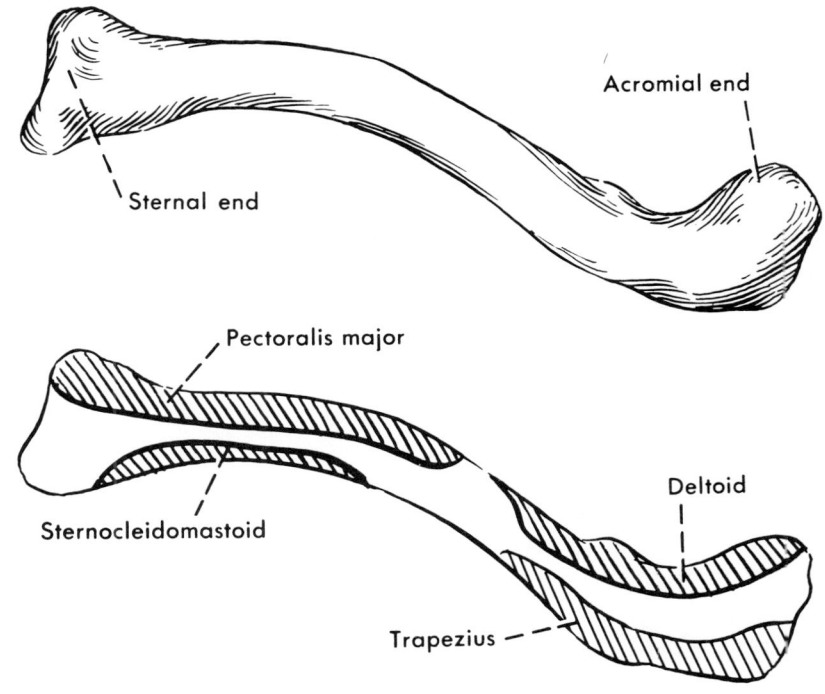
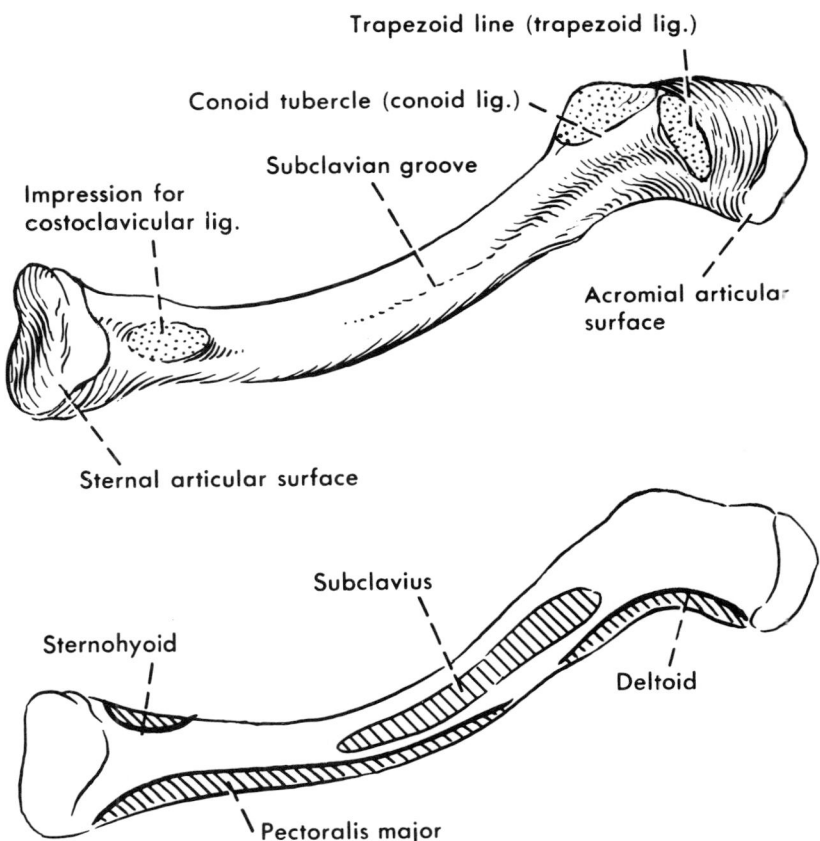

FIGURE 12–1. Muscular attachments and insertions of the clavicle from above (*A*) and below (*B*). (From Hollinshead, H. W.: Anatomy for Surgeons. Vol. 3, 2nd ed. New York, Harper & Row Publishers, Inc. pp. 266–267, 1969.)

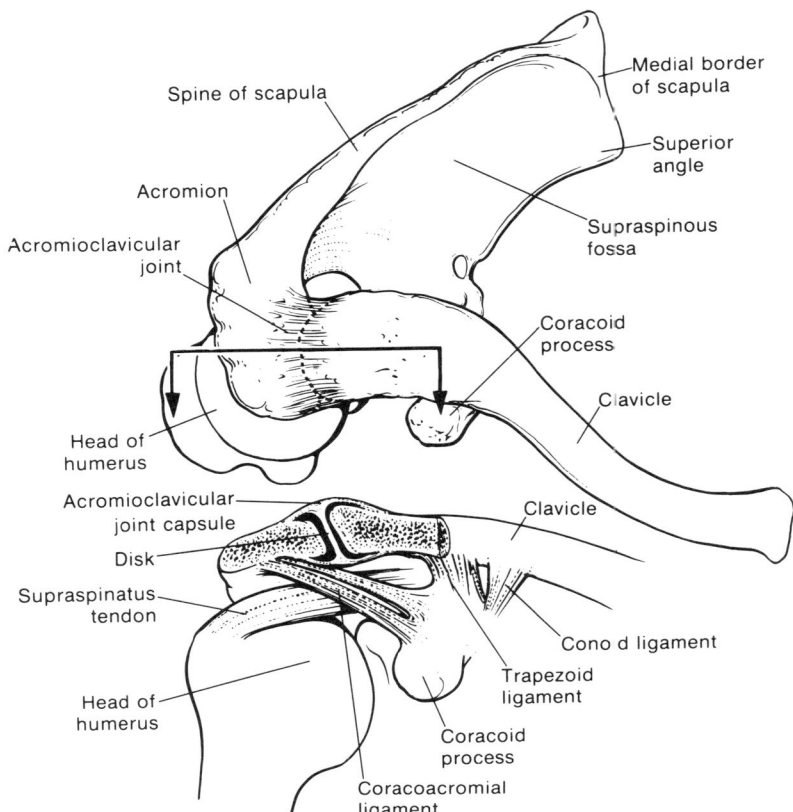

FIGURE 12–2. The superior and cross-section view of the shoulder. Note the two parts of the coracoclavicular ligament: the conoid and trapezoid. (From Hoppenfeld, S., DeBoer, P.: Surgical Exposures in Orthopaedics. Philadelphia, J. B. Lippincott Co., p. 933, 1984.)

that the acromioclavicular ligaments stabilize anterior and posterior displacement. Fukuda et al.[16] have shown in a biomechanical study of the AC joint that with smaller loads and displacements the AC ligaments are more important in preventing the AC joint from subluxing superiorly. With increased loads or displacement, the conoid ligament becomes the most important restraint to superior displacement. The trapezoid ligament tends to be more important in axial loading at the AC joint. The AC ligaments are the most important at small and large displacements in preventing posterior subluxation.

As shown by Bearn[3] and Rockwood,[42] the coracoclavicular ligaments do not function as restraining ligaments holding the clavicle downward but instead function as suspensory ligaments that hold up the scapula and attached upper extremity. This is important to keep in mind should ligament reconstruction be undertaken, as the reconstruction would have to be quite sturdy in order to suspend the forequarter.

CLAVICLE FRACTURES

CLINICAL PICTURE

The typical history given for a clavicle fracture is a fall on the point of the shoulder. Clavicle fractures can also occur with a direct anterior or superior blow to the shaft of the bone. A more unusual history would be a fall on the outstretched hand. The patient presents with extreme pain in the shoulder region. The forearm is often cradled in the contralateral arm and held splinted against the patient's thorax. Almost any motion whether of the trunk or the arm causes excruciating pain.

PHYSICAL AND RADIOGRAPHIC EXAMINATION

Physical findings are tenderness and deformity at the site of the fracture. It is important to palpate the clavicle to rule out a posterior displacement of one of the fragments. The skin should be carefully evaluated to make sure the injury is indeed closed. A thorough upper extremity neurovascular examination is mandatory. In the more violent injuries, it is pertinent to auscultate the ipsilateral lung field, owing to the very slight possibility of a pneumothorax.

Radiographic examination of a clavicle fracture involves simply an anterior-posterior (AP) clavicle view and also an AP view with a 15-degree cephalad tilt of the beam. The 15-degree tilt allows the clavicle to be seen free of the scapular shadow and also can more accurately give the clinician a clue to true displacement of the fracture fragments. In assessing posterior displacement, clinical examination is reliable. However, if radiographic correlation is needed, the radiographic examination to rule out posterior displacement of one of the fragments is the Alexander view. The Alexander view will be discussed in detail under acromioclavicular injuries. For medial third fractures, tomograms or perhaps even computerized tomography (CT) would be necessary to delineate the pathology completely, but clinical examination is nearly always adequate for choosing the proper treatment. In clavicle fractures, the lateral fragment is typically displaced inferiorly, and the medial fragment is displaced superiorly, with the ends of the bone tending to override.

DIFFERENTIAL DIAGNOSIS

Differential diagnosis for these injuries is extremely limited. A contusion without fracture is possible but easily ruled out by radiographic examination. An AC joint injury is part of the differential and will be considered at length later in the chapter. Also, a sternoclavicular joint injury rather than medial third fracture is another possibility. A blow to the top of the shoulder can result in a rotator cuff contusion or tear; however, the appearance of the athlete as he or she protects the arm and the clinical and radiographic examinations would differentiate a clavicle fracture from this entity.

CLASSIFICATION

Clavicle fractures are usually divided into those involving the middle, lateral, and medial thirds.[45] The middle third fractures account for 82 percent of the total number. Neer[35] has further divided the lateral third fractures into two types: type I, in which the coracoclavicular ligaments are intact, and type II, in which the coracoclavicular ligaments are torn. Others have added a type III, which represents intact coracoclavicular ligaments but also has an intraarticular component of the fracture that might lead to posttraumatic arthritis at a later date (Fig. 12–3). A special subgroup of the lateral one-third fractures concerns patients less than 13 and perhaps as old as 16 who incur an injury that is more properly termed a "pseudo AC dislocation."[15,37] This injury will be discussed at length later in the chapter. In addition to the above classification, standard fracture nomenclature can be applied—namely, *open* versus *closed*, *displaced* versus *nondisplaced*, *greenstick* versus *complete*, *comminuted* versus *simple*, and *plastic deformation without fracture*.[7]

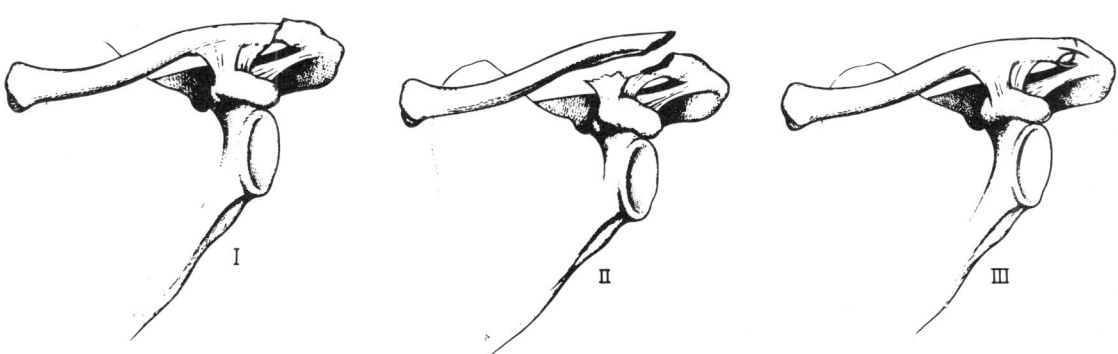

FIGURE 12–3. The classification of distal clavicle fractures, type I, II, and III. Type III shows intraarticular component. (From Rockwood, C. A., Green, D. P.: (eds.) Fractures in Adults. Vol. 1. 2nd ed. Philadelphia, J. B. Lippincott Co., p. 708, 1984.)

TREATMENT

Many different methods have been described to treat clavicle fractures. Basically, treatment can be divided into three broad categories: (1) use of a sling only, (2) treatment with a strap, harness, or even casting, and (3) internal fixation, either open or via percutaneous route. We will consider each section of the clavicle independently in terms of the treatment.

As noted, midshaft clavicular fractures account for the majority (82 percent)[44] of clavicular fractures. Operative intervention for these injuries has an extremely limited application. Neer states, "The most important causal factor in non-union fractures of the middle third has been improper open surgery."[34] Wilson believes that "open reduction of the clavicle in children is totally unnecessary and leads to disaster."[54] Even the AO/ASIF *Manual of Internal Fixation* stresses that "fractures of the clavicle heal with and without immobilization. The results of open reductions are less than satisfactory. The incisions spread, at times develop keloids and become ugly, and not infrequently the fractures themselves, after open reduction, go on to non-union."[32]

As stated above, the indications for an operative procedure for a midshaft clavicle fracture are extremely limited. One absolute indication would be for open fracture debridement or a vascular injury. Injury to the brachial plexus could be in the form of a stretch or a tear, and clinical judgment would need to be used to decide whether open exploration was indicated. Jablon et al.[23] reported on an irreducible midthird fracture that was caught in the trapezius in a 13-year-old girl. Open reduction and fixation of the fracture with a suture yielded a good result. Dameron and Rockwood[12] state that internal fixation is seldom necessary in a child, even with open debridement or reduction. Often, the posteriorly displaced fractures that one would think would need an open reduction can be reduced closed simply with a towel clip under general anesthetic. Should a pulsatile or expanding hematoma be diagnosed, emergent exploration should be performed. Should an open procedure be required, the question of fixation arises. Good results have been reported with Steinman pins and plates as well as simple suture fixation[45,57] (Fig. 12–4). The physician's judgment again would need to be utilized to decide whether an injury requires rigid internal fixation or whether, after open debridement is performed, routine closed treatment would be adequate. In the face of a vascular injury and repair, we tend to favor a more rigid form of fixation.

The vast majority of these injuries are treated closed. These injuries are notorious for not maintaining the reduction. There almost always will be some type of residual bump either owing to fracture callous or imperfectly reduced fragments. The amount of residual deformity depends on the number of years to maturity and the attendant capacity to remodel (Fig. 12–5). This type of deformity is of cosmetic concern only, causing no functional impairment. Our feeling is that even in a person to whom cosmesis is of great concern, late revision of the union with internal fixation can be performed electively and closed treatment should be followed rather than initial open reduction. Most orthopedists feel that the scar is as much of a cosmetic problem as the bump.

Although many orthopedists still favor some type of figure-eight bandage, either commercial or constructed with a padded stockinette, our experience has been that this device does not seem to provide any great improvement in final fracture position and can be associated with skin lesions, brachial plexus neuritis, and generalized discomfort. For this reason, we elect to treat our athletes with a simple sling for comfort and advise that they be prepared to sleep upright for the first 2 weeks following the injury, as this position seems to reduce their discomfort.

If an attempt is going to be made at reducing the fragments acutely, a hematoma block is often adequate for analgesia. In the first few days after the injury, a mild narcotic analgesic is much appreciated by these patients, as these injuries are quite painful.

As with many of the conditions presented in this text, we favor an aggressive program of rehabilitation. The patient generally will have enough decrease in pain that he or she can begin active grip strengthening and wrist flexion and extension within several days. These exercises should be performed with the elbow supported to avoid depressing the shoulder. The patient can begin on a stationary bicycle or walking in a shallow pool in order to maintain cardiovascular fitness as soon as the pain allows, which in our experience has been 5 to 7 days postinjury. Most can discontinue the sling at 3 to 4 weeks, and

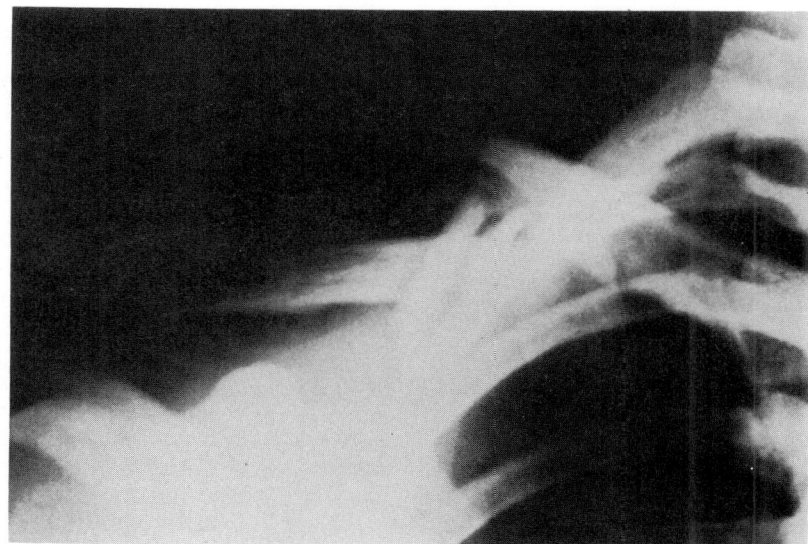
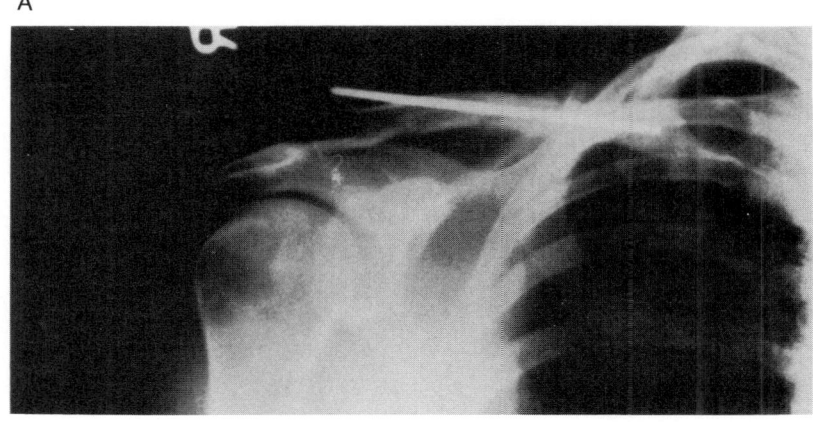

FIGURE 12–4. Unreducible displaced clavicle fracture threatening the skin integrity (A). Operatively reduced using Steinman pin (B). (From Zenni, E. J., Krieg, J. K., Rosen, M. J.: Open reduction and internal fixation of clavicular fractures. J. Bone Joint Surg. 63A:148, 1981.)

at this time, they can begin some lightweight/high-repetition exercise for the biceps and triceps. After the sling is removed, gentle active mobilization of the shoulder can begin and generally does not require a formal physical therapy program. After full range of motion has been established, we progress to the use of low-resistance isometric exercises and follow the isometrics with additional weight lifting with light weights and high repetition for shoulder strengthening. Return to noncontact sports, depending on the degree of upper extremity utilization in the sport, can be as quick as 5 to 6 weeks. Return to contact sports will generally take 12 to 16 weeks, and we ask the athlete to demonstrate full range of motion, normal strength, and clinical union. Radiographically, there should be signs of early union, but complete radiographic union may not be demonstrated at the time the athlete is ready to return to contact sports.

At any stage of rehabilitation, when pain signals too vigorous an activity level, we ask the athlete to return to the next lower level of rehabilitation. Special equipment for return to football is limited, but a donut-type pad may prevent irritation of the shoulder pads on a prominent callous or bone end.

For medial third fractures, diagnosis can be quite difficult and may require computed or routine tomography. For the majority of school-age athletes, these injuries represent a physeal injury. Treatment consists of the use of a sling until pain subsides and a rehabilitation program that follows the one outlined above. Physeal fractures remodel quite readily with little disability or deformity and require no special treatment in the vast majority of cases.

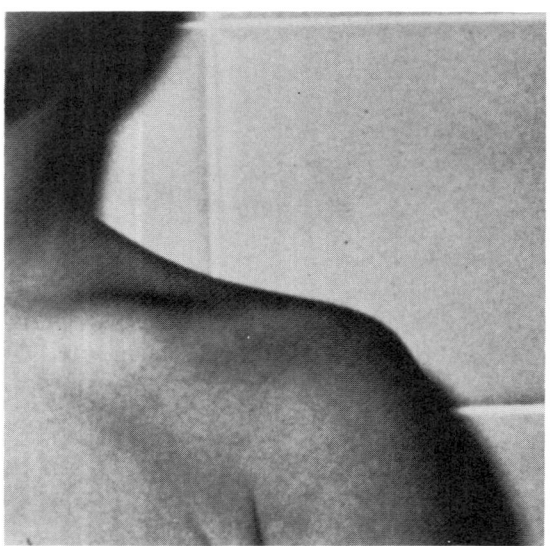

FIGURE 12–5. Residual bump seen in a young boy after a healed midclavicular fracture. (From Post, M.: The Shoulder, Surgical and Non-Surgical Management. Philadelphia, Lea & Febiger, p. 365, 1978.)

Lateral third fractures are quite uncommon and, as Rockwood states, can be "misdiagnosed or overtreated"[41] (Fig. 12–6). In young athletes, these fractures actually represent "pseudodislocations" of the AC joint. In children under the age of 16, the coracoclavicular ligaments remain attached to the periosteal sleeve, and the clavicle tears superiorly out of the periosteum.[15,37] Eidman et al. reported on 25 "AC separations" in children 5 to 16 years old treated surgically. There were no true AC dislocations below the age of 13, with these injuries actually being lateral third physeal fractures.[15] Rockwood has treated all of these injuries in all ages with figure-eight bandages since 1962 with good results and few complications.[41] Ogden treats these injuries conservatively unless there is significant displacement, when closed reduction and percutaneous pinning or open reduction and suture of the periosteal tube are performed.[37]

Neer has retrospectively reviewed a series of adults with a type II lateral third fracture in which he recommends pinning of the AC joint owing to the increased chance of nonunion.[35] In the older adolescent, the lateral third fracture may indeed be one of the adult pattern; however, there is little in the literature to guide the clinician on this point. Our feelings have been to treat these injuries with a sling and functional rehabilitation and, should nonunion develop, to proceed with an open procedure to obtain union.

Rehabilitation for these injuries proceeds in the same stepwise fashion as for midshaft fractures. Owing to the potential for nonunion, we tend to progress more slowly, perhaps delaying each of the stages by 1 week or so.

The prognosis for clavicle fractures (midshaft, lateral, and medial) is for these injuries to heal uneventfully with a full range of motion of the shoulder without residual pain. Accurate reduction of the fracture fragments is often not possible, but this does not impede a firm union and rarely causes symptoms. Complications of the fractures are

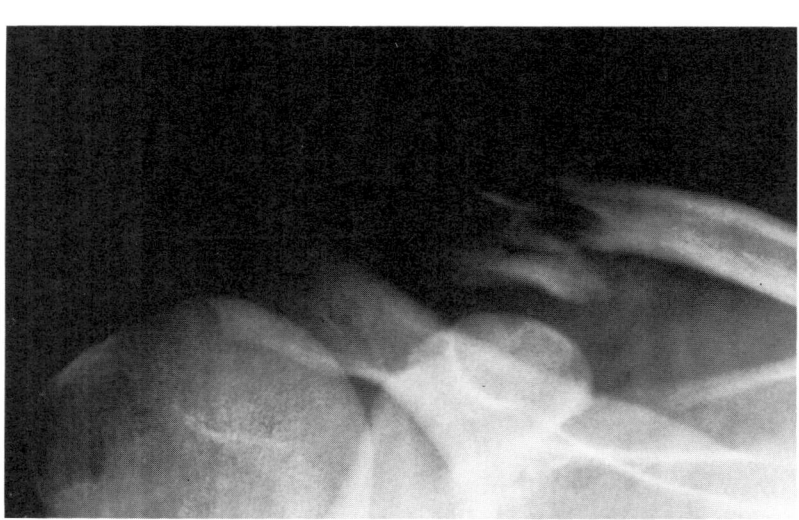

FIGURE 12–6. Lateral third fracture in a football player. This healed with closed treatment in 8 weeks.

rare but can include damage to adjacent structures including nerves, arteries, lungs, and skin (either early or late) and a poor cosmetic result.[40,55] We feel the use of the sling and the early functional rehabilitation outlined above provides the quickest way to return these athletes to safe participation in their sport.

ACROMIOCLAVICULAR JOINT INJURIES

CLINICAL PICTURE

The typical history for an acromioclavicular injury is an athlete who falls and lands on the point of his or her shoulder. The point of contact tends to be more posterior with an AC injury rather than the more anterior contact point for clavicular injuries. Another typical story is a football player or rugby player who lowers a shoulder in order to make a tackle and has contact on the top of this shoulder. As with the clavicle injury, the athlete will be cradling the arm and stabilizing it against the thorax.

PHYSICAL AND RADIOGRAPHIC EXAMINATION

The physical examination consists of palpation of the AC joint, which will be exquisitely tender. The entire clavicle needs to be palpated to rule out an associated fracture. Also, careful palpation of the distal end of the clavicle is necessary in order to evaluate the direction in which the dislocation has occurred.

An AP radiograph of the shoulder is an inadequate film because the amount of radiation necessary to penetrate the glenohumeral joint will often "burn out" the AC joint. The technician should be advised that the area of interest is the AC joint and distal clavicle. As with clavicular fractures, the technician may need to tilt the beam 15 degrees cephalad in order to prevent the AC joint and scapula from being superimposed, which would prevent complete evaluation. The comparison weight-bearing view has been well described. This consists of suspending weights from the patient's wrists and obtaining a film of both AC joints on one cassette in order to classify more accurately the injury as a type I, type II, type III, and so on. Although this view is always mentioned, in retrospect we have found that it seldom alters our treatment decisions. One additional view that is helpful is the Alexander view, which presents a lateral projection of the AC joint.[51] This view is obtained with the patient standing, holding the injured arm across the chest with the ipsilateral hand in his or her contralateral axilla. The patient then faces a 10 × 12 cassette and holds the cassette near the injured side with the contralateral hand pulling the injured shoulder against the film. If the position is correct, the uninjured shoulder should be 30 to 35 degrees angled away from the cassette. The X-ray tube is angled at 15 degrees caudad and aimed at the coracoid along the scapular spine (Fig. 12–7). This view is excellent for radiographically detecting posterior dislocation of the distal end of the clavicle, which on routine views might be interpreted as a partial dislocation, when in

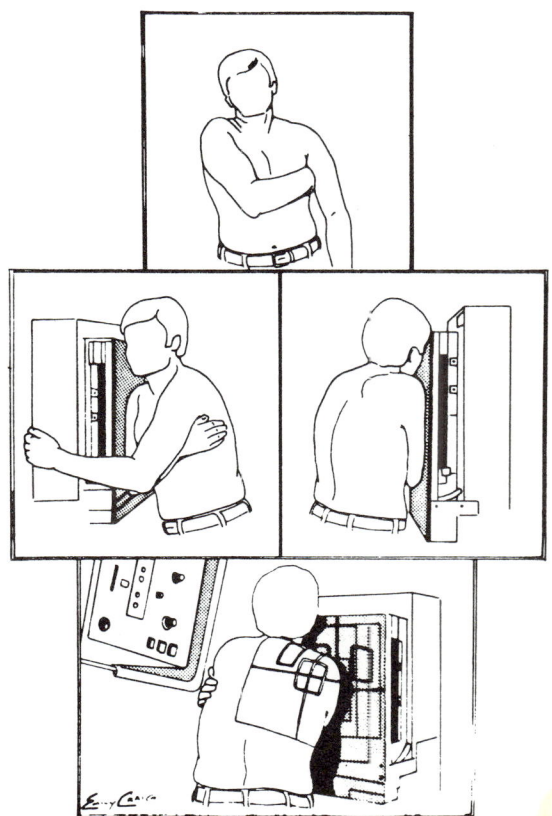

FIGURE 12–7. The Alexander view for evaluation of the acromioclavicular joint. (From Waldrop, J. I., Norwood, L. A., Alvarez, R. G.: Lateral roentgenographic projections of the acromioclavicular joint. Am. J. Sports Med. 9:338, 1981.)

reality it is a total dislocation, with the direction of the dislocation posterior rather than superior.

CLASSIFICATION AND DIFFERENTIAL DIAGNOSIS

The differential diagnosis for an acromioclavicular joint injury includes lateral third clavicle fractures as well as contusions without significant subluxation of the joint. The clinical picture of an athlete with a rotator cuff contusion is similar, having been the result of a direct fall on the shoulder. However, careful palpation of the injury usually is sufficient to differentiate these two diagnoses.

AC joint injuries are divided into six classification groups or types. A type I injury is a simple sprain of the AC joint. A type II injury is a disruption of the acromioclavicular ligaments without tear of the coracoclavicular ligaments and results in a subluxation of the AC joint. A type III injury represents complete disruption of the AC ligaments and the coracoclavicular ligaments with the clavicle displaced upward. A type IV injury is a complete dislocation with the distal clavicle displaced posteriorly; the coracoclavicular ligaments may be partially or completely torn. A type V injury is a severe type III with the distal end of the clavicle severely displaced up into the base of the neck with significant tearing of the deltoid and trapezius muscle attachments. A type VI injury is a dislocation of the AC joint with the distal end of the clavicle displaced down and under either the acromion or coracoid. The coracoclavicular ligaments may or may not be torn (Fig. 12–8). If one notes the interspace between the clavicle and the coracoid to be the same as the uninjured side but the AC joint is subluxed or dislocated, one should consider the possibility of a coracoid fracture, which

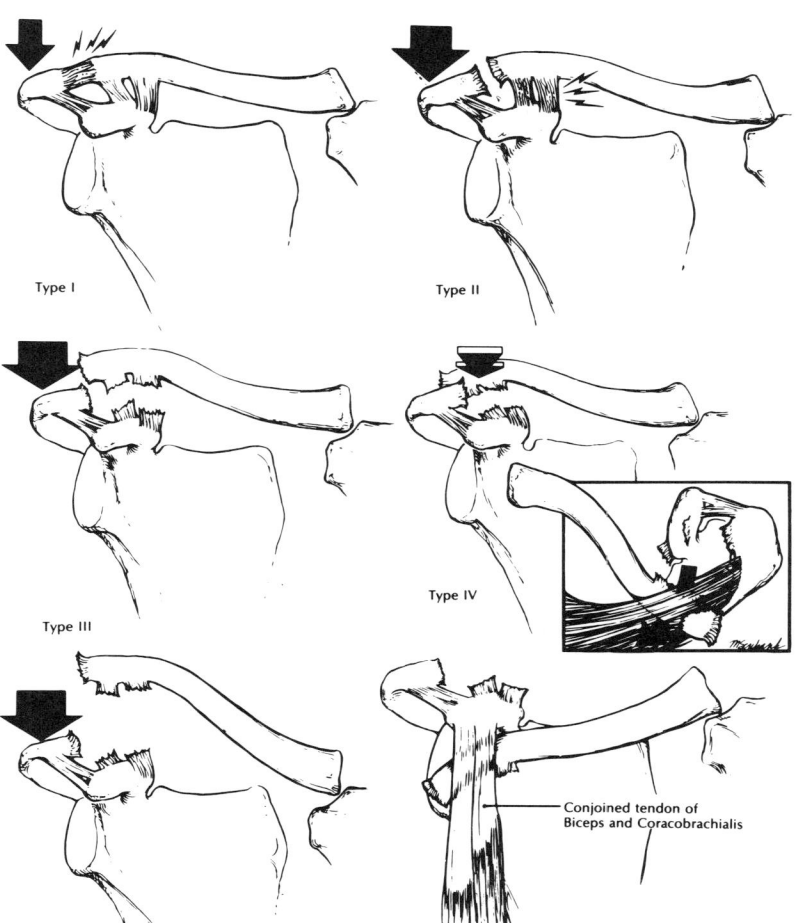

FIGURE 12–8. Classification of acromioclavicular joint injuries. (From Rockwood, C. A., Green, D. P. (eds.): Fractures in Adults. Vol. 1. 2nd ed. Philadelphia, J. B. Lippincott Co., p. 871, 1984.)

can be an epiphyseal injury in the young athlete.

TREATMENT

First, in children under 13 and perhaps as old as 16, a true acromioclavicular joint injury is extremely rare. As previously discussed, the actual pathology is an epiphyseal fracture with superior tearing of the periosteal tube and maintenance of the integrity between the coracoclavicular ligaments and the periosteum.[15,37] The reader is referred to the prior section to review these injuries.

In type I AC joint injuries, there is little controversy concerning treatment. The acute treatment consists of ice, rest in a sling, and medication for pain control. The sling can be discontinued as soon as the athlete can tolerate removal from a pain perspective, and gentle range-of-motion exercises are begun immediately. We usually see full painless motion at the end of 1 week. At this time, return to noncontact sports can occur. Return to contact sports generally takes another week or so, and we like to see minimal pain on direct palpation of the joint prior to returning the athlete to the field. Vigorous weight lifting or contact sports may cause some discomfort for up to 6 weeks, and this should not be cause for alarm. This is another situation where some additional padding, either foam or a donut, might be appreciated beneath the shoulder pads of a football player (Fig. 12–9).

Our treatment of choice for type II injuries is providing symptomatic treatment and emphasizing early functional rehabilitation. The athlete wears a sling for 2 weeks or so as needed and removes it several times each day to participate in some gentle active and passive range-of-motion exercises and also to begin using the extremity in activities of daily living as soon as tolerated. Ice and either a nonsteroidal antiinflammatory medication or mild narcotic compound are appreciated for their analgesic properties. Generally within 2 weeks, isometrics and light resistive exercises can be begun and are progressed as pain allows. Contact sports and heavy lifting are prohibited for 6 weeks to prevent a type II injury from being converted to a type III injury. Although the above statement is mirrored in many other discussions of this injury, we personally cannot recall seeing a type II injury converted to a type III injury and feel the surgeon must utilize his or her own judgment on a case-by-case basis when considering allowing an athlete to return to contact sports at an earlier date.

The Kenny Howard sling halter is a device that grasps the ipsilateral arm and attempts to elevate the humerus while at the same time depressing the clavicle to reduce the dislocation (Fig. 12–10). Generally, the joint is reduced with either oral or local analgesia and the splint is applied. The sling halter must be kept on at all times. A T-shirt should not be worn beneath this device. Showering or bathing is prohibited until the device has been removed. Radiographs are checked after the initial reduction at 24 and 48 hours and weekly.[1] After removal of the sling in 4

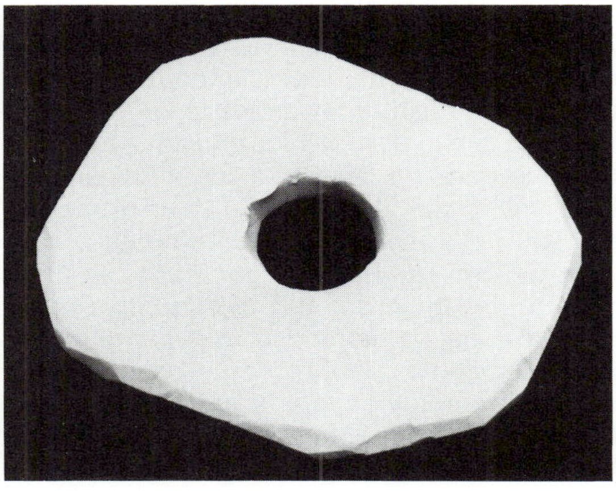

FIGURE 12–9. Padded "donut" to be worn under football padding, ensuring additional protection at the acromioclavicular joint.

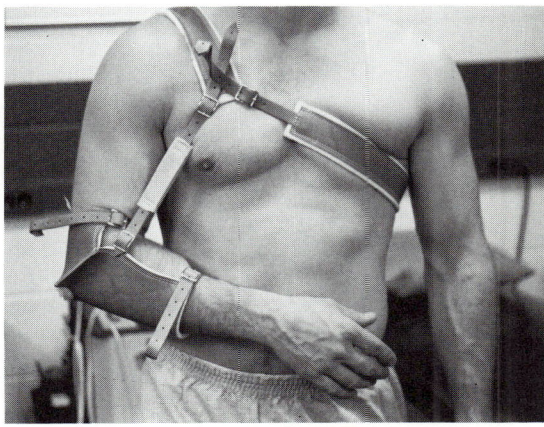

FIGURE 12–10. The Kenny Howard sling in place. Removal is at 4 weeks, and range of motion is begun.

weeks, gentle active and passive shoulder range of motion can be begun, followed with light resistive exercises as tolerated once near-normal range of motion has been attained in the shoulder.

Bergfeld et al.[4] and Cox[11] at the U.S. Naval Academy reported that 65 percent and 48 percent, respectively, of their population with type II injuries had later symptoms. Cox further showed that using the Kenny Howard splint halter decreased symptoms from 48 to 25 percent of the patients. However, the selection of patients to receive sling or immobilizer treatment was nonrandom. Major symptoms were present in 42 percent of Bergfeld's series and 13 percent of Cox's. However, only three patients required distal clavicular excision owing to symptoms, and this was in a patient population requiring quite vigorous physical use of their shoulder.

Walsh et al.[52] performed Cybex testing on eight patients treated symptomatically with type II sprains and found in 24 percent a strength deficit in high speed horizontal abduction. All the other strength differences were insignificant. No one has reported the incidence of complications with the Kenny Howard splint halter; however, skin sloughs, loss of reduction, and compliance problems are well recognized.

If the patient with an AC sprain were to develop severe, chronic symptoms, treatment would be activity modification when possible, a course of nonsteroidal antiinflammatories, or intraarticular steroid injection. If these fail, the surgical treatment would be the Mumford procedure: resection of the distal clavicle. The Mumford[33] procedure has a high degree of success at relieving symptoms, but there is concern that shoulder fatigue might occur postoperatively. Cook and Tibone[10] reported results in 23 athletes (6 professionals) that averaged 3.7 years follow-up after a Mumford procedure. The primary complaint was loss of maximum bench press strength, but Cybex testing demonstrated minimal weakness or fatigability in the operated limbs. Petersson[38] followed his patients with a Mumford procedure for an average of 9 years (3 to 30 years) with no deterioration of function.

In type II injuries, one can expect a significant percentage of symptomatic patients, but these patients rarely warrant surgical intervention. Should surgical intervention be required at a later date, an excellent outcome can be expected with distal clavicle excision.

Use of a harness might possibly reduce symptoms, but that question is unanswered at this time in a conclusive fashion. The success at the Naval Academy might be difficult to reproduce in a general, less disciplined population. For these reasons, we feel that symptomatic treatment with early functional rehabilitation is at this time the treatment of choice for type II acromioclavicular injuries in an athlete.

TYPE III ACROMIOCLAVICULAR INJURIES

Type III acromioclavicular injury still generates a considerable amount of controversy in sports medicine. Theoretically, there are three broad options for treating this injury: (1) symptomatic treatment with early functional rehabilitation; (2) strapping or use of a commercial harness, as mentioned in the type II section; and (3) operative treatment. In experience obtained from our own cases and those of other orthopedists, use of a sling halter or harness device tends to prolong disability and may lead to problems with skin irritation or outright ulceration, which causes poor patient satisfaction. In our eyes, that limits treatments to two broad options—early functional rehabilitation and surgery.

The nonoperative treatment for this injury is fairly similar to the method for type II injuries. Acutely, ice, use of a sling, and some type of analgesic either in the form of a nonsteroidal antiinflammatory medication or mild narcotic is utilized for pain control. As there is no concern about healing ligaments, rehabilitation can begin as soon as pain permits and progress as rapidly as the athlete can tolerate. The patient is encouraged to remove the sling and try activities of daily living within the first week and indeed should be encouraged to exercise the wrist and elbow out of the sling within the first day or two after the injury. Complete range of motion of the shoulder is generally attained within 2 to 3 weeks, and as soon as this occurs, we begin isometric exercises for the shoulder girdle and progress to resistive exercises with low weights and high repetitions. As with type II injuries, it is important to educate the patient and family that there will be a permanent bump on the shoulder. Depending on the individual athlete's tolerance for pain and enthusiasm for early rehabilitation, an athlete may return to noncontact sport within 4 weeks after this injury and to full contact in 6 to 8 weeks. A particularly motivated athlete may actually return to sport in a shorter amount of time.

The operative treatment of this injury has been much discussed, and there are many, many different procedures that have been described in the literature for an operative repair. There are several broad categories of operative procedures utilized. Fixation of the AC joint, usually with smooth or threaded pins, sometimes accompanied with a figure-eight wire, is well described. Most authors[43] recommend temporary fixation and removal of the device at about 6 weeks after surgery. It is also recommended that the wire be bent to prevent pin migration. Radiographic examination should occur at frequent intervals to monitor for pin migration. No real physical therapy can begin on the shoulder until the pins have been removed, owing to the risk of pin breakage. Some authors have even recommended keeping the patient in a sling until the fixation is removed. This operation has been described with and without ligament repair. A second broad category would concern fixation of the clavicle to the coracoid.[26] This can be a screw, as described by Bosworth,[6] or synthetic tape or wire. Some authors recommend temporary and others permanent fixation. This also can be accompanied by ligament repair. A third broad category concerns coracoclavicular (CC) ligament reconstruction, usually utilizing the coracoacromial (CA) ligament. Several techniques[25,47,53] are described, but all are a variation on the Weaver Dunn[53] technique. Others have also used the CA ligament to reconstruct the AC ligament.[36] Zaricznyj[56] uses a free tendon graft (from the fifth toe) to reconstruct both the AC and the CC ligaments. Others have used a free fascial graft as a biological type of fixation of the clavicle to the coracoid. Excision of the distal end of the clavicle[33] has been mentioned but has never gained wide acceptance for acute injuries. A fifth type of procedure involves a dynamic muscle transfer, generally involving the tip of the coracoid with the biceps and coracobrachialis[2] or biceps, coracobrachialis and pectoralis minor.[13] Most operative techniques described also recommended removing any intraarticular debris and repairing the deltoid trapezial fascia.

Before discussing the merits of operative versus nonoperative treatment, we again wish to emphasize that in student athletes under the age of 13 and perhaps until the age of 16, a true AC separation does not occur. This injury, as mentioned before, is simply a physeal fracture with maintenance of the integrity between the ligaments and periosteal tube. These injuries almost never would require an operative procedure.

However, in those student athletes who indeed have a true type III AC separation, there is some controversy. Operative procedures have a large number of complications associated with them, including pin breakage, pin migration, loss of reduction, clavicular fracture,[14] coracoid fracture,[29] neurovascular insult, infection, necessity of a second operation to remove hardware, scarring, loss of glenohumeral motion, and later arthritis of the AC joint. In prospective randomized studies in 1975 and 1986, Imatani et al.[21] and Larsen,[27] respectively, each reported superiority of nonoperative treatment. The patients were older than 18, however. Harris and Cox[20] surveyed orthopedic chairmen recently, noting that 60 percent favored nonoperative treatment for young athletes with type III separations. Larsen[27] suggests operation for people involved in heavy work, as does Rockwood.[42] However, Bjerneld et al.[5] followed conservatively treated patients for a mean of 5 years (minimum 2 years) and found good or excellent results in 30 of 33 patients, with 15 of these satisfactory results in patients involved in heavy labor. Jacobs and Wade[24] in an end-result study of operative versus nonoperative treatment with 5 to 33 years follow-up, averaging 10 years, concluded "results were quite similar . . . regardless of the type or degree of residual separation."

Others recommend operative care for the throwing athlete, but Eidman et al.[15] say, "We concur entirely [with Dr. Glick[19]] that athletes, particularly throwing athletes, probably do better with the joint unreduced than they do with an attempted reduction." A series of strength studies support nonoperative treatment. Walsh et al.[52] stated, "From the standpoint of objective strength, non-surgical treatment of Grade III injury is as effective as surgical treatment." MacDonald et al.[28] contend, "The non-surgical treatment of a third degree AC separation is superior in restoring normal shoulder function in the first year following injury." Galpin et al.[17] concluded that "non-operative treatment provided an equal, if not superior result, with an early return to activities, sports, and work."

The argument to operate on heavy laborers or throwing athletes does not seem to be supported by these objective strength studies. Perhaps the next step will be to add functional testing of injured athletes such as baseball velocity measurements or baseball, football, or javelin toss distance measurements. To be meaningful, careful standardization and patient selection would be required and quite difficult.

As more science and less conjecture are added to our knowledge base, it seems that the pendulum is swinging toward treatment of type III AC separations with nonoperative treatment. We must emphasize that where nonoperative treatment in the past has meant "skillful neglect," we feel that the concept of skillful neglect is inappropriate in our athletic population. We support contemporary early functional rehabilitation to facilitate an early return to sport for the athlete. It is of note that the closing comments from Urist's 1963 article[50] are still quite true today: "Entirely satisfactory treatment of complete dislocation of the acromioclavicular joint is rarely encountered with either conservative or open surgical methods. Further clinical investigations of this unsolved problem are clearly worthwhile."

TYPE IV, V, AND VI ACROMIOCLAVICULAR SEPARATIONS

Treatment of type IV, V, and VI acromioclavicular injuries is nearly always surgical, utilizing one of the techniques described in the type III section. A nonoperative approach to type IV injuries could be used if the clavicle could be disengaged from the trapezius in a closed fashion, thus converting it to a type III injury. Otherwise, this injury as well as types V and VI need surgical treatment owing to the gross anatomical displacement.[39,46]

A brief comment needs to be made on the acromioclavicular separations associated with a fracture at the base of the coracoid.[30] This is an unusual injury, and there is not extensive experience in dealing with it in the literature. However, if displacement is not significant, this injury can be treated with simple sling immobilization. As this represents a fracture, the time frame for return to sport is slightly different. We follow these injuries radiographically, and when early union is demonstrated, we consider returning the athlete to contact sports. This would be one instance where early aggressive mobilization of the shoulder girdle might be contraindicated and could lead to nonunion of this fracture. If the fracture is greatly displaced, some authors have recommended reducing the AC joint and cross pinning it. Obviously, this injury would be a contraindication to a Bosworth screw–type operative technique.

STERNOCLAVICULAR INJURIES

The sternoclavicular joint is only rarely injured, constituting 3 percent of all shoulder injuries in Cave's[9] series. The clinical picture may be of an injury caused by direct force or indirect force. A direct force injury might have occurred when an athlete was supine on the ground and another athlete landed on the medial aspect of his or her clavicle, producing a posterior dislocation. An indirect injury is a far more common mechanism: An athlete would be lying on his or her side, and a blow would compress his or her two shoulders toward the midline. A blow that forced the ipsilateral shoulder anteriorly would produce a posterior dislocation of the SC joint, whereas a force that pushed the shoulder girdle posteriorly would cause an anterior dislocation of the clavicle. This is an injury one might see in a football pileup. The patient presents with pain in the region of the sternoclavicular joint accentuated by any motion of the shoulder girdle.

PHYSICAL AND RADIOGRAPHIC EXAMINATION

Physical exam should start with palpation of the medial end of the clavicle, comparing the injured to the noninjured side. An anterior dislocation would obviously present with fullness of the injured clavicle, whereas a posterior dislocation would present with depression. This seemingly easy physical diagnosis can mislead the examiner, as noted by Rockwood.[41] A critical component of the physical examination, especially on a posterior injury, is assessment of concurrent injuries. The vascular tree must be evaluated, with confirmation of pulses and examination of the arm and neck for venous congestion. It

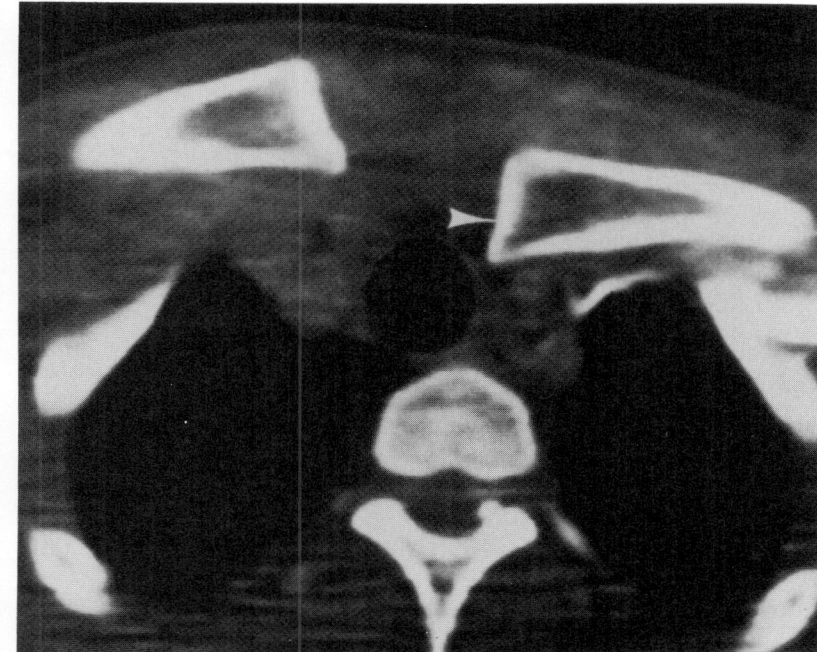

FIGURE 12–11. CT scan of a posterior dislocation of the sternoclavicular joint (*arrow*). Note its relationship to the trachea. (From Resnick, D.. Niwayama, N.: Diagnosis of Bone and Joint Disorders. Philadelphia, W. B. Saunders Co., p. 2845, 1988.)

is also critical to auscultate both lung fields to ensure pneumothorax has not occurred. The patient may complain of dysphagia, dyspnea, or tightness in the throat, and these should all be warning signs of injury to nearby structures.

Radiographically, an AP view of the clavicle or chest generally has too many interfering shadows to be useful. Several authors have recommended different views, but none of these views has come into common use. Rockwood[41] describes his "serendipity view," which involves placing the supine patient on a flat cassette and angling the X-ray beam 40 degrees from the vertical, with a cephalad tilt and the distance from subject to beam being 45 to 60 inches, depending on the size of the subject. On this view, a superiorly displaced clavicle indicates an anterior dislocation, and an inferiorly displaced clavicle indicates a posterior dislocation. Exact evaluation of the sternoclavicular joint quite often requires tomograms, and a CT scan also provides very accurate information (Fig. 12–11).

CLASSIFICATION AND DIFFERENTIAL DIAGNOSIS

Sternoclavicular injuries are normally divided into sprains, subluxations, or dislocations. The sprain represents a stable joint with no displacement of the clavicle in relation to the sternum, the subluxation represents a partial dislocation with damage to the ligamentous structures, and the dislocation represents complete disruption of the ligamentous structures and complete dissociation of the clavicle and sternum. A dislocation is further classified as being anterior or posterior.

The differential diagnosis of this injury includes a local contusion or injury to the insertion of the sternocleidomastoid muscle.

TREATMENT

In the patient population covered in this book, nearly all these injuries will in reality represent a fracture through the physis rather than a true joint dislocation. These injuries respond quite nicely to closed reduction. Operative intervention would only be indicated if a posterior dislocation were impinging on underlying neurovascular or respiratory structures.

In a mild sprain, treatment consists of applying ice, and consideration is given to providing medication for discomfort. Depending on the degree of the athlete's discomfort, a sling may or may not be used. Generally, the discomfort decreases within a week to allow fairly rapid return to sport, both contact and noncontact.

A subluxation may require application of a figure-eight clavicle strap with or without a sling, depending on the pain tolerance of the athlete. We recommend removing the sling within the first day to begin exercising the wrist and elbow, and if tolerated, some gentle isometrics about the shoulder girdle can be started. Again, depending on the discomfort that the athlete experiences, the figure eight is removed generally a week or 10 days after the injury, and the athlete is allowed to progress with upper extremity strengthening, with pain as a guideline.

An anterior dislocation generally represents an unstable situation. The surgeon can attain a closed reduction fairly easily, but it is an unstable reduction and the clavicle tends to redisplace anteriorly. The technique of reduction varies from surgeon to surgeon. Traction can be applied to the abducted arm with posterior pressure applied to the medial clavicle. Or several rolls of towels can be placed between the shoulder blades while an assistant applies pressure to the anterior point of each shoulder; and then again, the surgeon applies a posteriorly directed force to the medial clavicle. Should the clavicle redisplace, this is of no concern according to Rockwood,[41] as the remodeling capacity of the physis in this particular patient population is tremendous, and disability is generally minimal. For these injuries, a sling is utilized until the level of discomfort allows it to be discarded. This generally is 2 to 3 weeks. We would like to have the athlete begin to remove the sling and perform some gentle range-of-motion exercises of the shoulder girdle within 2 to 3 days after the injury, as pain allows. This may involve a trainer or the athlete himself or herself taking the shoulder through a passive range of motion, but early on, we do not proceed too vigorously. If the athlete can tolerate it, isometric exercises about the shoulder girdle are tried, and as pain decreases, he or she is progressed to light resistive exercises and finally to heavier weight work. The patient can generally return to noncontact sports in 2 weeks and to contact sports in 3 to 4 weeks, depending on how the athlete progresses in functional rehabilitation.

Treatment of the posterior dislocation starts with an extremely high index of suspension for concurrent injuries. As mentioned in the physical examination section, aggressive evaluation of the respiratory and vascular tree is mandatory. Should either pulmonary, bronchial, laryngeal, or vascular insult be identified, the appropriate subspecialist should be contacted prior to performing any reduction maneuvers to prevent any untoward consequences. Most posterior dislocations are reduced in a closed fashion. The reduction manuever is generally to extend and abduct the arm, the surgeon's fingers occasionally being utilized to manipulate the clavicle and reduce the medial end of it. At times, this can be difficult, and after sterilely prepping the patient, a towel clip placed around the medial clavicle can facilitate this maneuver (Fig. 12–12). Reduction occurs with a satisfying clunk. Rockwood[41]

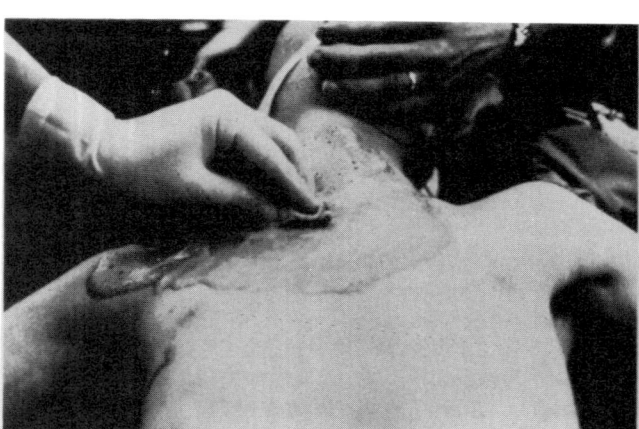
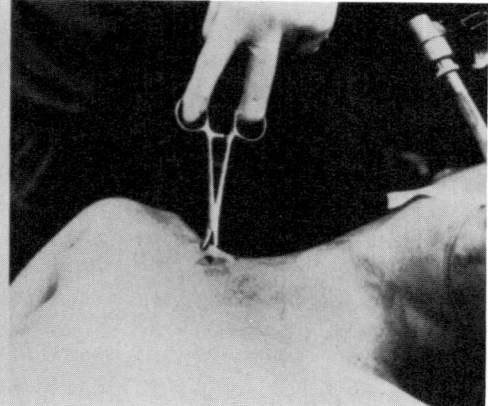

FIGURE 12–12. A towel clip being placed around the medial clavicle to facilitate reduction of a posterior dislocated sternoclavicular joint. (From Rockwood, C. A., Green, D. P. (eds.): Fractures in Adults. Vol. 1. 2nd ed. Philadelphia, J. B. Lippincott Co., p. 931, 1984.)

feels that a posteriorly dislocated clavicle that is unreducible in an athlete under the age of 20 with no concurrent symptoms can be managed with observation and with confidence that the physis can remodel the displaced bone so that no long-term sequelae occur.

Open reduction for these injuries in the athlete under age 20 is reserved only for that athlete who is having significant symptoms with a posterior dislocation. Should an open reduction be required, great caution is demanded if any method of fixation is used, as serious complications including death have been reported with the use of sternoclavicular transfixing pins.

Postreduction treatment consists of application of a figure-eight bandage that holds the shoulder back and up for a period of 3 to 4 weeks. Unlike the anterior dislocation, the reduction of the posterior injury generally provides a stable reduction, and the more prolonged downtime allows for ligamentous healing. After 3 to 4 weeks, the athlete is gradually weaned from the figure-eight splint and is begun on shoulder girdle range-of-motion and strengthening exercises. Prior to removal of the figure-eight strapping, the athlete can do some lightweight, high-resistive exercises for the wrist and elbow. The athlete should be able to return to noncontact sports within 4 to 5 weeks postinjury and to contact sports within 5 to 6 weeks postinjury.

In summary, injury to the sternoclavicular joint in the student athlete is unusual. We are fortunate in that this growth plate is one of the last to close, allowing closed reduction and early functional rehabilitation to provide these patients with an excellent outcome. The treating physician should be cautious if a posterior dislocation occurs, remembering that the mediastinal structures can be damaged with this injury.

OVERUSE INJURIES OF THE ACROMIOCLAVICULAR JOINT

One additional condition that needs to be mentioned in this chapter is the overuse injury of the AC joint. This does not represent an acute traumatic insult per se but is more likely the result of repeat microtrauma. It has been well described in the older population[8] but has begun to be seen in the younger athletes, especially those who are doing particularly heavy bench press work. This involves a diffuse discomfort or ache about the AC joint and can progress to frank distal clavicular osteolysis. Treatment consists of rest, particularly from weight lifting, and antiinflammatory medication. Very occasionally, an intraarticular steroid injection is required to gain control of the inflammatory process. With rest, this is generally a self-limiting condition, and most of our athletes have been able to return to their sport of choice with no long-term side effects. Specific alterations in resistance training that will help alleviate this condition are described in Chapter 2.

References

1. Allman, F. L.: Fractures and ligamentous injuries of the clavicle and its articulation. J. Bone Joint Surg. 49A: 777–784, 1967.
2. Bailey, R. W.: A dynamic repair for complete acromioclavicular joint dislocation. J. Bone Joint Surg. 47A: 858, 1965.
3. Bearn, J. G.: Direct observations on the function of the capsule of the sternoclavicular joint in clavicular support. J. Anat. 101(1): 159–170, 1967.
4. Bergfeld, J. A., Andrish, J. T., Clancy, W. G.: Evaluation of the acromioclavicular joint following first and second degree sprains. Am. J. Sports Med. 6: 153–158, 1978.
5. Bjerneld, H., Lennart, H., Thorling, J.: Acromioclavicular separations treated conservatively. Acta Orthop. Scand. 54: 743–745, 1983.
6. Bosworth, B. M.: Complete acromioclavicular dislocation. New Engl. J. Med. 241: 221–225, 1949.
7. Bowen, A.: Plastic bowing of the clavicle in children. J. Bone Joint Surg. 65A: 403–405, 1983.
8. Cahill, B. R.: Osteolysis of the distal part of the clavicle in male athletes. J. Bone Joint Surg. 64A: 1053–1058, 1982.
9. Cave, E. F. (ed.): Fractures and Other Injuries. Chicago, Year Book Medical Publishers, Inc., 1958.
10. Cook, F. F., Tibone, J. E.: The Mumford procedure in athletes. Am. J. Sports Med. 16: 97–100, 1988.
11. Cox, J. S.: The fate of the acromioclavicular joint in athletic injuries. Am. J. Sports Med. 9:50–53, 1981.
12. Dameron, T. B., Rockwood, C. A.: Fractures of the shaft of the clavicle. In: Rockwood, C. A., Wilkins, K. E., King, R. E. (eds.): Fractures in Children. Vol. 3. Philadelphia, J. B. Lippincott Co., pp. 608–623, 1984.
13. Dewar, F. P., Barrington, T. W.: The treatment of chronic acromioclavicular dislocation. J. Bone Joint Surg. 47B: 32–35, 1965.
14. Dust, W. N., Lencznerr, E. M.: Stress fracture of the clavicle leading to non-union secondary to coracoclavicular reconstruction with Dacron. Am. J. Sports Med. 17:128–129, 1989.
15. Eidman, D. K., Siff, S. J., Tullos, H. S.: Acromioclavicular lesions in children. Am. J. Sports Med. 9: 50–54, 1981.
16. Fukuda, K., Craig, E., An, K., Cofield, R. H., Chao, E. Y.: Biomechanical study of the ligamentous system of the acromioclavicular joint. J. Bone Joint Surg. 68A: 434–439, 1986.

17. Galpin, R. D., Hawkins, R. J., Grainger, R. W.: A comparative analysis of operative versus nonoperative treatment of grade III acromioclavicular separations. Clin. Orthop. 193:150–155, 1985.
18. Gardner, E.: The embryology of the clavicle. Clin. Orthop. 58:9–16, 1968.
19. Glick, J., Milburn, L., Haggerty, J., et al.: Follow-up study of 35 unreduced acromioclavicular dislocations. Am. J. Sports Med. 5:264–270, 1977.
20. Harris, T. J., Cox, J. S.: Acromioclavicular injuries and surgical treatment. In: Techniques in Orthopaedics. Vol. 4, Shoulder Surgery in the Athlete, pp. 119–124, 1985.
21. Imatani, R. J., Hanlon, J. J., Cady, G. W.: Acute, complete acromioclavicular separation. J. Bone Joint Surg. 57A: 328–332, 1975.
22. Inman, V. T., Saunders, J. B., Abbott, L. C.: Observations on the function of the shoulder joint. J. Bone Joint Surg. 26: 1–30, 1944.
23. Jablon, M., Sutlar, A., Post, M.: Irreducible fracture of the middle third of the clavicle. J. Bone Joint Surg. 61A: 296–298, 1979.
24. Jacobs, B., Wade, P. A.: Acromioclavicular-joint injury. J. Bone Joint Surg. 48A: 475–486, 1966.
25. Kawabe, N., Wantanabe, R., Sato, M.: Treatment of complete acromioclavicular separation by coracoacromial ligament transfer. Clin. Orthop. 185: 222–227, 1984.
26. Kennedy, J. C., Cameron, H.: Complete dislocation of the acromioclavicular joint. J. Bone Joint Surg. 36B: 202–208, 1954.
27. Larsen, E., Bjerg-Nielson, A., Christensen, P.: Conservative or surgical treatment of acromioclavicular dislocation. J. Bone Joint Surg. 68A: 552–555, 1986.
28. MacDonald P. B., Alexander, M. J., Frejuk, J., Johnson, G. E.: Comprehensive functional analysis of shoulders following complete acromioclavicular separation. Am. J. Sports Med. 16: 475–480, 1988.
29. Moneim, M. S., Balduini, F. C.: Coracoid fracture as a complication of surgical treatment by coracoclavicular tape fixation. Clin. Orthop. 168: 133–135, 1982.
30. Montgomery, S. P., Loyd, R. D.: Aulsion fracture of the coracoid epiphysis with acromioclavicular separation. J. Bone Joint Surg. 59A: 963–965, 1977.
31. Moseley, H. F.: The clavicle: its anatomy and function. Clin. Orthop. 68: 17–27, 1968.
32. Muller, M. E., Allgower, M., Schneider, R., Willenegger, H.: Manual of Internal Fixation. 2nd ed. New York, Springer-Verlag, New York, Inc., p. 166, 1979.
33. Mumford, E. B.: Acromioclavicular dislocation. J. Bone Joint Surg. 23: 799–802, 1941.
34. Neer, C. S.: Nonunion of the clavicle. JAMA 172: 1006–1010, 1960.
35. Neer, C. S.: Fractures of the distal third of the clavicle. Clin. Orthop. 58:43–50, 1968.
36. Neviasser, J. S.: Acromioclavicular dislocation treated by transference of the coracoacromial ligament. Clin. Orthop. 58: 57–68, 1968.
37. Ogden, J. A.: Distal clavicular physeal injury. CORR 188: 68–73, 1984.
38. Petersson, C. J.: Resection of the lateral end of the clavicle. Acta Orthop. Scand. 54: 904–907, 1983.
39. Post, M.: Current concepts in the diagnosis and management of acromioclavicular dislocations. Clin. Orthop. 200: 234–247, 1985.
40. Redmond, A. D.: Letter. Injury 13: 352, 1981.
41. Rockwood, C. A.: Fractures and dislocations of the ends of the clavicle, scapula and glenohumeral joint. In: Rockwood, C. A., Wilkins, K. E., King, R. E. Fractures in Children. Vol. 3. Philadelphia, J. B. Lippincott Co., pp. 624–682, 1984.
42. Rockwood, C. A.: Subluxations and dislocations about the shoulder joint. In: Rockwood, C. A., Green, D. P. (eds.): Fractures in Adults. Vol. 1. 2nd ed. Philadelphia, J. B. Lippincott Co., p 722, 1984.
43. Roper, B. A.: The surgical treatment of acromioclavicular dislocations. J. Bone Joint Surg. 64B: 597–599, 1982.
44. Rowe, C. R.: Fractures of the clavicle. In: Cave, E. F. (ed.): Fractures and Other Injuries. Chicago, Year Book Medical Publishers, Inc., pp 259–263, 1958.
45. Rowe, C. R.: An atlas of anatomy and treatment of midclavicular fractures. Clin. Orthop. 58: 29–42, 1968.
46. Sage, J.: Recurrent inferior dislocation of the clavicle at the acromioclavicular joint. Am. J. Sports Med. 10: 145–146, 1982.
47. Shoji, H., Roth, C., Chyinard, R.: Bone block transfer of coracoacromial ligament in acromioclavicular injury. Clin. Orthop. 208: 272–277, 1986.
48. Todd, T. W., DiErrico, J.: The clavicular epiphysis. Am. J. Anat. 41: 25–50, 1928.
49. Urist, M. R.: Complete dislocation of the acromioclavicular joint: the nature of the traumatic lesion and effective methods of treatment with an analysis of 41 cases. J. Bone Joint Surg. 28:813–837, 1946.
50. Urist, M. R.: Follow-up notes on articles previously published in the journal. J. Bone Joint Surg. 45A: 1750–1753, 1963.
51. Waldrop, J. I., Norwood, L. A., Alvarez, R. G.: Lateral roentgenographic projections of the acromioclavicular joint. Am. J. Sports Med. 9: 337–341, 1981.
52. Walsh, W. M., Peterson, D. A., Shelton, G., Neumann, R. D.: Shoulder strength following acromioclavicular injury. Am. J. Sports Med. 13:153–158, 1985.
53. Weaver, J. K., Dunn, H. K.: Treatment of acromioclavicular injuries, especially complete acromioclavicular separation. J. Bone Joint Surg. 54A: 1187–1194, 1972.
54. Wilson, J. C.: Fractures and dislocations in children. Pediatr. Clin. North Am. 14:659–662, 1967.
55. Yates, D. W.: Complications of fractures of the clavicle. Injury 7: 189–193, 1975.
56. Zaricznyj, B.: Reconstruction for chronic scapuloclavicular instability. Am. J. Sports Med. 11:17–25, 1983.
57. Zenni, E. J., Krieg, J. K., Rosen, M. J.: Open reduction and internal fixation of clavicular fractures. J. Bone Joint Surg. 63A: 147–151, 1981.

13
ELBOW DISLOCATIONS

FREDDIE H. FU
STEVE SALYERS

The elbow is second only to the shoulder as the most commonly dislocated major joint. It is the most commonly dislocated major joint in children under 10 years of age. Approximately one half of all elbow dislocations occur in patients under the age of 20.[1,2,3] In most series, sports injuries account for the largest group of etiologies. Typically, this injury involves the nondominant extremity.[1,2,3,5] A fall on the outstretched hand is far and away the most common history given. Any sport with the potential of a fall, especially a violent fall, places the athlete at risk of an elbow dislocation. Cycling, gymnastics, football, and wrestling have significant injury potential.

ANATOMY

The elbow joint is made up of three bones and three distinct articulations. The bones are the humerus, radius, and ulna, and the articulations are the trochlear-olecranon (or ulnohumeral), radiocapitellar (or radiohumeral), and proximal radioulnar. The bony architecture is demonstrated in the accompanying figures (Fig. 13–1). The intimate relationship of the nerves, arteries, and muscles about the elbow is best shown in cross section (Fig. 13–2).

The bony anatomy contributes far more to the stability of this joint than it does in the shoulder.[6] Morrey[7] refers to the elbow as "one of the most congruent and constrained joints in the body." However, most of the focus on the elbow joint stability has turned toward the collateral ligaments. The anatomy of the medial side has been well described for some time, but only recently has the importance of the medial structures in elbow stability surfaced.[6,7,8,9] There are three components to the medial ligaments: an anterior oblique (or bundle), a posterior oblique (or bundle) and a transverse oblique (or ligament). This pattern is very consistent (Fig. 13–3).

The humeral attachments of the anterior and posterior obliques are eccentrically located in relation to the axis of rotation of the elbow joint, producing variable laxity as the joint flexes and extends. Schwab[8] believes the anterior oblique has two bands, one that is tight in flexion and the other tight in extension, making the ligament functionally taut through all ranges of motion. Morrey and An[10] have demonstrated a change in the distance from origin to insertion of both the anterior and posterior obliques through a range of motion of the elbow, supporting the concept of medial laxity at certain ranges of motion. These authors agree, however, that the anterior oblique is the prime ligamentous stabilizer of the joint.

The anatomy on the lateral side of the joint has some variability from individual to individual. Most investigators agree on the anatomy of the annular ligament and a ligament from the humerus to the annular ligament (called lateral collateral by Tullos et al.[9] and radial collateral by Morrey[7]. Tullos et al.[9] and Wilkins[4] agree that there is no "true collateral" ligament stabilizing the humeroulnar articulation laterally, but Morrey[17]

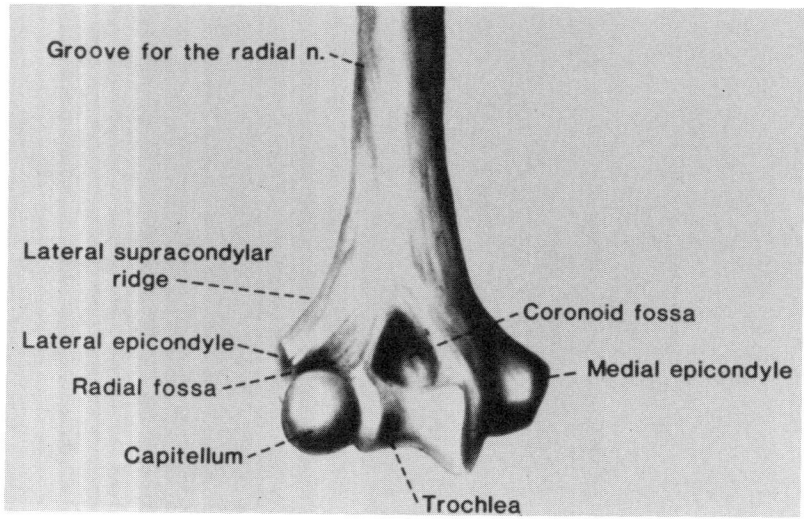
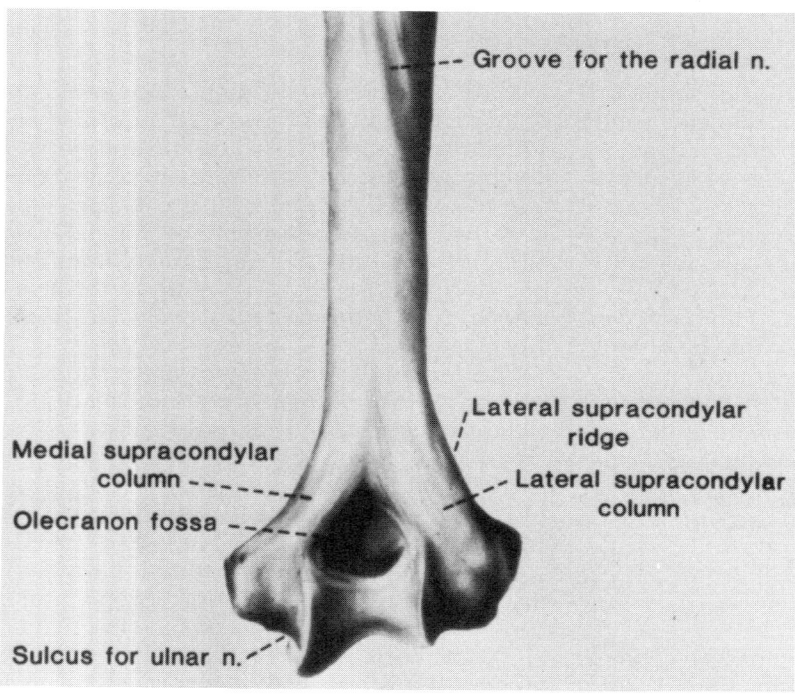
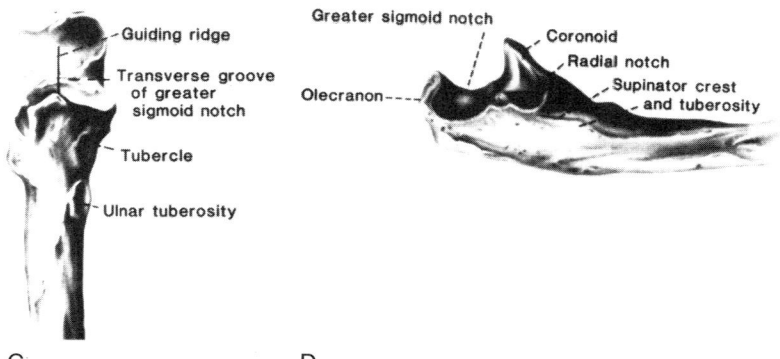

FIGURE 13–1. Bony architecture of the elbow. (A) The anterior humerus. (B) The posterior humerus. (C) The anterior ulna. (D) The lateral ulna. (From Morrey, B. F.: The Elbow and Its Disorders. Philadelphia, W. B. Saunders Co., pp. 11–13, 1985.)

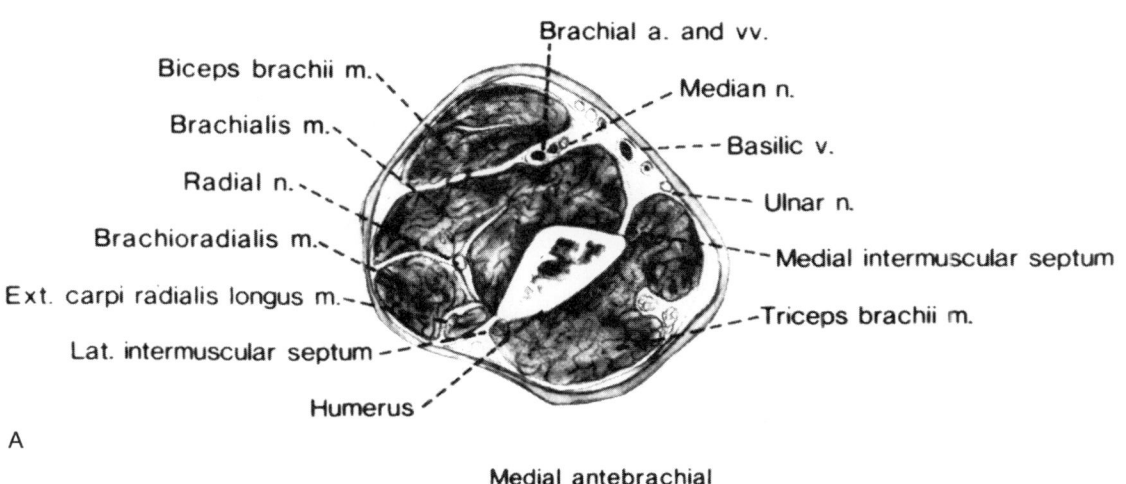
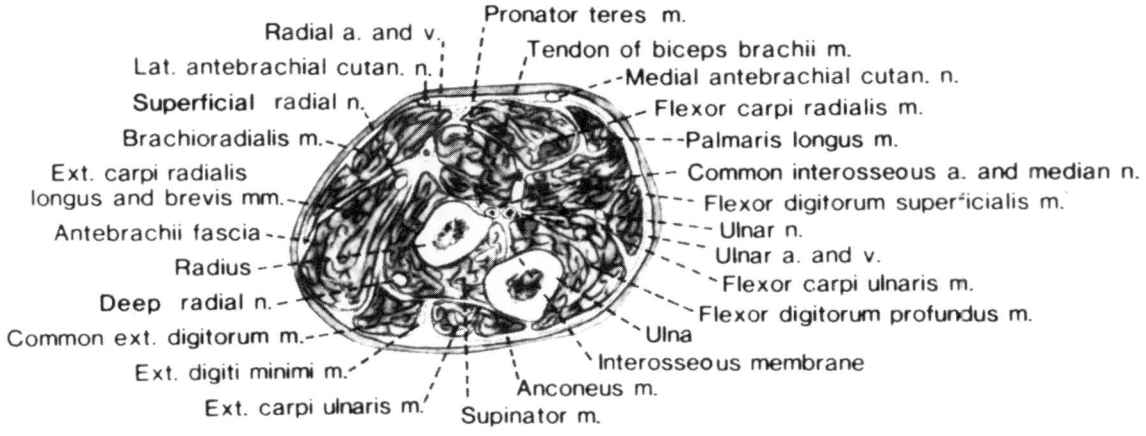

FIGURE 13–2. Cross-sectional anatomy of the muscles, nerves, and arteries in the region above (*A*), across (*B*), and distal (*C*) to the elbow joint. (From Morrey, B. F.: The Elbow and Its Disorders. Philadelphia, W. B. Saunders Co., p. 25, 1985.)

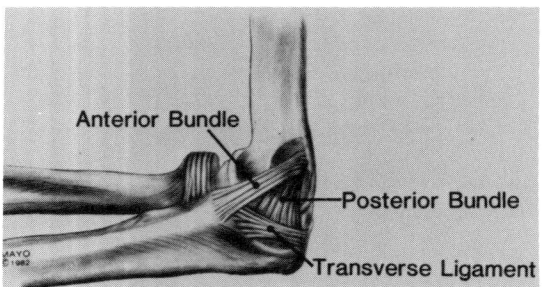

FIGURE 13-3. Ligamentous anatomy of the medial side of the elbow. (From Morrey, B. F.: The Elbow and Its Disorders. Philadelphia, W. B. Saunders Co., p. 19, 1985.)

has demonstrated an accessory collateral ligament running from the annular ligament to the ulna and a slip he calls the lateral ulnar collateral, running from the humerus to the christa supinatoris (Fig. 13-4). Several authors[11,12,13] felt the lateral ligament and capsule were the key structure preventing recurrent dislocation. However, the more recent biomechanical studies have shown this not to be true.

Morrey[17] has performed two experiments that more accurately reflect the anatomical contributions to elbow stability. The composite stability (varus/valgus, internal/external rotation, and anterior-posterior [AP] displacement) of the elbow was assessed with 0, 25, 50, 75, and 100 percent of the olecranon removed. This demonstrated a nearly linear decrease in stability, indicating a greater contribution by the olecranon than was initially thought. Also, a ligament cutting experiment[6] was performed that showed that the medial collateral ligament (specifi-

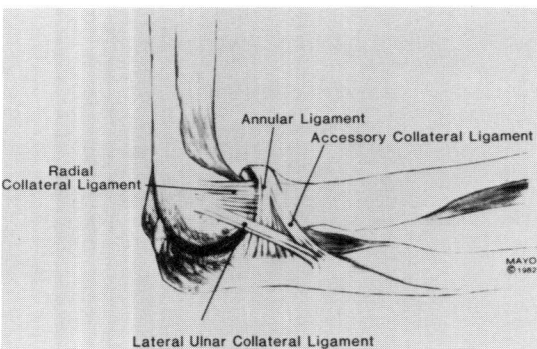

FIGURE 13-4. Ligamentous anatomy of the lateral side of the elbow. (From Morrey, B. F.: The Elbow and Its Disorders. Philadelphia, W. B. Saunders Co., p. 21, 1985.)

cally the anterior bundle) was the primary restraint to valgus laxity. The lateral ligament complex had a lesser contribution to resisting varus laxity than the bony articulation and the anterior capsule.

CLASSIFICATION

Dislocations are classified according to the displacement of the radius and ulna. This includes posterior (straight, posterolateral, or posteromedial), anterior, medial, and lateral. Divergent dislocations (where the proximal radioulnar joint is disrupted) are divided into anterior, posterior, or mediolateral. Posterior or posterolateral dislocations account for 80 to 90 percent of all dislocations of the elbow in the series reported.[1,2,3,5]

Isolated radial head dislocations are extremely rare, and the reader is referred to standard orthopedic texts[7] for further information. Most of what follows is directed toward posterior injuries, since the vast majority of athletic injuries are of this type.

MECHANISM OF INJURY

A fall on an outstretched hand is the typical history reported for posterior dislocations. There are two mechanisms described: (1) The olecranon levers on the olecranon fossa as the elbow hyperextends until the coronoid process slips posteriorly; a varus or valgus stress can create a posteromedial or posterolateral dislocation; or (2) the arm is slightly flexed with the lateral sloping surface of the trochlea acting as a cam, converting the vertical force to lateral rotation and valgus stress, which ruptures the lateral collateral, allowing the ulna to slip laterally and come to lie posteriorly or posterolaterally.

Most cases of anterior elbow dislocations reported were caused by a direct blow to the olecranon posteriorly with the elbow flexed.

Pure medial or lateral dislocations have not been reported in skeletally immature patients in the recent literature.

PATHOLOGY AND ASSOCIATED INJURIES

The soft tissue insult during posterior elbow dislocations is significant. The anterior capsule is torn, and the posterior capsule may be stripped off proximally along the distal humerus by the posteriorly driven radial head and olecranon.

The medial and lateral collateral ligaments are totally ruptured.[14] Rather than a direct tear of the ligaments, the medial epicondyle apophysis may be avulsed. The avulsed fragment can lie in an essentially nondisplaced position or can even come to lie within the joint. The incidence of medial epicondyle fractures varies from 0[5] to 30 percent[1] in the four major elbow dislocation series.[1,2,3,5] The lateral epicondyle fractures less frequently.

At the level of the joint, the brachialis is a large, fleshy muscle with a minimum of tendon compromising its thickness. Extensive rupture of this muscle is often seen.[14,15] A fracture of the coronoid may occur. This may be an avulsion injury or a shear injury as the coronoid impacts against the distal humerus. This is seen in 10 percent of elbow dislocations.[17]

Damage to the wrist flexor or extensor origins also occurs to a varying degree. With a medial epicondyle fracture, the flexor origin remains attached to the fragment and acts as a displacing force.

The radial head or neck can be fractured by the force of this injury. This occurs in 5 to 10 percent of elbow dislocations.[17]

The brachial artery can be torn. In certain situations, a tear in the brachial artery can be treated without surgery owing to the excellent collateral flow about the elbow. However, as Louis et al.[16] have shown, the collaterals about the elbow are consistently damaged with a dislocation, and brachial artery repair is strongly advocated. In Protzman's series of patients,[5] there were no brachial artery injuries, and this is consistent with what we have seen in athletic injuries.

The ulnar nerve can incur a traction injury during posterior dislocations. In children, entrapment of the median nerve within the joint has been reported. There are three types of entrapment: (1) with the median nerve displacing posteriorly to the humerus and passing through the joint, (2) bony entrapment between fracture surfaces, and (3) kinking of the nerve in the elbow joint.[18] The incidence of these injuries is quite low, as seen in the West Point series,[5] where there were no residual neurological deficits.

EVALUATION

When a posterior elbow dislocation is seen early, the diagnosis is easy. The extremity is held in flexion, with the forearm appearing shortened. The olecranon is prominent posteriorly. The athlete is generally in severe pain. Palpation reveals the antecubital fossa to be full and the olecranon and radial head prominent posteriorly. Above the olecranon, a palpable indentation in the triceps is noted. Slight flexion and extension of the elbow while palpating for crepitance can rule out a fracture with moderate certainty and can be performed if you plan a reduction attempt on the field prior to radiographic evaluation.

After the onset of swelling, difficulty occurs in differentiating this injury from a supracondylar fracture, lateral condylar fracture, and in the young child, transcondylar fracture. Excessive manipulation to aid the diagnosis is uncalled for as radiographic confirmation is easy and reliable.

Before moving to the radiographic evaluation, it is imperative to do a careful neurovascular examination. This takes only a few moments and can be performed without undue distress even in a young child.

Standard AP and lateral radiographs should be obtained. Occasionally, special views[19] or arthrography are required. Special views or arthrography are indicated if your clinical suspicions are not confirmed with routine radiographs. When an arterial injury is suspected, an arteriogram or digital subtraction studies should be performed without hesitation.

Interpreting films of a posterior, posterolateral, or divergent dislocation is not hard (Fig. 13–5). The rare medial or lateral dislocation can be overlooked on casual reading of the film, but the physical findings are not subtle. The hazards of radiographic evaluation lie in identifying the associated fractures. The radial head and neck, coronoid, and medial and lateral epicondyles must be carefully examined. After age 5 or 6, if the medial epicondylar ossific nucleus is not seen, it must be looked for in the joint, and comparison films are mandatory. All views are repeated and reevaluated after reduction.

When a child presents with a history of a fall and a swollen elbow, especially if there is no associated fracture, an elbow dislocation with spontaneous reduction should be considered and treated appropriately.

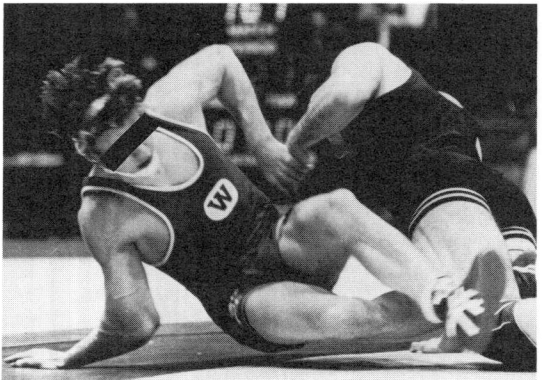

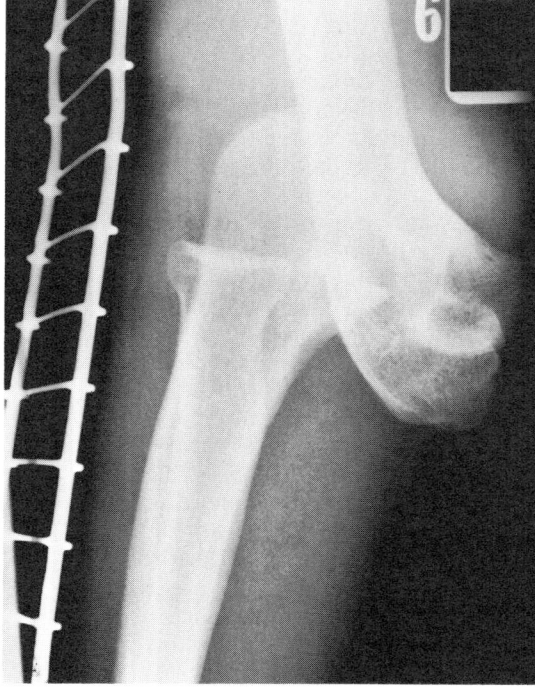

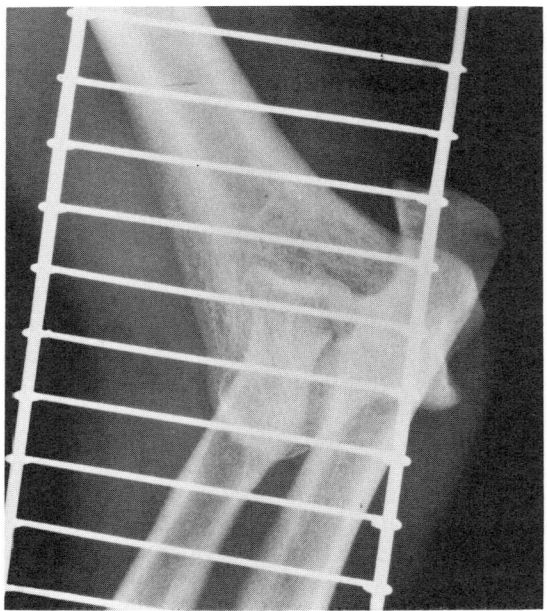

FIGURE 13–5. (A) A newspaper photographer caught this wrestler in the process of sustaining a posterior dislocation of the elbow. (B,C) A severely displaced posterior dislocation in another wrestler.

NONOPERATIVE TREATMENT

"All methods of reduction are directed toward sufficiently overcoming the muscle forces so that the coronoid process and radial head can slip from posterior to anterior past the distal end of the humerus."[4] In order to achieve this, adequate anesthesia is needed. This can be a general anesthetic, regional block, or sedation. If the diagnosis is reliably made at the time of the injury, a single attempt at gentle reduction can be tried on the playing field before muscle spasms become pronounced. This can lead to disaster if the injury is a supracondylar fracture rather than an elbow dislocation, so caution is advised.

Once adequate anesthesia is obtained, a closed reduction by gentle forces can nearly always be obtained. A number of methods have been described but fall into three main groups: (1) "pushers," (2) "pullers," and (3) combined pushing and pulling.

The pullers apply traction in two directions, one along the axis of the forearm and one along the axis of the humerus with the elbow flexed 75 degrees or so (Fig. 13–6). The methods differ in how the countertraction is applied. The pushers attempt to push the olecranon past the humerus with the elbow flexed (Fig. 13–7). Morrey[17] uses a combination of pushing and pulling. All authors correct medial or lateral displacements early in their reduction maneuver. The method of choice is the one with which the treating physician is most familiar.

Hyperextension is to be condemned as a method to "unlock" the coronoid; however, Morrey[17] feels safe extending the elbow to neutral to achieve this end in difficult reductions. Wilkins[4] believes the forearm should

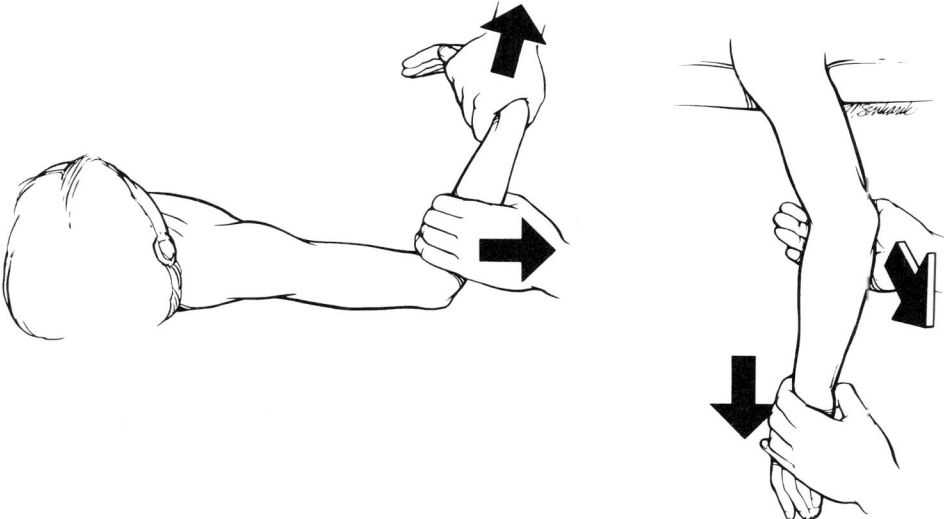

FIGURE 13–6. Puller technique for elbow reduction (see text). (From Rockwood, C. A., Green, D. P. [eds.]: Fractures in Adults. Vol. III, 2nd ed. Philadelphia, J. B. Lippincott Co. p. 540, 1984.)

stay supinated throughout the maneuver, but other authors do not specify forearm position.

Whichever method is used, it is absolutely critical to take the elbow through a full range of motion following reduction and test varus and valgus stability. The degree of stability helps determine how aggressive the rehabilitation can be. There also should be no grinding, mechanical block, or spongy feel with motion. If these occur, careful evaluation

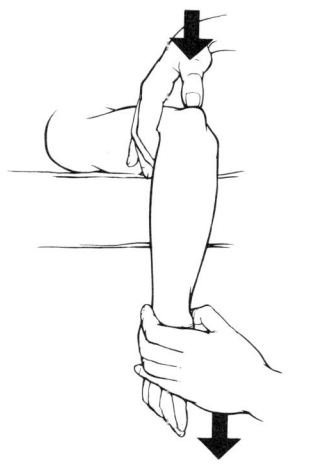

FIGURE 13–7. Pusher technique for elbow reduction (see text). (From Rockwood, C. A., Green, D. P. [eds.]: Fractures in Adults. Vol. III, 2nd ed. Philadelphia, J. B. Lippincott Co., p. 541, 1984.)

must rule out intraarticular entrapment of the median nerve or medial epicondyle. Aspiration of the hematoma may increase motion and decrease pain early in the rehabilitation process.

Careful and compulsive repeat radiographic and neurovascular evaluations must be undertaken prior to applying a splint. A long arm plaster splint with adequate padding is applied with the elbow flexed 90 degrees. If there is pronounced swelling, a questionable vascular exam, concern about a compartment syndrome, or an unreliable patient, hospitalization should be considered. Otherwise, instructing the parent how to observe the circulatory status is sufficient. Ice and elevation are useful, as always.

Protzman's[5] series at West Point contains a patient population most similar to that seen in a sports medicine practice. Although the study has several limitations, his conclusion that decreasing the period of immobilization leads to decreased loss of motion and a decreased period of disability seems to hold up in clinical practice and other studies.[23] With a simple posterior or posterolateral dislocation without associated fractures, hand, wrist, and shoulder motion can begin the day of injury. Flexion from within the splint can begin in 3 or 4 days, and the splint can be discarded in 10 days or so. The elbow should be supported in a sling for 2 to 3 weeks after this. Forced "passive" motion or manipu-

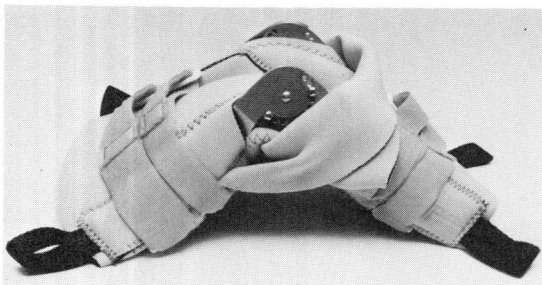

FIGURE 13–8. Single axis orthosis used for patients with elbow instability.

lation has no place in elbow dislocation treatment owing to the risk of loss of motion and increased heterotopic ossification. The risk for recurrent dislocation is very low with this protocol. Gentle strengthening exercises can begin 3 to 5 weeks after the injury and progress as pain allows.

If there is an associated fracture or gross instability, treatment must be altered. A single axis elbow orthosis may allow early motion in those elbows felt to be unstable to varus or valgus stress (Fig. 13–8).

OPERATIVE TREATMENT

The indications for open treatment of elbow dislocations are (1) open injury, (2) vascular injury, (3) fracture management, (4) median nerve entrapment, and (5) inability to obtain reduction (a situation that is quite rare) (Fig. 13–9).

Josefsson et al.[14] in a prospective randomized study of surgical versus nonsurgical managment in 30 consecutive patients, showed no advantage of operative treatment. This is in direct contrast to Norwood et al.[20] and Durig et al.[21] DeLee[25] concluded that "the incidence of recurrent dislocation is not sufficiently high nor the results of treatment by closed reduction sufficiently poor to warrant primary operative repair in pure elbow dislocations."

Management of open injury and vascular damage is beyond the scope of this text, but fracture management should be addressed. If the medial epicondyle is displaced greater than 1 cm, then it should be pinned in place utilizing a medial incision. Although selection of the distance of 1 cm is somewhat arbi-

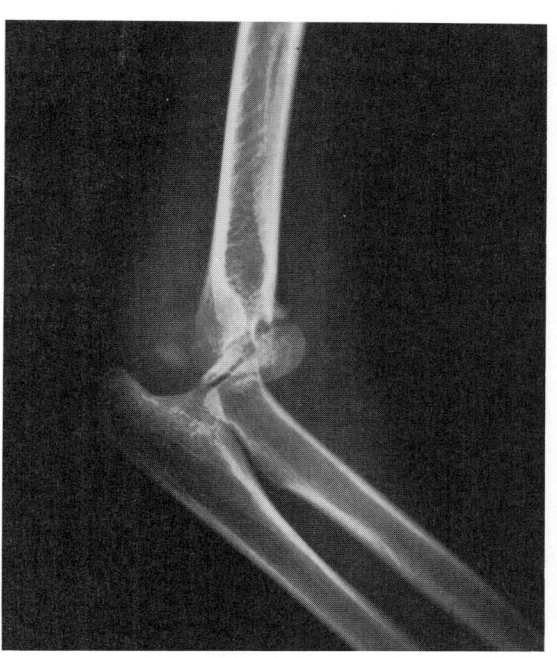
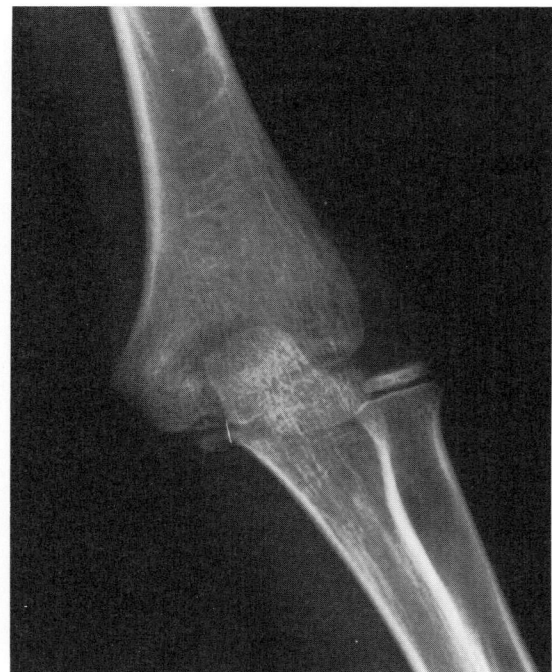

FIGURE 13–9. Incarceration of the medial epidondyle in the joint prevented closed reduction in this case.

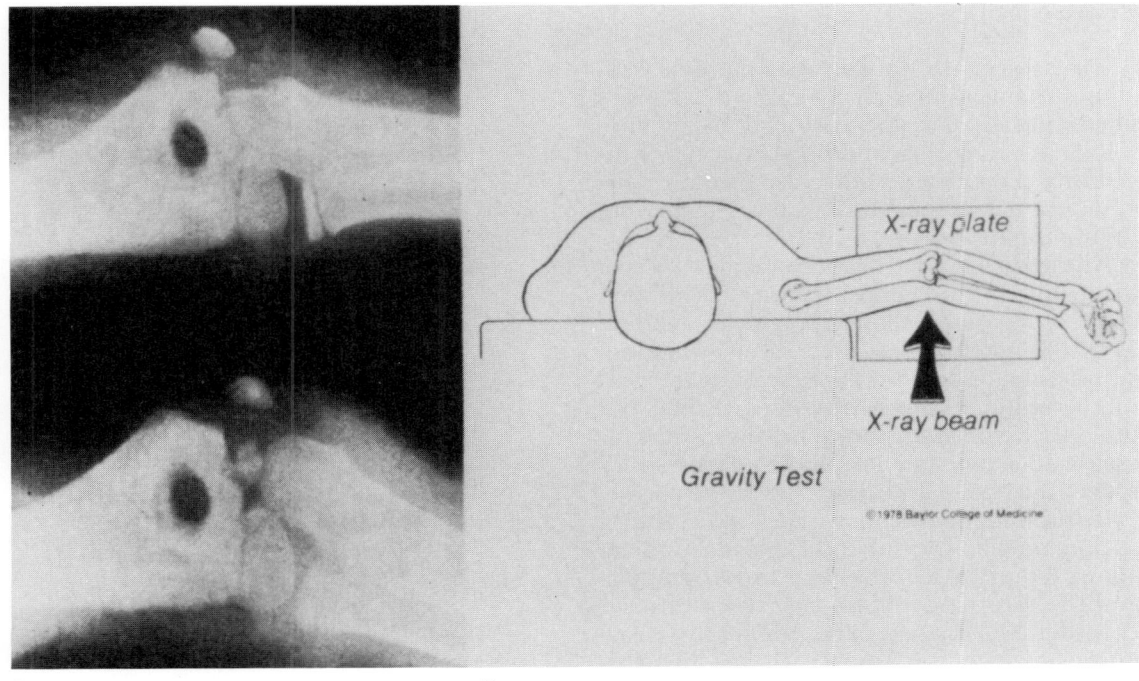

FIGURE 13–10. Gravity stress test for medial collateral ligament instability. (A) X-ray view. (B) Diagram. The injured arm is extended over the X-ray table, and the weight of the forearm stresses the medial collateral ligament. (From Schwab, G. H., Bennett, J. B., Woods, G. W., Tullos, H. S.: Biomechanics of elbow instability: the role of the medial collateral ligament. Clin. Orthop. 146: 46, 1980.)

trary, it is easy to see how malunion of this fracture could lead to functional medial ligamentous laxity, which would be potentially symptomatic in a throwing athlete. We therefore recommend being aggressive in obtaining an adequate reduction. Occasionally with an entrapped medial epicondyle fragment, closed manipulation with valgus stress and wrist extension can free the fragment and sometimes obviate the need to open the elbow. Minimally displaced medial epicondyle injuries can usually be managed closed.

In a throwing athlete with abnormal valgus laxity and a medial epicondyle fracture, strong consideration should be given to operative stabilization to prevent later valgus instability (Fig. 13–10). Assessment of the ulnar nerve clinically determines the need of exploring it, releasing it, or transposing it during the operative stabilization of the medial side.

If an associated fracture of the radial head or neck is noted, it should be addressed in routine fashion. Readers are referred to any standard fracture text[4] for details. Although not reported as an isolated problem, osteochondral fractures can occur.[24] If the joint is opened for any reason, it should be inspected to rule out intraarticular fragments.

COMPLICATIONS

Joint stiffness, specifically loss of extension, is the most common complication. Patients should be counseled that 5 to 10 degrees of extension loss is to be expected but that this motion loss is associated with few symptoms. Early institution of motion helps prevent this problem.

Nerve and vascular injuries have been alluded to. Early diagnosis is the key to preventing long-term sequelae from these injuries.

Heterotopic ossification in the ligaments is a common radiographic finding associated with few symptoms. This is less common in children. True myositis ossificans can lead to significant loss of motion, but it is a rare complication, especially in children.

Recurrent dislocation is also quite rare. Protzman[5] observed no recurrent dislocation in an active population with a minimum of postreduction immobilization. This is supported in other studies.[1,2,3,5,22,23]

PROGNOSIS

Josefsson et al.[22] looked at 52 patients with elbow dislocations, an average of 24 years postinjury. He had no redislocations, no neurological symptoms, and no symptoms of instability. There were eight patients with signs of abnormal valgus laxity, but these were asymptomatic.

Adult dislocators had an average loss of extension of 12 degrees, whereas childhood dislocators only lost an average of 4 degrees. There was essentially no loss of pronation, supination, or flexion. There were some mild radiographic findings of osteoarthritis, but the only associated symptom was a mild increase in extension loss. Other large series reflect the above findings.[1,2,3,5,23]

In the student athlete, we can expect return to noncontact sports in 2 to 3 weeks. Contact sports require at least twice as long for return, and the throwing athlete may not return for considerably longer. The long-term prognosis, however, is for most of these athletes to return to their sport with little disability.

CONCLUSION

Elbow dislocation in the student athlete can generally be managed by closed reduction and early motion. Long-term sequelae are usually mild with proper management of these injuries. Careful physical and radiographic examination pre- and postreduction are essential. Although loss of extension is the most common complication, the amount is generally not great enough to affect the patient's use of the extremity. Starting active range-of-motion exercises within a few days of the injury is the best way to prevent stiffness.

References

1. Neviaser, J. S., Wickstrom, J. K.: Dislocation of the elbow: a retrospective study of 115 patients. South. Med. J. 70 (2): 172–173, 1977.
2. Roberts, P. H.: Dislocation of the elbow. Br. J. Surg. 56 (11): 806–815, 1969.
3. Linscheid, R. L., Wheeler, D. K.: Elbow dislocations. JAMA 194 (11): 1171–1176, 1965.
4. Wilkins, K. E.: Fractures and dislocations of the elbow region. In: Rockwood, C. A., Wilkins, K. E., King, R. E. (eds.): Fractures in Children. Vol. 3. Philadelphia, J. B. Lippincott Co., pp. 363–575, 1984.
5. Protzman, R. R.: Dislocation of the elbow joint. J. Bone Joint Surg. 60A: 539–541, 1978.
6. Morrey, B. F., An, K.: Articular and ligamentous contributions to the stability of the elbow joint. Am. J. Sports Med. 11: 315–319, 1983.
7. Morrey, B. F.: Applied anatomy and biomechanics of the elbow joint. AAOS Instructional Course Lectures, 35: 59–68, 1986.
8. Schwab, G. H., Bennett, J. B., Woods, G. W., Tullos, H. S.: Biomechanics of elbow instability: the role of the medial collateral ligament. Clin. Orthop. 146: 42–52, 1980.
9. Tullos, H. S., Schwab, G. H., Bennett, J. B., Woods, G. W.: Factors influencing elbow instability. AAOS Instructional Course lectures, 30: 185–199, 1981.
10. Morrey, B. F., An, K.: Functional anatomy of the ligaments of the elbow. Clin. Orthop. 201: 84–89, 1985.
11. Hassman, G. C., Brunn, F., Neer, C. S.: Recurrent dislocation of the elbow. J. Bone Joint Surg. 57A: 1080–1084, 1975.
12. Osborne, G., Cotterill, P.: Recurrent dislocation of the elbow. J. Bone Joint Surg. 48B: 340–346, 1966.
13. Symeonides, P. P., Paschaloglou, C., Stavra, Z., Pangalides, T.: Recurrent dislocation of the elbow. J. Bone Joint Surg. 57A: 1084–1086, 1975.
14. Josefsson, P. O., Gentz, C. F., Johnell, O., Wendeberg, B.: Surgical versus non-surgical treatment of ligamentous injuries following dislocation of the elbow joint. J. Bone Joint Surg. 69A: 605–608, 1987.
15. Loomis, L. K.: Reduction and after treatment of posterior dislocation of the elbow. Am. J. Surg. 63(1): 56–60, 1944.
16. Louis, D. S., Ricciardi, J. E., Spengler, D. M.: Arterial injury: a complication of posterior elbow dislocation. J. Bone Joint Surg. 56A: 1631–1636, 1974.
17. Morrey, B. F.: The Elbow and Its Disorders. Philadelphia, W. B. Saunders Co., 1985.
18. Hallett, J.: Entrapment of the median nerve after dislocation of the elbow. J. Bone Joint Surg. 63B: 408–412, 1981.
19. Greenspan, A., Norman, A.: The radial head, capitellum view: useful technique in elbow trauma. AJR 138: 1186–1188, 1982.
20. Norwood, L. A., Shook, J. A., Andrews, J. R.: Acute medial elbow ruptures. Am. J. Sports Med. 9: 16–19, 1981.
21. Durig, M., Muller, W., Ruedi, T. P., Gauer, E. F.: The operative treatment of elbow dislocation in the adult. J. Bone Joint Surg. 61A: 239–244, 1979.
22. Josefsson, P. O., Johnell, O., Gentz, C. F.: Long-term sequelae of simple dislocation of the elbow. J. Bone Joint Surg. 66A: 927–930, 1984.
23. Mehloff, T. L., Noble, P. C., Bennett, J. B., Tullos, H. S.: Simple dislocation of the elbow in the adult. J. Bone Joint Surg. 70A: 244–249, 1988.
24. Selesnick, F. H., Dolitsky, B., Haskell, S. S.: Fracture of the coronoid process requiring open reduction with internal fixation. J. Bone Joint Surg. 66A: 1304–1305, 1984.
25. DeLee, J. C., Graen, D. P., Wilkins, K. E.: Fractures and dislocations of the elbow. In: Rockwood, C. A., Green, D. P. (eds.): Fractures in Adults. Vol. I. Philadelphia, J. B. Lippincott Co. pp. 559–652.

14

HAND AND WRIST INJURIES

DANIEL P. MASS
WILLIAM G. RAASCH

The hand is the most exposed part of the body during most athletic activities. Injuries to the hand can range from nuisance sprains to devastating long-term disabilities. Often what seems like a minimal injury to the athlete and coach can have long-term effects on the function of the hand. We believe that all injuries to the hand deserve thorough evaluation, both clinically and radiographically. With proper splinting and protection, many hand injuries may be well treated while allowing early return to sport. In the case of some injuries, however, the athlete and his or her family must understand that early return to play may compromise the ultimate result.

DISTAL PHALANGEAL INJURIES

TUFT INJURIES

The most common injuries to the hand are to the exposed distal phalanx.[5,28] Depending on the type of impact that is made during the sporting event, different injuries occur. In contact sports such as football and rugby, the distal phalanx is crushed between two objects, leading to a tuft or shaft fracture (Fig. 14–1). In ball sports such as softball and basketball, the distal phalanx is subjected to an axial load, often resulting in fractures with articular involvement.[7] (Fig. 14–2). Treatment is determined by fracture displacement and injury to the nailbed. If the fracture is nondisplaced or severely comminuted, protective splinting of the distal intraphalangeal (DIP) joint and the fingertip is required for 6 weeks, or until pain free (Fig. 14–3). In a minimally comminuted fracture with significant displacement, the fracture needs to be reduced under a digital block and pinned in place with either a Kirschner wire (K-wire) or a 21-guage needle (Fig. 14–4). We recommend performing the digital block through a volar approach. A skin wheel is made directly over the flexor tendon just proximal to the metacarpal head, and 2 to 3 ml of local anesthetic, without epinephrine, are injected on each side of the flexor tendon.[32] Because the wire or needle crosses the DIP joint, the joint and tip are protected with a splint. After 4 weeks, the pin may be removed and the athlete may return to sports if protective splinting is possible.

NAILBED INJURIES

If the nailbed is injured, the treatment must allow for optimum nailbed function. If the nail is not avulsed and the subungual hematoma is less than one third of the nail, then simply draining the hematoma and treating the fracture, if present, constitute adequate treatment. To drain the hematoma, a digital block is performed, and multiple holes are placed in the nail over the hematoma either with a hot paper clip or by spinning an 18-guage needle on a syringe. Care is taken not to damage the nailbed. The nail is covered with silver sulfadiazene or zinc oxide ointment (less expensive) and a dressing to maintain drainage.

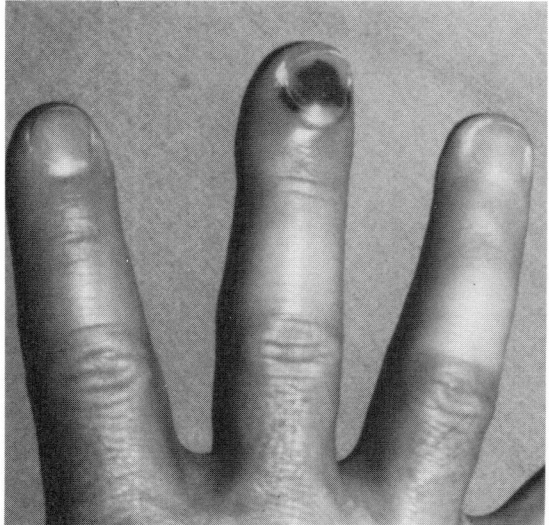
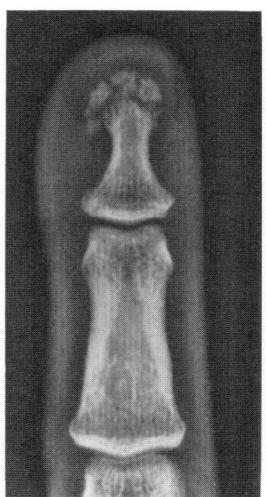
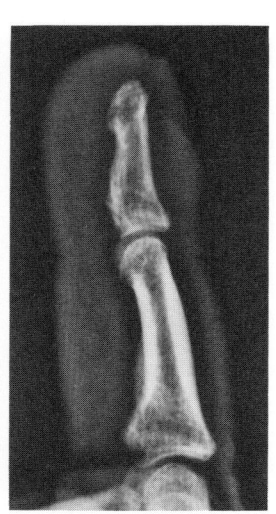

FIGURE 14–1. The clinical picture and radiographs of a comminuted distal phalanx fracture sustained when the finger was crushed between two free weights during weight training. Protective splinting is the treatment of choice for such a severely comminuted distal tuft fracture.

If the hematoma is greater than one third or the nail is partially avulsed, a significant tear in the nailbed is assumed. Under a digital block, a finger tourniquet is placed (either the finger of a sterile glove or a ½-inch penrose drain), the nail is removed, and the nailbed is repaired with fine chromic suture on an ophthalmic needle. The nail is then cleaned and

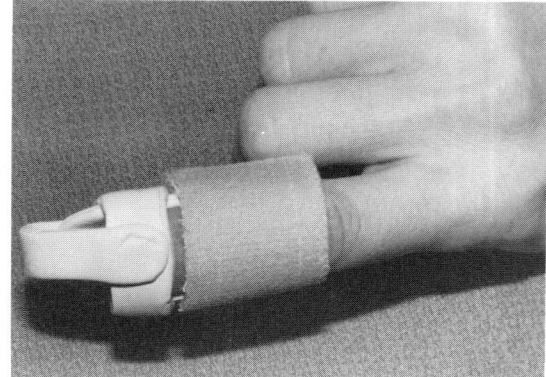
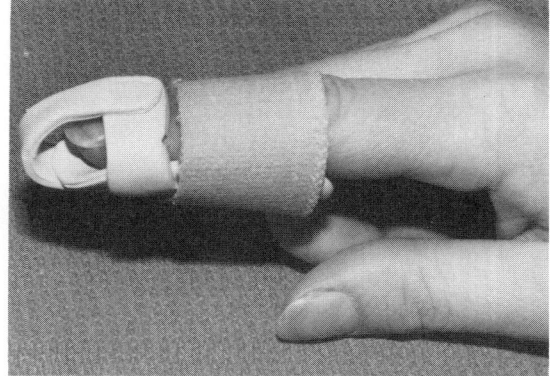

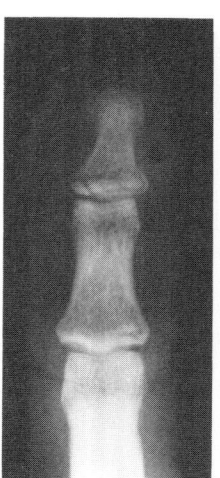
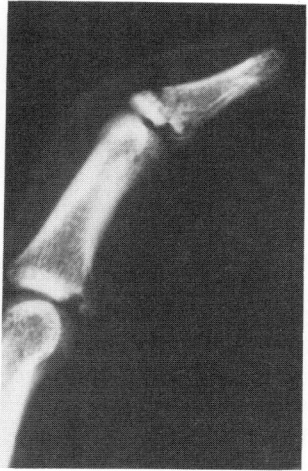

FIGURE 14–2. Radiographs of a intraarticular distal phalanx fracture sustained during a 16-inch softball game. The digit was subjected to an axial load when struck by the softball during an acrobatic catch.

FIGURE 14–3. Distal phalanx thermoplast splint providing protection to the distal phalanx while immobilizing the DIP joint.

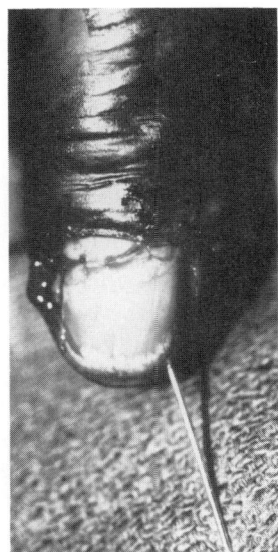

FIGURE 14–4. Percutaneous K-wire splinting of a distal phalanx provides fracture immobilization and access to soft tissue injuries.

several holes are made in it to allow for drainage. It is then placed back under the perionychium with a 4–0 dissolving mattress stitch at the base of the nail fold. The nail is the best protection for the bed and an excellent splint for the fracture. If the nail has been destroyed, then a silicone sheet or xeroform gauze can be used. The nail or other covering is dressed as described above to maintain drainage. The fracture is treated based on displacement and stability. Antibiotic coverage, consisting of erythromycin or an oral cephalosporin, should be used in all open fractures for at least 3 days.

Nail injuries and the associated fractures remain tender for 3 to 6 weeks. The patient should be told to expect some residual nail deformity, and that it takes 4 to 5 months for the nailbed to regrow fully. The athlete can return to training after the initial pain has resolved, but the tip must be protected so that the nail is not pulled off or the fracture displaced. If a pin has been placed through the joint, contact sports should not be played until the pin has been removed, usually after 3 to 4 weeks.

DISTAL INTERPHALANGEAL JOINT INJURIES

The most common cause of hand injury during sports is a direct blow to the extended finger. The position of the finger and the tension around the joint at the time of impact by either a ball or a body determine the injury.

MALLET FINGER

The most frequent injury is the common mallet finger, or extensor tendon avulsion, with or without a small fleck of bone from the dorsum of the distal phalanx[42] (Fig. 14–5). It is most commonly seen in athletes who are required to catch objects, such as the baseball fielder, football receiver, or the basketball player. This injury is caused by acute flexion of the extended DIP joint. The treatment for acute injuries with or without avulsion fractures is always conservative. Tendinous avulsions may be successfully treated conservatively when seen within 12 weeks of injury. Treatment consists of splinting the DIP joint in extension (not hyperextension) for 6 weeks with a fracture and 8 weeks with a tendon injury (Fig. 14–6). The proximal interphalangeal (PIP) joint should always be left free to move.[9, 10, 34, 40] Return to athletics depends on the position played, but most athletes can return with a padded splint after

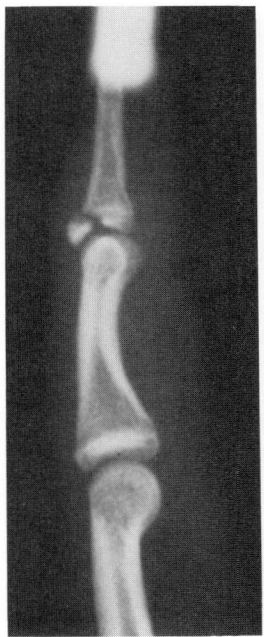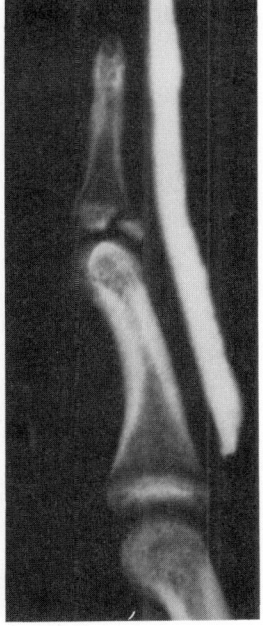

FIGURE 14–5. Radiographs of a bony mallet finger and the reduction film with the dorsal splint in place. The DIP joint is splinted in extension for at least 6 weeks.

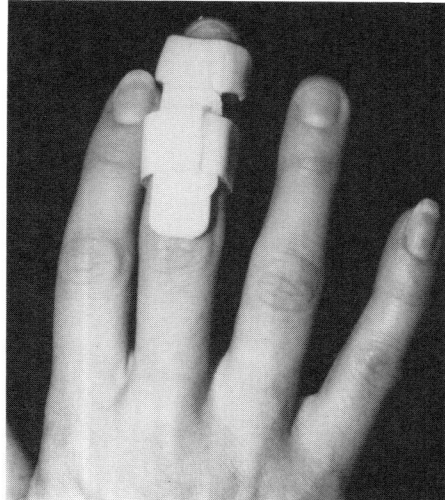
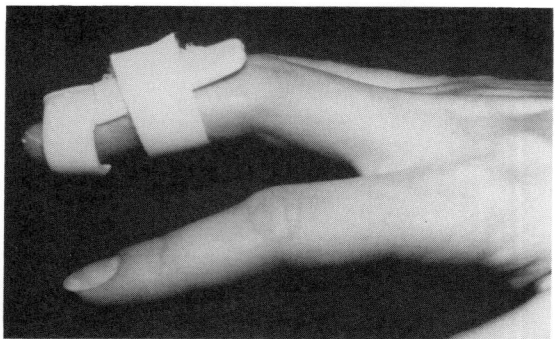

FIGURE 14–6. Dorsal DIP joint thermoplast splint with Velcro fasteners. The splint may be removed for washing, but care should be taken to maintain the DIP joint in extension.

the acute swelling and pain have dissipated. In the immature skeleton, this injury can lead to a Salter Harris IV fracture of the epiphysis. If treated acutely, this injury can usually be treated closed in the same manner. If closed reduction is not possible, then open reduction and 3 weeks of K-wire fixation are required. The athlete may return to sports in a splint after the K-wire is removed.

COMPRESSION FRACTURE

The compression fracture looks clinically like a mallet finger, with a flexed distal phalanx. Longitudinal compression of the distal phalanx into the middle phalanx often results in a large dorsal intraarticular fragment. This must be differentiated from the small avulsed fragment that occurs during sudden forced flexion in a bony mallet finger (Fig. 14–7). If this injury is not properly differentiated from a mallet finger, long-term problems can occur. The compression fracture is caused by the direct impact of a large ball, such as a 16-inch softball, a basketball, or a volleyball, on the tip of the extended finger. While initial treatment is an extension splint, the physician must recognize that there are significant forces acting at the fracture, which may result in an incongruous joint. The extensor tendon will tend to displace proximally and rotate the dorsal joint fragment, whereas the flexor profundus tendon will volarly sublux the main part of the distal phalanx. These injuries may require surgery[33, 40, 41] and K-wire pinning if closed reduction cannot be obtained or maintained. The patient with an adequate reduction must be watched closely during the first 3 weeks to look for loss of reduction. Whether treated by splinting or surgery, this injury prevents par-

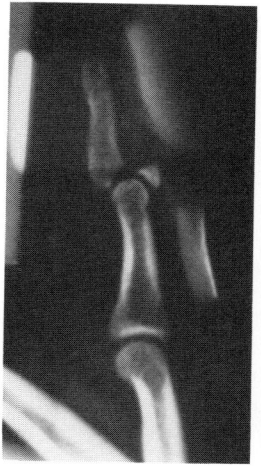
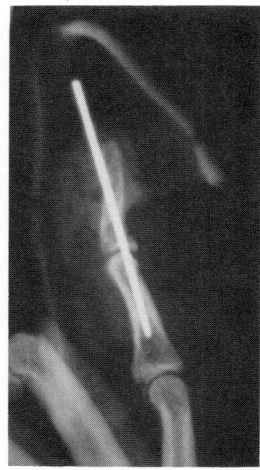

FIGURE 14–7. Radiographs of a compression fracture of the distal phalanx and the reduction film with the K-wire in place. This fracture may appear radiographically quite similar to the bony mallet finger, depending on the percentage of articular surface involved. When treated with splinting, this fracture requires close follow-up owing to its tendency to displace.

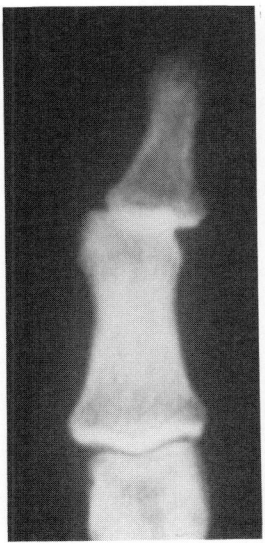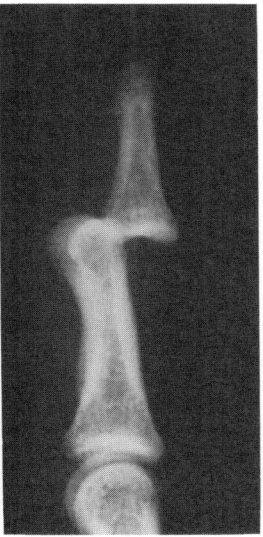

FIGURE 14–8. Radiographs of a dorsal dislocation of the DIP joint. After reduction, the DIP joint is splinted in slight flexion.

ticipation in contact and ball sports for at least 6 weeks.

DORSAL DISLOCATION

If the extended finger is impacted by a ball just volar to its tip, then a hyperextension force is imparted to the DIP joint. This causes the unusual DIP dorsal dislocation (Fig. 14–8). This injury is often an open dislocation because the stretching forces tear the skin and the flexor tendon sheath where they are tightly bound down at the volar crease.

Treatment of this injury, if closed, is a closed reduction under a digital block and 3 weeks of splinting the DIP joint in slight flexion. Athletics can be resumed when the patient is comfortable and can play with the splint. After 3 weeks, it is advisable to tape the joint during play.

If the dislocation is open, the joint is reduced under digital block, the skin edges are cleaned and debrided, and the flexor sheath and joint are irrigated with Ringer's lactate. If possible, the wound is loosely closed and the entire finger splinted for 2 days. The patient is given oral antibiotics and instructed to elevate the hand. After 2 days, the wound is inspected, and only the DIP joint is splinted. Return to athletics should wait until the sutures are removed.

PROFUNDUS AVULSION

The rarest injury around the DIP joint is a profundus tendon avulsion, usually in the ring finger[34] (Fig. 14–9). This football injury occurs during a tackle and is sometimes

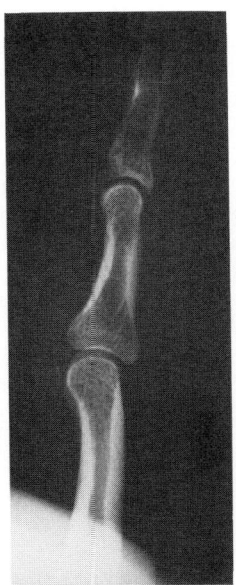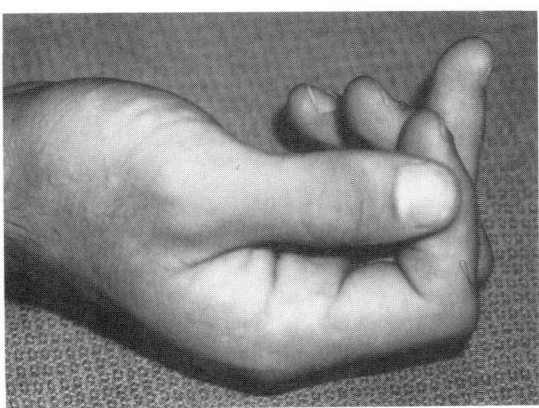

A B

FIGURE 14–9. (A) Radiograph showing the profundus avulsion fragment retracted to the level of the PIP joint. B shows the resting position of the involved hand on presentation. The extended DIP joint in the long finger is clinically obvious.

called "jersey finger." The runner is grabbed by the fingertips, and acute hyperextension occurs during a missed tackle. Because of the single tendinous origin of the profundus tendons, tethering occurs. This force is thought to be centralized on the ring finger causing an avulsion.

The treatment that yields the best result is early surgical reattachment. Because of the violence of the disruption, bleeding into the closed flexor sheath usually occurs, resulting in increased scarring in the sheath if surgery is delayed. The repair must be protected like any flexor tendon laceration. Vigorous therapy over 4 months will yield good, but usually not full, range of motion. In order to protect this repair, contact sports should be prohibited during these 4 months. If the athlete and his or her family are willing to accept a significantly compromised result, definitive treatment may be delayed until the end of the season. In this case, the ring and the long finger are taped together during play.

The delayed treatment depends on the functional goals of the athlete and on the retracted position of the tendon. If the retracted tendon is trapped at the PIP joint, motion may be limited. Further retraction of the tendon into the palm may result in a painful palmar lump. Both problems may be treated with excision of the profundus tendon. This will lead to a permanently floppy distal phalanx with reduced grip strength. The athlete may experience difficulty in throwing, tackling, or grabbing as a result. The reconstructive options include DIP joint fusion, which gives increased stability without improving strength, and flexor tendon grafting, a complex surgical procedure fraught with a high complication rate.

PROXIMAL INTRAPHALANGEAL JOINT INJURIES

The proximal intraphalangeal joint provides the greatest arc of motion of the finger. Therefore, loss of this motion can lead to significant disability, particularly in the adolescent. A stiff PIP joint can not only prevent athletic participation but can interfere with playing musical instruments and typing. These injuries must be treated carefully but aggressively to maintain a functional range of motion.

DORSAL DISLOCATION

The most common sports injury to the hand, dorsal dislocation of the PIP joint, is often called the "coach's finger." This hyperextension injury to the PIP joint can occur in almost any ball or contact sport. The degree of hyperextension, angulation, and longitudinal impact determine the stability of the joint after reduction. While many or most of these injuries are reduced on the field by the player or coach and come to no long-term harm, there is a small percentage of players who have long-term disabilities owing to continued instability (Fig. 14–10).

Treatment of the dorsal dislocation of the PIP joint is closed reduction and proper evaluation.[4, 23, 24, 31] First, X-rays are obtained to look for displaced fractures. Then, the joint is placed through an active range of function to see if redislocation occurs in full extension. Lateral stress testing is also preformed in both directions. Digital blocks are used during stability testing when there is significant pain.

In stable cases without associated fracture, the initial treatment is 2 to 3 days of PIP splinting in 30 degrees of flexion to allow for pain and edema control. This is followed by "buddy taping" during athletic activities for 6 more weeks to permit protected range of motion. A modern improvement on traditional buddy taping is the use of "traveling fellows," reusable Velcro straps that hold two adjacent fingers together Fig. 14–11. This treatment allows for return to normal motion within a few months.

If the athlete sustains a fracture-dislocation, an X-ray with the PIP joint splinted in 30 to 40 degrees of flexion determines reduction and congruity. If the joint is stable and the fracture fragments reduced, a dorsal splint is maintained until the patient is comfortable (3 to 4 days). A dorsal blocking splint is then made to start active range of motion while maintaining joint stability. After 3 weeks, the splint is brought into increasing extension. At 6 weeks, the splint is no longer needed, and buddy taping is started. Return to athletics is permitted when there is pain-free, nearly full range of motion.

UNSTABLE DISLOCATIONS

If, after reduction, the PIP joint is unstable, the athlete has sustained either (1) a com-

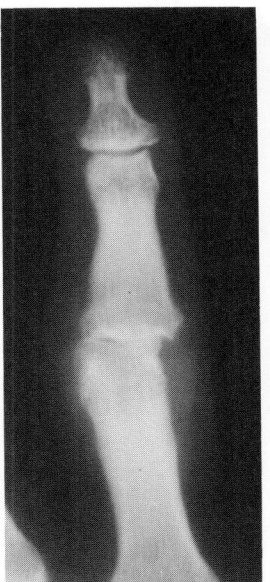
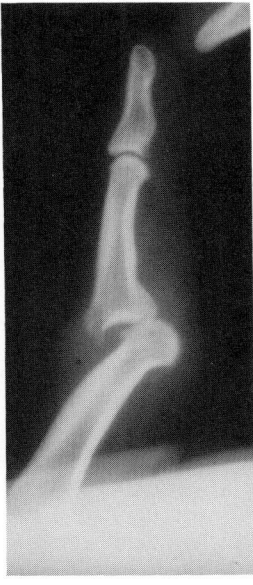
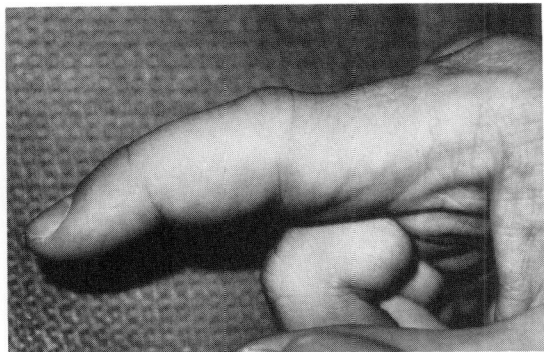

FIGURE 14–10. The radiographs and clinical picture of an athlete who sustained a dorsal dislocation of the PIP joint and went on to develop instability with arthritic changes. Early diagnosis with close follow-up may prevent such results.

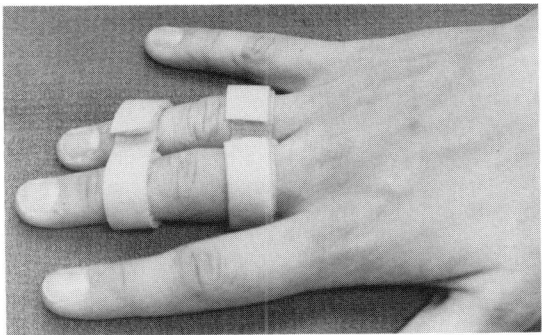
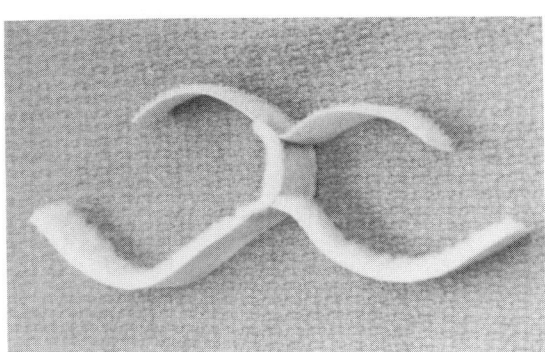

FIGURE 14–11. "Traveling fellows" provide a comfortable and removable alternative to buddy taping.

plete avulsion of the volar plate off the middle phalanx with an associated collateral ligament injury or (2) a fracture dislocation (compression fracture) with separated fracture fragments.

If the joint opens more than 30 degrees with lateral stress testing, the collateral ligament and the volar plate are completely torn. These injuries need to be reduced and the joint treated at least by buddy taping to the adjacent finger on the side of the collateral ligament tear. If there is pain with flexion after the swelling has subsided and the joint remains unstable, a collateral ligament repair or reconstruction is considered. Acute surgical repair and taping will allow for return to athletics after 2 weeks. Successful delayed reconstruction of the collateral ligament after the season is over is possible, but the operation has a high degree of complexity.

If the athlete has sustained a fracture dislocation and the fracture fragment is large with residual dorsal subluxation, then the treatment options are closed reduction and K-wire fixation of the joint or open reduction and internal fixation of the fragments via a volar approach. Either miniscrews or a pull-out suture may be used to maintain reduction. If this injury is seen late, with continued dorsal subluxation, then volar plate arthroplasty is the treatment of choice. The average range of motion of the PIP joint after volar plate arthroplasty is 30 to 80 degrees.

VOLAR DISLOCATION

In a small percentage of impact injuries, the middle phalanx is volarly dislocated on the proximal phalanx (Fig. 14–12). We have seen this from players of Ultimate Frisbee, football, and rugby. If this injury is reduced on the field without follow-up, or if the treating physician interprets the injury as a "standard dislocation" and splints the finger in 30 degrees of flexion, a boutonnière deformity will follow. This problem develops because of the disruption of the central extensor tendon slip at its insertion into the middle phalanx. The proper treatment of a volar dislocation is extension splinting of the PIP joint for 6 weeks.[43] Players can return to their sports only if they can wear the protective splint.

Traumatic contusions of the dorsum of the PIP joint can also lead to boutonnière deformities. If there is pain and swelling over the dorsum of the PIP joint despite the ability to extend the joint actively, the joint should be splinted in extension until the pain and swelling resolve, and then active extension should be reevaluated.

METACARPAL PHALANGEAL JOINT INJURIES

DORSAL DISLOCATIONS

Dorsal dislocation of the thumb metacarpal phalangeal (MP) joint is not an uncommon injury in the adolescent athlete. Finger MP joint dislocations however, are rare with the exception of the index finger.[35] Forced hyperextension of the digit is considered to be the mechanism of injury. This can occur during a fall in any noncontact sport or, more commonly, in a contact sport involving an impact that levers the digit dorsally. The pathophysiology was first and accurately described by Farabeuf in 1876.[11] Three grades of injury were identified: *incomplete, simple,* and *complex.* Incomplete injuries involve only the avulsion of the volar plate proximally. The collateral ligaments remain intact, and the metacarpal head does not sublux through the volar capsular defect. If the proximal phalanx continues its dorsal rotation about the metacarpal head, the collateral ligaments are partially torn or ruptured, owing to their eccentric insertion. The base of the proximal phalanx will eventually rest on the dorsum of the metacarpal head, creating a simple dislocation.

In the complex dislocation, the volar lip of the proximal phalanx rests on the dorsum of the metacarpal head with entrapment of the volar plate [18] (Fig. 14–13). In the thumb, the metacarpal head is circumferentially entrapped between the flexor pollicis brevis and the adductor pollicis.[26] Stener also describes the entrapment of the avulsed proximal end of the ulnar collateral ligament.[42] In the fingers, the metacarpal head buttonholes through the palmar fascia, with ulnar and radial displacement of the flexor tendons and the lumbrical, respectively.[18]

The treatment of simple and incomplete dislocations is closed reduction with splinting. Several authors [11, 16, 26] have advised against strong longitudinal traction, which may convert a simple into a complex dislocation. A closed reduction is performed by first hyperextending the proximal phalanx to 90 degrees on the metacarpal head and then applying dorsal pressure on the base of the

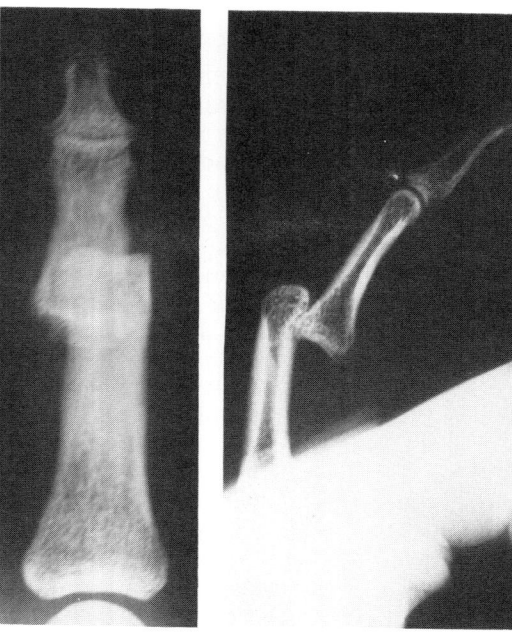

FIGURE 14–12. Radiographs of a volar PIP dislocation. Proper extension splinting of the PIP joint for 6 weeks will prevent a boutonnière deformity in this injury.

HAND AND WRIST INJURIES

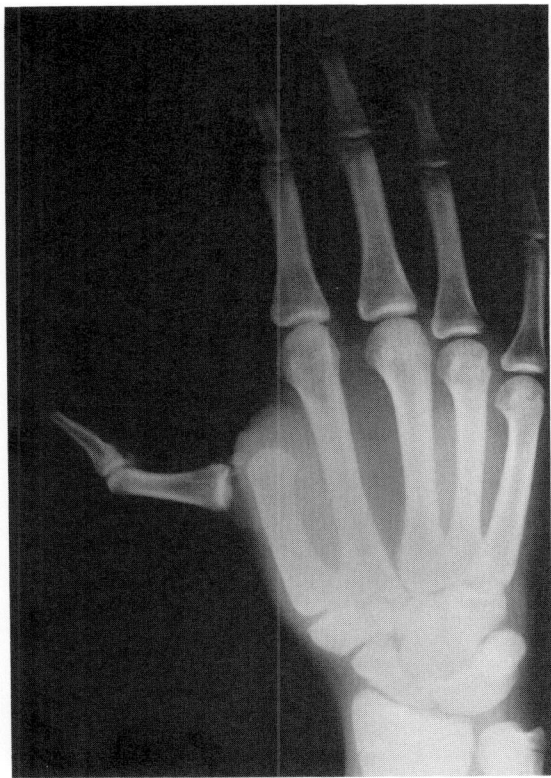 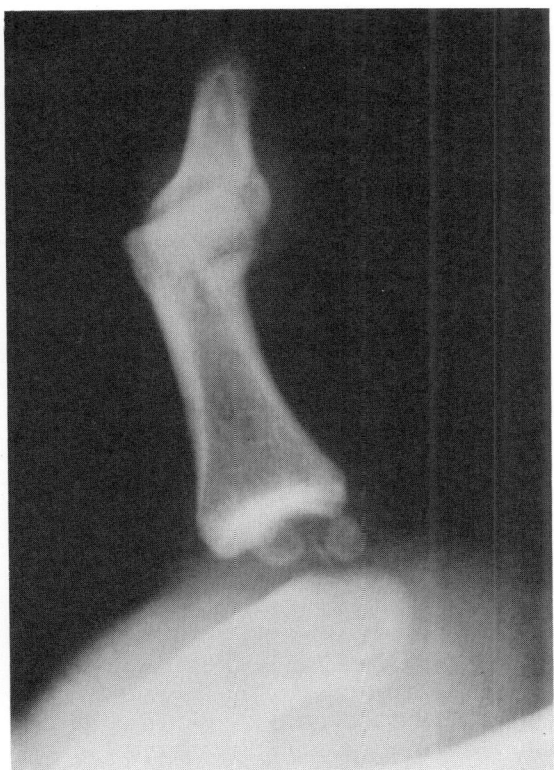

FIGURE 14–13. Radiographs showing an MP joint dislocation of the thumb. A single gentle attempt to closed reduction may be attempted; however, in complex dorsal dislocation, open reduction is often necessary.

proximal phalanx while flexing the joint into a reduced position. Extension block splinting is used initially and followed with buddy taping when the patient is comfortable (Fig. 14–14). The athlete may return to competition with splinting, the time frame dependant on the type of sport and risk of reinjury.

The term *complex dislocation* implies the need for open reduction. A single, gentle attempt at closed reduction of the thumb has been recommended by a few authors with the technique described above. It should be assumed, however, that a complex dislocation of a finger requires operative interven-

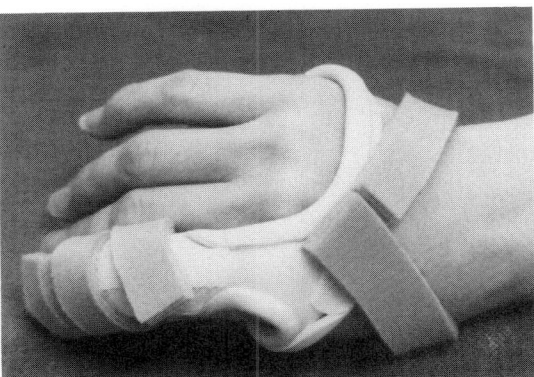 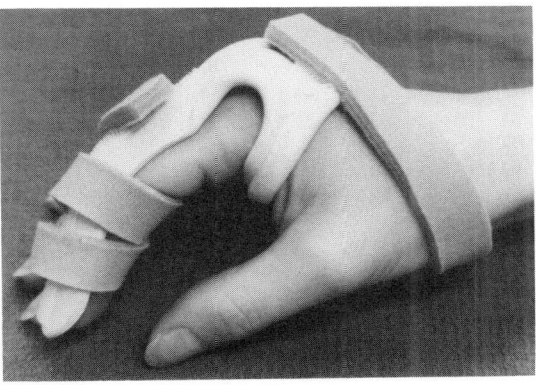

FIGURE 14–14. Removable dorsal block splinting of the index finger.

tion to extract the entrapped volar plate.[18] Farabeuf[11] and Weeks[46] recommended a dorsal approach; however, most authors advocate a volar approach. We recommend a volar approach, as it provides excellent surgical exposure to entrapped structures. We also recommend release of the A1 pulley, a structure that resists disengagement of the metacarpal head.[3] Care must be taken during surgery to avoid injury to the digital nerves that are stretched out over the metacarpal head. The joint is usually stable, allowing for early motion with a dorsal block splint. Cast immobilization may be required for 3 weeks if instability is present.

COLLATERAL LIGAMENT INJURIES OF THE FINGER MP JOINTS

The MP joints of the fingers lie in a relatively protected proximal position, decreasing the incidence of collateral ligament injury. Local tenderness at the metacarpal head and pain when stressing the joint medially or laterally suggest a collateral ligament injury. Because of the eccentric insertion of the collateral ligaments on the metacarpal head, the MP joint must be held in full flexion when stress testing. Splinting of the MP joint in flexion for 3 weeks has been the recommended treatment. This is followed with buddy taping until pain free. If there is significant pain with greater than 30 degrees of opening at the joint, a complete rupture is present. We believe that a complete rupture of the collateral ligament must be returned to its anatomical eccentric position.[37] This can only be accomplished with open reduction. If surgery is delayed until after the season, a ligament reconstruction is then necessary. This is a technically difficult procedure with the risk of increased stiffness. Return to athletics is possible 3 weeks after surgery with buddy taping of the injured finger to the adjacent finger on the side of the ligament injury.

LIGAMENT INJURIES OF THE THUMB MP JOINT

ULNAR COLLATERAL LIGAMENT INJURY

The term *gamekeeper's thumb* initially described a chronic laxity in the ulnar collateral ligament of the thumb MP joint. Campbell reported this occupational disability in the hands of British gamekeepers in 1955.[6] The term has now come to include the acute injury seen with forced abduction of the MP joint. This injury is often seen in downhill skiers when the ski pole is levered in the first web space. Football players are also susceptible to this injury when tackling an opponent with the hands.

The thumb is first evaluated radiographically for an avulsion fragment before lateral stability testing. If there is an avulsed fragment displaced less than 2 mm, casting in a thumb spica is the treatment of choice. If no fragment is present, lateral stress testing is performed by stressing the MP joint in the fully flexed position (Fig. 14–15). If stability testing demonstrates pain and laxity but less than 35 degrees of joint opening, the athlete may be treated with 6 weeks of thumb spica casting. If the joint opens more than 35 degrees in full flexion, the collateral ligament is completely disrupted. With complete collateral disruption, the lateral X-ray will often show volar subluxation of the proximal phalanx. A Stener lesion, interposition of the adductor aponeurosis between the two ends of the torn ligament, has been reported in 14 to 83 percent of patients with complete disruption.[20, 29, 30, 39, 47] Casting alone is insufficient when a true Stener lesion is present. Because there appears to be a high incidence of this lesion in complete disruptions, we agree with the literature that early operative intervention is justified. Following primary repair, the thumb is immobilized for 3 weeks in a thumb spica cast with the thumb inter-

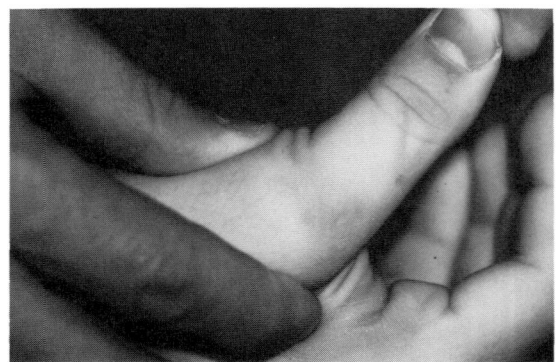

FIGURE 14–15. A positive clinical exam for a "gamekeeper's thumb." The thumb is examined with the MP joint in a fully flexed position to isolate the ulnar collateral ligament during testing.

phalangeal (IP) joint free to move. Protective flexion-extension splinting follows for an additional 3 weeks.

Return to athletics with protective thumb spica splinting is allowed after the pain and swelling are gone in nonsurgical cases and after 6 weeks in surgical cases. A silicone thumb spica splint is required during play. After the 6 weeks of splinting, taping for comfort is advisable.

RADIAL COLLATERAL LIGAMENT INJURY

Collateral ligament injuries on the radial aspect of the thumb MP joint are less common than the gamekeeper's injury. The patient usually presents late with a tender prominence on the radial aspect of the MP joint. The anatomy at the radial aspect of the joint precludes the possibility of a Stener lesion. Therefore, complete disruptions of the ligament should be more amenable to immobilization for 4 to 6 weeks in a thumb spica cast. If volar subluxation is present, however, surgical repair is recommended. Return to sports in a silicone thumb spica splint is possible during the first 6 weeks.

MIDDLE AND PROXIMAL PHALANGEAL FRACTURES

Fractures are the most common athletic hand injuries that require treatment.[38] As with any fracture, careful assessment of displacement, articular involvement, and stability must be made. With proper initial treatment, early return to sports and the prevention of long-term disability need not be mutually exclusive.

Fractures of the middle or proximal phalanges can usually be divided into four types: (1) shaft fractures, (2) distal intraarticular condylar fractures of the head, (3) phalangeal neck fractures, and (4) proximal lip fractures with varying degree of intraarticular involvement. This last group was previously discussed with PIP joint injuries.

THE MIDDLE PHALANX

The middle phalanx is the bone least likely to fracture in the hand, with crush injuries occurring more distally and pinch or twisting injuries more proximally. The most common types seen are the transverse and short oblique diaphyseal shaft fractures. They can usually be treated closed with two-finger splinting or buddy taping if stable. Long oblique or spiral fractures are inherently more unstable and often require closed reduction with K-wire fixation. Open reduction with screw fixation is another alternative that allows for early motion with decreased tendon adhesions. About 10 to 15 degrees of angulation in the plane of motion may be acceptable, but malrotation should not be accepted.

Condylar fractures with intraarticular involvement require anatomical reduction. If the fracture is nondisplaced, conservative management with two-finger splinting for 4 weeks is adequate. Because these fractures have a tendency to displace, close monitoring with weekly radiographs is required.[38] When taking radiographs, particular attention must be given to the positioning of the hand for true anterior-posterior (AP) view of the condyles. Displaced condylar fractures require reduction with fixation. Closed reduction, if possible, is preferable to reduce the inevitable stiffness associated with surgery at the DIP joint. If surgery is required, the dorsolateral approach between the central slip and lateral band or beneath the lateral band is recommended. The reduction is held with two small K-wires or a small 1.5 mm screw using standard AO technique. Early motion may be initiated if the reduction is stable; however, athletics are not allowed for 4 weeks, and the finger should be protected with taping or splinting.

Displaced transverse neck fractures require anatomical reduction to prevent rotation and allow for full flexion in the retrocondylar fossa. This can be accomplished with closed or open reduction followed with K-wire fixation.

THE PROXIMAL PHALANX

Fractures of the proximal phalanx are much more common than middle phalangeal fractures but many of the same principles described previously remain relevant. Transverse and short oblique neck and shaft fractures are treated the same except for incorporation of the MP joint and a second digit in all splinting. The immobilization of the MP joint can only be adequately performed if the

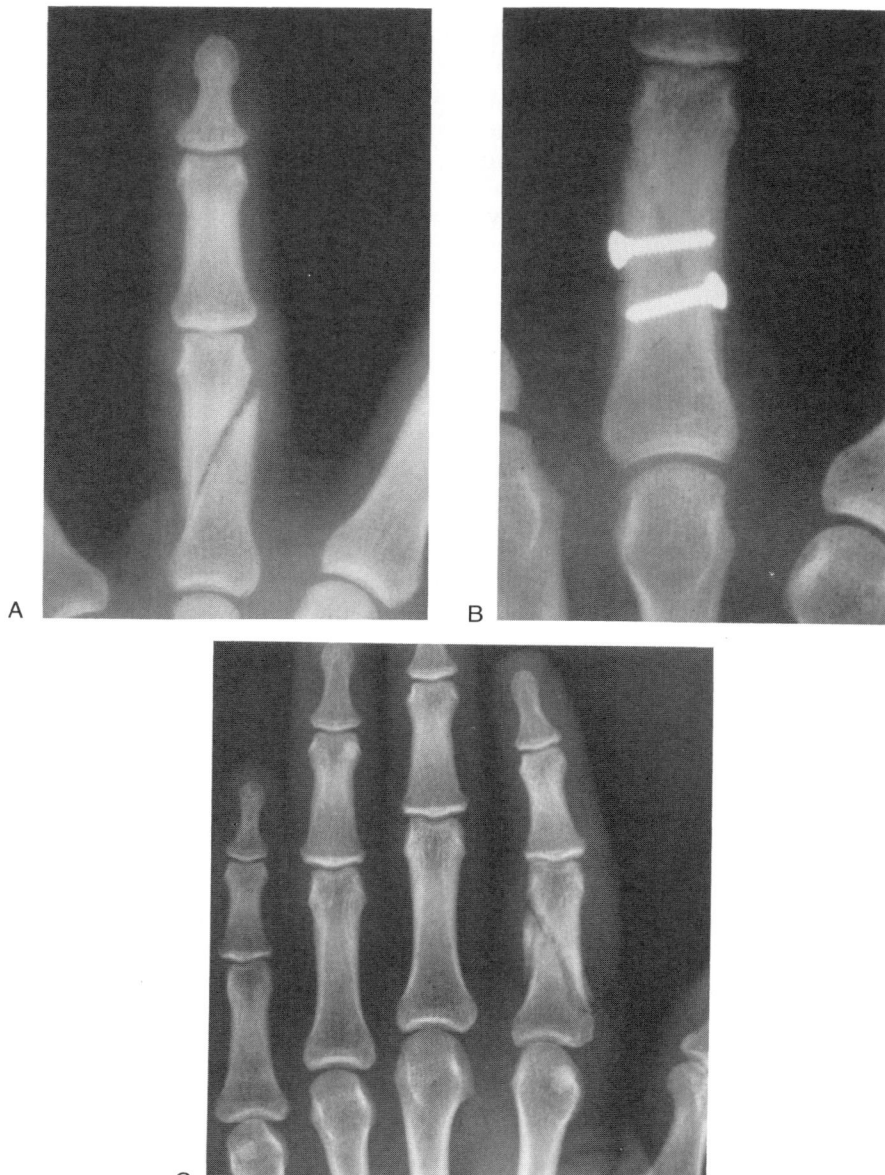

FIGURE 14–16. Radiographs of a long oblique proximal phalanx fracture before and after internal fixation with two 1.5-mm cortical screws. Internal fixation provided stable reduction and allowed for early return of motion. (C) When the fracture is stable and the reduction is acceptable, these injuries can be treated closed with splinting and early buddy taping.

splint is incorporated with a short arm cast. Unstable spiral and short oblique fractures require open reduction with internal fixation if displaced (Fig. 14–16). Any long spiral fracture extending into the retrocondylar fossa should be considered intraarticular, requiring open or closed anatomical reduction.

Treatment of distal condylar fractures can be very demanding because of the 110 degrees of motion required to maintain function at the PIP joint. Thus, any articular fracture must be treated aggressively to prevent loss of motion and function. Nondisplaced or stable reduced fractures are treated with PIP and MP joint immobilization, with a second digit included in the splint to prevent angulation and rotation. Displaced intraarticular fractures require reduction with K-wire or screw (1.5 mm) fixation. Abstinence from athletic activity is again required for 4 weeks, after which protective splinting for an additional 2 weeks is recommended.

METACARPAL FRACTURES

The most common metacarpal fracture is a neck fracture in the little finger, commonly known as a "boxer's fracture" (Fig. 14–17). Because of the increased mobility in the carpal-metacarpal joints of the ring and little fingers, greater angulation is accepted in these digits than in the long and index fingers. Hunter and Cowen[17] found 40 degrees of angulation acceptable in their series of 80 patients and recommended immediate splinting without reduction if angulation was less than 40 degrees. Rockwood and Green,[34] however, feel that immediate splinting without reduction should be restricted to acute fractures with less than 10 degrees of angulation or, if the fracture is more than a week old, with less than 40 degrees of angulation. The maximum acceptable angulation in the long and index fingers is 10 degrees because of their fixed carpal-metacarpal joints. With all digits, the amount of acceptable angulation decreases as the fracture becomes more proximal. Unacceptable angulation will displace the metacarpal head volarly into the palm, often causing a painful palmar bump during grasp.

Neck fractures can be treated closed if adequate reduction is obtained. Reduction is accomplished by flexing the MP and PIP joints 90 degrees and reversing the deforming force by pushing the metacarpal head dorsally through an axially applied force to the proximal phalanx. The digit is then immobilized with the MP joint in 70 degrees of flexion and the PIP joint in extension. A neighboring digit should be included in the cast. Because of volar comminution, many of these fractures are unstable. In unstable cases, reduction is obtained in the same manner and maintained with a K-wire driven through the metacarpal head. The K-wire is pushed through the skin and the extensor tendon displaced to one side; the K-wire is then driven in. Cast immobilization is required until the K-wire is removed in 3 weeks.

With shaft fractures, careful attention must

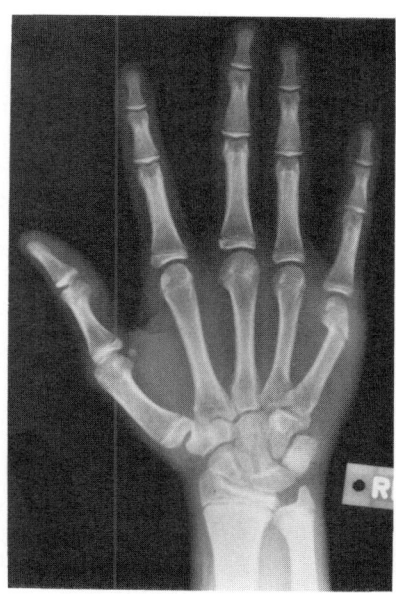
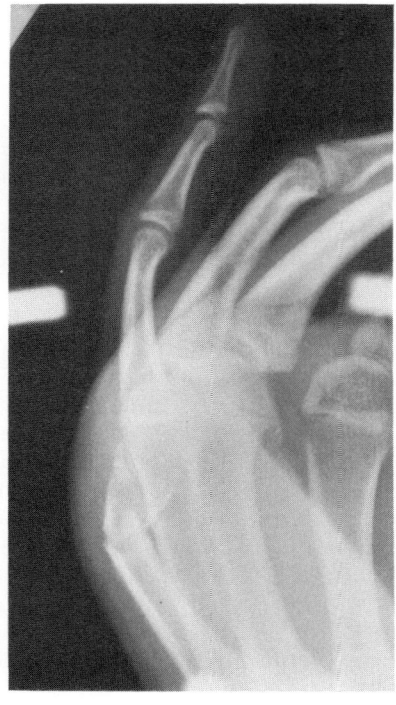

FIGURE 14–17. Radiographs of a "boxer's fracture." This fracture was successfully treated with closed reduction and an ulnar gutter cast.

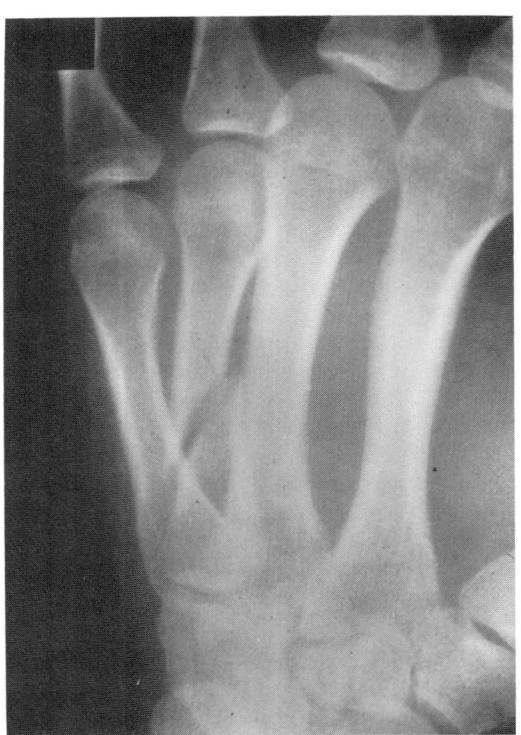 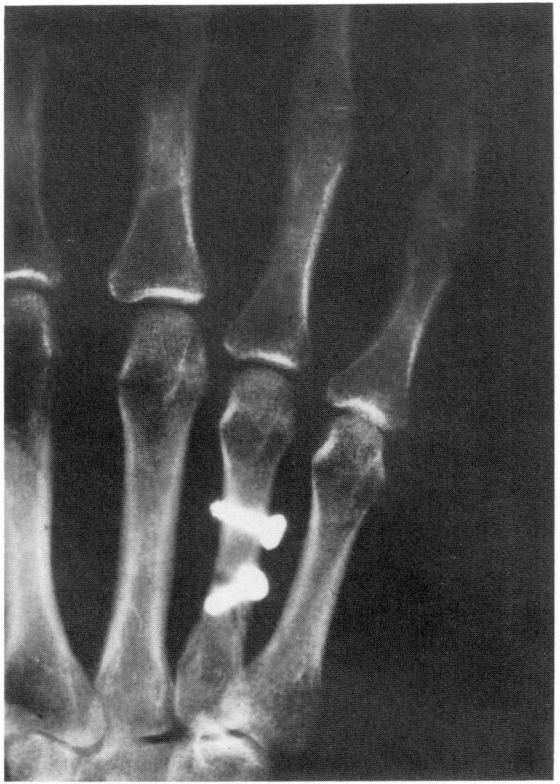

FIGURE 14–18. Radiographs of a spiral fracture to the ring finger metacarpal before and after internal fixation with two 2.7-mm cortical screws. Spiral fractures have a tendency to rotate and shorten and must be watched closely if casting is the method of immobilization.

be paid to rotation as well as angulation. Again, the deformity is amplified as the fracture moves proximally and less angulation is accepted in ring and long fingers. If stable, the fracture is treated with a molded cast, with the MP joint in 70 degrees of flexion. Spiral and oblique fractures are usually unstable with rotational deformity, shortening, and angulation. These fractures require a closed reduction with percutaneous K-wire pinning or open reduction with 2.7 AO screw fixation, which allows early postoperative mobilization (Fig. 14–18). Return to sports in a silicone protective splint is permitted after 3 weeks with stable or screw-fixed fractures.

Proximal carpometacarpal fractures are usually the result of crush injuries that include the carpometacarpal joints. The fractures are rarely displaced and are usually accompanied by considerable swelling. Casting is required only for comfort. With displacement of the fracture, open or closed K-wire pinning is performed. Of special interest is the proximal fifth metacarpal fracture, the "baby Bennett" fracture. Because of the peripheral position of this digit, the force can be transmitted from the metacarpal head down the shaft, resulting in a shear force and a lateral base fragment.

The extensor carpi ulnaris tendon inserts at the dorsal ulnar aspect of the base of the fifth digit metacarpal and causes proximal and ulnar displacement. Because the carpometacarpal joint is often obscured with routine radiographs, an AP film with the forearm in 30 degrees of pronation as recommended by Bora[2] will assist in the diagnosis of undisplaced or minimally displaced fractures. If missed, subluxation with reduced grip strength and eventual degenerative arthritis may occur. Treatment consists of closed reduction and K-wire or screw fixation with immobilization as described with the other metacarpal fractures.

THUMB METACARPAL FRACTURES

Shaft and distal metacarpal fractures are relatively rare in the thumb, and the treatment parallels similar fractures in the other digits. Because of the thumb's increased mobility, additional angular and rotational displacement can be accepted. The unique position of the thumb does, however, result in a predominance of metacarpal base fractures, with four distinct fracture patterns (Fig. 14–19).[15, 21, 27] Two of the fracture patterns are intraarticular, the so-called Bennett's and Rolando's fractures; the other two are transverse fractures with or without epiphyseal involvement, depending on the maturity of the athlete.

Bennett first described the small volar lip fracture at the base of the thumb in 1882[1] (Fig. 14–20). The mechanism of injury consists of an axial load to the partially flexed metacarpal. The volar lip fragment is anchored by the anterior oblique ligament, and the metacarpal shaft is displaced dorsally and radially by the concomitant pull of the

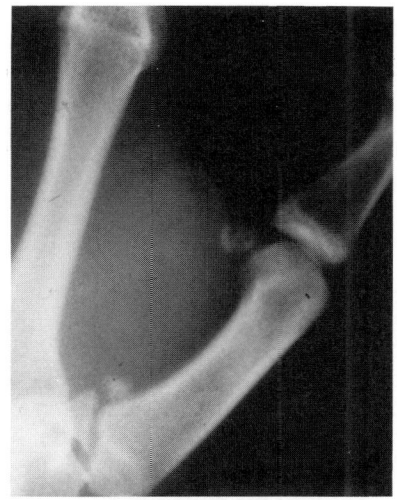

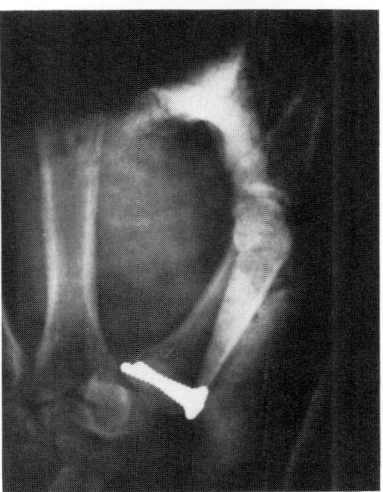

FIGURE 14–20. (*A*) Pre- and (*B*)postop radiographs of a "Bennett's fracture." Internal fixation is obtained with two 2.7-mm cortical screws.

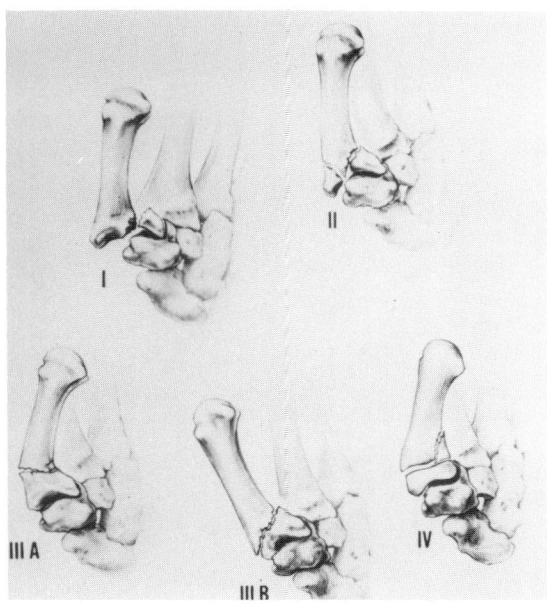

FIGURE 14–19. Four distinct fracture patterns may involve the base of the thumb metacarpal. Type I (Bennett's fracture-dislocation) and type II (Rolando's fracture) are intraarticular. These should be differentiated from the type III extra-articular fractures, which may be either transverse or oblique. Type IV fractures are epiphyseal injuries seen in children. (From Green, D. P., and O'Brien, E. T.: Fractures of the thumb metacarpal. South. Med. J., 65:807, 1972.)

abductor pollicus longus and the adductor pollicus.

A wide spectrum of treatment modalities has evolved in the orthopedic literature, a reflection of the difficulty often encountered in maintaining reduction. We recommend a single attempt at closed reduction with K-wire pinning before performing an open procedure. The K-wires are removed after 4 to 6 weeks, during which the athlete must refrain from athletic competition. Open reduction is required when interposed soft tissues prevent anatomical reduction and often when there is a delay in treatment. The importance of anatomical reduction needs to be stressed, as the alternative is an eventually painful arthritic joint requiring fusion. Open reduction can be preformed with 2.7-mm AO screws if the fragment is 5 mm in size (fragments are usually larger than they appear on X ray) (Fig. 14–20). If the fragment is smaller, K-wire fixation is used. Screw fixation allows for early mobilization and protected return to athletics in a silicone thumb spica cast after the surgical pain and swelling have resolved.

Silvio Rolando described the T- or Y-shaped intraarticular fracture at the base of the thumb metacarpal in 1910.[36] This fracture presents the same challenge to the modern orthopedic surgeon as that faced by Rolando. Fortunately, this is the least encountered of the metacarpal base fractures.[34] Treatment depends on the amount of comminution. With severe comminution, reduction is maintained through distraction. This is most commonly accomplished with a transverse K-wire through the first and second metacarpals for 3 to 4 weeks or until there is no clinical tenderness at the fracture site. Open reduction with internal fixation should only be attempted when large fragments are present.

The most common of the metacarpal base fractures are the extraarticular transverse or oblique fractures. Closed anatomical reduction can usually be obtained and held in place with a short arm thumb spica cast for 4 weeks. Because of the mobility of the thumb, failure to obtain exact anatomical alignment should not be considered an indication for open reduction.

WRIST INJURIES

One of the most devastating upper extremity injuries that can occur to an athlete is an injury to his or her wrist. These injuries usually occur with wrist hyperextension and impaction.[33] The compressive and rotational forces experienced at the time of impact will determine the involvement of ligamentous and osseous tissue. These injuries occur in many sports, from the football player falling while attempting a tackle to the gymnast mislanding a vault. For the athlete, the most devastating aspect of the wrist injury is the potential loss of months or years of competition often required for rehabilitation. The diagnostic challenge that the wrist injury presents to the physician can also prolong the time lost from competition.

INITIAL EVALUATION OF WRIST INJURIES

With the advent of systematic wrist evaluations and the addition of arthroscopy to our armamentarium, we have been able to increase our knowledge and therefore our diagnostic acumen in the problem wrist. First, a thorough examination of the wrist is performed to look for localized points of swelling or tenderness. This is followed by dynamic carpal instability testing: the Watson maneuver[13] for scapholunate dissociation and the "shear" test[19] as described by Kleinman to evaluate the lunatotriquetral joint. The location of most wrist injuries can be isolated by physical exam: radial versus ulnar, and distal radial ulnar joint versus carpal joint. Initial X rays should include AP, lateral, oblique, and ulnar and radial deviation views.

A painful, swollen wrist with no obvious fracture or intracarpal instability is treated with 3 to 4 weeks of splinting (Fig. 14–21). If disability remains persistent after the period of splinting, then further evaluation is undertaken. Special radiographic views based on clinical suspicion are helpful. For example, clenched fist and radial and ulnar deviation

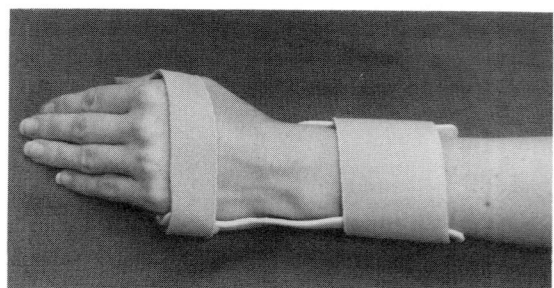

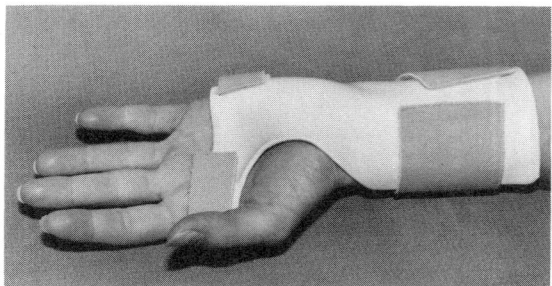

FIGURE 14–21. Thermoplast wrist splints with Velcro fasteners are comfortable and removable, resulting in good patient compliance.

films are useful for demonstrating scapholunate dissociation. Should plain radiographs prove undiagnostic, a triphasic bone scan with cone down views of the wrist is a logical next step. This may confirm a site of inflammation, demonstrate an occult fracture, or reveal an area of avascular necrosis. Based on the bone scan findings, a branch point is reached in the diagnostic work-up. Avascular necrosis problems can be best evaluated with magnetic resonance imaging (MRI), whereas occult fractures or degenerative changes are evaluated best with computerized tomography (CT) or trispiral tomography.[46] Arthrography is helpful when clinical suspicion is directed toward a triangular fibrocartilage complex (TFCC) tear or a dynamic carpal instability. Often, more than one exam in needed. Finally, arthroscopy[8] may be used to determine the extent of the problem or the predominant problem, as when the arthrogram demonstrates both a TFCC tear and a leak in the lunatotriquetral ligament (Fig. 14–22).

The evaluation of wrist injuries in gymnasts is discussed in detail in Chapter 24.

SCAPHOID FRACTURES

The most common fracture of the carpus is the scaphoid fracture. This injury occurs from a blow to the hyperextended wrist as when falling. This injury is seen frequently in football players, players of other contact sports, and gymnasts. If the patient is seen immediately after injury and has "snuff box" swelling and tenderness, he or she must be treated as having a scaphoid fracture and placed in a thumb spica cast even if radiographs are normal. After a minimum of 10 days, the cast is removed, the wrist is reexamined for tenderness, and repeat X rays are obtained. Usually, an occult fracture is visible at this time. If no fracture is seen but significant tenderness is still present, recasting for a few more weeks is indicated.

If on presentation a nondisplaced fracture is discovered, a minimum of 6 weeks of thumb spica casting is required to heal the fracture.[12, 25, 33, 44] A return to sports with protective casting is possible in sports in which a stiff wrist will not be a disability. In sports such as gymnastics, however, the healing bone is subject to excessive loads that may produce stress fractures through the original fracture site, resulting in delayed union or nonunion. These athletes, therefore, need to wait at least 3 months before returning to their normal activities.

Any displaced scaphoid fracture needs accurate reduction and long-term immobilization to allow for healing. This means long arm spica casting for 6 weeks, followed by short arm spica casting for a minimal of 6 more weeks. The proximal pole of the scaphoid should be monitored closely for the development of avascular necrosis. The fracture needs to be healed clinically and radiologically before discontinuing immobilization. At this point, protective splinting could be worn in some sports. If accurate reduction (alignment, within 1 mm, of all cortical margins on all X-ray views) is not obtainable by closed techniques, then open reduction and internal fixation, with or without bone grafting, should be performed[22, 45] (Fig. 14–23).

Improper treatment can lead to nonunion or to a malunion of the scaphoid with articular displacement or volar collapse (a humpback deformity). It should be noted that a nonunion can occur even with proper treatment. Both nonunion and malunion have been shown to lead to degenerative changes in the wrist over a 10- to 20-year period. For the teenage athlete, this may mean the development of arthritis during the "prime earning" years.

FRACTURE-DISLOCATIONS OF THE CARPUS

Fracture-dislocations of the carpus are unusual injuries that must be treated aggressively (Fig. 14–24). They require anatomical reduction and long-term immobilization. Most authors now recommend open reduction and internal fixation not only of the fractures but K-wire pinning of the joints in which the intraosseous ligaments have been torn.[14] Also recommended is the repair of both the dorsal and volar capsules. At surgery the patient is placed in a thumb spica splint until the swelling resolves. Then he or she is placed in a thumb spica cast for 8 weeks. At 8 weeks, the K-wires are removed, and a thumb spica cast is again placed for another 4 weeks. Rehabilitation is then started only if all the fractures have healed and there is no evidence of avascular necrosis.

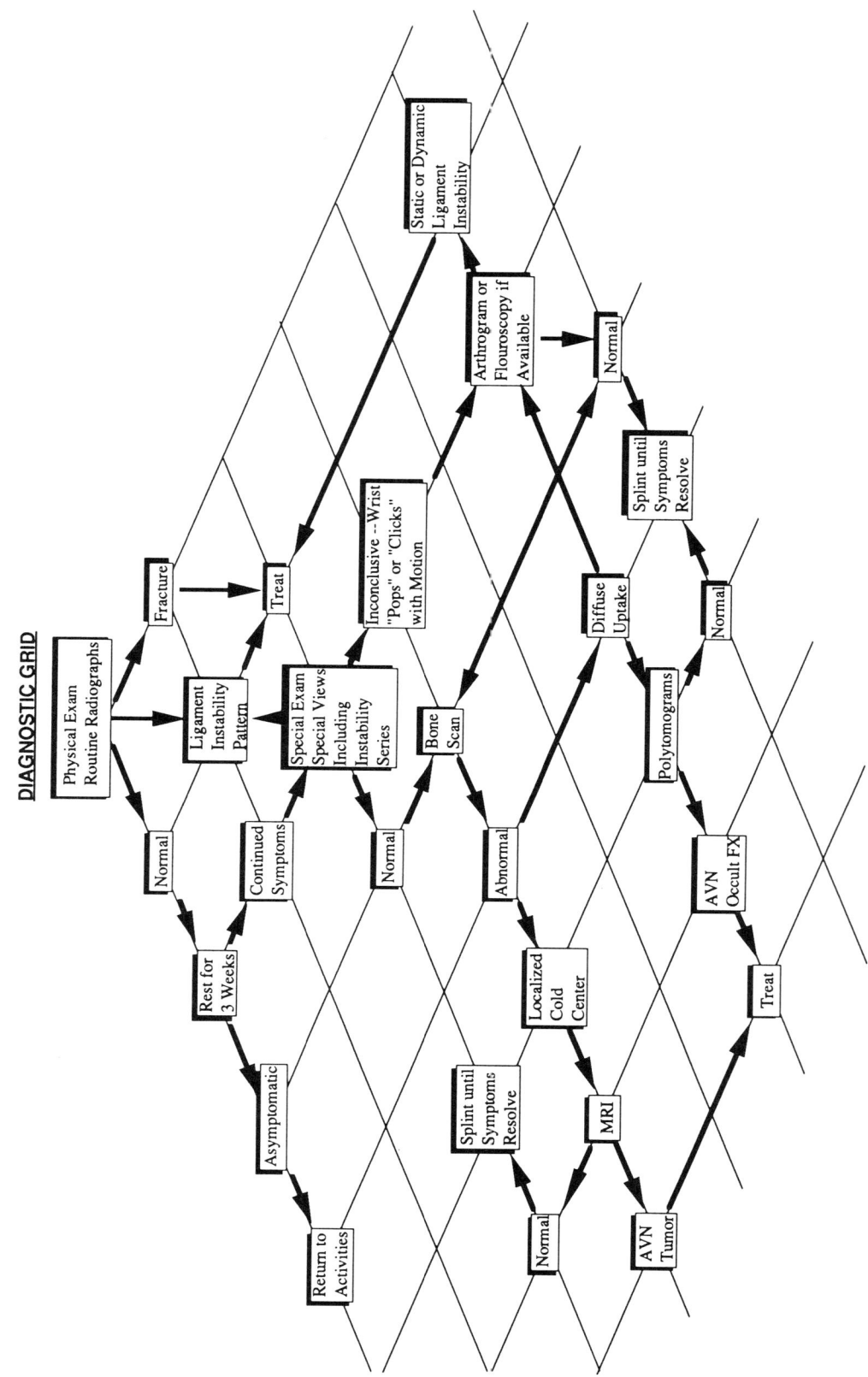

FIGURE 14–22. A diagnostic grid for the evaluation of wrist pain.

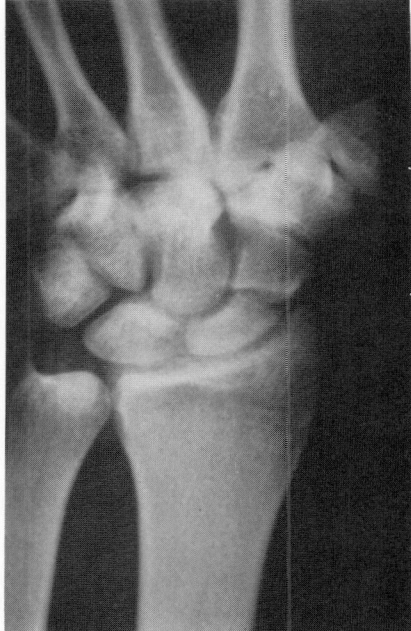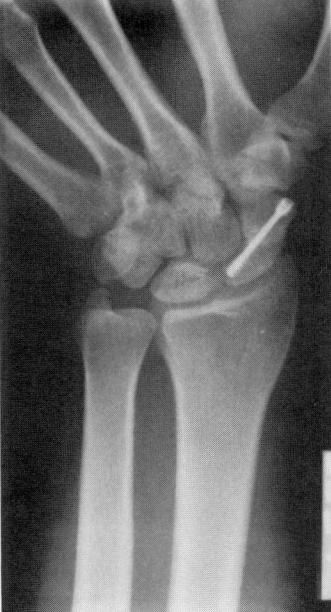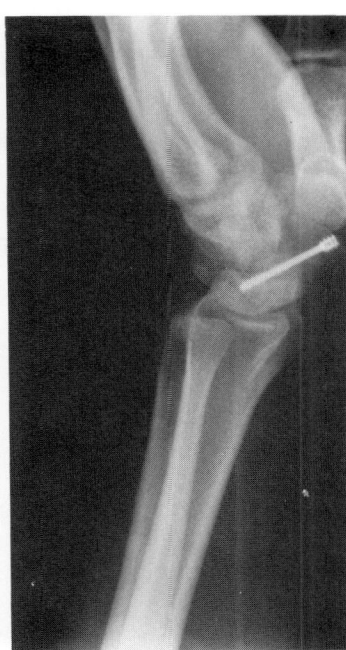

FIGURE 14–23. Radiographs of a scaphoid fracture that occurred in a young athlete while power lifting. The fracture did not heal with conservative casting and required internal fixation with a Herbert screw and bone grafting.

CARPAL INSTABILITIES

While carpal ligamentous injuries are unusual in the adolescent athlete, a combination of wrist hyperextension and intracarpal supination or pronation can produce intraosseous ligament injuries. The intraosseous ligaments in the wrist are short and taut, with little elasticity. Injury to these ligaments may range from intraligamentous tears to complete ruptures. If complete ligamentous disruptions occur, the injury is easily recognized in the acute stage. Dorsal intercalary segmental instability (DISI) or volar intercalary segmental instability (VISI) posturing may be present on plain radiographs and implicate the involvement of specific structures. In DISI posturing, the lunate is dorsiflexed and the scapholunate angle on a lateral radiograph is greater than 80 degrees (Fig. 14–25). This deformity results from a combined injury of the scapholunate intracarpal ligament and the volar radioscaphoid, radioscapholunate, and scaphocapitate ligaments. With VISI deformity, the lunate is volarflexed, and the lunatotriquetral angle decreases from its normal angle of 14 degrees to an average of minus 16 degrees.[47] This deformity is due to disruption of the lunatotriquetral ligaments and the volar ulnotriquetral ligament. Complete intraosseous ligament disruption is often recognized by intracarpal widening on the initial radiographs. For example, the "Terry Thomas sign," a widening of the space between the scaphoid and the lunate, is produced by disruption of the intracarpal scapholunate ligament (Fig. 14–26).

These injuries can be treated with either percutaneous pinning or open ligament repair and K-wire protection. As with fracture-dislocations, the immobilization takes 8 weeks with pins and 4 weeks of additional casting. Sports are obviously postponed until wrist motion returns.

The treatment of less severe wrist sprains is even more problematic than the treatment of obvious carpal instabilities. The patient with partial or complete interosseous rupture with intact volar ligaments will usually present with normal initial radiographs. The intact volar ligaments may stretch out over time in these cases, leading to eventual dynamic instability and ultimately degenera-

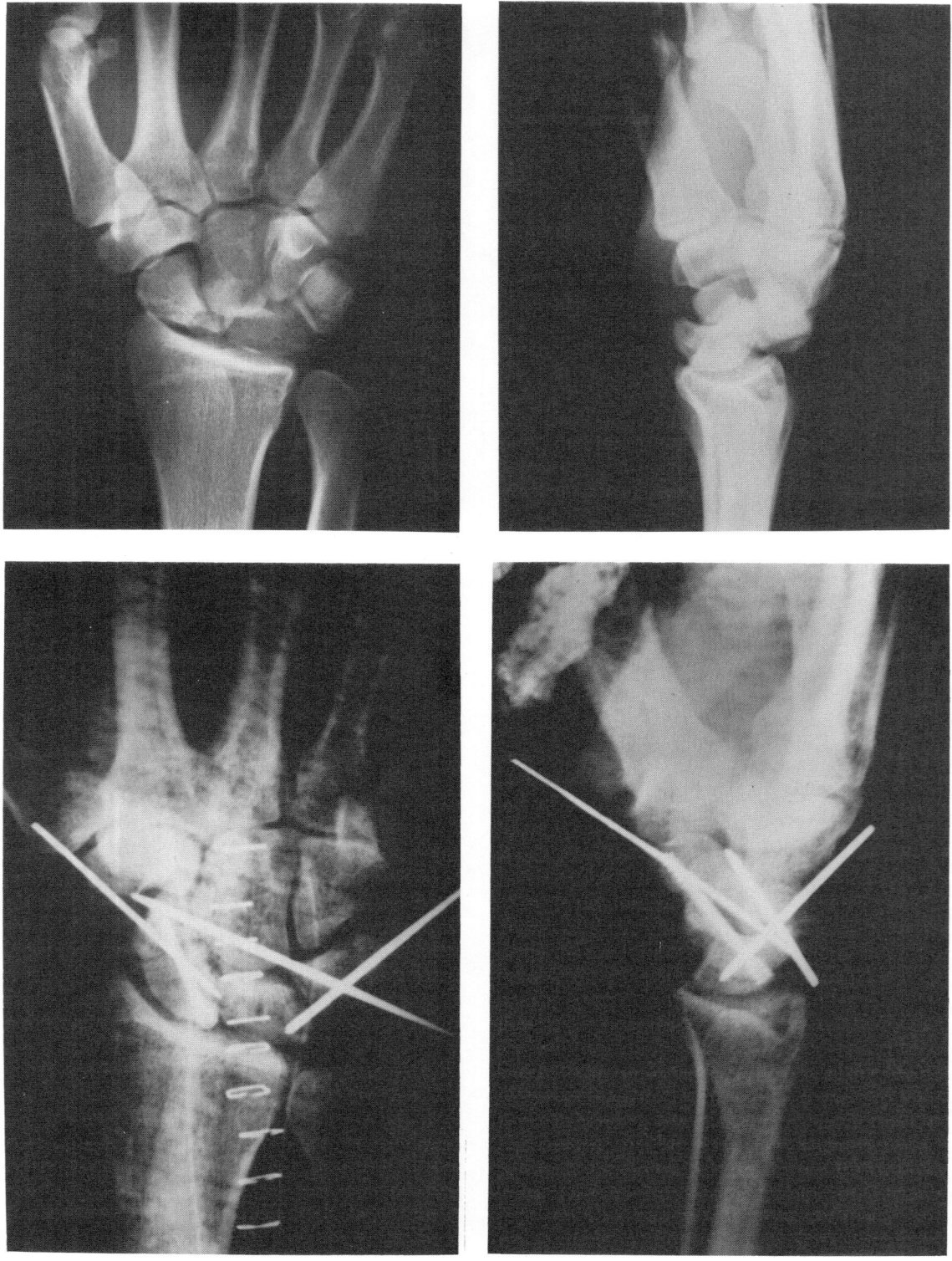

FIGURE 14–24. Radiographs of a transscaphoid perilunate fracture disloaction of the wrist. Postreduction films show internal fixation of the scaphoid fracture with a Herbert screw and reduction of the carpus with several K-wires.

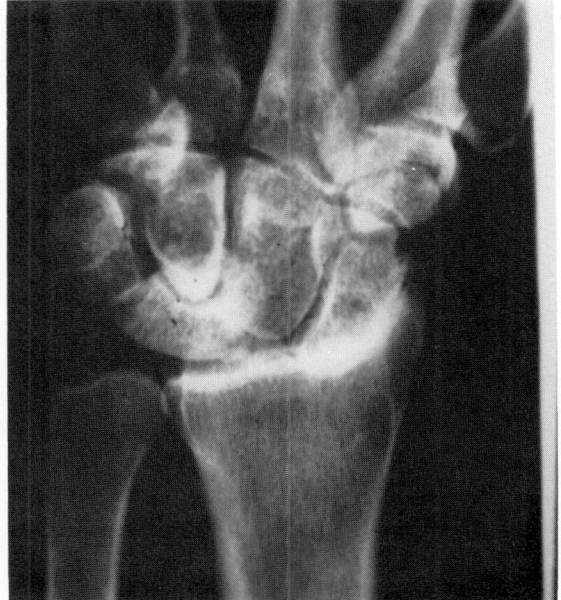
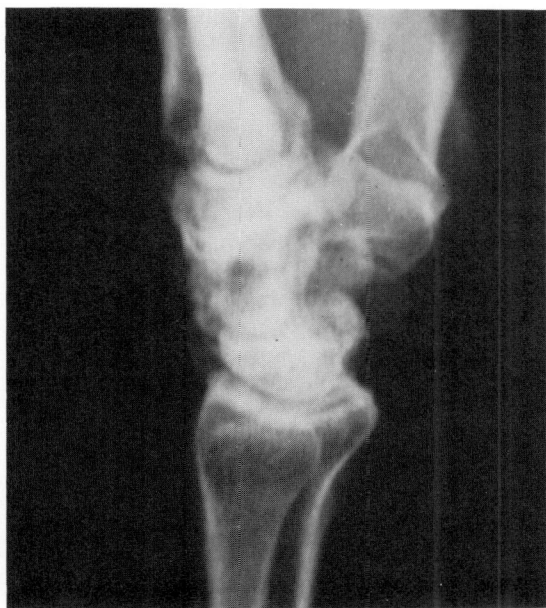

FIGURE 14–25. Radiographs of DISI posturing in a wrist. The dynamic rotatory instability of the scaphoid has led to the secondary arthritic changes over time. The pattern that is now seen has been termed scapholunate advanced collapse (SLAC).

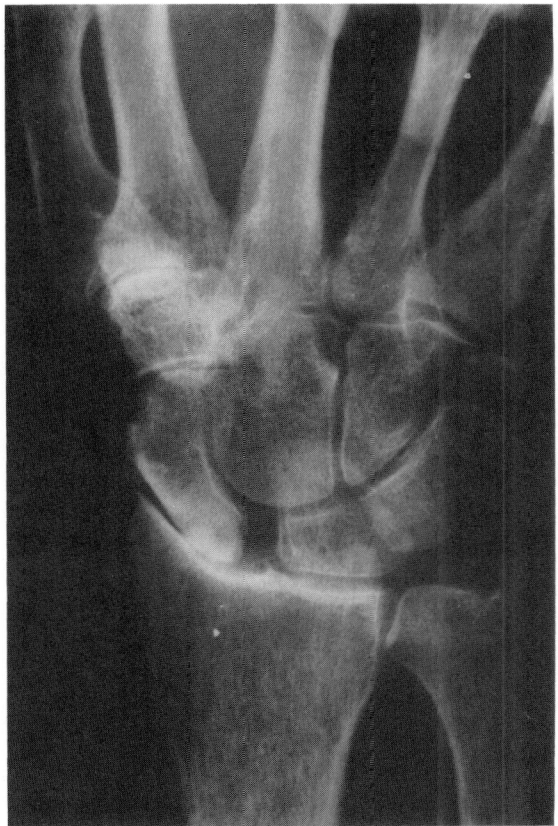

FIGURE 14–26. Radiograph showing the "Terry Thomas" sign in a wrist with a scapholunate dissociation and the secondary degenerative changes (SLAC wrist) that occur as a result of this injury. A scapholunate gap greater than 3 mm is considered diagnostic for scapholunate dissociation. Comparison wrist films may provide a more definitive diagnosis when widening of the scapholunate gap is in question.

tive changes. It is these "sprained wrist" injuries that need to be rested and reevaluated after 3 to 4 weeks. If the wrist is still tender at this time, and an arthrogram demonstrates a ligament tear consistent with the clinical findings, then our treatment of choice in the young athlete is to attempt a ligament repair and pinning of the joint. This surgery is difficult, however, and its long-term benefits are so far unproven. If the diagnosis is delayed, treatment becomes more difficult. There is no uniformity of opinion among the major authors for chronic dynamic carpal instability, and no routine intracarpal fusion has long enough follow-up to be recommended for use in teenagers.

It is our belief that no wrist sprain may be assumed benign. It is difficult, if not impossible, to distinguish between a partial rupture of a ligament and a lesser injury at the time of initial evaluation. Continued athletic stress on an injured avascular ligament could lead to progressive instability and disability. We feel that all "sprained" wrists with normal radiographs need to be rested and evaluated in 3 to 4 weeks. If there is no localized discomfort at this time, return to athletic activities can be allowed if the patient is followed closely. If pain continues, a thorough work-up is warranted before deciding on treatment and return to sports. Athletes who persist in playing with a sprained wrist risk the possibility of late carpal instability and subsequent degenerative arthritis.

References

1. Bennett, E. H.: Fractures of the metacarpal bones. Dublin J. Med. Sci., 73:72–75, 1882.
2. Bora, F. W., and Didizian, N. H.: The treatment of injuries to the carpometacarpal joint of the little finger. J. Bone Joint Surg., 56A:1459–1463, 1974.
3. Brunet, M. E., and Haddad, R. J.: Fractures and dislocations of the metacarpals and phalanges. Clin. Sports Med., 5(4):773–793, 1966.
4. Burton, R. I., and Eaton, R. G.: Common hand injuries in the athlete. Orthop. Clin. North Am. 4:809–838, 1973.
5. Butt, W. D.: Fractures of the hand: I. Description. Can. Med. Assoc. J., 86:731–735, 1962.
6. Campbell, C. S.: Gamekeeper's thumb. J. Bone Joint Surg., 37B:148–149, 1955.
7. Degroot, H., and Mass, D. P.: Hand injury patterns in softball players using a 16 inch ball. Am. J. Sports Med., 16(3):260–265, 1988.
8. Eddeland, A.; Eiken, O.; Hellgren, E.; and Ohlsson, N. M.: Fractures of the scaphoid. Scand. J. Plast. Reconstr. Surg., 9:234–239, 1975.
9. Elliot, R. A.: Injuries to the extensor mechanism of the hand. Orthop. Clin. North Am., 1:335–354, 1970.
10. Elliot, R. A.: Splints for mallet and boutonnière deformities. Plast. Reconstr. Surg., 52:282–285, 1973.
11. Farabeuf, L.H.F. (as quoted by Barnard, H. L.): Dorsal dislocation of the first phalanx of the little finger. Reduction by Farabeuf's dorsal incision. Lancet, 188–190, 1901.
12. Gasser, H.: Delayed union and pseudarthrosis of the carpal navicular: Treatment by compression-screw osteosynthesis: A preliminary report of twenty fractures. J. Bone Joint Surg., 47A:249–266, 1965.
13. Green, D. P.: The sore wrist without a fracture. AAOS Instructional Course Lectures, Vol. 34. C. V. Mosby Co., St. Louis, pp. 300–313, 1985.
14. Green, D. P.: Operative Hand Surgery, Vol. 2. New York, Churchill Livingstone, Inc., 1988.
15. Green, D. P., and O'Brien, E. T.: Fractures of the thumb metacarpal. South. Med. J., 65:807–814, 1972.
16. Green, D. P., and Terry, G. C.: Complex dislocation of the metacarpophalangeal joint. J. Bone Joint Surg., 55A:1480–1486, 1973.
17. Hunter, J. M., and Cowen, N. J.: Fifth metacarpal fractures in a compensation clinic population. J. Bone Joint Surg., 52A:1159–1165, 1970.
18. Kaplan, E. B.: Dorsal dislocation of the metacarpophalangeal joint of the index finger. J. Bone Joint Surg., 39A:1081–1086, 1957.
19. Kleinman, W. B.: The "Shear" test. Am. Soc. Surg. Hand Corr. Newsl., 51, 1985.
20. Lamb, D. W.; Abernethy, P. J.; and Fragiadakis, E.: Injuries of the metacarpophalangeal joint of the thumb. Hand, 3:164–168, 1971.
21. Macey, M. B., and Murray, R. A.: Fractures about the base of the first metacarpal with special reference to Bennett's fracture. South. Med. J., 42:931–935, 1949.
22. Maudsley, R. H., and Chen, S. C.: Screw fixation in the management of the fractured carpal scaphoid. J. Bone Joint Surg., 54B:432–441, 1972.
23. McCue, F. C.; Baugher, W. H.; Kulund, D. N.; et al.: Hand and wrist injuries in the athlete. Am. J. Sports Med. 7:275–286, 1979.
24. McCue, F. C., and Garroeay, R. Y.: Sports injuries to the hand and wrist. In Schneider, R. C. (ed.): Sports Injuries: Mechanisms, Prevention and Treatment. Baltimore, Williams & Wilkins, 1985.
25. McLaughlin, H. L.: Fracture of the carpal navicular (scaphoid) bone: Some observations based on treatment by open reduction and internal fixation. J. Bone Joint Surg., 36A:765–774, 1954.
26. McLaughlin, H. L.: Complex "locked" dislocation of the metacarpophalangeal joints. J. Trauma, 5:683–688, 1965.
27. McNealy, R. W., and Lichtenstein, M. E.: Bennett's fracture and other fractures of the first metacarpal. Surg. Gynecol. Obstet., 56:197–201, 1933.
28. McNealy, R. W., and Lichtenstein, M. E.: Fractures of the bones of the hand. Am J. Surg., 50:563–570, 1940.
29. Mogensen, B. A., and Mattsson, H. S.: Post-traumatic instability of the metacarpophalangeal joint of the thumb. Hand, 12:85–90, 1980.
30. Parikh, M.; Nahigian, S.; and Froimson, A.: Gamekeeper's thumb. Plast. Reconstr. Surg., 58:24–31, 1976.
31. Posner, M. A.: Injuries to the hand and wrist in athletes. Orthop. Clin. North Am., 8:593–617, 1977.

32. Ramamurthy, S.: Operative Hand Surgery, Vol. 1. New York, Churchill Livingstone, Inc., 1988.
33. Reagan, D. S.; Linscheid, R. L.; and Dobyns, J. H.: Lunotriquetral sprains. J. Hand Surg., 9A:502–514, 1984.
34. Rockwood, C. A., and Green, D. P. (eds.): Fractures in Adults, Vol. 1, 2nd ed. Philadelphia, J. B. Lippincott Co., 1984.
35. Rockwood, C. A., and Green, D. P. (eds.): Fractures in Children, Vol. 3. Philadelphia, J. B. Lippincott Co., 1984.
36. Rolando, S.: Fracture de la base du premier metacarpien: Et principalement sur une variété non encore decrite. Presse Med., 33:303, 1910.
37. Schubiner, J. M., and Mass, D. P.: Operation for collateral ligament ruptures of the metacarpophalangeal joints of the fingers. Br. Ed. Soc. Bone Joint Surg., 71B:388, 1989.
38. Simmons, B. P., and Lovallo, J. L.: Hand and wrist injuries in children. Clin. Sports Med., 7(3):495–510, 1988.
39. Smith, R. J.: Post-traumatic instability of the metacarpophalangeal joint of the thumb. J. Bone Joint Surg., 59A:14–21, 1977.
40. Stack, H. G.: Mallet finger. Hand, 1:83–89, 1969.
41. Stark, H. H.; Boyes, J. H.; and Wilson, J. N.: Mallet finger. J. Bone Joint Surg., 44A:1061–1068, 1962.
42. Stener, B.: Hyperextension injuries of the metacarpophalangeal joint of the thumb—rupture of ligaments, fracture of sesamoid bones, rupture of flexor pollicis brevis. An anatomical and clinical study. Acta Chir. Scand., 125:275–293, 1963.
43. Thompson, J. S., and Eatonm, R. G.: Volar dislocation of the proximal interphalangeal joint (abst.). J. Hand Surg., 2:232, 1977.
44. Vahvanen, V., and Westerlund, M.: Fracture of the carpal scaphoid in children: A clinical and roentgenological study of 108 cases. Acta Orthop. Scand., 51:909–913, 1980.
45. Verdan, C.: Fractures of the scaphoid. Surg. Clin. North Am., 40:461–464, 1960.
46. Weeks, P. M.: Acute Bone and Joint Injuries of the Hand and Wrist. A Clinical Guide to Management. St. Louis, C. V. Mosby Co., 1981.
47. Zilberman, Z.; Rotschild, E.; and Krauss, L.: Rupture of the ulnar collateral ligament of the thumb. J. Trauma, 5:477–481, 1965.

15

OSTEOCHONDRITIS DISSECANS

BEN K. GRAF
RICHARD H. LANGE

Osteochondritis dissecans is a condition resulting in partial or complete separation of a segment of normal hyaline cartilage from its supporting bone. The plane of separation may be superficial to the subchondral bone, creating a purely cartilaginous lesion, or more commonly, just deep to the subchondral plate, creating an osteochondral fragment. Initially, the cartilage of the lesion may be contiguous with the adjacent joint surface and abnormal only in its lack of firm bony support. Later, that lack of support may result in an unstable fragment that causes mechanical symptoms such as catching and locking. Finally, the fragment may completely separate from its bed and create a loose body within the joint.

ETIOLOGY

Although it has been more than 100 years since König[1] coined the term *osteochondritis dissecans*, there is still little agreement about the etiology of this disease. The four theories that are commonly suggested are ischemia, genetic predisposition, abnormal ossification, and trauma.

ISCHEMIA

The ischemic theory was first proposed in 1920 by Rieger[2] and in 1922 by Axhausen,[3] the latter suggesting that tubercle bacilli blocked subchondral end arteries and the former proposing that fat emboli could have a similar effect. More recently, Watson-Jones[4] described how thrombosis of end arteries resulted in the avascular necrosis of subchondral bone and the formation of an osteochondritic lesion. Several authors,[5,6,7] however, have found that osteochondritic lesions are not always necrotic. Some lesions of the medial femoral condyle that are in the classic location will maintain a blood supply from the intercondylar notch and contain no necrotic bone. Furthermore, these lesions can grow at nearly the same rate as the surrounding condyle.[8] Rogers and Gladstone[9] found the blood supply of the distal femur to be so luxuriant that ischemia was unlikely. Finally, Milgram[7] found many osteochondritic lesions that contained no bone, a situation unlikely to occur if bone necrosis is the key etiologic event.

GENETIC PREDISPOSITION

There have been numerous reports of families in whom more than one member was affected by osteochondritis dissecans.[10, 11, 12, 13, 14, 15, 16] Mubarak and Carroll[17] reported on 31 members of one family with osteochondritis dissecans. They found that the inheritance was due to an autosomal dominant trait with 100 percent penetrance in the second generation, 75 percent in the third, and thus far, 6 of 14 members in the fourth.

Petrie,[18] however, examined 34 patients with osteochondritis dissecans and 86 of their first-degree relatives; only 1 relative had osteochondritis dissecans, and no other forms of osteochondrosis, endocrine abnormalities, or dwarfism were found. Therefore, while some cases are genetically predisposed, the majority do not have a hereditary basis.

ABNORMAL OSSIFICATION

In 1941, Sontag and Pyle[19] first noted that irregular epiphyseal outlines and even calcified areas beyond the border of the epiphysis were common in children. They felt this was due to disseminated provisional calcification of areas of the epiphyseal cartilage. Such changes were found to occur in 67 percent of boys and 90 percent of girls by 18 months of age. Usually, the irregularities were gone within 2 years of onset. Caffey et al.[20] evaluated 147 children between the ages of 3 and 13 who had no symptoms of knee problems and found that irregularities at the margins of the distal femoral epiphysis were extremely common in normal children and that often the irregularities were indistinguishable from osteochondritis dissecans. Like Sontag and Pyle, they identified epiphyseal irregularities in nearly 90 percent of 4-year-olds but in less than 20 percent of 12-year-olds. Ribbing[21] noted similar changes in the knee joints of 291 normal children under the age of 10 years. He found the location and sex distribution of these abnormalities to be similar to that of osteochondritis dissecans.

In summary, epiphyseal irregularities are extremely common in young children, can be radiographically indistinguishable from osteochondritis dissecans, and yet only rarely develop into true osteochondritic lesions. It may be that, as Ribbing postulated, an accessory bony nucleus constitutes a "locus minoris resistentiae" that later, as a result of even minor trauma, may become an osteochondritic lesion.

TRAUMA

Since Konig's[1] description in 1888, trauma has been the most popular explanation for osteochondritis dissecans. Fairbank[5] felt that direct trauma could be ruled out, since the most common sites of occurrence were well protected from direct blows. He noted that the patella comes in contact with the classic site of an osteochondritic lesion (the lateral aspect of the medial femoral condyle) when the knee is fully flexed. Fairbank also found that with forced internal rotation of the tibia the medial tibial spine impinged on the lateral aspect of the medial femoral condyle. Additional support for the traumatic theory came when Kennedy[22] created osteochondral fractures in human cadavers through a combination of axial loading and rotational forces.

Numerous animal experiments have also suggested that trauma can induce lesions similar to osteochondritis dissecans. Rehbein[23] found that in dogs repetitive trauma produced a fibrous demarcation of the cartilage but no loose bodies. Langenskiold[24] gouged the epiphysis of 4- to 7-day-old rabbits so that a 2-mm fragment of cartilage was left attached to the femur by a narrow bridge of synovial tissue from the intercondylar notch. After 33 to 116 days, lesions with a bony nidus developed that histologically and radiographically resembled osteochondritic dissecans. Aichroth,[25] using adult rabbits, found that unstable osteochondral fractures did not heal and produced fragments similar to those of osteochondritis dissecans.

Clinical support for the traumatic theory is incomplete. About 40 percent of patients who have osteochondritis dissecans have a history of prior trauma.[26, 27, 28, 29] In Mubarak and Carrol's[29] series, however, half of the patients with a history of trauma had bilateral lesions, raising questions regarding the traumatic etiology. In addition, they found a tall medial tibial spine in only 30 percent of the children in their series, and half of those had lateral rather than medial condylar lesions.

In summary, a literature review fails to support a single etiology for all the lesions we now call osteochondritis dissecans. It appears likely that multiple factors, acting either singly or in combination, are involved.[30, 31]

CLINICAL PRESENTATION

INCIDENCE

As shown in Figure 15–1, osteochondritis dissecans is most likely to become symptomatic during the second decade of life. The youngest reported case, however, involves a 5-year-old,[32] so this entity must be con-

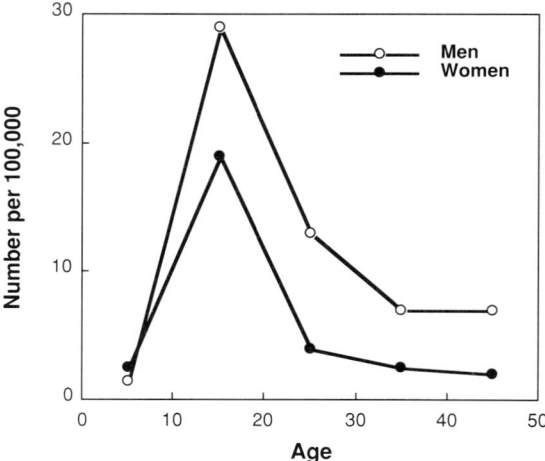

FIGURE 15–1. The age distribution of osteochondritis dissecans of the femoral condyles. (After Linden B: The incidence of osteochondritis dissecans in the condyles of the femur. Acta Orthop Scand 47:665, 1976.

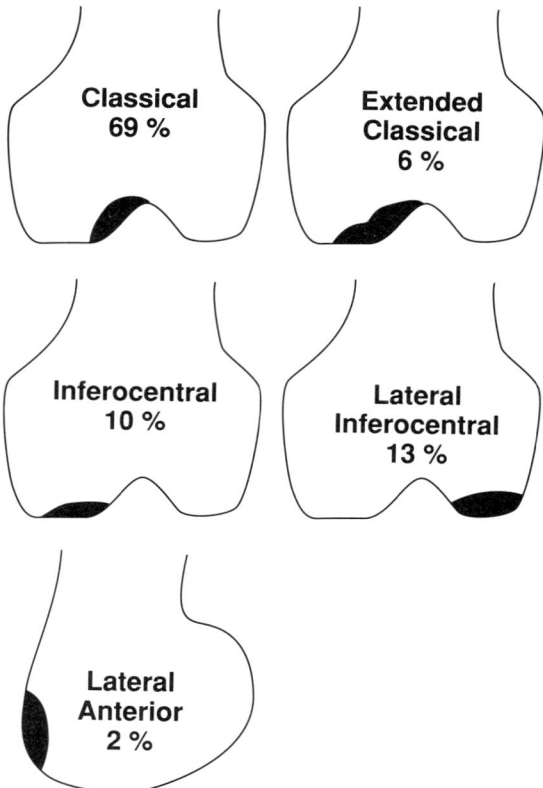

FIGURE 15–2. The site distribution of osteochrondritis dissecans of the femoral condyles. (After Aichroth P: Osteochondritis dissecans of the knee. A clinical survey. J Bone Joint Surg 53(B):440, 1971.

sidered even when evaluating young patients. It occurs most commonly in the knee, although the talus and capitellum of the humerus can also be affected. Within the knee, there has been one reported case of osteochondritis of the tibial plateau[33] and numerous reports of lesions of the patella.[34, 35, 36, 37] The vast majority of cases, however, involve the distal femur. As seen in Figure 15–2, the most common location is the so-called classic site on the lateral aspect of the medial femoral condyle. Involvement can also extend further onto the weight-bearing surface (Fig. 15–3) and less frequently may involve only the inferocentral region of the medial femoral condyle. Lateral femoral condylar lesions occur in approximately 15 percent of cases (Fig. 15–4).[36] Males develop this condition approximately twice as often as females.[26, 38] The incidence of bilateral involvement has not been firmly established. Mubarak and Carroll[29] reported bilateral involvement to be as high as 47 percent among 73 children under the age of 18. In 100 patients, Aichroth[26] found that 26 percent had a lesion in the opposite knee and 7 percent had a lesion at a site other than the knee. Green,[27] however, found only three bilateral lesions among 40 patients.

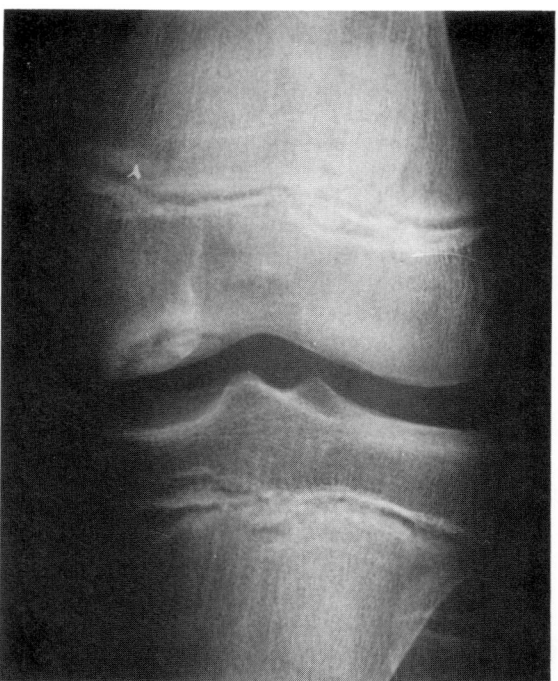

FIGURE 15–3. Extended classic lesion of the medial femoral condyle in the left knee of a 13-year-old male.

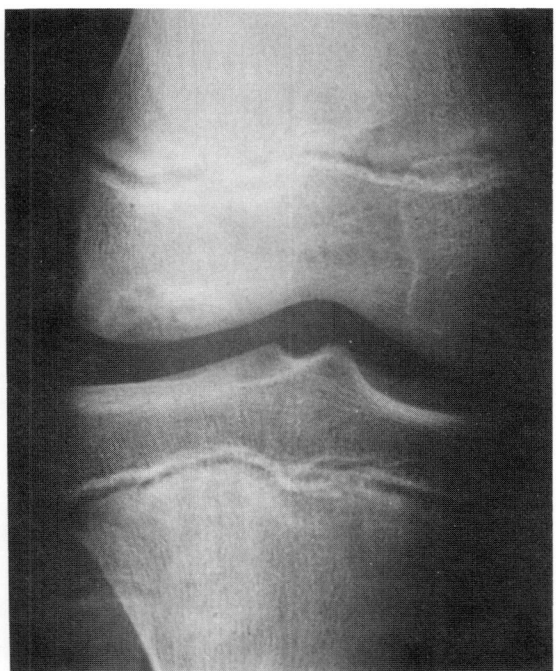

FIGURE 15–4. Lateral femoral condyle lesion in the right knee of this same patient.

that patients may walk with external rotation of the involved tibia. Once mechanical symptoms have appeared, there may be a joint effusion, catching, or even locking. If the fragment has completely separated, a loose body may be palpable.

RADIOGRAPHIC EXAMINATION

With such nonspecific historical and physical findings, radiographic evaluation is the key to diagnosis. In addition to the standard anterior-posterior (AP), lateral, and patellar radiographs, a notch or tunnel view should also be obtained. This is necessary because the classic location of the lesion on the lateral aspect of the medial femoral condyle is often not visible on the standard AP but is easily seen on the tunnel view (Figs. 15–5 and 15–6). The lateral radiograph should also be closely examined, especially in the area between a line extending along the roof of the intercondylar notch and a line drawn along the posterior border of the femur[40] (Fig. 15–7).

HISTORY

Initial symptoms of osteochondritis dissecans are often vague. The patient's chief complaint is usually pain, and its intensity is often related to the patient's activity level. Once a lesion becomes loose, mechanical symptoms may arise. Patients may note catching, locking, or giving way, and a joint effusion may develop.

PHYSICAL EXAMINATION

Early in the course of the disease, the physical examination may be entirely normal. There may be tenderness when the knee is flexed and pressure applied just medial or lateral to the patellar tendon. Wilson's test,[39] performed by flexing the knee 90 degrees, internally rotating the tibia, and then extending the knee gradually, is positive when anterior knee pain is produced at 30 degrees short of full extension and relieved when the tibia is externally rotated. In the author's experience, this test is often but not consistently positive in patients with classic lesions of the medial femoral condyle. Wilson also noted

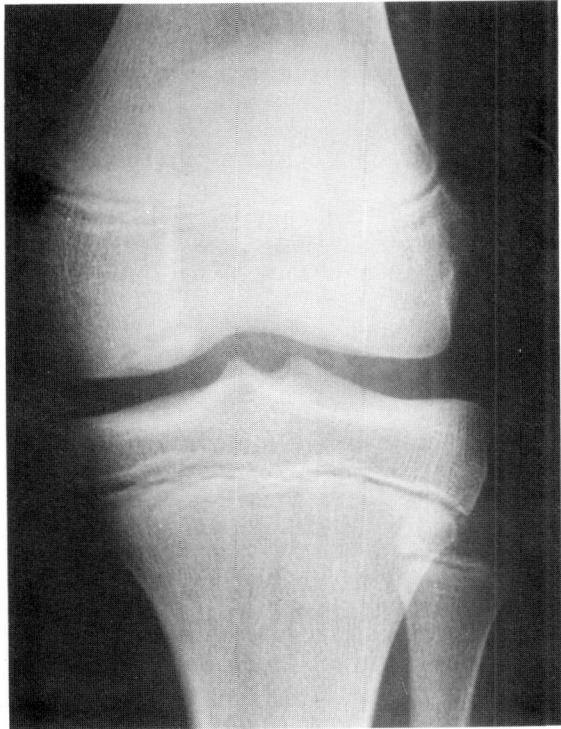

FIGURE 15–5. This classic lesion of the medial femoral condyle is visible on the AP radiograph.

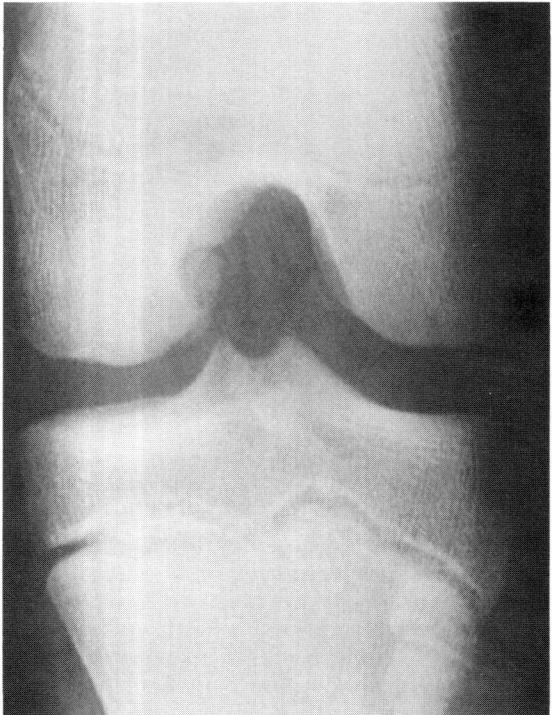

FIGURE 15–6. The notch view better defines the area of involvement.

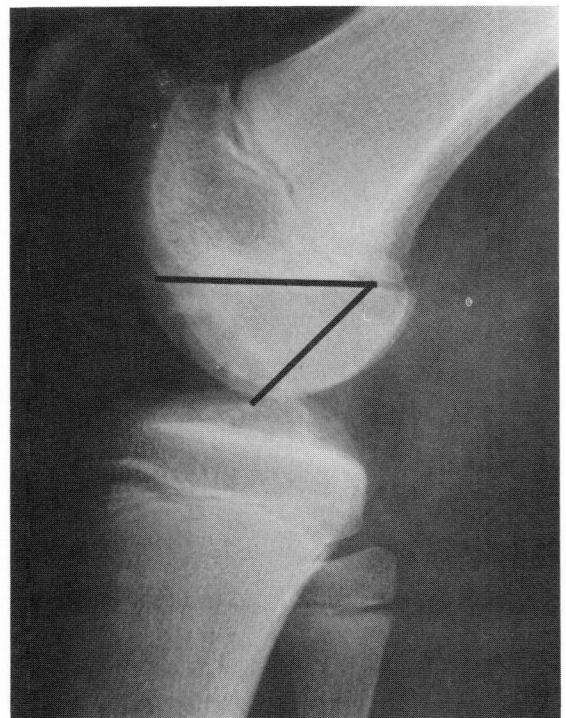

FIGURE 15–7. On the lateral radiograph, the lesion can be seen to lie in the area defined by the roof of the intercondylar notch and an imaginary extension of the posterior femoral cortex.

The lesion may appear as an empty crater if the fragment is not ossified or has broken free, but more commonly, it will be filled with one or more bony fragments. As noted by Milgram,[7] radiodensity in the lesion may be secondary to subchondral bone within the fragment, calcification of degenerative articular cartilage, new bone formation following attempted repair, or calcification in new layers of bone and cartilage deposited around the nidus after it became a free loose body.

Once the diagnosis of osteochondritis is made, additional information can be obtained from the radiographs that will help in planning treatment. First, the skeletal maturity of the patient should be assessed, since the prognosis for healing is more favorable in patients with open growth plates. Second, signs of displacement of the fragment provide important clues about the lesion. If the calcified portion of the fragment is clearly displaced, then it is almost certain that the articular cartilage has been broken and the lesion is unstable. Third, the characteristics of the crater may provide some prognostic information. Mesgarzadeh et al.[41] have shown that lesions greater than 0.8 cm^2 are likely to be loose, and those smaller than 0.2 cm^2 are likely to be stable. He also noted that a sclerotic margin of greater than 3 mm correlated with instability of the lesion.

SPECIAL STUDIES

In many cases, further studies are indicated to investigate the stability of the lesion. Arthrography, once the preferred technique for evaluating the integrity of the articular surface, is gradually being replaced by magnetic resonance imaging (MRI). A good quality MRI shows not only the breaks in the articular surface but also fluid underneath unstable lesions. Such fluid will appear as an area of extremely high signal with T2 weighting, and it often will communicate with the surface. The high signal indicating fluid should not be confused with the moderate-intensity signals that can occur with fibrosis and edema beneath stable lesions (Figs. 15–8, 15–9, 15–10, 15–11).

OSTEOCHONDRITIS DISSECANS   245

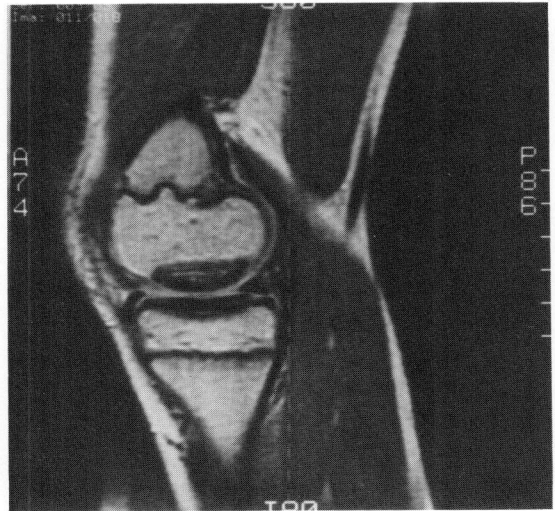

FIGURE 15–8. This MRI of the knee shown in Figure 15–3 shows extensive involvement of the medial femoral condyle on the T1 weighted image.

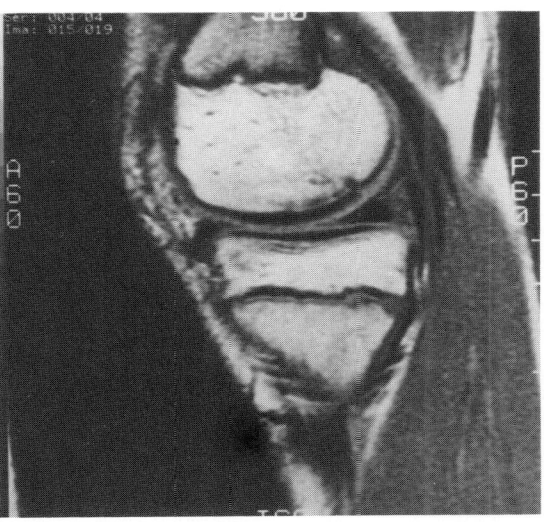

FIGURE 15–10. Two years after drilling there is nearly complete healing on T1 images.

Bone scans have also been recommended as predictors of stability.[42, 43] Mesgarzadeh[41] found all lesions with grade III or IV uptake on the late phase to be unstable and lesions with grade O or I uptake to be stable. Grade II uptake was not predictive. Cahill and Berg,[44] however, using technetium scans to monitor the progress of healing, thought that the initial scintigraphic activity lacked prognostic value.

Computerized tomography (CT) has been shown to be helpful in diagnosing patellar involvement,[36] whereas polytomography is valuable in defining the osseous component of femoral lesions. Lateral tomograms specifically aid surgical planning by determining whether a fragment contains sufficient bone to allow screw fixation (Fig. 15–12).

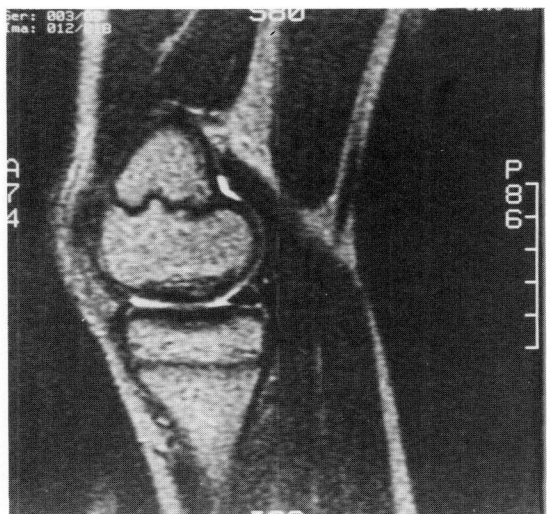

FIGURE 15–9. On the T2 image, there is increased signal in the depths of the crater but not the high signal that would be associated with a loose fragment. This was confirmed arthroscopically, with the articular surface noted to be entirely intact and the lesion stable.

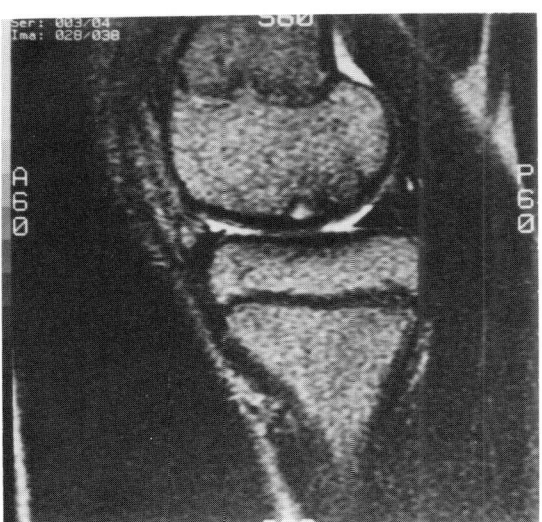

FIGURE 15–11. T2 shows only one small remaining area of increased signal, suggesting near complete healing. The patient was entirely asymptomatic at this time, and plain radiograph also suggested complete healing.

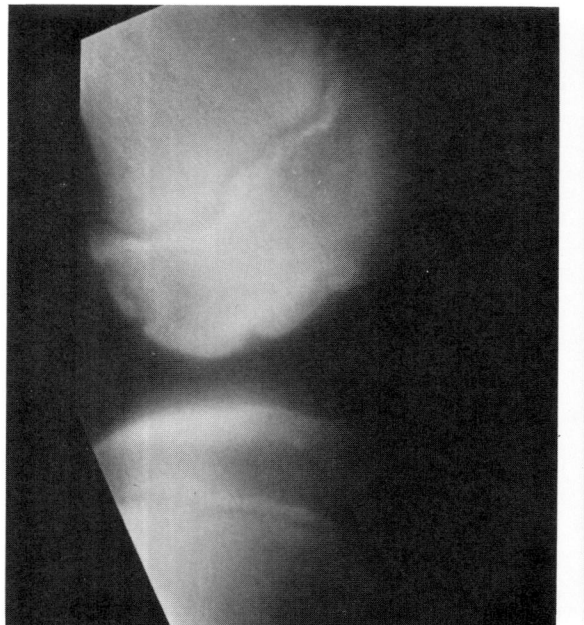 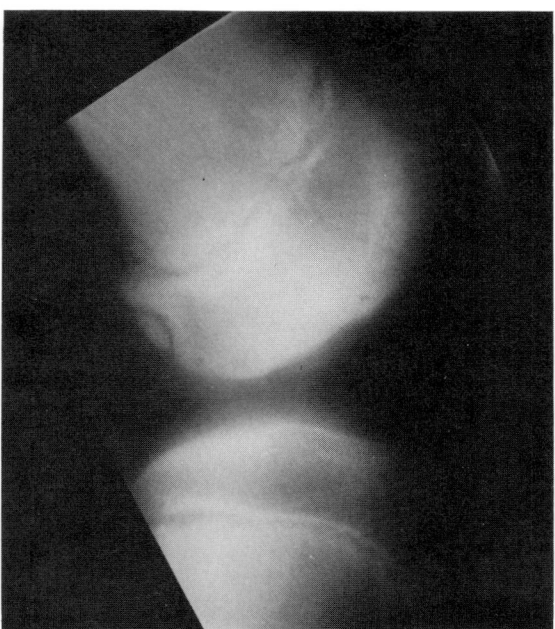

FIGURE 15–12. These lateral tomograms define two distinct areas of involvement in the lateral femoral condyle of this patient.

ARTHROSCOPY

Arthroscopic examination provides the definitive evaluation of integrity of the articular surface and the stability of an osteochondritic lesion.[45, 46, 47] Both visual and tactile (probe) examination should be used to assess the lesion. Arthroscopic techniques can also be used to treat many patients, as will be discussed later.

TREATMENT

The treatment of osteochondritis dissecans depends on the patient's age, the degree of symptoms, and the stability and location of the lesion. The goal of treatment of osteochondritis dissecans is to produce union of the fragment with restoration of a congruous joint surface. In situ lesions should be treated to encourage union, unstable lesions should be stabilized, and whenever possible, loose bodies should be replaced in their bed and stabilized. Most of the techniques outlined below are indicated in specific situations. These techniques include nonoperative treatment by observation, immobilization, or non–weight-bearing and operative treatment by removal of the fragment and curettage or abrasion of the bed, drilling, bone grafting, and fixation with either bone pegs, pins, or Herbert screws.

NONOPERATIVE

Nonoperative treatment has its greatest likelihood of success in patients with open growth plates. Wiberg[48] reported six cases of spontaneous healing of osteochondritic lesions in patients under the age of 16, whereas Van Demark[49] reported two cases, ages 11 and 13. Green[50] reported on 18 knees in patients under the age of 15 that were treated with either a weight-bearing cast or a brace; 17 of these knees healed after an average of approximately 4 months. Unfortunately, even in young patients, conservative treatment is not uniformly successful. In Cahill's[46] series of 34 skeletally immature patients with osteochondritic dissecans, four lesions detached while under observation, and six others required surgery because of worsening symptoms.

OPERATIVE

Operative treatment is often indicated in patients who have failed nonoperative management, have loose fragments, or who are skeletally mature at presentation. Surgical options range from simple debridement of the unstable cartilage to more demanding techniques for grafting and internal fixation.

Fragment Removal

Several authors have recommended removal of loose bodies or unstable lesions with curettage or abrasion of the bed. Although the short-term results of the arthroscopic form of this treatment have been good,[51, 52] the long-term results of the equivalent open procedure have been less encouraging. Degenerative changes are more commonly seen when the osteochondritis dissecans involves a large area of the weight-bearing surface.[53] It has also been found that concurrent or subsequent meniscectomy leads to further deterioration of the long-term results.[53, 54] Removal of the fragment does, however, appear to be better tolerated when it is done prior to growth plate closure rather than after skeletal maturity.[28]

Pin Fixation

Concern about the late effects of removal of the osteochondritic fragments led Smillie to recommend operative fixation of loose fragments to promote their healing.[55] He noted healing in 7 of 10 patients who were treated with drilling and pin fixation. Lipscomb et al.[56] recommended fixation of loose fragments with Kirschner wires combined with drilling of the bed and/or bone grafting. The wires were placed antegrade through the lesion and advanced until the tips penetrated the metaphysis of the femur. In this way, they could be removed in a retrograde manner, without opening the knee joint, 3 to 6 weeks after surgery. Weight bearing was delayed until fragments united, 6 to 16 weeks postoperatively. Union was obtained in seven of eight knees. Hughston et al.[53] and Guhl[57] have also reported encouraging results using similar techniques.

Bone Peg Fixation

Bone peg fixation has been used both to reattach free fragments and to provide stability to unstable in situ fragments.[58, 59, 60, 61, 62] This technique, which does not require a second operation to remove hardware, has been successful in uniting the fragments in all the cases reported. Healing times averaged 5 months in the various series. However, in spite of these high union rates, not all fragments were anatomically reduced. Lindholm and Osterman[60] reported that 68 percent of cases had a smooth joint surface, 19 percent had a depressed fragment, and 13 percent had a raised fragment.

Screw Fixation

Screw fixation offers the advantage of providing more consistent compression of the fragment in its bed than pins or Kirschner wires. In the past, the prominence of the screw head has been a significant disadvantage of this technique. The recent development of the Herbert screw allows fixation under compression while burying the proximal portion of the screw within the subchondral bone of the fragment[63, 64] (Figs. 15–13 and 15–14). Thomson[63] reported Herbert screw fixation and drilling to be successful in 16 of 18 cases, and Lange et al.[64] have also had encouraging early results. Removal of the buried implant after healing is difficult and may not be necessary.

Bone Grafting

Bone grafting may be combined with fixation of loose or free fragments or used alone when the articular cartilage is entirely intact. Guhl[57] and Lee and Mercurio[65] reported on retrograde drilling and grafting of in situ osteochondritic lesions. This technique offers

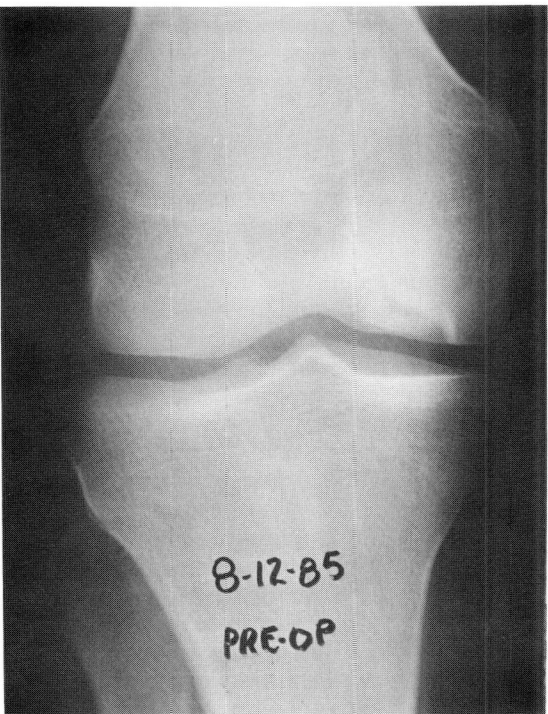

FIGURE 15–13. Preoperative lesion of the medial femoral condyle.

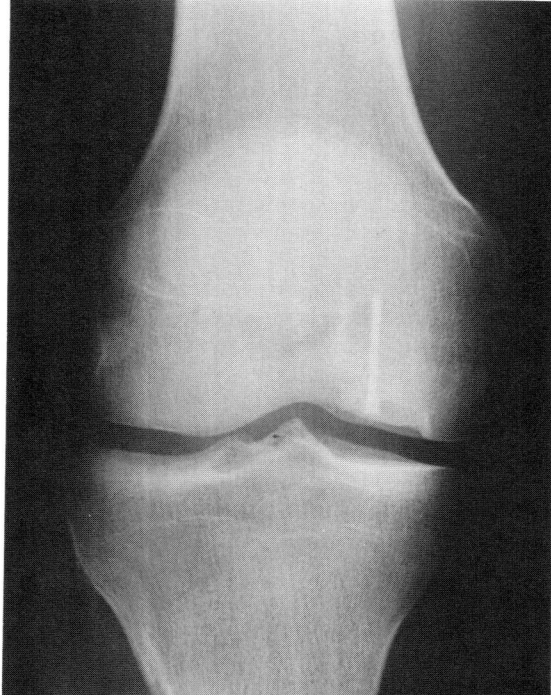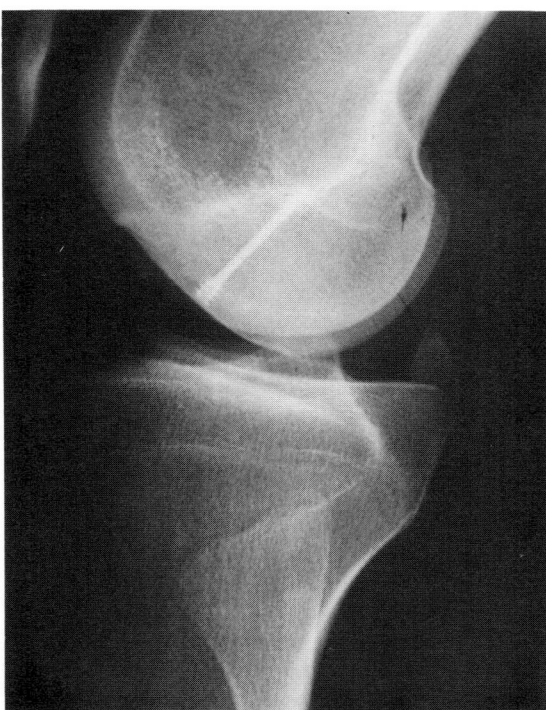

FIGURE 15–14. Six months after treatment by drilling and Herbert screw fixation, the lesion has completely healed and the patient is asymptomatic. The fragment is, however, somewhat depressed, and this patient may have been better treated by elevation by retrograde grafting and fixation.

the advantage of breaking the continuity of a sclerotic base and delivering bone graft to the bed without violating the articular surface. If the fragment is depressed, it can also be elevated through the retrograde channel by using a small tamp to compress the grafted bone under the fragment. Lee and Mercurio used this technique successfully with union at 6 to 7 months in three femoral lesions, whereas Guhl reported union in 9 of 12 cases. At the authors' institution, retrograde grafting has been combined with Herbert screw fixation with good preliminary results (Figs. 15–15, 15–16, 15–17, 15–18), suggesting that Guhl's three failures may have been the result of inadequate fixation.

Drilling

Antegrade drilling with a small Kirschner wire (K-wire) has been recommended for stable lesions with intact articular cartilage. Smillie[55] performed open drilling in 17 such patients, and after 12 to 16 weeks of postoper-

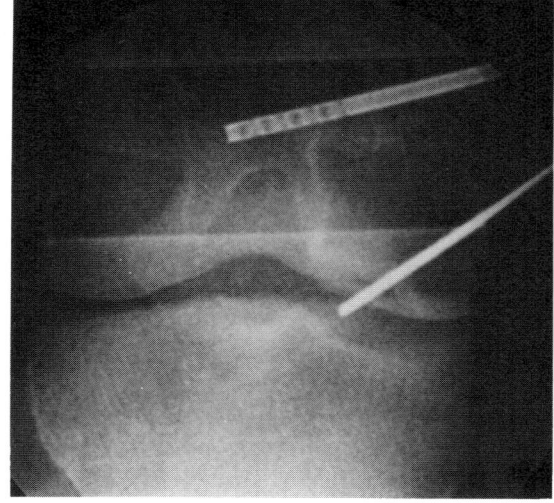

FIGURE 15–15. Retrograde grafting of a lesion of the medial femoral condyle begins with arthroscopic localization of the lesion and placement of a Kirschner wire through the lesion, exiting at the medial femoral condyle.

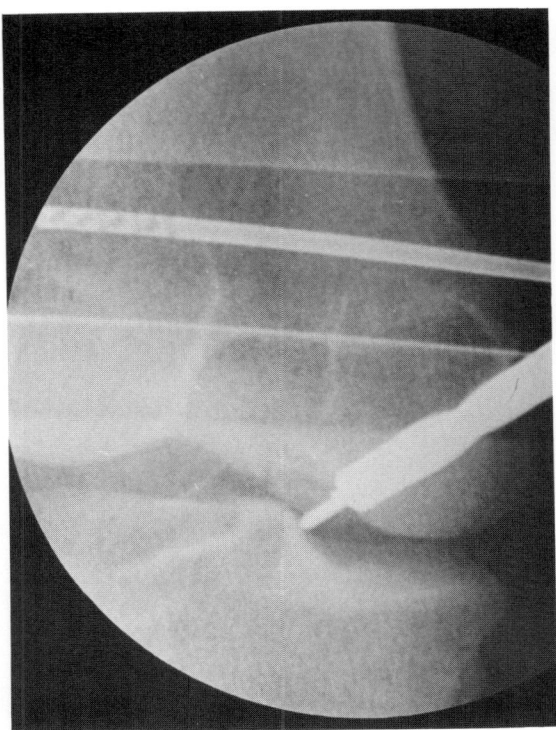

FIGURE 15–16. A small incision is then made to expose the K-wire on the medial aspect of the femur, and a cannulated reamer is used to retrograde drill to the base of the lesion.

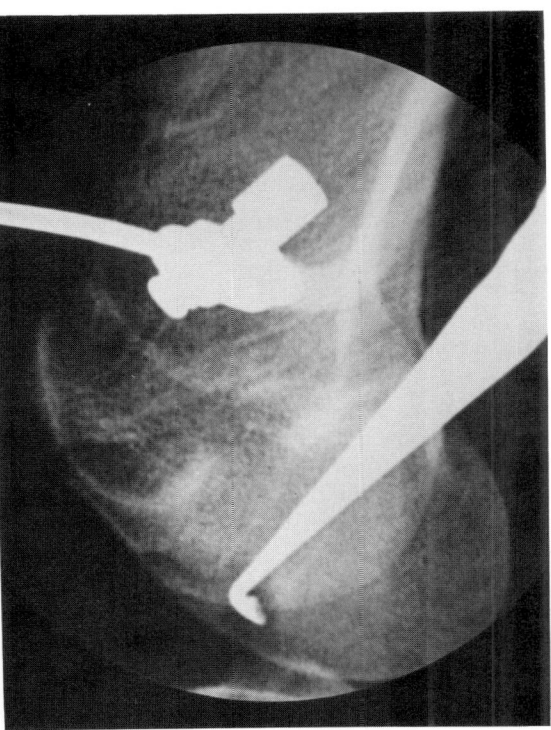

FIGURE 15–17. The base of the lesion is curretted under fluoroscopic control.

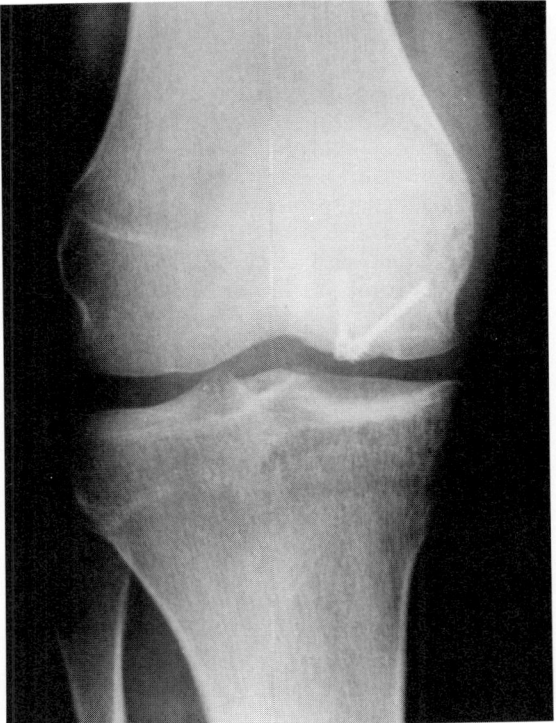
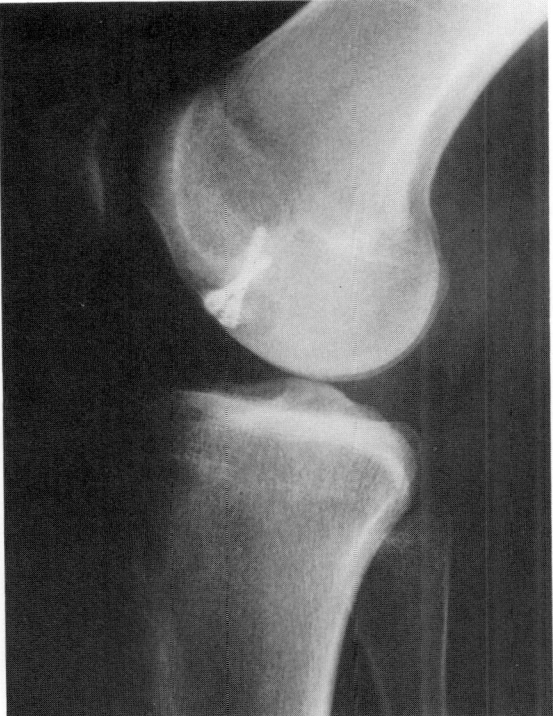

FIGURE 15–18. After retrograde cancellous bone grafting has elevated the fragment to a reduced position, it is fixed with two Herbert screws.

ative immobilization, 16 lesions united. Guhl[57] arthroscopically drilled lesions in 15 patients and obtained union in 14. Although the age issue is not specifically addressed in the literature, this technique appears to be most successful in patients with open growth plates (Figs. 15–19 and 15–20).

TREATMENT PROTOCOL

As the preceding discussion indicates, the literature has yet to define clearly the best treatment for each clinical situation. Therefore, the following protocol is put forth as one way, though certainly not the only way, to deal with this challenging disease (Figs. 15–21 and 15–22).

SKELETALLY IMMATURE PATIENTS

Patients with open growth plates are carefully questioned about the symptoms of

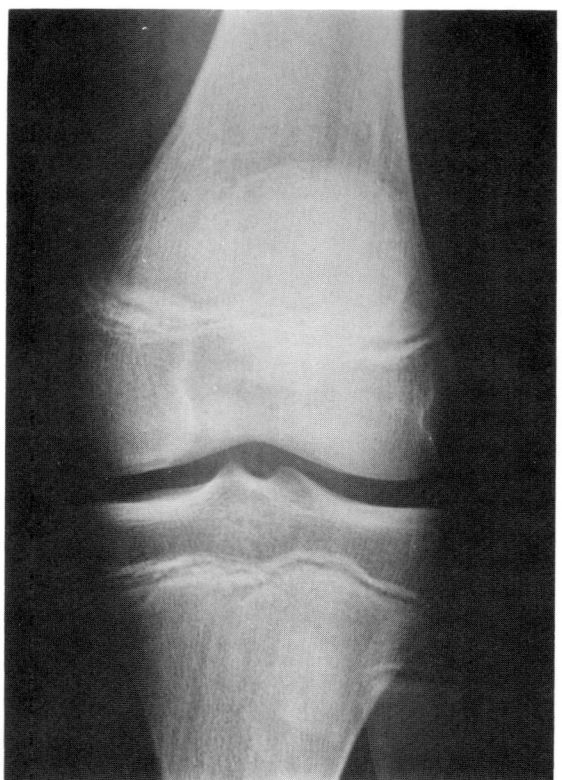

FIGURE 15–20. In this patient, complete healing was obtained.

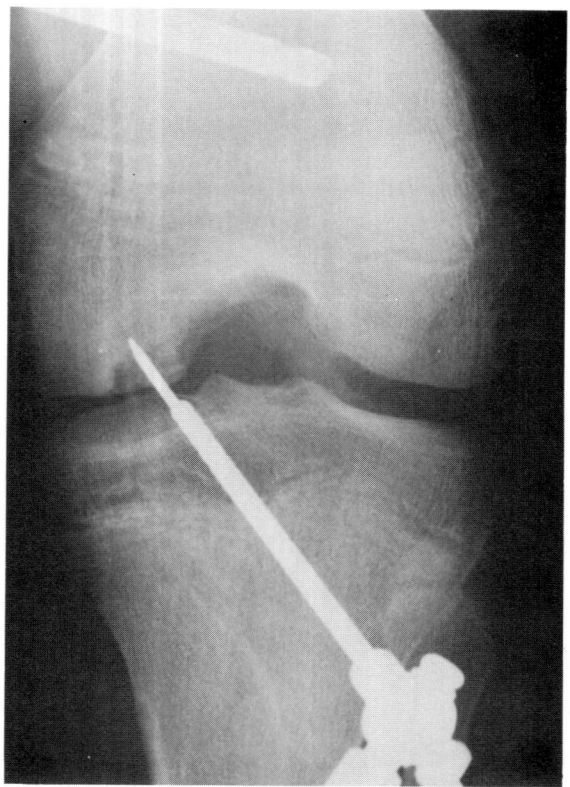

FIGURE 15–19. Drilling of osteochondritic lesions can usually be accomplished arthroscopically. This radiograph confirmed that the K-wire used for drilling was located in the center of the radiographic lesion.

catching, locking, swelling, and giving way. Any patient who is experiencing these symptoms is considered likely to have an unstable lesion and is evaluated further. At the present time, we prefer to use MRI to determine joint surface integrity. Individuals with either no mechanical symptoms (hence no MRI) or an intact articular surface (by MRI) are treated by activity modification and careful clinical and radiographic follow-up in 6 weeks. If pain persists, they are placed in a knee immobilizer and on crutches for an additional 6 weeks. If the patient becomes asymptomatic, activities can be gradually resumed, but radiographic follow-up remains essential until complete healing has occurred.

We consider symptomatic lesions that are unstable by MRI criteria, the recurrence of symptoms, or the failure to heal as skeletal maturity approaches as indications for surgical management. While asymptomatic lesions are followed in the skeletally immature patient, once growth plate closure approaches, surgery is recommended for all le-

OSTEOCHONDRITIS DISSECANS   251

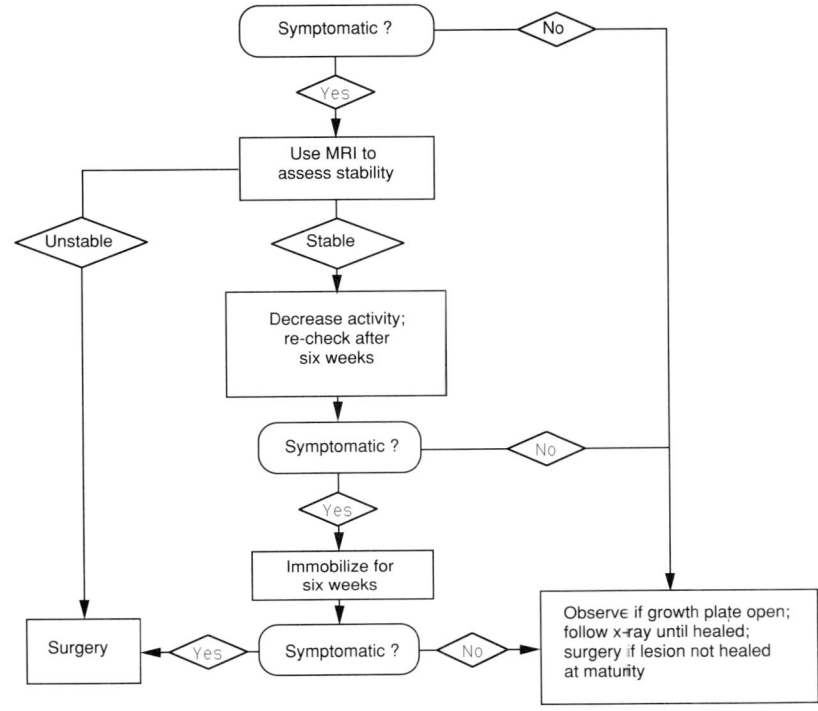

FIGURE 15–21. Algorithm for treatment of osteochondritis dissecans in the skeletally immature.

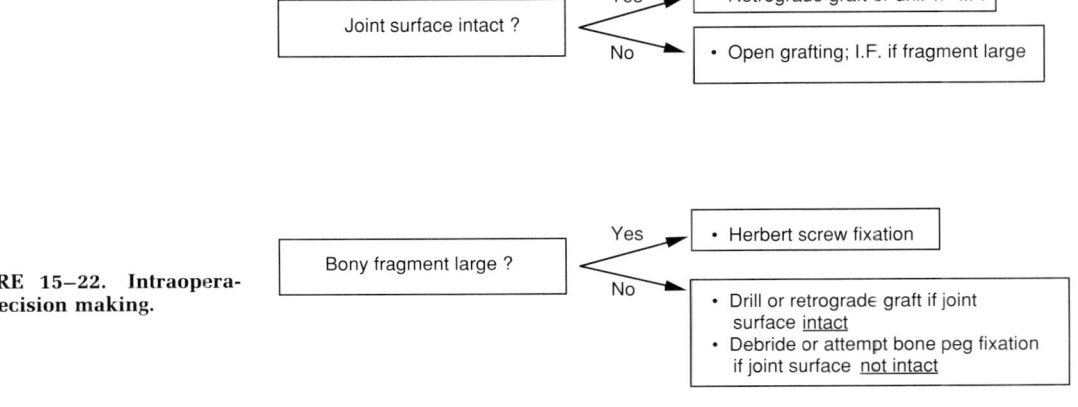

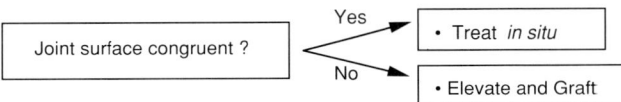

FIGURE 15–22. Intraoperative decision making.

sions that have not united radiographically. Such aggressive surgical management is predicated on the belief that in the adult only surgery offers the possibility of obtaining union of the osteochondritic fragment and thus allowing the integrity of the joint surface to be maintained over the long term.

Whenever surgery is planned and fixation is a possibility, tomograms are obtained to evaluate the osseous component of the fragment. At the time of the arthroscopic surgery, we evaluate the lesion size and location, joint surface integrity, and condylar contour. Stable lesions with intact articular surfaces are drilled. Postoperatively, these patients are kept on crutches but allowed intermittent motion for 6 weeks following surgery.

Osseous lesions with intact joint surfaces but instability to ballotment (the elevation and depression of a fragment that occurs with palpation or probing, indicating a lack of bony support) are drilled and fixed with a Herbert screw if compression does not result in depression of the fragment. If the fragment sinks below the normal contour of the condyle when compressed with a probe, retrograde grafting is performed to elevate the fragment; screw fixation is added if the osseous portion of the fragment is large enough to accommodate it. Those lesions with insufficient bone to allow screw fixation are treated by retrograde grafting alone.

Loose bodies or unstable lesions with partial joint surface disruption are grafted and fixed if at all possible. Grafting is generally done as an open procedure since retrograde grafting is difficult once the articular cartilage has been violated. In lesions with little or no bone, fixation is very difficult. In these cases, one alternative is debridement and abrasion of the bed. Preliminary data suggest that osteochondral allografts or autografts may be useful for large, unsalvageable lesions on the weight-bearing surface.[66, 67]

SKELETALLY MATURE PATIENTS

Patients who present with closed growth plates, or who reach maturity before union has been achieved, will usually not benefit from conservative treatment. Otherwise, the protocol in these patients is identical to that stated previously with the exception that drilling is replaced by retrograde grafting.

SUMMARY

Although it has been over 100 years since the term *osteochondritis dissecans* was first used, the etiology of this entity remains unclear. It is likely that indirect trauma to a susceptible area causes many of the cases, but hormonal and genetic factors may also play a role. The treatment of the young individual should generally be nonoperative, whereas patients at or near skeletal maturity are more likely to require surgical management. Regardless of its form, the goal of treatment should be the restoration of a congruous articular surface with normal bony support.

References

1. Konig F.: Über freie Korper in den Gelenken. Dtsch Z Chir 27:90–109, 1888.
2. Rieger M.: Zar Pathogenese von gelenkmausen Munchener. Med Wochensch 67:719, 1920.
3. Axhausen G.: Die Aetiologie der Kohler'schen Erkrankung der Metatarsalkopfchen. Bruns' Beitr Klin Chir 126:451–476, 1922.
4. Watson-Jones R.: Fractures and Joint Injuries. Volume I. 3rd ed. Baltimore, MD: Williams & Wilkins Co., pp. 106–107, 1944.
5. Fairbank H. A. T.: Osteo-chondritis dissecans. Br. J Surg 21:67–82, 1933.
6. Chiroff R. T. and Cooke C. P.: Osteochondritis dissecans: A histologic and microradiographic analysis of surgically excised lesions. J. Trauma 15:689–696, 1975.
7. Milgram J. W.: Radiological and pathological manifestations of osteochondritis dissecans of the distal femur. A study of 50 cases. Radiology 126:305–311, 1978.
8. Lindholm, T. S., Vankka E. and Osterman K.: Radiographically observed growth of fragment in juvenile osteochondritis dissecans. Acta Orthop Belg 48(3):504–509, 1982.
9. Rogers W. M. and Gladstone H.: Vascular foramina and arterial supply of the distal end of the femur. J. Bone Joint Surg 32A(4):867–874, 1950.
10. Phillips H. O. and Grubb S. A.: Familial multiple osteochondritis dissecans. J Bone Joint Surg 67A(1):155–156, 1985.
11. Pick M. P.: Familial osteochondritis dissecans. J Bone Joint Surg 37B(1):142–145, 1955.
12. Stougaard J.: Familial occurrence of osteochondritis dissecans. J Bone Joint Surg 46B(3):542–543, 1964.
13. Stougaard J.: The hereditary factor in osteochondritis dissecans. J Bone Joint Surg 43B(2):256–258, 1961.
14. Fraser W. N. C.: Familial osteochondritis dissecans. Proc J Bone Joint Surg 48B:598, 1966.
15. Hanley W. B. McKusick V. A. and Barranco F. T.: Osteochondritis dissecans with associated malformations in two brothers. A review of familial aspects. J Bone Joint Surg 49A(5):925–937, 1967.

16. Gardiner T. B.: Osteochondritis dissecans in three members of one family. J Bone Joint Surg 37B(1):139–141, 1955.
17. Mubarak S. J. and Carroll N. C.: Familial osteochondritis dissecans of the knee. Clin Orthop 140:131–136, 1979.
18. Petrie P. W. R.: Aetiology of osteochondritis dissecans. J Bone Joint Surg 59B(3):366–367, 1977.
19. Sontag L. W. and Pyle S. I.: Variations in the calcification pattern in epiphyses: Their nature and significance. AJR 45(1):50–54, 1941.
20. Caffey J., Madell S. H., Royer C. and Morales P.: Ossification of the distal femoral epiphysis. J Bone Joint Surg 40A(3):647–654, 714, 1958.
21. Ribbing S.: The hereditary multiple epiphyseal disturbance and its consequences for the aetiogenesis of local malacias—particularly the osteochondrosis dissecans. Acta Radiol 25:286–299, 1954.
22. Kennedy J. C., Grainger R. W. and McGraw R. W.: Osteochondral fractures of the femoral condyles. J Bone Joint Surg 48B(3):436–440, 1966.
23. Rehbein F.: Die Entstehung der Osteochondritis Dissecans. Arch Klin Chir 265:69, 1950.
24. Langenskiold A: Can osteochondritis dissecans arise as a sequel of cartilage fracture in early childhood? An experimental study. Acta Chir Scand 109(4):204–209, 1955.
25. Aichroth P.: Osteochondral fractures and their relationship to osteochondritis dissecans of the knee. An experimental study in animals. J Bone Joint Surg 53B:448–454, 1971.
26. Aichroth P.: Osteochondritis dissecans of the knee. A clinical survey. J Bone Joint Surg 53B(3):440–447, 1971.
27. Green J. P.: Osteochondritis dissecans of the knee. J Bone Joint Surg 48B(1):82–91, 1966.
28. Linden B.: Osteochondritis dissecans of the femoral condyles. A long-term follow-up study. J Bone Joint Surg 59A(6):769–776, 1977.
29. Mubarak S. J. and Carroll N. C.: Juvenile osteochondritis dissecans of the knee: Etiology. Clin Orthop 157:200–211, 1981.
30. Barrie H. J.: Hypothesis—a diagram of the form and origin of loose bodies in osteochondritis dissecans. J Rheumatol 11(4):512–513, 1984.
31. Barrie H. J.: Osteochondritis dissecans 1887–1987. A centennial look at König's memorable phrase. J Bone Joint Surg 69B(5):693–695, 1987.
32. Strange T. B.: Osteochondritis dissecans. Case report. Am J Surg 63(1):144–145, 1944.
33. Towbin J., Towbin R. and Crawford A.: Osteochondritis dissecans of the tibial plateau. A case report. J Bone Joint Surg 64A(5):783–784, 1982.
34. Desai S. S., Patel M. R., Michelli L. J., Silver J. W. and Lidge R. T.: Osteochondritis dissecans of the patella. J Bone Joint Surg 69B(2):320–325, 1987.
35. Stougaard J.: Osteochondritis dissecans of the patella. Acta Orthop Scand 45:111–118, 1974.
36. Howie J. L.: Computed tomography in osteochondritis dissecans of the patella. J Can Assoc Radiol 36:197–199, 1985.
37. Edwards D. H. and Bentley G.: Osteochondritis dissecans patellae. J Bone Joint Surg 59B(1):58–63, 1977.
38. Linden B.: The incidence of osteochondritis dissecans in the condyles of the femur. Acta Orthop Scand 47:664–667, 1976.
39. Wilson J. N.: A diagnostic sign in osteochondritis dissecans of the knee. J Bone Joint Surg 49A(3):477–480, 1967.
40. Harding W. G.: Diagnosis of osteochondritis dissecans of the femoral condyles. The value of the lateral X-ray view. Clin Orthop 123:25–26, 1977.
41. Mesgarzadeh M., Sapega A. A., Bonakdarpour A, et al: Osteochondritis dissecans: Analysis of mechanical stability with radiography, scintigraphy, and MR imaging. Radiology 165(3):775–780, 1987.
42. McCullough R. W., Gandsman E. J., Litchman H., et al: Computerized blood-flow analysis in osteochondritis dissecans. Clin Nucl Med 11(7):511–513, 1986.
43. Litchman H. M., McCullough R. W., Gandsman E. J. and Schatz S. L.: Computerized blood flow analysis for decision making in the treatment of osteochondritis dissecans. J Pediatr Orthop 8(2):208–212, 1988.
44. Cahill B. R. and Berg B. C.: 99m-Technetium phosphate compound joint scintigraphy in the management of juvenile osteochondritis dissecans of the femoral condyles. Am J Sports Med 11(5):329–335, 1983.
45. Bots R. A. and Slooff T. J.: Arthroscopy in the evaluation of operative treatment in osteochondrosis dissecans. Orthop Clin North Am 10(3):685–696, 1979.
46. Cahill B.: Treatment of juvenile osteochondritis dissecans and osteochondritis dissecans of the knee. Clin Sports Med 4(2):367–384, 1985.
47. Clanton T. O. and DeLee J. C.: Osteochondritis dissecans. History, pathophysiology and current treatment concepts. Clin Orthop 167:50–64, 1982.
48. Wiberg: Spontaneous healing of osteochondritis dissecans in the knee-joint. Acta Orthop 14(4):270–277, 1943.
49. Van Demark R. E.: Osteochondritis dissecans with spontaneous healing. J Bone Joint Surg 34A(1):143–148, 1952.
50. Green W. T. and Banks H. H.: Osteochondritis dissecans in children. J Bone Joint Surg 35A(1):26–47, 1953.
51. Denoncourt P. M., Patel D. and Dimakopoulos P.: Arthroscopy update #1. Treatment of osteochondrosis dissecans of the knee by arthroscopic curettage, follow-up study. Orthop Rev 15(10):53–58, 1986.
52. Ewing J. W. and Voto S. J.: Arthroscopic surgical management of osteochondritis dissecans of the knee. Arthroscopy 4(1):37–40, 1988.
53. Hughston J. C., Hergenroeder P. T. and Courtenay B. G.: Osteochondritis dissecans of the femoral condyles. J Bone Joint Surg 66A(9):1340–1348, 1984.
54. Almgard L. E. and Wikstad I.: Late results of surgery for osteochondritis dissecans of the knee joint. Acta Chir Scand 127:588–596 1964.
55. Smillie I. S.: Treatment of osteochondritis dissecans. J Bone Joint Surg 39B(2):248–260, 1957.
56. Lipscomb Jr. P. R., Lipscomb Sr. P. R. and Bryan R. S.: Osteochondritis dissecans of the knee with loose fragments. J Bone Joint Surg 60A(2):235–240, 1978.
57. Guhl J. F.: Arthroscopic treatment of osteochondritis dissecans. Clin Orthop 167:65–74, 1982.

58. Lindholm S. and Pylkkanen P.: Internal fixation of the fragment of osteochondritis dissecans in the knee by means of bone pins. Acta Chir Scand 140:626–629, 1974.
59. Lindholm S., Pylkkanen P. and Osterman K.: Fixation of osteochondral fragments in the knee joint. A clinical survey. Clin Orthop 126:256–260, 1977.
60. Lindholm T. S. and Osterman K.: Long-term results after transfixation of an osteochondritis dissecans fragment to the femoral condyle using autologous bone transplants in adolescent and adult patients. Arch Orthop Traumat Surg 97:225–230, 1980.
61. Johnson E. W. and McLeod T. L.: Osteochondral fragments of the distal end of the femur fixed with bone pegs. Report of two cases. J Bone Joint Surg 59A(5):677–679, 1977.
62. Gillespie H. S. and Day B.: Bone peg fixation in the treatment of osteochondritis dissecans of the knee joint. Clin Orthop 143:125–130, 1979.
63. Thomson N. L.: Osteochondritis dissecans and osteochondral fragments managed by Herbert compression screw fixation. Clin Orthop 224:71–78, 1987.
64. Lange R. H., Engber W. D., and Clancy W. G.: Expanding applications for the Herbert scaphoid screw. Orthopedics 8:1393–1397, 1986.
65. Lee C. K. and Mercurio C.: Operative treatment of osteochondritis dissecans in situ by retrograde drilling and cancellous bone graft. A preliminary report. Clin Orthop 158:129–136, 1981.
66. Rinaldi E.: Treatment of osteochondritis dissecans and cartilaginous fractures of the knee by osteocartilaginous autografts. Ital J Orthop Traumatol 8(1):17–21, 1982.
67. Yamashita F., Sakakida K., Suzu F. and Takai S.: The transplantation of an autogeneic osteochondral fragment for osteochondritis dissecans of the knee. Clin Orthop 201:43–50, 1985.

16
MENISCUS TEARS

KENNETH E. DEHAVEN
WAYNE J. SEBASTIANELLI

This chapter focuses on meniscal injury, but evaluation and management of these injuries must also include consideration of the ligaments and articular cartilage.

Clinical symptoms and disability are produced by meniscus lesions in several different ways. Locking and giving way are noted in displaceable or displaced meniscus tears, such as the common bucket handle tear. The pain associated with a nondisplaced tear of the meniscus does not originate from the tear of the meniscus but is believed to develop from altered meniscus mobility, which places abnormal traction stresses on the richly innervated capsule and synovium.

The work of Walker and Erkman,[59] Bullough et al.,[5] Krause et al.,[31] and others,[6,21,41] has documented the role of the meniscus in load transmission, joint stability, and articular cartilage lubrication and nutrition. Increased understanding of these important functions, coupled with the disappointing long-term results of total meniscectomy due to an increased incidence of subsequent osteoarthritis, particularly in children, has led to a more conservative approach.[10,20,22,38,58,63] The development of arthroscopy and arthroscopic surgery of the knee not only has paralleled but has also contributed significantly to this trend. Low morbidity associated with precision diagnosis has made diagnostic and operative arthroscopy invaluable in the treatment of meniscal lesions. Tears in menisci cannot only be identified but also classified as to their type, extent, and exact location. Arthroscopic surgery techniques permit partial meniscectomy to be carried out under direct visual control and also permits recognition of candidates for spontaneous healing or meniscus repair of lesions at or within the vascular zones.

With the increasing understanding of the physical properties of the meniscus as it relates to ultrastructure being developed by Bullough et al.,[5] Clark and Ogden,[9] and Mow et al.,[41] the rationale of therapeutic conservatism indeed has scientific basis. The removal of the mobile fragment to treat the mechanical symptoms of the meniscus tear while retaining as much functional meniscus tissue as possible will hopefully decrease the late sequelae of instability and degenerative changes associated with total meniscectomy.

DEVELOPMENT OF THE MENISCI OF THE HUMAN KNEE JOINT

The work of Clark and Ogden,[9] Scapinelli,[50] and Arnoczky and Warren[2] have documented the anatomy and vascularity of the human meniscus. Composed primarily of hypocellular fibrocartilage, the human meniscus with its predominantly circumferentially arranged collagen fibers is well designed to withstand the large tension loads applied in weight-bearing activities. Some of the collagen fibers are also radially oriented. In the surrounding capsular and synovial tissues about each meniscus, a perimeniscal capillary plexus is found. This plexus receives its blood flow from the medial, lateral, and middle geniculate arteries.[2] The peripheral 10 to

30 percent of the meniscus is penetrated by this plexus.

Human menisci reach their semilunar configurations at approximately 14 weeks of gestation.[9] These menisci have markedly increased cellularity and vascularity compared with adult specimens. Following birth, a gradual decrease in cellularity and vascularity takes place, with the adult appearance reached by age 10. As the cellularity and vascularity of the menisci decrease, the collagen fiber content rises. With the tension and shear stresses applied across the knee as one becomes more active, the collagen fibers organize into the circumferential and radial fibers of the adult meniscus substructure.

Extrapolating from these studies, meniscal injuries in the pediatric population may have a greater potential for healing. Unfortunately, the majority of meniscal injuries in the skeletally immature patient occur during adolescence, when the menisci have already assumed the vascular and histological characteristics of skeletally mature individuals.[9]

Statistically, meniscal tears are seen more frequently with increasing age in children. The youngest reported case of a meniscal tear in an otherwise normal medial meniscus is age 4.[49] Meniscal tears overall are exceedingly rare in children under 10 years of age. Congenitally abnormal menisci, however, are at increased risk for injury, and several series document young patients with meniscal tears in lateral discoid menisci.[22, 26, 27] As children reach adolescence, there is a sharp increase in the frequency of traumatic tears of normal menisci. This is felt to be associated with increased forces placed across the knee secondary to strength and weight gains and with participation in more sophisticated athletic events, increasing the relative risk of knee injuries.

CLINICAL ASSESSMENT

HISTORY

Most meniscal injuries occur with noncontact stress. Acceleration, deceleration, change in direction, and angular momentum are points often elicited from a patient's history of his or her knee injury. Meniscus tears can also occur with contact injuries, when the involved leg is subjected to a blow (most frequently from the lateral or anterolateral aspect) that adds a violent valgus, varus, or hyperextension element in addition to flexion and rotation. Anatomically, the sine qua non of meniscal injury is flexion and femoral tibial compression coupled with rotation, which creates shear stresses to the menisci, resulting in their ultimate failure.

Children and adolescents often cannot accurately describe the mechanism of injury. Witnesses or game films can often be helpful. The physician should be aware of the high incidence of collateral and cruciate ligament injuries associated with meniscus tears in young athletes. The history of a popping or tearing sensation as the knee gave way with the inability to extend the knee fully or bear weight can be indicative of such injury. In addition, there should always be a high index of suspicion of possible epiphyseal injuries about the knee in these skeletally immature patients. Because some meniscal injuries may produce intermittent symptoms, and because anterior cruciate ligament tears can predispose to recurring meniscus injuries, inquiries should be made by the physician about previous ligament or meniscal injuries.

A careful history should be taken regarding the appearance of intraarticular swelling. The typical synovial fluid effusion seen in isolated meniscal injuries usually develops gradually over a 48- to 72-hour period. Acute effusions occurring within hours after the injury are indicative of hemarthrosis, which is usually associated with anterior cruciate ligament tears, osteochondral fractures, patellar dislocations, and epiphyseal/physeal fractures. As an effusion itself can lead to inhibition of full extension, the history should attempt to ascertain whether full extension was possible immediately after the injury.

Locking and giving way can often be elicited from patients who have meniscal injuries. One must be certain, however, that reflex inhibition of the quadriceps musculature itself is not responsible for the giving way sensation. This could be due to any of the above-mentioned injuries. Associated chronic injuries should also be excluded such as previously unrecognized cruciate instability or patellofemoral disorders. The young patient with a chronic meniscal tear will often recall an acute episode followed by gradual improvement. These patients often attempt to return to full activity but are limited by joint line pain on the side of meniscal injury. They may also be plagued by periodic locking and giving way, which can be secondary to displacement of meniscal tissue or quadriceps weakness.

PHYSICAL EXAMINATION

Examination of the patient should be systematic and precise. As collateral ligament injuries can cause joint line tenderness, one should be certain to palpate the entire course of the ligament. Assessment of cruciate stability and patellofemoral joint problems should be made. Physeal injuries should be suspected whenever tenderness is at the level of either the distal femoral or proximal tibial physeal plates. The presence or absence of an effusion must be carefully determined. The range of motion should be measured and compared with the uninjured extremity. While some loss of flexion is common even after trivial injuries, the absence of even a few degrees of extension is significant. Subtle differences can be detected by having the patient lie prone on an examining table with the lower extremities only being supported from the midthigh proximally (Fig. 16–1). Remember that full extension may be prevented by pain and spasm, hemarthrosis or joint effusion, or a mechanical block from displaced meniscal or osteochondral tissue.

Careful palpation of the medial and lateral joint lines from anterior to posterior should be performed. Circumduction maneuvers of the McMurray type with the knee flexed can demonstrate pain or elicit a click, unmasking otherwise occult posterior horn tears.[65] Thigh circumference should be measured from a standard reference point to document the level of quadriceps atrophy.

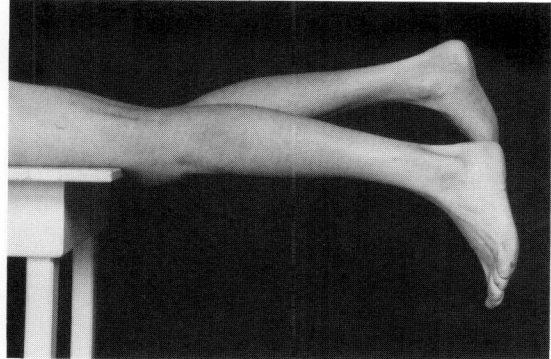

FIGURE 16–1. Photo of knee flexion contracture as visualized by prone examination position.

DIAGNOSTIC STUDIES

In addition to history and physical examination, roentgenographic studies can be helpful. Plain radiographs (including AP [anterior-posterior], lateral, Merchant, and tunnel views) will be normal or nondiagnostic for meniscus tears but should be performed routinely to exclude other associated skeletal pathology. Stress X-rays can be helpful in differentiating collateral ligament from growth plate injuries.

Many studies have documented the difficulty in properly assessing meniscal injuries in the skeletally immature patient.[7, 12, 24, 40, 57, 63] Sophisticated radiographic studies including double contrast arthrography, computerized tomography (CT) scanning, and magnetic resonance imaging (MRI) techniques have been used to help the clinician improve his or her diagnostic acumen. Studies from DeHaven and Collins[15] and Nicholas et al.[44] have reported the accuracy of arthrography to vary between 60 and 97 percent. Lateral meniscus tears are particularly difficult to assess with this technique because of shadows created by the popliteus tendon as it crosses the joint line through the popliteal hiatus. Cooperation of the patient and the skill of the arthrographer also play a very important role in the accuracy of this technique.

Manco et al.[35] have reported an accuracy of 91 percent with CT of the knee. Polly et al.[46] reported 90 percent accuracy for assessment of tears of the lateral meniscus and 98 percent accuracy for assessment of tears of the medial meniscus by MRI. Silva and Silver,[54] however, reported only 45 percent accuracy of MRI in evaluating meniscal injuries. As with double contrast arthrography, variability in results can be quite dependent on the sophistication of the scanning equipment and the overall interpretative skill and experience of the radiologist.

These diagnostic studies can still be quite helpful despite their inability to be accurate 100 percent of the time. Injuries inappropriate for either aggressive rehabilitation or a trial of conservative therapy can be very easily seen with these more sophisticated diagnostic tests (repairable tears of menisci, osteochondral fractures, and cruciate ligament injuries). In these particular instances, the diagnostic study can assist greatly in the decision-making process.

THE ROLE OF ARTHROSCOPY IN CHILDREN

Several authors—Morrissey et al.,[40] Suman et al.,[57] and Bergstrom et al.[4]—have documented that arthroscopy is a useful modality to help assist the clinical acumen of the orthopedic surgeon with respect to knee injuries in the skeletally immature patient. As children often tend to minimize their symptoms and frequently fail to communicate efficiently with the physician, arthroscopic intervention is often required for diagnosis in those patients whose knee injuries do not resolve with conservative treatment. Suman et al.[57] and Morrissey et al.[40] show the accuracy of clinical diagnosis of meniscal injuries as documented by diagnostic arthroscopy to be approximately 40 percent in patients under age 13 and 56 percent in patients over 13 years of age. Bergstrom et al. reported a clinical accuracy of 20 percent[4] (see Table 16–1).

The studies of Morrissey et al.[40] and Bergstrom et al.[4] support the clinical usefulness of arthroscopy in this age group and suggest that it may be quite advantageous to use arthroscopy earlier in the course of treating younger children. These studies emphasize that significant internal derangements of the knee can and do occur in these children and that serious articular cartilage damage often associated with chronic meniscal injuries might be prevented or minimized by earlier intervention.

The complete relaxation afforded by anesthesia allows for a thorough ligamentous examination, which frequently is very difficult in awake youngsters with acute injuries. One must be careful to rule out full thickness capsular injuries, which can lead to considerable amounts of extravasated irrigation fluid and cause neurovascular compression syndromes. Visualization can be achieved by completely draining the knee of bloody fluid and establishing a high flow system. The use of the tourniquet should be avoided if possible whenever an open procedure is anticipated.

Arthroscopic technique in children is quite similar to that in adults.[18, 19] In spite of the smaller size of their knee joints, the use of a standard 5-mm arthroscope is usually not a problem. The entire knee should be systematically inspected. Probing of both menisci to demonstrate any tears or instability should be routinely performed. Appropriate inspection of the posteromedial and posterolateral compartments can be carried out by passing the arthroscope through the intercondylar notch and using a 70-degree telescope. The use of an O'Donoghue probe can also assist in the evaluation of a peripheral posterior meniscal tear.

TYPES OF MENISCAL TEARS

O'Connor[52] described four basic patterns of meniscal tears. These include vertical longitudinal, horizontal, oblique, and radial tears. An individual meniscal lesion may be a combination of these patterns. Variations of these include complex tears and degenerative tears.

A *longitudinal tear* occurs when the circumferential fibers parallel to the periphery of the meniscus are split (Fig. 16–2). A full thickness longitudinal tear of sufficient length results in instability of the innermost fragment. The peripheral rim is usually intact but may be involved with a second tear. Partial thickness tears can originate from either the superior or inferior meniscus surface (Fig. 16–3). In addition to recognizing the fact that a vertical longitudinal tear is present, it is important to identify accurately how far from the meniscal capsular junction the tear occurred. If the tear has occurred within the vascular zone—that is, the pe-

TABLE 16–1 Comparison of Adolescent and Preadolescent Children

Age of Patient	History or Trauma	Number of Diagnoses Incorrect	Number of Diagnoses Correct	Delay in Diagnosis
Patients 13 years old and over	17/21 80%	8/21 39%	13/21 61%	9 months
Patients less than 13 years old	7/11	8/11	3/11	18 months

Source: From Morrissey, R. T., Eubanks, R. G., Park, J. P., and Thompson, S. B., Jr.: Arthroscopy of the knee in children. Clin. Orthop. 162:103–107, 1982.

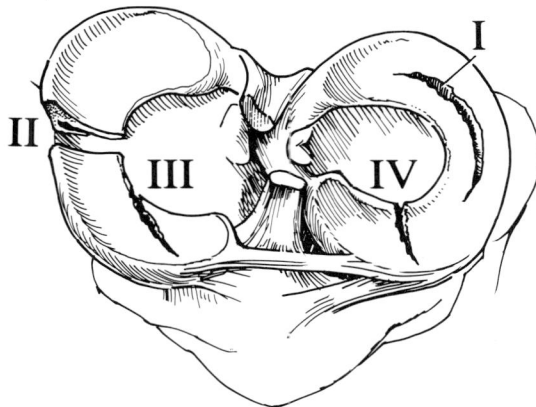

FIGURE 16–2. This sketch illustrates the four basic types of tear as described by O'Connor.[52] *I*, longitudinal tear, *II*, horizontal cleavage tear, *III*, oblique tear, *IV*, radial tear. (From Kalenak, A., Hanks, G. A., and Sebastianelli, W. A.: Arthroscopy of the knee. In Evarts, C. M. (ed.): Surgery of the Musculoskeletal System, Vol. 4, Ed. 2. Churchill Livingstone, Inc., chap. 114, 1990.)

ripheral one third of the meniscus as described by Arnoczky and Warren[2]—then this tear may be suitable for repair rather than excision. Vertical longitudinal tears often result in classic bucket handle tears if they extend through a significant portion of the meniscus and displace the inner fragment into the intercondylar notch.

Horizontal cleavage tears occur on a plane parallel to the superior and inferior surfaces of the meniscus. These tears are most commonly associated with the older patient and degenerative changes and are rarely, if ever, encountered in children (Fig. 16–2). They occur most commonly in the posterior horn of the medial meniscus and the middle third of the lateral meniscus. They are often associated with flap or radial tears.

The *oblique tear* is a full thickness vertical tear extending from the inner free margin of the meniscus into the body of the meniscus (Fig. 16–2). This particular variant may represent a continuation of a vertical longitudinal tear to the inner free margin of the meniscus, producing the loose fragment. If the oblique tear has a horizontal cleavage component in addition to the vertically oriented failure of the tissue, a true flap in then created (Fig. 16–2).

The *radial tear*, most commonly located in the middle third of the lateral meniscus, is another type of vertical tear (Fig. 16–2). These tears may extend for varying lengths from the inner edge to the periphery.

The incidence of complex tears and degenerative tears is obviously greater in the older patient and therefore will not be emphasized in this discussion.

TREATMENT

The goal of treatment is to relieve the symptoms caused by meniscus tears and at the same time to retain as much meniscus tissue as possible. Four basic treatment options should be considered: (1) leave certain tears alone, (2) repair, (3) partial meniscectomy, and (4) total meniscectomy. The first step in the decision-making process is to obtain precise definition of the type, location, and extent of the tear from a detailed and comprehensive diagnostic arthroscopy.

The next step is to determine whether the lesion needs to be treated surgically or not. Casscells[7] was among the first to recognize that not all meniscus tears cause symptoms or are associated with articular cartilage damage and advocated leaving such tears alone. Tears suitable for leaving alone are partial thickness split tears arising from either the femoral or tibial surfaces of the meniscus that can be demonstrated to be stable to probing. In addition, short (5 mm or less) complete peripheral vertical tears can be left alone since acute lesions will usually heal spontaneously. A third type of tear that can

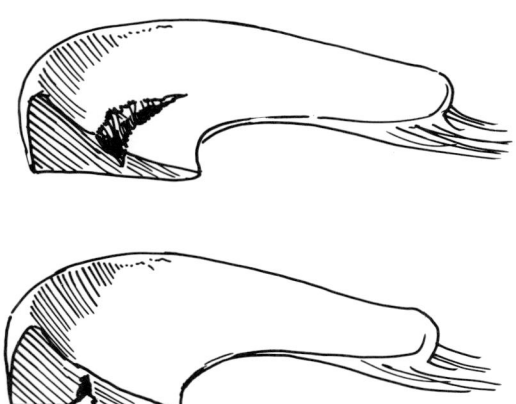

FIGURE 16–3. Incomplete longitudinal tears may occur on either the superior or inferior surface of the meniscus. (From Kalenak, A., Hanks, G. A., and Sebastianelli, W. A.: Arthroscopy of the knee. In Evarts, C. M. (ed.): Surgery of the Musculoskeletal System, Vol. 4, Ed. 2. Churchill Livingstone, Inc., chap. 114, 1990.)

be considered for leaving alone is a short (5 mm or less) radial tear. These general guidelines have been followed for the past several years in our center and by Gillquist and coworkers in Linkoping, Sweden. Our combined experiences have recently been published[61] and document that only 12 percent of such meniscus tears left alone required surgical treatment through a 2- to 8-year follow-up time. Two thirds of these required partial meniscectomy and the other third meniscus repair. In most cases, stable meniscus tears are associated with other more significant injuries that require surgical treatment, and it is not difficult to leave these tears alone. In cases in which meniscus tears appear suitable for leaving alone but represent the only pathological finding and correlate with the clinical symptoms that led to arthroscopy, the decision whether to leave alone or to treat surgically becomes a matter of judgment. In young athletes without mechanical symptoms, a period of conservative treatment and rehabilitation is warranted before exposing the child to the risk of even partial meniscectomy.

If the meniscus tear is found to be unsuitable for leaving alone and therefore needs surgical treatment, the next step in the decision-making process is to determine if it is a candidate for repair. Vertical longitudinal tears at or near the periphery (within the vascular zone) without significant damage to the body of the meniscus have been documented to be definitely suitable for repair.[8, 14, 25, 30, 51] The tear should be of significant length (over 6 mm or unstable, typically 15 to 25 mm). Tears that are clearly in the avascular zone or with extensive damage to the body of the meniscus are of questionable suitability. Vascular enhancement techniques and the use of fibrin clot are under development and might prove to be reliable means to extend the indications for repair. It should also be reemphasized that in these skeletally immature patients the extent of vascular penetration is greater than in the adult. This increases the potential for repair in children.

Meniscus tears that are not suitable for leaving alone or repair are treated by partial or total excision. In keeping with the philosophy of retaining as much meniscus tissue as possible, partial meniscectomy is the preferred approach, reserving total meniscectomy only for those rare lesions where even partial meniscectomy is not appropriate.[36]

PARTIAL MENISCECTOMY

Arthroscopic surgical technique has become sophisticated enough to permit advances in surgical approaches and also revolutionize the treatment of meniscus tears. Techniques described by O'Connor,[52] Jackson and Dandy,[28] Metcalf,[39] and Johnson[29] have made it possible to remove the affected portion of the meniscus quite expeditiously with minimal postoperative morbidity. The authors would like to stress, however, that tiny incisions do not always lead to the best result. The surgeon should be quite adept at triangulation techniques and quite honest with his or her own ability. A partial meniscectomy using arthroscopic instrumentation through a small arthrotomy, or even a well-done traditional meniscectomy, is better than a poor attempt at arthroscopic partial meniscectomy that is left unfinished.

Resection of meniscal lesions can be partial, subtotal, or total. Through the work of Jackson and Dandy,[28] McGinty et al.,[37] and others, partial meniscectomy appears to be preferable to total meniscectomy with respect to prevention of chronic degenerative changes. Two more recent studies,[34, 45] however, have noted that partial meniscectomy results are not different from total meniscectomy in anterior cruciate ligament (ACL) deficient knees. Removal of the torn portion of the meniscus as well as a smaller amount of normal meniscus tissue adjacent to the tear leads to the production of a contoured smooth surface in the remaining intact meniscal tissue. Disruption of the circumferential fibers produced by injury to the peripheral rim of the meniscus alters the normal transmission of force. This may lead to subtotal excision. Total meniscectomy involves removal of the complete meniscus. This is only necessary in very severe complex tears or vertical longitudinal tears in which the meniscus body has sustained irreparable damage. A horizontal tear associated with a large meniscal cyst may also require treatment by total meniscectomy. Fortunately, this lesion is quite rare. Smaller meniscal cysts can be treated by arthroscopic partial excision of the meniscal tear, and the cyst should spontaneously resolve. Occasionally, the mucoid material can then be expressed in the joint and removed arthroscopically. The authors have no experience with this technique but believe its principles are sound.

TECHNIQUES FOR EXCISION OF TEARS

Treatment of longitudinal tears requires a clear understanding of the extent and type of the tear. An acute complete tear in the peripheral one third of the meniscus shorter than approximately 1 cm in length can be treated by 4 weeks of immobilization alone. Stable partial thickness longitudinal tears can be observed without any further treatment other than immediate postoperative rehabilitation. Unstable vertical longitudinal tears occurring in the avascular zone of the body of the meniscus should be excised.

While others have been successfully employed, our preferred technique for resection of a vertical longitudinal or bucket handle tear of the medial meniscus is a two-puncture technique developed by Sprague.[56] The arthroscope is placed in the anterolateral portal. An anteromedial portal is made for instruments, and a valgus stress is applied to the knee (Figs. 16–4, 16–5, 16–6, 16–7, 16–8). The fragment is reduced with a probe. The posterior axilla of the tear is palpated and, using a basket forceps, partially transsected, preserving the remaining posterior rim and leaving a thin shred of meniscal tissue attached to the displaceable fragment. The anterior axilla of the tear is then identified and completely transsected flush with the anterior meniscus rim. This step sometimes requires changing portals for the telescope and cutting instrument to gain the proper angle of attack. The displaceable fragment that is now free anteriorly is grasped via a grasping forcep through the anteromedial portal. The fragment is then twisted on its long axis to tighten up any slack in the re-

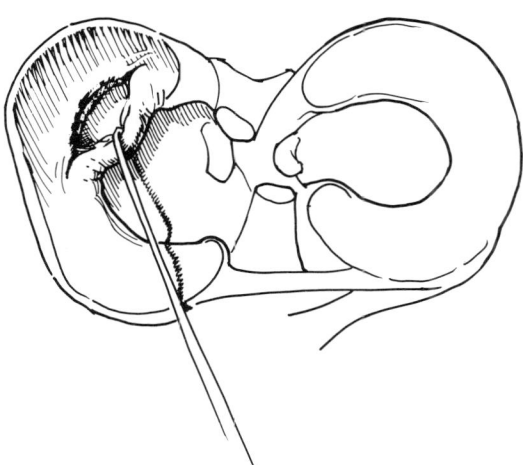

FIGURE 16–5. An arthroscopic probe displacing the bucket handle component toward the intercondylar notch. (From Kalenak, A., Hanks, G. A., and Sebastianelli, W. A.: Arthroscopy of the knee. In Evarts, C. M. (ed.): Surgery of the Musculoskeletal System, Vol. 4, Ed. 2. Churchill Livingstone, Inc., chap. 114, 1990.)

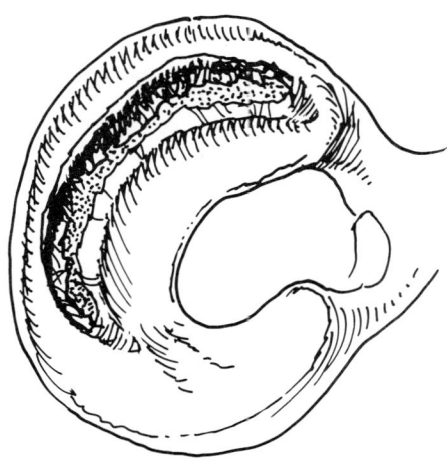

FIGURE 16–4. A longitudinal tear of the classic bucket handle type that can be displaced into the intercondylar notch. (From Kalenak, A., Hanks, G. A., and Sebastianelli, W. A.: Arthroscopy of the knee. In Evarts, C. M. (ed.): Surgery of the Musculoskeletal System, Vol. 4, Ed. 2. Churchill Livingstone, Inc., chap. 114, 1990.)

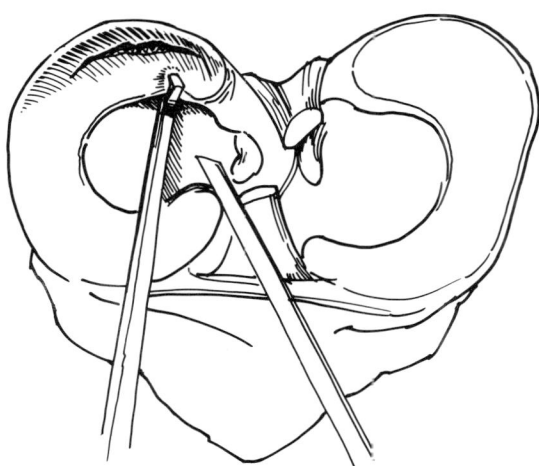

FIGURE 16–6. An arthroscopic basket rongeur initiating the transsection of the posterior limb of the bucket. With this technique, a small bridge of intact meniscal tissue is left so that the fragment will not become free upon complete release of the anterior limb. The posterior limb should be small enough so that the meniscal fragment may be avulsed with gentle traction. (From Kalenak, A., Hanks, G. A., and Sebastianelli, W. A.: Arthroscopy of the knee. In Evarts, C. M. (ed.): Surgery of the Musculoskeletal System, Vol. 4, Ed. 2. Churchill Livingstone, Inc., chap. 114, 1990.)

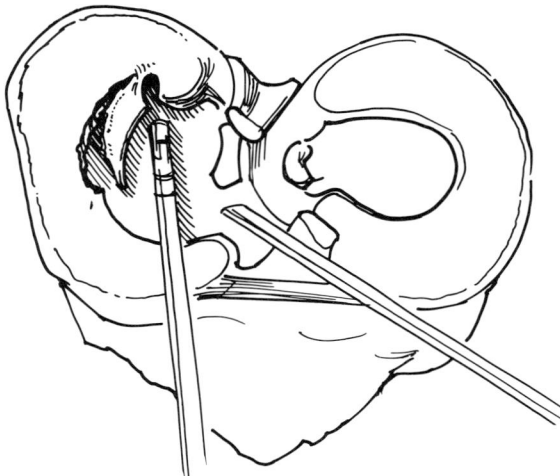

FIGURE 16–7. Note the small meniscal bridge holding the bucket handle fragment in place. The anterior limb has already been completely transsected with a basket rongeur. (From Kalenak, A., Hanks, G. A., and Sebastianelli, W. A.: Arthroscopy of the knee. In Evarts, C. M. (ed.): Surgery of the Musculoskeletal System, Vol. 4, Ed. 2. Churchill Livingstone, Inc., chap. 114, 1990.)

ful for cases when it is not possible to make the posterior cut under direct vision after reduction of the displaced fragment or when the fragment cannot be reduced. With this technique, the first step is to transsect the anterior attachment completely. The free meniscal fragment anteriorly is then grasped through the lateral portal with a grasping forceps and is displaced into the intercondylar notch, maintaining traction on the fragment. The posterior attachment is then divided with the use of a cutting forceps or knife through the accessory portal (Figs. 16–9 and 16–10). The free fragment is then removed from the joint and the remaining rim inspected, probed, and trimmed. Care must be taken to fashion a stable and contoured rim. We prefer to complete any operative procedure with power shaving and vacuuming to remove free fragments (Fig. 16–11).

Shahriaree[52] has described treatment of horizontal cleavage tears as being best handled by piecemeal excision. This will preserve the largest peripheral rim possible. Despite being tedious and time-consuming, this piecemeal excision will avoid unnecessary resection of healthy meniscal tissue. Care must be taken to ensure that the superior and inferior leaves of the horizontal tear are balanced and contoured to the vascular zone of the peripheral one third of the meniscus. This will encourage healing between the re-

maining small attachment posteriorly, avulsed, and removed from the joint. The remaining rim is then carefully inspected, probed, and trimmed as necessary to ensure that it is intact, stable, and well contoured.

A three-puncture technique utilizing an accessory anteromedial portal has been help-

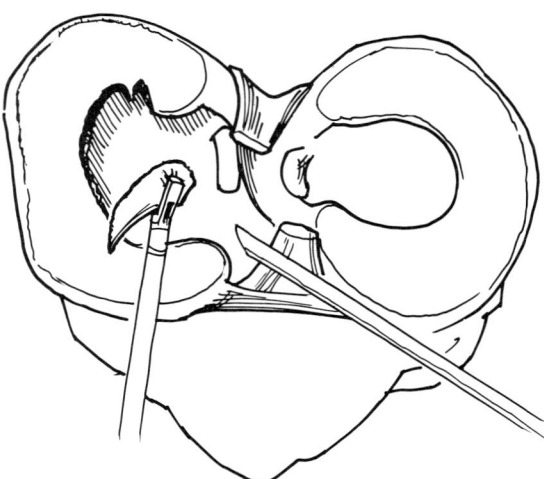

FIGURE 16–8. Following grasping and traction, the fragment is avulsed and removed from the knee joint. (From Kalenak, A., Hanks, G. A., and Sebastianelli, W. A.: Arthroscopy of the knee. In Evarts, C. M. (ed.): Surgery of the Musculoskeletal System, Vol. 4, Ed. 2. Churchill Livingstone, Inc., chap. 114, 1990.)

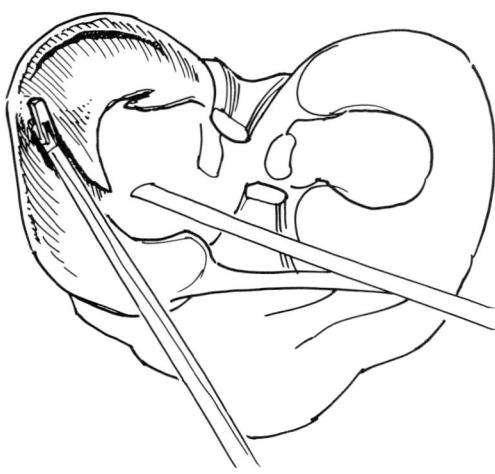

FIGURE 16–9. Partial meniscectomy technique utilizing an accessory anteromedial portal. The anterior limb is completely transsected. (From Kalenak, A., Hanks, G. A., and Sebastianelli, W. A.: Arthroscopy of the knee. In Evarts, C. M. (ed.): Surgery of the Musculoskeletal System, Vol. 4, Ed. 2. Churchill Livingstone, Inc., chap. 114, 1990.)

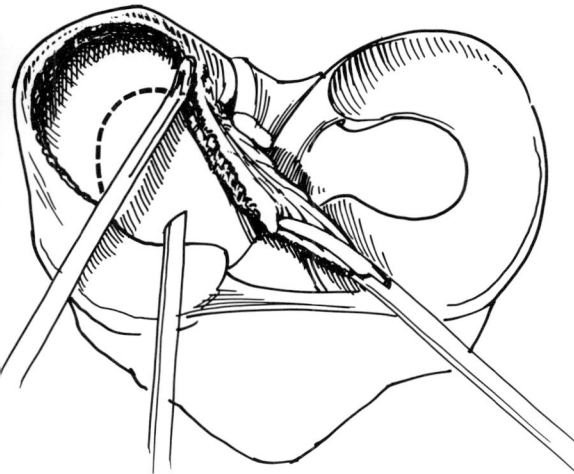

FIGURE 16–10. The grasping forceps, inserted through an accessory portal, are displacing the meniscal fragment into the intercondylar notch. The basket rongeur is then used to complete the detachment of the posterior limb. The fragment is then removed from the joint. (From Kalenak, A., Hanks, G. A., and Sebastianelli, W. A.: Arthroscopy of the knee. In Evarts, C. M. (ed.): Surgery of the Musculoskeletal System, Vol. 4, Ed. 2. Churchill Livingstone, Inc., chap. 114, 1990.)

maining portions of the superior and inferior leaves.

Surgical treatment of an oblique or flap tear is quite similar to resection of the longitudinal vertical tear or the bucket handle tear. Guhl[23] and others have pointed out that a thorough inspection and probing of the superior and inferior surfaces of the torn meniscus should be made to ensure that an additional flap of meniscal tissue has not become incarcerated between the meniscus and tibial plateau or femoral condyle.

Seen most commonly in the lateral meniscus, radial tears are best treated by saucerization (Fig. 16–12). The resection should be performed by angling the instrument at approximately a 45-degree angle toward the apex of the tear. In the rare instance of a radial tear completely transsecting the whole meniscus and traveling to the periphery, a much wider resection would be necessary. This would place the extent of the resection in the subtotal category. An alternative to such an extensive excision would be partial excision with arthroscopic repair of the peripheral one third.

Excision of lateral meniscus tears is best performed by placing the lower extremity in the figure-of-four position, with the arthroscope being placed in the anterolateral portal and operative instruments through the medial portal. At times it may be necessary to reverse one's perspective and place the arthroscope in the anteromedial portal, with instruments being used via the anterolateral portal. The surgeon must be familiar with improving the angle of attack by periodically switching the arthroscope/instrument portals and/or choice of instruments. The leg can also be placed in varying degrees of flexion and with varying degrees of varus stress to improve visualization and access of intraarticular structures.

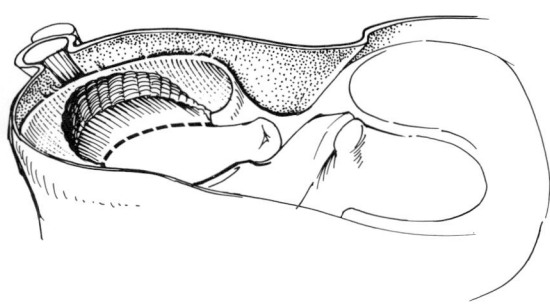

FIGURE 16–11. The completely contoured, stable, balanced rim following a arthroscopic partial meniscectomy of a longitudinal tear. (From Kalenak, A., Hanks, G. A., and Sebastianelli, W. A.: Arthroscopy of the knee. In Evarts, C. M. (ed.): Surgery of the Musculoskeletal System, Vol. 4, Ed. 2. Churchill Livingstone, Inc., chap. 114, 1990.)

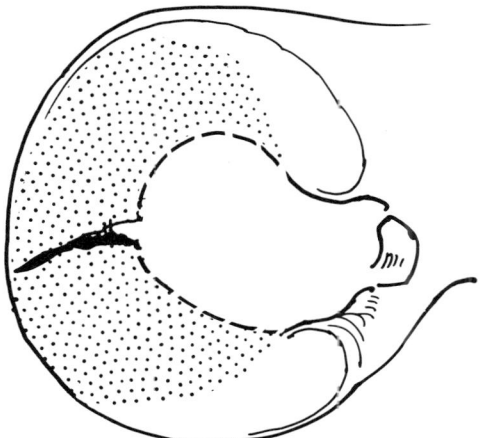

FIGURE 16–12. Artist's rendition of a radial tear requiring subtotal meniscectomy. Note the amount of normal meniscal tissue that must be removed to provide a stable contoured balanced rim. (From Kalenak, A., Hanks, G. A., and Sebastianelli, W. A.: Arthroscopy of the knee. In Evarts, C. M. (ed.): Surgery of the Musculoskeletal System, Vol. 4, Ed. 2. Churchill Livingstone, Inc., chap. 114, 1990.)

MENISCUS REPAIR

Multiple techniques have been developed to permit safe meniscus repair, and both open and arthroscopic techniques can lead to successful results. Current concepts of meniscus repair are primarily based on the experience with open techniques since 1976, whereas arthroscopic techniques have been developed more recently and continue to evolve. Initially, arthroscopic meniscus repair was associated with major complications (injuries to the peroneal and saphenous nerves, popliteal artery and vein, and deep sepsis), but through the work of Henning and others it has been established that arthroscopic meniscus repair can be performed safely using posteromedial-lateral incisions for protection of neurovascular structures and needle retrieval. This also helps prevent infection, as sutures are tied over the capsular layer protected by subcutaneous tissue and skin closure.

Theoretically, the major concern with arthroscopic repair is that rim preparation cannot be performed as well as with a purely open technique. In addition, vertical orientation of sutures is also difficult, if not impossible, using arthroscopic techniques. However, tears not purely within the meniscosynovial junction may be very difficult or impossible to repair with an open technique. Therefore, one must be adept at performing both open and arthroscopic repairs. The surgeon must be very meticulous about enhancing vascularity to permit a healing response for meniscus lesions whose blood supply is in question. Rasps, curettes, and motorized instruments have all been effective in preparation of the meniscus and synovium in these cases. Techniques to provide vascular access to clearly avascular zones and the use of fibrin clot injection to stimulate avascular healing remain under active investigation. The potential for increased application of meniscal repair techniques in the future is indeed exciting. However, additional laboratory and clinical studies are required to establish the efficacy of meniscal repair in the avascular zone and repairs associated with extensive damage to the meniscus body. Recent animal research by Newman et al. has shown that healing of radial tears did not restore normal biomechanical function to the meniscus.[43]

Criteria for repair must be specific. Not all tears need to be repaired, as spontaneous healing of acute peripheral tears can occur. As already mentioned, fresh tears less than 1 cm in length in the periphery of the meniscus that are *stable* to probing do not need to be sutured. Simple protection by immobilization in slight flexion and nonweight bearing of the limb for 4 to 6 weeks usually results in a healed meniscal lesion. The aftercare and rehabilitation are essentially the same as that described for formal meniscus repair below. Acute tears between 1 and 2 cm in length are more likely to require suturing, as spontaneous healing is much less likely to occur because of meniscal instability. The lag time between injury and treatment also has a significant role in selecting the best treatment for a given tear. Unstable peripheral vertical tears in an otherwise intact meniscus that are more than 6 weeks old will not heal spontaneously but can be successfully repaired. The authors have noted that preoperative arthrography has been helpful in identifying these potentially repairable chronic lesions, particularly in the medial meniscus. A timely arthrogram or MRI may identify a potentially repairable lesion and help the surgeon psychologically prepare the athlete for a procedure that may require 6 months before returning to agility sports (Table 16-2).

The details of meniscus repair have been described elsewhere[12, 15] but the authors

TABLE 16–2 Postoperative Rehabilitation Protocol for Meniscus Repair

Postop Time	Protocol
0–2 Weeks	Hinged splint; hinges locked at 45 degrees
2–4 Weeks	Hinged splint; limited motion of 30 to 70 degrees
4–6 Weeks	Splint removed Gentle range of motion Isometric thigh exercise Continue on crutches
6 Weeks	More aggressive motion exercises to regain remaining range of motion Begin progressive resistance exercise: quadriceps and hamstrings Continue crutches until lifting 15 pounds quads
3–6 Months	Bicycling and swimming Straight-ahead jogging to one-half speed running No hard running, agility maneuvers, or full squats
6 Months	Gradual return to unrestricted activities as tolerated

would like to state that careful exposure, freshening of the capsular bed to ensure vascularity on the capsular side of the repair, and trimming of any secondary tears in the rim or body of the meniscus should be performed routinely. A vertically oriented suture technique is preferred, especially with open techniques. The authors prefer to use small 4–0 absorbable sutures and to tie the sutures inside the joint, but others have advocated bringing the sutures out through the capsule. Sutures are placed approximately 3 mm apart. The number of sutures is determined by each specific anatomical situation, and complete reattachment of the capsular bed back to the rim of the meniscus is necessary. (Figs. 16–13, 16–14, 16–15, 16–16, 16–17, 16–18).

Arthroscopic repair techniques have varied with time. The authors strongly agree with the use of posterior protective incisions so that the needles can be safely passed and retrieved. At the present time, there has been no clear evidence that either permanent or absorbable suture material produces a higher ratio of success. Outside-in techniques such as the one described by Arnoczky et al.[3] are particularly useful in anterior tears, whereas inside-out techniques are preferred for posterior segment repairs. There are several types of inside-out cannulas on the market— some even zone specific to provide easy suture placement in the posterior medial or posterior lateral of the meniscus.

Whether repair is performed as an open or arthroscopic technique, details of aftercare are important. The principles are to provide maximal early protection to help encourage a successful healing response by protection from weight bearing and limiting motion to the 30- to 80-degree range for the first 4 to 6 weeks, followed by continued protection from heavy stresses during the maturation phase of healing to minimize risk of rerupture. Standard rehabilitation to regain range of motion and muscular strength is initiated at 6 weeks, with increasing weight bearing so that crutches are usually discarded by 7 to 8 weeks. Progressive resistance exercises for the quadriceps and hamstrings are initiated with either full range isotonic or isokinetic techniques unless there are patellofemoral symptoms or changes that would dictate modification of the quadriceps exercises (isometric at or near full extension or short arc terminal extension). Squats and leg presses are avoided, but hamstring curls are not restricted in any way. Swimming, cycling, and jogging are initiated at approximately 3 months, but full-speed running, squats, and agility activities are delayed until approximately 6 months. To date, we have not encountered any meniscus retear that required surgical treatment (repeat repair or partial meniscectomy) that did not present clinical symptoms and signs usually associated with meniscus tears. Accordingly, we recommend very close and careful clinical follow-up of meniscus repair cases but do not recommend routine arthrography and/or arthroscopy merely to document healing.

Because of the frequent association of repairable meniscus tears and anterior cruciate ligament injuries (80 percent of cases with repairable menisci have an associated acute or chronic ACL tear in the authors' experience), no discussion of meniscus repair is complete without considering treatment of

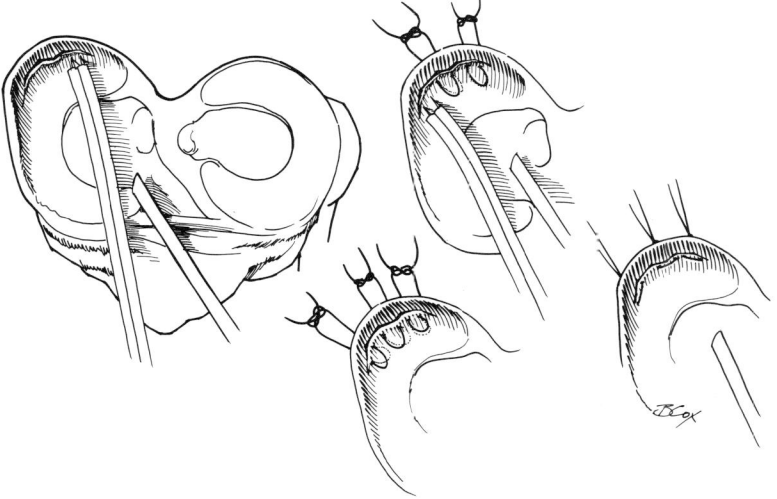

FIGURE 16–13. Artist's rendition of inside-out meniscus repair technique using double cannulated needle passers. Meticulous preparation of the capsule side of the meniscal bed is required to promote healing. (From Kalenak, A., Hanks, G. A., and Sebastianelli, W. A.: Arthroscopy of the knee. In Evarts, C. M. (ed.): Surgery of the Musculoskeletal System, Vol. 4, Ed. 2. Churchill Livingstone, Inc., chap. 114, 1990.)

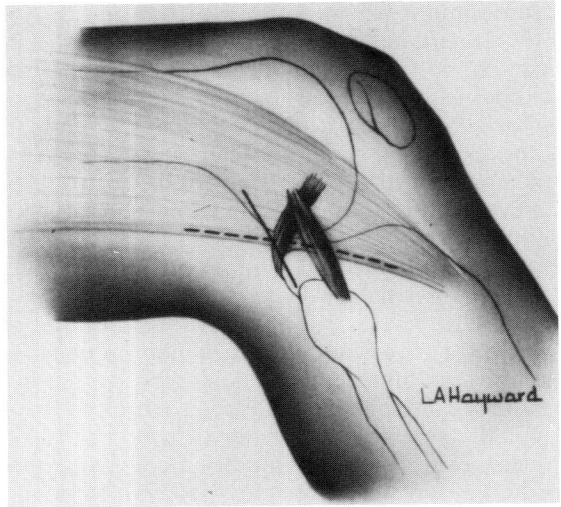

FIGURE 16–14. The lateral exposure for the open meniscus repair technique. The skin incision is marked by a *solid line,* and the iliotibial band splitting incision is marked by a *broken line.* (From DeHaven, K. E., Black, K. P., and Griffiths, H. J.: Open meniscus repair: Technique and two to nine years results. Am. J. sports Med. Vol. 17(6):788–795, 1989.)

FIGURE 16–15. Artist's rendition of peripheral detachment of the lateral meniscus. Note the popliteus tendon traversing the depths of the sketch at a 45-degree angle in the *bottom right-hand* corner of the intra-articular view. (From DeHaven, K. E., Black, K. P., and Griffiths, H. J.: Open meniscus repair: Technique and two to nine years results. Am. J. Sports Med. Vol. 17(6):788–795, 1989.

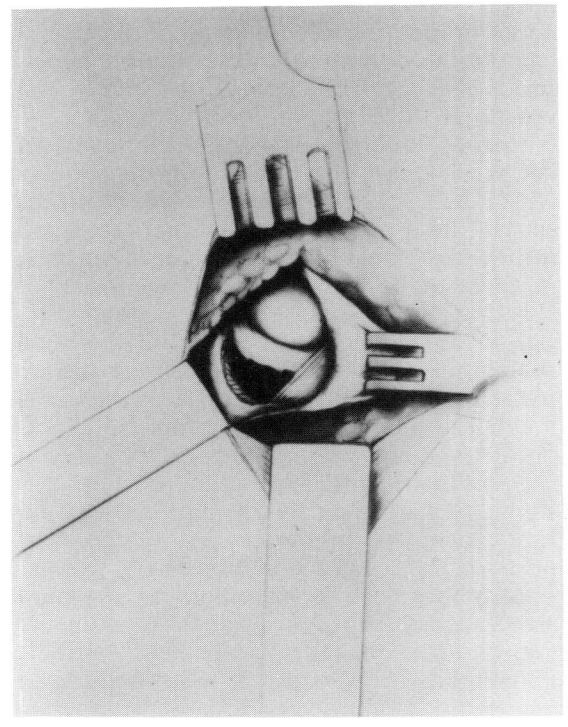

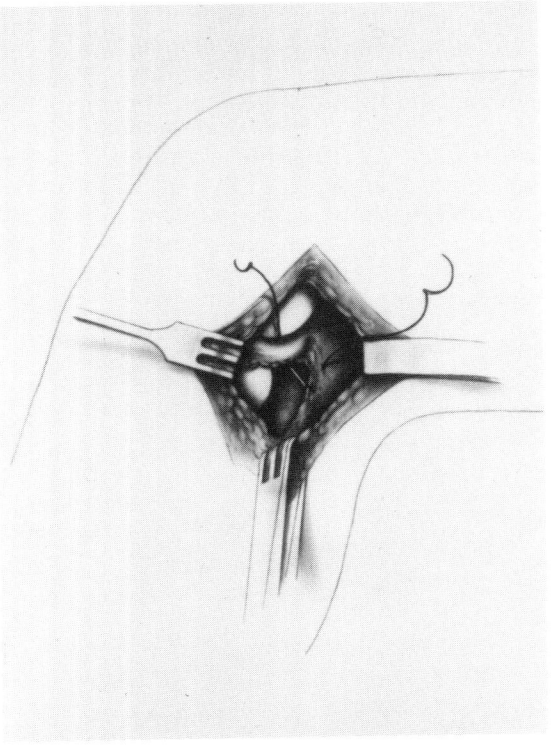

FIGURE 16–16. Care must be taken to get entire thickness bites on both the meniscal and capsular sides. The use of a smaller needle for the meniscal suture allows easier passage and grasping of the needle. This drawing depicts the repair of a right medial meniscus. (From DeHaven, K. E., Black, K. P., and Griffiths, H. J.: Open meniscus repair: Technique and two to nine years results. Am. J. Sports Med. Vol. 17(6):788–795, 1989.

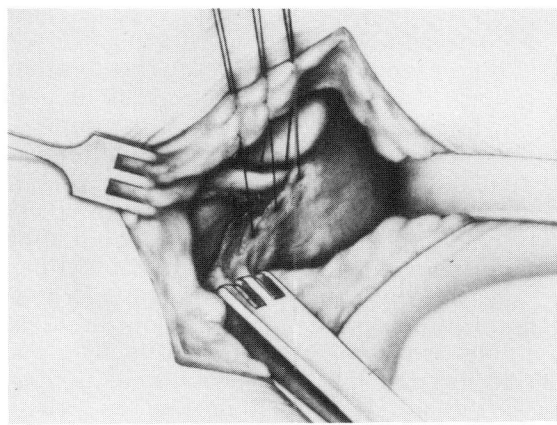

FIGURE 16–17. After the vertical capsular incision is made, the meniscal rim is sutured to its detached synovial bed using vertically placed absorbable 4–0 mattress sutures. A double armed suture is used, first passing the small needle from the inferior to superior surface of the meniscus; then the larger needle is passed from inferior to superior through the capsular bed. Individual sutures are placed 3 to 4 mm apart and tied intracapsularly, using as many sutures as necessary to achieve a strong repair. (From DeHaven, K. E., Black, K. P., and Griffiths, H. J.: Open meniscus repair: Technique and two to nine years results. Am. J. Sports Med. Vol. 17(6):788–795, 1989.

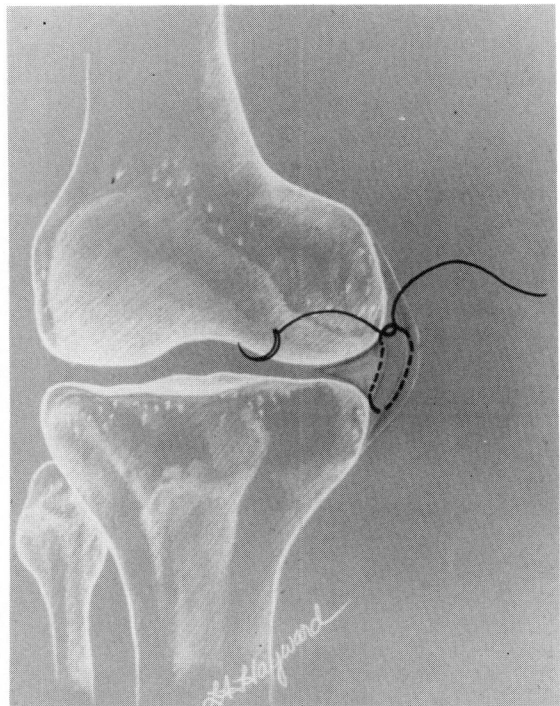

Figure 16–18. Sketch showing the vertical nature of these full thickness sutures when viewed in the coronal plane.

the ACL lesion. ACL insufficiency has been associated with a higher rate of rerupture following meniscus repair (38 percent versus 5 percent in ACL stable knees).[14] These data support the concept of ACL stabilization in conjunction with meniscus repair, particularly in young patients who wish to be athletically active. However, in skeletally immature patients, the treatment of ACL tears is complicated by concerns of affecting future growth of the distal femoral and proximal tibial epiphyses. This is discussed in detail in Chapter 18. We have encountered several patients with symptomatic, repairable meniscus tears in whom open epiphyses have represented a contraindication to ACL reconstruction. In these cases, we have proceeded with meniscus repair and activity modification until the patient reached sufficient skeletal maturity to permit standard ACL reconstruction. In other patients who were deemed to be incapable of reliably restricting their activities, extraarticular lateral tenodesis was carried out in conjunction with meniscus repair, anticipating future intraarticular reconstruction of the anterior cruciate ligament, if necessary, after skeletal maturity had been reached.

TOTAL MENISCECTOMY

Although an extremely rare procedure in the present state of the art, a few indications for total meniscectomy do remain. Large meniscal tears with associated large parameniscal cysts still may require open, en bloc resection of the meniscus and cyst. Circumferential fiber disruption producing two large separate pieces in a young individual also will likely lead to total meniscectomy. One must also remember that in young individuals with normal articular surfaces and very competent ligaments, arthroscopic total meniscectomy may be difficult, especially on the medial side. Open traditional meniscectomy, with protection of the articular cartilage, might be better in the long run for such an individual than arthroscopic technique that produces significant damage to the articular surfaces, even though the initial morbidity would be greater. The choice between these two techniques will depend on the experience of the surgeon.

The plane of resection during a total meniscectomy should be on the meniscus side of the meniscosynovial junction to avoid damage to the deep capsular layer of the collateral ligament complex.[11] Medially, two incisions are preferred to ensure adequate removal of the posterior horn. This will also minimize the risk of trauma to the articular cartilage. Details of the preferred technique for medial and lateral meniscectomy have been previously published.[12]

Because long-term follow-up studies of total meniscectomy patients have documented a significant incidence of radiographic degenerative changes, most orthopedic surgeons are justifiably hesitant to perform total meniscectomy in a young patient.[1, 37] Attention to detail in each particular case will lead one to make the best decision. Other factors that may contribute to degeneration following total meniscectomy include overall alignment of the limb, associated trauma to the articular cartilage, the presence of associated ligamentous laxity and functional instability, and the time from injury to treatment. For example, a varus knee with articular cartilage injury and associated ligamentous laxity will do very poorly following a total medial meniscectomy.

DISCOID MENISCUS

Young[62] was the first to describe a lateral discoid meniscus in an anatomical specimen circa 1889. Kroiss[32] in 1910 described the clinical snapping syndrome associated with a discoid meniscus. As many patients remain asymptomatic, the true incidence of discoid meniscus is difficult to determine. Based on meniscectomy data, it has been estimated to be about 2.4 percent of 1200 meniscectomies performed by Nathan and Cole.[42] Smille[55] reported discoid lesions in 4.2 percent of 8000 meniscectomies. Medial lesions are much less common than lateral, with an incidence of 0.3 percent as described by Resnick et al.[47] and Dickason et al.[16]

Internal derangement in the skeletally immature knee is difficult to assess. However, a discoid meniscus should be considered in the differential diagnosis. The clinical presentation is often confusing. The onset of symptoms or mechanism of injury often cannot be elicited. Symptoms of intermittent or persistent pain, effusions, or giving way may be absent when the major symptoms are clicking or catching. The most consistent physical findings include a palpable clicking, joint line tenderness, and restricted range of motion. Occasionally, there will be a joint effusion.

Routine roentgenograms are most often normal. Resnick et al.[47] and Nathan and Cole[42] have reported lateral joint widening, hypoplastic lateral femoral condyle, elevation of the fibular head, and hypoplasia of the lateral tibial spine as roentgenographic abnormalities that may be present. Plain radiographs should be obtained to exclude other causes of knee pain such as fractures, osteochondritis dissecans, growth plate injuries, osteoid osteoma, or osteomyelitis. The authors also urge that the possibility of hip disease with referred pain to the knee be kept in mind. Vahvanen[58] has questioned the usefulness of arthrography in discoid menisci. The recent advent of the MRI may be more helpful. The role of arthroscopy as a diagnostic and therapeutic tool for discoid lesions has been well documented by Eilert[18] and Ziv and Carroll.[64]

Watanabe[60] has described a classification of discoid menisci that is based on the arthroscopic appearance. Three types are described: (1) complete, (2) incomplete, and (3) Wrisberg ligament type. A complete discoid meniscus has meniscal tissue extending to the base of the tibial spine. The incomplete type has an inner edge of meniscus extending past the free edge of a normal meniscus but stopping short of the tibial spine. The meniscal capsular attachments are quite normal in both the complete and the incomplete types of discoid menisci. The Wrisberg ligament type has a congenital absence of the posterior meniscal capsular attachment and is attached posteriorly only by the meniscal femoral ligament of Wrisberg.

When first encountered, the arthroscopic appearance of a discoid meniscus can be quite confusing. In a complete discoid meniscus, one may inspect the medial or lateral compartment of the knee and conclude that the meniscus is absent. One must carefully inspect the base of the tibial eminence and search for the inner edge of the disk, which can also be mistaken for the displaced fragment of a bucket handle tear. A tear in a discoid meniscus can be difficult to demonstrate arthroscopically. The overabundance of meniscal tissue can interfere with arthroscopic visualization. Tears most frequently occur in the central zone of the discoid meniscus. If the superior surface is found to be intact, the inferior surface should be viewed from the contralateral portal while lifting the meniscus up with a nerve hook placed through the ipsilateral portal. In some cases, the tear is still intrameniscal and can be recognized only by abnormal "wrinkling up" of the central zone during probing.

The standard treatment of discoid lesions in the past was open complete meniscectomy. Kurosaka et al.[33] presented acceptable long-term clinical results in greater than 90 percent of patients following total meniscectomy. However, they noted moderate to severe radiographic degenerative changes in nearly 70 percent. As a result, Rosenberg et al.[48] and Dickhaut and DeLee[17] have advocated partial meniscectomy or saucerization for symptomatic complete or incomplete types. We concur with this approach. In addition, Rosenberg et al.[48] have presented data for repair of the Wrisberg ligament type discoid lesion associated with some debulking if excess body tissue of the meniscus is present. Needless to say, long-term studies will be required to determine whether these techniques will be better than total meniscectomy.

Recommended treatment for discoid meniscal lesions is as follows. If the patient presents with occasional snapping but without locking or joint effusion, observation is recommended. If the patient is more symptomatic with effusions, mechanical symptoms, or pain, then partial meniscectomy of the central portion of the discoid meniscus is recommended. Resection of the anterior portion of the free margin should be initiated with a side cutting basket forceps. Excision is then continued through the middle third, using scissors or a curved meniscal blade inserted from the anteromedial portal while viewing from the anterolateral portal. A second anteromedial portal is then made, and the freed meniscal fragment is grasped with a forceps. The meniscal tissue is then retracted into the intercondylar notch to improve visualization of the posterior portion of the meniscus. A basket forceps or scissors can then be used to complete the excision of the posterior fragment. The arthroscopic surgeon must not forget that it is often advantageous at certain points to change one's visualization and instrumentation from one portal to the other. Contouring of the remaining meniscal tissue is then performed so that the width of the body of the meniscus that remains is approximately the width of a normal meniscus. The overall objective is to create a stable, intact, and balanced rim. Care must be taken to ensure that the posterior horn indeed has a competent meniscocapsular attachment. As stated above, Rosenberg et al.[48] in 1987 reported successful arthroscopic peripheral attachment after central partial meniscectomy of a Wrisberg ligament type of discoid lateral meniscus, and successful open repair of an incomplete discoid lesion has been performed by the senior author.

In conclusion, arthroscopy is an invaluable tool not only for the diagnosis but also for the treatment of discoid meniscal lesions. Extrapolation of the data for partial meniscectomy in the "normal" meniscus to the discoid meniscus suggests that partial central meniscectomy of the discoid meniscus may prevent long-term degenerative changes. We await with great interest the required follow-up to see if this proves to be true.

References

1. Allen, P. R., Denham, R. A., and Swan, A. V.: Late degenerative changes after meniscectomy, J. Bone Joint Surg. 66B:666–671, 1984.
2. Arnoczky, S. P., and Warren, R. F.: Miscrovasculature of the human meniscus. Am. J. Sports Med. 10:90–95, 1982.
3. Arnoczky, S. P., Warren, R. F., and Spivak, J. M.: Meniscal repair using an exogenous fibrin clot. J. Bone Joint Surg. 70A:1209–1217, 1988.
4. Bergstrom, R., Gillquist, J., Lysholm, J., and Hamberg, P.: Arthroscopy of the knee in children. J. Pediatr. Orthop. 4:542–545, 1984.
5. Bullough, P. G., Munera, L., Murphy, J., and Weinstein, A. M.: The strength of the menisci of the knee as it related to their fine structure. J. Bone Joint Surg. 52B:564–570, 1970.
6. Cameron, H. W., and MacNab, L: The structure of the meniscus of the human knee joint. Clin. Orthop. 89:215–219, 1972.
7. Casscells, S. W.: The place of arthroscopy in the diagnosis and treatment of internal derangements of the knee. Clin. Orthop. 151:135–142, 1980.
8. Cassidy, R. E., and Shaffer, A. J. Repair of peripheral meniscus tears. A preliminary report. Am. J. Sports Med. 9:209, 1981.
9. Clark, C. R., and Ogden, J. A.: Development of the menisci of the human knee joint. J. Bone Joint Surg. 65A:538–547, 1983.
10. Cox, J. S., Nye, C. E., Schaefer, W. W., and Woodstein, I. J.: The degenerative effects of partial and total resection of the medial meniscus in dogs' knee. Clin. Orthop. 109:179–183, 1975.
11. DeHaven, K. E.: The knee. In Goldstein, L. A., and Dickerson, R. C. (eds.): Atlas of Orthopaedic Surgery, Ed. 2. C. V. Mosby Co., St. Louis, 1981.
12. DeHaven, K. E.: Injuries to the menisci of the knee. In Nicholas, J. A., and Hershman, E. B. (eds.): The Lower Extremity and Spine in Sports Medicine. C. V. Mosby Co., St. Louis, 1986.
13. DeHaven, K. E.: Role of the meniscus. In Bristol

Myers/Zimmer: Articular Cartilage and Knee Joint Function. New York, Raven Press.
14. DeHaven, K. E., Black, K. P., and Griffiths, H. J.: Open meniscus repair: Technique and two to nine years results. Am. J. Sports Med. 17(6):788–795.
15. DeHaven, K. E., and Collins, H. R.: Diagnosis of internal derangements of the knee. J. Bone Joint Surg. 57A:802–810, 1975.
16. Dickason, J. M., DelPisso, W., Blazina, M. E., Fox, J. M., Friedman, M. J., and Snyder, S. T.: A series of ten discoid medial menisci. Clin. Orthop. 168:75–79, 1982.
17. Dickhaut, S. C., and DeLee, J. C.: The discoid lateral meniscus syndrome. J. Bone Joint Surg. 64A:1068–1073, 1982.
18. Eilert, R. E.: Arthroscopy of the knee joint in children. Orthop. Rev. 5(9):61–65, 1976.
19. Eiskjaer, S., and Larsen, S. T.: Arthroscopy of the knee in children. Acta Orthop. Scand. 58:273–276, 1987.
20. Fairbanks, T. J.: Knee joint changes after meniscectomy. J. Bone Joint Surg. 30B:664–670, 1948.
21. Frankel, V. H., Burstein, A. H., and Brooks, D. B.: Biomechanics of internal derangement of the knee. Pathomechanics as determined by analysis of instant centers of motion. J. Bone Joint Surg. 53A:945–962, 1971.
22. Fujikawa, K., Iseki, F., and Mikura, Y.: Partial resection of the discoid meniscus in the child's knee. J. Bone Joint Surg. 63B:391–395, 1981.
23. Guhl, J. F.: Excision of flap tears. Orthop. Clin. North Am. 13:387, 1982.
24. Harway, R., and Handker, S.: Internal derangement of the knee in an infant: Case report. Contemp. Orthop. 17:49–51, 1988.
25. Hamberg, P., Gillquist, J., and Lysholm, J.: Suture of new and old peripheral meniscus tears. J. Bone Joint Surg. 65A:193–197, 1983.
26. Hayashi, L. K., Yamaga, H., Ida, K., and Miura, T.: Arthroscopic meniscectomy for discoid lateral meniscus in children. J. Bone Joint Surg. 70A:1495–1499, 1988.
27. Ikeuchi, H.: Arthroscopic treatment of the discoid lateral meniscus. Clin. Orthop. 167:19–28, 1982.
28. Jackson, R. W., and Dandy, D. J.: Partial meniscectomy. J. Bone Joint Surg. 58B:142, 1976.
29. Johnson, L. L.: Arthroscopic Surgery: Principles and Practice, Ed. 3. C. V. Mosby Co., St. Louis, 1986.
30. King, D.: The healing of semilunar cartilages. J. Bone Joint Surg. 28:333–342, 1936.
31. Krause, W. R., Pope, M. H., Johnson, R. J., and Wilder, D. G.: Mechanical changes in the knee after meniscectomy. J. Bone Joint Surg. 58A:599–604, 1976.
32. Kroiss, F.: Die Verletzungen der Kneigelenkszwischenknorpel und ihrer Verbindungen. Beitr. Klin Chir. 66:598, 1910.
33. Kurosaka, M., Yoshiya, S., Ohno, O., and Hirohata, K.: Lateral discoid meniscectomy. A 20 year follow-up. Presented at the American Academy of Orthopaedic Surgery Meeting, San Francisco, January 1987.
34. Lynch, M. A., Henning, C. E., and Glick, K. R.: Knee joint surface changes. Clin. Orthop. 172:148, 1983.
35. Manco, L. G., Kavanaugh, J. H., Lozman, J., Colman, N. D., Bilfield, B. S., and Fay, J. J.: Diagnosis of meniscal tears using high resolution computed tomography. J. Bone Joint Surg. 69A:498–502, 1987.
36. Manzione, M., Pizzutillo, P. D., Peoples, A. B., and Schweizer, P. A.: Meniscectomy in children. A long term follow-up study. Am. J. Sports Med. 11:111–115, 1983.
37. McGinty, J. B., Geuss, L. F., and Marvin, R. A.: Partial or total meniscectomy. J. Bone Joint Surg. 59A:763–766, 1977.
38. Medlar, R. C., Mandiberg, J. J., and Lyne, E. D.: Meniscectomies in children. Am. J. Sports Med. 8:87–92, 1980.
39. Metcalf, R. W.: Operative arthroscopy of the knee. In American Academy of Orthopaedic Surgeons: Instructional Course Lectures, Vol. 30. C. V. Mosby Co., St. Louis, 1981.
40. Morrissey, R. T., Eubanks, R. G., Park, J. P., and Thompson, S. B., Jr.: Arthroscopy of the knee in children. Clin. Orthop. 162:103–107, 1982.
41. Mow, V. C., Mak, A. F., Lai, W. M., et al.: Viscoelastic properties of proteoglycan subunits and aggregates in varying solution concentrations. J. Biomech. 17:325–338, 1984.
42. Nathan, P. A., and Cole, S. C.: Discoid meniscus. Clin. Orthop. 64:107–113, 1969.
43. Newman, A. P., Anderson, D. R., et al.: Mechanics of the healed meniscus in a canine model. Am. J. Sports Med. 17(2):164–175, 1989.
44. Nicholas, J. A., Freiberger, R. H., and Killoran, P. J.: Double-contrast arthrography of the knee. J. Bone Joint Surg. 52A:203–220, 1970.
45. O'Brien, W. R., Warren, R. F., Friederich, N. F., Muller, W., Jackson, R. W., James, P. H., Henning, C. E., and Lynch, M. A.: Degenerative arthritis of the knee following anterior cruciate ligament injury: A multi-center, long-term follow-up study. Presented at the 6th International Congress of the Society of the Knee, Rome, Italy, 1989.
46. Polly, D. W., et al: The accuracy of selective magnetic resonance imaging compared with the findings of arthroscopy of the knee. J. Bone Joint Surg. 70A:192–198, 1988.
47. Resnick, D., Goergen, T. G., Kay, J. J., Ghelman, B., and Woody, P. R.: Discoid medial meniscal. Radiology 121:575, 1976.
48. Rosenberg, T. D., Paulos, L. E., Parker, R. D., Harner, C. D., and Gurley, W. D.: Discoid lateral meniscus: Case report of arthroscopic attachment of a symptomatic Wrisberg-ligament type. Arthroscopy 3:227–282, 1987.
49. Saddawi, N. D., and Hoffman, B. K.: Tear of the attachment of a normal medial meniscus of the knee in a four-year-old child. J. Bone Joint Surg. 52A:809–811, 1970.
50. Scapinelli, R.: Studies on the vasculature of the human knee joint. Acta Anat. 70:305–331, 1968.
51. Scott, G. A., Jolly, B. L., and Henning, C. E.: Combined posterior incision and arthroscopic intraarticular repair of the meniscus. J. Bone Joint Surg. 68A:847–861, 1986.
52. Shahriaree, H.: The menisci in *O'Connor's Textbook of Arthroscopic Surgery*. J. B. Lippincott Co., Philadelphia, PA, 1984.
53. Shim, S. S., and Leung, G.: Blood supply of the knee joint. Clin. Orthop. 208:119–125, 1986.
54. Silva, I., Jr., and Silver, D. M.: Tears of the meniscus as revealed by magnetic resonance imaging. J. Bone Joint Surg. 70A:199–202, 1988.

55. Smille, I. S.: The congenital discoid meniscus. J. Bone Joint Surg. 30B:671–682, 1948.
56. Sprague III, N. F.: The bucket handle meniscal tear: A technique using two incisions. Orthop. Clin. North Am. 13:337–348, 1982.
57. Suman, R. K., Stother, I. G., and Illingworth, G.: Diagnostic arthroscopy of the knee in children. J. Bone Joint Surg. 66B:535–537, 1984.
58. Vahvanen, V., and Aalto, K.: Meniscectomy in children. Acta Orthop. Scand. 50:791–795, 1979.
59. Walker, P. S., and Erkman, M. J.: The role of the menisci in force transmission across the knee. Clin. Orthop. 109:184–192, 1972.
60. Watanabe, M.: Arthroscopy of the knee joint. In Helfet, A. J. (ed.): Disorders of the Knee. J. B. Lippincott Co., Philadelphia, PA, 145, 1974.
61. Weiss, C. B., Lundberg, M., Hamberg, P., DeHaven, K. E., and Gillquist, J.: Non-operative treatment of meniscal tears. J. Bone Joint Surg. 71A:811–822, 1989.
62. Young, R. T.: The external semilunar cartilage as a complete disc. In Cleland, J., Mackay, J. Y., and Young, R. B. (eds.): Memoirs and Memoranda in Anatomy. Williams and Norgate, London, 179, 1889.
63. Zaman, M., and Leonard, M. A.: Meniscectomy in children: A study of fifty-nine knees. J. Bone Joint Surg. 60B:436–437, 1978.
64. Ziv, I., and Carroll, N. C.: The role of arthroscopy in children. J. Pediatr. Orthop. 2 243–247, 1982.
65. McMurray, T. P.: The semilunar cartilages. Br. J. Surg. 29:407, 1942.

17
COLLATERAL LIGAMENT INJURIES

BRUCE REIDER

ISOLATED MEDIAL COLLATERAL LIGAMENT INJURIES

Although isolated sprains of the medial collateral ligament (MCL) are very common—perhaps the most common ligamentous knee injury in sports—their treatment remains somewhat controversial. Compared with the cruciate ligament tears, they are relatively benign injuries. It is probably accurate to state that more morbidity has resulted from the overtreatment to these injuries than from their neglect. The treatment program recommended here is an aggressive one. For this treatment to be safe and effective, however, the diagnosis must be confidently established, and the concomitant occurrence of other more serious injuries, such as tears of the cruciate ligaments, must be ruled out.

CLINICAL PICTURE

The majority of isolated medial collateral ligament sprains are contact injuries, produced by an acute lateral blow about the knee while the foot is braced by contact with the ground. This may occur in sports where the contact is intentional, such as football, or incidental, such as in basketball or soccer. The athlete may feel a pop or a tearing sensation at the medial aspect of the knee. Frequently, he or she will vividly describe the sensation of the medial side of the knee "opening up" and feeling loose afterward. Less commonly, the medial collateral may be sprained during a noncontact injury, such as a skiing fall during which the skis diverge and the body itself provides the requisite valgus stress. In the case of a noncontact injury, the clinician must have a higher index of suspicion of anterior cruciate ligament (ACL) tear. It is common for an athlete who has sustained an anterior cruciate ligament tear to state, "My knee went in," mistaking an axial rotation for a valgus one.

The initial pain is often intense, with the athlete remaining down on the field or court. This intensity often moderates within a few minutes. In the case of the first-degree medial collateral ligament sprain, the unsupervised athlete may actually resume play following the injury. As hemorrhage and edema take place, the pain again increases, and stiffness will set in during the first 12 hours.

PHYSICAL EXAMINATION

As mentioned above, the pain of the inciting injury temporarily decreases and the ligament may be minimally tender for the first hour or so. After this, point tenderness is usually found directly over the damaged portion of the ligament. Injury occurs most commonly in the proximal portion of the ligament or over the joint line. In a lean individual, the examiner may actually be able to palpate the torn ends of the ligament. The key to palpating the medial collateral ligament is locating the medial epicondyle and remembering that the ligament pro-

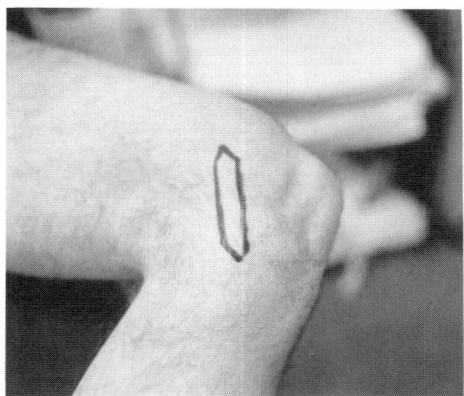

FIGURE 17–1. The medial collateral ligament begins at the medial epicondyle and courses distally to its insertion beneath the pes anserinus.

gresses distally and anteriorly along an oblique course until it passes under the pes anserinus (Fig. 17–1).

If the athlete is examined the day after the injury, local edema and some degree of effusion will usually have set in. In the lean athlete, an area of boggy thickening and point tenderness can usually be felt in the damaged portion of the medial collateral ligament. The effusion may vary from nonexistent to massive. The larger the effusion, the more the clinician should suspect concomitant injury to the anterior cruciate ligament. Stability testing is extremely important in establishing the correct diagnosis. As in all stability testing, the patient must be fully relaxed for testing to proceed easily and reliably. The technique that I prefer is one in which the clinician supports the full weight of the injured leg with one hand beneath the athlete's heel (Fig. 17–2). The patient is adequately relaxed when the examiner feels that the leg would fall to the table if it were released. The examiner then applies a mild valgus stress by pushing gently inward at the knee while reciprocally pushing outward at the heel with the knee in full extension. In virtually all normal knees, essentially no valgus opening will be felt in this position. When the test is abnormal, the clinician will feel the tibia and femur separate as he or she stresses the knee

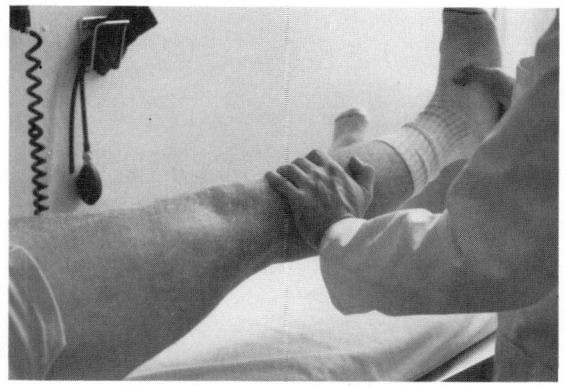

A

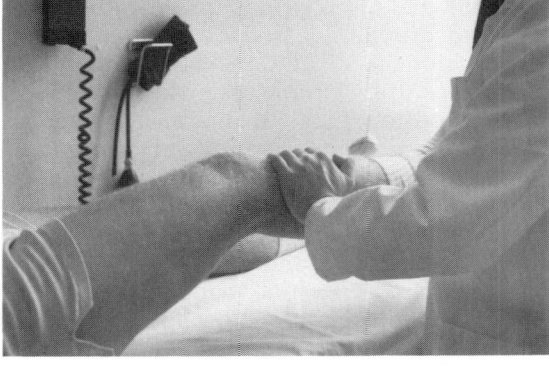

B

FIGURE 17–2. The laxity of the medial complex is first assessed in full extension (A) and then slight flexion (B). If the knee is flexed too far, uncontrollable hip rotation will prevent the examiner from applying an effective valgus torque to the knee (C).

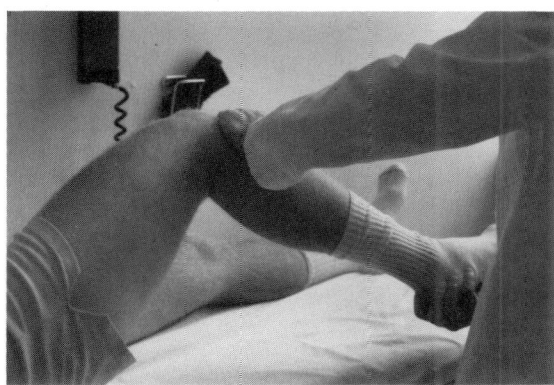

C

and come back together with a clunk as he or she relaxes. This opening in full extension is an ominous sign, as it usually indicates rupture of the medial collateral ligament, medial and posteromedial capsule, and one or both cruciate ligaments.[7, 9]

If the knee is stable in full extension, it is then flexed 5 or 10 degrees and the test repeated. This will relax the posterior capsule, allowing the medial collateral ligament to be tested in greater isolation.[7, 9] I do not recommend flexing the knee more than 5 or 10 degrees. The more the knee is flexed, the more the intended valgus stress will produce internal rotation of the extremity at the hip and confuse the examiner. Again, when the test is abnormal, the tibia and femur are felt to separate with valgus stress and to "clunk" back together with relaxation. Because some knees will open up slightly to valgus stress in this position, it is important to compare with the uninjured side.

Two systems of clinical classification of abnormal valgus laxity exist. The traditional classification is based on the *anatomical* classification of ligament injuries. In this anatomical classification, grade I sprains are those in which tenderness is present in the ligament, but no significant elongation has occurred; grade II sprains are those in which plastic elongation of the ligament has occurred, resulting in increased laxity but not total disruption; grade III sprains are those in which the ligament is completely ruptured. The *clinical* application of this anatomical classification defines grade I sprains as those marked by tenderness over the medial collateral ligament but no abnormal laxity, grade II sprains as those in which tenderness over the ligament is accompanied by valgus laxity but a "firm end point," and grade III sprains as those in which no definite end point is felt in response to valgus stress. The problem with this sytem of clinical classification is that pain and muscle spasm may prevent the examiner from accurately assessing the end point, making the differentiation between grade II and III sprains rather questionable. I personally feel that the alternative clincial classification offered by John Marshall[7] is easier to use and more prognostically valuable. In this system, grade I sprains remain the same, but grade II sprains include all those in which valgus stability in full extension is normal but valgus laxity in flexion is increased. Grade III sprains include only those in which valgus laxity is increased in both full extension and flexion (Table 17–1). This distinction is easier to make than trying to assess the end point to valgus stress. It is also helpful prognostically, since almost all knees with abnormal valgus laxity in extension will have an associated cruciate ligament injury and therefore fall into a different prognostic and treatment category than those with isolated medial collateral injuries.

TABLE 17–1. Clinical Grading of Isolated MCL Sprains

	Marshall Grading	Traditional Grading
Grade I	MCL tender; no abnormal laxity	MCL tender; no abnormal laxity
Grade II	Any amount of increased valgus laxity in flexion; normal valgus stability in full flexion	Increased valgus laxity with a "firm end point"
Grade III	Increased valgus laxity both flexion and full extension	Increased valgus laxity with a "soft end point"

RADIOGRAPHIC EXAMINATION

Radiographs are usually normal in the acute MCL injury, although they are usually done, especially in the adolescent, to rule out fracture. Occasionally an avulsion fracture will be seen. Ectopic calcification in the torn ligament, the Pellegrini-Stieda sign, may develop following this injury.[32]

DIFFERENTIAL DIAGNOSIS

Conditions most commonly confused with medial collateral sprains include contusion of the medial side of the knee, subluxation of the patella, and medial meniscus tear. Because the *medial contusion* will have been produced by a direct medial blow, an exact description of the mechanism of injury should help distinguish between contusions and medial collateral ligament sprains. The patient may be mistaken in his or her history, however, so the clinician must never completely rely on the history of a valgus torque to make the diagnosis of medial collateral sprain. Since contusions are successfully treated with the same functional rehabilitation approach used for medial collateral sprains, this distinction is not a vital one.

Patellar subluxation may also be confused with isolated medial collateral sprain. Both may be produced by a real or imagined valgus torque, and patellar subluxation may also be accompanied by medial pain. In the case of patellar subluxation, this medial pain is due to avulsion of a portion of the origin of the vastus medialis obliqus at the medial intermuscular septum, so the tenderness will start at the adductor tubercle and course proximally. Because the patient may not realize that a patellar subluxation has occurred, it is important to distinguish tenderness at the vastus medialis obliquus origin and tenderness distal to it in the substance of the medial collateral ligament (Fig. 17–3). Occasionally, patellar subluxation and medial collateral sprain may occur together.

Periodically, the clincian may experience some difficulty distinguishing between a *medial meniscus tear* and a sprain of the medial collateral ligament. This should not be a problem in second- and third-degree sprains, because the abnormal valgus laxity present verifies the existence of injury to the medial collateral ligament. Because the isolated medial collateral sprain is usually caused by a valgus torque that separates the medial femoral condyle and medial tibial plateau, a medial collateral ligament sprain may be associated with injury to the meniscofemoral or meniscotibial ligaments but almost never with a true tear of the body of the medial meniscus.[24] The primary difficulty in diagnosis will therefore arise in the patient who exhibits medial knee tenderness but no abnormal valgus laxity. In these cases, careful palpation to localize the site of the most exquisite tenderness will often make the diagnosis. When the principal tenderness is along the course of the ligament, either proximal or distal to the joint line, a tear of the meniscus is unlikely. Conversely, exquisite tenderness along the posteromedial joint line in the area posterior to the medial collateral ligament favors the diagnosis of medial meniscus tear (Fig. 17–4). In cases in which the maximum tenderness is at the point where the medial collateral ligament crosses the medial meniscus, it may not be possible to differentiate between a first-degree medial collateral sprain and medial meniscus tear at the time of the first examination. In these cases, the early postinjury course usually makes the diagnosis obvious. Since most athletes will recover from a first-degree medial collateral sprain within 10 days of the injury,[5] the persistence of significant tenderness or pain after this period of time should make the clinician suspect a medial meniscus tear.

It should always be remembered that an unstable *fracture through the distal femoral physis* may be mistaken for a knee ligament injury in the skeletally immature athlete. In general, such a fracture will produce more pain and swelling than an isolated MCL injury, and the femoral physis will be circumferentially tender. A stress radiograph may be necessary to rule out a physeal fracture in equivocal cases.

It is extremely important to rule out a *concomitant injury to the anterior cruciate ligament* when a medial collateral sprain is diagnosed. As noted, the anterior cruciate

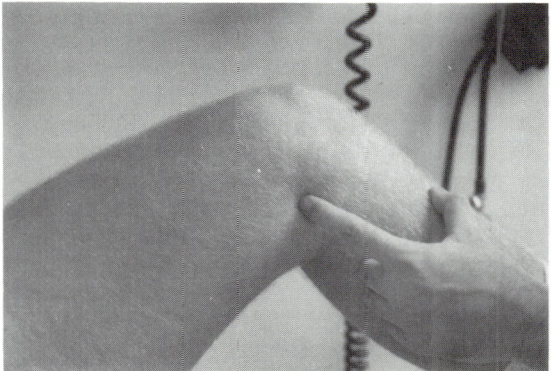

FIGURE 17–4. A medial meniscus tear will usually produce tenderness at the medial joint line posterior to the medial collateral ligament.

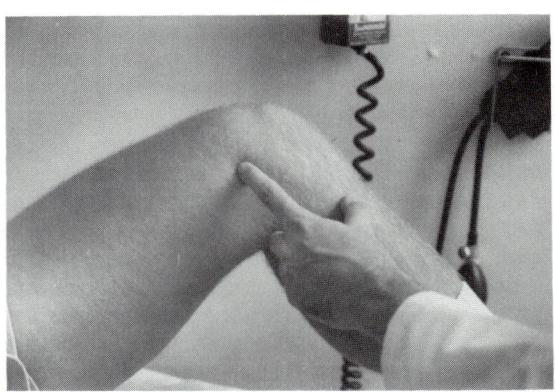

FIGURE 17–3. A primary episode of patellar subluxation or dislocation may produce tenderness at the vastus medialis obliquus origin proximal to the medial epicondyle.

ligament is virtually always torn in the presence of third-degree medial collateral sprains and may be torn in the presence of second-degree medial collateral ligament sprains.[7] When the anterior cruciate ligament is also ruptured, the medial collateral sprain becomes an injury of secondary importance. In such a case, concentrating on the medial collateral ligament injury and overlooking the anterior cruciate rupture will lead to inappropriate treatment decisions. Usually, a carefully performed Lachman test will be sufficient to rule out anterior cruciate ligament tear. In the case of more severe second-degree medial collateral ligament sprains, a certain amount of anteromedial laxity may be present to confuse the Lachman test results.[13] In severe second-degree medial collateral ligament sprains, an arthroscopy will occasionally be necessary to verify the integrity of the anterior cruciate ligament.

It should be emphasized that the typical history of a medial collateral ligament sprain is that of an acute injury accompanied by moderate or severe pain that gradually diminishes over the ensuing few weeks. With few exceptions, such as symptoms produced by the "whip kick" in breast strokers,[14, 15, 25, 29] pain attributable to the medial collateral ligament does not develop gradually or persist chronically. Therefore, the clinician should suspect another injury in cases in which medial knee pain has developed gradually or persists for more than a month following an acute knee injury.

TREATMENT

Accepted treatments for isolated medial collateral ligament injuries have undergone considerable evolution, from surgery to strict immobilization to aggressive rehabilitation and early return to sports. Even now, surgical or cast treatment of these injuries appears to have many adherents, although no objective studies have ever shown that these techniques produce superior results. Objective studies by Fetto and Marshall in 1978[7] and Indelicato[12] in 1983 have both shown that immobilization with casts or cast braces produces results comparable with those obtained with surgery. Even before these objective studies were published, Ellsasser et al.[6] published an article recommending aggressive rehabilitation without immobilization for these injuries in professional football players. Ellsasser and subsequent authors have emphasized that the diagnosis of an isolated medial collateral ligament sprain must be definitely made for such a program to be successful. A subsequent study by Derscheid and Garrick[5] showed that such a program could return college football players to competition in 10 to 20 days without an increased risk of reinjury to the knee. Longer-term studies at the University of Chicago[24] have shown that an aggressive rehabilitation program produces results comparable with those of surgery or immobilization but with a tremendous decrease in morbidity and a much more rapid return to competition. This treatment program is just as applicable to the school-age athlete as it is to the collegiate or professional competitor. Recent research by Woo[31] has added basic science support to these clinical studies by showing that active mobilization actually aided healing and maturation of transsected medial collateral ligaments in the rabbit model.[31] Complementary biomechanical research by Inoue et al. suggests that functional rehabilitation programs work because the ACL is a more important restraint to valgus torque than previously appreciated. They state that earlier biomechanical research overemphasized the role of the MCL in resisting valgus torque by restricting axial rotation of the knee during testing. This research also provided evidence that concomitant ACL injury dramatically affects the significance of an MCL tear.[13]

If a physician or athletic trainer is present at the time of injury, the knee should be packed in ice for about one-half hour initially and then every 3 to 4 hours for the first 24 hours. This ice regimen has two potential benefits. First, because it induces initial vasoconstriction, the immediate application of ice may limit the amount of initial hemorrhage. This benefit will pertain only if the ice is applied within minutes following the injury. Second, by lowering tissue temperature and thus slowing tissue metabolism, icing may limit the secondary extension of cell injury caused by swelling and edema. These benefits are achieved in the first 24 to 48 hours following injury. After this, the role of ice is primarily as an analgesic to facilitate therapeutic exercise.[16]

It should be explained to the patient at the outset that the functional rehabilitation program is a goal-oriented one. Each time the patient passes a functional goal, he or she is allowed to proceed to the next phase of rehabilitation. In the medial collateral ligament treatment program, the principal goals are (1) walking without a limp, (2) achieving 90 degrees of flexion in the knee, (3) achieving full range of motion in the knee, and (4) passing the functional running test. It should be emphasized to the athlete that he or she will not be withheld from sports for any arbitrary period of time but for as short or long a period of time as it takes him or her to achieve all functional goals. The athlete may be informed that the *average* time for return to sports such as football is 10 days for grade I medial collateral ligament injury and 21 days for a grade II injury. The athlete should be given a printed copy of the full rehabilitation program at the time of the first treatment. This procedure takes the responsibility for allowing for the return to competition from the clinician and places it squarely on the shoulders of the athlete.

Although it has been shown that motion may actually improve collateral ligament healing,[31] much of the benefit of the functional rehabilitation program is probably achieved by minimizing the secondary debilitation caused by other treatment programs. Since immobilization is deleterious to muscle, ligament, and cartilage, it should be minimized. Patients with grade I sprains usually feel comfortable without any specific support and often will disdain the use of crutches from the outset. Athletes with a grade II sprain, however, will usually experience an unsettling feeling of their joint opening abnormally and will be considerably reassured by the application of a valgus support. We have found that the lateral hinge braces initially developed as "prophylactic knee braces" fulfill this function ideally. Models made in a neoprene sleeve with Velcro closures allow for easy removal and reapplication by the patient. Except for washing and physical therapy treatments, these braces are worn night and day for the first 3 weeks following the injury. It is not recommended that knee immobilizers or double upright postoperative braces be substituted in this role (Fig. 17–5). They are more restrictive than the limited lateral hinge brace and tend to inhibit the use of the leg and encourage atrophy and prolonged disability.

From the beginning, weight bearing is encouraged, but crutches are usually used to ensure normal gait. If an athlete is allowed to force himself or herself to walk with a marked limp, he or she may develop an ab-

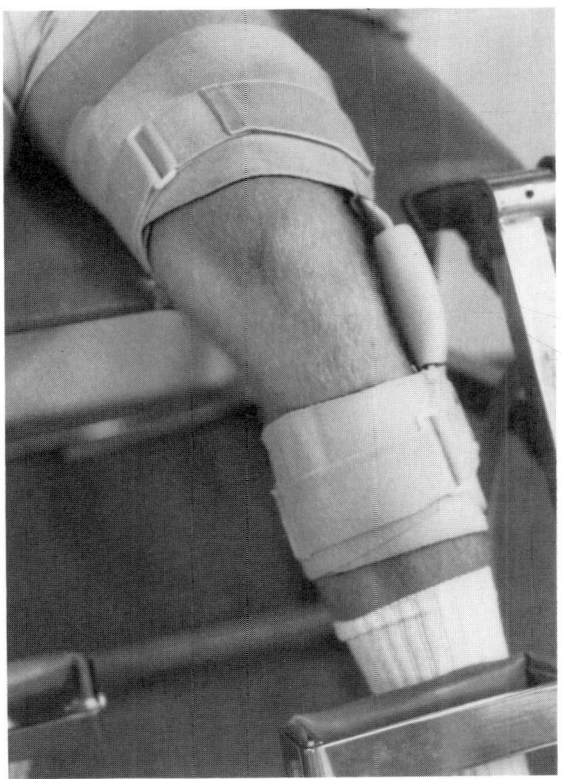

FIGURE 17–5. Braces such as these have not been shown to prevent knee injuries, but because they provide a gentle valgus restraint with minimal restriction of motion, we have found them to be very useful in the rehabilitation after MCL sprains.

normal gait pattern that is difficult to break. When the athlete can walk with minimal or no limp, he or she has reached the first functional goal and is allowed to discard the crutches.

As mentioned above, the primary benefit of cold after the first 24 hours is an adjunctive analgesic medium that can facilitate therapeutic exercise. This is ideally accomplished through daily or twice daily treatments with active range of motion in a cold whirlpool beginning the first day after injury. A water temperature of 15° to 18° C (61° to 64° F) is probably optimal for this purpose.[16] If a whirlpool is unavailable, the application of ice packs followed by active exercise while the knee is still numb is an acceptable substitute.

Dramatic loss of muscle strength following knee injuries may be caused by involuntary splinting, voluntary immobilization, or neural reflexes not completely understood. To allow safe early return to competition, this atrophy must be prevented with early aggressive treatment. In situations in which electrical muscle stimulation is available, (see Chapter 5), it can be helpful in combating reflex muscle inhibition. Frequent quadriceps setting (Fig. 17–6) is a simple technique that is available to all patients. Straight leg raising with weights in the supine, prone, and lateral decubitus positions is begun immediately with light weights. Adduction exercises, which would stress the medial collateral ligament, are avoided. (Fig. 17–7).

For an early return to competition to be realisitc, the athlete's cardiovascular conditioning must be maintained during the rehabilitation program. If a pool is available, swimming or lap walking in chest deep water or with a flotation vest is an excellent way to maintain conditioning. Upper body ergometers (Fig. 17–8) are found with increasing frequency at health clubs and gymnasiums and are an excellent resource for the athlete with a knee injury. Until range of motion in the injured knee is sufficient to allow for normal use of an exercise bicycle, one-legged bicycling using the healthy extremity, with the injured one propped out of the way, is another technique for maintaining cardiovascular fitness.

When the athlete has achieved 90 degrees of flexion in the knee, he or she has achieved the second goal and is allowed to begin progressive resistive exercises through a range of motion. Quadriceps exercises, such as knee extensions or leg presses, and hamstring exercises, such as leg curls, should both be included. These are usually begun with ankle

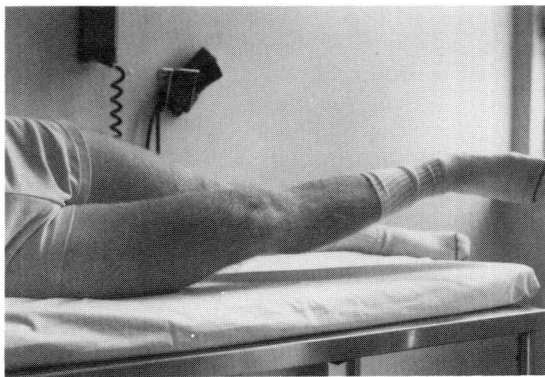

FIGURE 17–7. Adduction exercises such as this stress the injured MCL and should be avoided.

weights and progress to the use of an isotonic weight bench. Variable resistance, isokinetic, and computerized machines may be used but are not essential. The athlete also begins to use both legs for bicycling at this time. Because flexion in the knee is still limited, the athlete will generally begin bicycling with

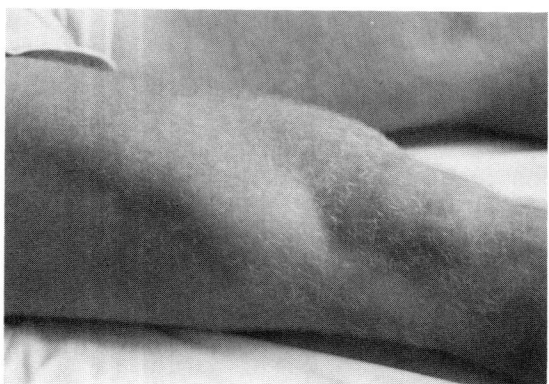

FIGURE 17–6. Quadriceps setting is begun immediately following injury. It may be supplemented with electrical muscle stimulation (see Chapter 5) if available.

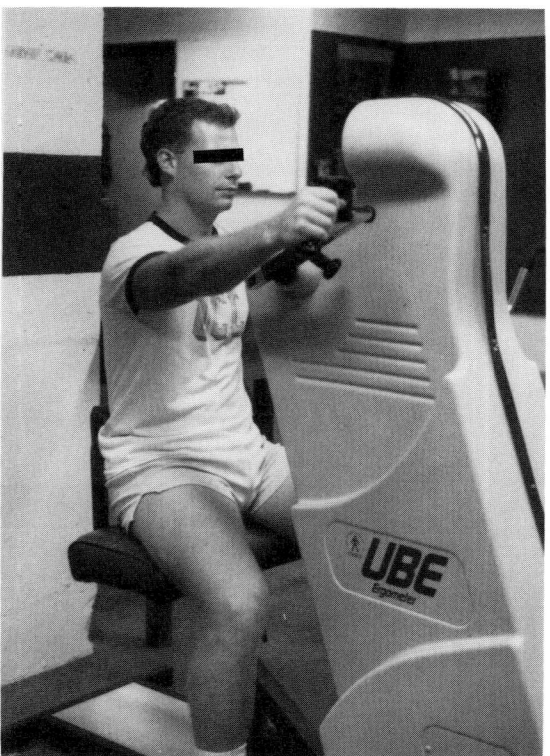

FIGURE 17–8. Upper body ergometers are one way of maintaining cardiovascular fitness during the early postinjury period.

the seat as high as possible. Gradually lowering the seat is an excellent way to increase flexion.

The third goal is the achievement of full motion in the knee. When this goal has been reached, the athlete is allowed to begin the functional running program while continuing to increase the weight in the progressive resistive exercises. The running program is actually a functional test of progressive difficulty. The athlete is first required to jog a mile. When he or she can complete this, the athlete progresses to a series of sprints, first at half, then quarter, and finally full speed (see Table 17–2). Finally, the athlete progresses to a series of zigzag sprints, executing sharp cuts. To complete the test successfully, the athlete must progress through the entire program in one session. If at any point during the test, he or she begins to limp or must stop because of pain, the test is discontinued and the athlete must start again from the beginning the next day. The exact details of the running program may be varied for different sports. The most important principle is that the athlete progresses from mild endurance work to speed work and finally to agility drills.[3, 27] Other tests such as figure-eight sprints and cariocas may be included if desired. Some athletes may balk at the rigor of the test, but this rigor is crucial to ensuring that the rate of reinjury on return to sport will be low.

Before the athlete is allowed to return to full practice and competition, the athlete must pass the functional running test. At this time, the athlete should also have minimal pain, no effusion, and full range of motion in the knee.

TABLE 17–2. Goal-Oriented Rehabilitation Program for Isolated Collateral Ligament Sprains

Initial Treatment
Apply ice immediately for 30 minutes and then every 3 to 4 hours for first 24 hours
Apply minimally restrictive hinge brace for grade II or III sprains
Instruct in use of crutches; weight bearing as tolerated
Active ROM exercises in cold whirlpool
Straight leg raising; EMS if available
Maintain cardiovascular conditioning with pool exercises, upper body ergometer, well-leg bicycling, etc.

**Goal One:
Athlete Walks Unassisted Without a Limp**
Discard crutches
Continue ROM, strengthening, conditioning

Goal Two: 90 Degrees of Knee Flexion
Begin two-legged bicycling; gradually lower seat
Begin isotonic PREs for quads and hamstrings
Continue ROM, conditioning

Goal Three: Full Knee Motion
Begin functional running program
Jog 1 or 2 miles
Five successive 50 to 100-yard sprints at one-half speed
Five successive 50 to 100-yard sprints at three-quarters speed
Five successive 50 to 100-yard sprints at full speed
Five zigzag sprints at one-half speed
Five zigzag sprints at full speed
Other agility drills appropriate for sport
Continued conditioning

Goal Four: Complete Entire Running Program in One Session; Minimal Pain; No Effusion; Full Strength
May return to competition
Discontinue use of brace for daily activities; may continue to use brace for sports if desired

ROM = Range of motion
EMS = Electrical muscle stimulation
PREs = Progressive resistive exercises

PROGNOSIS

The studies of Derscheid and Garrick[5] and Reider[24] have shown that a functional rehabilitation program such as the one described above is capable of returning an athlete quickly to competition without increased risk of knee injury. Thus, an isolated sprain of the medial collateral ligament should not be a career-ending or even a season-ending injury. Although the athlete is usually able to return to competition about 3 weeks following a grade II medial ligament sprain, most report that it is 2 to 4 months before they feel that the knee has fully recovered. This is consistent with the experimental findings of Woo et al.[31] who noted that 12 weeks were required to restore normal stability to the canine knee after MCL injury. During the period of initial return to sports, the athlete may wish to continue wearing the lateral hinge brace. Although these braces have not yet been shown to prevent injuries to the medial collateral ligament,[4, 8, 11, 23, 26, 29] they often reassure the athlete and give him or her a sense of security.

Our own follow-up study has indicated that the quality of results persists with time, at least over the first 3 to 5 years. Severe recurrent symptoms, such as the functional instability associated with anterior cruciate ligament tears, do not occur. Minor annoyance symptoms, such as occasional soreness, stiffness, or popping in the knee, are common. It remains to be seen whether longer-term follow-up will reveal more serious symptoms or arthritic deterioration after medial collateral ligament injury.[24]

ISOLATED SPRAINS OF THE LATERAL COLLATERAL LIGAMENT

Isolated sprains of the lateral collateral ligament (LCL) are quite rare compared with injuries to the medial collateral ligament. Their incidence is somewhat increased in wrestling, where the combatants' legs are frequently entwined, thus increasing the possibility of varus torque being applied to the knee. Because isolated lateral collateral sprains are rare, a physician should be very cautious about making this diagnosis. Lateral meniscus tears are much more common than sprains of the lateral collateral ligament. Many lateral meniscus tears, especially radial tears, do not produce an effusion but may be associated with localized synovitis and swelling of the lateral joint line (Fig. 17–9). This local swelling, combined with the normal varus laxity present in most knees, may cause a lateral meniscus tear to be confused with a lateral collateral sprain.

In most individuals, the lateral collateral ligament can easily be palpated by placing the extremity in the figure-four position. The normal lateral collateral ligament can be felt and sometimes seen running between the lateral epicondyle and the fibular head (Fig. 17–10). When evaluating the lateral collateral, keep in mind that most normal knees

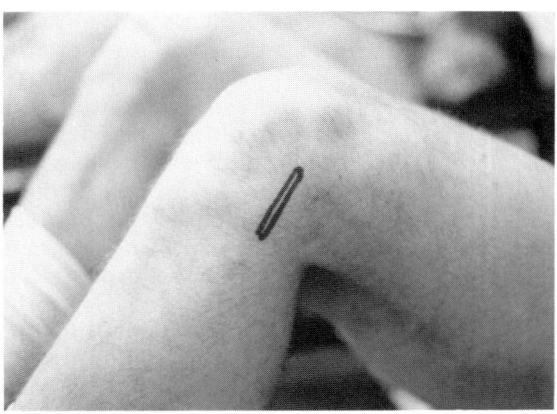

FIGURE 17–10. The course of the lateral collateral ligament is between the lateral epicondyle and fibular head.

have noticeable varus laxity in the flexed position (Fig. 17–11). It is extremely important to rule out the presence of a concomitant cruciate ligament injury when a lateral collateral ligament sprain is diagnosed. Once the diagnosis of an isolated lateral collateral ligament sprain is confidently made, the athlete may be treated just like the one with a sprain of the medial collateral ligament.

SURGICAL REPAIR AND RECONSTRUCTION OF MEDIAL COLLATERAL LIGAMENT INJURIES

As stated above, isolated medial collateral ligament injuries have been shown to heal well spontaneously. There is no evidence

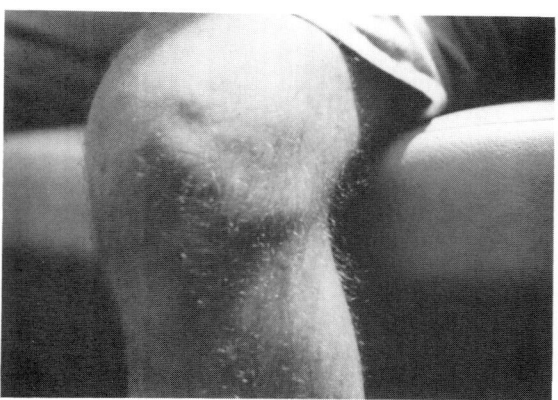

FIGURE 17–9. Most isolated lateral meniscus tears are marked by a subtle transverse band of swelling at the lateral joint.

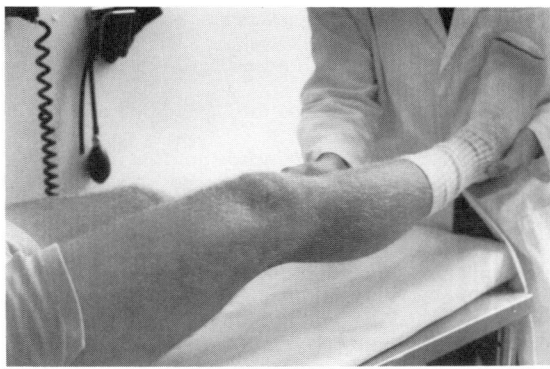

FIGURE 17–11. Like the MCL, the LCL is tested both in full extension and flexion. It is important to keep in mind that most normal knees have some varus laxity in flexion.

that surgical treatment will give better results than closed methods. Furthermore, Shelbourne and Nitz have shown that grade II medial collateral ligament tears associated with anterior cruciate ligament rupture will heal well without direct surgical repair as long as the anterior cruciate ligament is reconstructed primarily (see Chapter 18). As mentioned above, Inoue et al.[13] have shown that the anterior cruciate ligament is an important secondary restraint to valgus laxity; reconstructing the anterior cruciate ligament with a strong graft reestablishes this restraint and reduces the combined injury to a situation similar to the isolated collateral medial sprain. In contrast to the decreased scarring and postoperative morbidity associated with modern anterior cruciate ligament reconstructive techniques, concomitant exploration of the medial collateral ligament significantly increases surgical exposure and the potential for postoperative scarring and stiffness.

It is still my practice to repair directly the medial side in grade III "blowout" injuries in athletes. These are knees that open freely when valgus stress is applied to the fully extended knee. Rupture of the long fibers of the medial collateral ligament, the deep medial capsule and posteromedial capsule, and one or both cruciate ligaments is found in these cases.

In the case of grade III medial collateral ligament injury associated with anterior cruciate ligament rupture, the first step is to perform an arthroscopic reconstruction of the anterior cruciate ligament. The medial side is repaired after the anterior cruciate graft has been threaded in place and anchored at one end but before it has been fixed at the other end. The marked rotational laxity present in these cases makes isometric measurement of the anterior cruciate ligament graft exceedingly difficult; the surgeon usually has to forgo routine isometricity testing and rely on familiarity with the normal anatomical location of the anterior cruciate ligament when placing bone tunnels.

The repair of the medial side depends on the knowledge of the three-layer structure of the medial knee as described by Warren et al.[30] If a significantly long incision has already been made to harvest the patellar tendon graft, the medial exploration can be done through this excision by extending it proximally and curving it moderately posteriorly, elevating a flap as far posterior as the medial epicondyle. If there is no significant anterior incision, a longitudinal incision can be made directly over the course of the medial collateral ligament. The most superficial of the three deep layers is then incised along the fibers of the medial collateral ligament from the epicondyle to the pes anserinus. The long fibers of the medial collateral ligament and the site or sites of their tear should be easily identifiable. Deep to the medial collateral ligament, the injury to the capsular layer can be identified. It most commonly involves the meniscofemoral ligament and extends into the posterior capsule. In all but the most severe cases, it will stop medial to the posterior cruciate. If the capsule is torn within its substance, care must be taken to match up the two sides of the tear. Proceeding from posterior to anterior, horizontal mattress sutures of 0-gauge long-lasting resorbable suture are placed across the tear in line with the fibers of the capsule. Slight imbrication may be planned to allow for the plastic elongation that has inevitably occurred. Frequently, the capsule has been avulsed directly from the bone. In these cases, the exact site of anatomical attachment must be identified. If there is insufficient soft tissue on the bone to allow for the anchoring of reattachment sutures, oblique drill holes are placed in pairs to allow for the anchoring of heavy permanent suture into the bone using a stout needle. There is usually only enough space for one or two pairs of these holes. The permanent suture is then used to anchor the most substantial segment of the capsular ligaments using horizontal mattress or tendon repair suture techniques. Screws and staples provide fixation over too broad an area and are not recommended for capsular reattachment. After all the capsular sutures have been placed, they are then tied from posterior to anterior. The knee is then taken through a full range of motion to make sure that the placement has been anatomical.

Repair of the medial collateral ligament itself is then carried out. If it has been avulsed from the tibia or femur, it may be fixed using a small fragment AO screw with toothed washer as described by Mueller.[20] Exact anatomical placement of the screw is extremely important, especially on the femur.[1] The avulsed ligament should be preliminarily held in place using a 2-mm Kirschner wire and the knee taken through a range of motion to verify that the placement is correct. The wire can then be drilled into the bone and replaced by the AO screw and toothed washer. If the ligament is torn in its substance but is still substantial, tendon repair suturing techniques such as those of Kessler or Bunnell may be used to repair it. Enough imbrication should be performed to restore the ligament to its normal length but not overtighten it. Again, the knee should be taken through a full range of motion to verify proper placement of the repair.

Occasionally, the medial collateral ligament will be so severely damaged that it appears impossible to place sutures of any strength in it. In this case, it may be reinforced with a semitendinosus graft. Techniques utilizing the semitendinosus to reconstruct the medial collateral ligament have been described by McMurray,[19] Bosworth,[2] Helfet,[10] and others. Since the normal distal attachment of the semitendinosus at the pes anserinus overlies the distal medial collateral ligament, the distal attachment is left in place and the semitendinosus is freed proximally. Freeing the semitendinosus as far proximally as possible will usually yield just enough tendon to reach the anatomical proximal attachment of the medial collateral ligament at the epicondyle. The isometric site for attachment of this graft is extremely small;[1] again, the graft should be held in place with a 2-mm Kirschner wire and the knee taken through a range of motion until the most isometric attachment point is located. The graft is then fixed using a small fragment AO screw with tooth washer. The proximal portion of the graft may be sutured to adjacent soft tissue at the medial epicondyle to allow for further anchorage.

After the deep capsule and medial collateral ligament have been repaired, the superficial layer of the deep fascia is closed using a running suture. The anterior cruciate ligament is then fixed in place. As noted above, this additional exploration of the medial side increases the danger of postoperative stiffness compared with an isolated anterior cruciate ligament repair or reconstruction. It is recommended that the knee be placed in full extension in the immediate postoperative period to prevent the development of a disabling flexion contracture. After a period of 5 to 7 days, an aggressive, active range-of-motion program is begun to prevent the occurrence of stiffness. Early postoperative weight bearing, as described by Shelbourne and Nitz for anterior cruciate ligament reconstruction, is permitted in these cases as well.

References

1. Bartell, D. L., Marshall, J. L., Schieck, R. A., Wang, J. B.: Surgical repositioning of the medial collateral ligament. J. Bone Joint Surg. 59A:107–116, 1977.
2. Bosworth, D. M.: Transplantation of the semitendinosus for repair of laceration of medial collateral ligament of the knee. J. Bone Joint Surg. 34A:196, 1952.
3. Clancy, W., Bergfeld, J., O'Connor, G., et al.: Symposium: Functional rehabilitation of isolated medial collateral ligament sprains. Am. J. Sports Med. 7(3):206–213, 1979.
4. Cowell, H. R. (Editorial): College football: To brace or not to brace. J. Bone Joint Surg. 69A:1, 1987.
5. Derscheid, G. L., Garrick, J. G.: Medial collateral ligament injuries in football: Nonoperative management of grade I and grade II sprains. Am. J. Sports Med. 9(6):365–368, 1981.
6. Ellsasser, J. C., Reynolds, J. C., Omohundro, J. R.: The non-operative treatment of collateral ligaments injuries of the knee in professional football players. J. Bone Joint Surg. 56A:1185–1190, 1974.
7. Fetto, J., Marshall, J.: Medial collateral ligament injuries of the knee: A rationale for treatment. Clin. Orthop. 132:206–218, 1978.
8. France, E. P., Daniels, A. W., Goble, E. M., et al.: Simultaneous quantitation of knee ligament forces. J. Biomech. 16:553–564, 1974.
9. Grood, Edward S., Noyes, Frank R., et al.: Ligamentous and capsular restraints preventing straight medial and lateral laxity in intact human cadaver knees. J. Bone Joint Surg. 63A:1257–1269, 1981.
10. Helfet, A. J.: Disorders of the knee. J. B. Lippincott Co. Philadelphia, p. 230, 1974.
11. Hewson, G. F., Jr., Mendini, R. A., Wang, J. B.: Prophylactic knee bracing in college football. Am. J. Sports Med. 14:262–266, 1986.
12. Indelicato, P. A.: Non-operative treatment of complete tears of the medial collateral ligament of the knee. J. Bone and Joint Surg. 65A:323–329, 1983.
13. Inoue, M., McGurk-Burleson, E., Hollis, J. M., et al.: Treatment of the medial collateral ligament injury: The importance of anterior cruciate ligament on the varus-valgus knee laxity. Am. J. Sports Med. 15:15–21, 1987.
14. Kennedy, J. C., Hawkins, R. J.: Breast stroker's knee. Phys. Sports Med. 2:33–38, 1974.
15. Kennedy, J. C., Hawkins, R. J., Knssoff, W. B.: Orthopaedic manifestations of swimming. Am. J. Sports Med. 6:309–322, 1978.
16. Knight, K.: Cryotherapy: Theory, Technique and Physiology. Chattanooga, TN, Chattanooga Corp. Publishers, 1985.
17. Lemaire, M.: Carbon fibre IV: Ligamentous reconstruction. In Jenkins, H. R. (ed.): Ligament Injuries and Their Treatment. Rockville, MD, Aspen Systems, 1985.
18. Lemaire, M., Mirmad, C.: Les instabilities chroniques anterieures et internes du genou. Traitement. Rev. Chir. Orthop. 69:591, 1983.
19. McMurray, T. P.: The operative treatment of rup-

ture internal lateral ligament of the knee. J. Bone Joint Surg. 67:377, 1918.
20. Mueller, W.: The Knee. Springer-Verlag, Berlin, Heidelberg, New York, p. 157, 1983.
21. Noyes, F. R., Grood, E. S.: Biomechanical precepts and diagnosis and classification of knee ligament injuries. In Feagin, J. A. (ed.): The Crucial Ligaments. New York, Churchill Livingstone, Inc., 1988.
22. Noyes, F. R., Grood, E. S., Butler, D. L., et al.: Clinical laxity tests and functional stability of the knee: Biomechanical concepts. Clin. Orthop. 146:84, 1980.
23. Paulos, Lonnie E., France, E. P., et al.: The biomechanics of lateral knee bracing. Part I: Response of the valgus restraints to loading. Am. J. Sports Med. 15:419–429, 1987.
24. Reider, B.: Functional rehabilitation technique for the treatment of isolated medial collateral ligament sprains. Tech. Orthop. 2:47–52, 1987.
25. Rovere, G. D., Nichols, A. W.: Frequency associated factor and treatment of breaststroker's knee in competitive swimmers. Am. J. Sports Med. 13(2):99, 1985.
26. Rovere, G. D., et al.: Prophylactic knee bracing in college football. Am. J. Sports Med. 15:111–116, 1987.
27. Steadmen, J. R.: Rehabilitation of first- and second-degree sprains of the medial collateral ligament. Am. J. Sports Med. 7(5):300–302, 1979.
28. Stulberg, S. D., Shulman, K., Stuart, S., et al.: Breast-stroker's knee: Pathology etiology, and treatment. Am. J. Sports Med 8(3):164, 1980.
29. Teitz, Carol C., et al.: Evaluation of the use of braces to prevent injury to the knee in collegiate football players. J. Bone Joint Surg. 69A:1–9, 1987.
30. Warren, L. Fiske, and Marshall, J. L.: The supporting structures and layers of the medial side of the knee. J. Bone Joint Surg. 61A:56–62, 1979.
31. Woo, Savio L.-Y., and Masahiro, Inoue, et al.: Treatment of the medial collateral ligament injury. Part II: Structure and function of canine knees in response to differing treatment regimens. Am. J. Sports Med. 15(1):22–28, 1987.
32. Nachlas, I. W., and Olpp, J. L.: Para-articular calcification (Pellegrini-Stieda) in affections of the knee. Surg. Gynecol. Obstet. 81:206, 1945.

18

ANTERIOR CRUCIATE LIGAMENT INJURIES

K. DONALD SHELBOURNE
PAUL A. NITZ

In recent years, much has been written regarding the anterior cruciate ligament (ACL)–deficient knee, and varying recommendations for treatment have been given based on analysis of the available data. In spite of the concerted effort to establish a universal protocol for diagnosis and treatment of an ACL rupture, the clinical approach to this injury remains largely an enigma: Surgical procedures and therapeutic regimens abound, with no consensus regarding their application. Furthermore, most of the literature views the ACL-deficient knee in a "general" sense and includes *all* age groups when discussing clinical recommendations. Contrary to this approach, an ACL injury in a young, school-aged athlete must be regarded as a separate clinical entity, and it should be treated accordingly. The adolescent athlete is not merely a "young adult." The problems associated with a serious knee injury in this group are different. These athletes have different goals and desires that are often short term; they reflect a social structure quite different from similarly injured adults, who are generally employed full-time—perhaps supporting a family—and who participate in sports on a part-time, recreational basis only.

In our practice, we deal with many athletes at the high school and college level with ACL-deficient knees. Based on our experience in dealing with these patients, we have developed an approach to school-aged athletes that stresses the needs of the individual, while maintaining sight of long-term functional goals. The enthusiasm for our methodology in the treatment of ACL tears, both on the part of physician and athlete, leads us to believe that progress is *indeed* being made in the treatment of this significant injury in a very demanding population.

PATIENT HISTORY

Ligamentous injuries of the knee are accompanied by characteristic patient histories regarding the circumstances and mechanism of injury. Unfortunately, the clinician frequently glosses over the patient's history, relying instead on the physical exam, diagnostic studies (radiographs, arthrogram, magnetic resonance imaging (MRI), arthrometry), or as an extreme, examination under anesthesia and arthroscopy to provide the diagnosis. Attentiveness to the patient's version of events, *prior* to examining the knee, is rewarded in the majority of cases with a correct diagnosis. Even if a precise diagnosis cannot be made after obtaining the history, it should establish a focal point for subsequent examination, thereby allowing the physician to avoid inappropriate diagnostic tests and painful maneuvers. Simply stated, thoroughness in extracting the history of the injury and its sequelae cannot be overemphasized if one is to initiate the *proper* course of diagnosis and management.

The following paragraphs describe the typical presentation of an athlete who has sustained an acute ACL tear. Most athletes who tear their ACL will relate one or more of these "typical" historical details. Eliciting any of them should make the clinician very suspicious of an ACL tear. Nevertheless, the physician should always keep in mind that exceptions to these generalizations abound. For example, an occasional patient will describe very little initial swelling or disability but later develop disabling symptomatic instability. The examining clinician should always look for "typical" symptoms but should not feel that an acute ACL tear is definitively ruled out if they are not found.

The events resulting in a tear of the ACL often can be described vividly by the patient.[64] Examples include the basketball player who states, "I was coming down from a rebound, and when my foot landed on another player's foot, my knee twisted and it felt like it shifted to the side and then popped back into place," and the football player who volunteers, "I was running straight ahead when my leg was blocked from the front, and I felt my knee hyperextend and slide to the side with a loud 'pop.'" The clinician must allow the patient an opportunity to present these details, noting particularly the position of the extremity and foot in relation to the rest of the body at the time of injury.[88] Reconstructing or reenacting the events in a controlled manner in the office may clarify specific details, allowing for better appreciation of the forces and mechanism of injury. The patient's description of a "pop" at the time of injury, whether heard or felt, is also helpful: Studies have shown a 35 to 65 percent association of such impressions with ACL disruption,[28, 79, 84] although a pop can occur *without* ACL injury as well.[32]

The patient's perception of the severity of injury is an important clue when making the diagnosis of an ACL rupture; he or she will frequently convey history of an unwillingness to depart without assistance from the field of play at the time of injury. In addition, most individuals recount an inability to resume participation secondary to pain and a sensation of knee instability. In the unlikely event that the athlete returned to competition after a brief interlude, he or she invariably notes that the knee did not "feel right," leading to renewed withdrawal from the activity.

The subsequent history will include comments regarding pain, swelling, and stiffness in the knee, with associated difficulty walking on the extremity. Swelling generally occurs within the first several hours after the injury. The subjective quality of pain will vary with factors related to the mechanism of injury and associated injuries to the knee. An inability to extend the knee fully, resulting in ambulation with a mildly flexed knee, is often noted by the patient.

All too often the history of an acute knee injury includes a trip to the local emergency care facility, where, after posing for a set of radiographs, the patient is reassured that the knee is "fine, probably just sprained." A knee immobilizer and/or crutches are prescribed for the injured athlete, and a recommendation to ice the knee and elevate the extremity is provided, with a suggestion to "call the doctor if the knee does not feel better in about a week."

After following the emergency room instructions, the knee often does feel comparatively better, and follow-up is delayed for a variable amount of time, depending on how quickly the athlete attempts to return to the previous level of sports involvement. In this respect, the in-season athlete is at an advantage in comparison with the out-of-season athlete sustaining a similar knee injury: The former may attempt a return to competition in the first few weeks following ACL injury, soon realizing that there has been a marked loss in the ability to twist, turn, and cut. The in-season athlete's desire to "rejoin the team" motivates a rather urgent request for additional professional opinions as to the nature of, and treatment recommendations for, the present knee difficulty. In contrast, the out-of-season athlete (or the in-season athlete who makes no attempt at early return) may proceed for a period of time with little or no significant difficulty. The activities of daily living alone may not produce critical stresses in the unstable joint.

Upon attempted return to a competitive level, the athlete will realize that the knee is not dependable. At such time, the patient may seek medical counsel because the knee is giving way ("buckling") with cutting-, turning-type maneuvers. There may be a history of recurrent pain and swelling. In addition to having the patient recall the original knee injury, detailing the injury events and mechanism as meticulously as possible, it is important to ascertain how many, how frequently, and under what conditions episodes of giving way and swelling have occurred. A history of episodic catching or locking of the knee suggests meniscal damage, osteochondral lesion(s), and/or loose body(ies). Knowledge of potentially associated pathology has specific implications in the planning of treatment of the athlete's unstable knee.

In conclusion, while the history given by a patient with an ACL tear is familiar to most orthopedic surgeons,[25, 36] the diagnosis is frequently missed or delayed owing to an overdependence on the examination or diagnostic studies. Rectification of this clinical error begins with the physician's consistent, thoughtful evaluation of the patient's comprehensive history of the knee injury, thereby establishing an "index of suspicion."

MECHANISM OF INJURY

While no single mechanism has been identified that is common to *all* athletes sustaining ACL injury,[64, 84] careful questioning of those who have torn this ligament has repeatedly pointed out certain specific patterns. Even when the precise mechanism cannot be recalled, description of the events at the time of injury can provide important clues to the likely cause.

Team sports and individual sports both contribute to the pool of athletes with ACL-deficient knees. While both contact and noncontact sports participation may result in ACL damage, the majority of these injuries appear to be noncontact in nature.[83, 84, 93] ACL injury occurs most often in sports such as football, basketball, soccer, volleyball, and gymnastics, where twisting, cutting, jumping, and sudden changes in velocity (primarily deceleration) routinely occur. Less commonly, the ACL is ruptured as a direct result of an anterolateral blow to the knee.[112]

Mechanisms of ACL injury, whether occurring as an isolated event or in combination with damage to other soft tissue structures about the knee, have been classified using various methods. One descriptive categorization focuses on the forces that the body transmits to the knee. Examples from this perspective include hyperextension (landing from a jump, sudden deceleration); twisting or cutting maneuvers; and hyperflexion (attempting to prevent a backwards fall).[26, 28, 43, 57, 84] Another method for defining the mechanism of ACL disruption relies on defining the position of the tibia with respect to the body and thigh at the time of injury. This classification includes tibial displacement with varus angulation and internal rotation (ACL stretched over posterior cruciate ligament [PCL]); displacement with valgus angulation and external rotation (ACL stretched over lateral femoral condyle); and straight anterior displacement (massive quadriceps contraction).[32, 43, 79]

All mechanisms of ACL injury share one thing in common: The foot must be fixed or firmly anchored to the playing surface (i.e., weight bearing) at the time of injury. Various studies have evaluated the significance of the interface between shoe and playing field, and its contribution to knee injuries. The length of cleat used in football, soccer, and baseball has been cited as a potential factor—longer cleats are felt to contribute to an increase in the number of knee injuries. Torg et al. studied the adhesiveness of the turf-shoe interface, utilizing a measured "release coefficient"; they concluded that a level could be established for the release coefficient above which injury was more likely to occur.[109] Factors such as the type of turf, wear or condition of the surface, and the moisture content (humidity/rain) affect the coefficient, as does the type of shoe sole. This value can be checked readily when selecting acceptable shoes for playing on synthetic turf: A 25-pound weight is placed on the shoe, which is attached to a modified fish scale; a force of less than 50 pounds should be required to cause the shoe-weight combination to slide across the turf surface. Although adherence to these guidelines may result in less traction for the athlete on the turf, it more importantly leads to a reduced incidence of severe knee injuries.

An "enhancement factor"[22] has been identified for skiing-related ACL injuries. In such cases, the ski, when firmly attached to the foot (i.e., as a result of binding failure), acts as a lever arm on the leg. Resultant torques are markedly increased, leading to ligament damage.

Occasionally, an individual will present with an ACL rupture as a result of experiencing seemingly minor trauma, such as when landing from a jump. In these cases, the injury is probably the result of mistiming by the athlete: The "unsuspecting" extremity is in a compromised or "at-risk" position with the various muscle groups relaxed and unprepared to absorb the application of load adequately; instead, all the energy is absorbed by the ligament and associated soft tissue structures. Such a mechanism, while certainly not violent or impressive, can be considered analogous to several other orthopedic injuries (e.g., lumbar vertebral or calcaneal fracture resulting from falling only a short vertical distance or a comminuted fracture of the phalanx or metatarsal from stubbing the toe on a piece of furniture). These low-energy ACL tears can appear benign at presentation—there is little pain and minimal effusion in the acute period—in contrast to more violently injured knees with considerable associated damage.

FACTORS CONTRIBUTING TO ACL RUPTURE

Both the familial occurrence of ACL injury and the documented 3 to 4 percent incidence of bilateral ligament tears observed in one sports medicine practice (a figure that exceeds the expected value, based on the population risk) suggest that genetic and/or developmental factors interplay in the epidemiology of cruciate pathology.[104] Several specific variables have been proposed as contributors to this phenomenon.

The literature has made reference to the variability of femoral notch dimensions; narrow-notched femurs seem more likely to result in ligamentous injury.[3,42] Indeed, most knee surgeons have noted the wide range of notch sizes and shapes seen during ACL reconstruction. It is the "relative" width of the notch that appears to impact on the ACL in twisting injuries. We define a *narrow notch* as one where the PCL occupies greater than 50 percent of the available space in the anterior aspect of the notch; the ACL is more likely to be placed under adverse tension in this setting.

Another predisposing factor may be the presence of decreased or abnormal mechanoreceptors in the substance of the ligament itself.[101] Both familial incidence and the unexpectedly high occurrence of bilateral ACL disruption might, in part, be explained by such an underlying anomaly/variant of normal.[100] Theoretically, decreased proprioceptive feedback from the knee predisposes the individual to mistiming-type events, placing the knee at increased risk for ligamentous injury.

A hypoplastic tibial eminence may contribute to excess laxity in the knee as related to the "screw-home" mechanism as the knee approaches full extension. In such individuals, the ACL may be subjected to increased stress during the normal, anatomical rotation of the tibia.[26]

Feagin has implicated muscle fatigue as a contributor to increased risk for ACL injury.[26] His premise is straightforward: Tired muscles are not capable of controlling the extremity to the degree they normally do. If continued demand is placed on the fatigued extremity, such as seen late in the day after prolonged snow skiing, injury rates may climb. Further support for the role of muscle strength and conditioning comes from a study by Cahill and Griffith demonstrating decreased incidence of severe in-season injuries in athletes who underwent a specific preseason lower extremity conditioning program.[11]

In summary, although it would be difficult to isolate these variables scientifically and prove conclusively the importance of each in ACL disruption, there remains the impression that some significant factor(s) makes certain athletes more susceptible to this potentially debilitating injury.

PHYSICAL EXAMINATION

The role of the physical examination in the process of making the diagnosis should be to confirm that which is suspected from the athlete's history and stated mechanism of injury. These clinical parameters should all integrate cohesively in providing the correct answer. When the physician is presented with an athletic knee injury, the highest priority should be given to determining the status of the patient's cruciate ligaments. With respect to the ACL, a simple determination is sought: Is it intact or nonfunctional? The immediate sideline assessment of the injured athlete's knee *must* determine the status of the ACL with certainty.

Provided the ACL is intact and functional, the management of any other ligamentous injury about the knee is generally nonoperative. Most capsular, non-ACL knee injuries will heal satisfactorily owing to the preservation of the knee's center of rotation. On the other hand, if the joint has become ACL deficient, it is at risk for recurrent instability with inherent meniscal and chondral injuries and their recognized long-term sequelae. While the identification of various planes of abnormal motion about the knee, as eloquently described by Noyes, Hughston, and others,[39, 40, 46, 47, 69, 70, 80] is helpful in the scientific assessment of injuries and surgical results, the acute ACL rupture calls only for the reestablishment of the appropriate restraints to *primary* instability. This does not deny the importance of damage to secondary restraints. Our experience has shown that reconstruction of the primary restraint will allow secondary structures to heal without specific surgical intervention.

It is imperative that the patient be in loose-fitting shorts for the physical examination, thereby allowing thorough visualization and unobstructed examination of the lower extremity. Even before the examination, a clinician can learn valuable information regarding the injury by noting the patient's active (functional) range of motion. Observe carefully as the patient walks into the room and note the effort expended in getting onto the examination table, especially the manner in which the injured leg is lifted onto the table. The presence of effusion and any sites of ecchymosis about the injured knee should be noted, as well as the position in which the patient holds the knee while lying supine on the examination table. A traumatic knee effusion is presumed to be a hemarthrosis, and if the history and mechanism of injury correlate, one should statistically suspect an ACL injury. It is important for the clinician to recognize that the hemarthrosis may *not* be a result of the ligament tear itself but may rather be a manifestation of the trauma occurring to the knee at the time of injury. This statement is substantiated by the observation that patients with a *chronic* ACL deficiency who experience an episode of giving way *also* present acutely with a traumatic hemarthrosis. Therefore, the extent of the effusion is more a reflection of the overall energy level involved in the inflicting event rather than the result of bleeding from the substance of the torn ACL itself.

Determine whether the patient can obtain full extension with the injured knee. Apprehension or passive resistance on the part of the patient when attempting to extend the knee fully, in association with the stated mechanism of injury, is a consequence of ACL disruption until proven otherwise. The differential diagnosis in this situation is brief, and certain clues will point toward ACL injury: It is rare for the athlete who sustains an isolated acute bucket handle meniscus tear (and has a truly "locked" knee) to present with a history mimicking ACL injury; similarly, the patient experiencing patellofemoral joint dislocation (which has spontaneously reduced) should be able to extend the knee fully if given the opportunity and encouraged to do so—in addition, the recently dislocated patella should be point tender medially.

A typical scenario for misdiagnosis is the patient with a spontaneously reduced patellar dislocation who presents with what appears to be a "locked knee" (secondary to apprehension). If the clinician fails to evaluate the nature of this extension lag carefully, the preoperative diagnosis of a bucket handle meniscus tear may be made. When the patient is taken for arthroscopy, the knee fully extends as soon as anesthesia is induced and the patient is relaxed.

In contrast, an ACL injury may truly prevent full extension: The normal ACL fills the notch of the fully extended knee so tightly that when the ligament has been disrupted and lies loosely in, or anterior to, the notch, it can literally effect a mechanical block to full extension. *Voluntary* reluctance to extend the knee fully in the presence of ACL disruption has a biomechanical basis as well: By holding the knee in a mild degree of flexion, the patient unknowingly maintains the tibia in the "reduced position" (of the pivot shift phenomenon), thereby affording stability and comfort to the knee.

Examination of the normal, uninjured knee should be performed prior to assessment of the painful extremity. This allows the patient to experience and appreciate the various portions of the knee exam and provides for improved compliance and extremity relaxation when attention is turned to the injured knee. It is essential that the clinician appreciate the normal amount of laxity for a given patient prior to examining the potentially ACL-deficient knee. A small percentage of "normal" individuals have knees that demonstrate impressive anteroposterior laxity on stress evaluation and have a physiological pivot shift as well.

Throughout the examination, it is helpful to explain to the patient what is occurring during diagnostic manipulation in order to allay patient anxiety.

In the patient with an acute and painful knee injury, the Lachman test is performed first to determine the severity of ligamentous damage. This is in contrast to the pain-free knee with a chronic injury, where other structures may be examined prior to evaluation of the ACL. Several points need to be made regarding the Lachman maneuver. First, the result is compared with the opposite knee and should be classified as either positive or negative—not "partial" or "in-between." On completion of the test, there should be no question in the examiner's mind as to the result; an equivocal exam is the result of either suboptimal mechanics on the part of the clinician or poor patient cooperation; it is not due to "stretching" or partial disruption of the ACL. The key to performing the test is getting the patient to relax the injured leg *completely*. He or she must be supine with the head on a pillow and both heels on the examination table. The knee is supported gently by the examiner with both hands, while the joint is maintained in a slightly flexed position. Hip flexors are relaxed by externally rotating the hip. The patient is encouraged to relax the leg as the clinician discusses the events of the exam and what information is being sought through the test. It frequently takes time for the acutely injured athlete to relax the musculature sufficiently for a valid Lachman maneuver to be performed. The examiner must respond by being patient and reassuring—this time is critical for building the athlete's confidence in the physician. It is senseless to attempt the test if the extremity is not completely relaxed. Gentle flexion and extension of the injured knee while supporting it with both hands, along with gentle internal and external rotation of the hip, may help the patient to relax. Once the leg has become limp in the examiner's hands, he or she can proceed with the maneuver: While still supporting the knee, the examiner slides one hand down onto the proximal aspect of the leg in a posteromedial position and the other hand just above the knee on the lateral aspect of the distal thigh. The Lachman maneuver is then done in a quick, smooth motion, pulling the tibia firmly forward while restraining the femur and thigh, noting the amount of tibial translation and whether there is a firm end point when the anterior tibial translation stops (Fig. 18–1).

If the Lachman is positive, a flexion-rotation drawer test is performed to demonstrate rotational instability. This stress test has the advantage over other pivot-type maneuvers in that the flexion-rotation test does not require impingement of the lateral side of the knee and, as such, usually can be performed painlessly.[64] A dramatic jump during the flexion-rotation drawer does not have to

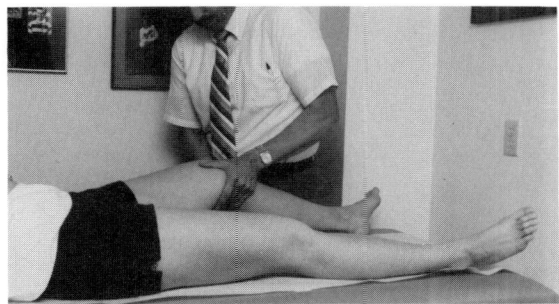

FIGURE 18–1. The Lachman test. Patient is pictured here lying supine, with heels fully supported on the table. External rotation and heel support used to promote relaxation, which allows the examiner to obtain a more accurate result with the Lachman test. Note hand position of the examiner.

be appreciated to confirm instability. Because anterolateral subluxation of the tibia normally occurs near full extension in the ACL-deficient knee, the exam can generally be performed through a very limited arc of knee motion. This maneuver requires that the patient lie supine, with the leg relaxed and the calf cradled in the examiner's hands. Beginning at about 10 degrees of knee flexion, the examiner gently flexes the knee while applying posteriorly directed pressure over the proximal anterior tibial surface. At 25 degrees of flexion, the subluxed tibia should reduce, resulting in posterior translation of the tibia and derotation of the femur from its externally rotated position into neutral alignment with the tibia.[79] It is important for the patient to realize the differences between normal and injured knee examinations when demonstrating the flexion-rotation drawer test (Fig. 18–2).

Once the status of the ACL is determined, the exam proceeds, checking for other instabilities or injuries. Joint line tenderness to palpation may be suggestive of meniscal pathology. The medial and lateral sides of the knee are evaluated by firm, rocking valgus and varus stresses in both 30 degrees of flexion and full extension, once again being sure that the extremity is relaxed and that the exam is performed in a gentle manner. In the event that both the ACL and a collateral ligament have been injured, it is important to check the condition of the posterior cruciate ligament by performing a posterior drawer test; in the acutely injured patient, there is added urgency in this exam to rule out a dislocated knee and associated injury involving the vascular structures of the popliteal fossa.

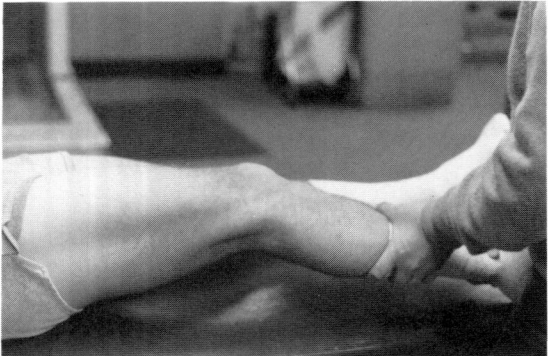

A

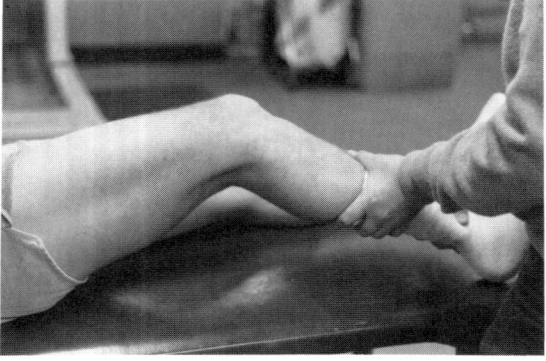

B

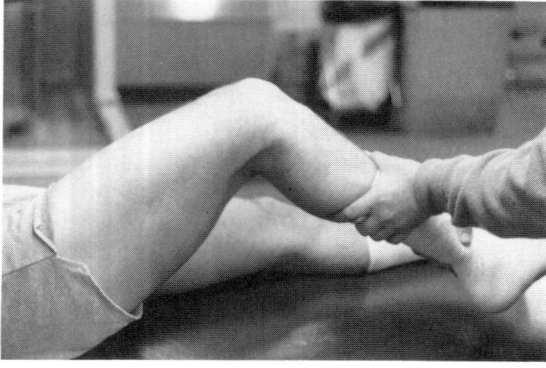

C

FIGURE 18-2. There are many variations on the pivot-shift maneuver. This version of the flexion-rotation drawer is relatively simple to perform and less anxiety-provoking for the patient than the classic pivot-shift test. (A) The leg is supported distally with the knee in slight flexion. The patient's limb should feel totally relaxed and limp in the examiner's hands. In the ACL-deficient knee, the tibia is subluxed anteriorly in this position. (B, C) As the knee is gently flexed, the tibia will be seen and felt to reduce suddenly. If the result is uncertain, small amounts of internal rotation and valgus stress may be added to the leg to accentuate the reduction phenomenon.

Grading of the Lachman and pivot-shift phenomena has not proven to be clinically helpful in patient management. The subjective grade of laxity has not reliably predicted which patients will have a functional instability requiring surgical intervention. Furthermore, varying grades of laxity may be perceived by different examiners on the same patient. This is especially appreciated when comparing the degree of laxity or pivot that a medical student or resident may demonstrate for a given patient to that displayed by the experienced attending physician. Such observations lead one to suspect that the degree of abnormal motion seen is as much a function of the examiner's skill and effort in getting the patient to relax as it is a function of the pathology present in the knee.

A variety of other tests have been described to assist the clinician in demonstrating abnormal knee motions or functional instability. While such tests may provide further insight regarding the injured knee, they need not be performed if adequate knowledge of the status of the various structures about the knee has already been gathered.

Reexamination of the knee is important in the individual who has incurred an apparently significant knee injury by history yet has an equivocal Lachman test on initial exam. As stated previously, the diagnosis of a partial ACL tear should not be based on an inadequate examination. Confirming the presence of a negative Lachman early in the clinical course allows the patient without serious injury to be reassured and permits better guidance in the rehabilitation of the knee. The physician should not rely on examination under anesthesia, MRI, or arthrometer values to provide the assessment of ACL status; rather, these tools should be utilized merely to confirm what is already known or suspected. MRI has not been as dependable for providing sensitive analysis of the ACL as it has for the PCL, primarily because of difficulties with the orientation of the magnetic coils with respect to the alignment of the normal ACL fibers.[67, 92, 102] Although MRI will undoubtedly be more accurate in the future, it is an expensive modality and should not be thought of as a substitute for adequate physical examination. Nevertheless, increasing confidence in the capabilities of MRI and the reliability of this imaging technique in depicting bone, cartilage, and ligamentous tissues points toward continued advancement in its utility for the evaluation of knee injuries.[53]

INJURIES ASSOCIATED WITH ACL TEARS

Considerable controversy has existed historically regarding the "isolated" ACL injury. Prior to the advent of improved arthroscopic equipment and technique, there was conjecture that injury to the ACL without associated soft tissue damage was not possible. The consensus now holds that if thorough examination under anesthesia and arthroscopic assessment fail to reveal additional pathology, then the ACL rupture may indeed be considered an isolated clinical event. As discussed previously, however, the examination of the injured athlete's knee must be comprehensive in looking for other ligament/cartilage injuries that might have occurred in conjunction with the ACL tear.

The ligament injury most commonly associated with ACL deficiency is tearing of the medial collateral ligament (MCL). The incidence of this combination ranges from 18 to 41 percent, depending on the series examined.[85, 86, 87, 98] This variablity probably reflects factors such as the patient population, sport involvement, and technique for recognizing the MCL injury. For example, the inclusion of patients with grade I (medial tenderness only) MCL damage versus only those with demonstrable medial laxity might significantly alter such statistics. Grade II injury (gaping of the medial joint line *with* an end point upon application of valgus stress at 30 degrees of flexion) may or may not have associated cruciate ligament damage, depending on the mechanism of injury. Complete medial ligamentous disruption (grade III) is generally associated with ACL rupture. The typical grade III injury is the result of a violent blow to the lateral side of the knee with the foot anchored firmly to the playing surface, such as occurs with an illegal block in football. Grade II MCL injury may occur from a similiar, less violent mechanism; it may also result from a twisting valgus stress in the *absence* of contact or extreme force applied to the lateral aspect of the knee.

A much less common injury occurring in conjunction with an ACL tear is lateral collateral ligament disruption, resulting in posterolateral rotary instability of the knee. Fortunately, this combination is rare—there is a disturbingly high incidence of associated peroneal nerve injury. The mechanism for this type of injury is usually a blow to the medial side of the knee (or a body falling against the medial aspect of the knee) with the athlete's foot planted on the playing surface.

A more serious combination of ligamentous knee injuries is the ACL-PCL combined deficiency; this injury generally occurs along with complete disruption of either medial or lateral capsuloligamentous structures and is the sports equivalent of the dislocated knee. While extremely severe, the forces resulting in this athletic injury rarely approach those seen in knee dislocations from other causes such as motor vehicle accidents. Nevertheless, steps must be taken by the physician to rule out damage to the neurovascular structures of the leg.

A major area of interest regarding injuries associated with ACL deficiency concerns the status of the medial and lateral menisci. With improvements in arthroscopy, more consistent and reliable statistical information can be anticipated that will solidify our understanding of this pathology. Several representative studies have confirmed a high incidence of meniscus tears with ACL injury, both acutely and chronically.[19, 26, 27, 49, 64, 79, 107] These surveys point out several trends worthy of comment. First, any knee sustaining an ACL injury—with or without associated ligamentous damage—has a high probability of meniscal injury.[96] Lateral meniscus tears outnumber those of the medial meniscus by approximately 2 : 1 in the acute setting. Second, with the passage of time, the unstable knee invariably accrues additional meniscal damage—nearly 100 percent of knees left untreated will develop such changes.[66] Finally, there is a change in the ratio of lateral to medial meniscal tears if the knee remains chronically unstable; the lateral side shows virtually no change in the number of tears, whereas the medial meniscus develops increasing damage, with many of these tears becoming complex in nature—and as a result, no longer amenable to repair.

A combination of injuries called the "unhappy triad" or "O'Donoghue's triad" has been long recognized. It is particularly seen by those caring for football players, both at the paraprofessional/trainer level and among physicians.[86, 87] Reports have mentioned this combination of ACL–MCL–medial meniscal tear occurring in up to 25 percent of surgically managed ACL inuries. However, the advent of skilled arthroscopy has led to an appreciation that *medial* meniscal injuries are less common with the ACL-MCL pattern than previously thought. In a review of patients with acute ACL-MCL tears who underwent arthroscopy and ACL reconstruction, we have found *lateral* meniscal damage far more often than medial side derangement (Table 18–1). Furthermore, it was observed that grade II MCL disruptions, when occurring with an ACL tear, had a higher incidence of associated meniscal pathology than did grade III MCL injuries. Historically, many "suspected" medial meniscus tears in association with MCL disruption may more accurately have been detachments of the medial meniscus from the joint capsule. Such injuries will uniformly heal without further intervention. *True* medial meniscal tears are an unusual finding in the acute ACL-MCL injury combination. A more likely triad consists of ACL–MCL–*lateral* meniscus tear. Overall, the incidence of all associated meniscal damage in conjunction with an acute ACL-MCL injury remains less than 50 percent (Table 18–2).

Another entity associated with ACL rupture is the lateral tibial capsular avulsion fracture (Segond fracture), found in approximately 10 percent of cases. Radiographic identification of such a defect gives the clinician an idea of the amount of torque applied to the knee at the time of injury (Fig. 18–3).

Chondral injuries are a major long-term concern; these have been reported in up to 23 percent of acute[26, 27, 48, 79] and 69 percent of chronic[19, 48] ACL injuries. In our experience, medial compartment chondral fractures occur twice as frequently as those of the lateral side in the acute setting. Damage to the articular surfaces of the chronically ACL-deficient knee is often impressive when reviewed arthroscopically, in spite of the frequent absence of radiographic clues that might correlate with such findings.

In attempting to understand the mysteries of the ACL, much has been written regarding the anatomy of this ligament and potential functional correlations of such observations. Subdivision of the ACL into "bundles" was touted as a means for greater insight into the problems of diagnosis and management. The delineation of types of ACL tears based on anatomical location followed, with discussion of "midsubstance tears," "avulsion tears," and the like. While these theoretical approaches have been of academic interest and import, they have not had significant impact on *clinical* patient management. The chief issue with any knee that has sustained a suspected ACL injury is whether there are normal functional restraints to tibial translation in the sagittal plane and to the pivot shift.

TABLE 18–1. Injuries Associated with ACL Tears

	ACL Reconstructions	
	Chronic	*Acute*
Number of reconstructions	423	336
Neither meniscus torn	99 (23%)	109 (32%)
Only lateral meniscus torn	70 (17%)	103 (31%)
Only medial meniscus torn	130 (31%)	59 (18%)
Both menisci torn	124 (29%)	65 (19%)
Grade III or IV chondromalacia	124 (29%)	31 (9%)

TABLE 18–2. Meniscus Tears Associated with Combined ACL-MCL Injuries

MCL Grade	n	Lateral Meniscus Tears	Medial Meniscus Tears
Second degree	39	26	5
Third degree	28	8	2

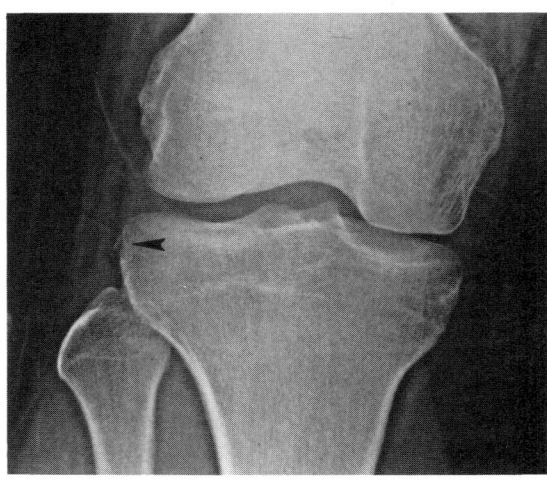

FIGURE 18–3. This Segond fracture represents a lateral capsular avulsion.

NATURAL HISTORY OF THE KNEE WITH AN ACL INJURY

Confusion and controversy have long prevailed regarding the natural history of the patient with an ACL-deficient knee have long prevailed. In attempting to define the clinical course following the injury, some studies have noted only minor difficulties, with the majority of patients returning to strenuous sports.[14, 34, 72, 73] The majority of retrospective analyses, however, depict a much more ominous scenario for the knee left with instability secondary to ACL disruption.[28, 41, 54, 68, 86] Ultimately, osteoarthritis requiring osteotomy or arthroplasty is the final sequela in the most unlucky patients with chronic ligamentous deficiency.[30, 54]

Documentation of the natural history in an ACL-deficient knee has acknowledged difficulties. Retrospective studies that have no uniformity of patient populations, a wide spectrum of associated injuries, and different rating systems have compounded this problem. Noyes et al. point out that such analyses are biased toward the symptomatic patient—the asymptomatic individual with a ligament deficiency rarely presents for medical care.[81, 82] Therefore, the problem of providing a true depiction of the natural history centers around an inability to accrue prospectively a representative group of patients with an isolated ACL injury, which then remains the *only* pathology present in the knee for the duration of the study period.

Various clinical studies have been designed with the objective of predicting which patients will have the greatest functional difficulty and morbidity resulting from ACL deficiency. In one retrospective study of 103 patients, Noyes et al. devised a "rule of thirds": One third of the patient population with a torn ACL experienced minimal symptoms, one third had mild symptoms requiring some activity restriction, and one third had pronounced difficulty with knee instability, pain, and swelling, requiring marked modification of life-style or ligament reconstruction.[83] Sixty-four percent of the 103 patients sustained a significant reinjury to the knee within the first 2 years following original injury, whereas 50 percent underwent meniscectomy during the same time frame. An alarming 44 percent demonstrated moderate to severe radiographic changes by 5 years after ACL rupture.

A clearer understanding of the natural history can be appreciated if one views the ACL-deficient knee as a syndrome complex, with patients falling somewhere along a clinical continuum.[26, 81, 82] Hawkins et al. provide a prospective study with an average follow-up of 4 years from the time of injury.[41] Their patient population is relatively nonbiased: Patients were not referred because of symptoms, nor were they selected for study owing to instability. In this study of young athletes treated nonoperatively for ACL tears, 86 percent rated their knee function as fair or poor. Only 14 percent of these conservatively managed individuals could ultimately return to their pre-injury level of sports participation, whereas 35 percent required surgical procedures during the study period for management of instability or meniscal pathology.

The identification of factors that predictably influence functional impairment and subsequent disability of the ACL-deficient knee has been of great interest to sports medicine physicians and athletic trainers alike. Patients experiencing the greatest increase in knee symptoms following initial ligament injury are those who incur reinjury, suffer recurrent joint effusions, have associated meniscal pathology, and are least compliant with the rehabilitation protocol.[81, 82] However, the *single* factor that has been most reliable when attempting to predict further difficulty with an ACL-deficient knee is the age at which the original injury is sustained. Those patients who are less than 20 years old at the time of injury will usually reinjure the knee, with worsening symptomatology (such as pain, swelling, and giving way), regardless of other factors. Patients greater than 20 years of age will have a less-predictable outcome; the clinical course in such patients is more related to activity level, the choice of sport, and intensity of participation.

Objective functional testing has been implemented by various investigators to assist the physician in the selection of those patients with a poorer prognosis.[105, 108] Tibone et al. found that the running cross-cut maneuver was the most valuable predictor of impaired function.[108] Noyes et al. have evaluated the comparative performances of injured and noninjured extremities in drills such as the one-legged hop for distance, timed one-leg hop, crossover hop, and the triple jump.[83] At our sports medicine clinic, patients with chronic ACL-deficiency were asked to perform a battery of functional tests; the results were then compared with each patient's subjective knee score. With the exception of the vertical jump, there was no correlation between performance and the patient's subjective assessment; nor did objective knee laxity (as measured by arthrometry) correlate with functional ability. Furthermore, in contrast to previously published data[32, 75] we found no correlation between hamstring-quadriceps strength ratios and either extremity performance during functional testing or subjective knee score. In conclusion, the functional assessment of various knee maneuvers does not appear to be able to select those unstable knees that, if treated conservatively, will do poorly in events requiring sudden and unexpected twists, cuts, or deceleration.

Literature reviewing the natural history of the ACL-deficient knee has illustrated a close association between the chronicity of the ligament rupture and the incidence of symptomatic meniscal tears.[96] Giove et al.'s report of conservatively (i.e., nonoperatively) managed patients who demonstrated only "mild" initial instability found that 55 percent underwent meniscectomy over time, 12.5 percent of whom had *both* medial and lateral involvement.[34] McDaniel and Dameron's 14-year average follow-up of nonrepaired/nonreconstructed ACL deficiency cites an 86 percent occurrence of uni- or bicompartmental meniscectomy.[73] In Lynch et al.'s retrospective study of patients undergoing ACL reconstruction, 98 percent of those in whom ACL injury had occurred greater than 1 year previously also had meniscal damage by the time of surgery.[66] Through continued follow-up of these patients, the authors were able to make some important radiographic correlations by examining serial sets of knee films for Fairbank changes (articular surface ridging/flattening, sclerosis, squaring of the tibial margins, and joint space narrowing)—findings associated with degenerative arthritis. Three percent of those patients with intact menisci at the time of ACL reconstruction developed two or more Fairbank changes. Individuals with meniscal tears that were considered stable, and were neither excised nor repaired, subsequently demonstrated a 7 percent incidence of similar radiographic derangement. A striking 35 percent of those requiring coincident meniscectomy (partial or total) at the time of ACL reconstruction progressed to greater than two Fairbank changes on later radiographs. In this study, then, articular cartilage damage correlated directly with the status of the menisci, rather than with the functional capability of the ACL.

Degenerative joint disease is clearly one possible result in a chronically ACL-deficient knee, a result that is exacerbated by the secondary loss of the menisci.[30, 54, 66] The physician periodically encounters a patient with chronic ACL injury but no meniscal damage. Such a patient usually follows a restricted life-style, maintains ideal body weight, and is not involved in sports or recreational activities where the knee would experience twisting, cutting, or sudden deceleration. He or she is unlikely to be an aggressive athlete who continues to compete in sports requiring such maneuvers.

The patient's ability to "return to sports" is not a valid method for assessing the natural history of ACL injury. This statistic often fails to clarify which sport(s), the level of participation, and any injury-related difficulties that occur. In the Giove et al. study, the sports most commonly returned to were swimming, golf, weight lifting, and bicycling. The sports participated in least were basketball, volleyball, and football. While the ability to participate in sports following ACL rupture is one clinical goal, the maintenance of joint surfaces over time must be considered of utmost importance. The avoidance of further meniscal injury is paramount in protecting the important articular surfaces following ACL injury.

DECISION MAKING

After making the scientific diagnosis of an ACL tear, the "art of medicine" must be practiced by the physician. He or she must have a clear appreciation of the athlete's particular social and recreational history, goals and ambitions, and any unique concerns. Any treatment decision must integrate all the particular factors in the student athlete's life; therapy cannot be guided by pathology alone. Additionally, the clinician should be prepared for a wide range of emotions upon announcing the diagnosis—one may anticipate initial reactions such as grief, anger, or denial. The emotions of the injured individual must be respected, and the physician must be sincerely sympathetic if rapport with the patient is to be maintained.

Patient education regarding anatomy, associated pathology, and natural history of the

ACL injury can be initiated at this time, if the patient appears prepared for such dialogue. On the other hand, if the circumstances and emotional setting are unfavorable, postponing the in-depth discussion for a couple of days is preferable. Regardless of the approach taken, the patient should begin physical therapy immediately to assist in maximizing patient comfort and restoring knee range of motion (ROM).

It is imperative that the student athlete understand that the torn cruciate ligament will not heal on its own. Without surgical treatment, the patient cannot anticipate restoration of a reliably functional knee. Likewise, the patient's comprehension of the goal of any selected treatment plan is important to the success of the program—largely resulting from improved patient compliance. For the individual with an ACL disruption, that goal is to avoid developing a "trick knee." The ideal treatment plan will ultimately provide the athlete with a knee that meets the youthful demands placed on the lower extremities without jeopardizing comfort and function of the knee in later years. Because patient attitude is so important to the success of any protocol, ensuring patient acknowledgment and acceptance of his or her appropriate responsibility in achieving the stated goal is critical. Patients and/or their families must never feel as if a given treatment plan has been forced on them but, rather, that they have taken an active role in selecting a course of therapy that will satisfy the present and future demands anticipated at the time such decisions are made.

The school-aged athlete who presents with a chronically unstable ACL-deficient knee should be counseled differently than the acutely injured individual. One major difference between these two groups of patients lies in the "experience" of those with a chronic deficiency: They are mentally better prepared for making treatment decisions based on subjective personal assessment of knee function. In addition, there is a predictably higher incidence of meniscal and articular surface pathology in athletes with a chronic ACL injury as a result of recurrent instability episodes. To offset future degenerative changes in the knee, this patient must be more emphatically advised to either undergo ACL reconstruction or effect a significant change in life-style in an attempt to avoid episodes of instability.

Radiographs of the knee can reveal some important pieces of information. First, the finding of open physes about the knee requires modification of treatment with regard to the proper timing of surgical management. The significance of the physis must be discussed with the patient and family; the importance of waiting until growth has virtually ceased prior to undergoing a reconstructive procedure is explained. Initial management emphasizes activity modification, extremity rehabilitation, and knee bracing until sufficient maturation occurs. Another radiographic finding that may influence decision making in the acute setting (when present) is a displaced tibial spine avulsion fracture. In this case, the recommendation should be to reduce the displaced fragment of bone and ensure its stability, either with or without fixation. Anatomical healing of an avulsed ACL will prevent pathological anterior laxity and obviate the need for ligament reconstruction.

Simplistically, there are two primary choices available in outlining a treatment plan for the school-aged athlete with an unstable ACL-deficient knee: nonsurgical management or surgery. One may initially elect the former approach and allow an intervening observation period to see how the patient functions prior to committing to a definitive protocol. This "wait-and-see" method then reveals one subset of athletes for whom surgical management is clearly the proper choice and another group that may appropriately be treated nonoperatively.

Generally speaking, the younger and more athletically inclined a patient is, whether at the recreational level or in interscholastic competition, the more at risk he or she is for sustaining additional injury to the knee. A highly motivated athlete will predictably experience the greatest benefit from surgical stabilization of the knee. Such individuals are frequently underclassmen in either high school or college with multiple sport involvement and the desire to continue this vigorous participation. Senior students, on the other hand, pose a more difficult problem: These adolescents are at a crossroads in life and may have no plans to continue the type or level of athletic endeavor that would place the knee at risk for sustaining recurrent trauma.

Similarly, the school-aged individual who suffers an ACL injury during an activity that is uncharacteristic for that person may have no desire to engage in future events that might compromise the knee; these patients may also do well with nonoperative management. The broad continuum of patient profiles again points out the significance of the maxim "In matters of treatment, it is more important to know the patient than merely to know the diagnosis."

In situations where the student athlete is clearly at risk for experiencing recurrent episodes of knee instability with giving way, it is appropriate for the physician to project a bias for surgical intervention. It is important to convey to patient and family that athletes sustaining ACL damage with intense, aggressive involvement in sports such as basketball, volleyball, football, soccer, wrestling, and gymnastics predictably do poorly with nonsurgical management. The converse is true as well: Those who do not participate in such sports may be advised that—provided giving-way events can be avoided—the patient may do very well with rehabilitation only.

During the decision-making process, it is emphatic that the patient and family understand and acknowledge that treatment is aimed at preventing a *functional problem,* or potential difficulty, *not* an anatomical abnormality.

NONOPERATIVE MANAGEMENT

In recognition of the distinct possibility for associated meniscal injury in the patient with a torn ACL, the physician must be prepared to manage such pathology as well. For those patients in whom surgical reconstruction is not anticipated, one must be careful to evaluate fully for the presence of meniscal tears before embarking on a rehabilitation program and before the onset of meniscal symptoms. In years past, the arthrogram was the diagnostic tool of choice. Increasing confidence in the value of MRI has brought this imaging technique to the fore in recent years. One disadvantage of MRI in the clinical setting has been the finding that these studies can actually be "oversensitive"; this is manifested by the demonstration of meniscal tears that appear quite impressive on the image and yet turn out to be insignificant, stable, or incomplete tears when viewed intraoperatively. As an alternative to imaging, arthroscopic assessment of the menisci and articular surfaces may be offered to the student and family.

Regardless of the method chosen, it is preferable to assess the menisci early in the course of treatment if there is suspicion of damage, allowing for appropriate further management. Identification and treatment of a surgically repairable meniscus injury will help prevent further trauma that might make the cartilage less amenable to repair. Arthroscopy can be performed at the convenience of the student and family, as long as it is relatively prompt. In addition, the postoperative protocol used by these authors for arthroscopic partial meniscectomy or meniscus repair is essentially the same as that used in ACL rehabilitation, utilizing early knee motion and lower extremity muscle strengthening.

In the event that a potentially repairable meniscal lesion is found, it should be made clear to the patient and family that ACL reconstruction is strongly recommended at the time of the meniscus repair. Only upon exclusion of meniscal pathology should the physician accept nonoperative management as an alternative when treating an ACL-deficient knee in the school-aged athlete (see Chapter 16).

If the decision has been made to manage the unstable knee nonoperatively, there must be substantiated belief on the part of both physician and athlete that the knee can be kept from giving way. This implies a willingness by the patient to avoid all activities that would put the knee at risk for instability episodes. The student should acknowledge that any activity associated with sudden starts and stops or quick, unanticipated turns must be avoided. Modification of perfomance may allow participation in such events as cheerleading, baseball, and softball; here again, the importance of avoiding certain maneuvers must be fully understood. Athletic endeavors that can be considered "safe" for the injured patient include running, bicycling, weight lifting, and swimming.

In the acute setting, the first goal prior to beginning any formal therapy is to make the patient comfortable with the injured knee. Pain medication, nonsteroidal antiinflammatory drugs, and ice are recommended initially, with the possible use of a knee immobilizer—depending on the patient's need. Follow-up is scheduled for 1 or 2 weeks to check on symptoms and progress. By this time, it is hoped that the athlete will have discontinued the immobilizer and any other ambulatory aids.

With satisfactory progress, physical therapy can next be recommended for the purpose of improving knee ROM and strengthening the musculature of the involved extremity. The therapist can demonstrate methods for maximizing ROM and establish a program based on closed-kinetic exercises (e.g., step-ups, wall squats, and calf raises) that will build strength and endurance. Much of the regimen can be performed at home without special or expensive equipment. This type of exercise lessens the shear stress across the unstable knee joint by using body weight to compress and stabilize the joint, in contrast to open-kinetic maneuvers such as leg extension and leg curls in which the tibial and femoral joint surfaces are not compressed. Follow-up in 4 to 6 weeks includes KT-1000 laxity measurements and Cybex dynamometer quadriceps and hamstring testing to provide an objective measurement of lower extremity strength and joint laxity.

When managing the athlete with chronic ACL deficiency who first presents to the office months or years following initial injury, a diligent search for anticipated meniscal pathology should first be undertaken—as with the acute injury. Here again, the presence of a potentially repairable meniscal tear may influence the choice of treatment schemes: An ACL reconstruction should be strongly considered in conjunction with a meniscus repair.

If meniscal injury is excluded and nonoperative management is chosen, emphasis is again placed on extremity strength and endurance. In the chronic injury scenario, the patient usually is able to begin rehabilitation immediately, obtaining arthrometer and dynomometer measurements at the first visit. However, if the patient with a chronic injury has presented as the result of a recent instability episode, there may be associated pain, effusion, and limited ROM, which must be managed as in an acute injury.

Dynamometer testing provides a consistently reproducible method for objectively following the progress of rehabilitation parameters. The desired goal is attainment of quadriceps-hamstring strengths in the injured extremity equal to 90 percent (or better) of those in the well leg at all speeds tested.[76, 111]

In follow-up appointments, in addition to monitoring the progress of therapy, it is important to verify whether the patient has been successful in preventing instability episodes. Should there be any history of inability to control giving way with activities of daily living, or within the constraints of acceptable life-style restrictions, the wisdom of nonoperative treatment should be reconsidered.

The issue of bracing is commonly raised by the student or family. In the subgroup of school-aged individuals who have opted for a trial of nonoperative management of the unstable knee (the wait-and-see approach), a discussion of bracing is germane to the treatment protocol. Although the patient who has chosen the nonoperative route has elected to avoid activities that would knowingly cause giving way, the pervading mentality is that a disabled extremity should be supported or protected. This is a topic that requires careful discussion with the patient, as there are certain misconceptions about the role of bracing and its alleged benefits.[75, 97, 106] Frequently, the athlete and/or family member knows someone whose "trick knee" lives in a large contraption with all sorts of hinges and straps, allowing that individual to lead a "normal" life. Any approach taken to bracing the ACL-deficient knee must include acknowledgment that while some control of sagittal tibial translation may be afforded by the brace, prevention of the pivot phenomenon is much less successful, especially with the high speeds and forces crossing the knee in competitive sports requiring rapid deceleration, cutting, and twisting.[8, 31, 75, 89] Laboratory studies have not shown current braces to stabilize the knee mechanically against the forces and accelerations that occur clinically. Nevertheless, clinical studies that show them to be effective in reducing the incidence of giving way in the unstable knee imply that they may work by other mechanisms, perhaps by enhancing proprioception or merely reminding the athlete that he or she has an unreliable joint.

As long as the patient and family understand the capabilities and limitations of knee bracing, a functional device may be prescribed for the patient, assuming there is enthusiasm for its use and that there are no treatable meniscal tears present. The snugly fitting, well-designed functional knee brace for ACL deficiency provides benefit in the acutely injured knee by controlling minor, low-energy instability during the period while the secondary stabilizing structures heal. Additionally, with chronic usage, the brace functions to "assist" in proprioceptive feedback, reminding the wearer of the knee's functional inadequacy. Combined with the possible effect of "slowing" the athlete slightly, the brace may provide a stabilizing benefit.

Another indication for bracing arises in the individual who desires to avoid or delay surgery yet is experiencing instability episodes with the activities of daily living. In this case, a clinical trial with a knee brace is an appropriate "next step" in the patient's management.

In summary, nonoperative management for the school-aged individual with an ACL-deficient knee follows no specific protocol. This patient must be approached with as much diligence and tenacity as an operative case. Top priority is given to patient education regarding the ACL injury and its natural history; knowledge and a proper attitude will further the athlete's commitment to, and sense of responsibility for, caring for the unstable knee. Meniscal pathology must either be ruled out or treated appropriately—the diagnostic algorithm should be pursued to this end. Rehabilitation of the extremity is emphasized whether the instability is acute or chronic, realizing that there is no specific exercise that will ultimately alter the underlying tendency toward giving way. The goal of physical therapy is a painless knee with full range of motion and leg strength equal to at least 90 percent of that measured in the uninjured extremity, allowing the patient to complete a functional running program. The ultimate clinical goal is to minimize the risk of reinjury, with or without use of a functional knee brace, through appropriate lifestyle changes and activity modification.

SURGICAL MANAGEMENT

Should the patient with an ACL-deficient knee opt for surgical reconstruction, then the educational process of explaining knee anatomy and function using a knee model and diagrams is initiated. All procedures—including examination under anesthesia, arthroscopy with possible meniscal resection or repair, and anterior cruciate ligament reconstruction—are presented in detail. The location of skin incisions, the technique of constructing a new ligament, and fixation of the graft are all thoroughly explained. Of course, the risks and potential complications of the surgery are presented as well. The perioperative course and rehabilitation schedule are outlined utilizing a preprinted handout describing the protocol. Patients with a chronic injury obtain dynamometer and arthrometer evaluations and complete a modified Noyes questionnaire. The family and patient are given time alone to go over the handout and to speak with patients who have previously undergone ACL reconstruction and happen to be in the office for various phases of follow-up. Emphasis is placed on the patient's ability to name and identify the injured structure(s) in the knee, to describe satisfactorily the reconstructive procedure, and to outline the postoperative course. The patient and family should not leave the office without comprehension of the planned course of events and a conversant knowledge of the pertinent anatomy and scheduled procedures. It is our feeling that an informed and knowledgeable patient will be more compliant and experience a less-eventful postoperative rehabilitation course.

Since the results of ACL reconstruction are generally not affected by the delay between time of injury and date of surgery,[99] the physician can put the patient and family at ease knowing that surgery can be scheduled at the convenience of all involved. The date chosen for reconstruction must be individualized according to the patient's academic responsibilities, the availability of support from family and friends for the initial convalescent period, and anticipated sport involvement, with special consideration given to in-season versus out-of-season timing of the injury. In general, delaying the surgery is ideal, as it allows for better patient preparation. The surgery can be arranged around times of heavy classroom load or during a holiday/semester break—thereby minimally conflicting with the student's schedule.

One marked disadvantage in delaying surgery occurs if the patient's injured knee becomes stiff and the extremity undergoes significant muscle atrophy with associated loss of strength prior to the reconstruction. It is therefore important that in the interim between the injury and surgery the patient work on knee range of motion and leg muscle strengthening. Enlisting the expertise of physical therapists to assist the patient in achieving full extension and maximizing strength during the time allotted before surgery provides for a smoother postoperative course. For the college student away from home, delaying surgery often allows for the patient's family to be present on the day of surgery and during that short period of time postoperatively when personal assistance is beneficial to the convalescing individual.

There are occasions where surgical reconstruction as soon after the injury as possible is of benefit to the student athlete. A definite indication for near-immediate intervention exists in the patient who has sustained a severe knee injury with disruption of both ACL and lateral support structures: Ligament reconstruction and primary repair of these lateral structures should be performed concomitantly, at the earliest possible date. Similarly, grade II and III medial collateral ligament injuries occurring in conjunction with ACL disruption will heal more predictably when cruciate reconstruction is undertaken with relative urgency, although good results can still be obtained if delay is necessary.[98]

An additional situation that requires consideration for ACL reconstruction in the immediate postinjury period involves the management of the competitive interscholastic athlete. In this scenario, the time of year during which the athlete has sustained the knee injury (in season versus out of season) does not impact on the timing of surgery. The realization that a full calendar year may be required before the athlete with a reconstructed knee is once again performing at the interscholastic-intercollegiate level give impetus for expedient management: If the athlete is to compete in next season's campaign, then the sooner the "rehabilitation clock" starts ticking, the better. Interscholastic or intercollegiate athletes will experience less inconvenience because many institutions have resources available to aid these individuals (tutors, student trainers).

One of the drawbacks to reconstructing the ACL-deficient knee urgently is that the athlete may experience greater difficulty adjusting to the consequences of the injury and its treatment in the initial postoperative period. In such cases, the patient often has not been able to experience the grief and depression so commonly witnessed after sustaining a major knee injury. As a consequence of not having lived through the full course of pain and functional instability due to the injury, the athlete may tend to blame the surgeon and the operation for the demise of the extremity, rather than accepting the injury itself as the precipitator of the inevitable postoperative soreness, weakness, and muscle atrophy. The patient may even become hostile toward the surgeon. These attitudinal and emotional difficulties may interfere with the patient's ability to rehabilitate satisfactorily following the reconstruction. By anticipating such setbacks, the astute physician can prevent long-term problems with rehabilitation and the physician-patient relationship.

Another potential setback following urgent reconstruction may occur in the initial rehabilitation period: Progress in the return of a desired range of motion may be delayed, and pain control may be more difficult than if there had been a greater time interval between time of injury and surgical reconstruction. The patient should be forewarned of this possibility. The physician must not only be aware of this possibility but also allow extra time for closer supervision and encouragement in the early postoperative period.

A review of our own surgical cases has shown that knees reconstructed three or more weeks following an ACL tear recover strength and motion faster and more easily than those reconstructed sooner. We would therefore recommend waiting at least 3 weeks from the time of injury before performing surgery unless this is contraindicated by concomitant injuries or other factors. If the athlete is in a controlled situation where aggressive postoperative rehabilitation can be ensured, this waiting period can be shortened from 3 weeks to 1.

The operative procedure itself consists of two phases. The initial portion involves arthroscopic assessment of the injured knee and appropriate management of associated damage. Systematic arthroscopic examination allows comprehensive evaluation of the joint's articular surfaces and menisci, along with confirmation of cruciate ligament status. During arthroscopy, the knee should be placed through its complete range of motion in order to view the entire articular surface of both femoral condyles. The origin of any chondral loose bodies must be identified. Video recording of the procedure permits improved documentation of the nature and extent of damage; it also aids patient counseling postoperatively. For example, the athlete who has developed grade III or IV chondral defects over a significant portion of the articular surfaces would be advised to avoid or modify impact-type activities in the future. Allowing the patient to witness the extent of articular damage on videotape helps to underscore the severity of the knee injury in that individual's mind. This realization may induce greater patient responsibility in subsequent selection of activity involvement and lifestyle.

Perhaps the greatest contribution of arthroscopy to the operative regimen is the assessment and management of associated meniscal injuries. The type and location of tears in the medial and lateral menisci can be visualized readily with proper technique. The lateral meniscus, when injured, typically exhibits either an avulsion tear of the posterior horn, a radial tear, or both.[13] The medial meniscus most often incurs an acute vertical tear, either incomplete or full thickness; these tears are generally located in the posterior half of the cartilage.

The lateral meniscus posterior horn avulsion is rarely treated; it is a stable injury that is asymptomatic in the vast majority of cases. Radial tears of the lateral meniscus are generally located in the midcoronal aspect of the cartilage; these are resected to provide a smooth contour along the central rim of the meniscus, thus preventing propagation of the damage, should additional twisting injuries occur to the knee.

ACL-associated medial meniscus injuries are aggressively managed (see Table 18–3). At one time, stable medial meniscal tears were completely ignored when identified in patients undergoing ACL reconstruction. However, since in the authors' experience approximately 5 percent of these patients have subsequently developed symptomatic difficulties with the meniscus requiring another procedure (excision or repair), initial stabilization with nonabsorbable suture has become the routine. This is, admittedly, in contrast to recommendations in the literature.[20] However, since beginning to place sutures in medial meniscus tears that had previously been left alone, there have been no occurrences of symptomatic reinjury to the same. Furthermore, from personal experience, there has been minimal morbidity associated with suturing these meniscal tears.

Stabilization of these seemingly benign medial meniscal lesions has proven beneficial in preventing further demise of the cartilage. Likewise, following the repair of unstable meniscal tears, there have been few recurrences of symptomatic meniscal injury requiring surgical intervention. While the repair of unstable meniscal lesions has become less controversial, the percentage of these tears that actually *heal* following a repair is unknown. The real benefit from stabilization of the unstable meniscus is the probable prevention of propagation of the tear in a manner similar to the aforementioned stable tears, as determined by a significant decrease in the development of clinical symptoms following repair.

TABLE 18–3. Management of Meniscal Tears at the Time of ACL Reconstruction

Acute	n	June 1982–December 1986 149 Reconstructions		January 1987–April 1989 187 Reconstructions	
Medial meniscus tear	125	45		80	
Left alone	52	25	(56%)	27	(34%)
Repaired	51	9	(20%)	42	(52%)
Removed	22	11	(24%)	11	(14%)
Lateral meniscus tear	172	66		106	
Left alone	56	27	(41%)	29	(27%)
Repaired	36	2	(3%)	34	(32%)
Removed	80	37	(56%)	43	(41%)

Chronic	n	June 1982–December 1986 193 Reconstructions		January 1987–April 1989 230 Reconstructions	
Medial meniscus tear	235	93		142	
Left alone	30	16	(17%)	14	(10%)
Repaired	93	55	(59%)	57	(40%)
Removed	112	22	(24%)	71	(50%)
Lateral meniscus tear	199	84		115	
Left alone	46	16	(19%)	30	(26%)
Repaired	33	5	(6%)	28	(24%)
Removed	120	63	(75%)	57	(50%)

Following arthroscopic evaluation, the surgical phase of the reconstruction is undertaken. In selecting a reconstructive procedure, one must recognize that primary repair of the ACL, whether acutely or chronically torn, is not a dependable procedure. The usual interstitial shredding of this ligament at the time of rupture makes it a less-than-ideal functional structure even if it can be placed in the correct anatomical location during repair. In longer-term follow-up studies of the acutely repaired ACL in athletes, it has been shown that there is a predictable poor functional outcome.[26]

The procedure chosen for ACL reconstruction should meet several criteria. Of course, it should be a procedure yielding a result that will stand up to the demands of the student athlete. Also, the surgery must have a guaranteed high success rate for the young person, that is, functional stability with a knee that has full range of motion and in which the patient has complete confidence. An early return to sports following ACL reconstruction is also an important priority. Many of these athletes can expect a limited career in interscholastic competition; enabling them to return to their former level of participation as soon as possible carries great significance for the patient. Lastly, the procedure should entail a minimum of inherent possible complications.

The autogenous patellar tendon graft for intraarticular reconstruction of the ACL has remained our preferred procedure for *both* the acute and chronically unstable knee in the school-age population. Continued success with such a procedure has led these authors to abandon the surgical alternatives of extraarticular reconstruction and allograft or prosthetic replacement for the ACL. Augmentation of the intraarticular graft with a lateral extraarticular tissue procedure, as is often done in cases of chronic instability, has also been discontinued. Patient complaints about lateral knee discomfort associated with such surgery, as well as the implementation of a more aggressive rehabilitation protocol that decreased the effectiveness of a lateral augmentation, were inducements to do so. Furthermore, many extraarticular procedures are nonisometric and potentially change the center of rotation about the knee. Orthopedic surgery and sports medicine are indebted to the research and clinical studies performed during the development of these extraarticular procedures; this work added tremendously to our knowledge of the intricacies of knee joint function.[4, 23, 35, 48, 51, 59, 65, 103, 110] However, either as an isolated procedure or in combination with intraarticular reconstruction of the ACL, an extraarticular augmentation has not proven to be the best surgical alternative for meeting the demands of the student athlete.

Intraarticular reconstruction of the ACL-deficient knee has been performed with various autogenous structures about the knee, including the iliotibial band,[50, 77] menisci,[18, 52] semitendinosus[15, 63] and/or gracilis muscles,[74, 115] and portions of the extensor mechanism.[16, 24, 55, 61] The patellar tendon with accompanying bone from both patella and tibial tubercle has been used as an ACL substitute by a number of authors.[16, 24, 55, 71, 96] The strength of this autogenous tissue has been documented to be superior to all other substitutes tested,[79] and clinical experience appears to substantiate its long-term viability. The donor tissue is readily available and technically not difficult to obtain. By including bone at either end of the tendon graft, bone-to-bone healing (which is more predictable than tendon-bone healing) can occur in the femoral and tibial bone canals. Morbidity resulting at the donor site is low: The bone fragments obtained when reaming the tunnel are used to fill in the bony defects in both patella and tibial tubercle, presumably expediting healing at these sites. Furthermore, the patellar tendon hypertrophies with time, reestablishing its original width. Extensor mechanism problems,[29, 38, 45, 91] including patellar maltracking, quadriceps weakness, and postoperative donor site pain, have been minimized through performance of a lateral capsular release at the time of surgery and the incorporation of appropriate measures into the rehabilitation program. Attention to technical detail can virtually eliminate complications such as patellar fracture or patellar tendon rupture following ACL reconstruction utilizing this methodology.

SURGICAL PROCEDURE

The success of any surgical protocol depends on precise technique. It is appropriate, then, to highlight those areas of the ACL reconstruction procedure that these authors consider most critical to its success.

The anterior aspect of the femoral notch is carefully assessed intraoperatively. The surgeon must determine how much of the available space anteriorly is occupied by the *posterior* cruciate ligament. If the PCL takes up more than half of the space in this anterior portion of the notch, a lateral notchplasty is performed. The purpose of the notchplasty is to provide both adequate space for the ACL substitute and better visualization of the posterior recesses of the notch. The surgeon should be careful not to extend the notch superiorly, as more than a few millimeters change in this direction can create problems with patellofemoral articulation as the knee approaches full flexion.

Successful isometric graft placement is contingent on proper location of the intraarticular femoral and tibial graft fixation sites. Regardless of the method used, the surgeon must consistently obtain isometric placement of the ACL substitute. The tibial guide pin should be placed such that its opening into the tibial plateau is located just anterior and lateral to the midaspect of the tibial eminence.[16] The authors prefer drilling the tibial channel from outside in. Ideally, the femoral bone channel is made as far posteriorly in the intercondylar notch as possible without causing breakthrough of the posterior cortex; it is reamed from inside out. The opening of this tunnel into the joint should be located just superior and posterior to the original ACL femoral insertion site to ensure isometric graft location.[16]

Various techniques and devices have been developed to aid the surgeon in obtaining correct placement of the bony canals. Whether these channels are created after arthrotomy or with arthroscopic assistance, it is imperative that adequate visualization be obtained ensuring their precise placement. While tunnels for tibia and femur should be created independently, the surgeon should be able to pass a Steinmann pin in a straight line through both canals simultaneously with the knee flexed approximately 30 degrees. This guarantees that the graft will not be passed around bony corners. If the bony canals are accurately placed, the graft will lie in the posterior aspect of the tibial tunnel and the anterior inferior portion of the femoral tunnel—essentially re-creating the anatomical location of the ACL.

A 10-mm graft is used consistently, regardless of the size or physical demands of the patient undergoing the reconstruction. Despite theoretical arguments for using various-sized grafts depending on the individual parameters, there have been no graft failures in our experience in spite of our uniform use of a 10-mm graft. Furthermore, tunnel placement is more consistent when using the same-sized drills for every patient.

Chamfering the intraarticular entrances to tibial and femoral tunnels with a curette eliminates sharp edges that might create stress risers or cause deterioration of the graft. Once the bone-patellar tendon-bone graft is obtained and sized, three evenly spaced 0.054-inch drill holes are made in an anterioposterior fashion along the midline longitudinal axis of each bony end of the graft. A #2 nonabsorbable braided suture is then passed through each hole and divided evenly (Fig. 18–4).

The patellar bone fragment has a more convex configuration and is more easily passed through the *tibial* bone tunnel, in an inside-out fashion, using the sutures to pull the bone plug into position; it should fit snugly in the bone canal. A tighter fit may be obtained by using bone shavings from prior drilling to pack the tunnel. The nonabsorbable sutures are then divided into anterior and posterior groups (three ends each), and each group is passed through a separate hole in an 18-mm semirigid convex plastic button. The groups of suture are then tied over the button, securing it (convex side toward bone) over the distal opening to the tibial bone tunnel. The tibial tubercle bone plug is next passed through the femoral tunnel from inside out. After placing the knee in approximately 30 degrees of flexion, this end of the graft is anchored to the lateral surface of the distal

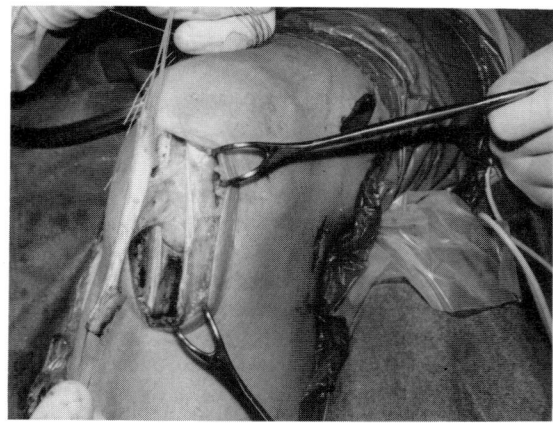

FIGURE 18–4. Bone-patellar tendon-bone graft with sutures in bone ends.

femur by tying the sutures over a second convex plastic button.

The loosest anatomical position of the graft occurs at 30 degrees of knee flexion; tension increases with full extension and with flexion greater than 90 degrees.[5, 56, 91, 111, 114] Consequently, the knee is now placed through its full range of motion to allow graft adjustment and ensure that the substitute ligament does not hinder full knee motion. Observation of the anterior notch during knee extension is critical, as there must be no impingement of the graft within the bony confines of the notch. Occasionally, additional excision of the anterior- and superior-most portions of the notch ceiling is required to eliminate such interference.

Graft placement should be lax enough to allow the full range of knee motion without placing excessive tension on the graft (Fig. 18–5). Securing the graft too tightly may cause more problems clinically than does permitting slight laxity. Subjectively, patients with a slightly increased Lachman in the reconstructed knee (when compared with the opposite extremity) but who have a negative pivot shift and a full, painless range of motion are more pleased with knee function than those patients whose grafts are "too tight." The latter group will demonstrate an initial decrease in range of motion, joint stiffness and recurrent knee pain, once full range of motion is established. Furthermore, the potential for graft disruption is heightened by overtightening.

Interference fit screw fixation of the bony portion of the graft in both tibial and femoral tunnels has been shown to provide the greatest strength-to-failure values in comparison with staple fixation or sutures tied over buttons.[60] However, the authors have found that button fixation provides advantages over other means of securing the graft. Because the buttonholes are closely spaced, the button permits excellent locking of the traction sutures. The convex shape of the button allows for slight tension cycling of the graft with knee motion and reduces the chance of the graft sliding in the bone tunnels. The presence of a slight "give" in the ligament complex allows any "micromotion" postoperatively to occur at the bone-bone interface rather than in the ligament. These dynamics prevent the ligament from "capturing the joint" and producing a stiff, painful knee postoperatively. Extraosseous placement of the buttons permits the bone tunnels to fill in completely with new bone. In the event of button removal for reasons of focal discomfort or surgical failure, there is, then, no resulting bone hole. An esthetic advantage is provided by the radiolucent nature of the buttons: The radiographic appearance of the reconstructed knee returns to near normal as the bone channels heal. Should long-term follow-up films be obtained, subjective patient approval and confidence might be improved on viewing a knee that has no staples, screws, or washers. All this aside, the greatest single advantage of button fixation is that the tautness of the graft can be adjusted easily, should it appear suboptimal or loosen with intraoperative manipulation of the knee: One need simply retie the sutures (the

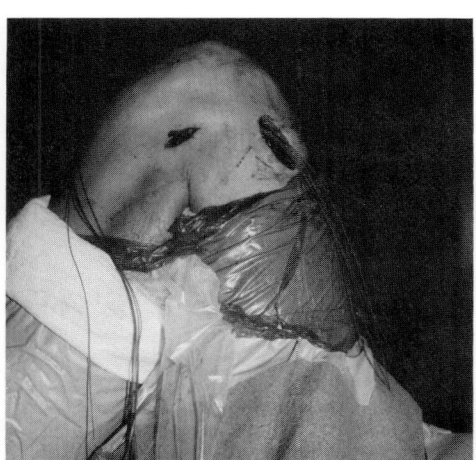
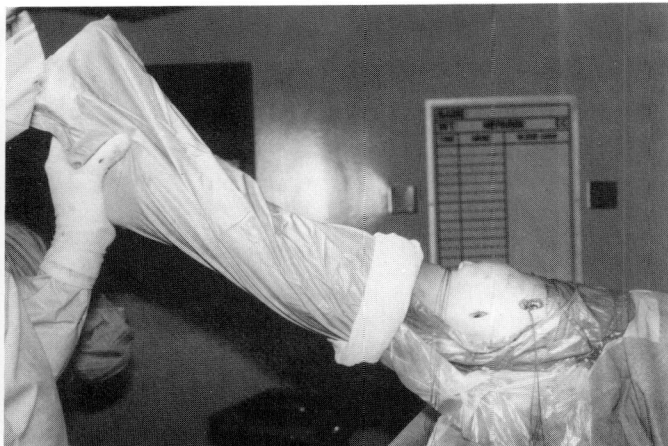

FIGURE 18–5. Knee range of motion in operating room after securing graft.

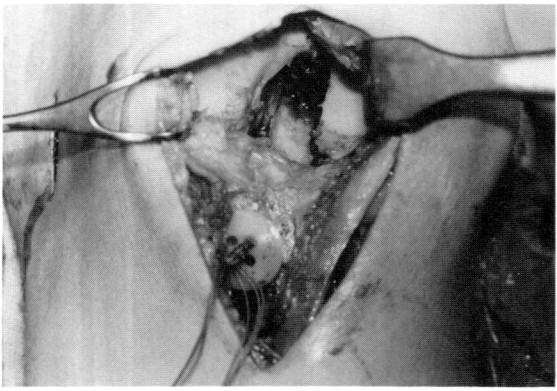 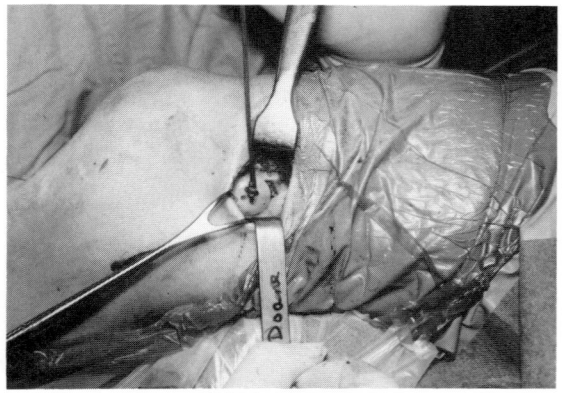

FIGURE 18–6. Tibial (A) and femoral (B) fixation with flexible buttons.

ends are not cut until just prior to incision closure for this reason). Most important, it has been our experience that, contrary to published opinion,[60] the buttons have more than adequate strength for their temporary role in fixation until bone healing is completed. To date, there have been no surgical failures resulting from button failure in greater than 800 ACL reconstructions so performed (Fig. 18–6).

Arthroscopically assisted techniques for ACL reconstruction have become popular, largely out of a desire to reduce the postoperative morbidity formerly associated with ACL reconstruction.[7, 12, 33] These techniques must not be considered a panacea for all potential postoperative problems. It has been our experience that much, if not most, of the morbidity attributed to the use of arthrotomy for ACL reconstruction has been the result of overly restrictive postoperative rehabilitation programs. An aggressive rehabilitation program, as described below, is more important than the surgeon's choice of "open" or "closed" technique. Cosmetic results with open technique may be as good or better than those produced by most arthroscopic techniques: We have routinely performed the procedure through the same incision used by most surgeons for patellar tendon harvest, utilizing a small arthrotomy without dislocation of the patella (Fig. 18–7). Whichever technique is chosen, it is extremely important that the surgeon is able to visualize the femoral and tibial ACL attachment sites reliably in order to obtain consistent results.

As reported in the literature, reconstruction of the ACL has increasingly involved the use of allografts or prosthetic devices.[6, 78, 95, 116] Short-term successes in small series have been demonstrated using the various substitutes, but these are tempered by acknowledgment of failure rates approaching 20 percent by some reports. These techniques, while potentially valuable for certain patient populations, are clearly not viable primary surgical alternatives for the school-aged athlete who requires long-term functional performance from his or her reconstructed knee. Such grafts may indeed have a role in repeat reconstruction cases, in whom it would be inadvisable to obtain the customary autogenous graft, or for an older individual who is not planning on long-term participation in athletic endeavors.

One subset of school-aged individuals requires modification of the above format for surgical reconstruction: Preadolescents with an ACL-deficient knee who have several

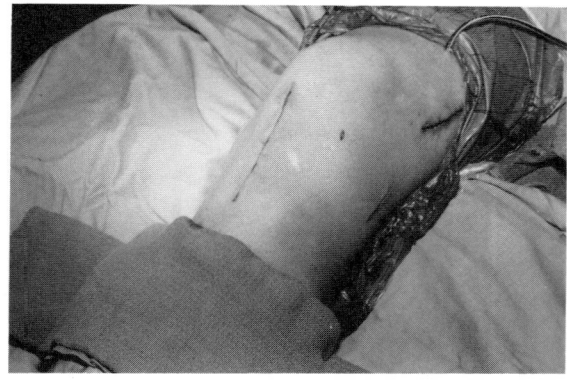

FIGURE 18–7. Closure of skin incisions.

years of anticipated growth remaining prior to epiphyseal closure (as determined by radiographs and family history) present a dilemma for the clinician. Over the past decade, various reports have appeared in the literature regarding ACL injuries in skeletally immature individuals.[9, 17, 21, 62, 71] Intraarticular reconstruction techniques have yielded apparent success in the early postoperative time frame, without development of limb length discrepancy or angulation. In general, however, these studies all involved individuals who, while still demonstrating open physes about the knee on radiographs, had nearly completed longitudinal growth and were, for all practical purposes, at adult height prior to surgery.

The preadolescent with significant growth remaining presents a different problem. For such patients, intraarticular reconstruction involves considerable risk of postoperative morbidity resulting from both graft harvest and drilling across the physeal plates. Harvesting bone from the ununited tibial tubercle may result in anterior tibial growth arrest with development of an attendant recurvatum deformity. Furthermore, bone obtained from this site is deficient of mature bone in the skeletally immature individual. Trauma to either femoral or tibial growth plate could precipitate growth arrest about the knee or initiate an angular growth deformity. These possible consequences are an obvious deterrent to elective intraarticular reconstruction.

Fortunately, athletes younger than 12 or 13 years of age rarely generate enough force about the knee to cause ACL disruption. In addition, apparent ACL damage (as ascertained through a positive Lachman test) may result from tibial spine avulsion more frequently in this population. This fracture can be adequately reduced, with predictably good resulting ligament stability. However, these facts may bias the physician adversely, causing an intrasubstance ACL tear to be overlooked. If the presence of ligament damage is indeed determined, counseling the patient and family again plays a major role in the ultimate outcome of treatment. Here, such education must involve not only the nature of the injury and its possible consequences but also the rationale for delaying definitive surgical treatment until the patient is approaching skeletal maturity. Activity modification—that is, avoidance of activities that would place the knee at risk for giving way—must be clearly emphasized. Participation in sports such as football, basketball, volleyball, gymnastics, and soccer is strongly discouraged. It is important for the young person to realize that the stated restrictions and limitations should only be temporary: If upon approaching skeletal maturity there remains a desire to participate in such sports, the athlete may undergo surgical reconstruction and the necessary rehabilitation at that time.

After embarking on this "delayed approach" to treatment of the ACL-deficient knee in a very young athlete, it is important to have periodic follow-up with the patient and parents to determine how successful the patient has been at preventing the knee from giving way. Here again, the importance of assessing meniscal status with either MRI or arthroscopy during the inital period of patient management cannot be overemphasized. A torn, repairable meniscus should prompt an emphatic recommendation for operative treatment (of the meniscus lesion) from the physician. At each clinic visit, the clinician must encourage the appropriate functional limitations. If there is noncompliance on the part of the patient, or if in spite of adhering to the activity recommendations, he or she is experiencing recurrent instability and knee effusions, then management must be altered.

A functional knee brace may be recommended but only with the strong caveat that the device in no way condones more aggressive and stressful activities. As mentioned previously, the knee brace may slow the youngster down enough to prevent further instability episodes, and it may also serve as a reminder that the knee is not functionally normal and needs to be protected.

As a last resort, an extraarticular procedure may be recommended. The criteria for such management, in review, include skeletal immaturity, clear noncompliance, and a predilection toward continued noncompliance prior to the time at which an intraarticular reconstruction might safely be performed. Another indication for such a procedure is the individual who continues to experience giving-way episodes despite complying with reasonable physical restrictions and utilizing functional knee bracing. In these unusual settings, a lateral extraarticular stabilizing procedure is preferred.

Under no circumstances should an extraarticular procedure be recommended for the purpose of facilitating the adolescent's return to competitive athletics, especially when a more definitive intraarticular procedure is anticipated upon attainment of skeletal maturity. In such a case, it is best to limit athletic participation and plan for the appropriate intraarticular reconstruction at the proper time. This scheme will generally permit resumption of competitive sports by the latter high school years and provide the athlete with the best knee possible for both short- and long-term considerations.

The limitations of extraarticular procedures in terms of joint stability must be recognized: Their usefulness is primarily due to a temporizing effect. By slowing the young patient's activity down, both during the recovery and rehabilitation phases, and by providing some measure of mechanical stability, effective management of the injury is achieved. The combination of the extraarticular procedure and subsequent functional knee bracing will hopefully allow the patient to progress toward skeletal maturity, at which time a more definitive intraarticular reconstruction can be recommended. This approach should provide the young person with the best knee possible for the greatest period of time: acceptable functional capability without accelerated degenerative changes in the short term, along with the possibility for additional long-term management. The focus when managing the preadolescent patient with an ACL-deficient knee, then, is to *endure* whatever temporary hardships are necessary in order to achieve ultimate long-term success.

There is one additional group of school-aged patients for whom extra precautions need to be taken: Many adolescents experience some degree of tibial tubercle apophysitis (Osgood-Schlatter disease) during the early teen years. This is especially true for those individuals involved in jumping sports such as basketball and volleyball. As a consequence of the inflammatory process, a bony ossicle may appear in the inferior aspect of the patellar tendon near its tibial insertion. A lateral radiograph of the knee is usually required for visualization of such anomalies. When such an ossicle is present, the surgeon must modify the harvest of the tibial aspect of the patellar tendon graft: A longer bone plug must be obtained from the tibia such that a full 2 cm of *normal* tibial bone is incorporated into the graft. Intraoperatively, it is helpful to identify the ossicle within the tendon and ascertain the true site of proximal tendinous insertion into the tibia before obtaining the measured bony portion of the graft. Once the graft is harvested, the bony fragment should be dissected sharply from the posterior aspect of the tendon graft. Depending on the size of this anomalous bone, its removal from the tendon may result in an excessively-lengthy tendinous portion of the graft. Accommodation can then be made by placing the lateral opening of the femoral canal slightly proximal to its normal location, thus lengthening the tunnel and assuring proper graft fit. Here again, attention to detail is necessary for a predictably good surgical outcome.

REHABILITATION

The rehabilitative course following ACL reconstruction has been a confusing topic for clinicians. Early literature regarding primary ACL repair and extraarticular reconstructions clearly dictated that adequate time be incorporated into the protocol to allow the tissues to heal. All efforts focused on preventing "stretching" of the reconstructed tissues in the early postoperative period by protecting the knee from all mechanical stresses.[23, 35, 51, 103] Initial protocols for postoperative management of intraarticular reconstructions honored historical precedent and followed the same cautious clinical course, further extrapolating the principles involved to include time for the graft to revascularize and "mature."[1, 2, 16, 90] Such philosophy, with its inherent delay in mobilization, resulted in significant knee stiffness and extremity weakness, thereby prolonging the patient's functional recovery and subsequent time before return to sports.[38, 45, 91] Early exercises for the operated extremity encouraged only the hamstring muscle group.[5, 56, 94, 111] Weight bearing, quadriceps strengthening, and progression to full knee extension began *months* after surgery.[10, 26, 37, 44, 58, 113, 114]

With time and experience, rehabilitation protocols for ACL reconstruction were accelerated—most began to permit full weight bearing at 9 to 12 weeks postoperatively. Also at this time, such activities as stationary bicycling and cautious pool training commenced. Allowable exercises were then slowly expanded to include skipping rope and jogging at 5 to 6 months. Full knee extension was first attempted at this juncture, and a running program was added, along with cautious agility exercises, in hopes of returning the patient to light sports training by 8 to 9 months postoperatively. Successful completion of this type of rehabilitation schedule permitted the athlete to return to full competition, wearing a functional knee brace with a 5- to 10-degree extension stop, by 12 to 18 months after surgery.[10, 26, 44, 58, 90]

The recent development of prosthetic ligaments and ligament augmentation devices prompted further change: Surgeons utilizing such methods became comfortable with more rapid rehabilitation progress. Indeed, use of prosthetic augmentation eliminated the fear of graft stretching, loosening, or failure. As no reports were on record demonstrating that accelerated postoperative rehabilitation could not be accomplished when a patellar tendon autograft alone was utilized for reconstruction, we undertook a clinical study to examine this issue. Over the course of several years and several hundred patients, steps were taken in an attempt to minimize the postoperative difficulties of knee stiffness, extensor weakness, and prolonged time to functional return. During the study, which included only patients undergoing a nonaugmented, central-third patellar tendon ACL reconstruction as described above, the rehabilitative protocol was gradually accelerated by decreasing the non–weight-bearing time, increasing progression of knee ROM, and directing earlier strengthening of the extremity. By following objective parameters, including serial arthrometer and dynamometer tests, ROM measurements, and repeat physical examinations, the impact of this progressively accelerated rehabilitation program was assessed. The results conclusively showed that stability of the reconstructed knee was not compromised, in spite of obtaining range of motion and strength of the extremity at a pace previously felt to jeopardize the graft.

Eventually, weight bearing on the operated extremity was allowed immediately after surgery, guided by the patient's tolerance to discomfort. Patient compliance with this less restrictive protocol was markedly improved, and subjective knee ratings by the patient (modified Noyes questionnaire) were equal to, or better than, scores obtained from patients following a more conventional rehabilitation protocol at similar times postoperatively. Safe, effective return to recreational and competitive sports has been remarkably accelerated without incurring graft failures while simultaneously *decreasing* the incidence of flexion contracture and prolonged muscle weakness, complications that previously accounted for significant patient dissatisfaction.

With the adoption of this accelerated protocol, (Table 18–4) postoperative rehabilitation is no longer a deterrent to surgical management of the ACL-deficient knee. Prior to this time, athletes would often opt for nonoperative management of a torn ACL to avoid the inconvenience of prolonged immobilization, non–weight bearing, and slow return to both everyday functional activities and, more important, sports. Thus, the athlete was accepting nonoperative management, with its attendant risk of reinjury and resultant long-term sequelae, rather than endure the perceived objectionable rehabilitation course.

While the surgeon's main concern in the rehabilitation phase has been to prevent activities that would injure the graft, the athlete's focus has been to return to "normal" as quickly as possible. Although the 2-year follow-up results after a slower, conventional rehabilitation protocol are acceptable, it has only been through accelerated protocols that surgical management has come more into line with the goals of athletes The safety of this rehabilitation format has been demonstrated in our clinical studies, thereby justifying the enthusiastic utilization of this protocol.

The current rehabilitative goal is to minimize "downtime" after reconstruction while working toward a *safe* return to normal activities as quickly as the patient desires. Full range of knee motion (with emphasis on full extension), return of injured extremity strength (when compared with the contralateral leg), and confidence in the operated knee (gained through completion of a running and agility program) are prerequisites for the athlete's return to competitive sports.

After the first 5 or 6 weeks following surgery—during which time a stricter protocol is followed—the pace of rehabilitation is largely left up to the patient. The keys to success in this accelerated protocol can be identified as follows:

1. Allow the patient to progress with weight bearing and muscle strengthening as tolerated.
2. Insist that the patient obtain full knee extension (equal to the opposite knee) in the

TABLE 18-4. Rehabilitation Following ACL Reconstruction

2 to 3 Days

CPM
PROM 0 to 90 degrees; let leg *fully* extend three times daily for 30 minutes
WB as tolerated with or without crutches and Dobi splint (rigid plastic immobilizer)

7 to 10 Days

Discontinue CPM
ROM; terminal extension 90 to 100 degrees flexion
Prone hang and towel extension
Wall slides for flexion
Partial squat 2 - to 4-inch step-up; calf raises
PWB to FWB without crutches; attempt to decrease use of the Dobi around the house but continue to use it when away from home
CPM; patellar mobilization

2 to 3 Weeks

ROM; terminal extension to 110 degrees
Partial squats on involved leg
Increased height of step-ups; calf raises; leg press
0 to 90 degrees; one-quarter squats and calf raises in squat rack
Bicycling and swimming
FWB with IKO (functional brace); always use brace when away from home

5 to 6 Weeks

ROM; terminal extension 120 to 130 degrees flexion
Continue with previously prescribed strengthening exercises
Cybex test at high speeds with 20 degrees extension block; if strength is greater than 70 percent, you will begin a functional progression that includes light jogging, agility drills, lateral shuffles, and jumping rope
KT1000
Discontinue IKO if muscle tone is sufficient

10 Weeks

Continue with previous strengthening exercises
Cybex test at high speeds
KT1000
Increase intensity level of functional progression

4 to 6 Months

Cybex at all three speeds
KT1000
Full functional progression back to activity to include cutting (must have near-normal strength, full motion, no swelling, good stability, and complete running program)

CPM	=	Continuous passive motion
PROM	=	Progressive range of motion
WB	=	Weight bearing
ROM	=	Range of motion
PWB	=	Partial weight bearing
FWB	=	Full weight bearing
IKO	=	Indiana knee orthosis

first few days postoperatively and *maintain* this extension thereafter.

3. Emphasize closed-kinetic (weight-bearing) exercises for the lower extremity in the initial period following surgery (Fig. 18-8).

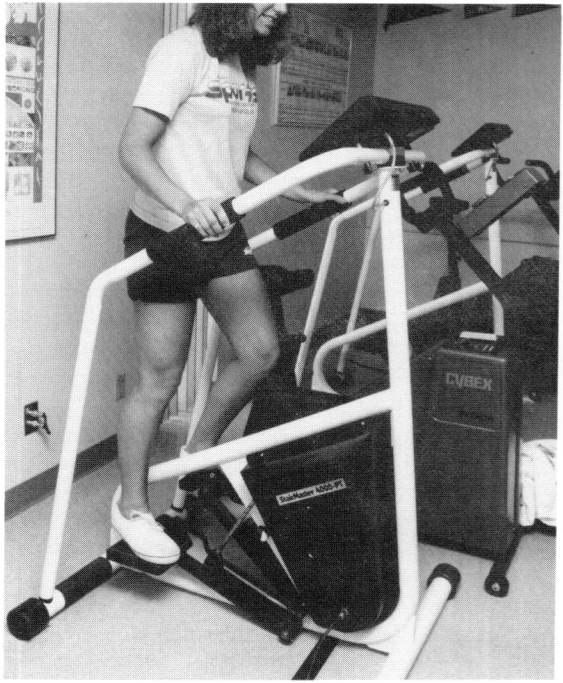

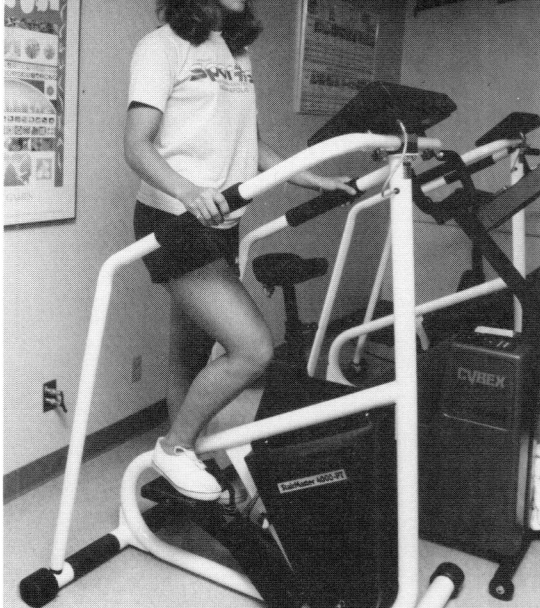

FIGURE 18-8. One example of the closed kinetic exercises that we use to minimize patellofemoral joint forces is the StairMaster 4000. In the initial period following surgery, patients can perform full knee extension (*A*) and mild knee flexion (*B*).

4. Incorporate functional and agility-type activities into the early rehabilitation once the injured extremity's hamstring/quadriceps strengths (based on isokinetic muscle testing) have surpassed 70 percent of the values for the nonoperated leg.

5. Dictate a graduated return to sports well in advance of participation in competitive athletics at the patient's prior ability level.

The benefit of obtaining full knee extension is manifested by greater patient satisfaction and performance and a decreased incidence of extensor mechanism complications. As this aspect plays such a dominant role in the ultimate success of the reconstructed knee, several points bear reiterating. Foremost, full knee extension must be pursued fanatically from the outset if one is to guarantee success in obtaining a knee with range of motion equal to the opposite extremity. Delaying full extension only makes eventual attainment of the desired range more difficult for the patient. This is especially true in the knee that is reconstructed shortly after the acute injury, in which a slight flexion contracture may already have developed in the short time between injury and surgery. Allowing a flexion contracture to persist or develop postoperatively, with eventual attempts at manipulating knee extension, has been less successful. In fact, such management may lead to further knee injury by marring or deforming the femoral condyles. Progress toward full extension must begin on the first postoperative day: Continuous passive motion (CPM), in a range from full extension to a comfortable degree of flexion, begins immediately (Fig. 18–9). When not in the CPM device, the heel of the operated extremity is elevated on pillows (or other supports) so that the leg and thigh make no contact with the bed; thus, the knee is allowed to sag into full extension, assisted by a plastic bag containing 2 or 3 pounds of crushed ice resting on the anterior aspect of the knee (Fig. 18–10). This maneuver is performed several times daily for as long as necessary and tolerated in order to get the operated knee out to full extension. Placing the nonoperated knee in a similar elevated position provides the patient a comparison with which to establish a goal for measuring progress. Active leg lifting by the patient encourages early quadriceps control (Fig. 18–11).

By the start of the second postoperative

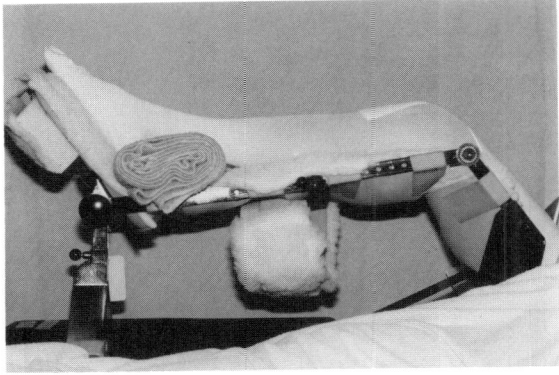

A

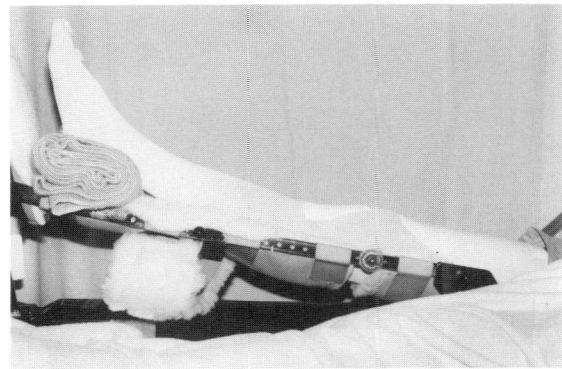

B

FIGURE 18–9. The continuous passive motion (CPM) machine allows the patients to work on flexion to tolerance and to maintain full extension. The heel is propped on a towel to ensure full extension.

week, once greater patient comfort has been obtained, prone hangs can be started (Fig. 18–12). To perform this exercise, the patient lies prone on a table or bed and allows his or her knees and lower legs to extend over the end; a 1- to 2-pound weight (such as a purse or handbag) is hung over the heel of the operated extremity. Performing this exercise for a few minutes each day will further ensure that the knee is achieving terminal extension. Emphasis is placed not on how often or how much time should be spent on extension exercises but rather on understanding the desired end point and working the length of time necessary to achieve and maintain this goal. Initial follow-up clinic visits should focus on the patient's ability to extend the knee with repeated encouragement to equal or exceed extension of the noninjured leg. Complacency will result in rapid loss of previously attained range of motion.

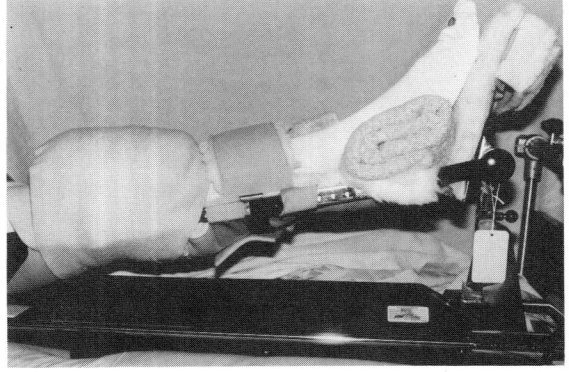
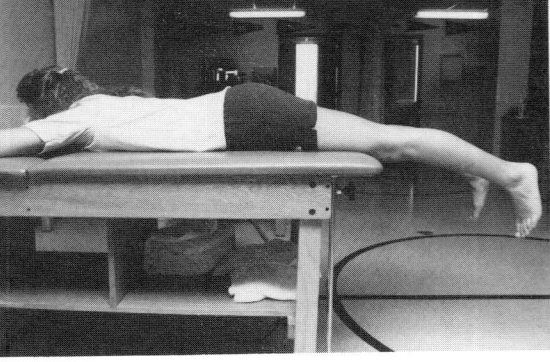

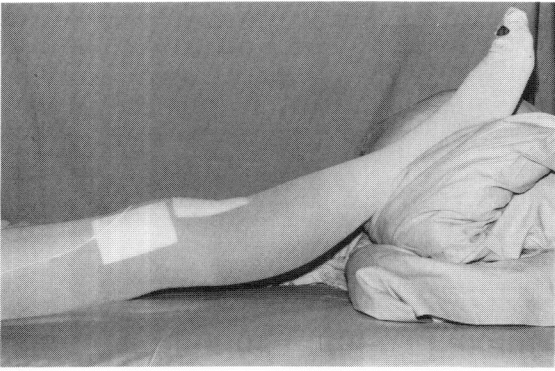
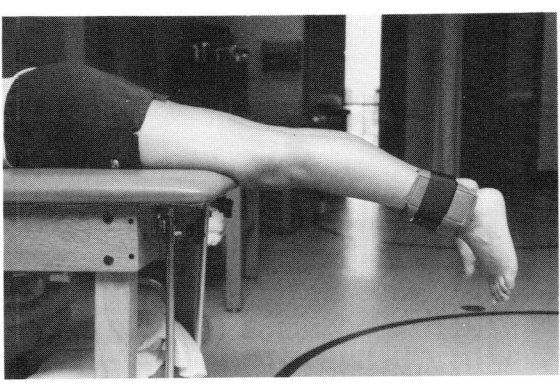

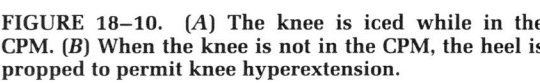

FIGURE 18–10. (A) The knee is iced while in the CPM. (B) When the knee is not in the CPM, the heel is propped to permit knee hyperextension.

FIGURE 18–12. (A) Prone hangs are used to achieve/maintain full extension and are performed with the patient in a relaxed prone position. (B) Weights can be utilized to attain extension equal to the opposite knee.

Patient stance and ambulation can aid in the pursuit of extension. Accordingly, there must be a concerted effort to avoid flexed-knee posturing; this is achieved through con-

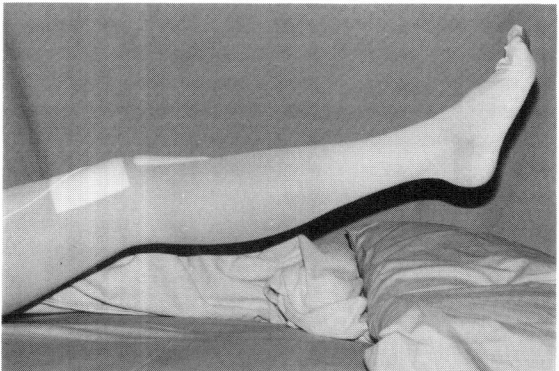

FIGURE 18–11. Reeducation of leg control is started while the patient is still in the hospital. The patient must demonstrate adequate leg control prior to discharge from the hospital.

centration on the extensor thrust of the knee with standing and walking. The patient is encouraged to remain out of the functional knee brace as much as possible, since the device prevents knee hyperextension, thereby hindering maintenance of previously accomplished terminal extension.

Athletes preparing to undergo ACL reconstruction will often try to obtain verbal guarantee from the surgeon as to when a return to sports will be permitted. While the individual is seeking a specific month, day, and perhaps hour in response to this query, the valid answer is conditional: It depends on several variables, most of which rely on patient motivation. Certain criteria should be fulfilled prior to returning to full athletic activity, including near-normal strength, full knee motion, functional knee stability, absence of appreciable effusion, and completion of a progressive running/agility program. The *earliest* one can reasonably expect to accomplish these goals is 3 to 4 months postoperatively. The patient who is highly motivated and experiences no setbacks during rehabilitation may indeed progress this rapidly. However, merely satisfying the aforementioned criteria will not guarantee reasonable performance when returning to competitive athletics.

In anticipation of this problem, sport-specific activities should be incorporated into the individualized rehabilitation program. For example, a basketball player may begin shooting baskets at 3 to 4 weeks, followed by ball dribbling and subsequently more specific cutting drills as confidence in the reconstructed knee is acquired. A football player may begin throwing the ball at 5 to 6 weeks, with the gradual addition of timing maneuvers such as dropping back, coming out of the stance, or performing specific cutting and running drills pertinent to the position played. The return of one's timing and confidence in the extremity truly dictates when a reasonably safe return to full sports, with a personally satisfying performance, can occur.

Clearly then, many of the factors controlling return to athletics rest with the athlete alone; these parameters are, in turn, influenced by level of competition involved. A superior athlete may achieve an earlier successful return if his or her preinjury talents and skills significantly exceeded the demands of the competition, whereas a marginal athlete may struggle. The type of sport and position played are also important. Participation in sports that are less stressful to the knee (e.g., tennis, swimming, and racquetball) may result in a quicker return than sports such as basketball, volleyball, or soccer. Similarly, an interior lineman in football may be able to return more readily than might a linebacker or running back at the same level of competition, simply because more predictable demands are placed on the knee by the former position, with less chance of sudden, unexpected cuts.

When discussing the timetable for return to sports, the athlete's degree of satisfaction with his or her performance is an important issue. While the clinician's concern is to get the patient *safely* back to competition at the level desired, the athlete is focused on a *performance level* equal to that experienced before the injury. If one is to maintain a wholesome relationship with the patient and prevent discouragement, it is essential for the physician to present this difference in perspective to the student athlete at the appropriate time during the rehabilitation period. This is most important in the extremely motivated athlete who has progressed quickly through the various phases of therapy postoperatively. Sensing that the clinical course is ahead of schedule, this athlete may fail to realize the extent of rehabilitation required for a safe return to sports: The proprioceptive skills necessary to perform "naturally," without feeling mechanical, require much longer to develop than extremity strength and range of motion. The return of confidence fostered by such "innate" ability can only be gained through *gradual* incorporation of experiences in which the extremity is tested at progressively more competitive and intense levels of activity. This segment of the rehabilitation program requires patience on the part of the athlete; there will be frustrating moments when he or she appreciates the limitations of the body, which is unable to accomplish what the mind is already prepared to do.

The transition from rehabilitation to competition will be smoother if the athlete first engages in activities other than the desired event or sport. For example, a basketball or football player may benefit tremendously from playing racquetball several times each week. Competition in another sport, such as a softball league or track and field, is helpful in acquiring confidence in the operated extremity prior to the first competitive postinjury season in the athlete's primary sport. Another way to diminish frustration during the first season back after injury is through preliminary involvement in the desired activity at a lower level of competition, without the intensity and external pressures of being "in season." Prior to returning for the interscholastic campaign, the school-aged basketball player might play in a summer league, assuming rehabilitation has progressed to this stage. Spring practice has equal value for the injured football player anticipating a return for the coming season. These approaches permit a more gradual return to normal or expected level of performance.

As mentioned, frequent postoperative follow-up visits are critical to the success of the patient's rehabilitation. The purpose of each visit is to monitor patient progress;

there should be satisfactory advancement in physical therapy and related endeavors such that the patient's goals are met in a timely fashion. By performing frequent checks, the clinician can identify potential complications early on and take appropriate measures.

Setbacks can occur at any time. Delay in attainment of joint motion must be identified immediately. While progression in knee flexion may proceed as patient comfort allows, full extension must be accomplished early and maintained as previously discussed. Occasionally, in spite of concerted efforts by both patient and therapist, the knee does not regain the desired extension. In such cases, repeat arthroscopy and performance of additional notchplasty with fat pad and scar tissue debridement, followed by serial extension casting for a few days, permit improvement in extension such that it equals that of the opposite extremity.

Knee swelling can persist for months following surgery; it must be managed aggressively if quadriceps inhibition and delay in functional recovery are to be minimized. Icing the knee frequently, especially after therapeutic exercise, should effectively eliminate this problem. Occasionally, one may be required to reduce patient activity temporarily and/or add a nonsteroidal antiinflammatory drug to control the effusion.

Overuse or "stress" injuries can occur during the course of rehabilitation.[38, 45] Patellar tendinitis or quadriceps tendinitis, while variably symptomatic, can be severe enough to delay strength recovery. Here again, icing the involved area and reducing both the amount and intensity of aggravating activity are important; additional management may require the avoidance of concentric exercise while emphasizing eccentric strengthening (see Chapter 2). More frequent follow-up visits are recommended if such problems are encountered, both to monitor progress and to provide encouragement to the frustrated patient.

Throughout the management of the student athlete with an ACL-deficient knee, the patient's attitude is vitally important. This is especially true during the lengthy period of rehabilitation. The patient's attitude and level of motivation are more significant in predicting a speedy recovery than age, sex, athletic ability, or any socioeconomic variable. Throughout the customary ups and downs following reconstruction, the physician and professional staff must be vigilant for any change in the patient's demeanor or attitude. Occasionally, the patient who was initially enthusiastic and seemingly motivated to undergo the reconstruction and rehabilitation will experience a marked depression, accompanied by significant weight loss and sleep derangement. One must not underestimate the impact of such changes and should be prepared to treat the patient accordingly. Referral to a sports psychologist may be very effective in these cases.

A particular subset of patients undergoing ACL reconstruction in whom problems with attitude and motivation during rehabilitation predictably occur includes interscholastic competitors who are seniors in high school. As a consequence of the timing of injury and elected treatment with respect to life events, these patients may be devoid of short-term goals and, as such, tend to "flounder" during the recovery process. Those student athletes in whom such difficulties are anticipated should be observed closely for motivational changes during rehabilitation. Proper management calls for frequent encouragement; the clinician must spend more time with such individuals in order to help them project ahead and set realistic goals beyond the senior year.

CONCLUSION

Use of the aggressive rehabilitation program outlined here has had a profound impact on decreasing the once-feared morbidity of intraarticular ACL reconstructions. While our surgical technique itself has not changed significantly in recent years, these modifications in postoperative protocol have markedly improved the prognosis for anterior cruciate disruption in the school-aged athlete. While sustaining such an injury and undergoing surgical treatment/rehabilitation remains a major event in the patient's life, we have been increasingly successful in preventing the circumstances from becoming a life-changing event. The goal of management of an ACL-deficient knee in this population is to afford the athlete an opportunity to pursue short-term athletic and recreational goals while maintaining the prospects for a comfortable, stable knee in the decades to come.

References

1. Amiel D., Ing D., Kleiner J. B., et al: The natural history of the anterior cruciate ligament autograph of patellar tendon origin. Am J Sports Med 14:449–462, 1986.
2. Amiel D., Kleiner J. B., Roux R. D., et al: The phenomenon of "ligamentization": anterior cruciate ligament reconstruction with autogenous patellar tendon. J Orthop Res 4:162–172, 1986.
3. Anderson A. F., Lipscomb A. B., Lindahl K. J., et al: Analysis of the intercondylar notch by computed tomography. Am J Sports Med 15:547–552, 1987.
4. Andrews J. R., Sanders R.: A minireconstruction technique in treating anterolateral rotatory instability (ALRI). Clin Orthop 172:93–96, 1983.
5. Arms S. W., Pope M. H., Johnson R. J., et al: The biomechanics of anterior cruciate ligament rehabilitation and reconstruction. Am J Sports Med 12:8–18, 1984.
6. Arnoczky S. P., Warren R. F., Minci J. P.: Replacement of the anterior cruciate ligament using a synthetic prosthesis. Am J Sports Med 14:1–6, 1986.
7. Bach B. R.: Arthroscopy-assisted patellar tendon substitution for anterior cruciate ligament insufficiency. Am J Knee Surg 2:3–20, 1989.
8. Beck C., Drez D., Young J., et al: Instrumented testing of functional knee braces. Am J Sports Med 14:253–256, 1986.
9. Bradley G. W., Shives T. C., Samuelson K. M.: Ligament injuries in the knees of children. J Bone Joint Surg 61A:588–591, 1979.
10. Brewster C. E., Moyens D. R., Jobe F. R.: Rehabilitation for anterior cruciate reconstruction. J Orthop Sports Phys Ther 5:121–126, 1983.
11. Cahill B. R., Griffith E. H.: Effect of preseason conditioning on the incidence and severity of high school football injuries. Am J Sports Med 6(4):180–184, 1978.
12. Caspari R. B., Meyers J. F., Whipple T.: A technique for arthroscopic reconstruction of the anterior cruciate ligament. Contemp Orthop 12:49–57, 1986.
13. Cerabona F., Sherman M. F., Bonamo J. R., et al: Patterns of meniscal injury with acute anterior cruciate ligament tears. Am J Sports Med 16:603–609, 1988.
14. Chick R. R., Jackson D. W.: Tears of the anterior cruciate ligament in young athletes. J Bone Joint Surg 60A:970–973, 1978.
15. Cho K. O.: Reconstruction of the anterior cruciate ligament by semitendinosus tenodesis. J Bone Joint Surg 57A:608–612, 1975.
16. Clancy W. G. Jr, Nelson D. A., Reider B., et al: Anterior cruciate ligament reconstruction using $\frac{1}{3}$ of the patellar ligament, augmented by extraarticular tendon transfers. J Bone Joint Surg 64:352–359, 1982.
17. Clanton T. O., DeLee J. C., Sanders B., et al: Knee ligament injuries in children. J Bone Joint Surg 61A:1195–1201, 1979.
18. Collins H. R., Hughston J. C., DeHaven K. E., et al: The meniscus as a cruciate ligament substitute. J Sports Med 2:11–21, 1974.
19. DeHaven K. E.: Diagnosis of acute knee injuries with hemarthrosis. Am J Sports Med 8:9–14, 1980.
20. DeHaven K. E.: Meniscus repair in the athlete. Clin Orthop 198:31–35, 1985.
21. DeLee J. C., Curtis R.: Anterior cruciate ligament insufficiency in children. Clin Orthop 172:112–118, 1983.
22. Ellison A. E.: Skiing injuries. Ciba Found Symp 29:2–40, 1977.
23. Ellison A. E.: Distal iliotibial band transfer for anterolateral rotatory instability of the knee. J Bone Joint Surg 61A:330–337, 1979.
24. Eriksson E.: Reconstruction of the anterior cruciate ligament. Orthop Clin North Am 7:167–179, 1976.
25. Eriksson E.: Sport injuries of the knee ligaments. Their diagnosis, treatment, rehabilitation and prevention. Med Sci Sports 8:133, 1976.
26. Feagin J. A.: The syndrome of the torn anterior cruciate ligament. Orthop Clin North Am 10:81–90, 1979.
27. Feagin J. A., Lambert K. L.: Mechanism of injury and pathology of anterior cruciate ligament injuries. Orthop Clin North Am 16:41–46, 1985.
28. Fetto J. F., Marshall J. L.: The natural history and diagnosis of anterior cruciate ligament insufficiency. Clin Orthop 147:29–38, 1980.
29. Fullerton L. R. Jr, Andrews J. R.: Mechanical block to extension following augmentation of the anterior cruciate ligament: case report. Am J Sports Med 12:166–169, 1984.
30. Funk F. J.: Osteoarthritis of the knee following ligamentous injury. Clin Orthop 172:154–157, 1983.
31. Garrick J. G., Requa R. K.: Prophylactic knee bracing. Am J Sports Med 15:471–476, 1987.
32. Gersoff W. K., Clancy W. G. Jr: Diagnosis of acute and chronic anterior cruciate ligament tears. Clin Sports Med 7:727–738, 1988.
33. Gillquist J., Odensten M.: Arthroscopic reconstruction of the anterior cruciate ligament. Arthroscopy 4:5–9, 1988.
34. Giove T. P., Miller S. J., Garrick J. G.: Nonoperative treatment of the torn anterior cruciate ligament. J Bone Joint Surg 65A:184–192, 1983.
35. Girgis F. G., Marshall J. L., Al Monajem A. R. S.: The cruciate ligaments of the knee joint. Anatomical, functional and experimental analysis. Clin Orthop 106:216–231, 1975.
36. Gollehon D. L., Warren R. F., Wickiewicz T. L.: Acute repairs of the anterior cruciate ligament—past and present. Orthop Clin North Am 16:111–125, 1985.
37. Gollnick T. D., Ericksson E., Harmark T., et al: Rehabilitation of the knee following surgery. Med Sci Sports 8:133–134, 1987.
38. Graf B., Uhr F.: Complications of intraarticular anterior cruciate reconstruction. Clin Sports Med 7:835–848, 1988.
39. Grood E. S., Noyes F. R.: Diagnosis and classification of knee ligament injuries: Part I. Biomechanical precepts. In The crucial ligaments. J. Feagin, editor. Churchill Livingstone, Inc., 245–260, 1987.
40. Grood E. S., Noyes F. R., Butler D. L., et al: Ligamentous and capsular restraints preventing straight medial and lateral laxity in intact human cadaver knees. J Bone Joint Surg 63A:1257–1269, 1981.

41. Hawkins R. J., Misamore G. W., Merritt T. R.: Followup of the acute nonoperated isolated anterior cruciate ligament tear. Am J Sports Med 14:205–210, 1986.
42. Houseworth S. W., Mauro V. J., Mellon B. A., et al: The intercondylar notch in acute tears of the anterior cruciate ligament: a computer graphic study. Am J Sports Med 15:221–224, 1987.
43. Howe J., Johnson R. J.: Knee studies in skiing. Clin Sports Med 1:277–288, 1982.
44. Huegel M., Indelicato P. A.: Trends in rehabilitation following anterior cruciate ligament reconstruction. Clin Sports Med 7:801–812, 1988.
45. Hughston J. C.: Complications of anterior cruciate ligament surgery. Orthop Clin North Am 16:237–240, 1985.
46. Hughston J. C., Andrews J. R., Cross M. J., et al: Classification of knee ligament instabilities. Part I. The medial compartment and cruciate ligaments. J Bone Joint Surg 58A:159–172, 1976.
47. Hughston J. C., Andrews J. R., Cross M. J., et al: Classification of knee ligament instabilities. Part II. The lateral compartment. J Bone Joint Surg 58A:173–179, 1976.
48. Hunter S. C., Andrews J. R., McLeod W. D., et al: Surgical reconstruction of chronic anteromedial rotatory instability of the knee. A review with computer analysis of 149 cases. Am J Sports Med 7:165–168, 1979.
49. Indelicato P. A., Bittar E. S.: A perspective of lesions associated with anterior cruciate ligament insufficiency of the knee. Clin Orthop 198:77–80, 1985.
50. Insall J., Joseph D. M., Aglietti P., et al: Bone block iliotibial band transfer for anterior cruciate ligament insufficiency. J Bone Joint Surg 63A:560–569, 1981.
51. Ireland J., Trickey E. L.: MacIntosh tenodesis for anterolateral instability of the knee. J Bone Joint Surg 62B:340–345, 1980.
52. Ivey F. M., Blazina M. E., Fox J. M., et al: Intraarticular substitution for anterior cruciate ligament insufficiency. A clinical comparison between patellar tendon and meniscus. Am J Sports Med 8:405–410, 1980.
53. Jackson D. W., Jennings L. D., Maywood R. M., et al: Magnetic resonance imaging of the knee. Am J Sports Med 16:29–38, 1988.
54. Jacobsen K.: Osteoarthrosis following insufficiency in the cruciate ligaments in man. A clinical study. Acta Orthop Scand 48:520–526, 1979.
55. Jones K. G.: Reconstruction of the anterior cruciate ligament. A technique using the central ⅓ of the patellar ligament. J Bone Joint Surg 45A:929–932, 1963.
56. Jurist K. A., Otis J. C.: Anteroposterior tibial femoral displacement during isometric extension efforts. Am J Sports Med 13:254–258, 1985.
57. Kennedy J. C., Fowler P. J.: Medial and anterior instability of the knee. An anatomical and clinical study using stress machines. J Bone Joint Surg 53A:1257–1270, 1971.
58. King S., Butterwick D. J., Cuerrier J. P.: The anterior cruciate ligament: a review of recent concepts. J Orthop Sports Phys Ther 8:110–122, 1986.
59. Krackow K. A. W., Brooks R. L.: Optimization of knee ligament position for lateral extraarticular reconstruction. Am J Sports Med 11:293–302, 1983.
60. Kurosaka M., Yoshiga S., Andrish J. R.: A biomechanical comparison of different surgical techniques of graft fixation in anterior cruciate ligament reconstruction. Am J Sports Med 15:225–229, 1987.
61. Lambert K. L.: Vascularized patellar tendon graft with rigid internal fixation for anterior cruciate ligament insufficiency. Clin Orthop 172:85–89, 1983.
62. Lipscomb A. B., Anderson A. F.: Tears of the anterior cruciate ligament in adolescents. J Bone Joint Surg 68A:19–28, 1986.
63. Lipscomb A. B., Johnston R. K., Snyder R. B., et al: Secondary reconstruction of anterior cruciate ligament in athletes by using the semitendinosus tendon. Preliminary report of 78 cases. Am J Sports Med 7:81–83, 1979.
64. Losee R. E.: Diagnosis of chronic injury to the anterior cruciate ligament. Orthop Clin North Am 16:83–97, 1985.
65. Losee R. E., Johnson T. R., Southwick W. O.: Anterior subluxation of the lateral tibial plateau. A diagnostic test and operative repair. J Bone Joint Surg 60A:1015–1030, 1978.
66. Lynch M. A., Henning C. E., Glick K. R.: Knee joint surface changes. Long term follow-up meniscus tear treatment in stable anterior cruciate ligament reconstructions. Clin Orthop 172:148–153, 1983.
67. Mandelbaum B. R., Finerman G. A., Reicher M. A., et al: Magnetic resonance imaging as a tool for evaluation of traumatic knee injuries: anatomical and pathoanatomical correlations. Am J Sports Med 14:361–370, 1986.
68. Mariani P. P., Puddu G., Ferretti A.: Hemarthrosis treated by aspiration and casting. Am J Sports Med 10:343–345, 1982.
69. Markolf K. L., Bargar W. L., Shoemaker S. C.: In vivo knee stability. J Bone Joint Surg 60A:664–674, 1978.
70. Markolf K. L., Mensch J. S., Amstutz H. C.: Stiffness and laxity of the knee—the contributions of supporting structures. J Bone Joint Surg 58A:583–593, 1976.
71. McCarroll J. R., Rettig A. C., Shelbourne K. D.: Anterior cruciate ligament injuries in the young athlete with open physes. Am J Sports Med 16:44–47, 1988.
72. McDaniel W. J., Dameron T. B.: Untreated ruptures of the anterior cruciate ligament. A followup study. J Bone Joint Surg 62A:696–705, 1980.
73. McDaniel W. J., Dameron T. B.: The untreated anterior cruciate ligament rupture. Clin Orthop 172:158–163, 1983.
74. McMaster J. H., Weinert C. R. Jr., Scranton P. Jr.: Diagnosis and management of isolated anterior cruciate ligament tears: a preliminary report on reconstruction with the gracilis tendon. J Trauma 14:230–235, 1974.
75. Millet C. D., Drez D. J.: Principles of bracing for the anterior cruciate ligament–deficient knee. Clin Sports Med 7:827–833, 1988.
76. Murray S. M., Warren R. F., Otis J. L., et al: Torque-velocity relationships of the knee extensor and flexor muscles in individuals sustaining inju-

ries of the anterior cruciate ligament. Am J Sports Med 12:436–440, 1984.
77. Nicholas J. A., Minkoff J.: Iliotibial band transfer through the intercondylar notch for combined anterior instability (ITPT procedure). Am J Sports Med 6:341–353, 1978.
78. Nikolau P: Anterior cruciate ligament allograft transplantation. Am J Sports Med 14:348–355, 1986.
79. Noyes F. R., Bassett R. W., Grood E. S., et al: Arthroscopy in acute traumatic hemarthrosis of the knee. J Bone Joint Surg 62A:687–696, 1980.
80. Noyes F. R., Grood E. S.: Diagnosis and classification of knee ligament injuries: Part II. Clinical concepts. In *The crucial ligaments*. J. Feagin, editor. Churchill Livingstone, Inc, 261–285, 1987.
81. Noyes F. R., Matthews D. S., Mooar P. A., et al: The symptomatic ACL deficient knee. Part II: The results of rehabilitation, activity modification, and counseling on functional disability. J Bone Joint Surg 65A:163–174, 1983.
82. Noyes F. R., McGinniss G. H.: Controversy about treatment of the knee with anterior cruciate laxity. Clin Orthop 198:61–76, 1985.
83. Noyes F. R., McGinniss G. H., Grood E. S.: The variable functional disability of the anterior cruciate ligament–deficient knee. Orthop Clin North Am 16:47–67, 1985.
84. Noyes F. R., Mooar P. A., Matthews D. S., et al: The symptomatic anterior cruciate–deficient knee. Part I: The long term functional disability in athletically active individuals. J Bone Joint Surg 65A:154–162, 1983.
85. Odensten M., Hamberg P., Gillquist J., et al: Surgical or conservative treatment of the acutely torn anterior cruciate ligament. Clin Orthop 198:87–93, 1985.
86. O'Donoghue D. H.: Surgical treatment of fresh injuries to the major ligaments of the knee. J Bone Joint Surg 32A:721–738, 1950.
87. O'Donoghue D. H.: Surgical treatment of injuries to the ligaments of the knee. JAMA 169:1423–1431, 1959.
88. O'Donoghue D. H.: Treatment of acute ligamentous injuries of the knee. Orthop Clin North Am 4:617–645, 1973.
89. Paulos L. E., Drawbert J. P., France E. P., et al: Lateral knee braces in football: do they prevent injury? Phys Sports Med 14:119–124, 1986.
90. Paulos L., Noyes F. R., Grood E. S., et al: Knee rehabilitation after anterior cruciate ligament reconstruction and repair. Am J Sports Med 9:140–149, 1981.
91. Paulos L. E., Rosenberg T. D., Drawbert J. P., et al: Intrapatellar contracture syndrome. An unrecognized cause of knee stiffness with patella entrapment and patella infera. Am J Sports Med 15:331–341, 1987.
92. Polly D. W., Callaghan J. J., Sikes R. R., et al: The accuracy of selective magnetic resonance imaging compared with findings of arthroscopy of the knee. J Bone Joint Surg 70A:192–198, 1988.
93. Ray J. M.: A proposed natural history of symptomatic anterior cruciate ligament injuries of the knee. Clin Sports Med 7:697–713, 1988.
94. Renstrom P., Arms S. W., Stanwick T. S., et al: Strength in the anterior cruciate ligament during hamstring and quadriceps activity. Am J Sports Med 14:83–87, 1986.
95. Roth J. H., Kennedy J. C., Lockstadt H., et al: Polypropylene braid augmented and nonaugmented intraarticular anterior cruciate ligament reconstructions. Am J Sports Med 13:321–336, 1985.
96. Rovere G. A.: Anterior cruciate–deficient knees: a review of the literature. Am J Sports Med 11:412–419, 1983.
97. Rovere G. A., Haupt H. A., Yates C. S.: Prophylactic knee bracing in college football. Am J Sports Med 15:111–116, 1987.
98. Shelbourne K. D., Baele J. R.: Treatment of combined anterior cruciate ligament and medial collateral ligament injuries. Am J Knee Surg 1:56–58, 1988.
99. Shelbourne K. D., Whitaker H. J., McCarroll J. R., et al: Anterior cruciate ligament injury: evaluation of intraarticular reconstruction of acute tears without repair. Presented at the American Orthopedic Society of Sports Medicine, Las Vegas, NV, February 12, 1989. Am J Sports Med (In press).
100. Sherman M. F., Bonamo J. R.: Primary repair of the anterior cruciate ligament. Clin Sports Med 7:739–750, 1988.
101. Shultz R. A., Miller D. L., Kerr C. S., et al: Mechanoreceptors in human cruciate ligaments: a histologic study. J Bone Joint Surg 66A:1072–1076, 1984.
102. Silva I. Jr., Silver D. M.: Tears of the meniscus as revealed by magnetic resonance imaging. J Bone Joint Surg 70A:199–202, 1988.
103. Slocum D. B., Larson R. L.: Pes anserine transplantation. A surgical procedure for control of rotatory instability of the knee. J Bone Joint Surg 50A:226–242, 1968.
104. Souryal T. O., Moore H. A., Evans J. P.: Bilaterality in anterior cruciate ligament tears: associated intercondylar notch stenosis. Am J Sports Med 16:449–454, 1988.
105. Tegner Y., Lysholm J., Gillquist J., et al: A performance test to monitor rehabilitation and evaluation of anterior cruciate ligament injuries. Am J Sports Med 14:156–159, 1986.
106. Teitz C. C., Hermanson B., Kronmall R. A., et al: Evaluation of the use of braces to prevent injury to the knee in collegiate football players. J Bone Joint Surg 69A: 2–9, 1987.
107. Terry G. C., Hughston J. C.: Associated joint pathology in the anterior cruciate ligament–deficient knee with emphasis on a classification system and injuries to the meniscocapsular ligament–musculotendinosis unit complex. Orthop Clin North Am 16:29–39, 1985.
108. Tibone J. E., Antich T. J., Perry J., et al: Functional analysis of anterior cruciate ligament instability. Am J Sports Med 14:276–284, 1986.
109. Torg J. S., Quedenfeld T. C., Landau S.: The shoe-surface interface and its relationship to football knee injuries. J Sports Med 2:261–269, 1974.
110. Unverferth L. J., Bagenstose J. E.: Extraarticular reconstructive surgery for combined anterolateral-anteromedial rotatory instability. Am J Sports Med 7:34–39, 1979.
111. Walla D. J., Albright J. P., McAuley E., et al: Hamstring control and the unstable anterior cruciate

ligament deficient knee. Am J Sports Med 13:34–39, 1985.
112. Wang J. B., Rubin R. M., Marshall J. L.: A mechanism of isolated anterior cruciate ligament rupture. J Bone Joint Surg 57A:411–413, 1975.
113. Yasuda K, Sasaki T.: Exercise after anterior cruciate ligament reconstruction: the force exhibited on the tibia by separate isometric contractions of the quadriceps or hamstrings. Clin Orthop 220:275–283, 1987.
114. Yasuda K., Sasaki T.: Muscle exercise after anterior cruciate ligament reconstruction: biomechanics of the simultaneous isometric contraction method of the quadriceps and the hamstrings. Clin Orthop 220:266–274, 1987.
115. Zarins B., Rowe C. R.: Combined anterior cruciate ligament reconstruction using semitendinosus tendon and iliotibial tract. J Bone Joint Surg 68A:160–177, 1986.
116. Zoltan D. J., Reinecke C., Indelicato P. A.: Synthetic and allograft anterior cruciate ligament reconstruction. Clin Sports Med 7:773–784, 1988.

19

POSTERIOR CRUCIATE LIGAMENT INJURIES

K. DONALD SHELBOURNE
PAUL A. NITZ

Although posterior cruciate ligament (PCL) injuries are not nearly as common as anterior cruciate ligament (ACL) tears, they are not as rare as sometimes thought. DeHaven identified PCL tears in 3 percent of all knees evaluated for acute hemarthrosis.[10] In various comprehensive knee ligament injury studies, PCL injury has been noted in 8 to 23 percent of all cases.[7, 28, 34, 39] Kennedy reported that in his practice one patient with PCL insufficiency came to surgery for every six who required surgical management for ACL deficiency.[29]

The mean age at the time for patients acquiring the PCL damage has been reported to generally be in the early to midtwenties[22, 38, 40] A sizable proportion of patients cited in these studies sustained their knee injury during their teenage years.[9, 22, 38, 40] Therefore, the possibility of PCL injury must always be considered in the evaluation of knee injuries in the school-age athlete.

Unfortunately, confusion and controversy have prevailed in the discussion of PCL injury. Most of the data regarding this ligament injury have been obtained from small retrospective patient studies. Contributing to the confusion have been diagnostic inconsistencies and the inclusion of diverse associated ligament injuries in reports about PCL trauma.[3, 22, 29] Additionally, a lack of uniformity in the method of reporting results has dominated the PCL injury literature. The current uncertainty regarding the long-term natural history of the isolated or combined PCL is reflected in the treatment recommendations for the school-age athlete. The principles and concepts presented here are a distillation of previously published sources on PCL injuries balanced with present trends and personal impressions.

MECHANISM OF INJURY

PCL injuries have often been associated with severe and violent trauma.[8, 28, 33, 36] Other series have identified a subset of individuals with PCL damage as a consequence of seemingly minimal trauma.[12, 35, 49] Some reports have attributed greater than 90 percent of the PCL injuries to motor vehicle accidents,[34, 49] whereas other investigators have identified athletic trauma as the cause of approximately 50 percent or more of the PCL injuries in their reported series.[8, 22, 29] These apparent discrepancies are caused by the fact that athletic injuries tend to cause isolated PCL tears, whereas motor vehicle accidents tend to produce more severe multiple ligament injuries. Series from major trauma centers tend to contain more multiple injuries and probably more occult knee dislocations. The mixing of isolated PCL tears with multiple ligament injuries and athletic injuries with vehicular trauma has confused the mechanism of injury as well as the natural history of the injury. Therefore, in the assessment of PCL injury mechanisms, it is important to recognize the potential variety of structural injuries and to separate the isolated PCL tears from multiple ligament injuries.

Isolated PCL injuries in athletes are commonly the result of a fall on the flexed knee while the foot is plantar flexed (Fig. 19–1). This mechanism displaces the tibia posteriorly on the femur while the posterior capsule and other ligamentous structures are relatively relaxed.[35] PCL rupture may also occur if the foot is dorsiflexed but the tibial tubercle happens to strike a prominence on the playing field. A direct blow to the anterior tibia while the knee is flexed can produce a similar type of injury[14] (Fig. 19–2). Fowler and Messieh have maintained that PCL rupture from a fall during sports is caused by the acute hyperflexion of the knee and not by the contact of the tibia with the ground.[12]

The authors have identified one other mechanism of isolated PCL injury (Fig. 19–3). Two athletes separately sustained this ligament injury, one while playing softball and the other while playing football, when the upper body and femur anteriorly translated and externally rotated over the fixed weight-bearing leg while the knee was near full extension. These two interstitial tears were the result of the tibia being in effect posteriorly displaced, generating the injurious tensile force to the ligament over the anterior cruciate ligament.

PCL tears associated with additional knee ligament injuries are generally the result of more severe trauma. Forced hyperextension of the knee will normally rupture the ACL and posterior capsule prior to PCL rupture.[29, 36, 50] Cross and Powell found in their review of PCL injuries that 35% of such tears oc-

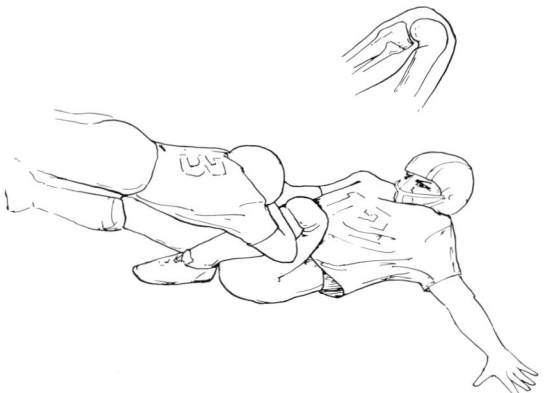

FIGURE 19–2. Forced hyperflexion of a flexed knee may also cause isolated PCL injury.

curred by a severe twist of the knee with a varus or valgus force.[8] A mechanism of rotation combined with either additional valgus stress[3] or an anterior pretibial blow to the flexed knee has been associated with complex injuries including the PCL.[1, 22, 50] The authors have identified combined PCL-MCL (medial collateral ligament) injuries occurring in those individuals who have experienced a significant valgus, external rotation stress to a flexed knee with the foot in a fixed yet non–weight-bearing position. (Fig. 19–4).[42] These injuries occur during a fall on

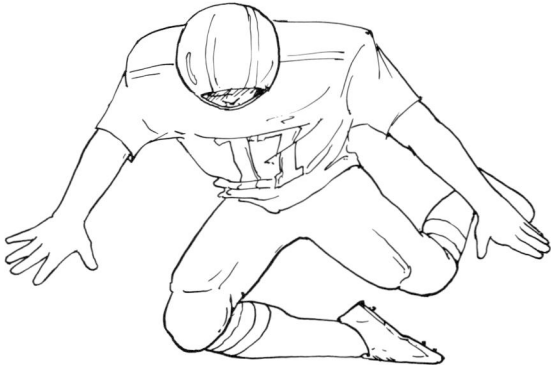

FIGURE 19–1. Falling on the knee while the foot is plantar flexed is a common method of isolated PCL injury in athletes.

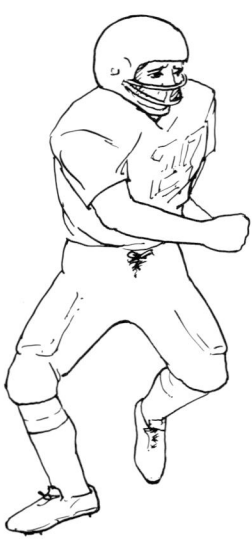

FIGURE 19–3. An unusual mechanism of isolated PCL injury is anterior translation and external rotation of the femur over the weight-bearing leg when the knee is near full extension.

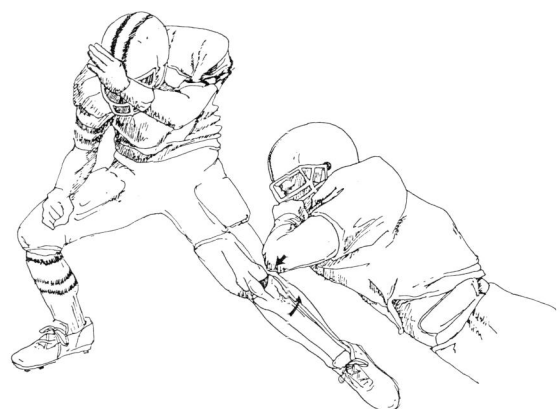

FIGURE 19-4. Rotation combined with additional valgus stress or an anterior pretibial blow to the flexed knee has been associated with complex injuries including the PCL.

the flexed knee while the knee is forced into a valgus or externally rotated position. This mechanism contrasts with the combined ACL-MCL injury that occurs when a similar valgus, external rotation stress is applied to a similarly flexed but weight-bearing knee.

Knowing the mechanism of injury can help the clinician direct the examination of the knee to the structures most likely to be injured. This is particularly important in posterior cruciate ligament injuries, since they are so easily overlooked.

HISTORY

Following an acute isolated PCL injury, the patient usually has a mild hemarthrosis and complains of posterior knee pain. The injured knee's range of motion is often limited from approximately 10 to 60 degrees.[33] Acutely, the patient often walks with a slightly flexed knee to avoid terminal extension and external rotation. It is not uncommon for the patient to report to the clinician that the knee feels like "something is just not right."

When PCL rupture is part of a multiple ligament injury, the swelling is usually much greater. If capsular disruption is severe, intra-articular hemorrhage may escape from the knee into the subcutaneous plane. Pain remains the patient's primary complaint, and it may be severe with consequent inability to bear weight. Edema and ecchymosis may be present in the injured extremity, again de-pending on the competence of the knee's capsule and the extent of the associated trauma to the limb.

Chronic PCL-deficient knees may range from completely asymptomatic to severely disabled. It is recognized that a significant percentage of such knees, especially those with isolated PCL tears, remain asymptomatic for an undetermined length of time.[40] It is not known when and how often these knees become symptomatic. Patients with chronic isolated PCL tears who present to physicians complain primarily of pain. Parolie and Bergfeld reported 25 patients with isolated PCL deficiency. Among these, 52 percent had knee pain and 48 percent had stiffness an average of 6.2 years following injury.[40] Dandy and Pusey also cited pain with walking in 14 of their 20 patients, who averaged 7.2 years following injury.[9] Symptoms of instability were only noted by 20 percent of Parolie and Bergfeld's and 45 percent of Dandy and Pusey's patients.

We have observed that some of our patients with chronic PCL deficiency experience pain only when running at full speed. Why is the PCL-deficient knee more likely to be symptomatic as the speed of running increases? One reason may be that the shorter period from heel strike to toe-off causes the knee's anterior-posterior translation to occur more abruptly. Also, the more complete knee extension during increased stride length at faster running speeds may produce a posterior tibial subluxation-reduction phenomenon near full extension similar to the dynamic posterior shift.[41]

In studies of combined PCL injuries, knee pain was most often retropatellar.[8] When instability is noted by the patient, it has been described as a straight anterior-posterior sliding of the femur on the tibia, which lacks the violent suddenness of the giving-way episodes associated with chronic ACL insufficiency.[8] The majority of patients with PCL deficiency are generally not functionally impaired by knee instability, however.[6]

PHYSICAL EXAMINATION

The purpose of examination of the injured knee is to confirm the diagnostic impression obtained from the stated mechanism of injury, symptoms, and cursory observation of the knee. Before proceeding with the stability examination, the clinician should take a moment to inspect the knee visually. Since most isolated PCL tears are the result of a fall on a flexed knee or a blow to the tibial tubercle, many patients will exhibit an ecchymosis or abrasion over the tubercle that suggests the diagnosis.[49] If the patient can flex the knee to 90 degrees, the clinician should compare the "profile" of the two knees when viewed from the side. In the chronic PCL-deficient knee, a "drop-back," or recession, of the tibial tubercle is usually visible (Fig. 19–5). In this case, the patella seems more prominent, creating a "ski slope" appearance. In acute or partial injuries, the drop-back may be very slight or absent.

In the past, some clinicians have disagreed over the clinical significance of the posterior drawer test.[19, 29, 38] However, more recent biomechanical studies have confirmed that isolated rupture of the PCL dramatically increases the posterior drawer laxity and that this increase is greatest in the 70- to 90-degree knee flexion range of the traditional posterior drawer test.[4, 13] Godfrey's posterior sag test[14] (Fig. 19–6) and Shelbourne's dynamic posterior shift test[41] (Figs. 19–7 and 19–8) are adjutant diagnostic maneuvers that when positive, confirm the posterior drawer test findings.

The posterior drawer test requires that the patient be capable of flexing the knee to 90 degrees while lying supine. The hip is flexed approximately 45 degrees, and the foot rests firmly on the evaluating surface. Following an acute PCL injury, initial muscle spasm and traumatic effusion may limit flexion of the knee. If the knee cannot be flexed to 90 degrees, a posterior Lachman test can provide useful qualitative information regarding anterioposterior translation of the knee (Figs. 19–9 and 19–10). Demonstrating that the Lachman test has a firm end point anteriorly while manifesting overall increased excur-

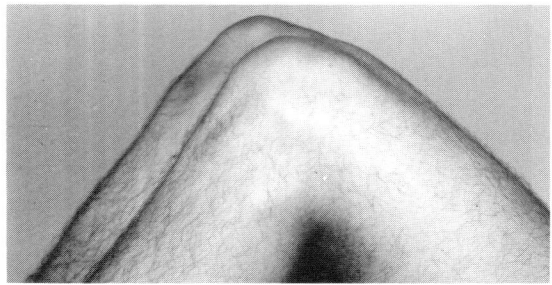

FIGURE 19–5. The knee in the foreground illustrates the "drop-back" usually seen in a PCL-deficient knee.

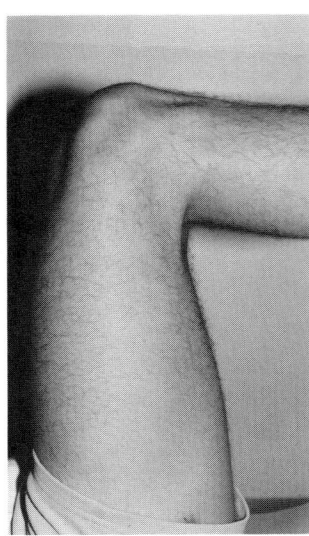

FIGURE 19–6. Godfrey test. With heels supported and leg relaxed, note the posterior position of the tibia.

sion in the sagittal plan in comparison with the contralateral knee should suggest to the clinician the probability of PCL deficiency. A subsequent posterior drawer reexamination a few days later when the patient's knee is more comfortable and range of motion (ROM) has improved would then permit definitive assessment of the PCL.

As with other ligament stability tests, the posterior drawer can only be properly interpreted if the patient's leg and knee are thoroughly relaxed. The examiner sits lightly on the patient's forefoot to stabilize the leg. The proximal calf muscles are cradled in the examiner's fingers medially and laterally, with the thumbs resting on the tibial articular landmarks on either side of the patellar tendon. The amount of anterior tibial plateau projecting anterior to the femoral condylar surfaces is appreciated by direct palpation (Fig. 19–11). Normally, the anterior tibial margin should project about 1 cm in front of the femoral condyles when the knee is flexed to 90 degrees. As mentioned, tibial drop-back due to gravity may alter this normal relationship before the examiner has even applied a posterior force to the tibia.

The proximal tibia is then pushed straight posteriorly with firm, smooth motion, palpating the change in alignment of the tibial plateau in reference to the femoral condyles (Fig. 19–12). Objective quantification of displacement can be accomplished with the posterior drawer test by noting the palpable displacement of the tibial plateau in respect

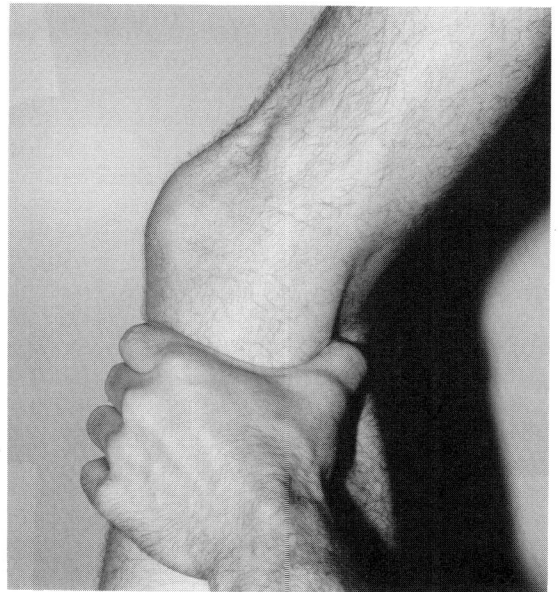

FIGURE 19–7. With the hip flexed 90 degrees and the heel supported in right hand, the knee is extended slowly, allowing passive hamstring tightness to accentuate the posterior tibial position of the tibia.

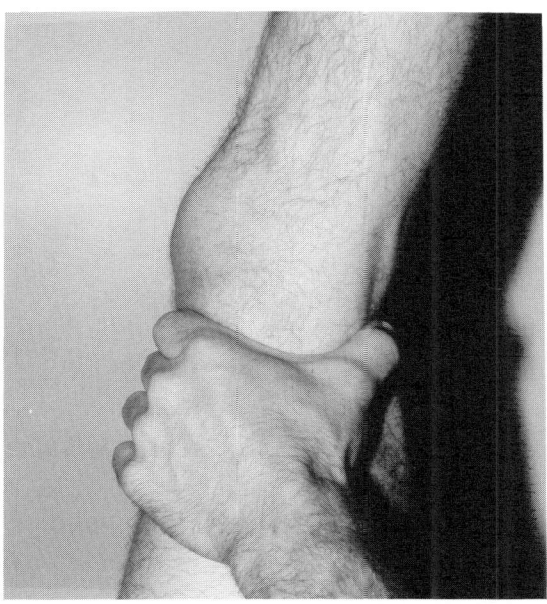

FIGURE 19–8. As the knee is fully extended, the tibia suddenly reduces on the femur dynamically.

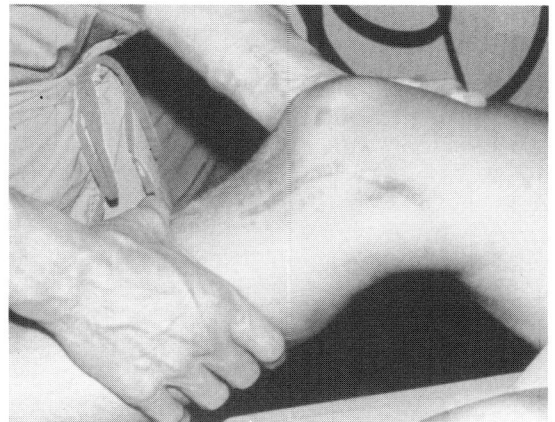

FIGURE 19–9. The posterior starting position for the Lachman test.

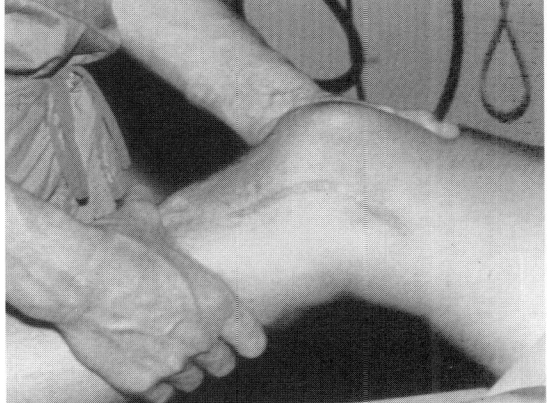

FIGURE 19–10. The tibia reduces to the normal position with a firm end point, indicating PCL laxity.

to the femoral condyles. Increased posterior translation in comparison with the contralateral knee, but with tibial plateau prominence remaining anterior to the femoral condyles, is assigned a 1+ posterior drawer (approximately 5 mm of increased posterior displacement). A tibial plateau that can be displaced posteriorly such that it is flush with the femoral condyles is graded as a 2+ posterior drawer (about 10 mm of increased posterior translation). Tibial plateau displacement posterior to the plane of the femoral condyles is graded as a 3+ posterior drawer (greater than 10 mm of abnormal posterior motion).

Grading this diagnostic test can provide valuable information about the structures that have sustained injury. A posterior drawer graded 2+ or less would most probably reflect as isolated PCL injury. A 3+ posterior drawer should cause one to suspect the probability of additional ligament and posterior capsular disruption.[13]

The clinician must be mindful that a posi-

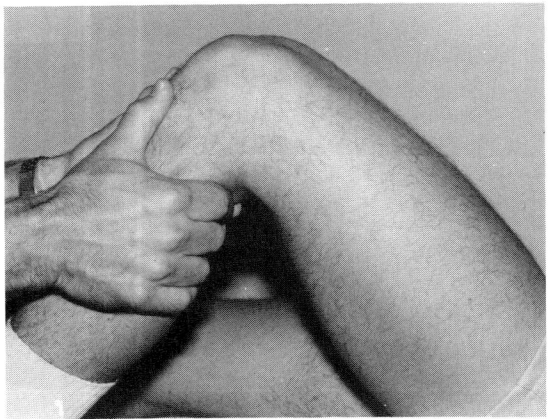

FIGURE 19–11. With a forward pull on the tibia, the normal step-off is palpated.

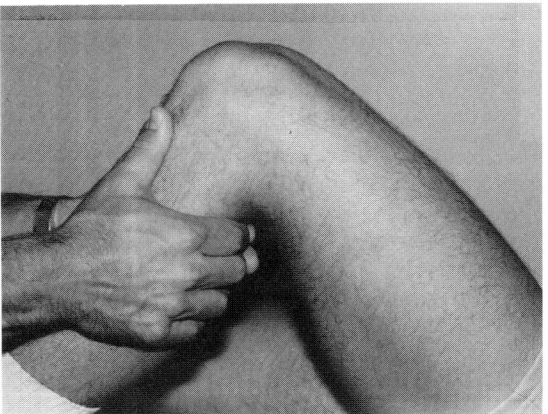

FIGURE 19–12. With a posterior drawer, the normal step-off of the tibia is lost, indicating PCL laxity.

tive posterior drawer may present subtly, especially when examining an isolated partial PCL tear. It is most important to verify that the tibia is in the reduced position rather than subluxed posteriorly before performing the posterior drawer maneuver. Failure to bring the subluxed tibia anteriorly prior to doing the posterior drawer test may confuse the examiner.

After testing with the tibia in a neutral position, the posterior drawer is repeated with the tibia internally rotated. Clancy and others[6, 40] have emphasized that this maneuver tightens the meniscofemoral ligaments of Wrisberg or Humphrey, present in 70 percent of knees,[17, 30] thus decreasing the magnitude of the posterior drawer by one grade in most patients with an isolated PCL rupture. A posterior drawer not decreased by internal rotation suggests the possibility of a more comprehensive posterior knee injury.

The dynamic posterior shift test uses the patient's own hamstrings to induce posterior subluxation of the tibia (Figs. 19–7 and 19–8). It will be positive in cases of isolated posterior laxity or combined posterior and posterolateral laxity. The dynamic posterior shift[41] is performed by first placing the supine patient's lower limb in 90 degrees of flexion at both the hip and the knee. The knee is slowly extended by the examiner lifting the leg upward with one hand while the other hand supports the distal thigh to maintain 90 degrees of hip flexion. As the knee approaches complete extension, a jerk or "clunk" occurs as the posteriorly subluxed tibia suddenly reduces anteriorly. The passively tightening hamstrings exert a dynamic axial load on the joint that accentuates the reduction phenomenon, thereby reproducing the instability episodes sometimes experienced by the patient with a PCL deficit.

Although PCL tears from sports are usually isolated injuries, the clinician should look carefully for signs of additional ligament damage. Hyperextension of the knee in excess of the contralateral knee prompts suspicion of ACL injury and the possibility of a spontaneously reduced dislocation. Associated collateral ligament injuries, especially when grade III, should also provoke consideration of a reduced knee dislocation. Because of the frequent association of arterial injury with knee dislocation, the clinician should evaluate the vascular status of all knees with multiple ligament injuries very carefully and perform arteriography when there is any question of arterial injury.

A positive posterolateral drawer test and external rotation recurvatum test as described by Hughston and Norwood strongly suggest injury of the knee's posterolateral corner (arcuate complex, popliteus, and lateral collateral ligament [LCL])[24] (Fig. 19–13). Equal posterior tibial translation (generally greater than 20 mm) at both 30 degrees and 90 degrees of knee flexion reflects injury to both the PCL and the LCL and popliteus tendon.[15]

Jakob et al. have described the reverse pivot-shift test for posteriolateral laxity.[26] It is similar to the classic pivot shift but is performed with the tibia externally rotated. The examiner supports the patient's leg with the knee fully extended by grasping and externally rotating the foot. A gentle valgus stress is applied to the tibia with the other hand as the knee is flexed. A sudden shift occurs at about 20 to 30 degrees of knee flexion as the

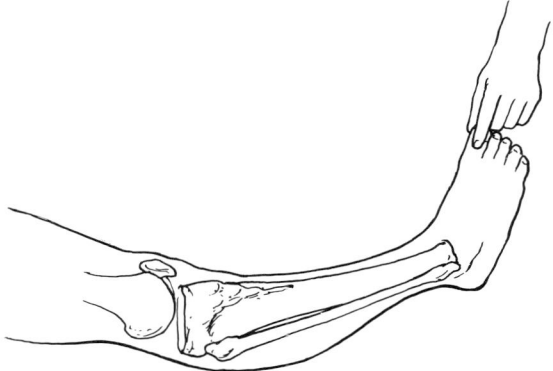

FIGURE 19–13. The Hughston external rotation recurvatum test is performed by lifting both legs by the greater toe. In the presence of posterior and posterolateral laxity, the knee will go into varus and recurvatum.

tibia externally rotates and subluxes posteriorly. In a knee with concomitant ACL insufficiency, it takes experience to distinguish this from the classic pivot shift.

Other diagnostic maneuvers such as the abduction and adduction stress tests in extension[20, 21] and the posterolateral drawer test and rotational recurvatum test[24] are primarily of importance in diagnosing associated ligamentous injuries.

Routine radiographs are usually normal in cases of isolated PCL rupture. However, an occasional isolated PCL injury will present as a bony avulsion, usually involving the tibial insertion (Fig. 19–14). These are usually clearly seen on lateral radiographs but may vary considerably in size.[31, 37, 47, 48]

ASSOCIATED INJURIES

It has been our experience that most PCL tears occurring during athletics are isolated structural injuries. While motor vehicle and similar accidents are more likely to produce combination injuries,[18] it is nevertheless the mechanism of injury that most determines the specific resultant abnormalities. In reviewing the incidence of associated injuries, it is important to remember that most series contain many injuries not caused by sports.

Various reports have identified a 46 to 90 percent incidence of medial collateral ligament (MCL) injuries with the acute PCL injury, often in combination with additional structural damage about the knee (ACL, posterolateral structures).[22, 29, 38] In a review of all acute PCL injuries presenting at the authors' sports medicine center, 24 percent of such injured knees were found to have an associated MCL disruption.[42] This injury is a result of a valgus, external rotation stress to the knee with a fixed but unloaded foot, as previously mentioned (Fig. 19–15). Upon initial assessment shortly after the injury, these patients were thought to have sustained

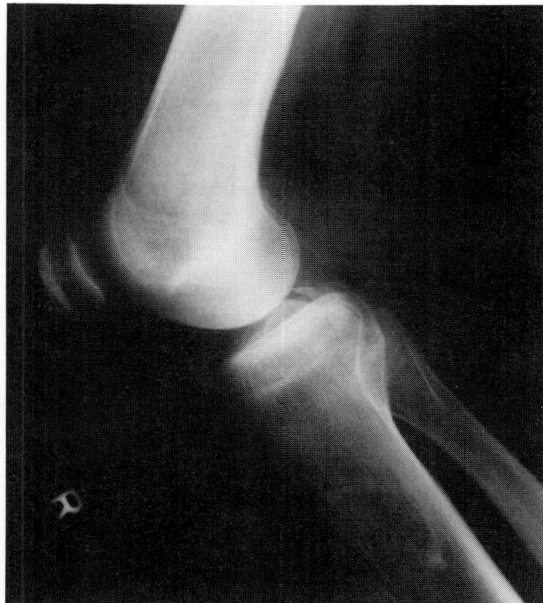

FIGURE 19–14. Occasionally, radiographs will reveal a bony PCL avulsion from the tibia.

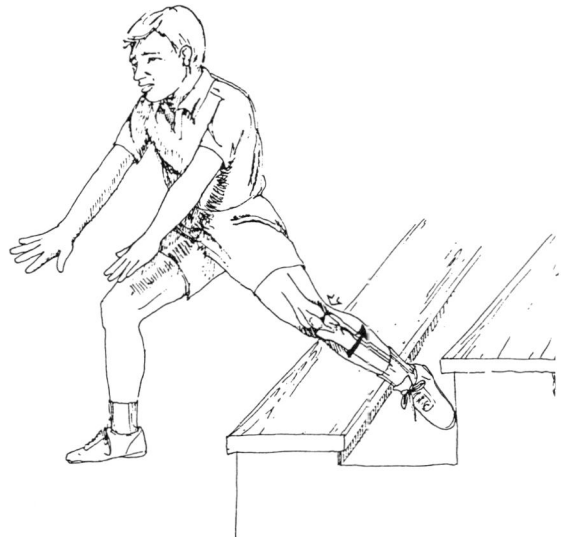

FIGURE 19–15. A valgus, external rotation stress to a fixed but unloaded limb will produce MCL injury in combination with PCL injury.

only an MCL injury. It was not until the patient's symptoms of pain and limited knee range of motion had abated that a more comprehensive exam could be performed and the PCL injury was identified. A heightened awareness of the possible association of these two injuries now causes us to assess carefully the status of the PCL in all MCL injuries, especially those with a suggestive mechanism of injury.

A number of other investigators have cited a frequent association of ACL tears with the PCL disruption (44 to 86 percent incidence). This combined injury may frequently be associated with collateral ligament damage.[22, 29, 33, 38]

In our experience, meniscal injuries are rarely associated with isolated PCL tears, although they have been reported as common in studies containing multiple ligament injuries.[38] Loos et al. found a 33 percent incidence of such lesions, with medial meniscal tears outnumbering lateral meniscal tears by a ratio of 7:1.[33] Cross and Powell discovered 86 knees with meniscal tears out of 116 PCL-deficient knees, with the medial side tears again outnumbering the lateral ones.[8] Because concomitant meniscus tears are unusual in the knee with a clinically isolated PCL tear, we do not recommend routine arthroscopy or magnetic resonance imaging (MRI) in these knees unless there is a specific reason to suspect a meniscus tear in a particular case.

The clinician must be aware of these complex injuries when managing the school-aged athlete with a suspected PCL tear. However, this information must be kept in perspective, as they truly are unusual injuries. Isolated PCL injuries occur far more commonly in the student's normal environment and athletic activities.

NATURAL HISTORY

The natural history of PCL injuries remains uncertain and controversial. There have been no truly prospective studies regarding this injury and its consequences. Most reported series to date have consisted of relatively few patients and have combined acute and chronic PCL injuries or have included a wide array of associated injuries. Recent studies by Parolie and Bergfeld[40] and Fowler and Messieh[12] have found that athletes with isolated PCL tears do well in the short term.

These findings have raised the question that sampling bias may have been responsible for the gloomy predictions of earlier reports, perhaps by including many patients with multiple ligament injuries or those who were referred for PCL reconstruction specifically because of disabling symptoms.

Clinicians are just beginning to elucidate the natural history of the PCL tear in athletes. As this information is accumulated, physicians will be better equipped to counsel student athletes who have sustained this injury and provide more authoritative management recommendations.

At present, several pieces of information are available regarding the progress of athletes with isolated PCL injuries.

1. Absolute static stability is not a requirement for acceptable function stability.[12] All 13 of Fowler and Messieh's patients returned to their former sports without limitations, although 10 of them rated only fair when assessed objectively. It should be noted that none of these patients had greater than a 1+ posterior drawer.

2. Patients having sustained PCL injuries as a result of athletic competition have historically functioned better and had fewer symptoms than those patients who acquired this ligament deficiency by other etiologies.[8]

3. Those patients with PCL-deficient knees who obtain and then maintain quadriceps strength equal to or greater than the contralateral extremity score higher functional ratings and consistently return to sports at the same preinjury level of competition.[8, 40] It is not clear whether the increased quadriceps strength is the cause of the better function or the result of it. However, Tegner et al. were able to demonstrate that patients with cruciate ligament deficiency were able to improve their knee rating scores markedly through completion of a quadriceps exercise regimen.[44] Cain and Schwab have also shown the importance of quadriceps function in the PCL-deficient knee by delineating the adaptive changes the extremity undergoes as a result of this ligament injury. Using electromyogram (EMG) techniques in one patient, they showed that the quadriceps muscle of the PCL-deficient knee contracts earlier in gait than that of the uninvolved extremity, thus providing a compensatory function of setting the knee in full extension prior to heel strike.[5] Tibone et al., however, found that the major EMG adaptation was early activation of

the triceps surae complex during stance phase and postulated that this was a compensatory mechanism to stabilize the foot-ankle tibia complex in the face of quadriceps weakness and posterior instability.[45]

4. There is disagreement whether or not the absolute amount of abnormal laxity in the PCL-deficient knee correlates with the patient's function. In Parolie and Bergfeld's study, the amount of knee laxity as measured by an arthrometer had no significant correlation with the patient's functional rating.[40] Cross and Powell concluded that "the posterior drawer sign was found to show poor correlation with the eventual functional result."[8] However, inspection of their data reveals a 6 percent incidence of fair and poor results in patients exhibiting a 1+ posterior drawer but 19 percent fair and poor results in patients with a 2+ posterior drawer and 43 percent fair and poor results in patients with a 3+ posterior drawer. It has also been our experience that patients with more dramatic posterior drawers are more likely to have symptoms and functional limitations.

5. The incidence of symptoms and degenerative changes tends to increase with time.[6, 8] Clinical, arthroscopic, and radiographic manifestations of articular arthritic changes, primarily of the medial knee compartment, have been demonstrated.[6] An early report by Kennedy and Grainger first notified clinicians of the possible progressive arthritic demise of the PCL-deficient knee.[28] Unfortunately, a high percentage of the knees in that series had sustained a more devastating injury of the knee suggestive of a dislocation. The subsequent arthritic degeneration of the knee cited by those investigators cannot be conclusively attributed to the PCL deficiency alone. Nevertheless, it appears that at least some patients will show progressive articular deterioration following PCL injury.

In our experience, straight posterior instability of the knee with a posterior drawer graded 2+ or less has not resulted in early disabling consequences. Athletes have been able to return to their former level of competition without a decline in their performance following rehabilitation of this knee injury. However, the long-term effect of this most common presentation of PCL deficiency in young athletes remains to be established. The definitive natural history of the knee with an isolated PCL deficiency will remain largely speculative until the results of present ongoing prospective studies of patients with acutely acquired PCL injuries are known. Until then, the clinician must continue to structure the treatment regimen for PCL-deficient knees based on the limited available information.

TREATMENT

The treatment of acute PCL injuries remains controversial, both because of the uncertainty about the natural history of such injuries and the recognition that no surgical procedure has been shown to provide consistently excellent results. It is not certain whether a less-than-anatomical result will prevent long-term articular deterioration. Within the past decade, clinicians have been advised to consider a diversity of management schemes. Hughston et al. recommended surgical treatment for PCL injuries when combined with injury to other knee ligaments.[18] Clancy et al. advised that acute PCL tears be repaired and augmented to prevent the potential medial compartment degeneration associated with this ligament's chronic deficiency.[6] Dandy and Bergfeld, however, recommended nonoperative treatment for isolated PCL tears in athletes.[9, 40]

Regardless of the subsequent management protocol selected, the school-aged individual sustaining a PCL injury must be counseled about the significance of the deficit. In the discussion, it should be emphasized that a choice of nonoperative treatment does not mean that the PCL is unimportant or that the knee will be normal without it. The uncertainty of the natural history of PCL deficiency must be explained so that the patient understands the clinician's inability to clearly predict the clinical course of this injury.

Risk factors that may potentially increase subsequent disability should be reviewed with the patient. Associated conditions that may increase the patient's risk of subsequent arthritis include (1) participation in strenuous sports such as football, basketball, and volleyball; (2) accentuated medial compartment stress (e.g., previous medial meniscus excision, genu varum); (3) weight in excess of ideal body weight; and (4) prior patellofemoral joint abnormality (e.g., chondromalacia patella).

While any one of these factors is not an absolute indication for surgical treatment, a combination of them may make the patient consider surgery more seriously. For example, the 18-year-old 250-pound basketball player with previous medial meniscectomy with 2+ posterior drawer who desires to continue competitive basketball may have a better long-term outcome with surgical reconstruction of the PCL than with a nonoperative program. The same 2+ posterior drawer in an 18-year-old equestrian with no prior knee problems or other stated risk factors may predictably do well with nonoperative management of the injured knee. In addition, patients with 3+ or greater posterior laxity or multiple ligament injuries are candidates for operative treatment.

The greatest problem confronting nonoperative management of the PCL-deficient knee is that there are no reliably predictable ways of identifying those patients who will deteriorate in the first few years following the PCL injury. Nonoperative treatment has been popular because of the satisfactory short-term results and the probability of returning athletes to the same level of competition. However, once the patient's knee becomes symptomatic, the "golden" period for reconstruction has been lost, with stabilization surgery then providing less satisfying results. On the other hand, because of the required lengthy postoperative rehabilitation, surgical reconstruction in the acute setting can force the school-aged athlete out of sports competition for a minimum of one, if not two, sports seasons. This may be psychologically and socially stressful to a high school athlete whose competitive career may already be short. Confronted with a long and difficult rehabilitation, the athlete may become resentful of his or her treatment experience. Clearly then, until a good comparative study contrasting surgical and nonsurgical management of the PCL-deficient knee with both short- and long-term results is performed, the clinician can only surmise what treatment will be best for each individual in the long term.

NONOPERATIVE TREATMENT

We recommend nonoperative management for most isolated PCL injuries. These patients will exhibit initially a posterior drawer of 2+ or less. Posterior tibial avulsion fractures associated with acute PCL injuries have previously been reported to be most amenable to surgical management with subsequent excellent results.[37, 47, 48, 49] However, despite the findings of Meyers,[37] we have found that these injuries can do well non-operatively and frequently have only a 1+ posterior drawer or less. It would seem that the inherent surgical risks associated with a posterior approach outweigh the proposed benefits of possibly eliminating the knee's minimal posterior tibial translation. We generally recommend, therefore, a nonoperative approach to this type of PCL injury as well.

The combined PCL-MCL knee injury also responds well to nonoperative treatment, once the MCL component of this injury has healed with less than 5 mm of increased valgus laxity. This knee is initially managed with supportive treatment as discussed below. A hinged brace is provided to protect the knee from valgus stress for a minimum of 6 weeks.

Rehabilitating the patient with an acute PCL injury initially involves minimizing the traumatic symptoms of pain, effusion, and decreased knee range of motion. Intermittent application of ice to the knee, antiinflammatory medication, immobilization if necessary, and the use of crutches are helpful for the first week following the injury. As comfort improves, the patient may progress to knee ROM exercises and extremity strengthening exercises with emphasis on quadriceps muscle tone.[8, 40, 44] We advocate closed kinetic exercises such as step-ups, one-quarter squats, and stair climbing in lieu of open kinetic exercises such as short arc quads and knee extension exercises, which exert increased forces across the patellofemoral joint. Completion of a running and agility program is a prerequisite to a return to competitive athletics. Most motivated athletes with isolated PCL injuries can return to the preinjury level of participation within 4 to 6 weeks of the date of injury. Extremity casting or other forms of rigid immobilization to allow "ligament healing" have not been practiced in our acute management of these injuries. The accelerated rehabilitation and lack of immobilization mentioned have resulted in no progression of the posterior drawer as judged by subsequent follow-up exams. The prognostic importance of obtaining and then maintaining lifelong quadriceps strength greater than or equal to the noninvolved extremity is emphasized.[5, 44] The athlete must understand that his or her commitment to the maintenance exercise program is no less important than a hypertensive patient faithfully taking medication or a diabetic patient complying with the recommended diet.

The decision as to whether or not the PCL-deficient knee should be braced is controversial owing to the small percentage of such knees that actually experience instability and the questionable capability of most braces to prevent posterior tibial translation. The properly designed functional knee brace that applies an anterior force on the leg, thereby diminishing posterior translation of the leg on the femur, has been beneficial for our patients in the initial rehabilitation phase (Fig. 19–16). Continuation of its use upon return to competitive athletics has been recommended, although compliance varies with the individual.

The school-aged athlete must realize that the PCL-deficient knee is a lifelong abnormality. Special care and attention for this extremity are encouraged, with yearly clinical follow-ups to ascertain whether the knee is symptomatic. The knee is reassessed by discussion of symptoms or functional changes, physical examination, strength evaluation, arthrometer measurements, and knee questionnaires. Annual knee radiographs and bone scans at 3- to 5-year intervals are utilized to look for signs of deterioration.

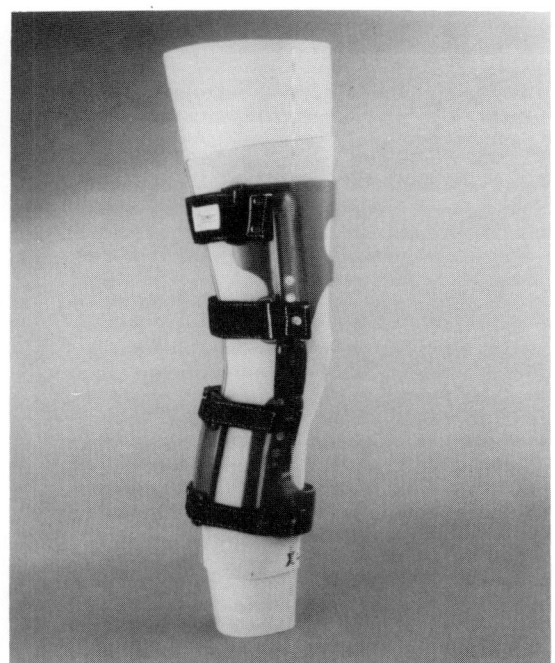

FIGURE 19–16. PCL brace with a rigid posterior calf pad and open anterior tibia.

These follow-up visits are good opportunities to modify the patient's activities and lifestyle when this is indicated by functional or symptomatic changes in the knee. The individual with the PCL-deficient knee should also understand that observing each patient's clinical course will provide valuable insight to improve the future management of PCL tears.

OPERATIVE MANAGEMENT

The current trend toward less frequent surgical management of PCL injuries[2] reflects the realization that no one procedure has provided consistently excellent results.[22, 23, 33] We do not know if a less-than-excellent result will prevent possible arthritic deterioration of the knee. Unfortunately, studies evaluating some of the recent surgical procedures for PCL replacement have reported objectively good results in only 33 to 65 percent of cases.[22, 23] Loos reported on a series of surgically managed PCL-deficient knees of which 62 percent required reoperation.[33] Clancy et al. published better surgical results, perhaps a consequence of refined patient selection and improved technique.[6]

We believe that acute surgery is indicated for the individual who desires to maintain an active life-style and who has a 3+ posterior drawer. Acute surgical treatment should also be considered for the knee with 2+ or greater posterior drawer and posterolateral laxity as manifested by reverse pivot shift or the dynamic pivot shift.[26, 41]

Relative surgical indications for the acute PCL injury would include those patients with 2+ or greater posterior drawer, significant prior patellofemoral symptoms, or medial compartment factors such as prior medical meniscectomy, medial osteochondritis dissecans, or marked varus alignment. The patient with an acute 2+ or greater posterior drawer and medial laxity who intends to continue competitive athletics such as football or basketball and who is above ideal body weight should also be considered for acute surgery.

It is our belief that a chronic PCL injury should have similar guidelines for surgical management. The symptomatic knee with 2+ or greater posterior laxity that is manually reducible on examination and is without advanced degenerative changes should be considered for PCL reconstruction if adequate attempts at rehabilitation as presented in the nonoperative management section fail to ameliorate the patient's knee symptoms. Again, the patient's activity level, knee alignment, body weight, and concomitant knee pathology would also affect the decision-making process.

Our insistence on a 2+ or greater posterior drawer before considering surgical treatment of acute or chronic PCL injury reflects the uncertainty that a knee with 1+ or less posterior drawer may be reliably improved with surgery. On the other hand, a knee with a 3+ posterior drawer may be markedly improved by PCL reconstruction if that laxity is reduced to 1+ or less and the dynamic posterior shift is eliminated.

TECHNIQUE

Surgical procedures espousing various tissues for augmenting or replacing the acutely or chronically deficient PCL have appeared in the literature. For the acutely torn PCL, surgical repair alone has been recommended.[22, 43] Replacing the PCL with the medial meniscus when the PCL was not amenable to repair has also been tried.[22] More recently, repair of the acutely torn ligament accompanied by augmentation has been advised. The augmenting tissues have included the gracilis and semitendinosus,[32] medial gastrocnemius,[7] and the bone-tendon-bone patellar tendon graft.[6]

The chronic PCL-deficient knee has also been surgically managed with various tissues of paraarticular etiology. Recent publications have recommended semitendinosus, with or without the gracilis,[28, 50] lateral meniscus,[44] medial gastrocnemius,[23, 25, 27] and the patellar tendon bone graft.[6]

Our current recommendation for acute or chronic PCL tears is intraarticular reconstruction using autogenous bone patellar tendon-bone graft with repair of the PCL if feasible. This has traditionally been done via an anteromedial "hockey stick" incision,[6] although arthroscopic or semiarthroscopic techniques are now advocated by some. An additional lateral incision is required for posterolateral repair with either technique. The utility of allograft tissue replacement of the PCL is also being explored enthusiastically at some centers, but only preliminary data are available at this time.

PCL reconstruction, especially in a young athlete, requires the strongest tissue available. We advocate the central patellar tendon (about 14 mm or up to 40 percent of the patellar tendon width) with attached bone at both ends because of its documented strength and proven reliability in ACL reconstructions. Studies by Grood et al.[16] and others have shown that the femoral attachment site is the most important factor in satisfactory ligament placement. The ideal location for the femoral attachment of the graft is toward the roof of the intercondylar notch, approximately 11 mm posterior from the junction of the trochlear groove with the notch. PCL drill guides and ligament tensiometers are available and are especially useful for the surgeon who performs this procedure infrequently or with arthroscopic techniques.

Knee dislocations are very rare in sports but may occur to the athlete during vehicular or other violent trauma. Nonoperative treatment of knee dislocation may yield satisfactory results in the older and more sedentary individual. Unless there are other contraindications to extensive surgery such as vascular compromise, we believe that the school-aged athlete who sustains a knee dislocation should undergo PCL reconstruction with patellar tendon graft and repair of the peripheral knee ligaments and capsular structures. While simultaneous surgical repair of both cruciate ligaments can achieve excellent static stability, it can also result in fixation of the tibia in a position of posterior subluxation if improperly done. This aberrant alignment of the tibia with the femur results in the knee having an abnormal center of rotation. The same outcome occurs if the ACL is reconstructed and the PCL is only repaired—the tibia is pulled back against the repaired PCL, resulting in a posteriorly fixed tibia. Reconstruction of both cruciates is too much surgery in the acute knee injury and has a high probability of postoperative stiffness. Reconstructing the PCL while leaving the ACL alone following a knee dislocation has provided most satisfactory results to date in our series of 20 knee dislocations sustained during athletic participation. These patients, some of whom have been followed for more than 5 years, have not presented in follow-up with symptomatic ACL instability postoperatively, yet have attained excellent knee range of motion, with usually only a trace to 1+ posterior drawer. However, despite these results, very few individuals recover from this injury to the point where they can return to stressful competitive sports. In most of these potentially devastating injuries, the appropriate goal is a knee that will allow routine daily activities without pain rather than a return to competitive athletics.

REHABILITATION

Rehabilitation following a PCL reconstruction should progress in a graduated fashion. Knee range of motion and quadriceps strength are emphasized initially, followed by a functional recovery program. Initially, the knee is immobilized in full extension to prevent drop-back of the tibia (Fig. 19–17). Weight bearing to tolerance with the immobilizer supporting the knee in full extension is begun shortly after surgery. This immobilizer is used for the first 2 to 3 weeks following the reconstruction. Thereafter, a hinged knee brace allowing motion from 0 to 60 degrees is substituted. This brace should be removed only for washing and controlled exercises for the next 4 to 6 weeks. By the sixth postoperative week, a PCL functional knee brace is provided that should be removed only for washing and exercises for the following 2 to 3 months. Use of the functional knee brace is recommended for all athletic activities for a minimum of 1 year after PCL reconstruction.

Active knee flexion should be obtained slowly, with maximum flexion of about 60 degrees for the first 4 weeks. Ninety degrees of knee flexion should be obtained by the sixth to eighth postoperative week. Stationary bicycle exercising is encouraged when that goal is obtained.

In contrast to knee flexion, knee extension must be equal to the opposite extremity within the first week following surgery. Full extension capabilities must be maintained throughout the rehabilitation course but should be particularly monitored during the first 4 postoperative weeks to make sure that a flexion contracture is not developing. Full knee extension in the first few postoperative weeks is encouraged by supporting the heel when the patient is lying supine and by lying prone with the foot overhanging the table.

Isometric quadriceps exercises and straight leg raising are emphasized during the first few weeks after surgery. Progressive muscle strengthening with emphasis on quadriceps strength is started after sets of straight leg raises are mastered. The inclusion of closed kinetic exercises (one-quarter squats, step-ups, stair climbing, etc.) should be a major part of the exercise protocol by the sixth postoperative week or sooner. Isokinetic quadriceps strength is periodically evaluated during follow-up examinations, the frequency depending on the patient's clinical progression as well as motivation and timetable for return to sports. The involved extremity should have quadriceps strength of 80 to 90 percent of the uninvolved extremity prior to beginning a functional program of running, jumping, and agility drills. The time at which the athlete can return to competitive sports is largely a function of the athlete's motivation and clinical course. Attaining sufficient quadriceps strength and satisfactorily completing the functional program can be accomplished as early as 4 to 5 months following the reconstruction. However, light recreational activities such as shooting baskets and throwing and catching a football can begin earlier when the patient feels comfortable doing so in the functional knee brace.

CONCLUSION

This chapter has emphasized the importance of recognizing the mechanism of injury and physical examination skills necessary to make the diagnosis of PCL injury. A recurrent theme in this chapter has been that PCL tear in the school-aged athlete is usually an isolated injury. The natural history of the PCL-deficient knee remains an enigma, but as this becomes clarified, management will become less controversial. Until then, clinicians must cautiously advise young patients and their parents about the prognosis and risks of the PCL-deficient knee. At this time, the ma-

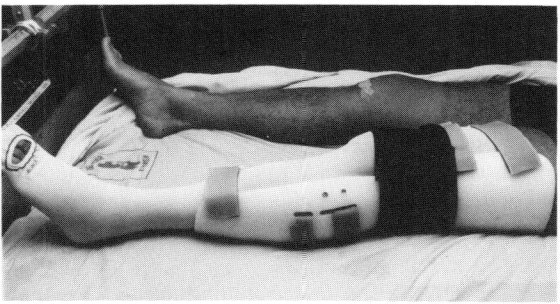

FIGURE 19–17. The postoperative PCL brace holds the knee in full extension to prevent drop-back of the tibia.

jority of sports-related PCL injuries can be managed nonoperatively, with return to the preinjury level of athletic participation upon completion of a directed rehabilitation program.

References

1. Baker C. L., Norwood L. A., Hughston J. C.: Acute combined posterior cruciate and posterolatral instability of the knee. Am J Sports Med 12:204–208, 1984.
2. Barton T. M., Torg J. S., Das M.: Posterior cruciate ligament insufficiency. A review of the literature. Sports Med 1:419–430, 1984.
3. Bianchi M.: Acute tears of the posterior cruciate ligament: Clinical study and results of operative treatment in twenty-seven cases. Am J Sports Med 11:308–314, 1983.
4. Butler D. L., Noyes F. R., and Grood E. S.: Ligamentous restraints to anterior-posterior drawer in the human knee. A biomechanical study. J Bone Joint Surg 62A:359, 1980.
5. Cain T. E., Schwab G. A.: Performance of an athlete with straight posterior knee instability. Am J Sports Med 9:203–208, 1981.
6. Clancy W. G. Jr., Shelbourne K. D., Zoellner G. B., et al: Treatment of knee joint instability secondary to ruptures of the posterior cruciate ligament. J Bone Joint Surg 65A:310–322, 1983.
7. Clendenin M. B., DeLee J. C., Heckman J. D.: Interstitial tears of the posterior cruciate ligament of the knee. Orthopaedics 3:765–772, 1980.
8. Cross M. J., Powell J. F.: Long term follow up of a posterior cruciate ligament rupture: a study of 116 cases. Am J Sports Med 12:292–297, 1984.
9. Dandy D. J., Pusey R. J.: The long term results of unrepaired tears of the posterior cruciate ligament. J Bone Joint Surg 64B:92–94, 1982.
10. DeHaven K. E.: Diagnosis of acute knee injuries with hemarthrosis. Am J Sports Med 9:107–113, 1981.
11. Fleming R. E. Jr., Blatz D. J., McCarroll J. R.: Posterior problems in the knee. Am J Sports Med 9(2):107–113, 1981.
12. Fowler P. J., Messieh S. S.: Isolated posterior cruciate ligament injuries in athletes. Am J Sports Med 15:553–557, 1987.
13. Fukubayashi T., Torzilli P. A., Sherman M. E., et al: An in vitro biomechanical evaluation of anteroposterior motion of the knee. J Bone Joint Surg 64A:258, 1982.
14. Godfrey J. D.: Ligamentous injuries of the knee. Curr Pract Orthop Surg 5:56, 1973.
15. Gollehon D. L., Torzilli P. S., Warren R. F.: The role of the posterolateral and the cruciate ligaments in the stability of the human knee. J Bone Joint Surg 69A:233–242, 1987.
16. Grood E. S., Hefzy M. S., Lindenfield R. N.: Factors affecting the region of most isometric femoral attachments. Part I. The posterior cruciate ligament. Am J Sports Med 17:197–207, 1989.
17. Heller L., Langman J.: The menisco-femoral ligaments of the knee. J Bone Joint Surg 46B:307–313, 1964.
18. Hughston J. C.: The posterior cruciate ligament in knee joint stability. J Bone Joint Surg 51A:1045–1046, 1969.
19. Hughston J. C.: The absent posterior drawer test in some acute posterior cruciate ligament tears of the knee. Am J Sports Med 16:39–43, 1988.
20. Hughston J. C., Andrews J. R., Cross M. J., et al: Classification of knee ligament instabilities. Part I. The medial compartment and cruciate ligaments. J Bone Joint Surg 58A:159–172, 1976.
21. Hughston J. C., Andrews J. R., Cross M. J., et al: Classification of knee instabilities. Part II. The lateral compartment. J Bone Joint Surg 58A:173–179, 1976.
22. Hughston J. C., Bowden J. A., Andrews J. R., et al: Acute tears of the posterior cruciate ligament. J Bone Joint Surg 62A:438–450, 1980.
23. Hughston J. C., Degenhardt T. C.: Reconstruction of the posterior cruciate ligament. Clin Orthop 164:59–77, 1982.
24. Hughston J. C., Norwood L. A.: The posterolateral drawer test and external rotation recurvatum test for the posterolateral rotatory instability of the knee. Clin Orthop 147:82–87, 1980.
25. Insall J. N., Hood R. W.: Bone block transfer of the medial head of the gastrocnemius for posterior cruciate insufficiency. J Bone Joint Surg 64A:691–699, 1982.
26. Jakob R. P., Hassler H., Staeubli H. U.: Observations on rotary instability of the lateral compartment of the knee. Acta Orthop Scand (Suppl) 191:1–32, 1981.
27. Kennedy J. C., Galpin R. D.: The use of the medial head of the gastrocnemius muscle in the posterior cruciate deficient knee. Indication-technique-results. Am J Sports Med 10:63–74, 1982.
28. Kennedy J. C., Grainger R. W.: The posterior cruciate ligament. J Trauma 7:367–377, 1967.
29. Kennedy J. C., Roth J. H., Walker D. M.: Posterior cruciate ligament injuries. Orthop Dig, August-September:19–32, 1972.
30. Last R. J.: Some anatomical details of the knee joint. J Bone Joint Surg 30B:683–688, 1948.
31. Lee H. G.: Avulsion fracture of the tibial attachments of the crucial ligaments. Treatment by operative reduction. J Bone Joint Surg 19:460–468, 1937.
32. Lipscomb A. B., Johnston R. K., Snyder R. B.: The technique of cruciate ligament injuries. Am J Sports Med 9:77–85, 1981.
33. Loos W. C., Fox J. M., Blazina M. E., et al: Acute posterior cruciate ligament injuries. Am J Sports Med 9:86–92, 1981.
34. Lysholm J., Gillquist J.: Arthroscopic examination of the posterior cruciate ligament. J Bone Joint Surg 63A:363–366, 1981.
35. McCarroll J. R., Ritter M. A., Schrader J., et al: The isolated posterior cruciate ligament. Phys Sportsmed 11:146–151, 1983.
36. McMaster W. C.: Isolated posterior cruciate ligament injury: literature review and case reports. J Trauma 15:1025–1029, 1975.
37. Meyers M. H.: Isolated avulsion of the tibial attachment of the posterior cruciate ligament of the knee. J Bone Joint Surg 57A:669–672, 1975.
38. Moore H. A., Larson R. L.: Posterior cruciate ligament injuries. Results of early surgical repair. Am J Sports Med 8:68–78, 1980.
39. O'Donoghue D. H.: Surgical treatment of fresh inju-

ries to the major ligaments of the knee. J Bone Joint Surg 32A:721–738, 1950.
40. Parolie J. M., Bergfeld J. A.: Long term results of nonoperative treatment of isolated posterior cruciate ligament injuries in the athlete. Am J Sports Med 14:35–38, 1986.
41. Shelbourne K. D., Benedict F.: Dynamic posterior shift test. An adjuvant in evaluation of posterior tibial subluxation. Am J Sports Med 17:275–277, 1989.
42. Shelbourne K. D., Mesko J. W.: Combined posterior cruciate–medial collateral ligament rupture: mechanism of injury. J Knee Surg 3(1):41–44, 1990.
43. Strand T., Molster A. O., Engesaeter L. B., et al: Primary repair in posterior cruciate ligament injuries. Acta Orthop Scand 55:545–547, 1984.
44. Tegner Y., Lysholm J., Gillquist J., et al: Two year follow up of conservative treatment of knee ligament injuries. Acta Orthop Scand 55:176–180, 1984.
45. Tibone J. E., Antich M. S., Perry J., Moynes D.: Functional analysis of untreated and reconstructed posterior cruciate ligament injuries. Am J Sports Med 16:217–223, 1988.
46. Tillberg B.: The late repair of torn cruciate ligaments using menisci. J Bone Joint Surg 59B:15–19, 1977.
47. Torisu T.: Isolated avulsion fracture of the tibial attachment of the posterior cruciate ligament. J Bone Joint Surg 59A:68–72, 1977.
48. Torisu T.: Avulsion fracture of the tibial attachment of the posterior cruciate ligament. Indication and results of delayed repair. Clin Orthop 143:107–114, 1979.
49. Trickey E. L.: Rupture of the posterior cruciate ligament of the knee. J Bone Joint Surg 50B:334–341, 1968.
50. Trickey E. L.: Injuries to the posterior cruciate ligament. Diagnosis and treatment of early injuries and reconstruction of late instability. Clin Orthop 147:76–81, 1980.

PATELLAR INSTABILITY AND PAIN

LONNIE E. PAULOS
PATRICIA A. KOLOWICH

Disorders of the patellofemoral joint, taken as a group, are the most common knee complaints among young athletes. Recent trends have encouraged youths to become more involved in intense athletics at an early age. In addition, many are choosing one particular sport and train for that activity year-round. The knees, and specifically the patellae, can be the object of significant impact force during these intense training sessions. Acute injury to the patella, the development of a chronic pain syndrome, or an instability pattern could alter or disrupt a training schedule or, in some cases, force an individual to give up a sport. A specifically designed examination should provide a physician with a specific diagnosis. This diagnosis will allow an individualized treatment plan to be determined that will facilitate the return of an athlete to his or her sport.

BIOMECHANICS OF THE PATELLOFEMORAL JOINT

A clear understanding of the biomechanical function of the patellofemoral joint forms the basis of a solid rehabilitation program that will strengthen the quadriceps muscle while not aggravating patellar symptoms. The articular cartilage on the median crest of the patella is the thickest of any joint in the body. This emphasizes its importance in load transmission across the patellofemoral joint.[28] Studies have documented the contact patterns of the patellofemoral joint from extension through flexion.[14] The patella does not contact the articular surface of the trochlea until 20 to 30 degrees of knee flexion. More knee flexion must occur before contact in patella alta. Patellofemoral contact is continuous from the medial to the lateral facet and begins distally on the patella at approximately 20 degrees of knee flexion and gradually progresses to the proximal pole of the patella by 90 degrees of flexion. Flexion past 90 degrees induces contact with the odd facet of the patella. As the contact zone moves proximal on the patella, the contact area increases.[20] Biomechanical studies and mathematical models[14] have shown that when the leg is in the weight-bearing position, the force across the patellofemoral joint increases as flexion increases.[20] However, increased contact area helps to distribute this force to maintain a joint force the articular surface can withstand. In addition to an increase in patellar contact area, the quadriceps tendon also assumes a load-bearing relationship after 90 degrees of knee flexion to help dissipate these increased forces. However, when the knee is loaded by applying resistance to the ankle or tibia as in most knee extension exercises, the necessary quadriceps force actually decreases as knee flexion angle increases. This causes the patellofemoral pressure to follow a parabolic curve, with peak pressure occurring at 36 degrees of knee flexion[46] (Fig. 20–1).

PATELLAR INSTABILITY AND PAIN

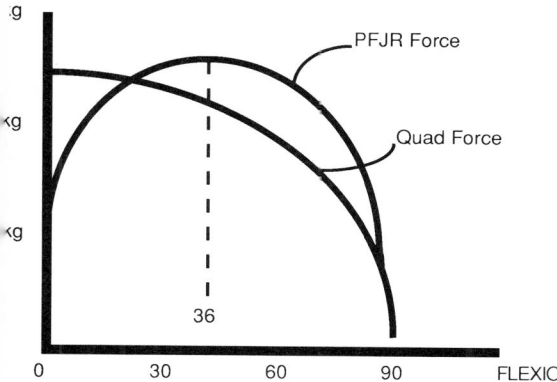

FIGURE 20–1. Because of the patellofemoral contact area changes with flexion, peak patellofemoral joint reaction force during a knee extension exercise actually occurs at about 36 degrees of flexion. (From Reilly, D. T., Martens, M.: Experimental analysis of the quadriceps muscle force and patello-femoral joint reaction forces for various activities. Acta Orthop. Scand. 43, p. 126, 1972.)

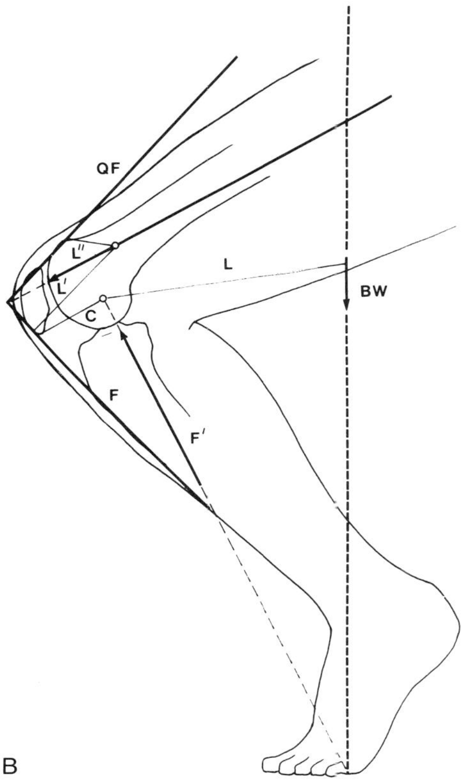

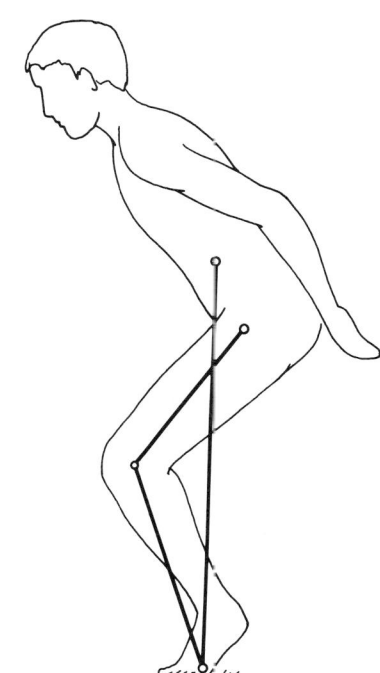

FIGURE 20–2. (A) During a forward knee bend (squat), the center of gravity moves posterior to the center of knee joint rotation. (B) The forces generated in the knee by the quad (QF) resist the moment created by body weight. (C) This results in a high patellofemoral contact force (*Resultant Force*) that increases as the depth of the squat increases. These results are in contrast to a seated knee extension exercise (Fig. 20–1).

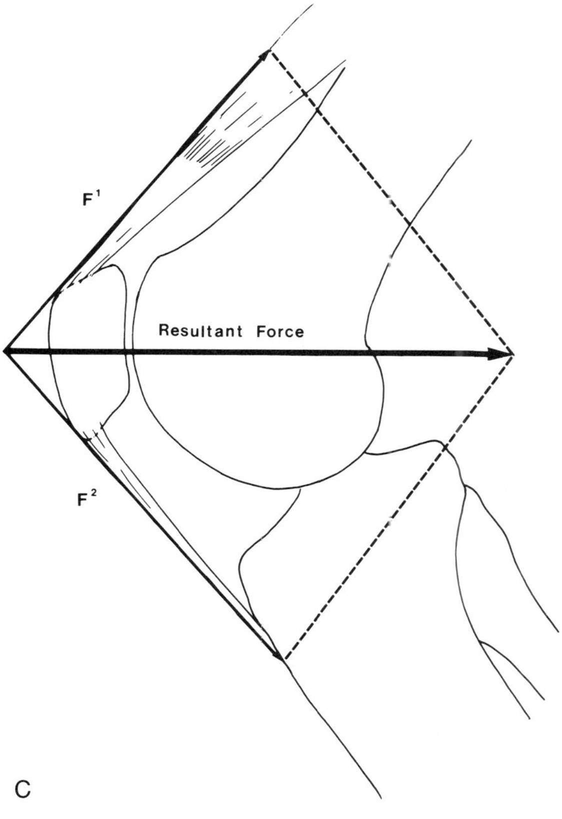

Maquet[36] has shown that forces transmitted across the patellofemoral joint at the beginning of the single stance support phase of gait reach three times body weight. These forces rapidly decrease as support of body weight is shared with the opposite limb. Other studies have shown that the patellofemoral joint reaction force reaches 7.0 times body weight with activities such as jogging and squatting.[9, 42]

A static representation of the patellofemoral joint reaction force reveals that as knee flexion increases, more force must be generated in the quadriceps muscle to maintain that position. The body's center of gravity moves more posterior to the center of the patellofemoral joint, increasing the moment arm, thus increasing the force required to maintain equilibrium (Fig. 20–2). Kaufer[29] emphasized the importance of the patella as a fulcrum by documenting that after patellectomy a 30 percent increase in quadriceps force is required to extend the leg fully.

CLASSIFICATION

The presenting symptoms of patellar disorders are usually pain or instability. *Patellar instability* may range from subtle subluxation to frank dislocation. Some cases of instability are clearly induced by trauma, whereas others are nearly atraumatic and related to dysplasia of the extensor mechanism. Full-blown patellar dislocation is usually easy to diagnose, but in milder cases of patellar hypermobility the athlete may complain of pain without realizing that instability is present. Primary episodes of patellar instability may be isolated or may lead to the repeated episodes characteristic of recurrent dislocation or subluxation.

Patellar pain syndromes can create mild annoyance or severe disability. Some cases of chronic pain are clearly related to chondral damage caused by direct trauma to the patella; many more are insidious in onset and are often thought to be induced by overuse or subtle malalignment. A few cases of pain are caused by clearly defined boney abnormalities such as *osteochondritis dissecans* or *bipartite patella*. *Osgood-Schlatter disease, Sinding-Larsen-Johannsen syndrome* and *patellar tendinitis* are causes of anterior knee pain related to the patellar tendon. They are discussed in Chapter 21.

Direct trauma to the knee is common and may produce a *chondral fracture*, which causes subsequent chronic pain and crepitus. *Prepatellar bursitis* and *patellar fracture* are other possible consequences of a direct blow to the kneecap.

PATELLAR INSTABILITY

Acute patellar dislocation usually presents as a distinct episode, either resulting from direct contact with an object or another player or from a cutting or pivoting noncontact maneuver. In most cases, the patient realizes that the patella has dislocated and may even reduce it himself or herself. Sometimes the patient may state that the "knee went out" without being aware that the patella was involved specifically. In these cases, it is important to distinguish patellar dislocation from ligament rupture by a careful physical examination.

Subluxations are generally less dramatic clinical episodes than dislocations and are accompanied by less swelling. The athlete may experience a sudden episode of pain or feel the knee unpredictably collapses when the patella subluxes as the knee goes into flexion. Often the patient will state that the knee feels "weak" or unreliable without realizing that the patella is specifically involved.

Knees that are subject to recurrent patellar dislocations or subluxations will have these episodes on a recurring basis at intervals that may vary from years to days. If the knee remains painful after the patient recovers from the acute episode, it usually signifies that there has been some significant damage to the articular surface of the patella. The nature of this pain is described later under "Patella Pain Syndromes."

PHYSICAL EXAMINATION

The physical examination (Table 20–1) is also extremely important in helping to isolate a diagnosis and propose a correct treatment program.[44] The physical examination should be performed with full visibility of the lower extremities with the patient preferably in shorts without shoes or socks. Weight-bearing alignment in the standing position should be determined with the feet pointing forward (Fig. 20–3). Excessive varus or valgus alignment can alter the distal pull on the patella. Excessive femoral anteversion or ex-

TABLE 20–1. Physical Examination of the Patellofemoral Joint

Standing
Weight-bearing alignment
Rotational alignment (femur, tibia)
Patellar position (? "squinting")
Foot alignment (? pronation)
Heel alignment (? valgus)

Sitting
Patellar position (alta, baja)
90-degrees tubercle-sulcus angle
Tenderness (inferior patella, tubercle)
Effusion
Crepitus

Supine
Passive patellar tilt
Lateral/medial patellar glides
Patellar facet tenderness
Apprehension
Active quadriceps vector
Effusion
Flexibility (hamstrings, iliotibial band)

Prone
Flexibility (Quadriceps)
Foot alignment

ternal tibial torsion can give the appearance of "squinting patella." Foot position is extremely important and best evaluated in the frontal standing position. Excessive foot pronation can lead to medial knee strain as well as patellar pain problems. Also, varus, valgus, or neutral heel alignment is evaluated from posterior in the standing position.

The position of the patella can be evaluated in the sitting position with the knees flexed 90 degrees over the edge of the examination table, with respect to patella alta (high patella), patella baja (low patella), and tubercle-sulcus angle. In a normal person, the patellae will face forward when the knees are flexed 90 degrees. If patella alta is present, the patellae will face obliquely toward the ceiling. The 90 degree tubercle-sulcus angle is also assessed while examining the seated patient from the front while the knees are flexed 90 degrees (Fig. 20–4). An imaginary horizontal line is drawn through the medial and lateral epicondyles, and a perpendicular to this line is drawn through the center of the patella. The angle between this vertical line and a line drawn from the center of the patella to the center of the tibial tubercle is the 90-degree sulcus angle. Normal is less than 8 degrees in females and 5 degrees in males. We feel that this is a more functional measurement than the traditional Q angle, which is measured with the knee in full extension, because the patella is engaged in the femoral trochlear groove when the measurement is done in flexion. Palpate the inferior pole of the patella and the tibial tubercle for tenderness indicative of Sinding-Larsen-Johannsen syndrome or Osgood-Schlatter disease. Palpation for an effusion can also be done in this position. Active flexion and extension with a hand over the anterior knee will allow grad-

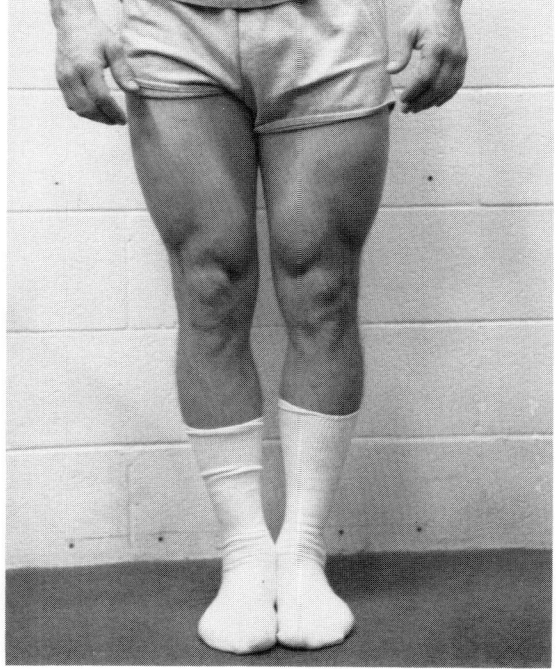

FIGURE 20–3. Weight-bearing alignment is assessed in the standing position with the feet pointing forward.

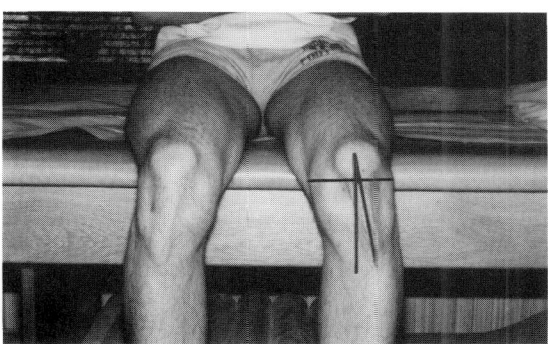

FIGURE 20–4. The 90-degree tubercle-sulcus angle is assessed in the seated position (see text).

ing of the crepitus that is present. (Grade 0 = no crepitus; I = minimal palpable crepitus; II = moderate palpable crepitus; III = constant palpable crepitus; and IV = audible crepitus.) Having the patient climb onto a small step stool while your hand is on the patella will bring out subtle degrees of crepitus.

The supine examination of the patella is also important. The patient must be completely relaxed to perform an adequate examination. The passive patellar tilt (Fig. 20–5) is determined with the examiner standing at the foot of the exam table. The index finger is placed on the lateral edge of the patella and the thumb on the medial edge. Attempt to elevate or tilt the lateral patellar facet away from the lateral femoral condyle. Care must be taken not to sublux the patella laterally when performing this test, as this may alter the final result. The test is recorded as a positive tilt, a negative tilt, or a neutral tilt in reference to a line parallel to the transcondylar axis. When the lateral edge of the patella remains below this line, the tilt is negative; if above the line, positive; and parallel to the line, neutral. Normally, males have a tilt of approximately +5 degrees and females +10 degrees. Also, younger individuals tend to have more patellar tilt than older ones.

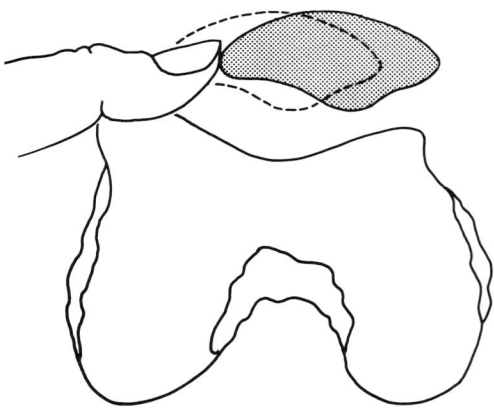

FIGURE 20–6. The passive medial and lateral patellar glides are measured at 30 degrees of flexion.

The next step in the examination is to measure the medial and lateral patellar glides (Fig. 20–6). The knee should be flexed approximately 30 degrees and relaxed by resting it on a small pillow or rolled towel. The patella is divided into imaginary longitudinal quadrants, and the glide is recorded as the number of quadrants displaced while performing the test. The patella is first pushed in a medial direction to determine the medial patellar glide, an indication of the competence of the lateral restraint. A tight lateral restraint will have a medial glide of one quadrant. The patella is then displaced in a lateral direction to determine the lateral patellar glide, an indication of the competence of the medial restraint. A lateral glide of one quadrant suggests a very competent medial restraint, whereas a lateral glide of three or four quadrants suggests an incompetent medial restraint. While performing the lateral glide test, note the presence or absence of patient apprehension, which may indicate patellar instability. The examiner may also perform an "apprehension test" by gliding the patella laterally and gently beginning to flex the knee. This will simulate a subluxation episode and bring out a negative response from the patient with patellar instability.

Palpate the articular surface of the medial and lateral facet for tenderness or evidence of inflammation. Determine the direction of the quadriceps pull or active quadriceps vector (Fig. 20–7) by having the patient contract the quadriceps muscles with the knee extended and observing the direction of pull on the patella. Normally, the patella should move

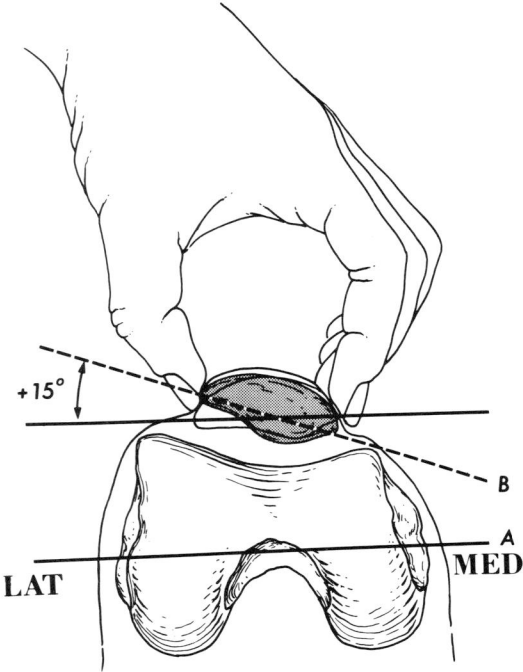

FIGURE 20–5. The passive patellar tilt is recorded in relation to a line parallel to the transcondylar axis (A).

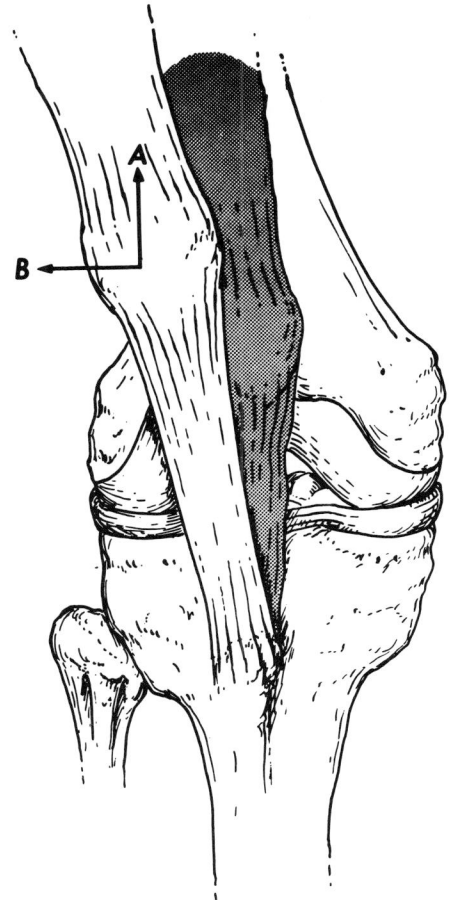

FIGURE 20–7. When the quadriceps is contracted, the patella should move straight superior or lateral and superior in a 1:1 ratio.

straight superior or lateral to superior in a 1:1 ratio. An abnormal lateral pull will move more lateral than superior—that is, subluxation in extension.

The most sensitive way to examine the knee for an effusion is to express the fluid into the suprapatellar pouch and then firmly compress the suprapatellar pouch and lateral gutter and watch medially for a "medial bulge sign" or evidence of fluid being forced into the medial gutter. Also, observe evidence of quadriceps atrophy or, more important, vastus medialis obliquus atrophy.

It is very important to determine the flexibility of maturing athletes. Individuals with patellar instability initiated by little or no trauma frequently have stigmata of generalized ligamentous laxity. Conversely, patients with patellofemoral pain syndromes may appear "tight jointed." As adolescents enter their rapid growth phase, bone growth can exceed muscle flexibility. Increases in strength also accompany the growth spurt. These strength increases may not be symmetrical for agonist/antagonist muscle groups, and this strength imbalance as well as lack of flexibility may predispose an athlete to injury.[41, 43] Quadriceps tightness limits knee flexion and can put an abnormal force across the patellofemoral joint. Tight hamstrings can limit knee extension. This can increase patella contact with the femur and thus affect the forces transmitted across the patellofemoral joint. An extremely tight gastrocnemius-soleus complex can also limit knee extension. Hamstring tightness is easily assessed in the supine position by performing a passive straight leg raise and determining the angle of hip flexion at which complete knee extension can no longer be maintained. Quadriceps flexibility is evaluated in the prone position. The thigh and anterior iliac crest should remain firmly flat on the exam table, and as the knee is flexed, the heel should reach the buttock.

The strong iliotibial band can act as a lateral tether and lead to overuse syndromes involving the greater trochanter and lateral femoral epicondyle. Many knees go through a "valgus phase" where the lateral structures are very tight.[41] This is frequently seen in ballet dancers that concentrate on abduction and external rotation exercises. Lateral knee pain can develop as a result of tightness in the lateral parapatellar structures.

The maturation phase of growth will produce a divergence between male and female athletes. While prepubescent male and female athletes have similar body fat composition, muscle mass, and skeletal structure, this can change dramatically for females at puberty. Body fat increases and is redistributed; the pelvis widens, resulting in hip varus and knee valgus; and strength is usually no longer equal to males.[22] Anatomical malalignment can predispose adolescent and maturing athletes to overuse problems. Leg length discrepancy, altered hip rotation such as excess femoral anteversion, or excessive genu varum or valgum can affect an athlete's performance during repetitive training.[43] It is essential in these young athletes that physical abnormalities are recognized and appropriately addressed and that early instructions in both proper technique and conditioning are given.

RADIOGRAPHIC EVALUATION

Radiographic evaluation of the patellofemoral joint always should include an anteroposterior (AP) or posteroanterior (PA) view, a lateral non–weight-bearing view with the knee flexed 45 degrees, and a skyline view of both patellae.[6] The AP or PA view will provide information pertinent to the presence of a bipartite patella (Fig. 20–8) and evaluation of the medial and lateral tibiofemoral compartments. The lateral view, as described by Insall and Salvati,[26] can be used to evaluate the presence of patella alta or baja (Fig. 20–9). According to Insall and Salvati, the ratio of the length of the patella (LP) to the length of the patellar tendon (LT) should be between 0.8 and 1.2. If the ratio is less than 0.8, it is indicative of patella alta, and if greater than 1.2, patella baja. Tangential or axial radiographs of the patellofemoral joint in various degrees of knee flexion have been described by several authors.[6] The most commonly used view is the Merchant view taken with the knees flexed 30 degrees.[39] Flexion less than 20 degrees will not engage the pa-

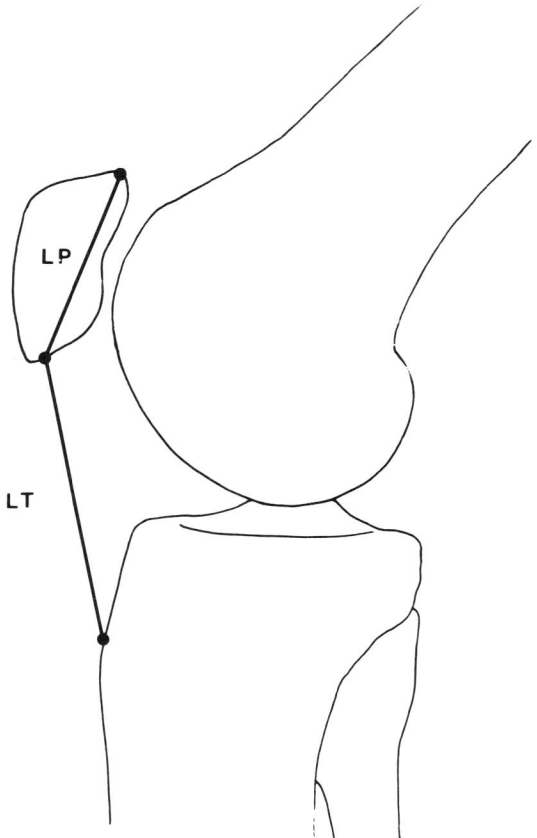

FIGURE 20–9. According to Insall, the ratio of **LP** to **LT** on a lateral radiograph with the knee flexed at least 30 degree to tense the patellar tendon should be between 0.8 and 1.2.

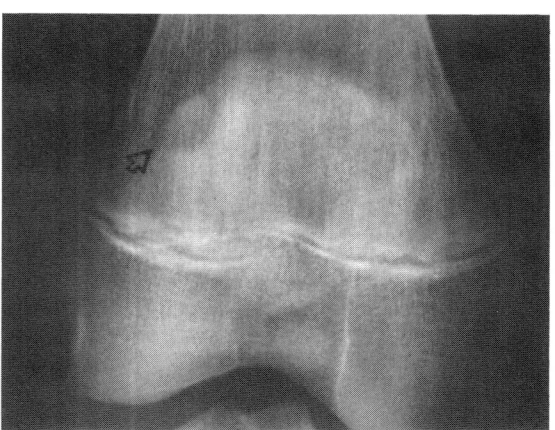

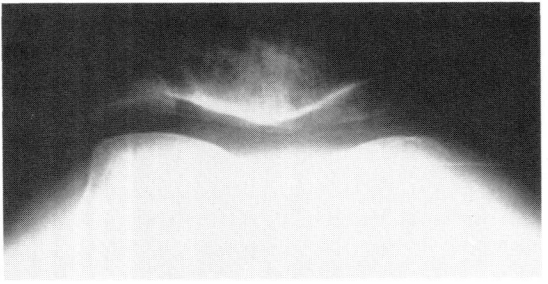

FIGURE 20–8. AP or skyline views may reveal a bipartite patella, most commonly in the supralateral quadrant.

tella in the trochlea, and with flexion greater than 45 degrees, most patellae will be well centered in the trochlear groove. For reproducible results, a wooden or plastic wedge should be used to position the knees for all tangential radiographs. The roentgenogram should expose both knees for comparison so that the knees are flexed the same amount on every set of radiographs. There have been several measurements described utilizing these studies. Although we do not believe treatment should be based solely on radiographic findings, they may be a useful adjunct in diagnosis.[1] The trochlear sulcus angle can be measured to identify a congenitally shallow sulcus.[6] Merchant et al.[39] described the patellofemoral congruence angle to document lateral patellar subluxation. A laterally opening angle is indicative of patellar subluxation. Knees with recurrent dislocation were found by Merchant to have an

PATELLAR INSTABILITY AND PAIN 339

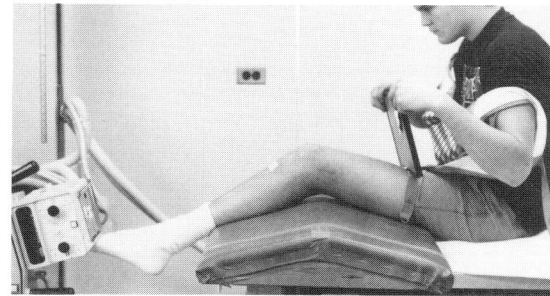

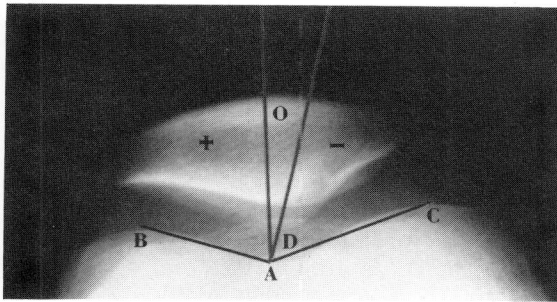

FIGURE 20–10. (A) For consistent results, skyline views should be taken in a standard position. (B) The Merchant congruence angle *DAO* is the angle between the line *AO*, which bisects the sulcus angle *BAC*, and the line *AD*, which connects the lowest point (A) of the intercondylar sulcus to the lowest point on the articular ridge of the patella. (D) Merchant's average normal congruence angle was −6 degrees, with a standard deviation of 11 degrees.

average congruence angle of +23 degrees, although a normal individual will occasionally fall into this range. A normal congruence angle should be −6 degrees (standard deviation [SD] 11 degrees) (Fig. 20–10). Laurin et al.[34] described the lateral patellofemoral angle to quantify lateral patellar tilt. The Laurin measurements require a skyline view taken with the knee in only 20 degree of flexion. Schutzer et al.[48] have used computerized tomography (CT) scans at varying angles of knee flexion to define patellofemoral contact radiographically. This has provided good reference information, but cost and scheduling problems usually prohibit this study from being used routinely on outpatients.

INITIAL EVALUATION AND TREATMENT OF ACUTE PATELLAR DISLOCATION AND SUBLUXATION

A *patellar dislocation* is defined as complete loss of contact between the patellar and trochlear articular surfaces. Spontaneous reduction may occur on occasion, but usually the patella is reduced by lateral manual pressure on the patella, accompanied by knee extension (Fig. 20–11). Patellar subluxation occurs when the patella is partially forced out

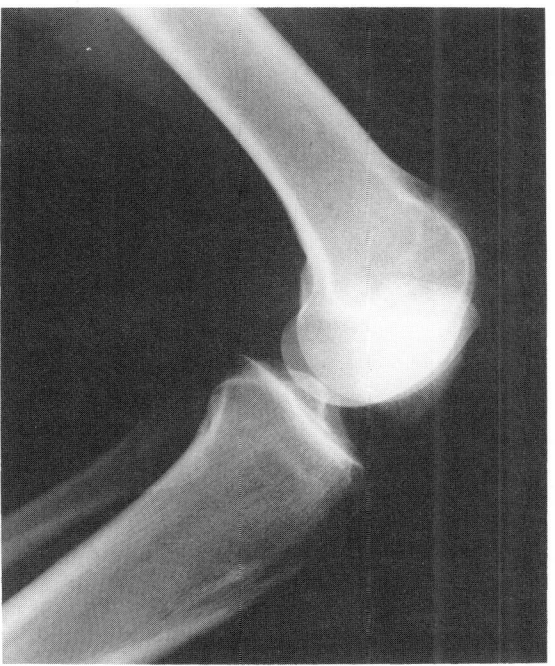

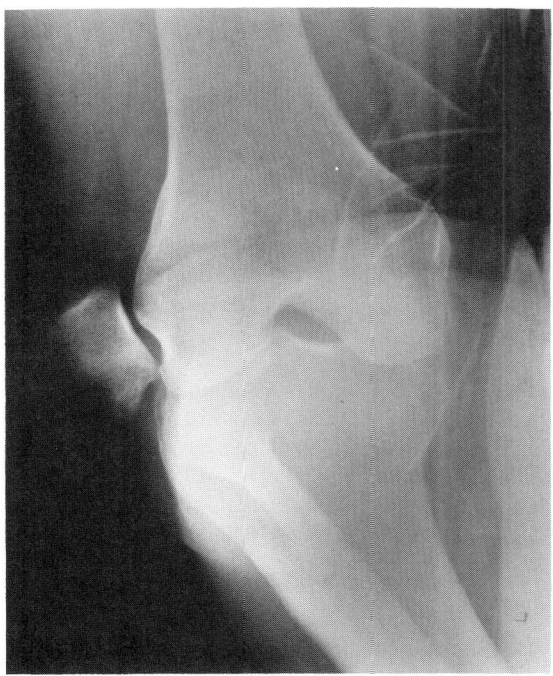

FIGURE 20–11. Acute dislocation of the patella.

of its normal articulating position in the trochlea, but complete dislocation does not occur. Spontaneous reduction occurs routinely.

Acute patellar dislocation can occur because of a direct blow forcing the patella out of the trochlear groove or as a result of a lateral force vector that develops when the quadriceps is contracted and a varus or valgus stress occurs such as during a cutting maneuver. In the acute setting, especially after an initial dislocation, there is a significant amount of pain and swelling. A hemarthrosis is usually present, and the athlete has pain with attempted knee motion. An active straight leg raise should be performed to verify an intact extensor mechanism.

A patellar dislocation disrupts the medial retinacular structures, which usually tear from the area of the adductor tubercle. If a straight leg raise cannot be performed after extensive encouragement, carefully evaluate the extensor mechanism for possible disruption. If the injury is seen several days later and the acute reaction has subsided, usually there will be a residual effusion and tenderness over the medial patellar facet, the medial retinaculum, and the adductor tubercle (not the medial femoral epicondyle, which is seen with a medial collateral ligament, [MCL] sprain). Frequently, the patient will experience discomfort with valgus stress, again leading to the possibility of confusion with an MCL sprain. Occasionally, patellar dislocation and MCL sprain may occur simultaneously. A major diagnostic finding on physical exam is a positive apprehension test as described above. Other predisposing stigmata such as hypermobile patella, quadriceps dysplasia with a deficient vastus medialis obliquus, or increased 90-degree tubercle-sulcus angle may be noted.

The diagnosis of patellar dislocation is unmistakable in the acute setting with the patella still dislocated. The knee is slightly flexed and the patella is prominent laterally in its dislocated position. Prompt reduction in the field will afford the patient a significant amount of pain relief. The reduction is accomplished by extending the knee while applying gentle medially directed pressure along the lateral patellar edge. Do not force the reduction. If the patella does not reduce easily, there is no harm in waiting for immediate transportation and evaluation in the emergency room to ensure the dislocation is not complicated by a fracture. Swelling or an effusion may develop fairly rapidly and is the result of a hemarthrosis due to tearing of the medial retinaculum. There is usually extensive tenderness in the medial parapatellar area down to the adductor tubercle, as mentioned. Evaluation of specific patellar parameters (lateral/medial glides, passive patellar tilt, 90-degrees tubercle-sulcus angle) is difficult owing to pain and apprehension. Examination of the opposite knee may provide a baseline.

In order to decide on the best initial treatment for each case of primary dislocation, it would be helpful to be able to predict with some certainty which patients will go on to have recurrent episodes. Larsen and Lauridsen[32] reported a follow-up study in an attempt to delineate predisposing factors to recurrent dislocation. Dysmorphology was assessed on radiographs and a physical examination was performed. Results revealed the only correlation with an increased risk of repeat dislocation was age less than 20 years at the time of the initial dislocation. The presence of dysplastic factors on radiographs did not influence rate of redislocation. Patella alta and clinical episodes of subluxation were found more commonly in patients whose dislocation was atraumatic.

Early textbooks described cylinder cast immobilization for 3 to 6 weeks after a patellar dislocation. This may well be the treatment of choice in selected patients. However, this promotes extensive quadriceps atrophy and has not been our treatment of choice.

A thorough physical examination is performed to ensure no concomitant ligamentous injuries have occurred. A Merchant view radiograph of both knees is obtained to ensure that the patella remains centralized and symmetric within the trochlea. Small bony fragments along the medial patellar facet may occur when the patella reduces and are usually embedded in soft tissue. The presence of a fragment is not an indication for surgical intervention.

A centralized patella is initially treated nonoperatively with a patellar stabilizing brace. A significant hemarthrosis may require initial use of a postoperative patellar stabilizing brace that wraps around with Velcro fasteners and a lateral horseshoe pad. As the effusion subsides, a pull-up neoprene sleeve with a patellar cutout and lateral pad may be utilized. An electric muscle stimulator may be used to initiate an active quadriceps contraction if none is present. Ice and nonsteroidal antiinflammatory medication are important adjuvants to minimize pain and swelling. Straight leg raises are initiated as soon as possible. The patient then advances through the four phases of rehabilitation described below.

A patella that does not centralize on the Merchant view but shows evidence of an asymmetrical lateral tilt and subluxation is considered for operative intervention. This position on the Merchant view indicates that the medial restraints have been substantially torn and would heal in a lax position. A nonoperative course as described above could be pursued; however, the incidence of recurrent dislocations is high in this group, and athletic individuals may particularly benefit from early surgical intervention.

The surgical procedure should encompass a brief arthroscopic evaluation to include a superolateral view of patella tracking through incremental flexion followed by a medial restraint repair and then a lateral release if necessary. The lateral release is done if the passive patellar tilt is negative after the medial restraints have been repaired. If this is difficult to assess because of the swelling and soft tissue trauma, the passive patellar tilt of the uninjured knee as measured preoperatively can be used as a guide for the necessity of lateral release. The extremity should be passively mobilized in a limited motion brace (0 to 60 degrees of flexion) for 4 to 6 weeks before full flexion is encouraged. Isometric contractions as well as straight leg raises in the brace may be performed starting the first day postoperatively.

Patellar subluxation is more difficult to recognize initially.[21] The patella is in a reduced position, and an effusion is slow to develop. Tenderness may be present along the medial parapatellar structures, and an apprehension test is usually positive. A complete knee examination should be performed to rule out other ligamentous or bony injuries.

Radiographs should be obtained of the knee in an anteroposterior and a lateral projection and a Merchant or tangential view of the patella. It would be very unusual to see a bony fracture of the medial patellar facet after a subluxation. The radiographs should be evaluated for the possible presence of a poorly developed sulcus or lateral femoral condyle and for evidence of patellar malposition by the lateral patellofemoral angle and congruence angle. A Merchant view of both knees allows comparison of the injured and uninjured knee for discrepancies. Patients with patellar subluxation will usually have normal radiographs.

Treatment is symptomatic and in the acute setting begins with ice and antiinflammatory medication and compression via a patellar sleeve. Patients may bear weight on the extremity as soon as tolerated. A structured rehabilitation program is necessary to gain or maintain adequate quadriceps strength prior to returning the individual to his or her sport. The amount of time prior to a return to sport varies between individuals. Surgical intervention after an initial acute episode of patellar subluxation is almost never necessary.

TREATMENT OF RECURRENT INSTABILITY OF THE PATELLA

Episodes of recurrent patellar instability (dislocation or subluxation) can follow an initial acute episode of traumatic instability. Physical examination may aid in predicting recurrence if the patella is hypermobile, if there is obvious disruption of the medial restraints, or if the 90-degree tubercle-sulcus angle is increased. The risk to the patient of recurrent episodes of instability is further damage to the medial restraints or medial patellar facet surface, lost time from a sport, time needed for rehabilitation, and of course, pain related to the episodes of instability.

Initial treatment should proceed as outlined above after an acute episode of dislocation. If a complete evaluation reveals normal patellar parameters, treatment should proceed conservatively as a nonoperative rehabilitation program. Conservative treatment initially depends on the patient's level of comfort. If they are extremely painful, a straight leg immobilizer may be used for 5 to 7 days, bearing full weight in extension as tolerated. Preferably, if tolerated, the patient may be placed in a patellar brace with a lateral pad and immediately bear weight on the affected extremity. Straight leg raises are instituted the same day. Progressive range of motion within pain tolerance follows. Usually within 2 weeks, the patient has enough comfort and motion to progress to an exercise bike for quadriceps strengthening. A routine rehabilitation program continues as outlined below. Ice is also an important component of treatment and is used liberally the first 72 hours and at least daily after exercise in the ensuing weeks. Emphasizing a good flexibility program and strength equilibrium for agonist/antagonist muscle groups is necessary for return to sports.

REHABILITATION PROGRAM FOR PATELLAR INSTABILITY

The initial rehabilitation program is performed with straight leg raises to avoid loads across the patellofemoral joint. Also, as the rehabilitation program proceeds, exercises can be added in the 70- to 120-degree knee flexion range, thus taking advantage of the increased joint contact area. The mainstay of rehabilitation is quadriceps strengthening and flexibility. The mechanism of strengthening is very important as work on isokinetic and/or knee extension isotonic machines may exacerbate patella problems. Strengthening should be initiated with a straight leg raise program. When three to four sets of 10 repetitions can be tolerated, add ankle weights in 1- or 2-pound increments. The ultimate goal for the total number of straight leg raises performed and pounds of ankle weight varies between authors.[15, 23] A realistic goal is three sets of 10 leg raises with 12 pounds of ankle weights.[41] This is a minimum goal, but patients may benefit by increasing their exercises to twice a day or performing more than three sets.

Bicycling is an excellent activity for quadriceps function. Patients with severe pain and atrophy (and/or patellar malalignment) may not be able to begin cycling until they have gained some quadriceps tone and strength through straight leg raises. This is not a rapid process. Depending on the amount of weakness, it may take 4 to 8 weeks before cycling is comfortable, but usually patients are able to cycle by 2 weeks after their injury. They must be both consistent and persistent with their program, performing some type of exercise on a daily basis. When patients have chronic instability with significant weakness, a supervised therapy program is often beneficial to allow them to reach the point of comfortable cycling before converting to an unsupervised home therapy program.

Bicycling is more controlled on an exercise bike than an outdoor bike. The program should begin with *no* resistance and be timed in minutes, rather than pedaling a set distance. Depending on tolerance, start with 5 to 10 minutes and increase the time in 5-minute increments once or twice a week until the patient can tolerate 45 minutes without stopping and with no resistance. Once this level of exercise is comfortable for the patient, the resistance may be increased very slowly. Also at this time, they may begin some outdoor biking on level ground in low gear with the seat raised to a high level. For additional resistance exercises to gain strength, terminal extensions from 0 to 30 degrees with increasing ankle weights may be done in sets of 10, assuming there is no pain. Also, a leg press program may be instituted (avoiding the 30- to 60-degree flexion arc) when sufficient strength has been gained to perform the exercise pain free. No limit need be placed on the amount of weight lifted as long as the exercise remains pain free. Occasionally, the motion is limited from 0 to 30 degrees to facilitate this. Most patients with anterior knee pain or patellofemoral pain should indefinitely avoid all isotonic knee extensions and any intense isokinetic knee flexion/extension workouts, at least in the range of motion around the 36 degrees of flexion predicted by Reilly and Martens[46] to cause peak patellar pressure during knee extension.

When access to a bicycle or leg press machine is not possible, substitutions can be made as long as several basic principles are followed. Unlike the bottom of the foot, the anterior tibia was not made to lift weights! This extensor moment creates extremely high contact pressure across the patellofemoral joint when the knee is in a flexed position. Higher repetitions and lower weight or resistance should always be the rule. Deep knee bends or knee flexion greater than 40 or 45 degrees should be avoided until later in the rehab program. A good substitute for a conventional resistance exercise program is to use a stretch cord to provide the resistance. Some of these are available in different strengths so that patients may progress from light resistance to a heavier resistance gradually. Exercise can include standing wall slides or minisquats (0 to 40 degrees) against the stretch cord. This provides concentric strengthening only.

Nonsteroidal antiinflammatories are a useful adjunct to decrease inflammation in a knee that shows evidence of an effusion or pain severe enough to affect activities of daily living. Some patients may initially respond to the therapy with a flare-up of their symptoms, and antiinflammatory medication can also help to alleviate this reaction. Ice packs or ice massage can also be used to relieve pain and facilitate exercise sessions.

To summarize, an all-inclusive rehabilitation program should include quadriceps and hamstring strengthening and stretching with avoidance of early bent-knee activities. A flexibility program is essential to maintain lower extremity flexibility during and after the growth spurt. Ice application is necessary to prevent the increased activity of the rehabilitation from causing increased inflammation and should be used after each exercise session on a daily basis. Nonsteroidal antiinflammatory medication can also be useful to decrease any inflammation that is present.

Patients with a history of patellar subluxation or dislocation frequently benefit from a patellar knee sleeve with a lateral pad to help hold the patella in a reduced position while proceeding with the strengthening program. Patients with a hypermobile patella will also experience some symptomatic relief from their pain and relate a feeling of "more stability" regarding their patella.

Before returning to a sport, patients should have no effusion, full range of motion without pain, and full recovery of normal strength, which is most reliably evaluated on a muscle testing machine (Cybex, Biodex, Merac). Because knee extension exercises may cause high patellofemoral pressures, these machines should be approached with caution. In the more symptomatic patient, it may be wise to avoid the 20- to 50-degree range of motion during such testing, limit testing to high speeds only, or avoid this testing altogether. Patellar stabilizing braces are worn on return to any sport that involves cutting maneuvers or physical contact.

RECURRENT DISLOCATION OR SUBLUXATION DESPITE CONSERVATIVE TREATMENT

Recurrent episodes of instability despite following the above parameters dictates failure of a conservative treatment program. At this point, an athlete needs to decide if it would be acceptable to give up the offending sport or activity or proceed with surgical intervention. If the instability episodes occur with activities of daily living, then activity modification alone is not going to be sufficient treatment. It is difficult to cite a specific number of instability episodes that should constitute an indication for surgery, but the surgeon and patient should remember that each episode carries the risk of irreversible articular damage; this risk should be balanced against the morbidity of the surgery itself.

Many surgical techniques for patellar realignment have been described in the literature.[8, 25, 40] These vary from (1) an isolated lateral release performed by either open[3, 7, 38] or arthroscopic methods[19, 37, 40] to (2) a proximal realignment as described by Insall et al.[25] or Hughston[21] or (3) a proximal and distal realignment that includes medializing the tibial tubercle[8] if the patient is near the end of growth or (4) a split patellar tendon transfer if the patient is still growing.[16, 33]

SURGICAL TREATMENT OF RECURRENT PATELLAR INSTABILITY

It is important to tailor surgery to the physical findings of each individual patient. The type of surgery performed is decided by a meticulous physical examination that identifies all patellar parameters. A tight lateral restraint indicated by a negative passive patellar tilt with normal or decreased medial and lateral patellar glides and a normal 90-degree tubercle-sulcus angle is an indication for an isolated lateral release. A lateral patellar glide of greater than or equal to three quadrants is indicative of a deficient medial restraint and may indicate the need for a proximal realignment (medial reefing) procedure. When the distal patellar vector, or 90-degree tubercle-sulcus angle, is increased (greater than 5 degrees), it may be necessary to perform a distal realignment or medialization of the tubercle.

Lateral Release

The lateral release is performed through an anterolateral arthroscopic portal. A brief arthroscopic exam of the knee is performed to ensure there is no other intraarticular pathology. Patellar tracking is then viewed through a superolateral portal during incremental flexion. A lateral patellar strike and failure to centralize the patella within the trochlea by 40 degrees of knee flexion is an arthroscopic indication to proceed with a lateral release. The Mayo scissors are used through the anterolateral portal to create a

344 PART II—COMMON SPORTS INJURIES

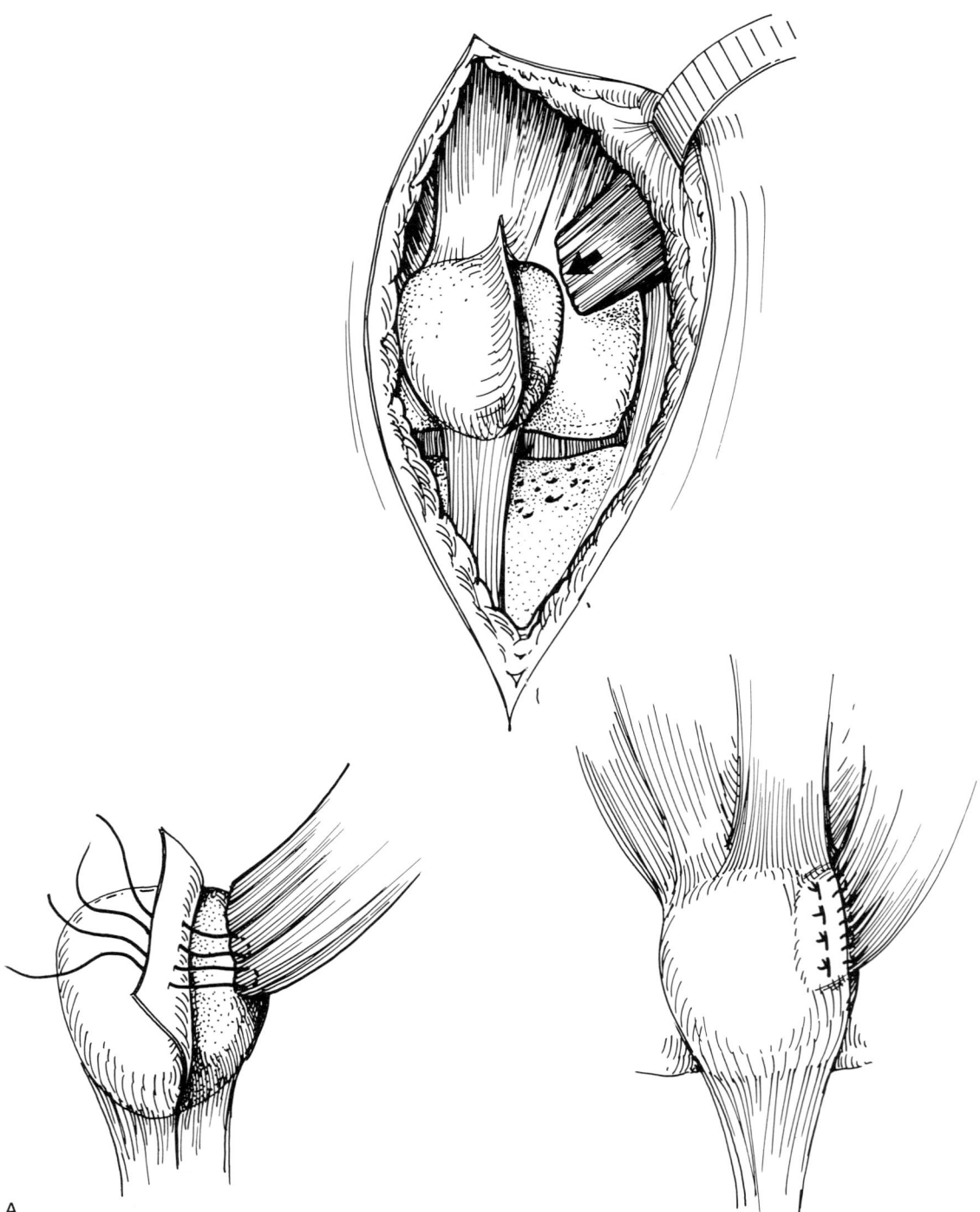

FIGURE 20–12. (*A*) The authors' preferred technique for proximal realignment. The VMO is mobilized and advanced under a flap of patellar periosteum and soft tissue.

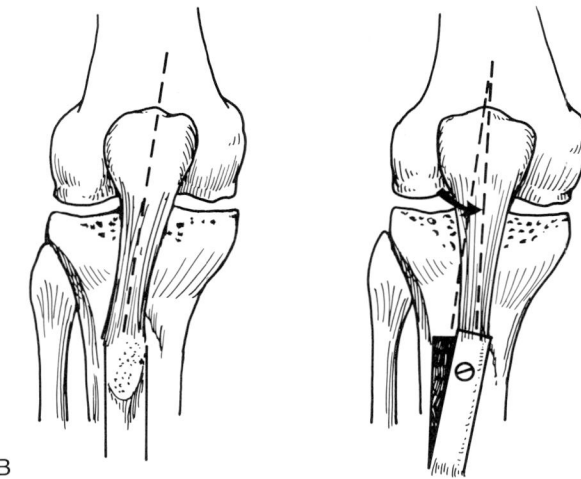

FIGURE 20–12. *Continued.* (B) The authors' preferred technique for distal realignment, the Cox modification of the Elmslie-Trillat procedure.

subcutaneous tunnel about 1 cm lateral to the patella. The lateral restraints are then transsected with one blade of the scissors in the subcutaneous space and one blade in the joint. The release is completed up to the level of the vastus lateralis but not into the vastus lateralis, as permanent strength deficit would result. The intraoperative passive patellar tilt should be increased to plus 45 to 60 degrees. Electrocautery should be used to cauterize the margins of the release and the geniculate vessels to prevent a hemarthrosis. The portals are closed with a buried absorbable suture. Postoperatively, the knee is held in extension in a straight leg knee immobilizer for 1 week. Straight leg raises are started on the day of surgery. At 1 week, the splint is removed and a passive patellar tilt is performed in the office to free any adhesions. The rehabilitation program is started and follows the rehabilitation program described at the end of this section. Patellar mobilizations should be performed three to five times per day by the patient. Range of motion begins when the splint is removed. Most patients have enough flexion to ride the stationary bicycle by the end of the second postoperative week. Rehabilitation does not cease until a strength test reveals less than a 10 percent deficit in the quadriceps and hamstring muscle groups as outlined in the rehabilitation protocol.

Proximal Realignment

When the preoperative physical exam demonstrates a lateral glide of greater than or equal to three quadrants, this indicates a deficient medial restraint. We then elect also to perform a medial VMO (vastus medialis obliquus) reefing procedure along with the lateral release.

The skin incision is lateral to the patella, incorporating the anterolateral arthroscopy portal. Incise down to fascia and elevate a medial skin flap by subcutaneous dissection. A lateral release is performed as an open procedure. The passive patellar tilt should be 45 to 60 degrees. Identify the VMO on the medial side. Mobilize the VMO by an incision along the medial aspect of the patella and dissect proximally up to the rectus femoris muscle. Next, elevate the suprapatellar soft tissue and periosteum sharply off the patella. Cottony-dacron #2 sutures are used to advance the VMO down over the patella (Fig. 20–12A). By using horizontal mattress sutures, the suprapatellar tissue overlaps the VMO. All sutures should be placed first and then tied individually. After tying every two to three sutures, the knee is put through a range of motion to ensure that none of the sutures are too tight. A running #1 or #0 Vicryl suture tacks down the border of the suprapatellar tissue over the nonabsorbable suture used to reef the VMO. Hemostasis, especially of the superior and inferior geniculate arteries, is meticulously obtained after tourniquet deflation prior to wound closure. The subcutaneous tissue and skin are closed in a routine fashion. The knee is placed in a straight leg knee immobilizer. Straight leg raises are performed immediately as well as passive motion (0 to 40 degrees). Motion is not advanced past this until 4 weeks postoperatively. Cycling is usually started by 6 to 8 weeks when flexion allows a full revolution. Rehabilitation progresses according to the authors' preferred protocol as outlined.

Distal Realignment

A distal realignment is not performed unless the 90-degree tubercle-sulcus angle is increased (greater than 5 degrees). In nearly mature adolescents, the preferred method of distal realignment is the Cox modification of the Elmslie-Trillat[8] (Fig. 20–12B). A parapatellar skin incision is made to expose the patella and tibial tubercle. Distally, the tibial tubercle is elevated with a saw from the lateral side on a long tongue of bone (4 to 5 cm) and left attached distally. This bony tongue is then medialized to the neutral position with the knee flexed 90 degrees. Care is taken to ensure there is no elevation or depression of the tubercle when it is medialized. Fixation with one or two cancellous screws is preferred. The tibial tubercle may be predrilled prior to the saw cut to facilitate placement of the screws for fixation.

When the distal realignment is completed, the proximal realignment is performed as described above. The knee should be put through a range of motion before and after the proximal realignment to ensure normal patellar tracking.

Adolescent patients that have not reached skeletal maturity should have a distal soft tissue realignment performed rather than a bony realignment, as problems with growth interruption at the tibial tubercle may occur. Our preferred method is that described by Larson in which the medial one half of the patellar tendon is transferred medially.[33]

AUTHORS' PREFERRED REHABILITATION PROGRAM

Our rehabilitation program can be broken down into three phases (Table 20–2). Each phase must be performed in its entirety, pain free or with minimal pain, before progressing to the next stage. Antiinflammatory measures are a very important component of each phase of the program. Phase I can be considered the initial phase of rehabilitation. Goals in this phase should include pain relief, time for rest and healing, and neuromuscular reeducation. Two 15-minute daily exercise sessions should be tolerated with minimal pain and effusion and progressive increases in range of motion before proceeding to phase II. Ice, compression, elevation (ICE), aspirin or other nonsteroidal antiinflammatory medication, and crutches and braces as necessary are used for pain control. Specific exercises included in phase I are isometrics for the quadriceps concentrating on the vastus medialis obliquus, cocontractions for the quadriceps and hamstrings, and "spectrum isometrics" (isometrics performed at a number of different flexion angles). Straight leg raises start without ankle weights with 10 repetitions twice a day. Increase the number as tolerated to fatigue. Active and passive range of motion should be performed to tolerance of motion with at least 10 repetitions of each twice per day. Patellar mobilization should be performed along with the range-of-motion program.

A good flexibility routine is an essential component of a well-rounded rehabilitation program and begins in phase I, the initial rehabilitation phase. The goal of a flexibility or stretching program is to stretch the muscles so that limb motion is not limited. For example, a tight hamstring muscle can limit complete knee extension with the hip flexed.

TABLE 20–2. Rehabilitation Following Patellar Injury or Realignment Surgery

Phase I
ICE (ice, compression, elevation)
Antiinflammatory medication
Flexibility
Strengthening—isometrics, straight leg raises
Goals—minimal effusion, minimal pain, improving range of motion

Phase II
ICE
Antiinflammatory medication
Flexibility
Strengthening—add functional activities (swimming, cycling)
Goals—gain muscular strength, tolerate 30-minute exercise program twice daily

Phase III
ICE only after exercise session
Strengthening—add isotonics (0 to 30 degrees leg press, terminal extensions)
Flexibility
Endurance training (high reps, low weight)
Isokinetics (high-speed only, after tolerating isotonic lift with 10 pounds through full range of motion)

Phase IV
Running program (when strength 75 percent normal)
Return to sport (when strength 90-plus percent normal)

A stretching program will eliminate these contractures and allow normal function of each joint through a full range of motion.

Patients may progress from phase I to phase II of the rehabilitation protocol if they exhibit (1) a minimal effusion, (2) minimal pain, and (3) improving range of motion. The goals of phase II are to (1) gain muscular strength, (2) protect the patellar surface from injury, and (3) tolerate a 30-minute exercise period twice daily. Antiinflammatory measures, ice, compression, and elevation are still continued, as in phase I, but nonsteroidal antiinflammatory medication is only used as necessary. Exercises progress from the isometric program in phase I now to include a progressive resistance program. These exercises include straight leg raises and terminal extension with ankle weights, toe raises, a light swimming program, and finally, low resistance cycling with the bike seat elevated. Flexibility and range of motion continue as described in phase I.

Phase III is the advanced rehabilitation phase. Progression to phase III occurs when straight leg raises and terminal extensions can be done with 10 to 15 pounds of ankle weights. The ice, compression, and elevation are continued only after each exercise session. Medication is seldom necessary. Isometric exercises are continued into phase III. Progressive resistance exercises are advanced to include isotonic workouts with weight machines for the hamstring and quadriceps muscle groups. Quadriceps workouts begin with one weight plate from 0 to 30 degrees of motion. Weight is advanced until reaching one-quarter body weight or a plateau in strength at 15 repetitions. This can be started eccentrically if a slight amount of pain is present with concentric contractions. When this is accomplished, increase motion 0 to 90 degrees and decrease the weight lifted by one half. Each advance in weight and motion should first be introduced through eccentric exercises.

A flexibility program continues as outlined in earlier phases and should be performed as a warm-up before other exercises; it is also a good "cool-down" activity.

Endurance training may begin in this phase. Initial training for quadriceps endurance may be rapid successive lifts with low weight to fatigue. Cardiovascular endurance may be increased by swimming, pool jogging, or bicycling. High-speed isokinetic exercises can be added after the patient can tolerate lifting 10 pounds isotonically through a full range of motion. More sophisticated exercise machines—for example, the Merac (Universal Inc., Iowa)—can be adjusted to reduce resistance through the 20- to 50-degree knee flexion arc. When other types of machines are used, it is usually wise to avoid the 20- to 50-degree arc to prevent overstressing damaged patellar articular cartilage. Phase IV is the final phase of rehabilitation and includes return to activity and maintenance of strength. Strength and endurance training continue throughout this phase. Flexibility is important during both warm-up and cool-down periods. When strength testing documents 70 to 75 percent quadriceps strength compared with the uninvolved extremity (or in bilateral cases, relative to expected force generated based on body weight), a straight running program is started. Sport-specific skill drills are slowly included for coordination and endurance. When strength increases to 90 to 95 percent, return to competition is allowed.

Activities that should generally be avoided in these patients include running steps, squatting, climbing excessive stairs or hills, or any activity that causes a significant amount of pain.

PATELLA PAIN SYNDROMES

There are several syndromes that are associated with anterior knee pain. Historically, these syndromes were placed in a group and called *chondromalacia*. Currently, chondromalacia is a term reserved for arthroscopically proven changes on the articular surface of the patella. Presently, by a detailed history and meticulous physical examination, an attempt is made to identify possible etiological factors for anterior knee pain. These may include lateral patellar compression syndrome (LPCS), patellar malalignment, lower extremity malalignment, foot malalignment, quadriceps dysplasia, hamstring and quadriceps tightness, plica syndrome, overuse, or a history of direct trauma.

HISTORY

An accurate and detailed history is extremely important when initiating an evaluation of adolescent knee pain. *Location* of the pain should first be identified. Most patients will describe the pain as being "in the front of the knee" or "right under the knee cap." Some will locate the pain anteromedially, whereas those with LPCS may localize it to the lateral facet. Others will say, "It hurts all over" but will usually point to the front of the knee. *Longevity* or duration of the complaint is important to document. Knowing the duration of pain will help the clinician decide on an appropriate treatment regimen. If the pain is of short duration, the physician may wish to hold off on prescribing an elaborate treatment program, knowing that many cases will subside; a chronic, recalcitrant pain is more likely to require a more concerted therapeutic effort. *Onset* of symptoms is important. A gradual, nontraumatic insidious onset is most common in this group of patients. A history of direct trauma may signal traumatic chondral damage to an otherwise normal knee. Overuse is a common etiological factor in adolescent anterior knee pain. In these cases, a careful history will reveal a recent change in the amount or duration of physical activities. Examples of typical aggravating factors include a rapid increase in mileage in runners or a drastic change in technique such as adding hill running to a workout program. Extensive jumping drills, squatting drills, or sudden increases in lower extremity weight lifting may all lead to anterior knee pain in normal individuals.

Identify activities that aggravate the pain. Specifically, ask about pain going up or down stairs or inclines. Frequently, the earliest patellar symptom will be pain going down stairs. Other activities that frequently bring out patellofemoral pain include squatting and kneeling. The presence of stiffness in the knee after sitting with the knee bent for long periods of time—that is, through a movie, long car ride, or during classes—is typical of a patellofemoral pain syndrome. Although this is a symptom, it has frequently been called "the movie sign." Direct trauma to a normal patellofemoral joint may initiate a cycle of anterior knee pain. Initially, an effusion may be detected, but chronic effusions are unusual. Frequently, the initial trauma and effusion result in some quadriceps weakness, which may then lead to chronic anterior knee pain. Patients may develop patellofemoral crepitus, which has been shown to correlate with the amount of chondromalacia or articular surface disruption that is present. Most patients with this subtype of patellofemoral pain syndrome will respond to a diligent physical therapy program that includes both stretching and strengthening.

It is important to ask specific questions regarding episodes of *giving way*, which might be related to pain or quadriceps weakness. Pain or weakness can cause giving way or collapsing of the knee on its own, although patellar instability or anterior cruciate ligament damage should also be considered if this symptom is present. The presence of *crepitus*, or crunching, behind the knee cap or swelling about the knee are also important symptoms to document, as they may signify actual chondral damage to the patella. Patients may complain of *"locking"* of the knee. This is usually pseudolocking that occurs with flexion rather than the mechanical locking associated with a meniscal lesion that blocks extension.

It is extremely important to assess the *severity* of the pain and the amount of disability it is creating for the athlete. This will help the physician avoid overtreating an annoying but minor problem. Some athletes will only need reassurance and advice on avoiding overuse, whereas others will be quite severely disabled by their pain and require a supervised physical therapy program.

It is frequently necessary to pose direct questions to obtain a good history, while trying not to lead the patient. A detailed history should be able to isolate a patellar problem from other problems about the knee. Hip pain can radiate to the knee in adolescents, and it is important always to examine the hip during the knee exam.

PHYSICAL EXAMINATION

The physical examination will provide information necessary to determine the etiology of the knee pain further. The major points of the extensor mechanism exam have already been described in the patellar instability section. In cases of patellar pain, the signs of dysplasia are often subtler than they may be in cases of gross patella instability. It is important to look for quadriceps weakness, which may cause patellar pain in the absence of other predisposing factors. Rotational malalignment in the femur and/or tibia may lead to "squinting patellae." Foot abnormalities such as forefoot pronation, flat feet, or heel varus may contribute to some cases of anterior knee pain. Muscle tightness in the quadriceps or hamstrings may incite patellofemoral pain, so these muscle groups should be carefully assessed.[43] The presence of cartilaginous crepitus should be noted, since it usually indicates actual chondral damage.

LPCS is a specific cause for anterior knee pain that is worthwhile distinguishing from other causes. The diagnosis of lateral patellar compression syndrome is made by a correlation with a history of anterior knee pain that is worse with bent knee activities and a physical examination that reveals a negative passive patellar tilt. These patients complain of knee pain usually with retropatellar crepitus and pain with functional bent knee activities. The pain is chronic in duration and usually gradual in onset. These patients usually do not complain of swelling or effusions. On physical examination, in addition to a negative passive patellar tilt, findings may include a medial patellar glide less than two quadrants, a normal or tight lateral patellar glide (two quadrants), and a normal 90-degree tubercle-sulcus angle. Severe cases frequently have referral of pain to the medial joint line.

REHABILITATION PROGRAM FOR PATELLOFEMORAL PAIN

The primary treatment for patellofemoral pain is a physical exercise program. An adequate trial of physical therapy consists of a minimum of 4 to 6 months. This means that the patient must actually be doing the exercises on a daily basis, not just instructed to do them without any follow-through! All components of the program are necessary to see any expected results.

A well-balanced rehabilitation program has been outlined earlier in this chapter. The nature and severity of the symptoms will determine the parameters of the individual program. An athlete with mild symptoms may need only some activity modification advice and an independent exercise program, whereas a youth with severe pain and disability will require close supervision. The amount of initial discomfort present will determine the need for antiinflammatory medication. If pain is constant, it is best to begin an antiinflammatory drug with the program to facilitate progress and prevent increased inflammation with the new activity. Patients who only experience pain with activities may not require medication to initiate a program. Ice should be an integral part of every program and should be applied after each daily workout session for 15 minutes. Each program will need to be individualized to each patient, but all must include a flexibility session that is usually incorporated into the warm-up period. Strengthening follows this and will be guided initially by the patient's strength and tolerance. Strengthening exercises should include spectrum isometrics, straight leg raises with progressive ankle weights, bicycling, and a leg press program. In general, isotonic knee extensions and isokinetic exercise programs should be avoided indefinitely. These two exercises often cause or aggravate anterior knee pain.

Ice is the most important modality that can be used on a patient. There is no need for ultrasound or phonophoresis in most patients. An exception to this would be patients with a component of patellar tendinitis with isolated inferior pole or tibial tubercle tenderness. Neoprene sleeves may be an adjunct to the therapy program. Although there is no proof as to their effectiveness, patients state that they "keep their knee warm" or "provide some support," and they seem to help some individuals progress in their therapy program (Fig. 20–13).

Orthotics may help the individual whose physical examination reveals a discrete abnormality that may be controlled with a specific orthotic. An example is a patient with a valgus knee and excessive foot pronation. This patient may benefit from a foot orthotic with a longitudinal medial arch support. Orthotics, however, do not substitute for a well-balanced rehabilitation program. Careful attention must be observed when prescribing orthotics. Patients must be seen in follow-up soon after they receive their orthotics to ensure against overcorrection, which may lead to further overuse symptoms. For example, a varus knee should not be fitted with an arch support that builds up the medial side; this may lead to a lateral overuse syndrome from increasing the varus moment.

Patients should be encouraged to avoid aggravating activities during their initial rehabilitation program. They may continue to participate in activities that are not painful. The most aggravating activities include jumping sports (basketball, volleyball) and sports that involve an extensive amount of bending or squatting (some racquet sports, some football positions, etc.).

Patients who continue to have intolerable symptoms after 6 months of therapy need to

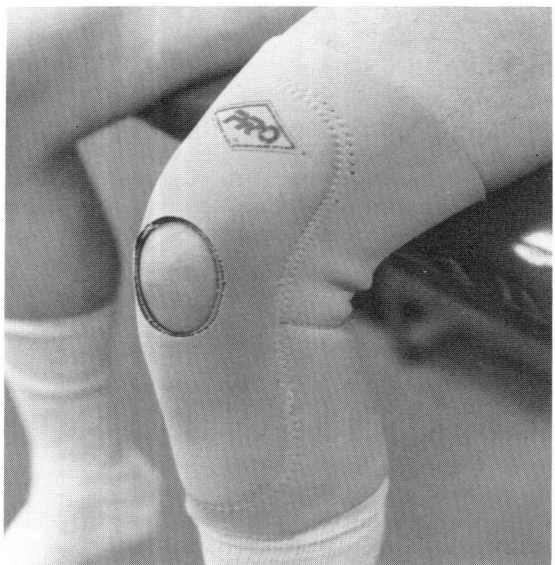

FIGURE 20–13. Although their mechanism of action is unclear, patellar knee sleeves appear to give many patients subjective relief while they are worn.

be critically reevaluated. First, the history is reviewed to ensure nothing is being missed such as recurrent patellar subluxation. The physical examination is reviewed and repeated to document the patellar parameters and ensure that a malalignment problem is not overlooked. The rehabilitation program is reviewed to document that no aggravating exercises such as isokinetics were inadvertently added to the program. Also, record the frequency and duration of exercise periods.

Surgical treatment should not be recommended until patients have failed an adequate trial of physical therapy as outlined above and are significantly disabled by their pain. Activity modification should be considered an alternative at this stage also. Patients who refuse to modify their activities and are avid athletes have less predictable results with surgical intervention,[15, 19, 23] since activity modification is usually still necessary after surgery. Occasionally, patients with significant patellofemoral crepitus may benefit from arthroscopy and patellar debridement. Pathological plical shelves are uncommon, but when encountered, patients usually experience significant relief of their pain with excision at the time of arthroscopy.[5] A lateral release should only be performed if the passive patellar tilt is a negative value or zero degrees, as in LPCS. Performing a lateral release in a patella that is hypermobile may lead to medial dislocation, which can be disabling. Open realignment procedures are more appropriately performed for patellar instability. Patients with anterior knee pain and no abnormal patellar parameters should not be considered for realignment procedures. Elevation of the tibial tubercle, described by Maquet, has come to be regarded as a salvage procedure for patients with anterior knee pain.[35] Biomechanically, elevating the tibial tubercle displaces the patellar tendon in an anterior direction that increases the lever arm. This allows the system to function with less force being transmitted across the patellofemoral joint.[36] Although the biomechanics favorably support this procedure, complication rates of 5 to 35 percent have been reported.[45] These complications include skin slough, osteomyelitis, anterior compartment syndrome, cosmetic deformity, and fracture. Careful attention to detail while performing this procedure may yield a lower complication rate. However, this is still regarded as a salvage procedure for patients with osteoarthritis of the patellofemoral joint and should not be considered as a primary operation for adolescent athletes with patellar pain syndrome.

CONCLUSIONS

Patellofemoral pain is common in adolescents. A thorough history and physical examination should aid in establishing the etiology of the patellofemoral pain. Although the etiology will provide some treatment guidelines throughout the patient's course, initial treatment in most every case begins with a diligent rehabilitation program that is pursued for 6 months before considering surgical alternatives. When a therapy program has failed, possible surgical alternatives should be evaluated based on the physical examination and abnormal patellar parameters. Surgery should be performed as a last resort to correct significant disability, never to prevent the "potential" of arthritis.

OTHER PATELLAR DISORDERS

PREPATELLAR BURSITIS

Direct trauma to the anterior aspect of the knee can result in a painful prepatellar hematoma or bursitis. A careful physical examination will usually distinguish between prepatellar swelling and an intraarticular effusion. The remainder of the knee examination is normal. Initial treatment should include ice, compression, immobilization (straight leg knee immobilizer or neoprene sleeve, depending on severity), and antiinflammatory medication. Active quadriceps contractions are initiated immediately with a straight leg raise program. Progression through a rehabilitation protocol proceeds as the swelling resolves. Rarely, surgical excision of a chronic bursa may be required for patient comfort if all attempts at conservative treatment fail (see Chapter 28).

CHONDRAL FRACTURE

The presence of an intraarticular effusion after a direct blow to the patella may be indicative of a chondral fracture. A significant amount of retropatellar crepitus that was not present prior to the injury is an unfavorable prognostic sign. The physical examination is usually normal with the exception of patellar facet tenderness, crepitus, and an effusion. Radiographs are almost always negative. The initial treatment consists of ice, antiinflammatory medication, early range of motion, and an early strengthening program with straight leg raises progressing slowly as tolerated. It is helpful to avoid further traumatizing the damaged cartilage by advising the athlete to avoid the crepitant arc during weight lifting. Enthusiastic resistive exercising through the crepitant arc may aggravate the patient's pain. Early arthroscopic intervention might be prompted by the presence of loose bodies on the radiograph. Severe, recalcitrant cases that fail a conservative therapy program of at least 6 months may be candidates for arthroscopy and patellar debridement. The longevity of this procedure is unproven, but it does seem to provide patients with symptomatic relief.

FRACTURE OF THE PATELLA

Rarely, a direct blow may result in a patellar fracture. Patients present with severe pain on attempting a straight leg raise, a significant hemarthrosis, and occasionally a palpable defect. Radiographs reveal the fracture and allow an assessment of displacement. Nondisplaced fractures may be immobilized and treated nonoperatively. Frequently, these are stable fractures with the medial and lateral retinaculum intact, and passive range of motion from 0 to 30 degrees can be initiated after 2 to 3 weeks. Weight bearing is allowed in extension. Fractures with 2 mm of displacement or greater are usually treated with open reduction and internal fixation. Most commonly, tension band wiring is performed. This allows stable fixation and early range of motion.[52]

There are two chronic bony abnormalities of the patella that can cause chronic pain with activities—osteochondritis dissecans and bipartite patella.

OSTEOCHONDRITIS DISSECANS

Osteochondritis dissecans of the patella is extremely rare (Fig. 20–14). Rombold reported the first case of osteochondritis dissecans of the patella in 1936.[53] The world's literature reflects just over 100 cases reported since then. Males predominate over females from 2.5:1 to 9:1. The average age range in which most patients presented was 14 to 18 years old, although ranges vary from 10 to 35 years old in the extremes. Up to 16 percent of the patients that were reported demonstrated bilateral lesions.[48] The most common presenting complaints were progressive knee pain frequently aggravated by bending activities and recurrent swelling. Many patients also presented with a history of locking or trauma occurring at the onset of their symptoms.[27, 51]

Physical examination most frequently reveals the presence of patellofemoral crepitus, patellar tenderness, and/or an effusion. Radiographs are necessary to document the diagnosis. The most sensitive method of detecting an osteochondritis dissecans of the patella is felt to be a slightly overexposed lateral view. The skyline view is used to localize the lesion to either the medial or lateral patellar facet. Most lesions abut the articular cartilage. The majority of lesions have been reported in the lower or inferior half of the patella. These were divided between median crest or medial facet followed by the lateral facet.[11, 13] Occasionally, a CT scan may be performed to localize a lesion better.

There has been a report of two cases of osteochondritis dissecans in the lateral patellofemoral groove, one in a 17-year-old, the other in a 47-year-old.[31] Both patients pre-

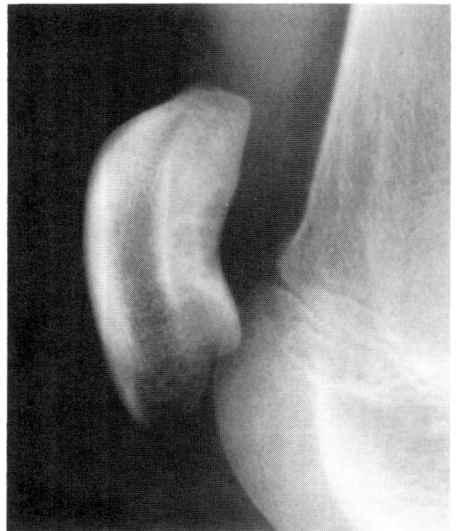

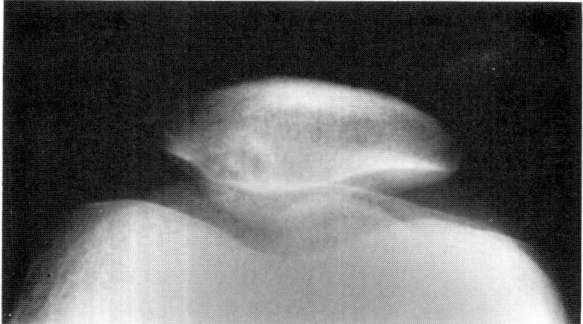

FIGURE 20-14. Osteochondritis dissecans of the patella.

sented with pain, and the 17-year-old had an effusion. Roetgenograms in both patients demonstrated a defect in the superior condylar surface on the lateral view which was not seen on the AP radiograph. A CT scan was performed on both patients that readily demonstrated the lesions. These were later confirmed at the time of arthroscopy, and the pathology reports documented the diagnosis of osteochondritis dissecans.

Osteochondritis dissecans of the patella should be treated as other patellofemoral pain syndromes with a rehabilitation program. The main indication for surgical intervention is a history of locking that may implicate a loose body, especially with a loose body seen on radiographs. Routine arthroscopy without these symptoms does not produce reliable results.[48]

BIPARTITE PATELLA

A bipartite patella is also a relatively rare cause of patellofemoral pain. Its incidence has been described as varying from 0.05 percent by Stucke to 1.66 percent by Blumensaat (from Ficat and Hungerford[14]). Patients present with anterior knee pain. The onset may vary from an acute presentation associated with a direct blow to the patella to a more insidious onset that mimics generalized patellofemoral symptoms. A physical examination will usually localize the area of tenderness to the superior and lateral patellar margin. Inspection with the knee flexed 90 degrees reveals a bony prominence in this superior lateral area. Roentgenograms are diagnostic and demonstrate the accessory ossification center (Fig. 20-8). A radiographic classification was proposed by Saupe (from Green[17]) in 1943 based on the location of the accessory ossification center. There were three types: type I (5 percent) at the inferior pole; type II (20 percent) at the lateral margin; and type III (75 percent) at the superior lateral pole. There has been a case report of painful medial bipartite patella[18] that is not included in Saupe's classification. There is controversy regarding the etiology of a bipartite patella as evident by three current hypotheses. Smillie (from Green[17]) felt the etiology in most cases was a "non-union of lateral margin fractures due to poor blood supply." Other possible etiologies include a congenital or developmental anomaly or a traction avulsion (type I). There is a documented case of an acute fracture simulating a symptomatic bipartite patella.[12] The patient was a 17-year-old who sustained a blow to his patella while playing soccer. Several days later, radiographs revealed what appeared to be a bipartite patella; however, a further search revealed normal radiographs taken several months earlier for probable patellar tendinitis. In 1921, Todd and McCally proposed that blunt trauma to the interface between the accessory and main ossification centers caused inflammation and subsequent limited healing owing to the fibrous nature of the interface, ultimately resulting in a painful syndrome with a nonunion of the fragment or an inflamed synchondrosis.

A bipartite patella that presents with pain should initially be treated with a rehabilitation program, nonsteroidal antiinflammatory medication, and ice massage. If symptoms do not lessen or resolve over 3 to 6 months of therapy, surgical excision may be recommended. Results from excision of the superolateral bipartite fragment have been very good with full return to pain-free activities if severe underlying chondromalacia is not seen at the time of surgery. A small (3- to 4-cm) longitudinal lateral incision is made, and the prepatellar tissue is sharply divided down to the bony fragment. The fragment is then sharply dissected and "shelled out" from its position adjacent to the patella. The articular cartilage is frequently in continuity and must be sharply divided, followed by beveling of the articular edges. The retinaculum is repaired, and a splint is used for immobilization for 1 week. Range of motion is then initiated, and quadriceps rehabilitation proceeds as tolerated according to the protocol. Full recovery is usually expected in 2 to 4 months.

References

1. Aglietti, P., Insall, J. N., Cerulli, G.: Patellar pain and incongruence. Clin. Orthop. 176, p. 218, 1983.
2. Aglietti, P., Insall, J. N., Walker, P. S., Trent, P.: A new patellar prosthesis. Clin. Orthop. 107, p. 175, 1975.
3. Betz, R. R., Magill, J. T., Lonergan, R. P.: The percutaneous lateral retinacular release. Am. J. Sports Med. 15, p. 477, 1987.
4. Bowers, K. Douglas: Patellar tendon avulsion as a complication of Osgood-Schlatter's disease. Am. J. Sports Med. 9, p. 356, 1981.
5. Broom, M. J., Fulkerson, J. P.: The plica syndrome: a new perspective. Orthop. Clin. North Am. 17, p. 279, 1986.
6. Carson, W. G., James, S. L., Larson, R. L., Singer, K. M., Winternitz, W. W.: Patellofemoral disorders: physical and radiographic evaluation: Part 2: Radiographic examination. Clin. Orthop. 185, p. 178, 1984.
7. Ceder, L. C., Larson, R L.: Z-plasty lateral retinacular release for the treatment of patellar compression syndrome. Clin. Orthop. 144, p. 110, 1979.
8. Cox, J. S.: An evaluation of the Elmslie-Trillat procedure for management of patellar dislocations and subluxations: a preliminary report. Am. J. Sports Med. 4, p. 72, 1970.
9. Dalquist, N. J., Mayo, P., Seedhom, B. B.: Forces during squatting and rising from a deep squat. Eng. Med. 11, p. 69, 1982.
10. DeHaven, D. E., Dolan W. A., Mayer, J. J.: Chondromalacia patellae in athletes. Clinical presentation and conservative management. Am J. Sports med. 7, p. 5, 1979.
11. Desai, S. S., Patel, M. R., Michelli, L. J., Silver, J. W., Lidge, R. T.: Osteochondritis dissecans of the patella. J. Bone Joint Surg. 69B, p. 320, 1987.
12. Echeverria, T. S., Bersani, F. A.: Acute fracture simulating a symptomatic bipartite patella. Am. J. Sports Med. 8, p. 48, 1980.
13. Edwards, D. H., Bentley, G.: Osteochondritis Dissecans patella. J. Bone Joint Surg. 59B, p. 58, 1977.
14. Ficat, R. P., Hungerford, D. S.: Disorders of the Patello-femoral Joint. Williams & Wilkins, 1977.
15. Fisher, R. L.: Conservative treatment of patellofemoral pain. Orthop. Clin. North Am. 17, p. 269, 1986.
16. Goldthwait, J. E.: Slipping or recurrent dislocation of the patella: report of eleven cases. Boston Med. Surg. J. 50, p. 169, 1904.
17. Green, W. T.: Painful bipartite patella: a report of three cases. Clin. Orthop. 110, p. 197, 1975.
18. Halpern, A. A., Hewitt, O.: Painful medial bipartite patellae. Clin. Orthop. 134, p. 180, 1978.
19. Henry, J. H., Goletz, T. H., Williamson, B.: Lateral retinacular release in patellofemoral reconstruction: indications, results, and comparison to open patellofemoral reconstruction. Am. J. Sports Med. 14, p. 121, 1986.
20. Huberti, H. H., Hayes, W. C.: Patellofemoral contact pressures: the influence of Q-angle and tendofemoral contact. J. Bone Joint Surg. 66A, p. 715–724, 1984.
21. Hughston, J. C.: Subluxation of the patella. J. Bone Joint Surg. 50A, p. 1003, 1968.
22. Hunter, L. Y., Andrews, J. R., Clancy, W. G., Funk, F. J.: Common Orthopaedic Problems of Female Athletes. Vol. 31. AAOS Instructional Course Lectures, 1982.
23. Insall, J.: Condromalacia patella: patellar malalignment syndrome. Orthop. Clin. North Am. 10, p. 117, 1979.
24. Insall, J. N., Aglietti, A., Tria, A J.: Patellar pain and incongruence. II—clinical application. Clin. Orthop. 176, p. 225, 1983.
25. Insall, J., Bullough, P. G., Burnstein, A. H.: Proximal tube-realignment of the patella for chondromalacia patella. Clin. Orthop. 144, p. 63, 1979.
26. Insall, J., Salvati, E.: Patella position in the normal knee joint. Radiology 101, p. 101, 1971.
27. Ireland, J., Trickey, E. L., Laysnon, A.: Osteochondritis patella. J. Bone Joint Surg. 63B, p. 292, 1981.
28. Johnson, R. S.: Anatomy and biomechanics of the knee. In Operative Orthopaedics, ed. M. Chapman. J. B. Lippincott Co., 1988.
29. Kaufer, H.: Mechanical function of the patella. J. Bone Joint Surg. 53A, p. 1551, 1971.
30. Kettlekamp, D. B.: Current concepts review: management of patellar malalignment. J. Bone Joint Surg. 63A, p. 1344, 1981.
31. Kurzweil, P. R., Zambetti, G. J., Hanulton, W. G.: Osteochondritis dissecans in the lateral patellofemoral groove. Am. J. Sports Med. 16, p. 308, 1988.
32. Larsen, E., Lauridsen, F.: Conservative treatment of patellar dislocations: influence of evident factors on the tendency to redislocation and the therapeutic result. Clin. Orthop. 171, p. 131, 1982.
33. Larson, R.: The unstable patella in adolescent and preadolescent. Orthop. Rev. 14, p. 156, 1985.
34. Laurin, C. A., Dussault, R., Levesque, H. P.: The tangential X-ray investigation of the patellofemoral joint: X-ray technique, diagnostic criteria and their interpretation. Clin. Orthop. 144, p. 16, 1979.
35. Maquet, P.: Mechanics and osteoarthritis of the patello-femoral joint. Clin. Orthop. 144, p. 70, 1979.

36. Maquet, P.: Biomechanics of the Knee. Springer-Verlag, 1984.
37. McGinty, J. B., McCarthy, J. C.: Endoscopic lateral retinacular release: a preliminary report. Clin. Orthop. 158, p. 120, 1981.
38. Merchant, A. C., Mercer, R. L.: A lateral release of the patella. Clin. Orthop. 103, p. 40, 1972.
39. Merchant, A. C., Mercer, R. L., Jacobsen, R. H., Coal, C. R.: Roentgenographic analysis of patellofemoral congruence. J. Bone Joint Surg. 56A, p. 1391, 1974.
40. Metcalf, R. W.: An arthroscopic method for lateral release of the subluxating or dislocating patella. Clin. Orthop. 167, p. 9, 1982.
41. Michelli, L. J.: Overuse injuries in children's sports: the growth factor. Orthop. Clin. North Am. 14, p. 337, 1983.
42. Nisell, R.: Mechanics of the knee. Acta Orthop. Scand. (Suppl.) 261(56), p. 30, 1985.
43. O'Neill, D. B., Michelli, L. J.: Overuse injuries in the young athlete. Clin. Sports Med. 7, p. 591, 1988.
44. Paulos, L. E., Drawbert, J. P., Rosenberg, T. D.: Knee and leg soft tissue trauma. Orthopaedic Knowledge Update. AAOS, 1987.
45. Radin, E. L.: Anterior tibial tubercle elevation in the young athlete. Orthop. Clin. North Am. 17, p. 297, 1986.
46. Reilly, D. T., Martens, M.: Experimental analysis of the quadriceps muscle force and patello-femoral joint reaction forces for various activities. Acta Orthop. Scand. 43, p. 126, 1972.
47. Schonholtz, G. J., Zahn, M. G., Magee, C. M.: Lateral retinacular release of the patella. Arthroscopy 3, p. 269, 1987.
48. Schutzer, S. F., Ramsby, G. R., Fulkerson, J. P.: Computed tomographic classification of patellofemoral pain patients. Orthop. Clin. North Am. 17, p. 235, 1986.
49. Schwartz, C., Blazina, M. E., Sisto, D. J., Hirsch, L. C.: The results of operative treatment of osteochondritis diesecans of the patella. Am. J. Sports Med. 16, p. 522, 1988.
50. Steiner, M. E., Grana, W. A.: The young athlete's knee: recent advances: problems of the extensor mechanism. Clin. Sports Med. 7, p. 534, 1988.
51. Stougaard, J.: Osteochondritis Dissecans of the patella. Acta Orthop. Scand. 45, p. 111, 1974.
52. Mueller, M. E., Allgöwer, M., Schneider, R., Willenegger, H.: Manual of Internal Fixation 2nd Ed. Springer-Verlag, Berlin, pp 248–253, 1979.
53. Rombold, C. Osteochondritis dissecans of the patella: A case report. J. Bone Joint Surg. 18, 230–231, 1936.

DISORDERS OF THE PATELLAR TENDON

BEN K. GRAF
C. KEITH FUJISAKI
BRUCE REIDER

Disorders of the patellar tendon are common in young athletes. Although they are often considered less "serious" than intraarticular knee problems, they may produce considerable disability and occasionally force the premature end of an athletic career. Osgood-Schlatter disease and Sinding-Larsen–Johannson disease occur in adolescents and are usually self-limited; patellar tendinitis occurs in the skeletally mature athlete and may be progressively disabling.

OSGOOD-SCHLATTER DISEASE

Osgood-Schlatter disease is commonly found in athletically active adolescents. It is usually a self-limited process involving the tibial tuberosity and rarely requires surgical intervention. The etiology remains controversial; however, recent studies tend to support Osgood and Schlatter's original hypothesis that trauma is the cause of this entity.

ETIOLOGY

Numerous causes of Osgood-Schlatter disease have been proposed, including avascular necrosis, infection, patellar tendon degeneration with heterotopic bone formation, and trauma.

Avascular Necrosis

Avascular necrosis as a cause of Osgood-Schlatter disease is unlikely because of the abundant blood supply to the tibial tuberosity. This vascular supply comes from medial, lateral, and inferior vessels around the tibial tuberosity. In addition, there are metaphyseal vessels that traverse the physis through communicating channels.[1, 2] as well as vascular contributions from the epiphysis and the patellar tendon insertion. Furthermore, radiographs of healing lesions of Osgood-Schlatter disease do not show the characteristic signs of avascular necrosis—namely, sclerosis, collapse, fragmentation, and remodeling.

Infection

Infection is also an unlikely cause of Osgood-Schlatter disease since patients do not present with leukocytosis and are not febrile. In addition, cultures taken from patients requiring surgery for failed conservative treatment have been negative.[3]

Degeneration

Patellar tendon degeneration with heterotopic ossification within the substance of the tendon has also been hypothesized as a cause of Osgood-Schlatter disease.[3] Histological studies, however, have shown that there is no tendon necrosis and a normal tendon insertion into the anterior portion of the ossicle in patients with Osgood-Schlatter disease.[4]

Trauma

Osgood and Schlatter, when they first independently described this lesion in 1903, theorized that trauma was the cause of the disease process. This hypothesis has been widely accepted as the cause of Osgood-Schlatter disease.[1, 4, 5, 6, 7, 8] Understanding the normal growth and development of the proximal tibia is necessary when proposing trauma as the etiology of Osgood-Schlatter disease. Growth of the proximal tibia is unique in that it involves two growth centers in close proximity: the proximal tibial physis and the tibial tuberosity apophysis. The growth of the tibial tuberosity can be divided into four stages as described by Ehrenborg: cartilaginous, apophyseal, epiphyseal, and bony.[9] The cartilaginous stage encompasses the period from birth until about 8 years of age. During this stage, the tibial tuberosity is an entirely cartilaginous anterior outgrowth of the tibia (Fig. 21–1A). The apophyseal stage begins when the secondary ossification center appears in this anterior outgrowth (Fig. 21–1B), whereas the onset of the epiphyseal stage is marked by the coalescence of the ossification centers of the proximal tibial epiphysis and the tibial tuberosity apophysis (Fig. 21–1C). The epiphyseal stage ends and the bony stage begins when physiological growth plate closure occurs between the proximal tibial metaphysis and the already consolidated epiphysis and apophysis (Fig. 21–1D).

The histology of the tibial tuberosity growth plate is also unique because it is composed of three tissue types: cartilage, fibrocartilage, and fibrous tissue.[2] Proximally, the cytoarchitecture is identical to that of the remainder of the proximal tibial growth plate. More distally, there is a gradual transition to fibrocartilage until the distal end, where fibrous tissue predominates. This unusual architecture may enable the tibial tuberosity to withstand the forces developed by the quadriceps mechanism, since fibrous tissue is better able to tolerate high tensile loads than cartilage or fibrocartilage.

Active adolescents generate forceful, repetitive contractions of the quadriceps muscles in sporting events and activities of daily living. During the apophyseal stage, the tibial tuberosity is susceptible to injury. Microavulsions can occur through the bone and cartilage of the secondary ossification center since it is weaker than the distal fibrous tissue and adjacent bone (Fig. 21–2). Since the trauma is repetitive, a local inflammatory reaction occurs at this site, and a continuum from acute to chronic inflammatory changes can be found.[5] The avulsed fragments of bone and cartilage may develop into a separate ossicle whose development parallels that of the ossification center of the tibial tuberosity.[9] Histological sections from the defect in the tibial tuberosity show vascular connective tissue and osteoid, both characteristics of a healing fracture.[4] In summary, all recent evidence supports Osgood and Schlatter's original hypothesis that the disease is traumatic in origin.

SIGNS AND SYMPTOMS

Adolescents who develop Osgood-Schlatter disease are usually between the ages of 11 and 15 years, with girls presenting earlier because the secondary ossification center of the tibial tuberosity usually appears 2 years earlier in females than in males. The ratio of

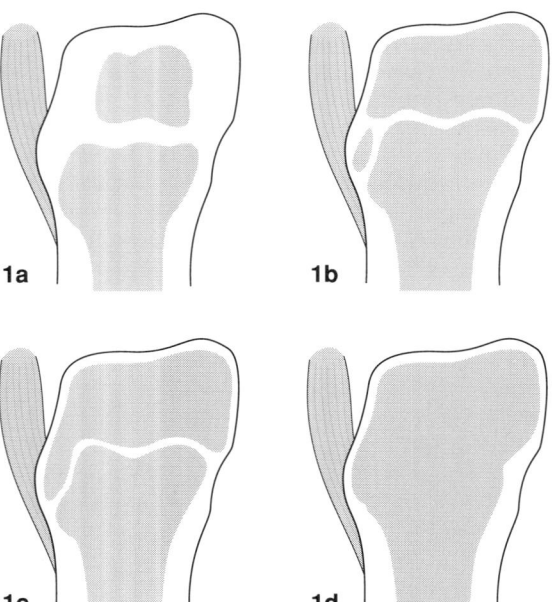

FIGURE 21–1. Stages of proximal tibial development. (A) Cartilaginous stage. (B) Apophyseal stage. (C) Epiphyseal stage. (D) Bony stage. (Adapted from Ogden, J. A., and Southwick, W. O., Osgood-Schlatters disease and tibial tuberosity development. Clin Orthop 116:180–189, 1976.)

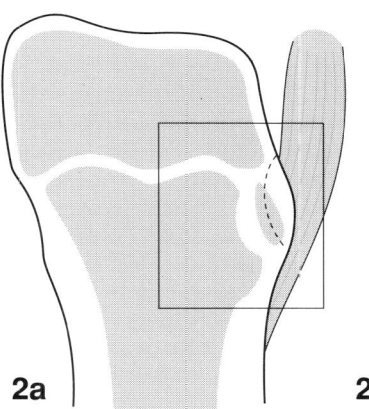 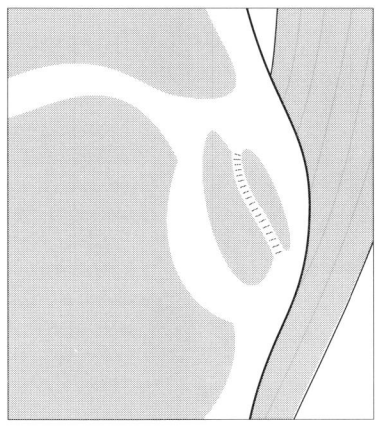 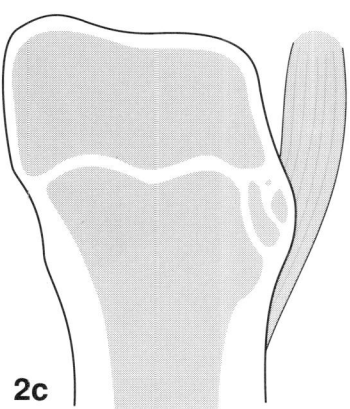

FIGURE 21–2. Avulsion injuries through the tibial apophysis seen in (A) and (B) can result in the formation of ossicles as noted in (C). (Adapted from Ogden, J. A., and Southwick, W. O., Osgood-Schlatters disease and tibial tuberosity development. Clin Orthop 116:180–189, 1976.)

affected males to females is approximately 3 : 2. The left side is more commonly affected than the right side, and up to 25 percent of cases may be bilateral.[6, 10] Many patients relate the onset of symptoms to one specific traumatic episode. Pain, which is typically described as a dull ache, is exacerbated by activities involving impact loading such as jumping or stair climbing and is relieved by rest. It is not unusual for patients to have symptoms for 6 to 12 months prior to seeking medical evaluation.

Physical examination usually reveals a prominent tibial tuberosity with soft tissue swelling and local tenderness (Fig. 21–3). A full active range of motion is present, and the pain is aggravated by knee extension against resistance, passive hyperflexion, and occasionally, medial or lateral subluxation of the patella. While straight leg raising is usually not painful, quadriceps atrophy may be present in long-standing cases.

Associated physical findings include genu valgum,[8] pronated feet, and increased external tibial torsion.[11] There has also been a reported association between Osgood-Schlatter disease and Sever disease.[10]

RADIOGRAPHIC FINDINGS

Because the tibial tuberosity is lateral to the midline of the tibia, lateral radiographs with the tibia in slight internal rotation are recommended (Fig. 21–4). Soft tissue radiographs will enhance identification of soft tissue swelling and bony ossicles. The radiographic findings include the following: loss of the homogeneity of the infrapatellar fat pad, obliteration of the inferior angle of the infrapatellar fat pad, irregularity and thickening of the tissues between the anterior surface of the tibia and the posterior margins of the fat pad, a thickened patellar tendon, and fragmentation of the tibial tuberosity.[12, 13] Of all the findings, the most obvious, fragmentation of the tuberosity, is also the most variable.[14]

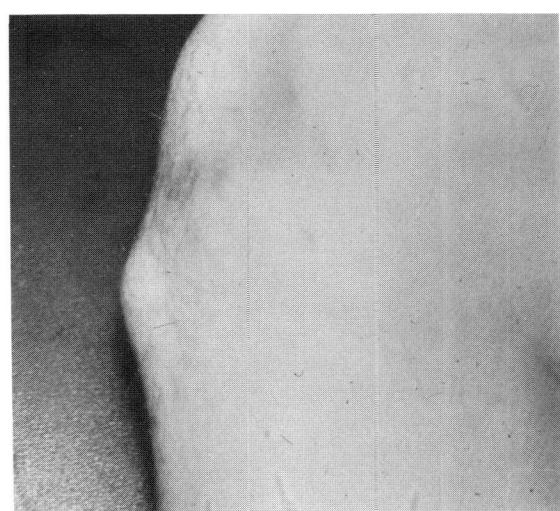

FIGURE 21–3. Lateral photograph of an adolescent with Osgood-Schlatter disease shows the prominent tibial tuberosity and soft tissue swelling.

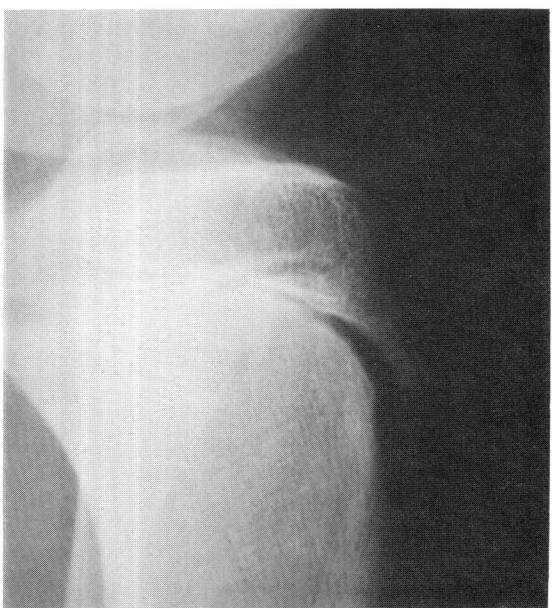

FIGURE 21–4. Later radiograph shows fragmentation of the tibial tuberosity in the patient with Osgood-Schlatter disease.

DIFFERENTIAL DIAGNOSIS

The differential diagnosis of Osgood-Schlatter disease includes contusion of the tibial tuberosity with subcutaneous hematoma formation, prepatellar bursitis, osteomyelitis of the proximal tibia, osseous or vascular tumors of bone, osteochondromatosis, patellar tendinitis, and Sinding-Larsen–Johansson disease.[15]

TREATMENT

The treatment of Osgood-Schlatter disease is generally nonoperative. Restriction of activity is essential in those patients who present acutely or in those with acute exacerbation of chronic symptoms. Immobilization in a cylinder cast for 6 to 8 weeks has been advocated for patients with severe symptoms.[16, 17] This may, however, lead to significant muscle atrophy and stiffness. We prefer the use of a knee immobilizer, which, when removed, allows the patient to complete range-of-motion exercises. Only occasionally is any immobilization necessary, as adequate pain relief can usually be obtained with rest, ice, and nonsteroidal antiinflammatory drugs. A gradual return to activity is allowed when there is minimal discomfort with direct palpation over the tuberosity. Those patients who have developed quadriceps atrophy are required to complete a rehabilitation program and demonstrate at least 90 percent of the quadriceps and hamstring strength of the uninvolved limb prior to returning to sports.

Patients with milder, more chronic symptoms often can continue their normal activities, though perhaps at a reduced level. Protective padding to the involved area to prevent direct trauma and orthotics to decrease lower extremity impact forces may be helpful. A routine quadriceps stretching program should be initiated to diminish stress on the patellar tendon insertion. Although an infrapatellar strap has been described,[18] the authors have found it to be of limited value. Methylprednisolone injections have been recommended but can result in subcutaneous atrophy and fat pad necrosis and are best avoided.[19] Rest, ice, and nonsteroidal drugs are usually sufficient to control pain and swelling. Symptoms generally subside when the tibial tuberosity apophysis fuses with the tibial metaphysis (the bony stage of development).

In those patients who remain symptomatic owing to a painful ununited ossicle in the patellar tendon, surgical excision is recommended.[20, 21] Generally, this is performed after skeletal maturity since prior to that time most patients respond to conservative measures and after that time there is no risk of a recurvatum deformity occurring as a result of surgery. However, there are skeletally immature patients who develop a painful ununited ossicle and remain symptomatic despite conservative treatment. In this situation, simple surgical excision of the fragment appears to be safe even prior to growth plate closure.[22, 23, 24, 25] The procedure is as follows: A 3-cm longitudinal incision is made just lateral to the tibial tubercle. The patellar tendon is exposed and incised longitudinally over the fragment. The ossicle is dissected free of the patellar tendon by sharp dissection and separated from the remaining tibial tubercle with a periosteal elevator. Once the fragment has been removed, the patellar tendon is reapproximated, and the wound is closed. Postoperatively, the patient is placed in a knee immobilizer that is removed to allow early range-of-motion exercises. Weight bearing is allowed as tolerated, and a formal rehabilitation program is initiated once the soft tissues have healed. Patients return to full activities when the pain has subsided, the range of motion is normal, and the quadriceps strength is at least 90 percent of that of the normal limb.

COMPLICATIONS

Patella alta is felt to be a potential consequence of Osgood-Schlatter disease.[26, 27, 28] The theory is that repetitive trauma to the tibial tuberosity causes proximal migration of the patellar tendon insertion. Others, however, have not found an association between these two conditions. When considering the possibility of patella alta, measurement of patellar height by the method of Blackburne and Peel[43] is preferable to that described by Insall and Salvati,[42] since the patellar insertion may be distorted by the fragmentation of the tibial tuberosity.

A permanently enlarged tibial tuberosity is a common sequela of Osgood-Schlatter disease and may be just a cosmetic deformity or contribute to the development of prepatellar bursitis. Other reported complications include genu recurvatum[29, 30] and avulsion fracture of the tibial tuberosity.[31, 32, 33] The latter is relatively uncommon, occurring in only a very small percentage of those patients with Osgood-Schlatter disease.

SINDING-LARSEN–JOHANSSON DISEASE

Sinding-Larsen and Johansson, in 1921–1922, independently described a syndrome in which adolescents present with tenderness and radiographic fragmentation of the inferior pole of the patella and yet do not relate any history of trauma.[34, 35] Initially, Sinding-Larsen and Johansson felt this represented an epiphysitis but in fact no epiphysis is involved. More reasonable hypotheses are that necrosis of tendon fibers occurs with subsequent calcification near the inferior pole of the patella or that avulsion of the periosteum of the patella occurs with resultant ossification. In either case, Sinding-Larsen–Johansson disease appears to be due to a repetitive traction phenomenon at the patellar tendon attachment site, like Osgood-Schlatter disease, but on the inferior pole of the patella.

Patients are usually athletically active and range from 10 to 13 years of age. Pain is exacerbated by running, stair climbing, and kneeling. Tenderness is present upon direct palpation of the inferior pole of the patella and made worse with resisted quadriceps contraction. Patients may have a concomitant history of Osgood-Schlatter or Sever disease.

Calcification near the inferior pole of the patella occurs within several weeks from the onset of acute symptoms (Fig. 21–5). Four radiographic stages have been identified: stage I, normal findings; stage II, irregular calcification at the inferior pole of the patella; stage III, coalescence of the calcification; stage IVa, incorporation of the calcification with the patella to yield a normal appearance; and stage IVb, a calcified mass separate from the patella.[36]

Patients with acute onset of pain or those with severe chronic pain may need to be placed in a knee immobilizer or cylinder cast for comfort. Those with chronic symptoms may only need restriction of activity and symptomatic treatment. Typically, it takes between 9 and 12 months before a patient is symptom free if they initially present with stage I radiographic findings. Like Osgood-Schlatter disease, this is usually a self-limited disease, and patients may return to activity when pain free, even if complete incorporation of the fragment to the patella has not occurred.

PATELLAR TENDINITIS

Patellar tendinitis is a painful condition of the patellar tendon found in skeletally mature athletes. It is often called "jumper's knee," a term that also includes the less common quadriceps tendinitis.[37] It is usually located in the proximal patellar tendon, like Sinding-Larsen–Johannson disease, but does not involve calcification in the tendon. Although frequently described in adults in their twenties, patellar tendinitis frequently begins in older teenagers.

PATHOGENESIS

Patellar tendinitis is a degenerative condition of the tendon thought to be caused by recurrent overload. Curwin and Stanish have hypothesized that this overload occurs in the eccentric phase of quadriceps action, such as when landing from a jump, because the ten-

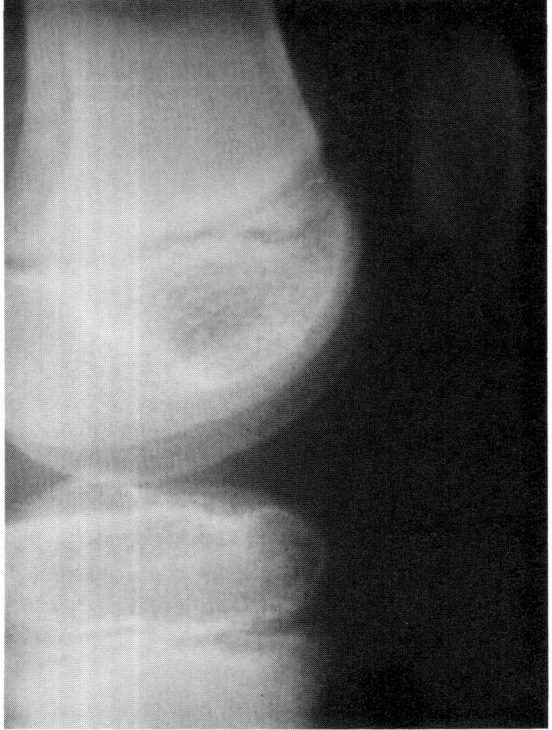

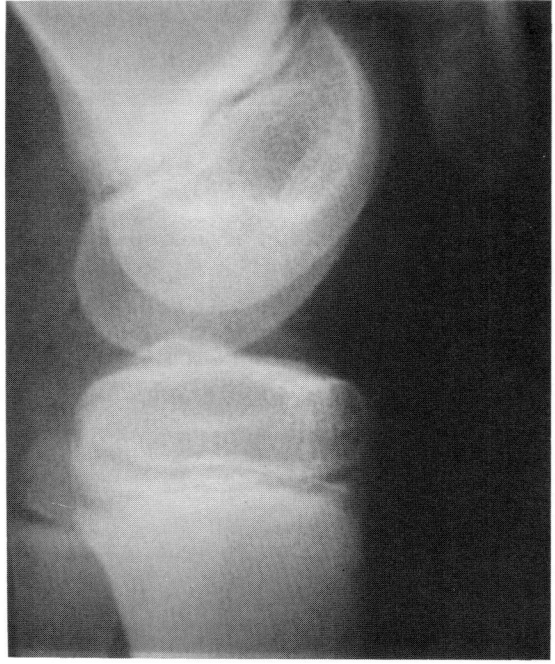

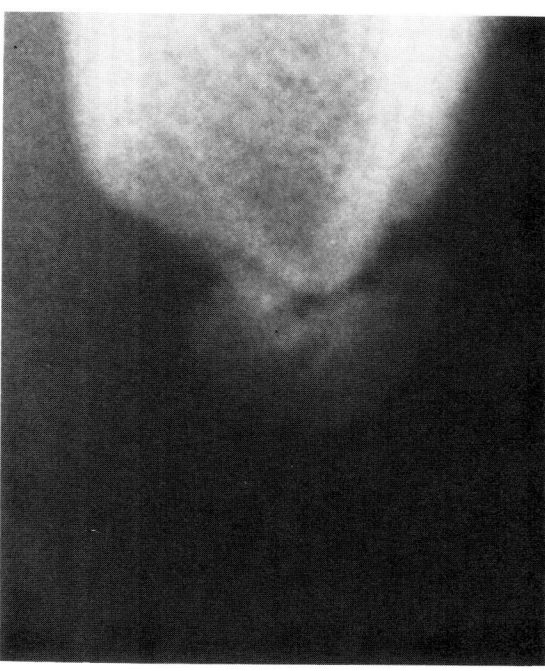

FIGURE 21–5. This patient presented with pain and tenderness localized to the distal pole of the patella. The initial radiographs (A) were unremarkable, but radiographs 3 months later (B) showed a calcified mass separate from the patella. (C) Close-up of the calcified mass.

sion generated during eccentric work far exceeds that which occurs during concentric contraction.[38] This overload causes collagen fibrils to slide past each other, with breakage of crosslinks and rupture of the weakest fibers. This concentrates the tensile load on the remaining fibers, thus perpetuating the process. In older patients, this may lead to macroscopic tendon rupture.

In young athletes, patellar tendinitis occurs at the proximal end of the patellar tendon near its attachment to the inferior pole of the patella. "Jumper's knee" may also present in middle-aged patients as quadriceps tendinitis proximal to the patella, but this is very rare in youngsters. The lesion usually involves the deep, central fibers of the tendon. Stanish[38] has hypothesized that the fibers in this area are less elastic and more subject to bending than in other areas of the tendon. Hypovascularity may also contribute to this localization by reducing the potential for healing.

Histopathology of the tendon includes local mucoid degeneration and fibrinoid necrosis mingled with areas of regeneration with fibroblast proliferation and thin-walled vessels.[41] Clefts, sometimes visible macroscopically, develop as the changes become more advanced.

CLINICAL PICTURE

As noted, patellar tendinitis normally presents as a progressive pain at the inferior pole of the patella in a skeletally mature athlete. Occasionally, the athlete will remember a specific inciting episode, but usually the onset is gradual. As the term "jumper's knee" implies, this problem is common in basketball players, but it is not limited to them, occurring in almost any sport requiring jumping or running.

The level of pain can vary from an annoyance to one that prevents athletic participation. The severity is usually graded along the lines suggested by Blazina et al.[37]

Phase 1. Pain after activity only; no undue functional impairment

Phase 2. Pain during and after activity; still able to perform at a satisfactory level

Phase 3. Pain during and after activity and more prolonged; patient has progressively increasing difficulty in performing at a satisfactory level

Roels et al.[41] also proposed a similar classification, with the addition of gross tendon rupture as Phase 4 of the scheme. Happily, complete tendon rupture is virtually unknown in the young athlete.

Physical examination will reveal point tenderness at the inferior pole of the patella and proximal patellar tendon (Fig. 21-6). Visible localized swelling in the tendon is often present, although this may wax and wane, depending on the current activity of the condition. Firm palpation of the involved tendon will reveal a characteristic spongy crepitant sensation. Resisted knee extension will usually aggravate the pain. Since the condition is extraarticular, the presence of an effusion should prompt the clinician to look for another cause.

The differential diagnosis includes prepatellar bursitis and the various causes of patellofemoral pain, although the characteristic point tenderness of patellar tendinitis will usually make this differentiation clear. Sometimes patellar pain syndromes and patellar tendinitis will occur in the same athlete.

RADIOGRAPHIC EVALUATION

In most cases, plain radiographs will be normal. However, elongation of the distal pole of the patella has been occasionally described.[40] A bone scan may show increased uptake at the distal pole of the patella. Recently, Fritschy and de Gautard have described the ultrasonographic changes seen in the patellar tendon[39] and divided them into three stages.

Stage 1: Pure inflammatory stage. This is the initial stage, characterized by edema of the tendon fibers. The tendon is swollen and thickened, but still presents a homogeneous appearance. This stage appears to be reversible with conservative treatment, but patients are usually past this stage when they present.

Stage 2: Irreversible anatomical lesions. The tendon has a heterogeneous appearance. There are hypoechoic zones corresponding to areas of inflammation, edema, fresh hematoma, or segmental microrupture and hyperechoic zones corresponding to fibrous scar or calcification. The tendinous envelope is more or less well defined but may have a variable appearance.

Stage 3: Final stage. The tendinous envelope is irregular and thickened, and the tendon fibers appear heterogeneous, but the swelling has disappeared. This is normally the picture in cases that have failed conservative treatment.

TREATMENT

The extent of treatment depends on the severity of the condition. Initial treatment includes quadriceps stretching, icing after activity, and eccentric quadriceps strengthening exercises. Curwin and Stanish[38] have reported great success utilizing eccentric strengthening exercises in many types of tendinitis. To load the knee extensor mechanism eccentrically, they describe a program that begins with slow partial squats. Ultimately, this progresses to the "drop and stop" ma-

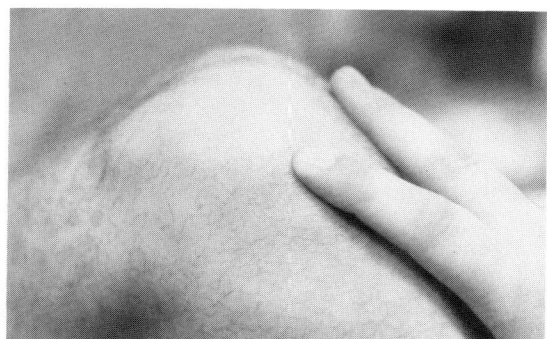

FIGURE 21-6. Patellar tendinitis usually presents with tenderness and often swelling of the proximal patellar tendon.

neuver, during which the athlete drops to a semicrouched position and stops the movement with an eccentric quadriceps contraction. Finally, resistance is added to this program. Because this technique requires considerable supervision, we have substituted eccentric quadriceps exercises using a traditional weight bench or knee extension machine. The athlete is instructed to select a low weight that will be appropriate for one leg. He or she is instructed to raise the weight with both legs but lower it with the involved leg only. This allows the athlete to concentrate the exercise on the eccentric phase of quadriceps action as the weight is being lowered (Fig. 21–7).

As the condition becomes more severe, activity modification may be necessary. The athlete may be forced to establish sports priorities. For example, a varsity athlete may need to give up out-of-season recreational sports to allow his or her knees a chance to recover. Within training sessions, certain offending activities may need to be avoided, or the length of training may have to be reduced. Nonsteroidal antiinflammatory drugs are useful for reducing an acute flare-up and controlling symptoms during the crucial part of the season. However, since the condition tends to be a chronic one, it is recommended that these drugs be reserved for such instances and not be given on a continuous basis. Although they definitely will decrease pain and make the condition more tolerable, they are unlikely to eradicate it once it is well established. Physical therapy techniques including transverse friction massage, ultrasound, or phonophoresis may also be helpful. Steroid injections have been described, but we do not recommend them for fear of contributing to a patellar tendon rupture.

The athlete must realize that patellar tendinitis can be controlled but rarely eradicated. The young athlete may find some slight consolation in the fact that symptoms will normally decrease when he or she retires from intense competition at the end of high school or college. Sometimes the severity of the pain itself will force an early retirement.

Surgery should be considered a treatment of last resort. It is only a consideration for the athlete who is severely disabled and who does not wish to give up competition. Described surgical techniques have varied from exploration of the tendon with excision of degenerated tissue to drilling of the patella and even complete disinsertion and reattachment of the tendon to the patella. The purpose of the surgery is to remove degenerative tissue and create a healing response. We have shied away from actual detachment of the tendon, although it may be a consideration for individuals who have failed to respond to more conservative surgery.

The area of involved tendon may be approached through a transverse or longitudinal incision. We normally place a longitudinal incision on the lateral border of the tendon so that it will not be knelt upon later. The tendon is incised longitudinally completely through its substance in the midline (Fig. 21–8). As noted, it is the deep portion of the tendon that is normally involved. The degenerative areas can normally be distinguished visually by a disorganized and pasty white appearance. Such tissue should be aggressively debrided. Normally, the superficial portion of the tendon is not involved and may be left in place, thus avoiding com-

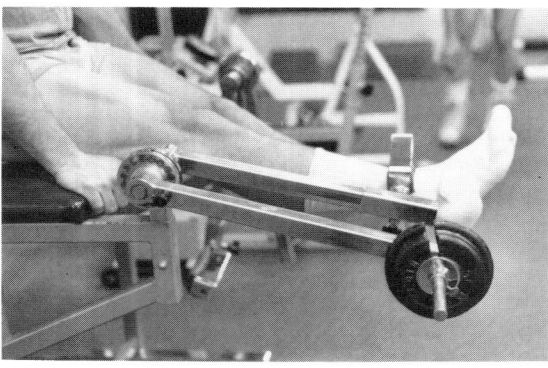
A

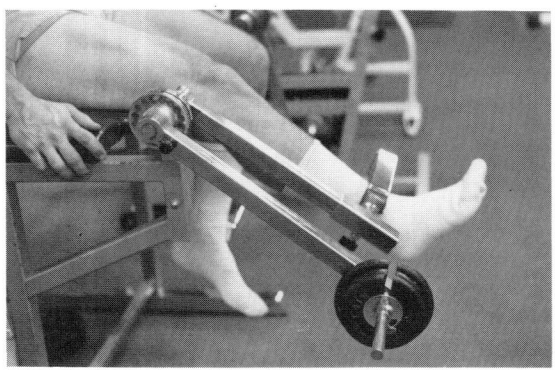
B

FIGURE 21–7. To emphasize eccentric quadriceps work, the athlete is instructed to select a weight appropriate for one leg, then raise it with both legs (*A*) and lower it slowly with the involved leg (*B*).

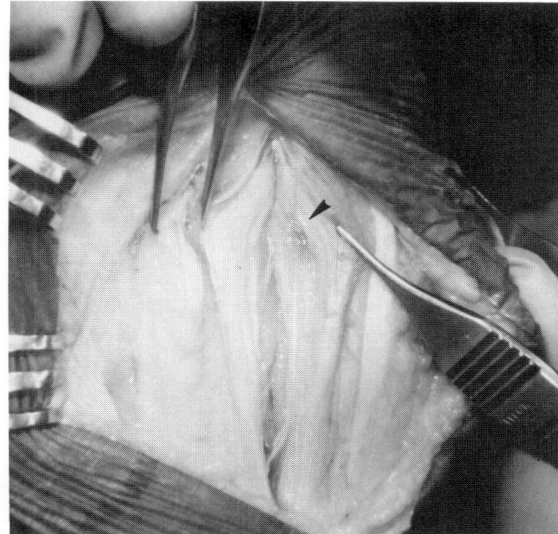

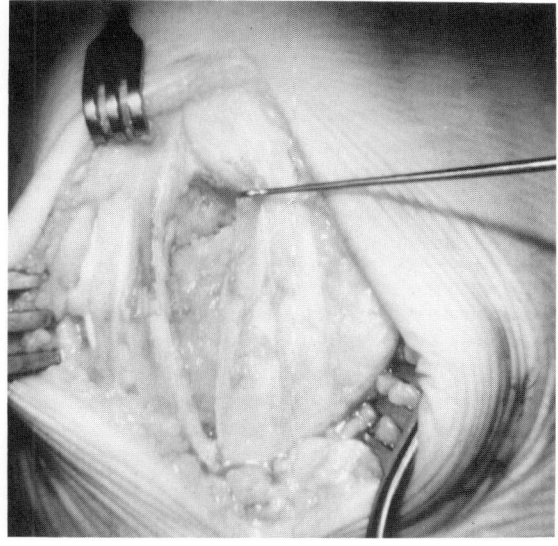

FIGURE 21-8. Exploration of the tendon will reveal areas of degeneration and sometimes macroscopic cyst formation. (A) Surgery includes excising such tissue, incising between fibers to encourage neovascularization, and currettage and drilling of any adjacent bone exposed in the process (B).

plete disinsertion of the tendon. The exposed bone at the tip of the patella should be curretted or rongeured until it is raw and bleeding. Small drill holes may also be used to encourage neovascularization. Additional incisions made between the fibers of the remaining tendon may also encourage vascular ingrowth. Postoperatively, the knee is only immobilized for a few days to discourage bleeding. Unless the tendon is felt to have been severely weakened, weight bearing may be allowed as soon as tolerated. The athlete is allowed to return slowly to eccentric weight training and ultimately sports activities over the next 4 to 6 months. The success rate of this surgery is below that achieved by excision of painful ossicles in cases of Osgood-Schlatter disease or Sinding-Larsen-Johannson disease, emphasizing that these are different conditions. Fritschy and de Gautard[39] have reported success after "carding" the tendon in four of six cases, and it has also been our experience that it succeeds about two thirds of the time. Martens et al. reported 16 excellent, 9 good (slight discomfort after physical activity), and 2 poor results in 27 similar cases.[40] Complete disinsertion and reattachment of the tendon has been described by Blazina et al.[37] and Fritschy and de Gautard[39] as curative in cases that did not respond to more conservative surgery.

References

1. Ogden J. A., Southwick W. O.: Osgood-Schlatter's disease and tibial tuberosity development. Clin Orthop 116:180-189, 1976.
2. Ehrenborg G., Lagergren C.: The normal arterial pattern of tuberosity tibiae in adolescents and growing dogs. Acta Chir Scand 121:500ff, 1961.
3. Cole J. P.: A study of Osgood-Schlatter disease. Surg Gynecol Obstet 65:55-67, 1937.
4. LaZerte G. D., Rapp I. H.: Pathogenesis of Osgood-Schlatter's disease. Am J Pathol 34(4):803-815, 1958.
5. Ehrenborg G., Engfeldt B.: Histologic changes in the Osgood-Schlatter lesion. Acta Chir Scand 121:328-337, 1961.
6. Ehrenborg G., Lagergren C.: Roentgenologic changes in the Osgood-Schlatter lesion. Acta Chir Scand 121:315-327, 1961.
7. Micheli L. J.: The traction apophysitises. Clin Sports Med 6(2):389-404, 1987.
8. Willner P.: Osgood-Schlatter's disease: etiology and treatment. Clin Orthop 62:178-179, 1969.
9. Ehrenborg G.: The Osgood-Schlatter lesion. A clinical study of 170 cases. Acta Chir Scand 124:89, 1962.
10. Kujala U. M., Kvist M., Heinonen O.: Osgood-Schlatter's disease in adolescent athletes. Retrospective study of incidence and duration. Am J Sports Med 13(4):236-241, 1985.
11. Turner M. S.: The effect of tibial torsion on the pathology of the knee. J Bone Joint Surg 63B:396-398, 1981.
12. Crigler N. W., Riddervold H. O.: Soft tissue changes in X-ray diagnosis of the Osgood-Schlatter lesion. Va Med 109:176-178, 1982.

13. Scotti D. M., Sadhu V. K., Heimberg F., O'Hara A. E.: Osgood-Schlatter's disease, an emphasis on soft tissue changes in roentgen diagnosis. Skeletal Radiol 4:21–25, 1979.
14. Woolfrey B. F., Chandler E. F.: Manifestations of Osgood-Schlatter's disease in late teenage and early adulthood. J Bone Joint Surg 42A(2):327–332, 369, 1960.
15. D'Ambrosia R. D., MacDonald G. L.: Pitfalls in the diagnosis of Osgood-Schlatter disease. Clin Orthop 110:206–209, 1975.
16. Ehrenborg G.: The Osgood-Schlatter lesion. A clinical and experimental study. Acta Chir Scand (Suppl) 288:1–36, 1962.
17. Roberts J. M.: Fractures and dislocations of the knee. In Rockwood CA, Wilkins K. E., King R. E. (eds): Fractures in Children. Vol. 3. Philadelphia: JB Lippincott Co, 957–966, 1984.
18. Levine J., Kashyap S.: A new conservative treatment of Osgood-Schlatter disease. Clin Orthop 158:126–128, 1981.
19. Rostron P. K. M., Calver R. F.: Subcutaneous atrophy following methylprednisolone injection in Osgood-Schlatter epiphysitis. J Bone Joint Surg 61A(4):627–628, 1979.
20. Mital M. A., Matza R. A., Cohen J.: The so-called unresolved Osgood-Schlatter lesion. A concept based on fifteen surgically treated lesions. J Bone Joint Surg 62A:732–739, 1980.
21. Cser I., Lenart G. Y.: Surgical management of complaints due to independent bone fragments in Osgood-Schlatter disease (apophysitis of the tuberosity of the tibia). Acta Chir Acad Sci Hung 27(3):169–176, 1986.
22. Thomson J. E. M.: Operative treatment of osteochondritis of the tibial tubercle. J Bone Joint Surg 38A(1):142–148, 1956.
23. Ferciot C. F.: Surgical management of anterior tibial epiphysis. Clin Orthop 5:204–206, 1955.
24. King A. G., Blundell-Jones G.: A surgical procedure for the Osgood-Schlatter lesion. Am J Sports Med 9(4):250–253, 1981.
25. Glynn M. K., Regan B. F.: Surgical treatment of Osgood-Schlatter's disease. J Pediatr Orthop 3:216–219, 1983.
26. Lancourt J. E., Cristini J. A.: Patella alta and patella infera. J Bone Joint Surg 57A(8):1112–1115, 1975.
27. Andrisana A., Mignani G., Mazzetti M.: Long-term results in Osgood-Schlatter's disease. Ital J Orthop Traumatol 11(4):483–486, 1985.
28. Jakob R. P., Von Gumppenberg S., Engelhardt P.: Does Osgood-Schlatter disease influence the position of the patella? J Bone Joint Surg 63B:579–581, 1981.
29. Jeffreys T. E.: Genu recurvatum after Osgood-Schlatter's disease. Report of a case. J Bone Joint Surg 47B:298–299, 1965.
30. Stirling R. I.: Complications of Osgood-Schlatter's disease. J Bone Joint Surg 34B:149–150, 1952.
31. Bowers K. D.: Patellar tendon avulsion as a complication of Osgood-Schlatter's disease. Am J Sports Med 9(6):356–359, 1981.
32. Ogden J. A., Tross R. B., Murphy M. J.: Fractures of the tibial tuberosity in adolescents. J Bone Joint Surg 62A:205–215, 1980.
33. Nimityongskul P., Montague W. L., Anderson L. D.: Avulsion fracture of the tibial tuberosity in late adolescence. J Trauma 28(4):505–509, 1988.
34. Johansson S.: En forut icke beskriven sjukdom i patella. Hygiea 84:161–166, 1922.
35. Sinding-Larsen M. F.: A hitherto unknown affection of the patella in children. Acta Radiol 1:171–173, 1921.
36. Medlar R. C., Lyne D.: Sinding-Larsen-Johansson disease. J Bone Joint Surg 60A(8):1113–1116, 1978.
37. Blazina M. E., Kerlan R. K., Jobe F. W., et al: Jumper's knee. Orthop Clin North Am 4:665–678, 1973.
38. Curwin S., Stanish W. D.: Jumper's knee. In Tendinitis: Its Etiology and Treatment. Lexington, MA: DC Heath & Co, 1984.
39. Fritschy D., de Gautard R.: Jumper's knee and ultrasonography. Am J Sports Med 16:637–650, 1988.
40. Martens M., Wouters P., Burssens A., Mulier J. C.: Patellar tendinitis: pathology and results of treatment. Acta Orthop Scand 53:445–450, 1982.
41. Roels J., Martens M., Mulier J. C., Burssens A.: Patellar tendinitis (jumper's knee). Am J Sports Med 6:362–368, 1978.
42. Insall J., Salvati E.: Patella position in the normal knee joint. Radiology 101:101, 1971.
43. Blackburne J. S., Peel T. E.: A new method of measuring patellar height. J Bone Joint Surg 59B:241–242, 1977.

ANKLE, HINDFOOT, AND MIDFOOT INJURIES

JOHN LARKIN
MICHAEL BRAGE

The ankle represents a highly constrained joint that distributes large forces across a very small surface area. Recent epidemiological studies in school-age children revealed that three of four sports injuries involved the lower extremity.[49] Of these lower extremity injuries, contusion and ankle sprains represent the most common injury involved in competitive and recreational sports.[50] This chapter discusses acute and chronic ankle and foot injuries that are commonly seen in the preadolescent and adolescent athlete. By defining the areas of anatomical weakness and the mechanics of injury, one can understand how the ankle is predisposed to injury and what forces can lead to recurrent injury.

ANATOMY

The bony anatomy of the ankle is composed of three articulations: the tibiotalar, talofibular, and tibiofibular joints (Fig. 22–1). The joint itself is often referred to as a *mortise joint*, owing to its geometric configuration. This term originates from carpentry to describe joinery, in which a square peg is placed into a square hole, increasing stability.[180]

The tibiotalar joint is a domed, wedge-shaped structure with the anterior portion often up to 25 percent wider than the posterior. The talar dome itself is convex, allowing it to fit into the concave surface of the distal tibial plafond. The posterior aspect of the joint is further stabilized by a small lip on the distal tibia that overhangs the posterior talus. Maximum stability occurs in dorsiflexion as the talus locks into the anterior portion of the distal tibia. Stability of the ankle is further increased owing to the joint's wedge shape. Stability decreases in plantar flexion as the narrow portion of the posterior talus rolls forward into the wider anterior tibia. Stability in this position is ligamentous rather than bony. This predisposes the ankle to ligamentous sprains in plantar flexion.

In addition, the bony support of the ankle is greater on the lateral side than the medial side. On the lateral aspect, the fibula extends down to the level of the subtalar joint. It functions as a bony buttress against the talus distally and laterally. The medial joint is not protected in this manner. With an inversion stress, the ankle collapses medially, resulting in stress of the lateral ligaments and secondary injury.

MEDIAL LIGAMENTS

The medial aspect of the ankle is stabilized by the deltoid or medial collateral ligament. This is a fan-shaped structure with both a superficial and deep component. The superficial portion is composed of four ligaments consisting of the tibionavicular, tibiocalcaneal, and anterior and posterior tibiotalar

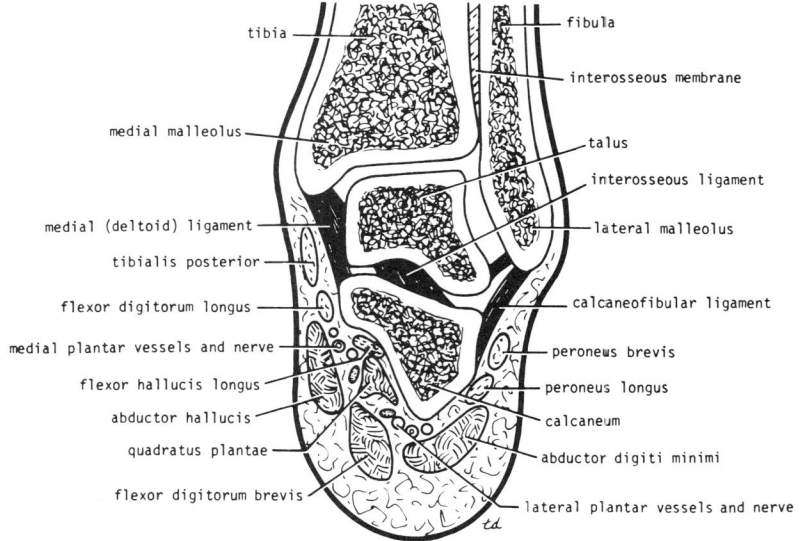

FIGURE 22–1. Right ankle as seen from posterior aspect in coronal section. (From Snell RS: Clinical Anatomy for Medical Students. Ed 2. Boston, Little, Brown & Co, Inc, p. 564, 1981.)

ligaments (Fig. 22–2). The deep portion is a transverse ligamentous connection running between the medial malleolus and the underlying talus. The principle function of the deltoid is to limit eversion. As a secondary function, it restricts external rotation.

Isolated tears of the superficial deltoid occur often with supination-external rotation injuries. However, an isolated tear of the deep ligament is rare. This is particularly true in a skeletally immature individual where supination-external rotation injuries can result in injury to the distal tibial physis.

The deep portion of the deltoid functions to prevent lateral subluxation of the talus. If torn, the deep ligament can impinge within the medial joint space. This results in widening of the medial joint, which may be seen on a mortise view radiograph. (Fig. 22–3).

LATERAL LIGAMENTS

The lateral ligament complex of the ankle functions to bind the fibula to the talus and calcaneus. The lateral complex is composed

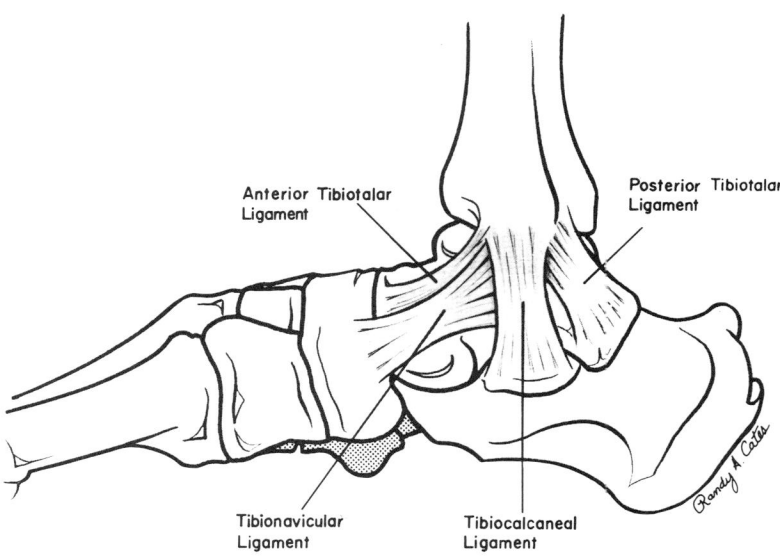

FIGURE 22–2. Medial aspect of the ankle showing deltoid ligament complex. The superficial portion of the deltoid ligament is composed of four ligaments: tibionavicular, tibiocalcaneal, and anterior and posterior tibiotalar ligaments. (From Leach RE, Schepsis AA: Acute injuries to the ligaments of the ankle. In Evarts CM (ed): Surgery of the Musculoskeletal System. New York Churchill Livingstone, p. 8:145, 1983.)

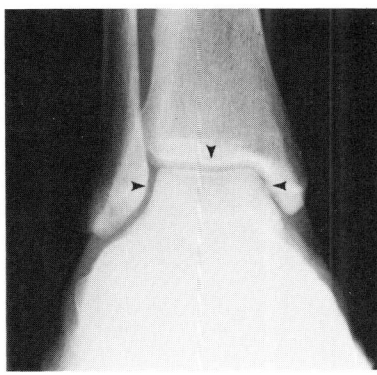

FIGURE 22-3. Mortise view radiograph demonstrating symmetrical tibial plafond. No more than 2 mm of difference between the joint spaces should be present on an intact mortise.

of three ligaments: the anterior talofibular ligament, the calcaneofibular ligament, and the posterior talofibular ligament (Fig. 22-4).

The anterior talofibular ligament is within the ankle capsule. It runs along the anterior border of the distal fibula to the lateral neck of the talus. Tension within the anterior talofibular ligament varies with ankle position. It is slack in dorsiflexion and tightest in plantar flexion. It functions to limit internal rotation and inversion of the talus. Since it is tightest in plantar flexion, its principle stabilizing effects are seen in this position. Although the anterior talofibular ligament anatomically is the broadest of the three lateral collateral ligaments, it is the weakest.

The calcaneofibular ligament is extracapsular, running from the distal lateral fibula to the lateral aspect of the calcaneus. It forms the floor of the peroneal tendon sheath. The ligament spans both the tibiotalar and the subtalar joints. It functions in plantar flexion as a secondary stabilizer to assist the anterior talofibular ligament. In dorsiflexion, it tightens to limit talar and calcaneal inversion. Isolated tears of the calcaneal fibular ligament

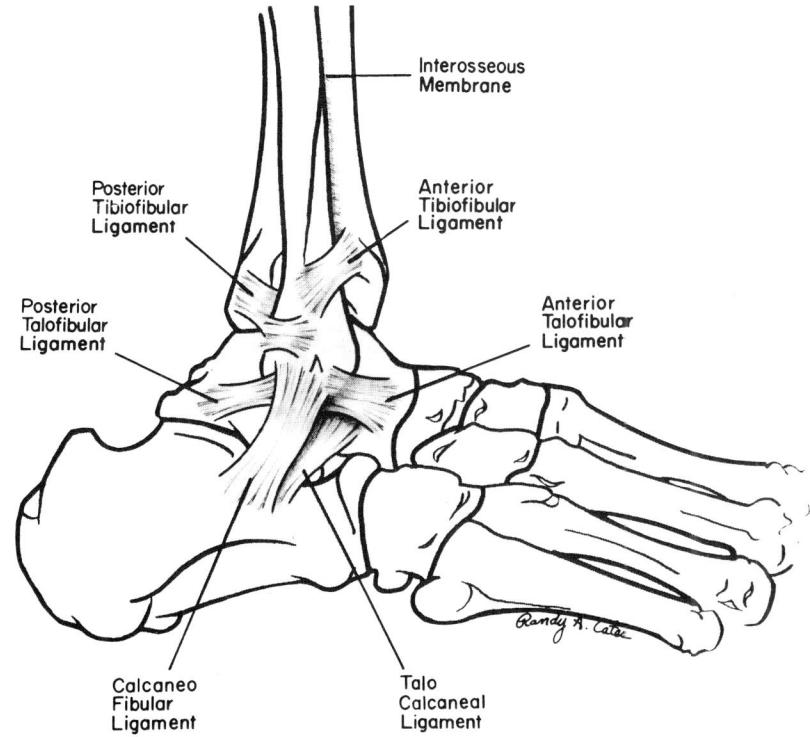

FIGURE 22-4. Lateral ligaments, composed of the anterior talofibular ligament, the calcaneofibular ligament, and the posterior talofibular ligament. (From Leach RE, Schepsis AA: Acute injuries to the ligaments of the ankle. p 8:144 In Evarts CM (ed): Surgery of the Musculoskeletal System. New York, Churchill Livingstone, p. 8:144, 1983.)

have not been reported. Most injuries of this ligament occur in association with anterior talofibular ligament disruption.[43]

The posterior talofibular ligament runs from the posterior fibular fossa to the posterior portion of the talus attaching to the lateral tubercle of the calcaneus. This ligament is the strongest of the three lateral joint ligaments and functions primarily to limit dorsiflexion.

A fourth structure, the talocalcaneal ligament, is also present.[94] This ligament in reality blends with the anterior talofibular ligament, originating on the anterior talus and running across the subtalar joint to insert on the calcaneus. It is on occasion mentioned in lateral reconstruction procedures of the ankle. Functionally, it is included in the anterior talofibular ligament, and injuries to it occur by the same mechanism as those of the anterior talofibular.

Although some authors consider the syndesmotic complex as part of the lateral ligaments, we will consider it separately. The syndesmotic complex is composed of four ligaments anchoring the fibula to the tibia (Fig. 22–5). The distal tibia is grooved along its lateral margin to allow recession of the distal fibula. The strongest connection is via the interosseous ligament, which attaches adjacent surfaces of the tibia and fibula. This represents the distal extension of the interosseous membrane between the tibia and fibula. Overlying the anterior and posterior ridge of the fibula are the anterior and posterior tibiofibular ligaments. Posteriorly, the inferior transverse ligament lies distal to the posterior tibiofibular ligament and represents the fourth ligament of the syndesmotic complex. These ligaments not only anchor the fibula to the tibia but also allow distal fibular rotation during gait.

BIOMECHANICS

Human gait is divided into two phases, *stance* and *swing*. In walking, the stance phase encompasses 60 percent of the total gait cycle, with the swing phase composing the remaining 40 percent.[67] The gait cycle, during walking, runs from heel strike to heel strike on the same extremity and lasts approximately 1 second.[103, 104, 126]

The stance phase consists of heel strike, foot flat, heel rise, and toe off. Swing is divided into acceleration, toe clearance, and deceleration[67, 126] (Fig. 22–6). As walking speed increases, the time spent in swing phase increases, and there is a corresponding decrease in stance. The loss of time in stance decreases the length of time spent in single foot support. During walking, at least one foot, at any given time, remains on the ground. With running, "float" develops, in which both feet are off the ground simultaneously.[7] As speed increases and float develops, forces across the ankle and foot increase.[105]

Initial heel strike during walking gait results in forces of approximately 80 percent of body weight across the ankle (tibiotalar) joint. Twenty percent of this force is directed anteriorly as a shear force. One third of the way through the gait cycle, the swinging leg passes the contralateral planted foot and heel rise begins to occur.

As the heel rises, forces are shifted anteriorly onto the ball of the foot. The load then rolls along the medial aspect of the foot, passing between the first and second metatarsal

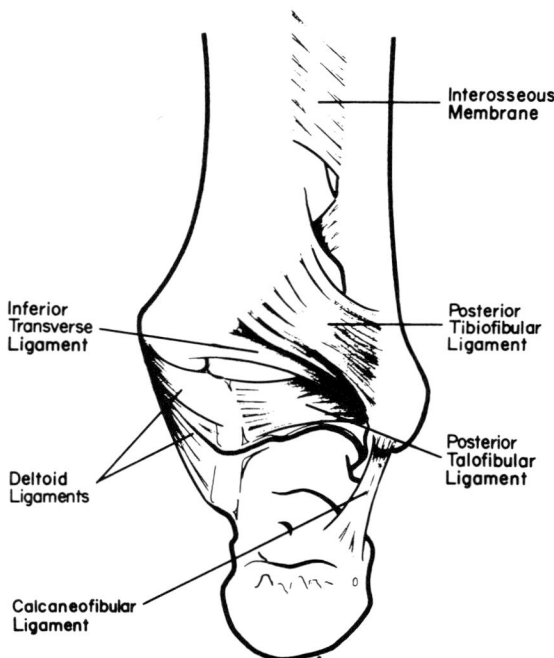

FIGURE 22–5. The syndesmotic complex as viewed posteriorly. It is composed of four ligaments: the interosseous ligament, the inferior transverse ligament, and the anterior and posterior tibiofibular ligaments. (From Leach RE, Schepsis AA: Acute injuries to the ligaments of the ankle. In Evarts CM (ed): Surgery of the Musculoskeletal System. New York, Churchill Livingstone, p. 8:144, 1983.)

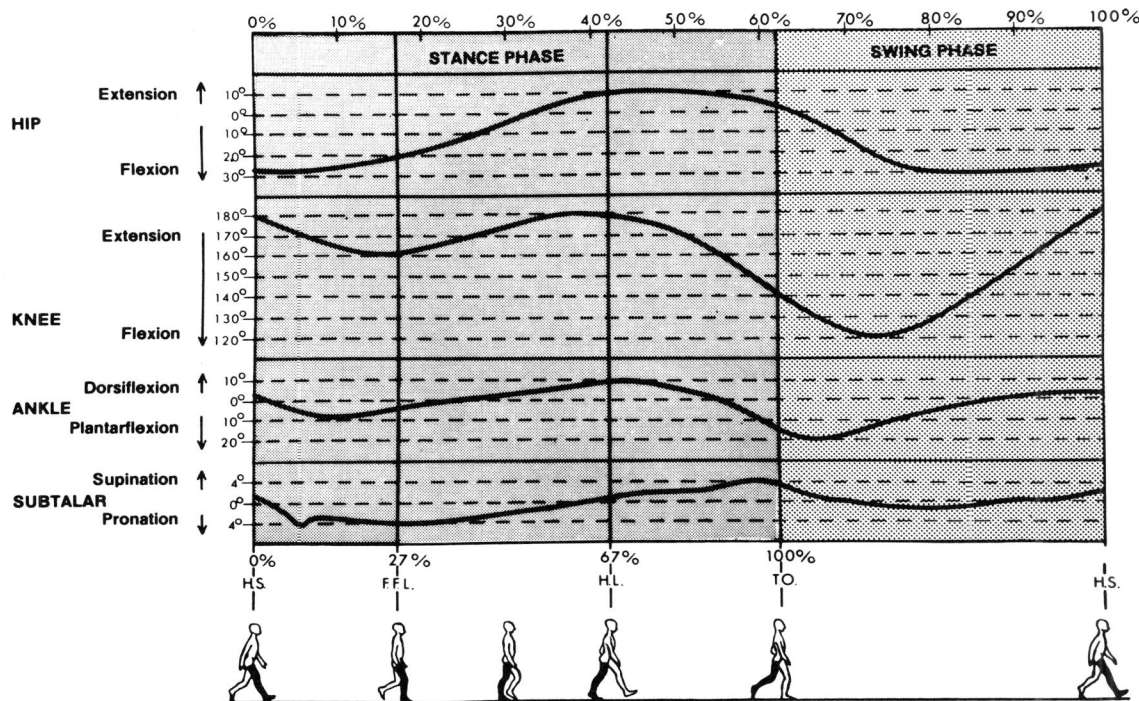

FIGURE 22–6. The gait cycle composed of stance phase (60 percent) and swing phase (40 percent). Stance consists of heel strike, foot flat, heel rise, toe off. Swing is composed of acceleration, toe clearance, and deceleration. From Root ML, Orien, WP Weed JH: Normal and Abnormal Function of the Foot. Los Angles Clinical Biochemics Corp., p. 145, 1977.

heads. Just before toe off, vertical loading on the ball of the foot increases up to 120 percent of the body weight. These forces are multiplied with running. Vertical forces with running are 2.5 to 3 times that of normal walking, occurring in one fifth of the time of stance phase.[98]

Clinically, maximum forces are loaded onto the ball of the foot prior to toe off. The ankle is in plantar flexion, where its principle support is limited to muscle and ligamentous structures. In this position, it is most unstable, and it is here that maximum loading is occurring. One can now see why injuries to the ankle occur during this phase of gait.

To allow ground contact to occur, the foot must undergo plantar flexion to become flat. Once the foot is flat, the tibia begins to rotate externally. The load shifts anteriorly, rolling toward the metatarsal heads. As the tibia externally rotates, the talus dorsiflexes and supinates. This results in locking of the transverse tarsal joint or midfoot. The transverse tarsal joint (Chopart's joint) must lock to allow weight to be transferred distally onto the ball of the foot. This is often referred to as the "screw home" mechanism. In addition, as the foot is shifted into a vertical position, it must become rigid to support the body's weight.

Clinically, this is important in a runner with a hyperpronated foot. With forefoot hyperpronation, the normal screw home mechanism that occurs from supination to pronation across the subtalar joint is prevented. This decreases the impact-absorbing capacity of the hind foot, placing increased stress across the midfoot. This may lead to midfoot pain and degeneration of the talonavicular joint.

The cavus foot, on the other hand, prevents adequate pronation. Without pronation, the midfoot does not lock at the transverse tarsal joint. The midtarsal joint therefore remains flexible. Stresses are distributed onto the midfoot, often leading to stress fractures most commonly seen in the navicular. Failure of forefoot rigidity has also been associated with distal metatarsal stress fractures, commonly seen in the second metatarsal of long-distance runners.

LIGAMENTOUS STABILITY OF THE ANKLE

Ligament stability varies with foot position. The anterior talofibular ligament tightens with plantar flexion and is slack in dorsiflexion (Fig. 22–7). With plantar flexion, the anterior talofibular ligament works primarily to resist inversion forces and internal rotation of the talus. The calcaneofibular ligament functions primarily in dorsiflexion. In this position, it assumes a near vertical alignment, functioning as a true collateral ligament. In plantar flexion, the calcaneofibular ligament rotates approximately 90 degrees into a more horizontal position (Fig. 22–7). Although it does help in preventing internal rotation of the talus in plantar flexion, it is primarily a secondary restraint to the anterior talofibular ligament for resisting talar inversion.[68] As the foot comes into dorsiflexion, the anterior talofibular ligament moves into a horizontal position, allowing the calcaneofibular ligament to become the primary restraint to talar inversion.

If an ankle is plantar flexed at the time it sustains an inversion stress, the principle ligament injured is the anterior talofibular. Inversion injuries, occurring when the foot is plantar flexed, represent the most common mechanism of ankle injury. Since this is the position in which the anterior talofibular ligament is under maximum tension, it follows that this represents the most commonly injured ligament in ankle sprains.

It is rare that forced inversion occurs when the ankle is in dorsiflexion.[68] In these rare cases, involvement of the calcaneofibular ligament may be more extensive. It should be reemphasized, however, that isolated tears of the calcaneofibular ligament without injury to the anterior talofibular ligament have not been reported.[43]

The posterior talofibular ligament is the strongest of the three lateral collateral ligaments. Although some authors have suggested its strength protects it from injury, in reality it is rare that this ligament is placed under maximum stress.[1, 3] Stress on the posterior talofibular ligament occurs with the ankle in dorsiflexion and inversion. This is also where stress is placed primarily on the calcaneofibular ligament. Like the calcaneofibular ligament, no isolated cases of posterior talofibular ligament disruption have been recorded in the literature. It is probable that the posterior talofibular ligament is protected by its anatomical position, preventing it from injury.

ANKLE SPRAINS

Garrick and Requa evaluated over 15,000 participants in 19 sports seen in a sports medicine office practice. These athletes competed at the high school, college, and recreational level. Foot and ankle injuries constituted 25 percent of all injuries.[50] In an attempt to ascertain type and frequency of ankle injuries in high school, Garrick and Requa studied 2,840 high school athletes in 14 sports. These individuals sustained 1,176 injuries, of which 14 percent involved the ankle. Thus, 1 in 17 high school athletes suffered an ankle injury; 85 percent of these injuries were sprains, and four out of five sprains involved the lateral ankle.[50]

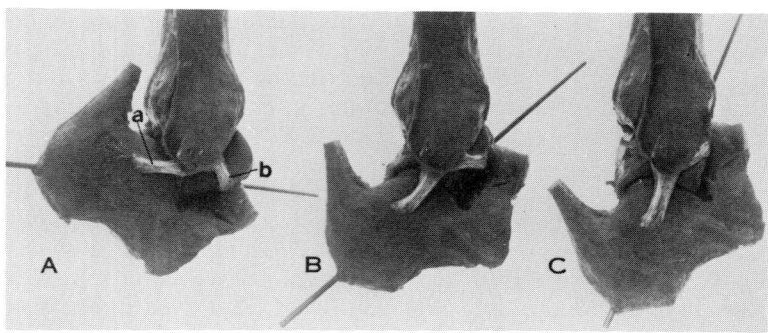

FIGURE 22–7. *a*, Anterior talofibular ligament; *b*, calcaneofibular ligament. (*A*) Ankle plantar flexion revealing maximum tension in the anterior talofibular ligament. The calcaneofibular ligament is shifted into a horizontal position. (*B*) Neutral position. (*C*) Ankle dorsiflexion revealing maximum tension on the calcaneofibular ligament. The anterior talofibular ligament shifts into a horizontal position. (From Inman VT: The Joints of the Ankle. Baltimore, Williams & Wilkins, p. 70, 1976.)

LATERAL ANKLE SPRAINS

Lateral ankle injuries typically result from an inversion stress in which the foot rolls under the ankle. Sports that require a cleated shoe often allow the foot to become planted to the ground and the body rotates over it. In most cases, the ankle is plantarflexed, which results in loss of bony stability as previously discussed. Only the ligaments and contracting muscles remain to resist the loading inversion force. If the peroneal muscles cannot resist the load, the ligaments are progressively loaded, often to failure.

Common mechanisms of injury include cutting, where push-off of the opposite foot places inversion stress on the plantarflexed foot, or landing on the foot that is slightly inverted at ground contact. Landing on an irregular surface may also result in the foot buckling under the ankle.

The patient may describe a "snap" or "crack" associated with severe pain and inability to weight bear. In general, the less weight that can be borne, the more serious the injury. Initial evaluation of ankle injuries must assess neurovascular status, with palpation of pulses (dorsalis pedis and posterior tibial) along with capillary refill and sensation. Bony tenderness may indicate a nondisplaced fracture.

Sprains are commonly classified as first, second, and third degree. In first-degree sprains, the ligament is partially torn, but no instability of the ankle is present on exam. Second-degree sprains result in further disruption of the ligament and may show increased laxity in the ankle. Functional integrity, however, is maintained. A third-degree sprain is the result of complete ligament disruption, and functional integrity of the ligament is lost.

The most common sprain of the ankle is a partial tear of the anterior talofibular ligament. This is a lateral injury resulting from an inversion stress. As noted, the anterior talofibular ligament is the primary stabilizer of the lateral ankle in plantar flexion. It is under maximum tension in a vertical position. The calcaneofibular ligament is shifted into a horizontal position in plantar flexion. It functions as a secondary stabilizer to resist inversion of the talus and calcaneus. With inversion stress, injury occurs first to the anterior talofibular ligament and then to the calcaneofibular ligament. Partial injuries to the anterior talofibular ligament do not lead to instability of the ankle; however, complete disruption may increase anterior translation, as demonstrated by the anterior drawer examination.

The anterior drawer examination demonstrates ankle instability by allowing the talus to sublux forward out of the mortise. It is performed by direct pressure from behind the heel with the foot in plantar flexion. (Fig. 22–8). The foot is pulled forward while the tibia is stabilized. Normal anterior excursion in the ankle is less than 5 mm. Cadaver experiments have shown anterior translation of 8 to 10 mm when the anterior talofibular ligament alone is sectioned. Up to 15 mm of increased anterior translation may be seen by sectioning all three ligaments (anterior talofibular, calcaneofibular, and posterior talofibular).[19] The anterior drawer examination must be performed in a relaxed patient. Comparison between the involved and noninvolved ankle is essential because of anatomical variability among individuals.

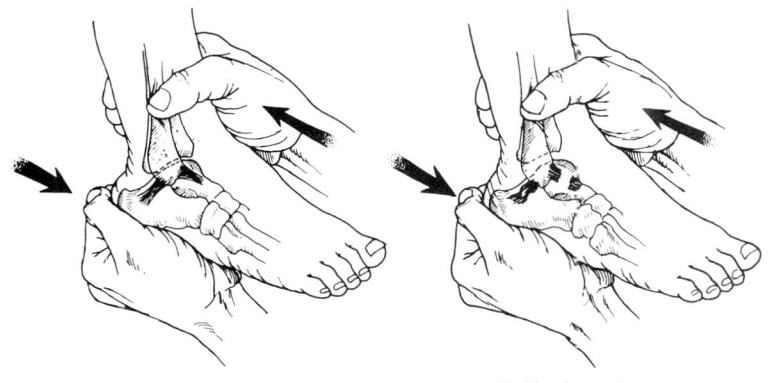

FIGURE 22–8. The anterior drawer examination. Increased anterior translation is seen as the talus subluxes forward out of the tibial plafond. (From Ellison, AE (ed): Athletic Training and Sports Medicine. Chicago, American Academy of Orthopaedic Surgeons, p. 318, 1984.)

Positive drawer sign

Anterior talofibular ankle sprains show tenderness in the region of the anterior talofibular ligament, often with ecchymosis distally and laterally. Injuries involving both the anterior talofibular and calcaneofibular ligaments occur commonly with internal rotation. The foot may be twisted during a football pileup or struck by an oncoming soccer player and twisted around the ankle.

Radiographic Findings

Routine radiographs include anteriorposterior, mortise views, lateral views, and inversion stress views. Stress radiographs demonstrating talar tilt have been described as one method to measure instability of the lateral ligaments. However, considerable variability exists as to the normal range of talar tilt.[31, 92, 161] Measurements between 0 and 25 degrees have been reported to be normal.[146] In addition, talar displacement can be blocked by muscle contraction evoked by pain.[98] Without anesthesia, both reliability and sensitivity of stress radiographs remain questionable. With appropriate anesthesia, whether applied locally or regionally, most authors would agree that a total talar tilt of 20 degrees or 10 degrees more than the uninjured side is consistent with a double ligament tear involving both the anterior talofibular ligament and calcaneofibular ligament (Fig. 22–9). Stress films should be done with the foot in internal rotation of 15 to 20 degrees, with inversion stress applied by heel grasp.

Ankle arthrography has been recommended by some as a diagnostic modality for ankle injuries.[33, 34] Disruption of the anterior talofibular ligament results in extravasation of dye into the anterior aspect of the lateral malleolus. This is best seen on AP radiographs. Involvement of the calcaneofibular ligament allows posterior dye extravasation, often tracking up the peroneal tendon sheaths, since the calcaneofibular ligament forms the floor of the peroneal tendon tunnel. Diagnosis of calcaneofibular ligament tears, however, may not be made if a large capsular tear accompanies the injury. In this case, dye extravasates out the capsular rent anteriorly and laterally before being forced up the peroneal tendon sheaths. At present, no arthrographic findings have been described for posterior talofibular ligament disruption. Because of variability of the exam, especially in the acute setting, we find ankle arthrography

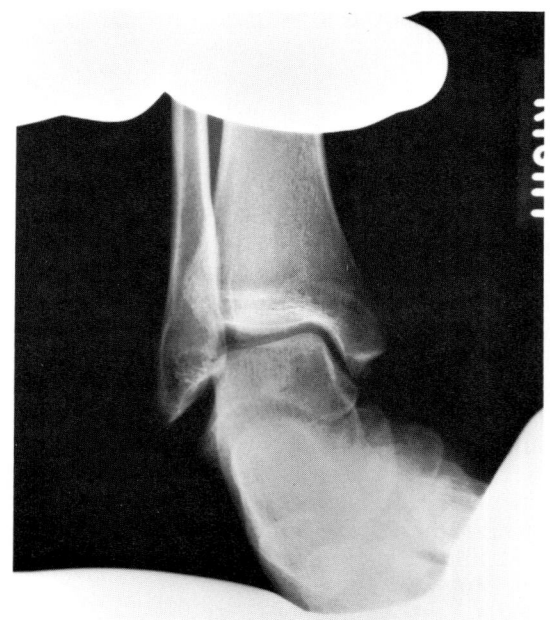

FIGURE 22–9. Stress radiographs demonstrating increased talar tilt. Ten degrees greater than the uninjured side or a total talar tilt of 20 degrees is considered evidence of injury to the anterior talofibular and calcaneofibular ligaments.

offers little additional information and is rarely indicated.

Treatment

Described treatments of lateral ankle sprains range from early mobilization with compressive dressings to primary repair.[37, 42, 46, 47, 59, 96, 122, 163, 166] Injuries showing no evidence of increased laxity of the ankle, either by anterior drawer examination or increased talar tilt radiographically, can be treated with a program of early return to weight bearing. In the acute setting, the overall goal is to decrease tissue edema and inflammation. Two methods, cryotherapy and compressive dressings, are used to minimize edema and swelling along with decreasing the inflammatory response. In the acute setting, cryotherapy, using a Jobst cryocompressive boot, is applied for 20 minutes three times a day. In settings where this device is not available, ice can be utilized but should not be placed directly on the exposed skin. In general, a maximum of 20 minutes of icing is recommended in order to prevent burning of the skin. Ice functions to decrease the inflammatory response and stimulates

ANKLE, HINDFOOT, AND MIDFOOT INJURIES

TABLE 22–1. Rehabilitation Protocol for Ankle Sprains

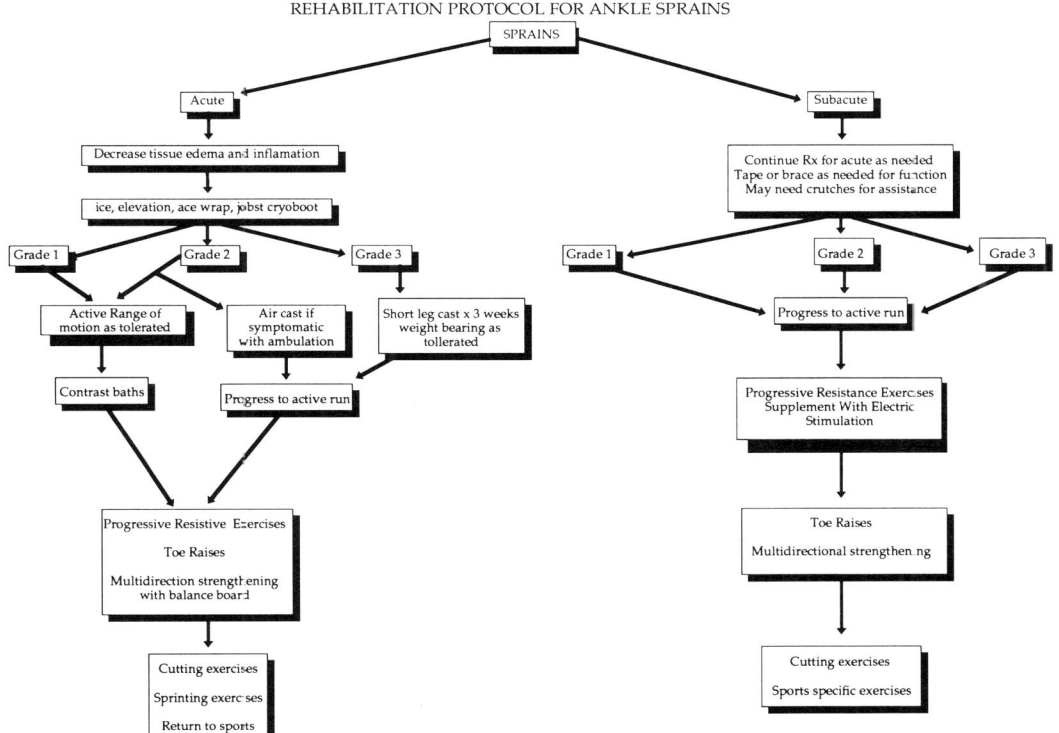

vasculature constriction, decreasing tissue edema. It is also beneficial from its anesthetic point in decreasing sensitivity to pain. The use of cryotherapy has been shown to be effective in yielding early recovery and return to activity.[65] Compressive dressings to minimize edema consist of an elastic bandage that is reinforced, depending on extent of injury, by an external air stirrup. We have found that the use of an Air Cast in the acute setting often allows earlier return to weight bearing without discomfort. The use of an assistive device such as an Air Cast prevents further injury until muscular strength is restored, allowing better ankle control and stability. (Table 22–1).

For grade I and grade II injuries, active range of motion followed by progressive resistance emphasizing the peroneal musculature is begun. Exercise is progressed within the limits of pain tolerance. At approximately 3 to 5 days, as swelling begins to resolve, contrast baths are begun, with range-of-motion (ROM) exercises encouraged in the whirlpool. The alteration of hot and cold contrast baths can be helpful in reestablishing vasomotor tone and decreasing edema. Gait training stresses normal heel to toe gait. As the normal pattern of gait returns, gait speed is increased.

As pain tolerance permits, strength training is advanced from isometric strengthening to progressive resistive exercises stressing the peroneal musculature laterally and the posterior tibial musculature medially. Toe raises against gravity are begun once the patient is able to control inversion and eversion of the foot in the plantar-flexed position. Multidirectional strength training is now commenced, beginning with multipositional isometrics emphasizing the posterior tibial and peroneal musculature. We have found that the use of the balance board is extremely effective in retraining multidirectional strength and proprioception. It is initially utilized with both feet, emphasizing unidirectional strengthening, specifically concentrating laterally if it is a lateral injury or medially if it is a medial sprain. This is then progressed to unilateral strengthening with one leg extended on the board and the other in a flexed non–weight-bearing position. Routine workout usually involves approximately 10 minutes per day until stability is demonstrated independently with the board.

By this time, range of motion should be painless and gait training has progressed from a jog to sprinting. Cutting exercises are begun with walking turns initially and progressed to running-cutting maneuvers. Unilateral toe raises on an incline are helpful in further strengthening the peroneal musculatures and enhancing cutting strength.

Once sprinting is tolerated, sports-specific exercises are begun. We have found the use of the hop test to be extremely effective in assessing one's ability to return to sport participation. The patient initially begins in a bilateral hop program on a 20-foot runway. This is then progressed to a unilateral vertical hop and ultimately to a unilateral horizontal hop. We require approximately 80 percent or greater return of strength in the injured extremity compared with the uninjured limb prior to return to sports.

With grade III ankle sprains, which demonstrate increased anterior ankle laxity as shown by an anterior drawer examination, or increased talar tilt demonstrated radiographically, initial immobilization is recommended. A short leg cast is utilized with the foot in neutral or in slight eversion. Weight bearing in the cast is encouraged within the limits of pain and swelling. At 3 weeks, the cast is removed and the rehabilitation program previously described begun. The use of limited immobilization is recommended at 3 weeks owing to the effects of disuse on the biomechanical properties of ligaments.[124, 125]

Injuries to the peroneal and posterior tibial nerves have been associated with lateral inversion ankle sprains. Nitz et al. showed that 17 percent of patients with grade II and up to 86 percent of grade III lateral ankle sprains may have an associated peroneal nerve injury. In addition, 10 percent of grade II sprains and 83 percent of grade III sprains show some posterior tibial nerve denervation.[123] These injuries were thought to be secondary to nerve traction at the time of initial inversion sprain. For this reason, our ankle rehabilitation program strongly emphasizes both peroneal and posterior tibial musculature strengthening to allow return to full vocational or competitive sports (Table 22–1).

Surgical Treatment

Although some authors have recommended surgical intervention for lateral ligament tears, conservative treatment with early rehabilitation remains our mainstay.[136, 150] The use of surgical repair in acute lateral ankle injuries has shown no greater long-term functional benefit compared with closed treatment.[42, 87] For chronic recurrent lateral ankle sprains that demonstrate clinical instability as shown by the anterior drawer examination and radiographic instability as seen by increased talar tilt, surgery may be indicated. These are individuals who suffer recurrent sprains despite extensive rehabilitation. In this group of patients, lateral reconstruction using the Chrisman-Snook operation provides an excellent anatomical reconstruction with good long-term functional results.[158]

We recommend Chrisman's own modification, which routes the tendon graft through a tunnel in the calcaneus rather than just subperiosteally as originally described (Fig. 22–10). The lateral malleolus and peroneal tendons are exposed with a longitudinal incision just posterior to the fibula, which curves distally toward the base of the fifth metatarsal while protecting the sural nerve. The peroneus brevis is identified and divided in half longitudinally as far proximal as possible. This should be done carefully so that a strong tendon is left for the peroneus brevis and yet a strong graft is obtained. A tunnel is made through the fibula in an AP direction at the level of the plafond using a cannulated reamer. A curved tunnel is made in the lateral calcaneus posterior and inferior to the lateral malleolus by aiming two oblique drill holes so that they converge within the body of calcaneus and enlarging the connection with a curved curette. These tunnels should be situated so that the resultant path of the graft mimics the anterior talo-fibular ligament (ATFL) and calcaneo fibular (CFL) ligament as closely as possible.

The free end of the tendon segment is secured with a Bunnell suture and threaded through both tunnels. A malleable wire loop is particularly helpful for pulling the tendon through the curved tunnel in the calcaneus.

It is extremely important to set the tension in each limb of the reconstruction separately to avoid overrestricting motion. The anterior limb is then tensioned with the ankle in full plantar flexion and slight eversion and the graft sutured to soft tissue where it enters and exits the fibula as well as to any remnants of the ATFL. The posterior limb is tensioned in a similar manner with the ankle in full dorsiflexion and slight eversion and sutured to both ends of the calcaneal tunnel. This limb also reconstructs the peroneal retinaculum. When tensioned in this fashion, the procedure will produce an ATFL substitute that is tight in plantar flexion and a CFL substitute that is tight in dorsiflexion. Overtightening these ligaments will lead to unnecessary overrestriction of motion. Some surgeons eschew the Chrisman-Snook procedure for fear of weakening the peroneus brevis or overrestricting motion. Although these are not normally a functional problem, the surgeon may wish to consider delayed primary repair of the ankle ligaments as described by

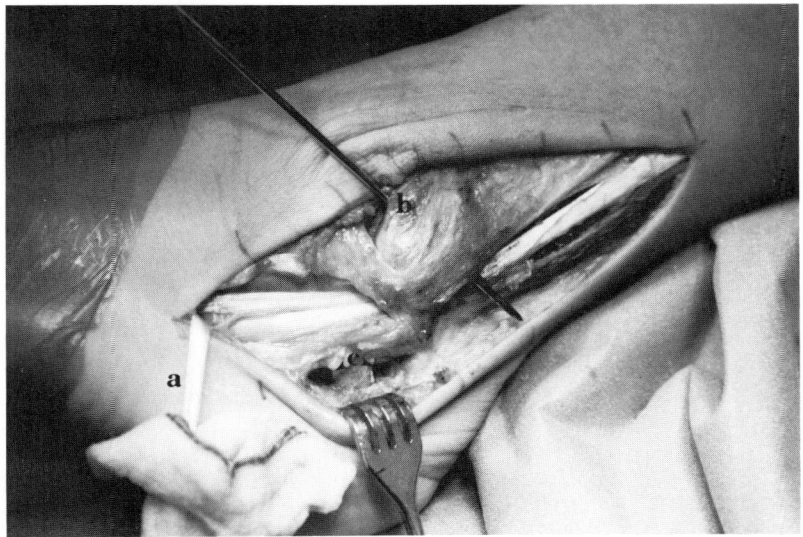

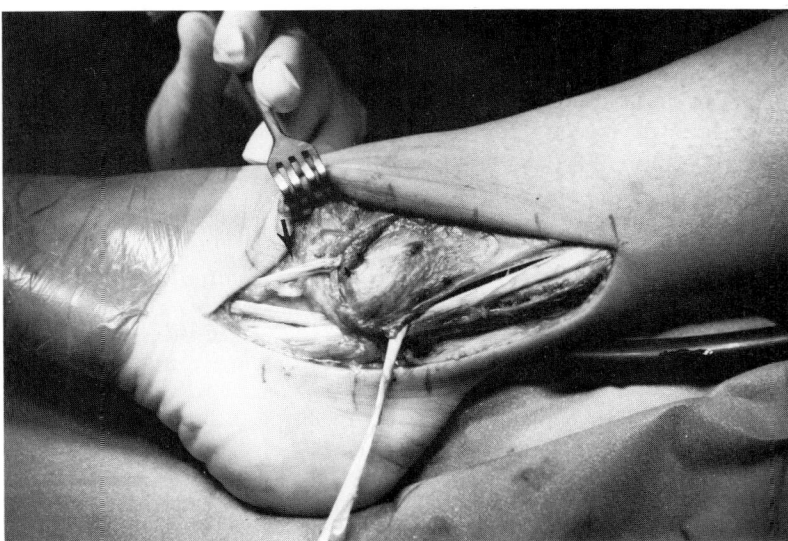

FIGURE 22–10. (*A*) The modified Chrisman-Snook ankle reconstruction routes one half of the peroneus brevis tendon (*a*) through tunnels in the distal fibula (*b*) and calcaneus (*c*). (*B*) The tension on the anterior limb is set when the ankle is maximally plantar flexed, and

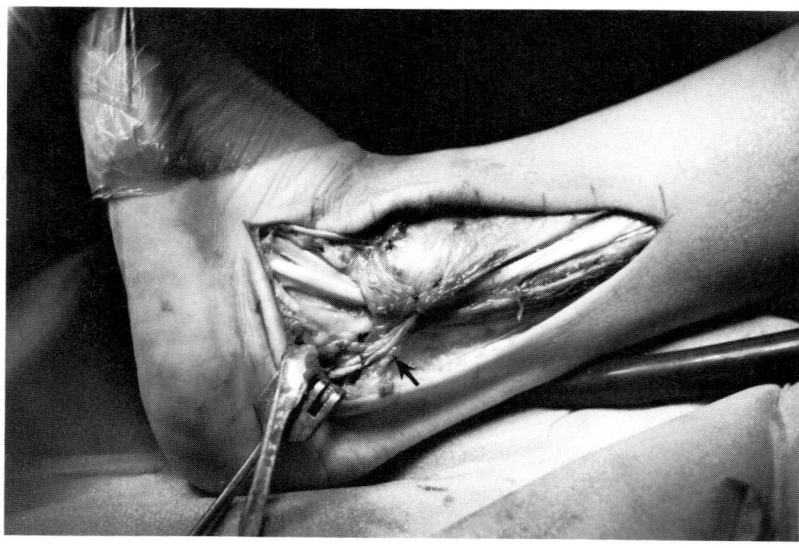

FIGURE 22-10. *Continued* (C) the tension on the posterior limb is set when the ankel is maximally dorsiflexed.

Brostrom et al.[13] in patients such as ballerinas for whom peroneal strength is particularly crucial (see Chapter 27).

MEDIAL ANKLE SPRAINS

Medial injuries in the skeletally immature patient that involve the deltoid ligament are rare without an associated tibial malleolar fracture. After skeletal maturity, isolated deltoid ligament injuries are still rare and usually have an associated injury to the lateral ankle ligaments. Injuries in the adolescent school-age athlete generally result from an external rotation force with the foot in neutral. In football, this most commonly occurs during a pileup, when an eversion stress with the foot in plantar flexion is not uncommon. Wrestlers also seem predisposed, owing to their wide-based stance, resulting in increased eversion stress while attempting to gain traction.[43] Most medial injuries in this population result in superficial deltoid ligament tears without underlying deep deltoid involvement. Ankle instability is not a problem.

Involvement of the deep deltoid is a severe injury and is almost uniformly associated with more extensive lateral injury, either ligamentous or bony. Ligamentous disruption of the syndesmosis usually occurs with external rotation. As the syndesmosis tears, the forces of external rotation are transmitted more proximally, resulting in a proximal fibular fracture as originally described by Maisonneuve (Fig. 22–11). Medial injuries should always include radiographs up to the level of the knee to prevent missing this fracture. In a skeletally immature athlete, these forces may result in a fracture of Tillaux, which is described later.

Isolated syndesmotic sprains are rare; most involve a deltoid ligament injury. Symptoms of syndesmotic injury include tenderness anteriorly and posteriorly along the distal tibiofibular joint (Fig. 22–12). The anterior talofibular ligament and calcaneal ligament usually are nontender. Pain with compression of both malleoli may be found, along with pain up the syndesmosis with ankle dorsiflexion.

If the ankle mortise is symmetrical on the AP mortise radiograph, treatment is symptomatic. The RICE principle of rest, ice, compression, and elevation is the general rule. A posterior splint may be used for comfort during the first week. Early weight bearing with crutches to assist in ambulation is recommended. Our standard ankle rehabilitation program as described for lateral ankle sprains is begun within the limits of pain tolerance. Emphasis with medial sprains, however, is on strengthening of the posterior tibial mus-

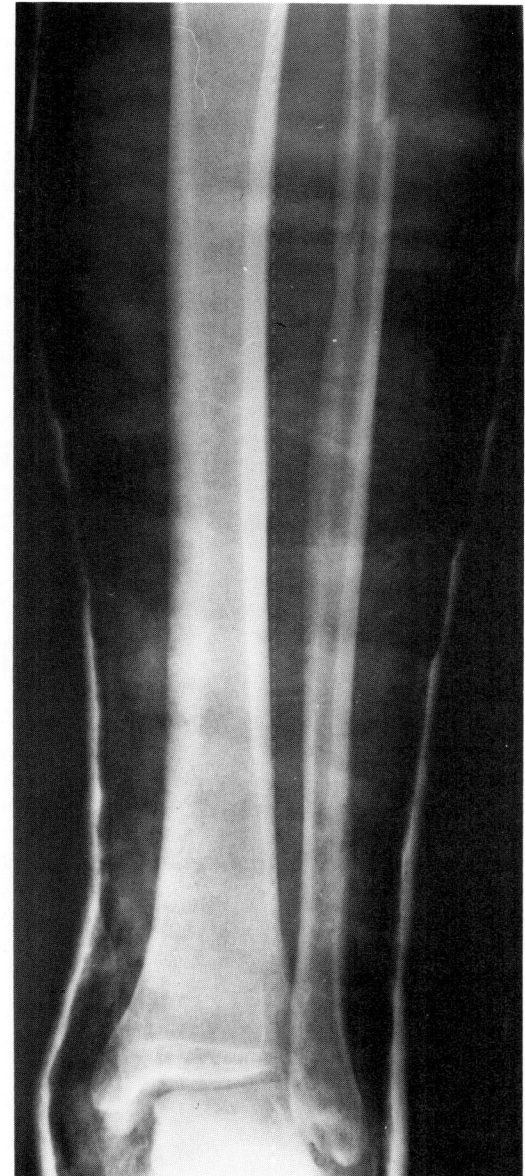

FIGURE 22–11. The Maisonneuve fracture in which the syndesmosis is torn, leading to proximal fibular fracture and deltoid ligament tear.

of greater than 4 mm medially between the talus and medial malleolus suggests deltoid ligament injury.[52] When disrupted, the tibiofibular syndesmosis must be reapproximated using a syndesmotic screw. This is a fully threaded cortical screw and should incorporate both tibial cortices. It is placed across the tibiofibular joint and should not be lagged, as this can result in narrowing of the anterior ankle mortise with resultant loss of ankle dorsiflexion. In most cases, this restores ankle mortise symmetry. Although recent reports indicate that early weight bearing with the syndesmotic screw is not harmful, we recommend non–weight-bearing ambulation for a full 6-week interval.[36, 44, 100, 114, 121] Once wound healing is complete, ROM exercises are begun, maintaining a non–weight-bearing status. At 6 weeks, the screw is removed under local anesthesia and progressive weight bearing commenced.

Controversy remains as to whether surgical intervention is necessary to fix the torn deltoid. Some authors have suggested that operative repair of the deltoid ligament allows stronger ligament healing. Long-term follow-up of the deltoid injuries treated conservatively once the syndesmosis injury has been reapproximated have shown no difference from primary open deltoid repair.[50] We therefore favor closed treatment if the mortise is symmetrically reduced following stabilization of an associated lateral fracture or syndesmosis injury.

If attempts at reduction fail to restore medial ankle symmetry once the lateral column has been reconstructed, deltoid ligament impingement within the medial mortise should be suspected. This warrants operative intervention to reduce the ankle mortise. Repair is by primary apposition of the torn deep and

culature, progressing to a multidirectional strengthening program including the peroneal musculature, along with dorsiflexion and plantar flexion.

In more severe injuries, lateral subluxation of the talus may result from medial deltoid ligament tears and syndesmosis disruption and/or fracture of the fibula. Lateral subluxation of the talus is demonstrated by widening of the medial mortise joint. Overall widening

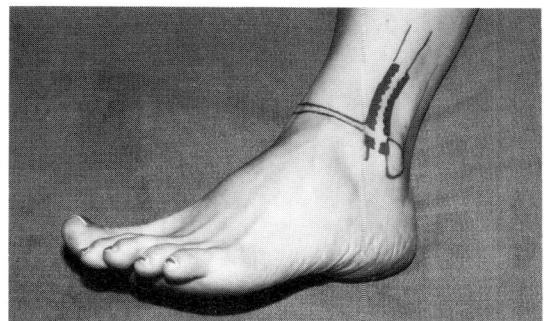

FIGURE 22–12. Syndesmotic injury results in tenderness anteriorly and posteriorly along the distal tibiofibular joint.

superficial deltoid ligament once it is removed from the medial ankle mortise.

Chronic medial ligament instability is rare unless corresponding lateral instability is present. Most chronic instability problems demonstrate radiographic medial widening associated with lateral talar subluxation. Reconstruction of the lateral column generally reduces the talus, resulting in a symmetrical mortise joint.

PERSISTENT PAIN FOLLOWING ANKLE SPRAIN

Chronic, persistent ankle pain only occurs after a small percentage of ankle sprains. However, since ankle sprains are so common, this clinical problem is not rare.

Depending on the severity of the original injury, most athletes with grade I or II ankle sprains are able to return to sports within 1 to 4 weeks of injury, although the ankle may be sore for months. Persistence of pain that is severe enough to prevent sports participation 6 weeks after the original injury warrants a clinical reassessment. Significant swelling is a cause for concern, especially if there is a band of swelling across the front of the ankle joint, indicating an effusion or intraarticular synovitis, rather than only over the injured ligaments. Radiographs should be repeated to look for a problem that might not have been seen on the first set of films, such as osteochondral fracture of the talar dome, fractured os trigonum, subtalar joint injury, or avulsion fractures with impingement of the fracture fragment (Fig. 22–13). If the patient is having recurrent injuries, rather than persistent pain, then persistent muscle weakness, ligamentous instability, or peroneal tendon instability are possible diagnoses.

Most of these ankles will continue to have normal radiographs and presumably have persistent local irritation or synovitis from small chondral fractures or impingement of torn ligament fibers. Many of these cases will improve with continued rest and nonsteroidal antiinflammatories (NSAIDS). If rehabilitation has not been adequate, then additional resistance exercises should be pursued.

Persistent disabling pain and swelling for 3 to 6 months following the initial injury warrants consideration for arthroscopy or surgical exploration. The exact length of conservative treatment will depend on the severity of the symptoms and the ability to identify a specific cause for the pain.

Many patients sustain small avulsion fractures in conjunction with an ankle sprain, and most of these become asymptomatic. Persistent pain despite treatment with NSAIDS with point tenderness directly over a radiographically visible avulsion fragment that corresponds to the site of the patient's pain will usually respond well to excision of

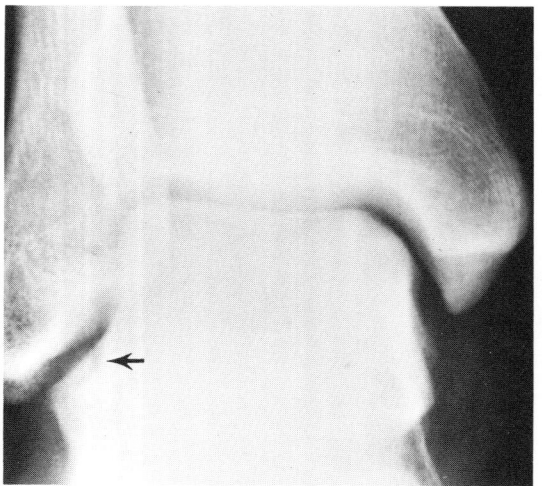
A

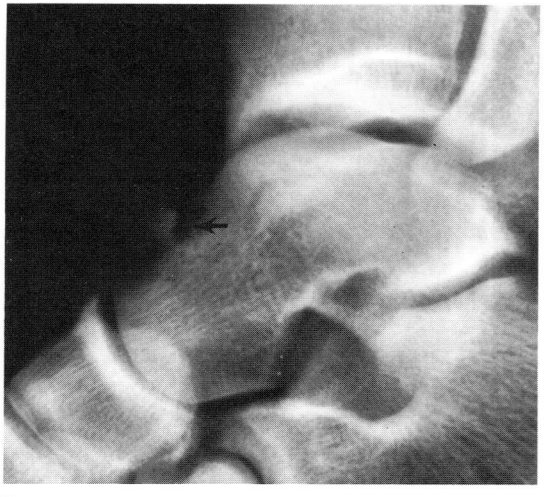
B

FIGURE 22–13. Avulsion fragments such as these may sometimes impinge and cause persistent pain following ankle sprains.

the fragment. Some of these fragments are intraarticular and can be removed arthroscopically; many are firmly attached to the piece of capsule or ligament that avulsed them and are easier to identify and remove directly via a small incision under local anesthesia. Sometimes these fragments can only be seen on radiographs taken from exactly the right angle, so the findings of point tenderness should prompt a careful radiographic search for such a fragment.

Arthroscopy is the procedure of choice for persistent swelling and pain in the absence of specific bony fragments. We have not found arthrography or computerized tomography to be helpful in these cases. We have not used magnetic resonance imaging (MRI) for them, but it so far has not been a good test for detecting small chondral fragments in the knee. Intraarticular anesthetic injection may be used as a diagnostic test to confirm that the symptoms are indeed intraarticular; we have not found intraarticular steroids to provide more than transient relief.

Occasionally, arthroscopy will reveal a significant chondral fragment that was radiolucent. More commonly, the area of tenderness corresponds to impingement of torn ligament ends or occasionally synovial fronds. Limited debridement of these tissues, if they correspond to the site of the patient's pain and tenderness, will yield substantial improvement or resolution in most cases.

TENDINITIS

Tendinitis represents an overuse injury of the dense connective tissue that composes a tendon. *Tenosynovitis, bursitis,* and *tendinitis* are often used interchangeably and incorrectly. Bursitis is an inflammation of a synovial sac that most commonly is interposed between skin and an underlying bone or tendon. Tenosynovitis is an inflammation of the synovial lining of the tendon sheath that encloses a tendon; not all tendons have a sheath. Tendinitis is an actual injury of the tendon itself related to overload failure.

Tendons are relatively avascular structures with a low metabolic turnover.[144] Tendinitis usually results from chronic repetitive trauma that leads to microscopic and even macroscopic tears. These tears cause an inflammatory response with the influx of inflammatory cells from both peritendinous tissues and within the tendon itself. The inflammatory response usually is present within the first 3 days of injury.[144]

The young athlete is most commonly affected at the site of tendon insertion into the bone. This often is in an area where the bone has a growth plate and is referred to as an apophysis. Differentiation of an apophysitis of the bone and tendinitis is often difficult. In reality, this is often a moot point since treatment for either an apophysitis or tendinitis will be the same.

As previously stated, overuse is the primary etiology of tendinitis. Most originate from trauma caused by eccentric overload. This occurs when the extremity or joint is decelerating. The tendon is placed on stretch when its muscle is contracting to slow down the extremity or resist the load of contact with the ground.

ACHILLES TENDINITIS

Achilles tendinitis does occur in the young athlete, although its incidence is much less than in the adult population. In the skeletally immature, the Achilles tendon inserts into the calcaneal apophysis. With overloading, apophysitis of the posterior calcaneus (Sever's disease) often develops before the body of the tendon becomes inflamed. Tendinitis of the Achilles is common, however, with skeletal maturity. In sports, it represents 20 percent of all cases of tendinitis involving the foot and ankle.[48, 97] In running athletes, it has been associated with up to 11 percent of all injuries.[72]

Inflammation of a tendon results from either improper biomechanics or overuse. In most cases, it is a combination of both. Foot deformities, such as forefoot pronation or excessive heel varus, increase the work the Achilles must perform. With excessive heel varus, the Achilles is placed on increased stretch along its lateral insertion site into the apophysis of the calcaneus. Repetitive trauma results in microtears within the tendon and secondary inflammation and tendinitis, or microfractures in the calcaneal apophysis with secondary apophysitis.

The primary clinical finding is tenderness along the tendon insertion. Signs of acute tendinitis may also include erythema or warmth along the tendon, although this is less common. In runners, findings of tight heel cords and hamstring muscles may be present. Limited ankle dorsiflexion is a frequent physical finding in long-distance runners. Pain initially presents after running but tends to become progressive, eventually occurring with walking or long periods of standing in chronic cases. Palpable crepitation may be felt as the ankle is taken through its range of motion in long-standing cases.

Risk factors leading to Achilles tendinitis include training errors, primarily resulting from "too much, too soon," which is common in runners who increase their distance at too rapid a pace. Running on uneven surfaces, especially hills, may also be a common etiology. Frequently, the runner travels a similar course with one leg always on the outside of a banked surface. Finally, and most frequently, inadequate warm-up without heel cord stretching contributes to this injury.

Athletic shoes may contribute to the problem of Achilles tendinitis. Shoes with inadequate heel counters or soft counters often lead to recurrent inflammation of the tendon insertion. In addition, a shoe with a "negative cant" in which the heel is lower than the toe increases stretch on the Achilles principally during midstance and push-off.

Treatment of Achilles Tendinitis

Initial treatment for most tendinitis involves rest. This is the key in the adolescent population. Initial treatment includes the use of a $\frac{3}{4}$-inch heel lift to decrease stretch across the Achilles tendon. To decrease inflammation, antiinflammatories are recommended for a 10-day initial course. In younger children, buffered aspirin or tolmetin can be used.[115] Modalities used in physical therapy consist of phonophoresis on either side of the tendon along with icing.

The approach to treatment should be to determine the etiology to prevent recurrence. If heel varus results in medial shortening with increased stretch laterally, then orthotics are prescribed to correct the heel into a neutral position.

Initially, stretching of the gastrocnemius and soleus muscles is begun with the knee flexed, then progressed to a straight knee stretching program. Emphasis is also placed on hamstring musculature stretching to address the entire lower extremity. Strengthening including concentric and eccentric training is utilized for both the anterior and posterior musculature.

In runners, attention to the running surface is important. Initial return to running is on a flat, even surface, with care taken to prevent running against hills or banked surfaces. Optimally, running is begun on a cedar track and progressed to a hard surface. Initially, interval running is recommended with an intervening day of rest between outings. If symptoms remain absent, milage is progressively increased in 20 percent increments.

SEVER'S DISEASE

Calcaneal aphophysitis represents an inflammation of the open calcaneal growth plate (Fig. 22-14). It is thought to occur owing to traction on the apophysis of the os calcis. In runners, strong shearing forces result across the calcaneal apophysis owing to the plantar fascia and triceps surae.[141] Symptoms include pain over the posterior calcaneus near the insertion site of the Achilles tendon. Soft tissue swelling and induration may be present. Initial onset of symptoms occurs with running activity and presents early in the season. Presentation is primarily in the 8- to 13-year-old age group.[171] This is a common injury associated with soccer players, especially those athletes playing on artificial surfaces.

Risk factors leading to Sever's disease include tight heel cords, internal tibial torsion, and forefoot varus or pronation. Forefoot pronation results in increased contact forces at heel strike owing to restricted subtalar joint pronation. In most patients, radiographs are unremarkable. In severe cases, however, fragmentation with sclerosis of the apophysis can occur. Treatment is primarily symptomatic. Use of a $\frac{1}{2}$- to $\frac{3}{4}$-inch height heel wedge (posterior to anterior) is recommended. In cases of forefoot varus or pronation, orthotics represent the mainstay of treatment. Physical therapy consists of a posterior strengthening program along with triceps surae and hamstring stretching. In recalcitrant cases, casting in neutral may be used for 1 to 2 weeks, followed by an aggressive physical therapy program.

PERONEAL TENDINITIS

The peroneal tendons function as strong ankle evertors and weak plantar flexors of the

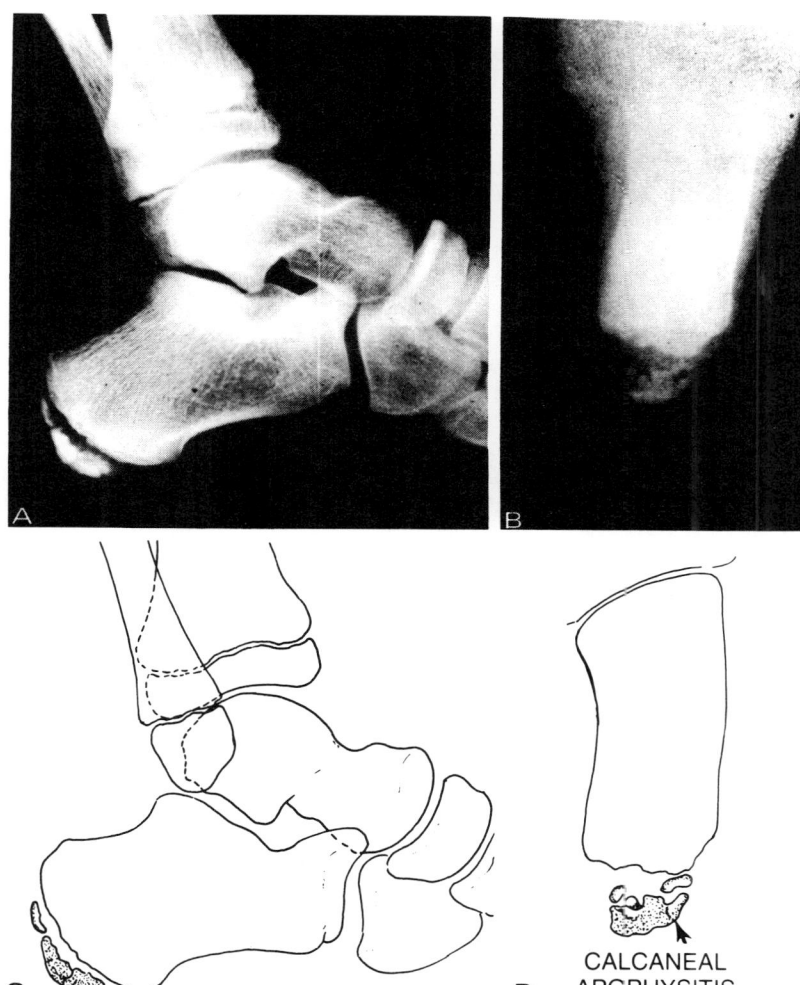

FIGURE 22–14. Sever's apophysitis. Revealing fragmentation of the posterior calcaneal apophysis resulting in posterior heel pain. (From Kelikian H: Disorders of the Ankle. Philadelphia, WB Saunders Co, p. 121, 1985.)

foot. They provide lateral stability to the ankle primarily during the stance phase of gait.[48] Individually the peroneus brevis provides an abduction force to the base of the fifth metatarsal, and the peroneus longus exerts a plantar flexion force to the first metatarsal–cuneiform joint.

The tendons run in a shallow groove on the posteroinferior surface of the distal fibula.[40, 60] In this groove, the retrofibular sulcus barely accommodates the peroneus brevis. The peroneus longus lies behind it. The tendons are held in place by the superior peroneal retinaculum, which with the fibula forms an osteofibrous tunnel for the tendons. Tendinitis results from recurrent friction and stress on the tendons as they run around the posterior fibula.

In most cases, the forefoot of these patients is pronated and the heel is in valgus or everted. The abnormal heel valgus results in increased tension on the tendons owing to the pulley effect around the distal fibula. Maximum stress occurs as the forefoot pronates to allow the foot to become flat in midstance. Recurrent stress results in microtears in the tendons, leading to tendinitis. Peroneal tendinitis is most common in long-distance and cross-country runners. It may, however, occur during the rehabilitation of lateral ankle sprains, since most rehabilitation programs stress strengthening of the peroneal musculature.

Symptoms are characterized by pain along the peroneal tendon sheath just posterior to the lateral malleolus. Associated signs may include swelling and tenderness. The pain may be aggravated by dorsiflexion of the first metatarsal, as this places the peroneal longus tendon on stretch. These symptoms may be chronic in nature or recurrent and relapsing, presenting like a lateral ankle sprain.

Treatment is aimed at correcting the heel valgus to prevent undue eversion of the calcaneus. Strong support of the second through fifth metatarsal heads in alignment with the hind foot is recommended. This allows the first metatarsal to remain in a relaxed plantar flexed position, preventing overcontraction of the peroneal longus as the foot rolls toward toe off. If heel valgus is prominent, orthotics to correct the hind foot to neutral are used. During the initial acute phase, nonsteroidal antiinflammatory medication may be employed, usually for the first 10 days of treatment.

PERONEAL TENDON INSTABILITY

Dislocation or subluxation of the peroneal tendons should always be included in the differential diagnosis of chronic lateral ankle pain. Because this represents an uncommon injury, the diagnosis is often missed. The proposed initial mechanism of injury is one of forced dorsiflexion of the foot associated with forceful contraction of the peroneal muscles.[64, 149, 169] This mechanism may occur during skiing, when both ski tips catch in the snow and the skier is pitched forward, producing a forced dorsiflexion of the ankle. As the peroneal musculature contracts, disruption of the superior retinaculum occurs with dislocation of the peroneal tendons over the lateral malleolus.[117, 120, 186] Peroneal tendon dislocation can also occur in football or basketball when the foot becomes planted or caught and the player is thrown forward with a resultant sudden violent dorsiflexion of the ankle.

Three grades of injury have been described. Grade I consists of separation of the retinaculum from the tip of the lateral malleolus. In grade II, the peroneus brevis pulls off the distal 1 to 2 cm of the superior peroneal retinaculum. Finally, in grade III, a thin, shell-like avulsion fracture of the distal lateral malleolus occurs that remains attached to the deep peroneal retinaculum and fascia.[39] In all grades, the superior retinaculum is torn from its fibular attachment. Radiographically, soft tissue swelling is usually seen. However, in grade III injuries, the small, shelllike fracture of the posterior fibula is sometimes visualized along the lateral ankle.[21]

Diagnosis of peroneal dislocations is often difficult in the acute setting. Swelling, ecchymosis, and pain along the lateral malleolus usually prevent adequate examination. Commonly, an ankle sprain is suspected when the radiographs are normal. Once swelling and ecchymosis resolve, the athlete may complain of a recurrent snapping or "pop" along the lateral malleolus, followed by a sense of giving way. On occasion, a snap may be heard or felt.[169]

Treatment of acute injuries remains conservative. Splinting or casting using taping with a crescent-shaped felt pad to hold the tendons reduced is recommended. Generally, 6 weeks of protected immobilization is required.[112] Chronic injuries, however, do not respond to conservative modalities, and surgical treatment is utilized.[135] Most of these chronic lesions represent grade II and III injuries. The surgical treatments fall into four categories: (1) periosteal flap procedures, (2) tendon slings, (3) rerouting procedures, and (4) bone block reconstruction.

Periosteal flap reconstruction uses a small flap of periosteum to create a pedicle that is sewn posteriorly over the displaced peroneal tendons.[149, 186] A posterior tendon sling was first proposed by Jones, using a portion of the Achilles tendon.[75] Rerouting procedures place the peroneal tendon under the reconstructed calcaneal fibular ligament. One disadvantage of the rerouting procedures is the required division of either the peroneal tendons or the calcaneofibular ligament to allow reconstruction.[149] The original bone block procedure was first described in 1920 and at present has undergone numerous modifications.[83] It is usually performed by creating a posterior sliding wedge from the distal fibula, which functions to deepen the peroneal groove.[60, 99] Other operations deepen the tendon groove by cutting a trough in the posterior fibular sulcus.[186] So far, no comparative series with a sufficient number of cases and long-term follow-up has shown one procedure to be beneficial over another.

However, we have found the Thompson procedure described by Zoellner and Clancy to be effective while not sacrificing any important structure or requiring internal fixation (Fig. 22–15).[186] This operation utilizes a trap-door osteoplasty of the posterior fibula

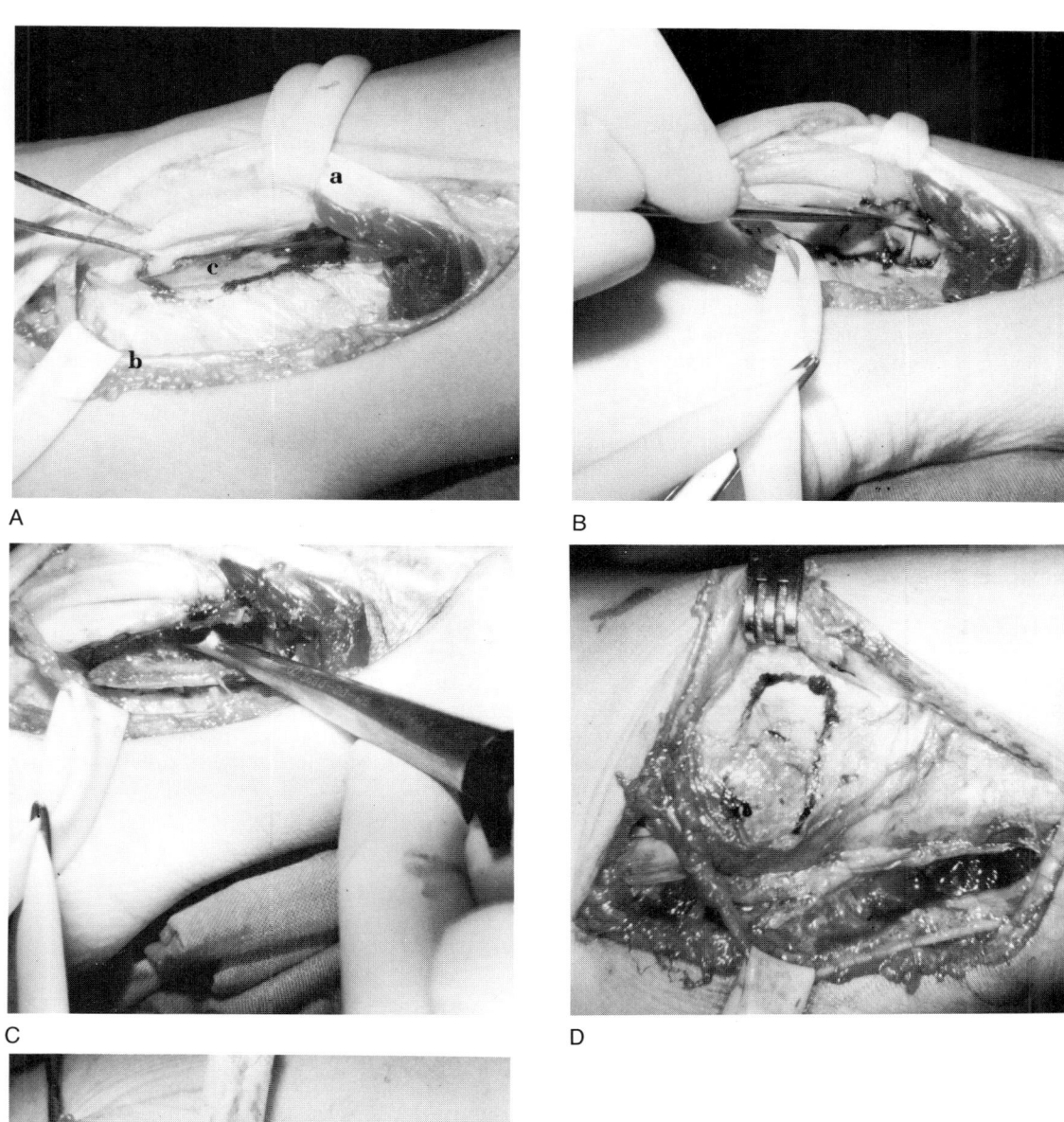

FIGURE 22-15. Thompson peroneal tendon stabilization as described by Zoellner and Clancy. (*A*) The peroneal tendons (*a*) are retracted anteriorly, and the sural verve (*b*) is protected. A trap door (*c*) is outlined on the posterior distal fibula. (*B*) The cortex is fully incised laterally, superiorly, and distally and perforated medially. (*C*) The trap door is hinged on its posterior edge. The underlying cancellous bone is curetted away, and the trap door is tamped back down, creating a deeper peroneal tendon groove. The tendons are relocated. (*D*) A flap of fibular periosteum is outlined. (*E*) It is carefully elevated, reflected posteriorly, and sewn to the adjacent deep tissue to create a new peroneal retinaculum.

to deepen the peroneal groove and reconstructs the retinaculum with a strip of periosteum from the lateral malleolus.

The peroneal tendons are approached through a longitudinal incision just posterior to the fibula, with care to protect the sural nerve. Whatever retinaculum remains is detached posteriorly to allow anterior dislocation of the peroneal tendons. A rectangle about 1 cm wide extending about 4 cm proximal to the tip is drawn on the posterior fibula. The fibular cortex is then incised along the superior, lateral, and inferior sides of the rectangle with an osteotome, and the medial side is perforated in postage stamp fashion using the corner of a small osteotome. The rectangle is elevated on the medial hinge and the underlying cancellous bone removed with a curette and rongeur. The rectangle of cortex is then sunk back in its original bed using a bone tamp, thus creating a deep peroneal groove with a smooth surface. An oblique strip of periosteum is then carefully elevated from the lateral surface of the distal fibula and reflected over the relocated tendons to create a new retinaculum. It is anchored firmly to the adjacent periosteum at both ends using resorbable sutures along with any remnants of the original retinaculum. The foot is immobilized in dorsiflexion and inversion for 2 weeks to use the peroneal tendons to help hold the trap door in place, then recasted in a neutral position for 4 more weeks.

POSTERIOR TIBIAL TENDINITIS

Not uncommon in the school-age athlete is posterior tibial tendinitis.[148] Symptoms consist of pain along the posterior tibial insertion onto the navicular, often tracking proximally to the medial malleolus. These symptoms are aggravated by placing the posterior tibial tendon on stretch via resisted inversion. In most cases, excessive forefoot pronation is seen, or flexible flat foot. Most athletes are involved in track, usually long-distance or cross-country. Pain may radiate proximally up into the medial calf. Although much has been written regarding acute rupture of the tibialis posterior tendon, it is a rare problem in adolescent sports.[58, 73]

Treatment of Posterior Tibial Tendinitis

Initial treatment involves rest and attention to medial arch support. We have found the use of over-the-counter shoe inserts, such as the Sorbathane or Spenco medial arch support, to be beneficial. Some Spenco can be heated and molded to the foot, which is especially helpful to runners who show evidence of increased forefoot pronation. If moderate or severe pronation is present in the forefoot, the patient most likely will need a custom-made orthotic for long-term use.

Physical therapy concentrates on both concentric and eccentric strengthening of the posterior tibialis musculature. A home program using surgical tubing for stretching of the posterior leg musculature is utilized. This is progressed to inversion and eversion resistance exercises using surgical tubing. As pain resolves, progressive resistive exercises are then begun along with a balance board strengthening program.

Attention to sports-specific problems, such as running, includes examination of the runner's surface. Posterior tibial tendinitis is often the result of a running surface that is too hard such as asphalt or concrete. If the athlete is training on a sloped track, the runner should alternate directions, running first in a clockwise and then a counterclockwise fashion to prevent recurrent eversion stress along the medial ankle. As pain resolves, distance is progressively increased.

CHRONIC ANKLE PAIN

THE ACCESSORY NAVICULAR BONE

Numerous supernumerary ossicles have been described in the foot and ankle. Approximately 22 percent of children less than 16 years of age demonstrate an accessory bone in the foot on plain radiographs.[153] Although most are clinically insignificant, an exception is the accessory navicular bone, which may be a source of medial ankle pain in young athletes.

First described by Bauhin in 1605, the accessory navicular is complicated by its multiplicity of names in the English literature. Terms such as *os externum tibiale, pre hallux, accessory scaphoid,* and *tarsal naviculari* are a few examples.[184] Estimates of the overall incidence of this bone vary between 2 and 14 percent.[10, 38, 55]

The accessory navicular is considered a congenital variant and has been shown to develop from a separate ossification center at the tuberosity of the navicular bone. Frequently, it fuses with the navicular in adolescents. It may be bilateral and can occur in a bifid form.

The accessory navicular is located at the medial end of the tarsal navicular bone. It lies within the tendon of the tibialis posterior muscle (Fig. 22–16). Three types have been classified.[151] Type I is a small accessory bone, with a well defined round outline without attachment to the body of the navicular. It essentially is a sesamoid of the posterior tibialis tendon. Approximately 30 percent of all accessory navicular bones are type I. Type II accessory naviculars are triangular in shape, attached to the body of the navicular by a fibrocartilaginous synchondrosis. In type III the accessory bone is partially fused to the body of the navicular by an osseous bridge. This is often termed a *cornuate navicular*, owing to the shape of the navicular on radiographs.

Although most accessory naviculars are asymptomatic, those patients presenting with symptoms most commonly are adolescents with well-localized complaints. The symptoms consist of a dull aching pain along the medial arch of the foot. Symptoms are often aggravated by shoe wear. Trauma, which is minor in nature, may often incite the onset of acute symptoms. The etiology of acute symptoms after trauma may be due to rupture of the fibrous or osseous union of the accessory bone to the navicular. In the acute setting, symptoms may consist of a sharp, sticking pain along the medial arch that limits weight bearing.

Other athletes present with chronic symptoms that consist of aching pain along the medial arch associated with increased physical activity. Sports involving running or jumping may aggravate the symptoms. In chronic cases, an inflamed bursa may develop over the prominent medial aspect of the navicular. Some individuals have been known to present with a nonspecific posterior tibial tendinitis.

Physical examination reveals a prominence of the medial aspect of the navicular. Often the examiner can palpate the ossicle in the soft tissues. Tenderness is usually present in symptomatic patients.

On routine radiographs, the accessory navicular bone is usually seen medial and proximal to the tarsal navicular. It may have a smooth, rounded outline or, in cases of synchondrosis or fracture, can be irregular at its interface with the navicular. In those cases in which it is partially fused (type III), the navicular bone will often present with a curved medial prominence. Increased uptake on technetium bone scan is found in symptomatic patients.[151] Asymptomatic patients will often have normal bone scans. It must be remembered, however, that the presence of an accessory navicular alone may not always be the cause of medial ankle pain. Differential diagnosis includes osteochondritis, tarsal coalition, avascular necrosis of the tarsal navicular (Kohler's disease), and osteoid osteoma of the navicular.

Initial treatment is always conservative.[102] Orthotics concentrate on supporting the medial arch. In severe cases where pain is acute and may be secondary to fracture or rupture

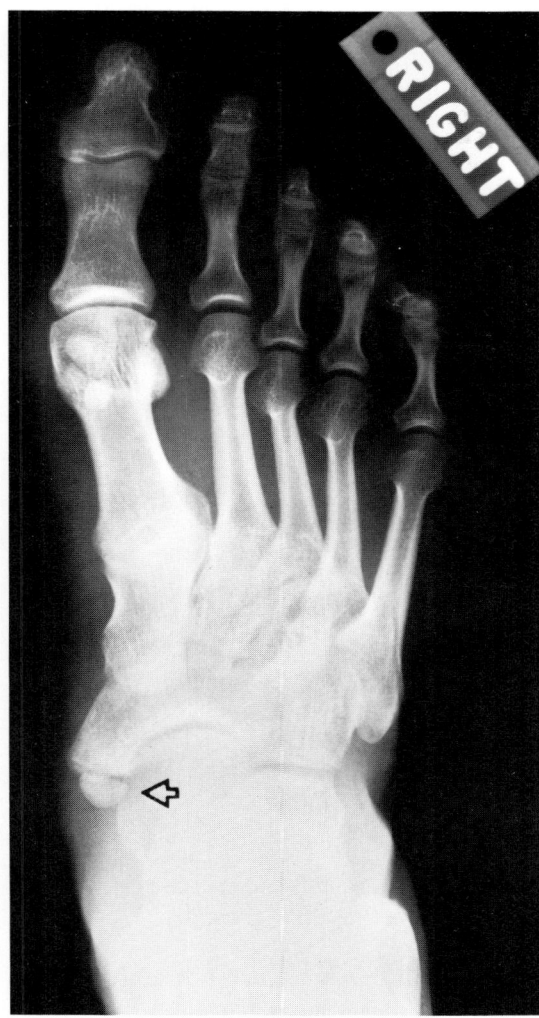

FIGURE 22–16. An accessory navicular located within the tendon of the tibialis posterior.

of the fibro-osseous bridge with the navicular, a below-knee walking cast may be used to relieve initial symptoms. Casting for 4 to 6 weeks, followed by a molded medial arch support, is used in these patients. Nonsteroidal antiinflammatory medication may be helpful during the initial 10 days of treatment.

Surgical intervention is warranted in those patients who fail conservative modalities.[138] The approach to surgery has changed with our understanding of the pathophysiology of this condition. In 1929, Kidner speculated that the accessory navicular bone resulted in displacement of the tibialis posterior tendon, weakening the dynamic support of the longitudinal medial arch of the foot.[84] It was his theory that the abnormal insertion of the tibialis posterior tendon eventually resulted in a planovalgus foot. His approach, therefore, was to reinforce the buttress mechanism of the spring ligament by rerouting the posterior tibial tendon into the plantar aspect of the navicular bone. Excellent results have been reported in relieving symptomatic planovalgus feet by this operation.[20, 84, 94]

Recent articles, however, negate the idea that displacement of the posterior tibial tendon secondary to an accessory navicular could weaken the medial longitudinal arch of the foot. The cause of pain in symptomatic accessory navicular patients is currently felt to be due to shear forces at the level of fibrous union or synchondrosis between the accessory navicular and navicular bone. The posterior tibial tendon does play a role in generating increased tension and shear at the junction of the accessory navicular and navicular bone.[179] Pes planus (flat foot) adds compression forces that may aggravate symptomology. The finding of pes planus, however, may merely be serendipitous.[167] Our current surgical recommendation is to split the peroneal tendon longitudinally to allow simple excision of the accessory navicular and its synchondrosis. The longitudinal incision in the posterior tibial tendon is then reapproximated. Postoperatively, a soft dressing is employed with non–weight bearing for 3 weeks, followed by partial weight for a subsequent 3 weeks. A general ankle rehabilitation program is then prescribed, similar to that utilized for medial ankle sprains.

OS TRIGONUM

Another supernumerary ossicle of clinical importance is the os trigonum (Fig. 22–17).

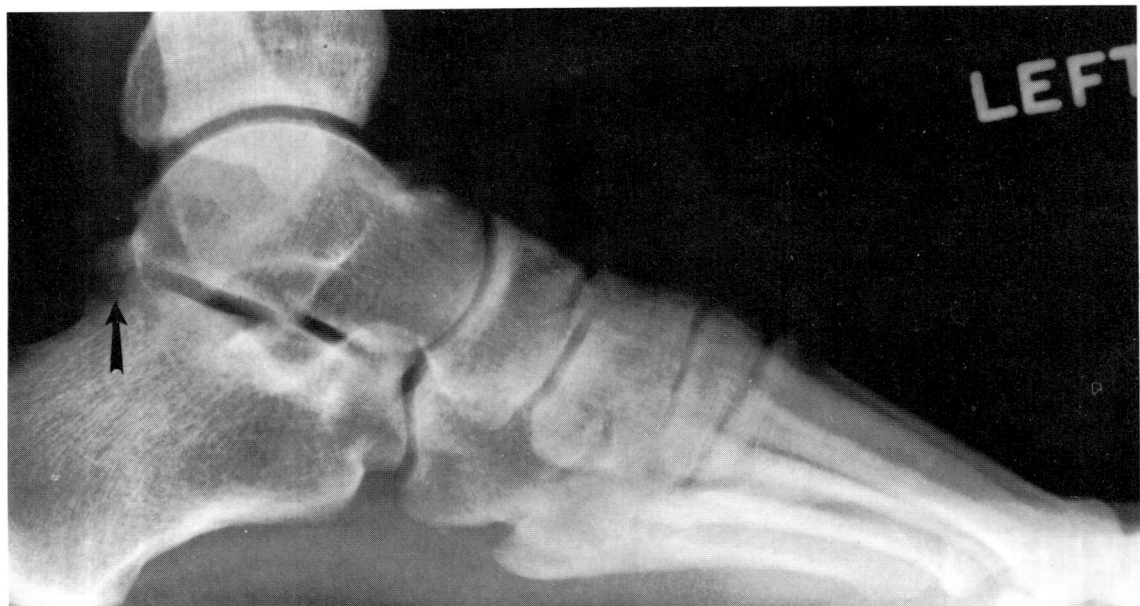

FIGURE 22–17. An os trigonum best seen on lateral radiographs along the posterior aspect of the talus.

This anomaly was first described by Rosenmueller in 1804.[142] Shepherd was the first to describe fracture of this ossicle. He felt the injury was an avulsion fracture of the peroneal tarsal ligament rather than an ununited apophysis.[154] Others have refuted this idea, believing the os trigonum results from an independent secondary center of ossification.[178]

The body of the talus ossifies at 7 months of age. Its posterior aspect has a rounded contour and is not as prominent as in the adult.[66] Secondary ossification centers of the posterior tubercles do not appear until between the ages of 8 and 11 years. They usually unite with the body within a year of their appearance.[111] Whether the os trigonum represents an actual fracture or merely a failure of the ossicle to unite with the posterior talus remains a source of debate. The os trigonum may be unilateral, bilateral, or bipartite.[181] At times, it can be united to the talus, calcaneus, or both via a fibrocartilaginous or osseous bridge.

Geist noted a 7 percent incidence of free os trigonums and a 12 percent incidence of fused ossicles in 100 cases.[54] Kleinberg revealed a 5 percent incidence of the unfused bone in 350 patients.[85] Burman and Lapidus reported a 6.4 percent incidence of the free ossicle with a 43 percent incidence of the fused bone.[15] In general, there appears to be a greater incidence of the fused ossicle than that of the free os trigonum.[15, 54, 85, 152, 153]

Symptoms from an os trigonum are thought to result from impingement of the posterior aspect of the talus as it abuts on the posterior margin of the tibia in maximum plantar flexion. Repeated minor impingement of an os trigonum may lead to an area of compression, with resultant fracture and separation of the tubercle from the talar body. If the injury is unrecognized, continued motion may lead to a painful nonunion.

The athlete will often present with a history of recurrent chronic ankle sprains. They complain primarily of posterior ankle pain or occasional giving way most commonly during running or cutting. The episodes of giving way of the ankle may occasionally be associated with swelling along the anterior aspect of the Achilles tendon. In most settings, the diagnosis is missed on initial evaluation.[132]

A common history is that of forced plantar flexion of the ankle such as sustained in a football pileup. Physical examination may reveal deep tenderness anterior to the Achilles tendon, with occasional swelling. Active and passive plantar flexion of the ankle usually results in pain, with limited motion and stiffness of the ankle due to associated muscle spasm. Painful dorsiflexion of the great toe can often be seen and is attributed to the proximity of the flexor hallucis longus tendon as it runs along the posterior talus. Anterior drawer and lateral talar tilt examination reveal no evidence of ankle instability.

Routine ankle radiographs, specifically lateral radiographs, usually identify the os trigonum. The free ossicle usually has a rounded, smooth border. Fracture of the fused bone will often show a narrow, jagged edge with occasional extension into the talar body.[86] When diagnosis is delayed, follow-up radiographs may show signs of ossification in the surrounding soft tissues. In symptomatic cases, a technetium bone scan is often definitive, revealing increased uptake in the posterior process of the talus. Asymptomatic os trigonums have normal bone scans.[132]

Acute fractures are best treated with plaster immobilization for 6 weeks. Generally, a non–weight-bearing splint or cast is used. Physical therapy is begun at 6 weeks using the ankle rehabilitation program described in the section on ankle fractures. Chronic injuries that demonstrate persistent pain should be treated conservatively with rest, nonsteroidal antiinflammatory medication, and occasional immobilization for 3 to 6 weeks if symptoms persist. Approximately one third of patients who have chronic symptoms respond to conservative therapy.[132] We concur with recommendations for surgical intervention in patients whose symptoms persist despite conservative therapy. Paulos et al. recommend surgical removal of the tubercle through either a posterior lateral or posterior medial approach without malleolar osteotomy.[132] We find that this is the most utilitarian approach, allowing the earliest return to sports participation. Postoperatively, the ankle is splinted in a posterior mold, and rehabilitation commences once the surgical incision demonstrates healing. Overall, return to full participation in sports may be anticipated within 2 months.

The role of the os trigonum in dance injuries is discussed in Chapter 27.

TARSAL COALITION

Tarsal coalition is the abnormal fusion between bones of the hind foot and midfoot. The first written description was by Buffon in 1750.[14, 64] Unions between the bones may be fibrous, cartilaginous, or osseous. Cruveilhier first described a calcaneonavicular coalition in 1829.[109] This was first demonstrated radiographically by Slomann in 1921.[156]

Tarsal coalitions must not be overlooked as a cause of ankle and foot pain in an active adolescent participating in sports. It is during the second decade of life that participation in organized athletics quickly increases. The patient may report intermittent diffuse ankle pain over several months that is aggravated with activity. Complaints of midfoot pain or stiffness of the hind foot should lead to suspicion of possible tarsal coalition. There may be a history of recurrent sprains.

The true incidence of tarsal coalition is unknown. Current literature considers it to be less than 1 percent.[62, 153, 164, 170] The most prevalent coalitions are calcaneonavicular, talonavicular, and talocalcaneal (Fig. 22–18). Of these, calcaneonavicular coalitions appear to predominate.[95, 164, 168] Approximately 50 percent of talocalcaneal fusions and 60 percent of calcaneonavicular bars are bilateral.

Historically, it was felt that accessory ossicles within the foot united together to produce tarsal fusions.[62, 134, 156] Currently, the etiology appears to be a failure of segmentation involving the primitive mesenchyme of the foot.[63] A familiar pattern has been demonstrated suggesting an autosomal dominant inheritance with nearly full penetrance.[63, 11, 22, 182] Leonard has shown 39 percent of first-degree relatives of patients with known tarsal coalition to exhibit some form of tarsal fusion.[95] In addition, an association with carpal coalitions, symphalangism, and other congenital limb anomalies has been reported.[53]

Symptoms depend on the location of the coalition.[107, 164] Painful talonavicular coalitions may present as young as 2 years of age. Most commonly, calcaneonavicular and talocalcaneal bars present between 8 and 16 years of age. The symptoms develop as the fibrous or cartilaginous union between the tarsal bones begins to ossify. Symptoms consist of dull aching pain that is aggravated by activity or prolonged standing. They often occur when activity is increased during the initial onset of track or basketball season.

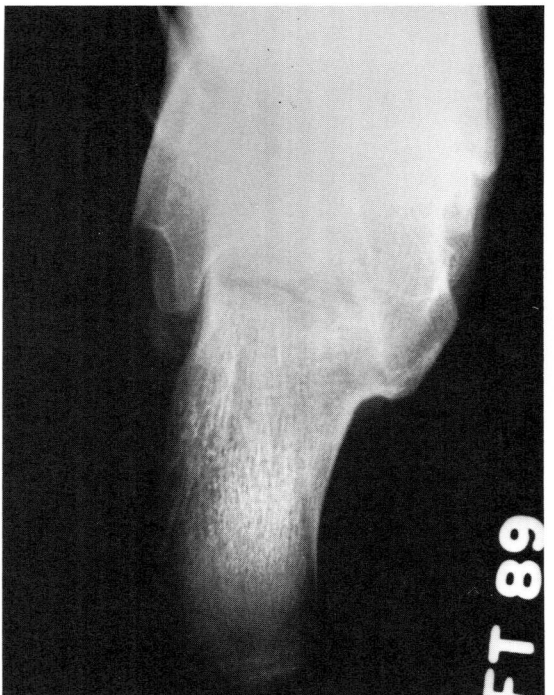

A

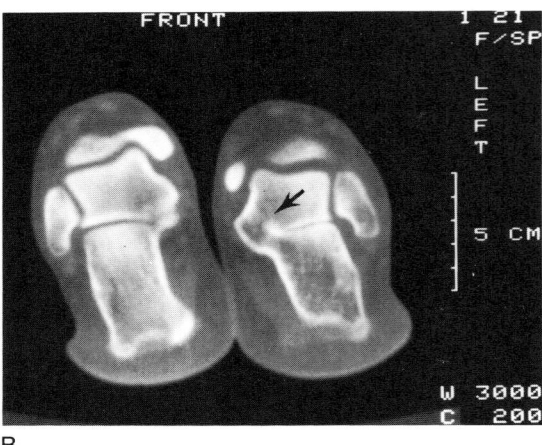

B

FIGURE 22–18. Tarsal coalitions. Most prevalent are the calcaneonavicular, talonavicular, and talocalcaneal lesions. A talonavicular coalition is shown here on plain radiographs (*A*) and computerized tomography (*B*).

Pain is concentrated in the midtarsal region, the sinus tarsi, or medially over the talonavicular joint.[107]

Examination usually demonstrates a stiff foot, often with decreased motion of the subtalar joint.[29] The association of peroneal spastic flat foot with tarsal coalitions is well documented historically[29] Clinically, there may be a loss of the longitudinal arch, limited subtalar motion, hind foot valgus, and forefoot abduction. The etiology of the peroneal spasm remains unknown.[73] The overall incidence of peroneal spastic flat foot with tarsal coalition is between 10 and 33 percent.[41, 107] It is theorized that inflammation around the tarsal coalition results in peroneal spasm. Kyne and Mankin report that peroneal tendons contract to pronate the foot in order to reduce subtalar interarticular pressure and decrease pain.[89] Adaptive shortening of the peroneal tendons can result from long-standing spasticity, leading to a fixed deformity.

Radiographic examination begins with standard AP, lateral, and oblique views of the foot. Tarsal coalitions are commonly missed on routine radiographs owing to bony superimposition and oblique orientation of the coalition. Certain secondary changes, however, that are suggestive of tarsal coalitions may be noted on initial plain radiographic views. These findings include talar beaking, rounding of the lateral talar process, and narrowing of the posterior talocalcaneal facet.[118, 127] These latter two changes are thought to be secondary to degenerative processes. The presence of talar beaking is believed to be secondary to a traction spur generated by increased stress at the insertion site of the talonavicular ligament.[25, 168] Other authors feel there is actual impingement of the navicular on the talar neck. This impingement is most frequently associated with talocalcaneal coalitions.[89, 168]

Descriptions of an "anteater nose" involving the superior calcaneal process has been associated with calcaneonavicular bars.[118] This radiographic description represents a tubular elongation of the anterior portion of the superior calcaneus as viewed on lateral radiographs (Fig. 22–19). The "nose" projects toward the middle of the tarsal navicular. Calcaneonavicular coalitions are best demonstrated by a 45-degree medial oblique radiograph.[118]

Radiographically, the diagnosis is often missed—especially when the union between the navicular and calcaneus is either cartilaginous or fibrous. Likewise, the talocalcaneal joint with its multiple facets often renders diagnosis of coalitions within the subtalar joint extremely difficult. In general, most talocalcaneal coalitions involve the middle facet, which is best demonstrated on the calcaneal axial view as described by Harris and Beath.[62] The X-ray beam is directed anteriorly toward the subtalar joint approximately 45 degrees from the horizontal. In reality, however, multiple roentgenograms may be necessary at 30, 35, and 40 degrees to demonstrate this facet. The posterior facet parallels the middle facet and is therefore also demonstrated with these views.

The anterior facet requires a lateral oblique view in order to decrease superimposition of the talar head.[69] Lateral tomograms are especially helpful in demonstrating coalitions involving the anterior facet.[91, 25] In patients whose plain films are "normal" with a history of chronic ankle pain, a bone scan is an excellent screening device. Increased technetium uptake will be demonstrated in symp-

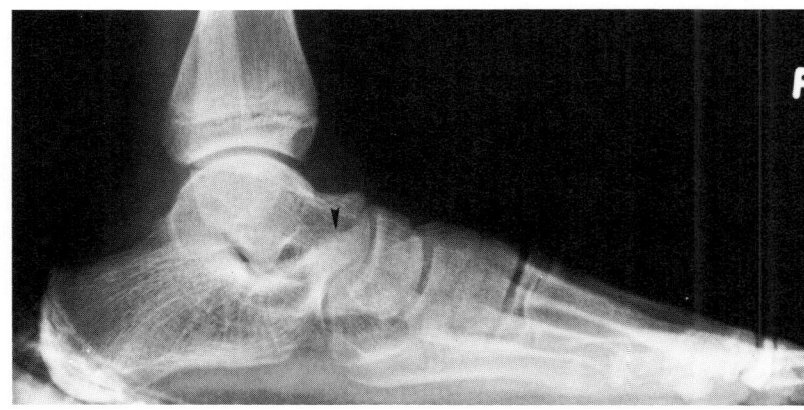

FIGURE 22–19. The "anteater" nose deformity represents a tubular elongation of the anterior portion of the superior calcaneus. It is best viewed on lateral radiographs.

tomatic areas.[58] Currently, computer tomography is the best radiographic modality to diagnose tarsal coalitions accurately. The coronal plane is optimal for the subtalar facets, whereas the talonavicular and calcaneocuboid joints are best exhibited in the transverse plane.[165]

Between 30 and 90 percent of patients have been reported to respond to nonoperative conservative treatment of tarsal coalitions.[5, 12, 23] Most patients with minor symptoms respond well to orthotics consisting of a medial heel wedge or molded heel cups correcting the hind foot into varus. Prior to the use of orthotics, a trial course of short leg casting correcting the hind foot into varus has proved successful in some cases.[27] It may also predict the success of more expensive molded orthotics. Persistent pain, despite orthotics or trial casting, is an indication for surgical intervention.

Surgical treatment varies depending on the type of coalition present. The current recommendation for a calcaneonavicular bar is surgical resection of the coalition and interposition of fat, muscle, or another inert material.[30, 116] This procedure is best reserved for children under the age of 14 years who demonstrate no arthritic changes. Postoperatively, these patients are immobilized in a short leg cast for 1 week. Physical therapy is then begun once adequate wound healing is demonstrated. Emphasis is on maximizing subtalar motion. Weight bearing is begun within 10 to 14 days or as tolerated by patient comfort. In cases where resection fails and a coalition reforms, or where the tarsus demonstrates degenerative changes, triple arthrodesis is used as a salvage procedure. Triple arthrodesis may restrict athletic participation by fusing the midfoot and thus blocking talar motion.

Surgical management of talocalcaneal coalitions remains controversial. Many authors feel that degenerative changes in talocalcaneal coalitions are often present at the time of initial diagnosis.[27] In addition, resection of these bars often requires surgical excision of the medial facet of the talocalcaneal joint. This results in considerable stress being distributed to the anterior and posterior facets.[25, 27, 73] Some believe that this leads to further degenerative arthritis. For this reason, many authors promote triple arthrodesis as an initial treatment.[25, 27, 73] Again, this severely restricts athletic potential. In addition, successful excisions of talocalcaneal bars have been reported.[4, 70, 168] For this reason, we attempt resection and use the triple arthrodesis for salvage in cases of failure. If triple arthrodesis is to be employed, the foot should be skeletally mature unless symptoms are disabling.[118]

Talonavicular and calcaneocuboid coalitions are usually congenital, bilateral, and in most cases, asymptomatic.[71] Symptomatic coalitions involving either the talonavicular or calcaneocuboid joint can be treated by surgical resection with supplemental muscle or fat interposition.

ANKLE FRACTURES

Ligaments are stronger than bone in the skeletally immature athlete. Thus, the athlete with an open physis will often suffer a growth plate fracture rather than a ligamentous rupture or sprain. The physis represents an area of inherent structural weakness in the ankle joint, and inversion stress or external rotation injury that would result in a sprain of the anterior talofibular ligament in the adult will manifest itself as a Salter Harris type II fracture in a skeletally immature athlete. By 15 to 16 years of age, the distal tibial and fibular growth plates begin to close and an adult injury pattern develops with a predominance of ligamentous sprains.

DISTAL FIBULA FRACTURES

The most common fracture of the ankle involving the skeletally immature athlete is a Salter-Harris type I or II fracture of the distal fibula.[97, 113] These injuries result from an adduction external rotation stress. This injury is typically sustained in either football or soccer, in which the athlete plays with a cleated shoe. In this setting, the shoe becomes planted and the body weight rotates over the foot, resulting in an external rotation force that is directed transversely across the tibial plafond to concentrate at the distal fibular physis. If one examines the ankle radiographically, it will be noted that the tibiotalar joint is roughly at the level of the distal fibular growth plate. Thus, forces that propagate along the tibial plafond, which commonly occur with external rotation, concentrate at the fibular growth plate. The fracture

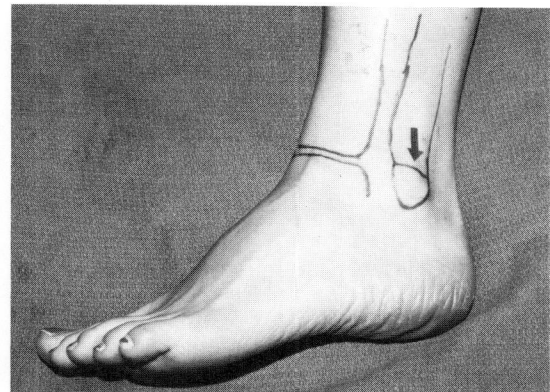

FIGURE 22–20. Tenderness over the distal fibular physis can indicate a nondisplaced physeal fracture of the fibula.

then occurs across the fibula along this inherent line of weakness.[128]

Most of these distal fibular fractures are nondisplaced. Plain radiographs are commonly unremarkable, allowing the diagnosis to be missed. The most accurate sign is tenderness over the distal fibular physis (Fig. 22–20). This area of tenderness is more proximal than that which is seen with a lateral ankle sprain.

TREATMENT

Nondisplaced fractures are treated with cast immobilization with the ankle in neutral for 3 to 4 weeks. A short leg cast is utilized and the patient is kept non–weight bearing for 3 weeks. At 4 weeks the cast is removed and the ankle examined for residual tenderness. Residual discomfort usually necessitates continued immobilization for a full 6 weeks. Weight bearing is permitted if continued immobilization in a short leg cast is necessary.

Those fractures demonstrating displacement can almost always be reduced by closed means. Reduction is by inversion and internal rotation of the foot. Postreduction immobilization in a short leg cast is recommended for the initial 3 weeks. At 4 weeks the cast is removed and the ankle examined for tenderness. If no tenderness is present, protected weight bearing in an air stirrup (Air Cast) is utilized during the final 3 weeks of immobilization. Growth arrest of the distal fibular physis is uncommon as a posttraumatic sequela in these patients.[79, 80, 81]

DISTAL TIBIA FRACTURES

Salter-Harris type I fractures of the distal tibia represent an unusual injury in athletics. They are rarely displaced and are often missed on initial radiographs.

The epiphyseal fragment of the fracture site often includes a horizontal flake of metaphyseal bone. This can represent a subtle finding radiographically.

Treatment of these fractures consists of closed reduction followed by a non–weight-bearing long leg cast for 3 weeks and a short leg weight-bearing cast for the final 3 weeks of immobilization. A total of 6 weeks of immobilization is recommended for these injuries.

Salter-Harris type II injuries of the distal tibia occur by a variety of mechanisms. These are common injuries in football and soccer. The mechanism is primarily the result of an eversion stress or external rotation force while the foot is in pronation. This mechanism of injury usually causes displacement of the metaphyseal fragment of the tibia laterally or posterolaterally. Frequently, there is a fibular component to this injury (Fig. 22–21). The fibula may exhibit a small, mini-

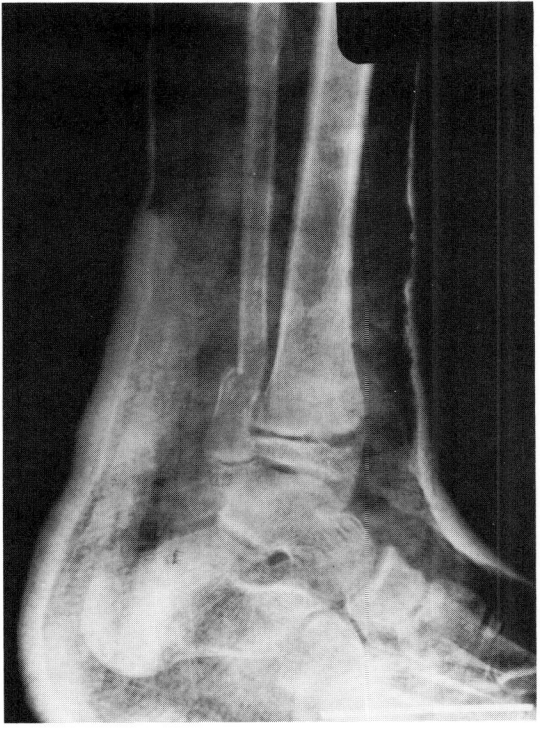

FIGURE 22–21. Salter Harris type II injury of the distal tibia. Note the associated compression fracture involving the distal fibula.

mally displaced greenstick fracture; although with significant force, the amount of unicortical compression laterally can be marked.

Signs of injury include diffuse swelling along with ecchymosis similar to that seen with a severe lateral ankle sprain. Tenderness is primarily concentrated along the anterior lateral portion of the ankle mortise.

Treatment of these fractures remains conservative, with closed reduction performed using longitudinal traction and internal rotation of the foot. In those cases in which closed reduction is unable to be performed, the periosteum may be stripped from the anterior tibia, resulting in interposition of the periosteum into the fracture site laterally. This requires open reduction to allow removal of the periosteum. A long leg non–weight-bearing cast is utilized for 3 weeks, then a short leg non–weight-bearing cast for the final 3 weeks of immobilization. Weight bearing is restricted for a full 6 weeks.

Salter-Harris type III and IV injuries involving the distal tibia may be thought of as extensions of Salter-Harris type I and II distal fibular fractures (Fig. 22–22). They are common in sports such as basketball and volleyball. The injury results from an adduction force with the foot in supination. This pattern of injury may be seen in a football or volleyball player who lands on the foot that is in slight inversion. This injury may also result in landing on an irregular surface in a sport such as the long jump. The foot is twisted under the ankle, with a resultant fracture of the medial malleolus medially and an associated lateral ligament sprain of the ankle.

In mild injuries, the athlete may only suffer a lateral sprain or fracture of the distal fibular epiphysis. As the force of injury increases, however, a Salter Harris type III or IV fracture develops in the distal tibia. One proposed traumatic mechanism of fracture is thought to be secondary to talar impingement on the lower medial half of the distal tibial plafond. In most cases, however, it is thought that a shear force is generated across the joint surface that propagates up into the distal tibial physis. A fracture then occurs along the hypertrophic zone of the physis and extends into the metaphysis of the distal tibia medially.[128]

In type III and IV Salter Harris fractures, closed reduction may be successful by everting the foot under longitudinal traction. Debate remains, however, as to how much angulation is acceptable. Although up to 20 degrees of angulation can demonstrate acceptable remodeling in the skeletally immature, anatomical realignment minimizes the complication of angular deformities.[137, 160] Most important, however, is realignment of the articular cartilage of the distal tibial plafond. Displacement over 2 mm involving the articular surface of the ankle is an indication for open reduction. Reduction of the medial malleolus is performed with care taken to respect the physis. A cancellous lag screw is placed parallel to the physeal growth plate through the metaphyseal portion of the fracture fragment. Following internal fixation, the patient is placed in a short leg non–weight-bearing cast for 6 weeks. Minimally displaced fractures are treated by closed reduction, followed by a non–weight-bearing long leg cast for 3 weeks, then a short leg non–weight-bearing cast for the final 3 weeks.

The incidence of Salter Harris type V compression injuries in athletics is unknown. The diagnosis of these injuries at time of original injury is commonly missed owing to unremarkable radiographs. If this injury is suspected, long-term follow-up is recommended since growth arrest can occur.

Medial malleolar fractures below the level of the tibial plafond occur secondary to an abduction force with the foot in pronation. This is similar to the mechanism seen in

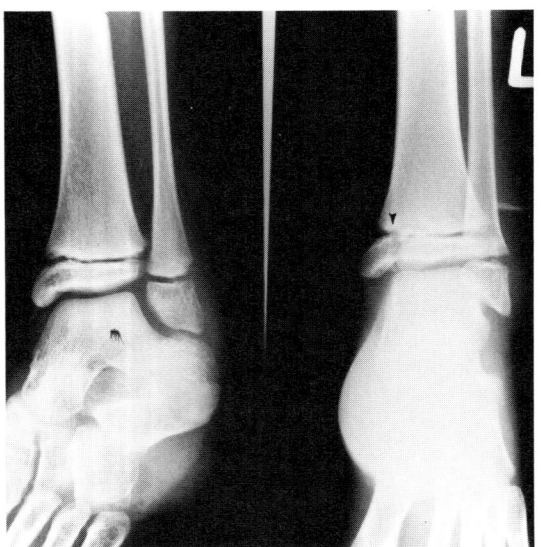

FIGURE 22–22. Salter Harris type III injury of the distal tibia with associated Salter Harris type I injury to the distal fibula.

Salter Harris type II fractures involving the distal tibia. These injuries, however, do not involve the articular weight-bearing surface of the ankle. They therefore can be easily reduced by closed reduction using an adduction force. Postreduction treatment with a short leg non–weight-bearing cast for 4 weeks is usually sufficient.

Notably, Stanitski and Micheli[162] have reported a number of children involved in long distance running who present with these fractures. They felt this injury was secondary to avulsion of the medial malleolus due to overuse in a foot which was biomechanically susceptible. This would be a foot in which forefoot pronation was predominant. Increased medial ankle stress would result due to the pronated forefoot leading to an eventual avulsion fracture or stress fracture of the medial malleolus.[174]

THE TILLAUX FRACTURE

Between the ages of 12 and 15 years, the distal tibial physis begins to close. This process occurs approximately 18 months before completion of tibial growth. The distal tibial physis closes asymmetrically—first closing in the central portion, then proceeding medially and lastly closing along the anterolateral aspect. The posterior lateral physis closes before its anterolateral counterpart. External rotation injury during this period can often fragment the physis. This occurs primarily along the anterior lateral portion of the distal tibial epiphysis owing to the attachment of the anterior tibiofibular ligament.[91, 137, 160] Avulsion of the anterior lateral fragment of the distal tibial epiphysis is known as a Tillaux fracture (Fig. 22–23), named for Paul Jules Tillaux (1834–1904). These fractures represent a Salter Harris type III injury. Despite involvement of the growth plate, angular deformity is rare since remaining growth in these individuals is limited owing to their age. However, anatomical reduction must be achieved since there has been disruption of the articular surface of the tibial plafond.

The majority of Tillaux fractures show minimal displacement, and no reduction is necessary. If displacement is present, gentle internal rotation of the foot, combined with direct pressure over the anterior lateral portion of the ankle joint, can be used to obtain reduction. Following reduction, the extremity is immobilized in a short leg non–weight-bearing cast for 4 to 6 weeks. A disruption of the articular cartilage, however, with greater than 2 mm of displacement or step-off is an indication for open reduction.[77] The surgical approach is through an anterior lateral incision to allow anatomical reduction of the fragment and fixation with a cancellous lag screw. This screw can cross the physis when

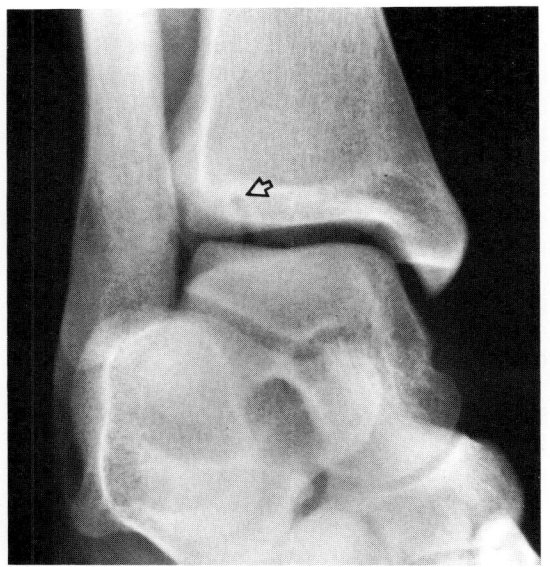
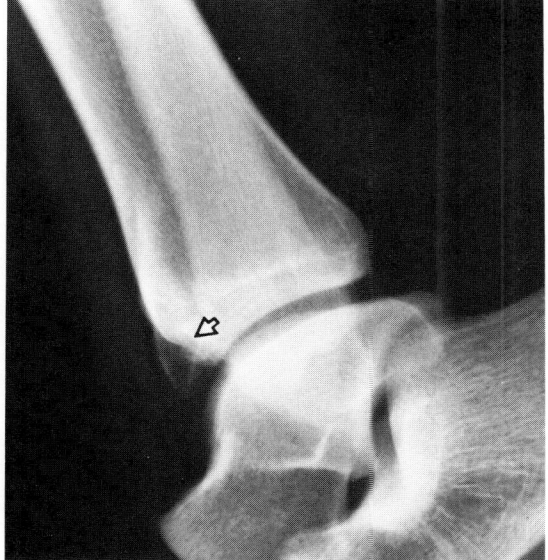

A B

FIGURE 22–23. The Tillaux fracture.

closure is almost complete or be placed parallel to the epiphysis in the more immature patient.

THE TRIPLANE FRACTURE

This represents an uncommon injury that occurs in the same age group as the Tillaux fracture. It is a combination of a Salter Harris type III fracture, like the Tillaux, and a Salter Harris type II fracture involving the distal metaphyseal portion of the tibia (Fig. 22–24). The pathomechanics of injury most commonly result from external rotation of the foot in supination. Both the triplane and the Tillaux fracture are commonly associated with skateboard injuries.

In the AP plane, the fracture propagates along the physis. It then extends up into the metaphysis either laterally or medially. This pattern often makes radiographic interpretation somewhat confusing. On AP radiographs, the fracture looks like a Salter Harris type III injury. On the lateral view, the metaphyseal fragment can be seen, giving it a Salter Harris type IV appearance.

Debate has persisted as to whether this represents a two- or three-part fracture as originally described by Marmor.[109] His original description included three fractures: an anterolateral fragment, like the Tillaux; a medial posterior lateral fragment, which included the metaphyseal spike; and finally, the remaining distal tibial metaphysis. Cooperman et al., however, in a retrospective review found no cases that revealed an isolated anterolateral fragment (like the Tillaux) as originally described by Marmor.[26] In reality, both two- and three-part fracture fragments have been documented in the literature. Most cases seen clinically, however, demonstrate two fragments, which may occur either medially or laterally along the distal tibial plafond.

These fractures require anatomical reduction. Displacement of the articular surface of the tibial plafond over 2 mm is considered unacceptable. Closed reduction can be attempted using internal rotation of the foot along with anterior lateral pressure at the level of the ankle mortise. Reduction should be confirmed by tomogram or computer tomography. Two-part fractures treated by closed reduction are immobilized initially for 3 weeks in a long leg non–weight-bearing cast, followed by a short leg non–weight-bearing cast during the final 3 weeks. In total, a full 6 weeks of non–weight-bearing status is recommended. Both casts should be applied with the foot in mild internal rotation.

Three-part fractures generally require open reduction and internal fixation. The surgical approach is first aimed at reducing the posterior medial fragment. This is best accomplished by placing the foot in internal rotation, followed by dorsiflexion. Two cancellous lag screws are then placed through the metaphyseal fragment of the fracture above the tibial physis. This fixes the metaphyseal portion of the bone to the intact distal tibial metaphysis. The anterolateral fragment is then reduced through a separate anterolateral incision and lagged with a cancellous lag screw that is placed parallel to the distal tibial physis to avoid crossing the growth plate. Postoperatively, these patients are treated with a short leg non–weight-bearing cast for a full 6 weeks.

Premature closure of the physis following these injuries is not uncommon. Most, however, do not result in an angular deformity since remaining growth is limited.[26] The highest morbidity associated with this fracture results from incomplete reduction of the articular surface of the tibial plafond, leading to secondary degenerative arthritis.

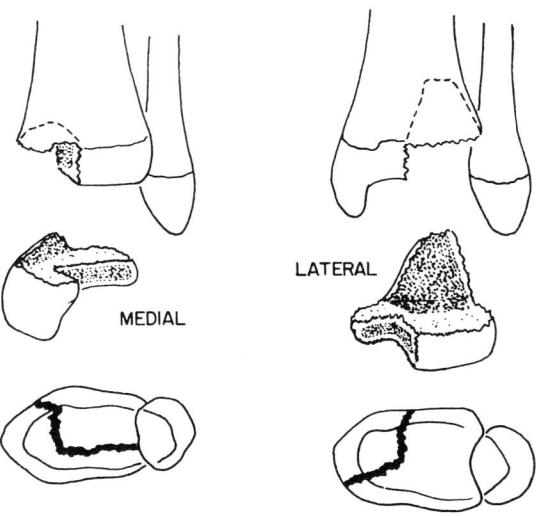

FIGURE 22–24. Medial and lateral triplane fractures. (From Ogden JA: Skeletal Injury in the Child. Philadelphia, Lea & Febiger, 1982.)

REHABILITATION OF ANKLE FRACTURES

Rehabilitation of the casted ankle is essentially limited to isometric contractions that are performed during the initial phase of treatment. Following removal of the cast, the overall goal of therapy is to restore full range of motion, decrease tissue edema, return strength to a normal range, and therefore restore normal gait.

Following immobilization, most ankles are painful as range of motion is instituted. Therapy can proceed in a progressive fashion despite pain, as long as edema and swelling do not result. Signs of edema and swelling should alert the therapist that overuse is occurring. We have found the use of a cryocompression boot following initial ROM exercises to be of some benefit in limiting the occurrence of swelling. Therapy concentrates on strengthening both medial and lateral ankle musculature. Emphasis is placed on restoring both full dorsiflexion and plantar flexion mobility. The modalities employed to restore both peroneal and posterior tibial strength are similar to those described for both medial and lateral ankle sprains. Once range of motion is restored, aggressive resistant exercise for strengthening, along with balance board training, is utilized.

TRANSCHONDRAL FRACTURES OF THE TALUS

The literature is replete with a plethora of diagnostic names for transchondral talar fractures. These include *osteochondritis dissecans*, *dome fractures*, and *aviator's astragalus*.[17, 23, 24, 108, 110, 119] The term *osteochondritis dissecans* was first used by König to describe loose bodies involved in the knee joint.[88] Kappis then used this term to describe similar findings involving the ankle.[78] Theories that this lesion resulted from trauma were slow to evolve and were not comfirmed until 1959 by Berndt and Harty.[9, 16, 140, 145, 159]

The initial diagnosis of a talar transchondral fracture is often missed by bony superimposition and poor visualization on standard radiographs.[8] Athletes who are initially diagnosed with an ankle sprain may then be reassessed because of inability to return to preinjury performance status. Persistent ankle pain and inability to regain full range of motion is often seen.

This lesion is thought to be traumatic in origin, owing to impingement of the articular surface of the tibia on the talus with resultant fracture of its articular cartilage down to underlying subchondral bone.[9] Lesions can be either medial or lateral (Fig. 22–25). Typically, medial transchondral fractures are located in the posterior one third of the articular surface. Lateral lesions are generally located in the anterior middle third of the talar dome. A classification of these lesions was described by Berndt and Harty (Fig. 22–26). Stage I is a small area of compression of the articular cartilage and underlying subchondral bone. In stage II, the osteochondral fracture is incomplete, with rupture of the lateral ligaments. Stage III lesions are present if the osteochondral fragment is completely detached but still located within the underlying subchondral bed. Finally, in stage IV lesions, the fragment is displaced within the joint.

The mechanism of injury with lateral lesions is thought to be primarily an inversion stress with dorsiflexion leading to compression of the anterior lateral talar dome. Medial lesions can be reproduced by inversion and plantar flexion along with external rotation. Despite the studies by Berndt and Harty as to a traumatic etiology, nontraumatic osteochondral lesions have been described.[108, 149, 183] Nontraumatic lesions appear to occur primarily on the medial side and may represent as many as 30 percent of all medial lesions. The etiology of these lesions remains unknown.

Acute transchondral fractures are often diagnosed initially as either medial or lateral ankle sprains. Swelling and ecchymosis are often present along with limited painful ankle motion. If undiagnosed, chronic cases are most commonly discovered owing to recurrent pain. Ankle stiffness and occasional swelling medially or laterally may be seen along with occasional crepitation with dorsi- and plantar flexion of the ankle. In general, symptoms are aggravated by activity and relieved with rest. At times, intermittent locking may occur, depending on the mobility of the osteochondral fragment.[1, 34, 183] Radiographically, routine ankle mortise views most commonly demonstrate the lesions. Plantar flexion is best to highlight medial lesions, with dorsiflexion allowing best visual-

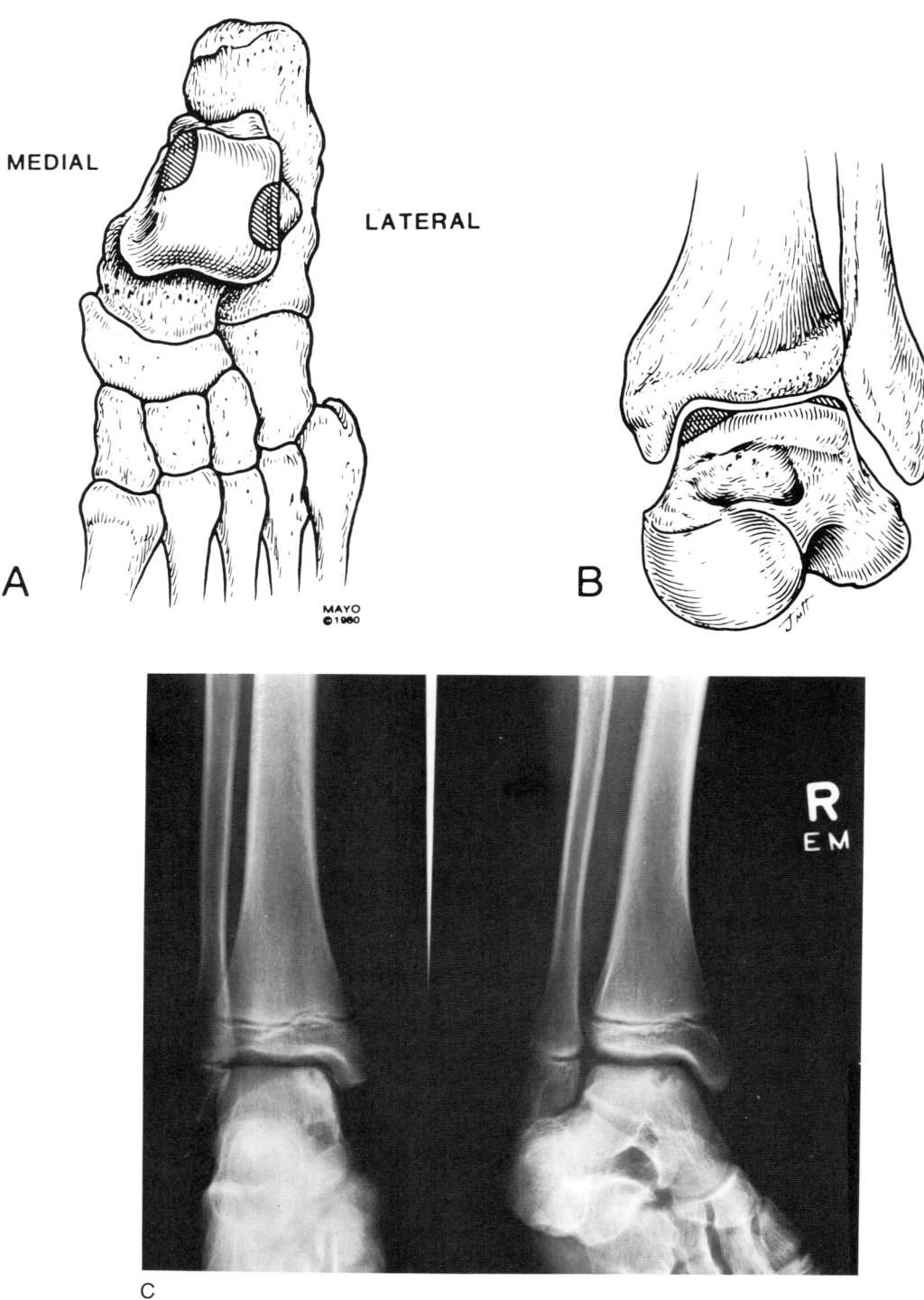

FIGURE 22–25. Transchondal fractures of the talus. Medial lesions tend to be posterior with lateral lesions lying more anterior. (From Leach RE, Schepsis AA: Acute injuries to the ligaments of the ankle. In Evarts CM (ed): Surgery of the Musculoskeletal System. New York, Churchill Livingstone, P. 8:116, 1983.) (*C*) Radiographic appearance of a medial lesion.

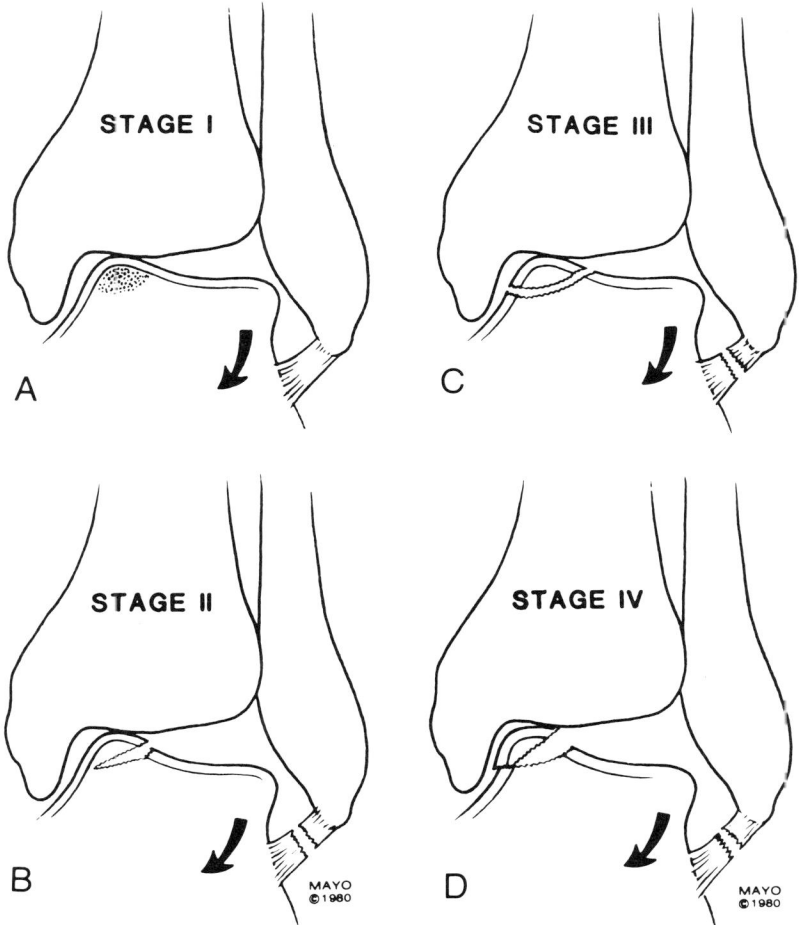

FIGURE 22–26. Berndt and Harty classification of osteochondral fractures. (A) Stage I. Compression fracture of the talar dome with intact articular cartilage. The underlying subchondral bone often undergoes necrosis. (B) Stage II. Partial fracture of the articular cartilage and underlying subchondral bone without displacement of the fragment. (C) Stage III. A complete osteochondral fracture without displacement of the fracture fragment from its bed. (D) Stage IV. Complete osteochondral fracture with displacement. (From Leach RE, Schepsis AA: Acute injuries to the ligaments of the ankle. In Evarts CM (ed): Surgery of the Musculoskeletal System. New York, Churchill Livingstone, 1983.)

ization of lateral lesions. Tomography may be helpful in defining the extent of pathology and determining the anteroposterior position. In patients with recurrent chronic ankle pain, the use of technetium bone scans will often highlight an undiagnosed lesion.

Potential for healing is present for stage I, stage II, and stage III lesions. Stage IV lesions have not been shown to heal. Multiple reports have shown these lesions can progress from a milder stage to a more severe one.[45]

In general, stage I and stage II lesions are treated conservatively regardless of location.[17, 133] Protected ankle movement is sufficient for stage I lesions until asymptomatic. Stage II lesions are immobilized in a short leg cast until evidence of reossification is seen, which will often take 2 to 3 months. Treatment of stage III lesions is based on location. Medial stage III lesions are initially treated conservatively with a short leg cast. Failure to demonstrate healing within 2 months of immobilization is a surgical indication.

The use of technetium bone scans can often determine the propensity for healing. If a lesion shows no evidence of uptake, then surgical excision of the fragment is recommended. Evidence of increased uptake lends credence to our recommendations for surgical drilling to stimulate ingrowth from the subchondral base.[157, 185]

In stage III medial lesions that demonstrate

increased uptake on bone scan, drilling is recommended and the fragment is left in place. A posterior medial arthroscopic approach is utilized. Immediate range of motion and strengthening is begun, although weight bearing is restricted, with crutches used for a full 6 weeks. In type III lateral lesions arthroscopic excision of the fragment, along with drilling of the subchondral bone, is performed. Immediate physical therapy to return full range of motion and strength to the injured ankle is begun. Weight bearing as tolerated is permitted.

In athletes with either medial or lateral acute type III lesions where prolonged immobilization may be unacceptable, we recommend arthroscopic drilling and removal of the fragment. Postoperative ankle rehabilitation is begun as soon as adequate wound healing is demonstrated. Weight bearing as tolerated is prescribed.

In stage IV lesions, the potential for healing is poor. Our approach is arthroscopic removal of the fragment and drilling, with immediate physical therapy to return full range of motion and strength to the injured ankle.

THE JONES FRACTURE

Robert Jones described four cases of fracture involving the base of the fifth metatarsal distal to the tuberosity[76] (Fig. 22–27). This fracture has a high probability of delayed union or nonunion and requires prolonged immobilization.[181] Refracture is often high in these injuries after union.[18, 33] In 1984, Torg et al. separated the Jones fracture into three radiographic types: (1) the acute fracture, (2) fractures with delayed union, and (3) nonunions with sclerotic bone obliterating the medullary canal.[174] Radiographically, acute fractures have sharp, fine borders with minimal corticle or periosteal reaction. Most important, there is no evidence of intramedullary sclerosis. Chronic fracture, or delayed union, often has an associated periosteal reaction around the bone resulting in widening of the fracture line with associated intramedullary sclerosis. In fractures that have gone on to complete nonunion, similar findings are found, but the medullary canal is completely obliterated by sclerotic bone.

Acute Jones fractures are best treated in a short leg non–weight-bearing cast for 6 weeks. Torg has demonstrated that weight bearing leads to higher rates of nonunion.[174] Some success has been demonstrated in delayed union by prolonged immobilization in a non–weight-bearing short leg cast. However, this prolonged immobilization can be very detrimental to the competitive athlete. Therefore, with both delayed union and nonunion, we recommend surgical intervention. Intramedullary screw fixation of the fifth metatarsal, as described by DeLee et al., is our recommended approach.[35] The screw is inserted at the tuberosity, with care taken to countersink the head and ensure that all screw threads are distal to the fracture site. Bone grafting is not needed. Gradual weight bearing is then commenced at approximately 2 weeks. On the average, return to sports can be anticipated between 7 and 14 weeks. Although the advantage appears to be shorter healing time, reports of screw breakage and painful hardware are included in the literature.

STRESS FRACTURES

The stress fracture is not a fracture that occurs from sudden violence or trauma. It represents a process in which fracture occurs after the reparative ability of the bone is exceeded. Repetitive cyclic loading by forces that are less than that required to produce an acute fracture are thought to lead to eventual fatigue failure within the bone and a subsequent stress fracture.[56]

Stress fractures are frequent findings in adolescent athletes. They constitute approximately 6 percent of all injuries to runners.[49] Commonly, the athlete will describe a recent increase in his or her training program. This

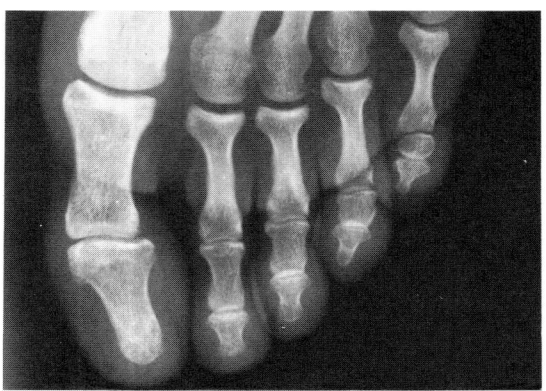

FIGURE 22–27. The Jones fracture.

may include either increasing distance or speed, changing to a harder running surface, or often a recent change in shoes. Pain from stress fractures initially begins at the conclusion of activity. With chronic injury, pain will begin to occur earlier during the training session. Ultimately, the pain increases to the point that it precludes running and may even cause limping during walking.

TARSAL NAVICULAR STRESS FRACTURES

Tarsal navicular stress fractures represent a commonly undiagnosed condition. Radiographs are often unremarkable, and physician suspicion is generally low.[176]

Symptoms include vague, dull, aching pain over the dorsal aspect of the midfoot, with occasional localized tenderness to palpation in the region of the navicular joint. Some athletes present with decreased subtalar joint motion. Often, these symptoms present in the long-distance or marathon runner. Biomechanically, some authors feel that runners with increased forefoot pronation are subject to increased stress at the level of the talonavicular joint. This stress is felt to lead to eventual stress fracture of the navicular.[172] In addition, decreased subtalar joint motion also appears to increase stress at the level of the tarsal navicular joint.[173] Contributing to this is the central avascular portion of the tarsal navicular bone itself, which has been documented by angiographic studies. This area may be predisposed to fracture, owing to its avascularity.[102, 175]

Athletes presenting with chronic, persistent middorsal foot pain with unremarkable radiographs should undergo technetium bone scan for diagnosis (Fig. 22–28). This represents the most accurate and sensitive means to diagnose navicular stress fractures. Tomography may be helpful in assessing the degree of fracture displacement.[57]

For partial fractures, or nondisplaced complete fractures, short leg non–weight-bearing casts should be applied for 6 weeks. Return to sports is then dependent on radiographic evidence of healing.[173] In general, patients exhibiting trabecular healing at 6 weeks with no evidence of tenderness on weight bearing may begin ankle rehabilitation. Guidelines for return to sports are the same as those of ankle sprains or fractures.

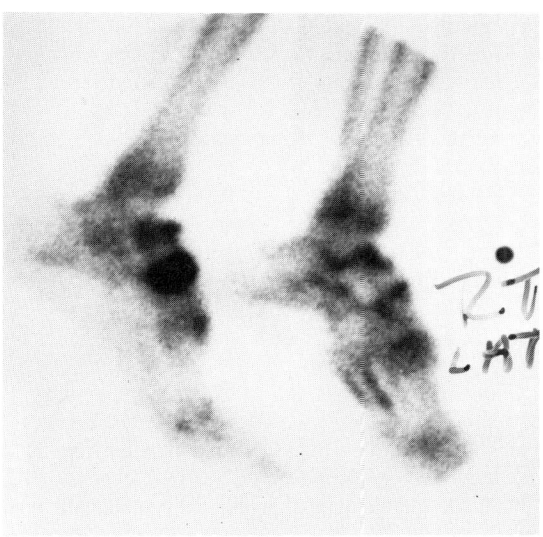

FIGURE 22–28. Bone scan of a patient with persistent midfoot pain and unremarkable radiographs revealing an occult tarsal navicular stress fracture.

Displaced fractures are best treated by internal fixation using a Herbert or cancellous lag screw. Postoperatively, the patient is again immobilized in a non–weight-bearing short leg cast for 6 weeks. In athletes presenting with delayed or nonunions, bone grafting with medullary curettage and internal fixation is utilized. Healing in these patients may be prolonged.

MEDIAL MALLEOLAR STRESS FRACTURES

Stress fractures of the medial malleolus have been only recently described in the English literature. Shelbourne et al. have reported six athletes presenting with recurrent medial ankle sprain during running and jumping.[154] All were runners. Their symptoms consisted of an insidious onset of dull, aching pain, occasionally associated with ankle effusions. Most did not give a definitive history of trauma. Symptoms were aggravated by activity and relieved by rest.

Three patients documented visible fracture of the medial malleolus on routine radiographs. These extended from the medial tibial plafond either obliquely or vertically to the medial malleolus. The other three patients had unremarkable plain radiographs but positive technetium bone scans. Those patients with visible fractures were treated with internal fixation using a malleolar screw and standard AO technique. Those demonstrating normal plain radiographs were treated by restriction of activity for 3 weeks or light immobilization using an air stirrup brace.

All fractures went on to healing. This lesion, although rare, represents a nondisplaced fracture of the medial malleolus (Fig. 22–29). Our approach, generally, is conservative, with light immobilization and protected weight bearing for 3 to 6 weeks until radiographic healing is demonstrated.

Recently, Reider et al. reported a case of stress fracture of the medial malleolus that presented as a chronic, painful nonunion.[139] This patient required open reduction and internal fixation to achieve fracture union. Although rare, such cases demonstrate the importance of obtaining a bone scan in cases of persistent ankle pain with bony tenderness.

FIBULAR STRESS FRACTURES

Persistent lateral ankle pain that is dull and aching in nature but recurrent with activity may indicate the presence of a fibular stress fracture. These injuries are most common in runners who increase their distance rapidly over a short period of time. Rarely are they associated with joint effusions. Soft tissue swelling, however, can be present with physical exam, demonstrating localized tenderness over the distal third of the fibular. Roentgenograms may or may not be positive during the acute phases of injury (Fig. 22–30). However, in athletes with consistent lateral ankle pain and normal radiographs, technetium bone scans may be extremely useful in establishing the diagnosis. Treatment is restriction from impact loading activities for 4 to 6 weeks. Occasionally, light immobilization using an air stirrup for those athletes with moderate to severe discomfort is recommended during this period. Ankle rehabilitation is begun at the time of diagnosis in order to ensure minimal loss of muscle strength during the restricted activity period. Once pain resolves, progressive resistive exercises are encouraged along with balance board training. As pain fully resolves, the program is progressed in a similar fashion as that described for lateral ankle sprains.

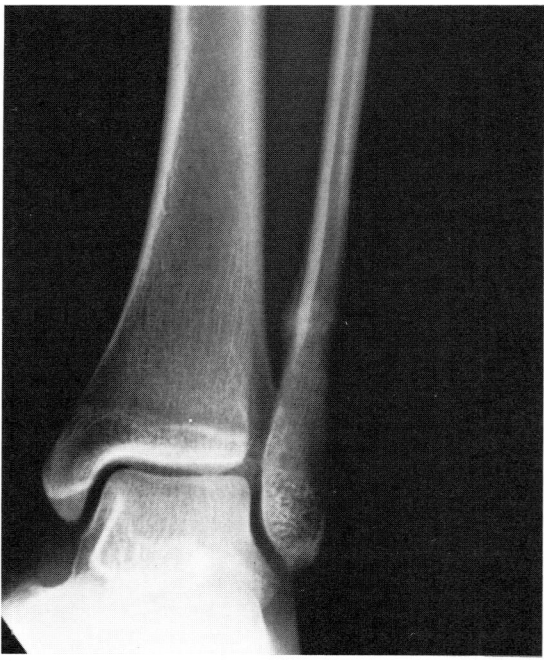

FIGURE 22–30. Fibular stress fracture in a 15-year-old female cross-country runner.

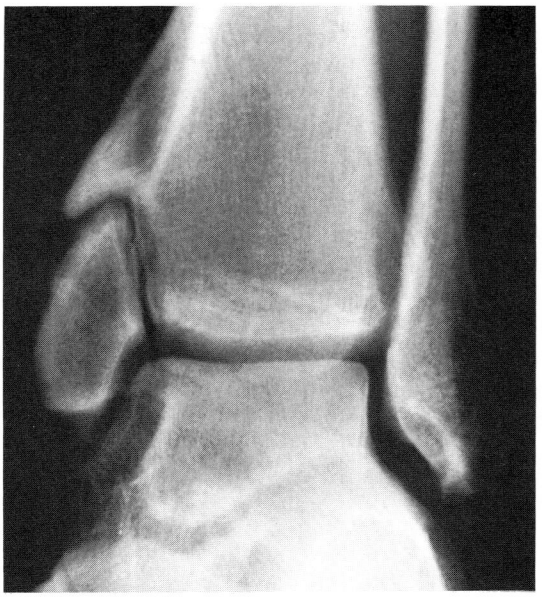

FIGURE 22–29. A rare case of a nonunion of a medial malleolus stress fracture.

References

1. Alexander A. H., Lichtman D. M.: Surgical treatment of transchondral talar dome fractures (osteochondritis dissecans) long term follow up. J Bone Joint Surg 62A:646–652, 1980.

2. Anderson K. J., LeCocq J. F.: Operative treatment of injury to the fibular colateral ligament of the ankle. J Bone Joint Surg 36A:825–832, 1954.
3. Ashhurst A. P. C., Bromer R. S.: Classification and mechanism of fractures of the leg bones involving the ankle. Based on a study of three hundred cases from Episcopal Hospital. Arch Surg 4:51–129, 1922.
4. Ashier M., Mosier K.: Coalition of the talo calcaneal middle facet: Treatment by surgical excision and fat graft interposition. Orthop Trans 7:149–150, 1983.
5. Badgeley C. E.: Coalition of the calcaneo and the navicular. Arch Surg 15:75–88, 1927.
6. Baird R. A., Jackson S. T.: Fractures of the distal part of the fibula with associated disruption of the deltoid ligament. J Bone Joint Surg 69A:1346–1352, 1987.
7. Bateman J. E., Trott A.: The Foot and Ankle. New York, Thieme-Stratton, Inc, 1980.
8. Bauer M., Johnson K., Linden B.: Osteochondritis dissecans of the ankle. A 20 year follow up study. J Bone Joint Surg 69B:93–96, 1987.
9. Berndt A., Harty M.: Transchondral fractures (osteochondritis dissecans) of the talus. J Bone Joint Surg 41A:988–1020, 1959.
10. Bizarro A. H.: On sesamoid and supernumerary bones of the limbs, J Anat 55:256, 1921.
11. Boyd H. B.: Congenital talonavicular synostosis. J Bone Joint Surg 26:682, 1944.
12. Braddock G. F. T.: A prolonged follow up of peroneal spastic flat foot. Clin Orthop 16:64, 1960.
13. Brostrom L., Liljedahl S. O., Lindvall N.: Sprained ankles II. KLJ arthrographic diagnosis of recent ligaments ruptures. Acta Chir Scand 129:485–499, 1965.
14. Buffon G. L. L.: Comte de Histoire Naturelle Avec La Description Du Cabinent du Roy. Tome 3:47, 1750.
15. Burman M. S., Lapidus P. W.: The functional disturbances caused by the inconstant bone and sesamoids of the foot. Arch Surg 22:936–975, 1931.
16. Campbell C. J., Ranawat C. S.: Osteochondritis disssecans: The question of etiology. J Trauma 6:201–221, 1966.
17. Canale S. T., Belding R H.: Osteochondral lesions of the talus. J Bone Joint Surg 62A:97–102, 1980.
18. Carp L.: Fracture of the fifth metatarsal bone with reference to delayed union. Ann Surg 86:308–320, 1971.
19. Castaing J., Delplace J.: Entorses de LaCheville. Interet de l'etude de la Stabilite dans le Plan Sagittal pour le Diagnostique de Gravite. Recherche Radiographique du Tiroir Astragalien Anterieur. Rev Chir Orthop 58(51):1665–1701, 1972.
20. Chaler E. H.: Foot pain and the accessory navicular bone. IR J Med Sci 442:471, 1962.
21. Church C. C.: Radiographic diagnosis of acute peroneal tendon dislocation. Am J Roentgenol 129:1065–1068, 1977.
22. Clessner J. R., Jr., Davis G. C.: Bilateral calcaneal navicular coalitions occurring in twin boys. A case report. Clin Orthop 47:73, 1986.
23. Coltrart W. D.: Aviators astragalus. J Bone Joint Surg 34B:545–566, 1952.
24. Convery F. R., Akeson W. H.: The repair of large osteochondral defects. Clin Orthop 82:253, 1972.
25. Conway J. J., Cowell H. R.: Tarsal coalition and roentgenographic demonstration. Radiology 92:799–811, 1969.
26. Cooperman D. R., Spiegel P. G., Laros G. S.: Tibial fractures involving ankle in children. J Bone Joint Surg 60A:1040, 1978.
27. Cowell H. R.: Talocalcaneal coalition and new causes of peroneal spastic flat foot. Clin Orthop 85:16, 1972.
28. Cowell H. R., Elener V.: Rigid painful flat foot 2° to tarsal coalition. Clin Orthop 177:54–60, 1983.
29. Cowell H. R.: Diagnosis and Management of Peroneal Spastic Flat Foot. In AAOS Instructional Course Lectures, Vol. 24. St. Louis, CV Mosby Co, pp 94–103, 1975.
30. Cowell H. R.: Tarsal Coalition Review and Update. In AAOS Instructional Course Lectures, Vol. 31. St. Louis, CV Mosby Co, pp 264–271, 1982.
31. Cox J. S., Hewes T. F.: Normal talar tilt angle. Clin Orthop 140:37–41, 1979.
32. Cruveilher J.: Anatomie, Pathologue due Corps Humain, Tome I: 1829.
33. Dameron T. B., Jr.: Fractures and anatomical variations of the proximal portion of the 5th metatarsal. J Bone Joint Surg 57A:783–792, 1975.
34. Davidson A. M., Steel H. D., Mackenzie D. A., Penny J. A.: A review of twenty one cases of transchondral fractures of the talus. J Trauma 7:378–415, 1967.
35. DeLee J. C., Evans S. P., Julian J.: Stress fracture of the 5th metatarsal. Am J Sports Med 5:349–353, 1983.
36. DeSouta L. J., Gostilo R. B., Meyer T. J.: Results of operative treatment of displaced external rotation-abduction fractures of the ankle. J Bone Joint Surg 67A:1066–1074, 1985.
37. Drez D., Young J. C., Douglas W., Shackleton R., Parmer W.: Non-operative treatment of double lateral ligament tears of the ankle. Am J Sports Med 10:197–199, 1982.
38. Dwight T.: Variations of the Bones of the Hands and the Foot: A Clinical Atlas. Philadelphia, JP Lippincott Co, pp 14–23, 1907.
39. Eckert W. R., Davis E. A.: Acute rupture of the peroneal retinaculum. J Bone Joint Surg 58A:670–673, 1976.
40. Edwards M. E.: The relations of the peroneal tendons to the fibula, calcaneus and cuboideum. Am J Anat 42:213–253, 1928.
41. Elkins R. A.: Tarsal coalition in the young athlete. Am J Sport Med 14:477–480 1986.
42. Evans G. A., Hardcastle P., Frenyo A. D.: Acute rupture of the lateral ligament of the ankle: To suture or not to suture. J Bone Joint Surg 66B:209–212, 1984.
43. Farins B.: Ankle injuries in athletics. Presented at the American Academy of Orthopaedic Surgery Meeting, Las Vegas, NV, February 9–14, 1989.
44. Finsen V., Saetermo R., Kiesgarrd L., Farran K., Engebretsen L., Dieter K., Benum P.: Early post operative weight-bearing and muscle activity in patients who have a fracture of the ankle. J Bone Joint Surg 71A:23–27, 1989.
45. Flick A. R., Gould N.: Osteochondritis dissecans of the talus (transchondral fractures of the talus): Review of the literature and new surgical

46. approach for medial dome lesions. Foot and Ankle 5:165–185, 1985.
46. Freeman M. A. R.: Treatment of ruptures of the lateral ligament of the ankle. J Bone Joint Surg 47B:661–668, 1965.
47. Freeman M. A. R., Dean M. R. E., Hanham I. W. F.: The etiology and prevention of functional instability of the foot. J Bone Joint Surg 47B:678–685, 1965.
48. Frey C. C., Shereff M. J.: Tendon injuries about the ankle in athletes. Clin Sports Med 7:103–118, 1988.
49. Garrick J. G.: Characterization of the patient population in a sports medicine facility. Physician Sports Med. 13:4–5, 1985.
50. Garrick J. G., Requa R. U.: Epidemiology of foot and ankle injuries in sports. Clin Sports Med 7(1):29–36, 1988.
51. Garrick J. G.: The frequency of injury mechanism of injury and epidemiology of ankle sprains. Amer J Sports Med 5(6):241–242, 1977.
52. Gasfon S., McLaughlin H. L.: Complex fracture of the lateral malleolus. J Trauma 1:69–78, 1961.
53. Geelhood G. W., Neil J. V., Davidson R. T.: Symphalangism and tarsal coalition: A hereditary syndrome. J Bone Joint Surg 51B:278, 1969.
54. Geist E. S.: Supernumerary bones of the foot—A roentgenographic study of the feet of one hundred normal individuals. Am J Orthop Surg 12B 403–414, 1914 to 1915.
55. Geist E. S.: The accessory scaphoid bone. J Bone Joint Surg 7:570, 1925.
56. Glad M., Ahronson Z., Stein M., et al: Unusual distribution and onset of stress fractures in soldiers. Clin Orthop 192:142–146, 1985.
57. Goergen T. G., Venn-Watson E. A., Rossman D. J., et al: Tarsal navicular stress fractures in runners. Am J Roentgenol 136:201–203, 1981.
58. Goldman A. B., Paulou H., Schneider R.: Radionuclide bone scanning in subtalar coalitions: Differential considerations. Am J Radiology 138:427–432, 1982.
59. Gross A. E., MacIntosh D. L.: Injury to the lateral ligaments of the ankle: A clinical study. Can J Surg 16:115–117, 1973.
60. Gudas C. J.: Sports-related tendon injuries of the foot and ankle. Clin Pod Med and Surg 3:303–319, 1986.
61. Hamilton W. C.: Traumatic Disorders of the Ankle. New York, Springer-Verlag, pp. 273–277, 1984.
62. Harris R. I., Beath T.: Etiology of peroneal spastic flat foot. J Bone Joint Surg 30B:624, 1948.
63. Harris B. J.: Anomalous structures in the developing human foot. Anat Rec 121:399, 1955.
64. Heiple K. G., Lovejoy C. O.: The antiquity of tarsal coalition. Bilateral deformity in a pre-Columbian skeleton. J Bone Joint Surg 51A: 979–983, 1969.
65. Hocutt J. E., Jaffe R., Rylander C. R., Beebe J. K.: Cryotherapy in ankle sprains. Am J Sports Med 10:316–319, 1982.
66. Ihle C., Cochran R. M.: Fracture of the fused os trigonum. Am J Sports Med 10:47–50, 1982.
67. Inman V. T., Ralston H. J., Todd F.: Human Walking. Baltimore, Williams & Wilkens, pp. 1–61, 1981.
68. Inman V. T.: The Joints of the Ankle. Baltimore, Williams & Williams, 1976, pp. 1–35.
69. Isherwood I.: A radiological approach to the subtalar joint. J Bone Joint Surg 43B(3):566–574, 1961.
70. Jack E. A.: Bone anomalies of the tarsus in relation to "peroneal spastic flat foot." J Bone Joint Surg 36B(4):530–542, 1954.
71. Jacobs A. M.: Tarsal coalitions, an instructional review. J Foot Surg 20:214, 1981.
72. James S. L., Bates B. T., Osternig L. G.: Injuries to runners. Am J Sports Med 6:40–50, 1978.
73. Jayakumar S., Cowell H. R.: Rigid flat foot. Clin Orthop 122:77–84, 1977.
74. Johnson R. A.: Tibialis posterior tendon rupture. Clin Ortho 75:140–147, 1983.
75. Jones E.: Operative treatment of chronic dislocation of the peroneal tendons. J Bone Joint Surg 14:574–576, 1932.
76. Jones R.: Fracture of the base of the 5th metatarsal bone by indirect violence. Ann Surg 35:697–700, 1902.
77. Joy G., Patzakis M. J., Harvey J. P., Jr.: Precise evaluation of the reduction of severe ankle fractures. J Bone Joint Surg 56A:979–993.
78. Kappis M.: Weitere Beitrage zur Traimatisch-Mechanischen Englehimg der "Spartmen" Knorpelabiosurgen. Dtsch Z Chir 171:13–29, 1922.
79. Karrholm J., Hansson L. I., Selvin G.: Roengen stereophotogrammetric analysis of growth pattern after supination—Adduction ankle injuries in children. J Ped Ortho 2:271–279, 1982.
80. Karrholm J., Hansson L. I., Selvik G.: Change in tibiofibular relationships due to growth disturbances after ankle fractures in children. J Bone Joint Surg 66A:1198, 1984.
81. Karrholm J., Hansson L. I., Selvik G.: Roentgen stereophotogrammetric analysis of growth pattern after pronation ankle injuries in children. Acta Orthop Scandinavica 53:1001–1011, 1982.
82. Kavanaugh J. H., Braver T. D., Mann R. V.: The Jones fracture revisited. J Bone Joint Surg 60A:776–782, 1978.
83. Kelly R. E.: An operation for chronic dislocation of the peroneal tendons. Br J Surg 7:502, 1920.
84. Kidner F. C.: The prehallux (accessory schaphoid) in its relation to flatfoot. J Bone Joint Surg 11:831, 1929.
85. Kleinberg S.: Supernumerary bones of the foot. Arch Surg 65:499–509, 1917.
86. Kohler A.: Roentgenology, 2nd Ed. London, Bailliere, Tindall and Cox, p 142, 1935.
87. Korkala O., Rusanen M., Jokipii P., Kytomaa J., Avikainen V.: A prospective study of the treatment of severe tears of the lateral ligament of the ankle. Int Orth 11:13–17, 1987.
88. König: Ueber Freie Körper in Den Gelenken, Deut Z Chir 27:90–109, 1888.
89. Kyne P. S., Mankin H. J.: Changes in intra-articular pressure with subtalar joint motion with special reference to the etiology of peroneal spastic flat foot. Bull Hosp Joint Dis 26:181, 1965.
90. Lauge-Hansen N.: Fractures of the ankle. III Genetic roentgenologic diagnosis of fractures of the ankle. Am J Roentgenol 71:456, 1954.
91. Lauge-Hansen N.: Fractures of the ankle II Combined experimental-surgical and experimental-roentgenologic investigations. Arch Surg 60:957, 1950.

92. Laurin C. A., Quellet R., St. Jacques R.: Talar and subtalar tilt: An experimental investigation. Can J Surg 11:170–179, 1968.
93. Leach R. E., Schepsis A. A.: Acute injuries to the ligaments of the ankle. In Evarts C. M. (ed): Surgery of the Musculoskeletal System. New York, Churchill Livingstone, Inc, pp. 8:143–170, 1983.
94. Leonard M. A., Gonzales S., Breck L. W., Basom C., Palafox M., Kosick Z. W.: Lateral transfer of the posterior tibial tendon in selected cases of pes plano valgus (Kidner operation) Clin Orthop 40:139, 1965.
95. Leonard M. A.: Inheritance of tarsal coalition and its relationship to spastic foot. J Bone Joint Surg 56B:520, 1974.
96. Lindstrand A., Mortensson W.: Anterior instability in the ankle joint following acute lateral sprain. Acta Radiol Diagn (Stoch) 18(5):529–539, 1977.
97. Lipscomb P. R.: Non-suppurative tenosynovitis and paratendinitis instructional courses of the American Academy of Orthopaedic Surgeons. XVI, 1966, p. 154–164.
98. Ljungquist R.: Partial tears of the patella tendon and achilles tendon. In AAOS Symposium on the Foot and Leg in Running Sports. St. Louis, CV Mosby Co, 1982.
99. Lowy A., Kruman N., Kanat I.O.: Subluxing peroneal tendons treatment with the use of an autogenous sliding bone graft. J Am Podiatric Med Assoc 75:249–253, 1985.
100. Lund-Kristensen J., Greiff J., Riegels-Nieisen P.: Malleolar fractures treated with rigid internal fixation and immediate mobilization. Injury 13:191–195, 1985.
101. Mann R. A., Moran G. T., Dougherty S. E.: Comparative electromyelography of the lower extremity in jogging, running, and sprinting. Am J Sports Med 14:501, 1986.
102. Mann R. A.: Biomechanics for Running. In Nicholas J (ed): The Lower Extremity and Spine in Sports Medicine. St. Louis, CV Mosby Co, pp. 396–411, 1986.
103. Mann R. A.: Biomechanics of running. In AAOS Symposium on the Foot and Leg in Running Sports. St. Louis, CV Mosby Co, pp. 30–44, 1982.
104. Mann R. A.: Biomechanics of the Foot and Ankle in Surgery of the Foot. St. Louis, CV Mosby Co, pp. 1–30, 1986.
105. Mann R. A.: Biomechanics of the Foot in American Academy of Orthopaedic Surgeons: Atlas of Orthotics. St Louis, CV Mosby Co, 1975.
106. Mann R. A.: Biomechanics. In Jahss M. H. (ed): Disorder of the Foot. Philadelphia, WB Saunders Co, pp. 37–67, 1982.
107. Marjom R. C., Crawford A. H.: Surgical management of tarsal coalition in adolescent athletes. Foot Ankle 7:183–193, 1986.
108. Marks K. L.: Flake fracture of the talus progressing to osteochondritis dissecans. J Bone Joint Surg 34B:90–92, 1952.
109. Marmor L.: An unusual fracture of the tibial epipysis. Clin Orthop 73:132, 1970.
110. McCallough C. J., Venugopal V.: Osteochondritis dissecans of the talus: The natural history. Clin Orthop Rel Res 144:264–268, 1979.
111. McDougall A.: The os trigonum. J Bone Joint Surg 37B:257–265, 1955.
112. McLennan J. G.: Treatment of acute and chronic luxations of the peroneal tendons. Am J Sports Med 8:432–436, 1980.
113. McManama G. B. Jr.: Ankle injuries in the young athlete. Clin Sports Med 7(3):547–562, 1988.
114. Meyer T. L., Kumler K. W.: ASIF technique and ankle fractures. Clin Orthop 150:211–216, 1980.
115. Micheli L. J.: Overuse injuries in children's sports: The growth factor. Ortho Clin N Am 14:337–360, 1983.
116. Mitchell G. P., Gibson J. M. C.: Excision of calcaneo-navicular bar for painful spasmodic flat foot. J Bone Joint Surg 49B(2):281–287, 1967.
117. Mortiz J. R.: Ski injuries. Am J Surg 98:493–505, 1959.
118. Moseir K. M., Archer M.: Tarsal coalitions and peroneal spastic flat foot. J Bone Joint Surg 66A:976, 1984.
119. Mukherjee S. K., Young A. B.: Dome fractures of the talus. A report of 10 cases. J Bone Joint Surg 55B:319–326, 1973.
120. Murr S.: Dislocation of the peroneal tendons with marginal fracture of the lateral malleolus. J Bone Joint Surg 43B:563–565, 1961.
121. Müller M. E., Allgower M., Schneider R., Willenegger H.: Manual of Internal Fixation. Techniques Recommended by the AO Group, 2nd Ed. New York, Springer-Verlag, 1979.
122. Niethard F. U.: Die Stabilitat des Sprunggelenkes nach Ruptur des Lateralen Bandapparates. Arch Ortho Unfallchir 80:53–67, 1974.
123. Nitz A. J., Dobner J. J., Kersey D.: Nerve injury and grade II and III ankle sprains. Am J Sports Med 13:177–182, 1985.
124. Noyes F. R., Torvim P. J., Hyde W. B., et al: Biomechanics of ligament failure II: An analysis of immobilization, exercise, and reconditioning effects in primates. J Bone Joint Surg 56A:1406–1418, 1974.
125. Noyes F. R.: Functional properties of knee ligaments and alterations induced by immobilization: A correlative biomechanical and histologic study in primates. Clin Ortho 123:210–239, 1977.
126. Nuber G. W.: Biomechanics of the foot and ankle during gait. Clin Sports Med 7(1):1–13, 1988.
127. Oestreich A. E., et al: The "anteater nose": A direct sign of calcaneo-navicular coalition on the lateral radiograph. JPO 7:709–711, 1987.
128. Ogden J. A.: Skeletal Injury in the Child. Lea & Febiger, pp. 555–620, 1982.
129. Olson R. W.: Arthrography of the ankle. Its use in valuation of ankle sprains. Radiol 92:1423–1446, 1969.
130. Outland T.: The pathomechanics of peronial spastic flat foot. J Bone Joint Surg 39:703, 1957.
131. Paul G. R.: Transchondral fractures of the talus. In Yablon I. G., Segal D., Leach R. E. (eds): Ankle Injuries. New York, Churchill Livingstone, pp. 113–130, 1983.
132. Paulos L. E., Johnson C. L., Noyes F. R.: Posterior compartment fractures of the ankle. A commonly missed athletic injury. Am J Sports Med 11:439–443, 1983.

133. Pettine K. A., Marrey B. F.: Osteochondral fractures of the talus. a long-term follow up. J Bone Joint Surg 69B:89–96, 1987.
134. Pfitzner W.: Die Varighimen in Aufbar des Fusselcelts Bertrage Zurkemtniss des Venschlichen Extreurita-Tenskelets VII. Wopphd. Arbeit 6:245, 1986.
135. Poll R. G., Duijfes F.: The treatment of recurrent dislocation of the peroneal tendons. J Bone Joint Surg 66B:98–100, 1984.
136. Prins J. G.: Diagnosis and treatment of injury to the lateral ligament of the ankle. Acta Chir Scand. (Suppl) 486:1–149, 1978.
137. Rang M.: Children's Fractures. Philadelphia, JB Lippincott Co, p. 198, 1974.
138. Ray S., Goldberg V. M.: Surgical treatment of the accessory navicular, Clin Orthop 177:61–66, 1983.
139. Reider B., et al: Non-union of a medial malleolus stress fracture: A case report. Am J Sports Med. Accepted for publication.
140. Rendu A.: Fracture Intra-Articulaire Parcellaire de la Pondie Astraglienne. Lyon Meds 150:220–222, 1935.
141. Rockwood C. A., Wilkens K. E., King R. E. (eds): Fractures in Children. Philadelphia, JB Lippincott Co, 1984.
142. Root M. L., Orien W. P., Weed J. H.: Normal and Abnormal Function of the Foot, Clinical Biomechanics. Vol. II. Los Angles, Clinical Biomechanics Corp. pp. 127–163, 1977.
143. Rosenmueller: quoted in Holland C. T.: On rarer ossifications seen during X-ray examinations. J Anat 55:235–248, 1921.
144. Rosse C., Clawson D. K.: The Musculoskeletal System in Health and Disease. New York, Harper & Row Publishers, Inc, p. 381, 1980.
145. Rödén S., Tillegard P., Unander-Scharin L.: Osteochondritis dissecans and similar lesions of the talus. Report of 55 cases with special reference to etiology and treatment. Acta Orthop Scand 23:51–66, 1953.
146. Rubin G., Witten M.: The talar tilt angle and the fibular collateral ligaments of the ankle. J Bone Joint Surg 42A:31–326, 1960.
147. Salter R. B., Harris W. R.: Injuries involving the epiphyseal pure. J Bone Joint Surg 45A:587–622, 1963.
148. Santopietro F. J.: Foot and foot-related injuries in the young athlete. Clin Sports Med 7:563–589, 1988.
149. Sarmtiento A., Wolf M.: Subluxation of peroneal tendons: Case treated by rerouting tendons under the calcaneofibular ligament. J Bone Joint Surg 57A:1115–1116, 1975.
150. Savastano A. A., Lowe E. B.: Ankle sprains: Surgical treatment for recurrent sprains. Am J Sports Med 8:208–211, 1980.
151. Sella E. J., Lawson J. P., Ogden J. A.: The accessory navicular synchondrosis. Clin Orthop 209:280–285, 1986.
152. Shands A. R., Jr., Durham N. C.: The accessory bones of the foot: An X-ray study of the feet of 1054 patients. South Med Surg 93:326–334, 1931.
153. Shands A. R., Jr., Wentz I. J.: Congenital anomalies, accessory bones and osteochondritis in the feet of 850 children. Surg Clin N Am 33:1643–1666, 1953.
154. Shelbourne D. K., Fisher D. A., Rettig A. C., McCandle J. R.: Stress fractures of the medial malleollus. Am J Sports Med 16:60–63, 1988.
155. Shepherd R. J.: A hitherto undescribed fracture of the astragalous. J Anat Physiol 17:79–81, 1882.
156. Slomann H. C.: On coalitio calcanio-navicularis. J Orthop Surg 3:586, 1921.
157. Smith G. R., Winquist R. A., Allan N. K., Northrop C. H.: Subtle transchondral fractures of the talar dome: A radiological perspective. Radiol 124:667–673, 1977.
158. Snook G. A., Chrisman D., Wilson T.: Long term results of the Chrissman-Snook operation for reconstruction of the lateral ligament of the ankle. J Bone Joint Surg 67A:1–7, 1985.
159. Spatt J. F., Frank N. G., Fox I. M.: Transchondral fractures of the dome of the talus. J Foot Surg 25:68–72, 1986.
160. Spiegel P. G., Cooperman D. R., Laros G. S.: Epiphyseal fractures of the distal ends of the tibia and fibula. J Bone Joint Surg 60A:1046, 1978.
161. St. Jacques R., Laurin C. A.: Normal variation of talar tilt of the ankle in children. Can Med Assoc J 93:695–699, 1965.
162. Stanitski C. L., Micheli J. J.: Medial malleolus avulsion injuries. Presentation at Pediatric Orthopaedic Study Group Meeting, San Diego, CA, April 1982.
163. Staples O. S.: Ruptures of the fibular collateral ligaments of the ankle: Result study of immediate surgical treatment. J Bone Joint Surg 57A:101–107, 1975.
164. Stormount D. M., Peterson H. A.: The relative incidence of tarsal coalition. Clin Orthop 181:28–36, 1983.
165. Stoskopf C. A., et al: Evaluation of tarsal coalition by computerized tomograph. J Ped Ortho 4:365, 1984.
166. Street F.: Footballers and ankle injuries. Medisport 1:32–35, 1979.
167. Sullivan J. A., Miller W. A.: The relationship of the accessory navicular to the development of the flat foot. Clin Orthop 144:233, 1979.
168. Swiontkowski M. F., Scranton P. E., Hansen S.: Tarsal coalitions: Long term results of surgical treatment. J Ped Ortho 3:287–292, 1983.
169. Szczukowski M., St. Pierre R. R., Fleming L. L., Somogyi J.: Computerized tomography in the evaluation of peroneal tendon dislocation. Am J Sports Med 11:444–447, 1983.
170. Tachdjian M. D.: The Child's Foot. Phildalphia. WB Saunders Co, 1985.
171. Tachdjian M. D.: Pediatric Orthopaedics. Philadelphia, WB Saunders Co, 1972.
172. Ting A., King W., et al: Stress fractures of the tarsal navicular in long distance runners. Clin Sports Med 7(1):89–102, 1988.
173. Torg J. S., Pavlov H., Torg E.: Overuse injuries in sport: The foot. Clin Sports Med 6(2):291, 1987.
174. Torg J. S., Baldkini F. C., Zelko R. R., et al: Fractures of the base of the fifth metatarsal distal to the tuberosity. J Bone Joint Surg 66A:209–214, 1984.
175. Torg J. S., Pavlov H., Cooley L. H., et al: Stress fracture of the tarsal navicular J Bone Joint Surg 63A(5);700–712, 1982.
176. Towne L. C., Blazina M. E., Cozen L. N.: Fatigue fracture of the tarsal navicular. J Bone Joint Surg 52A:376–378, 1970.

177. Tropp H., Gillquist J.: Factor affecting stabilometry recordings of single limb stance. Am J Sports Med 12:185–188, 1984.
178. Turner W.: A secondary astragalus in the human foot. J Anat Physiol 17:82, 1882.
179. Veitch J. M.: Evaluation of the Kidner procedure in the treatment of symptomatic accessory tarsal scaphoid. Clin Ortho 131:210, 1978.
180. Weber M. J.: Ankle fractures and dislocations. In Chapman M. W. (ed): Operative Orthopaedics. Philadelphia, JB Lippincott Co, pp. 471–475, 1988.
181. Weinstein S. I., Bonfiglio M.: Unusual accessory (bipartite) talus simulating fracture. J Bone Joint Surg 57A:1161–1163, 1975.
182. Wray J. B., Herndon C. N.: Hereditary transmission of congenital coalition of the calcaneus to the navicular. J Bone Joint Surg 45A:365–372, 1963.
183. Yvars M.: Osteochondral fractures of the dome of the talus. Clin Orthop 114:185–191, 1976.
184. Zadek I., Gold A. M.: The accessory tarsal scaphoid. J Bone Joint Surg 30A:957, 1948.
185. Zinman C., Resi N. D.: Osteochondritis dissecans of the talus: Use of the high resolution computed tomography scanner. Acta Orthop Scand 53:697–700, 1982.
186. Zoellner G., Clancy W.: Recurrent dislocation of the peroneal tendon. J Bone Joint Surg 61A:292–294, 1979.

23

GREAT TOE METATARSOPHALANGEAL JOINT PROBLEMS

ANGUS MCBRYDE, JR.

Injuries to the sesamoids are a potential concern in most sports since almost all of them require running or some other form of weight-bearing. During running, more than half of the weight-bearing load travels through the great toe complex, and forces up to three times body weight may be transmitted across the sesamoids.[1] The medial (tibial) sesamoid bears most of this force and thus is more prone to injury than the lateral (fibular) sesamoid.

While sesamoids elsewhere in the body are variable in occurrence, the hallux sesamoids are virtually constant, although the medial may present in a bipartite or multipartite form in 10 to 33 percent of feet.[2,3,7] The medial sesamoid tends to be larger and longer than the lateral, which is smaller and rounder.

The hallux sesamoids form an integral part of the first metatarsophalangeal (MTP) joint. They each have articular surfaces of hyaline cartilage that allow them to protect and articulate with the plantar aspect of the distal first metatarsal (Fig. 23–1). The great toe, MTP joint mechanism is complex, involving both intrinsic and extrinsic muscles.[2,4] Although the medial and lateral heads of the flexor hallucis brevis encompass the sesamoids, the adductor and abductor hallucis tendons also contribute attachments, producing a strong conjoint tendon that inserts into the proximal phalanx. The flexor hallucis longus lies securely between the sesamoids and provides push-off strength accentuated and finely tuned by the sesamoids and the entire metatarsophalangeal joint mechanism. It is obvious, then, that injury to this complex mechanism can be devastating to the young athlete involved in walking, running, jumping, dancing, or even cycling and skiing.[9]

CLINICAL PICTURE

It is usually clear when an athletic injury involves the first MTP joint complex.[1] However, identifying the specific injured structure and arriving at a precise diagnosis can be difficult. For example, a valgus stress can sprain the medial joint capsule, an injury marked by medial swelling, pain to valgus stress testing, and sometimes instability. However, the hemarthrosis that accompanies this injury makes diagnosis difficult. Sesamoiditis or even straightforward MTP joint synovitis can be primary or secondary and tough to define on examination. The problems of diagnosis are compounded by the small size of the joint and the proximity and mechanical integration of the structures that can be injured. An injury here causes pain, limping, and difficulty wearing shoes, all aggravated by repetitive stress. This clinical impact makes both acute traumatic and overuse injuries of the great toe MTP joint a major cause of competitive and recreational athletic disability in young athletes.[10]

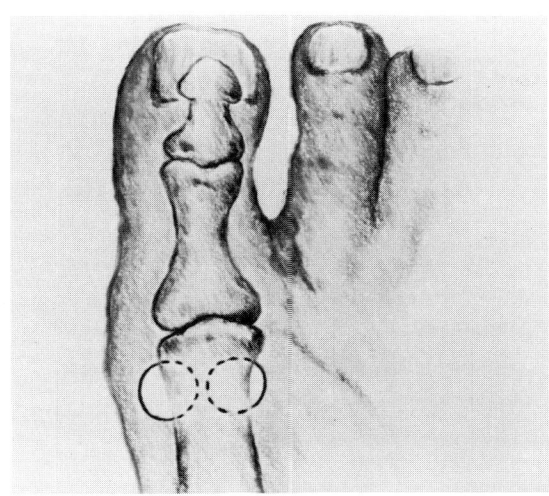

FIGURE 23–1. The great toe MP joint is a complicated joint. The medial (tibial) and the lateral (fibular) sesamoids lie beneath the first metatarsal head. They absorb and transmit forces with load bearing.

HISTORY

A good history is essential in defining the cause of the injury. Since 70 percent of great toe MTP joint problems are related to overuse produced by errors in training techniques or intensity, a detailed history may go a long way toward developing the treatment plan.

Sometimes the history is straightforward, relating the injury to a particular shoe or activity. Examples include a spike or cleat directly under the first metatarsal head of a high-jump takeoff foot, a soccer shoe with a malfitting upper that promotes great toe MTP joint impact with kicking, or a recent increase in a specific repetitive activity such as high-impact aerobics. Often, additional history from a coach, parents, or teammates will be helpful in uncovering habitual gait abnormalities or changes in training surface, footwear, or training techniques that may have contributed to the injury.

PHYSICAL EXAMINATION

The injured great toe MTP joint should be examined carefully for deformity, tenderness, restricted motion, instability, and pain with resisted flexion or extension. If the other foot is normal, careful comparison will allow for the detection of subtle abnormalities.

The examiner should first look for any gross deformities such as hallus valgus and related secondary abnormalities such as an inflamed bunion bursa or visible dorsal osteophytes. The joint should then be palpated very carefully for tenderness or subtle deformities. If medial tenderness is present, the examiner should try to determine whether the tenderness is at the joint margin, at the sesamoid metatarsal interface, or in the soft tissue itself. Careful lateral palpation should search for marginal spurring or tenderness in the deep attachment of the adductor hallus. Dorsally, the examiner should look for palpable exostosis formation or tenderness, which may be made worse with extension of the joint. Finally, the examiner should carefully palpate the plantar surface of the joint, trying to localize tenderness over the medial or the lateral sesamoid directly. Pushing the individual sesamoids distally will often bring out pain in an acute injury.

The examiner should look for stigmata of generalized ligamentous laxity and check the range of motion in the great toe MTP joint specifically. A minimum of 60 degrees of dorsiflexion and 25 degrees of plantar flexion are required for normal function of the joint; any loss of motion below this range should be noted. A flexion contracture of the interphalangeal joint should also be sought, since this can secondarily affect the MTP joint. Gently grasping the first metatarsal in one hand and the proximal phalanx in another, the examiner should perform a gentle Lachman test to detect abnormal anteroposterior (AP) laxity. Finally, the patient should be asked to flex and extend the joint against resistance and any resulting pain carefully noted. Although steroid injections are discouraged, local anesthetic injection into the joint can be a helpful adjunctive technique for differentiating intraarticular from extraarticular problems. Flexor hallus longus tenosynovitis, digital neuritis, and bunion bursitis are examples of extraarticular problems that would not be rendered painless by an intraarticular block.

RADIOGRAPHIC EXAMINATION

Adequate radiographs are essential in the diagnosis of great toe MTP joint problems. These should include routine AP, lateral, and oblique views of the foot as well as the special axial view for the sesamoids. Acute fractures and preexisting deformities such as hallux valgus, hallux rigidis (Fig. 23–2) with early joint space narrowing, and dorsal im-

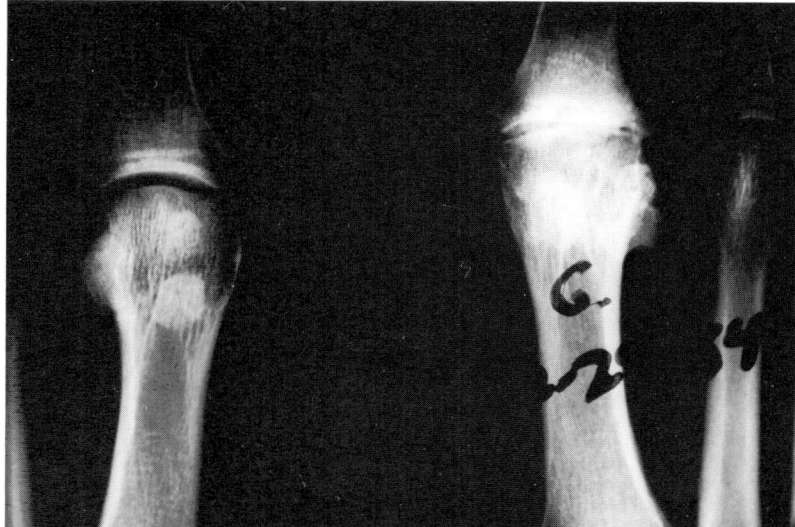

FIGURE 23–2. Hallux rigidus with loss of motion and gradual joint space narrowing, but with continued alignment, is a severe disability. An orthosis with a first metatarsal extension was helpful in this patient in his earlier stages when there was simple restriction of motion.

pingement exostosis can be easily identified. Sesamoid variants such as a bipartite or multipartite medial sesamoid can be difficult to differentiate from traumatic fractures or stress fractures on routine radiographs. A bone scan may be helpful in making this distinction. A bone scan may also be helpful in determining whether the MTP joint or sesamoids are involved in the pathological process and which sesamoid is particularly involved, but it will not indicate a specific diagnosis. In advanced cases of avascular necrosis, plain radiographs may demonstrate dramatic collapse or fragmentation of the involved sesamoid. Occasionally, linear tomography or computerized tomography (CT) may be necessary to differentiate between a sesamoid stress fracture and a bipartite sesamoid or to document the union of such a fracture following treatment.

TREATMENT

Sesamoid injuries can be divided into acute and chronic problems according to their mode of presentation. However, there is considerable overlap between the groups since acute injuries can go on to produce chronic pain, whereas chronic injuries of insidious onset can present with an acute crisis. Table 23–1 summarizes the diagnoses normally included in the acute and chronic categories.

TABLE 23–1. Classification of Great Toe MTP Joint Injuries

Acute Injuries	Chronic Injuries
Fracture	Synovitis
Undisplaced	Hallux rigidus
Severely displaced	
Avulsion displaced	Bursitis
Synovitis	Hallux valgus
Sprain	Sesamoids[7]
Medial	Stress fracture[3, 6, 7]
Lateral	Osteochondritis[3]
Plantar "turf toe"	Sesamoiditis
Sesamoids	(chondromalacia)
Sesamoiditis[8]	
Fracture	
Contusion	

ACUTE INJURIES

FRACTURES

Primary bony injuries with undisplaced acute fracture of any portion of the MTP joint, including the sesamoids, are treated in a standard fashion with 4 to 7 weeks of short leg cast immobilization. The cast should include a full toe platform and extension support distally. Displaced fractures require reduction if an unacceptable deformity is present. If the fracture involves an articular surface, then anatomical realignment should be the goal, using surgery if needed as a means to achieve anatomical reduction.

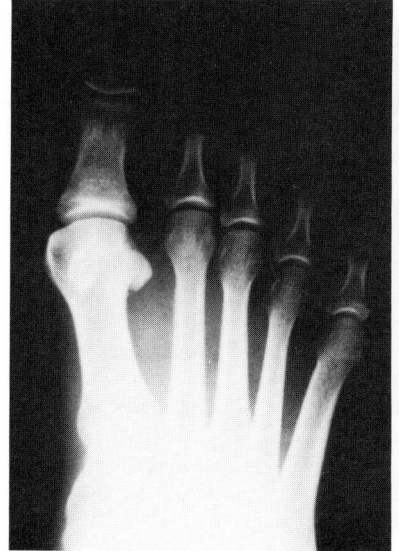
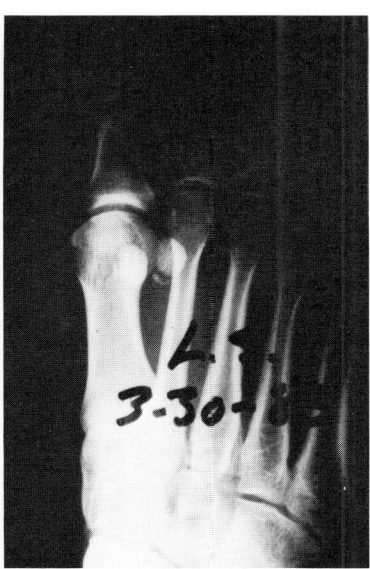
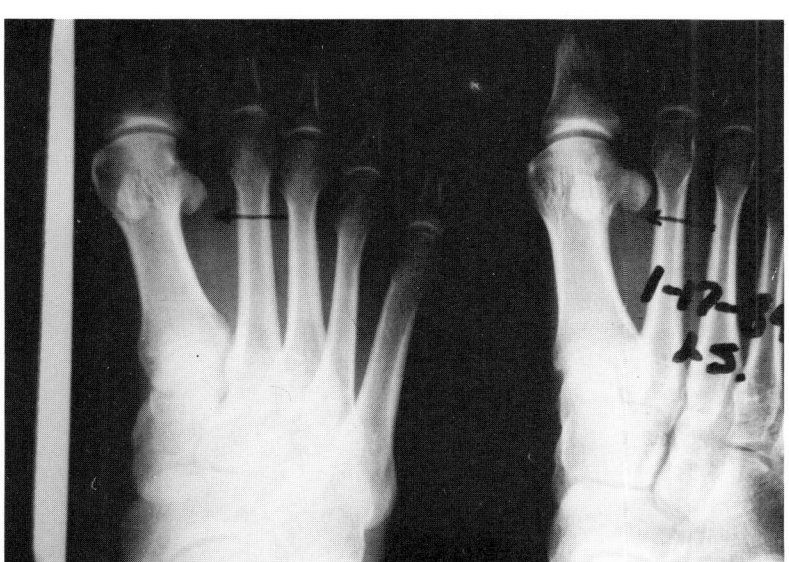

FIGURE 23–3. This is an avulsion fracture in a 30-year-old female aerobics participant (*A*) after 3 months of symptoms, then (*B*) after 6 weeks of casting with healing, no symptoms, and full return to use 9 months later.

Growth abnormalities are a potential problem in injuries to the physis of the proximal phalanx in the young child but should not be a concern in the nearly mature adolescent skeleton. Whether they involve sesamoids, first metatarsal, or proximal phalanx, most acute fractures of the great toe MTP joint are avulsion injuries. Prognosis is therefore usually good in these injuries, since the strong intact supporting tendinous expansion usually prevents wide displacement of the fragments (Fig. 23–3). The sesamoid fractures are usually transverse and most commonly involve the tibial sesamoid. MTP joint arthrofibrosis may result when a first metatarsal or proximal phalanx intraarticular fracture is present.

ACUTE SPRAIN AND RELATED INJURIES

Acute sprain of the medial or lateral aspect of the MTP joint, traumatic synovitis, and direct contusion of the joint are soft tissue injuries that may respond to similar treatments. They should be treated acutely with a program of icing and immobilization by taping or splinting to avoid the extremes of motion and to put the joint at relative rest. Wooden or rigid soled shoes or bunion splints are helpful for temporary support. Nonsteroidal antiinflammatory drugs are valuable for reducing the acute inflammatory reaction from these injuries. Modalities such as ultrasound, iontophoresis, and phonophoresis can be of additional help. An acute synovitis secondary to trauma but without major structural injury will require 3 weeks for resolution of acute symptoms and another 3 weeks of protection during a graduated return to sports participation.

TURF TOE

Despite its whimsical name, turf toe may produce considerable acute and chronic disability. The common mechanism is an acute hyperdorsiflexion injury. These injuries can involve sesamoid fracture or avulsions or may result in tearing of the entire plantar ligamentous complex without radiographic evidence of sesamoid injury. Many of these injuries are mild; however, the sesamoids may be partially or completely torn from their bed. In the most severe cases, rupture of the plantar complex at the level of the sesamoids leaves a mobile gap that makes healing difficult, especially if repetitive use of the toe continues.

Acute injuries with minimal soft tissue tearing leave no residual stiffness and have an excellent long-term prognosis. More severe injuries such as turf toe or sesamoid fractures may lead to chronic symptoms. In general, uncontrolled MTP joint symptoms can lead to prolonged disability.

CHRONIC INJURIES

Many of the chronic injuries listed in Table 23–1 are so classified because they result from repetitive stress rather than acute trauma. Others may represent lingering symptoms from an incompletely resolved acute injury. Finally, some chronic conditions may present with an acute crisis, such as when chronic loss of dorsiflexion due to dorsal impingement of distal metatarsal osteophytes is made acutely symptomatic by sudden forced dorsiflexion of the toe.

SESAMOIDITIS

Sesamoiditis is a clinical diagnosis usually related to repetitive stress and not acute injury. It tends to occur more frequently in the "high arch" or cavus foot. The diagnosis is a clinical one, marked by point tenderness on one of the sesamoids in the absence of radiographic evidence of a specific bony abnormality such as stress fracture or avascular necrosis. *Symptomatic partite sesamoid* is the term usually given to this condition when the sesamoid is noted to be bipartite or multipartite radiographically. It is probably a manifestation of chondromalacia of the articular surfaces of the sesamoids and may be complicated by chronic synovitis. Although it is difficult to document, we fear that young patients with such a chronic synovitis will ultimately develop loss of motion and hallux rigidus. For this reason, we feel that an aggressive approach to control the synovitis in such cases is important. Treatment options for cure or control are similar to those used in acute injuries and include icing, nonsteroidal antiinflammatory drugs, physical therapy modalities, and temporary rest with splinting

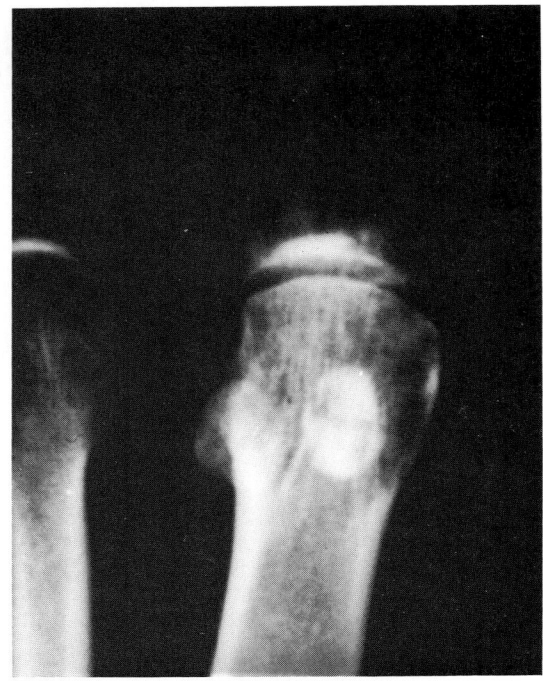

FIGURE 23–4. A sesamoid stress fracture is irregular and does not have rounded edges, as would a partitioned sesamoid. This AP view also shows varying width of the lucent fracture line. This runner eventually needed surgery.

GREAT TOE METATARSOPHALANGEAL JOINT PROBLEMS

and activity modification. Frequently, substitute training using swimming or water exercise with a flotation vest is necessary. Permanent orthoses with a built-in first metatarsal extension, a midsole load shift, or a stiffer last built into the athletic shoe may help. Fabrication of a custom shoe with a protective toe box roomy enough to permit splinting of the toe may be necessary. About 10 days to 3 weeks of rest by casting may be necessary to reduce symptoms to the point that use of the foot may be tolerated.

OSTEOCHONDRITIS

Osteochondritis or avascular necrosis of the sesamoids may occur as a primary disor-

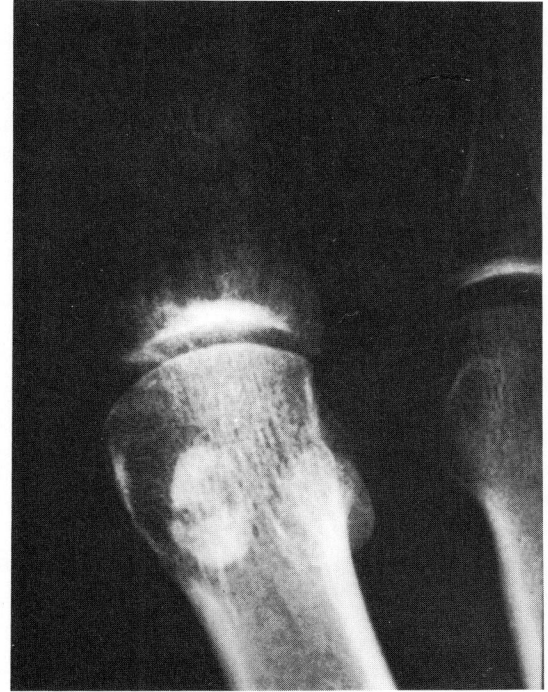

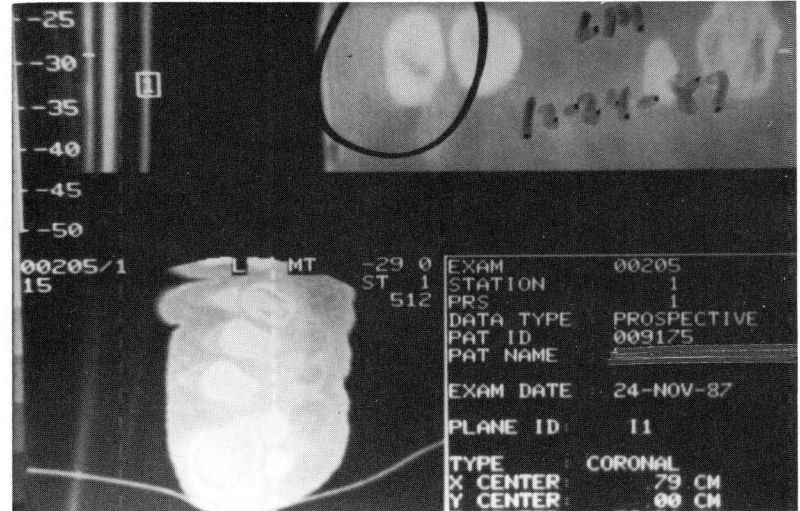

FIGURE 23–5. In older stress fractures, the lucent fracture line becomes wider and more irregular. Shown are (*A*) AP X-ray, and (*B*) CT scan. Osteochondritis can follow prolonged nonunion.

der, possibly related to recurrent stress, or as a secondary problem following stress fracture. We have not seen this as a complication of a traumatic fracture. In the case of a stress fracture, resulting avascular necrosis may lead to fragmentation and collapse of the sesamoid. Such lesions should be treated conservatively for at least 6 months using the methods described for sesamoiditis. If the symptoms continue to be disabling, and the sesamoid appears too collapsed and too fragmented to permit bone grafting, partial or complete excision may be necessary.

STRESS FRACTURES

Stress fractures of the sesamoid present with increasing pain and point tenderness of one of the sesamoids incited by a repetitive activity such as running, basketball, or dancing. A bone scan may be necessary to confirm the diagnosis accurately, as plain radiographs will not be abnormal until approximately 3 weeks after injury (Fig. 23–4). Treatment should consist of 6 weeks of casting in a short leg platform cast, followed by 6 weeks of protected weight bearing. If the fracture has not united after 6 months of treatment and symptoms are sufficiently severe, surgical treatment should be considered (Fig. 23–5). Single sesamoid excision has been used by many surgeons for such cases and may give good short-term results. However, we worry that such excision may increase stress on the other sesamoid, the flexor hallux longus tendon, and the MP joint itself and that the subsequent shift in alignment of the flexor mechanism may lead to chronic inflammatory and degenerative changes, especially in the athlete. Because of this, we have preferred to treat these ununited stress fractures with bone grafting in lieu of excision whenever possible. We usually prefer an intraarticular surgical approach, obtaining the bone graft from the adjacent first metatarsal. Postoperatively, the patients are immobilized for 6 to 8 weeks or until union occurs. Computerized tomography may be helpful in detecting early union before it is evident on plain radiographs.

SUMMARY

The great toe MTP joint, including its sesamoids, is subject to the same posttraumatic acute and repetitive stress injuries as any other bone or joint. Preexisting mobility or deformity is important in the intensity of treatment and in determining prognosis. Special efforts in differential diagnosis of the primary problem are necessary.

References

1. Drez, D.: Forefoot Problems in Runners. Symposium on the Foot and Leg in Running Sports. St. Louis, C. V. Mosby Co., pp. 73–75, 1982.
2. Hamilton, W. G.: Surgical anatomy of the foot and ankle. Clin. Symp. 37(3): 1985.
3. Kliman, M., Gross, A., Pritzker, P., Greyson, D.: Osteochondritis of the hallux sesamoid bones. Foot Ankle 3(4): 220–223, 1983.
4. Mann, R.: AAOS Instructional Course Lectures. Vol. 31. St. Louis, C. V. Mosby Co., pp. 167–200, 1982.
5. McBryde, A.: Stress fractures in runners. Clin. Sports Med. 4:737–752, 1985.
6. McBryde, A.: Stress fractures in runners. In D'Ambrosia, R., Drez, D. (eds.): Prevention and Treatment of Running Injuries. 2nd ed. Thoroughfare, NJ, Slack Inc., pp. 43–82, 1989.
7. McBryde, A., Anderson, R.: Sesamoid foot problems in the athlete. Foot and ankle injuries. Clin. Sports Med. 7(1):51–60, 1988.
8. McBryde, A., Jackson, D., James, C.: Injuries in runners and joggers. In Schneider, R., Kennedy, J., Plant, M., et al. (eds.): Sport Injuries. Baltimore, Williams & Wilkins, pp. 395–416, 1985.
9. Richardson, G.: Injuries to the hallucal sesamoids in the athletes. Foot Ankle 7(4): 229–244, 1987.
10. Van Hal, M. E., Keene, J. S., Lange, T. A., Clancy, W. G.: Stress fractures of the great toe sesamoids. Am J. Sports Med. 10:122, 1982.

Part III

SPORT-SPECIFIC SPORTS MEDICINE

24

GYMNASTICS

BERT R. MANDELBAUM

Gymnastics has evolved into an extremely popular and competitive sport in North America and around the world. The long hours of disciplined training during childhood that are required to master the risky and complex maneuvers of gymnastics produce a variety of characteristic medical problems. Physicians caring for young gymnasts must strive to help prevent injuries prior to their occurrence, minimize the morbidity of injuries that occur, and help the athlete to maximize his or her performance and personal development. The purpose of this chapter is to provide the reader with a historical perspective and understanding of the technical details of this demanding sport. Such an understanding of the "dose" of activity administered to the gymnast during training will help the clinician evaluate the "response" of the gymnast's body during the years of growth and development and will allow him or her to provide recommendations regarding optimal participation, performance, and competition.

HISTORICAL PERSPECTIVE

Gymnastics has been a sport handed down from civilization to civilization. The earliest versions were described by the Egyptians in 2000 B.C. Subsequently, it was the Greek civilization that further popularized the concept of integration of body and mind in gymnastics. Approximately 700 B.C., the Athenians signaled the merit of gymnastics by identifying it as a sport worthy of the Olympic competition. The Spartans titled the sport *gymnastics*, meaning "to perform exercises while naked." The Roman civilization, led by Claudius Galen, the first sports physician, defined gymnastics as a sport to maximize the quality of physical and mental life. With the end of the Roman Empire, the sport went through a transformation, as the only remaining gymnasts became entertainers.

Through the Renaissance, gymnastics became redefined as an essential component of physical and mental training. Frederick Jahn of early ninteenth-century Germany was referred to as the "Father of Gymnastics." His refinement of techniques was directed at improving general health and morale. In addition, Jahn further popularized the concept of the gymnast with respect to specific skills, maneuvers, and exercises.

Gymnastics in the United States had its initiation at Harvard College, where Charles Frollen, a direct descendant of Jahn, started a program in 1825. In recent years, there has been a crescendo of interest in the sport as it has grown to almost 2 million gymnasts on a club, school, and collegiate level. In retrospect, a significant growth and popularity of gymnastics in this country became obvious after the Olympics of 1972 and 1976 when such stars as Olga Korbut and Nadia Comaneci introduced the world, through the media, to the beautiful sport requiring grace, determination, discipline, and, in their cases, perfection! It is the performances and efforts of all involved that have led to the tremendous resurgence of the sport.

At the present time, children are beginning the sport at the age of 5 or 6 and training up to 24 hours per week, 365 days a year during the years of growth and development. Girls' and boys' gymnastics are distinctly different sports whose participants differ significantly in the ages of initiation, peak level of performance, and retirement.[9,10] The elite female gymnast initiates her sport at approximately age 6, reaches high-level maximal competitive levels by age 16, and retires at about 18. The male elite gymnast initiates the sport at about age 9, reaches peak level of competition by age 22, and usually retires sometime after age 24. Thus, the elite female and male gymnasts are training and competing at different stages of their physical and psychological development, with the female gymnasts maximally involved at a particularly vulnerable age. The current trend toward gathering young elite gymnasts in regional training centers has added the stress of isolation from their families to the physiological and psychological demands being placed on their developing bodies.

Men's gymnastics includes six different exercises: pommel horse, vault, floor exercise, parallel bar, high bar, and rings. Women's gymnastics is decidedly different. The four sports include uneven parallel bars, floor exercise, the balance beam, and vault (Fig. 24–1). These different events make different biomechanical and technical demands on the gymnast. The male gymnast is dependent on developing a powerful upper extremity and must compete with power, finesse, and extreme maneuverability to succeed in each of the six events. The female counterpart must include some power but requires a high level of grace, artistry, rhythm, and dance to succeed during those events. The differences in age of peak participation, training requirements, and performance demands lead to distinct differences in injury patterns between male and female gymnasts. Female gymnasts have been particularly subject to certain medical and orthopedic problems.

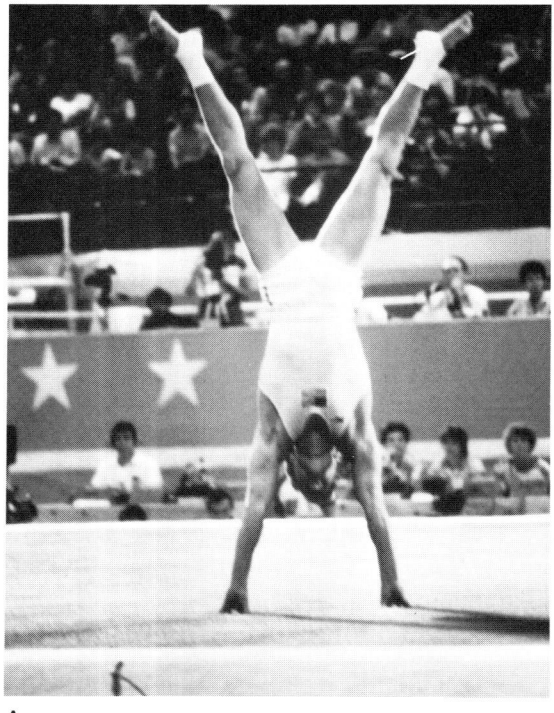
A

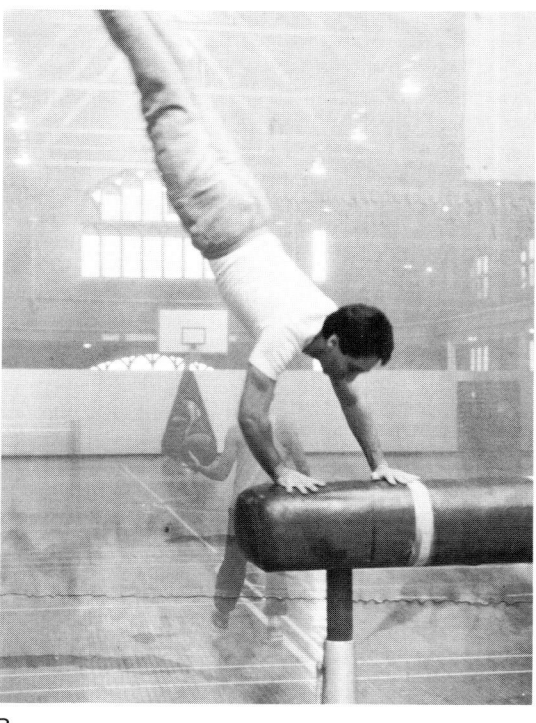
B

FIGURE 24–1. The six men's gymnastic events include (*A*) floor exercise, (*B*) vault, (*C*) parallel bars, (*D*) rings, (*E*) high bars, and (*F*) pommel horse. The four women's events include (*G*) vault, (*H*) floor exercise, (*I*) uneven parallel bars, and (*J*) balance beam.

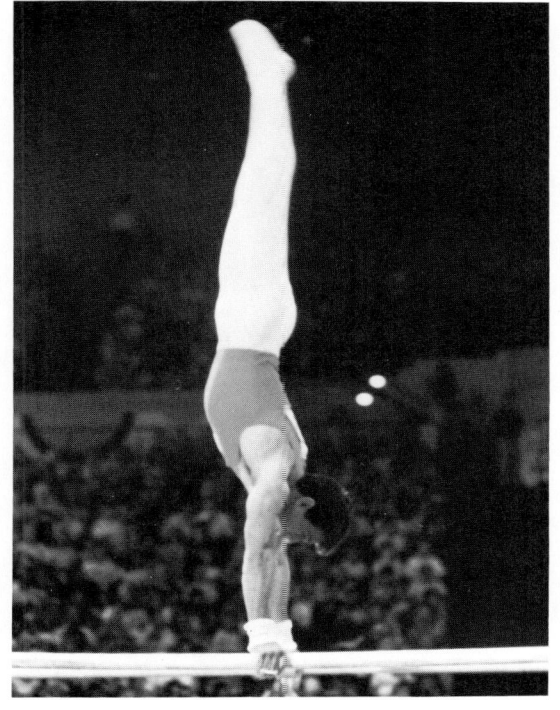

C

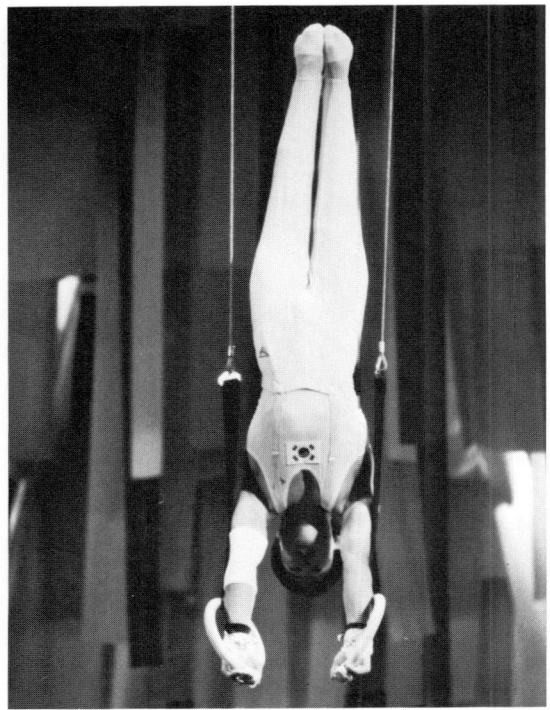

D

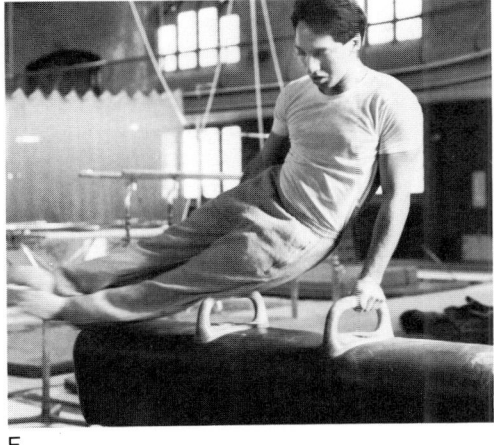

F

FIGURE 24–1. *Continued.*

E

Illustration continues on following page

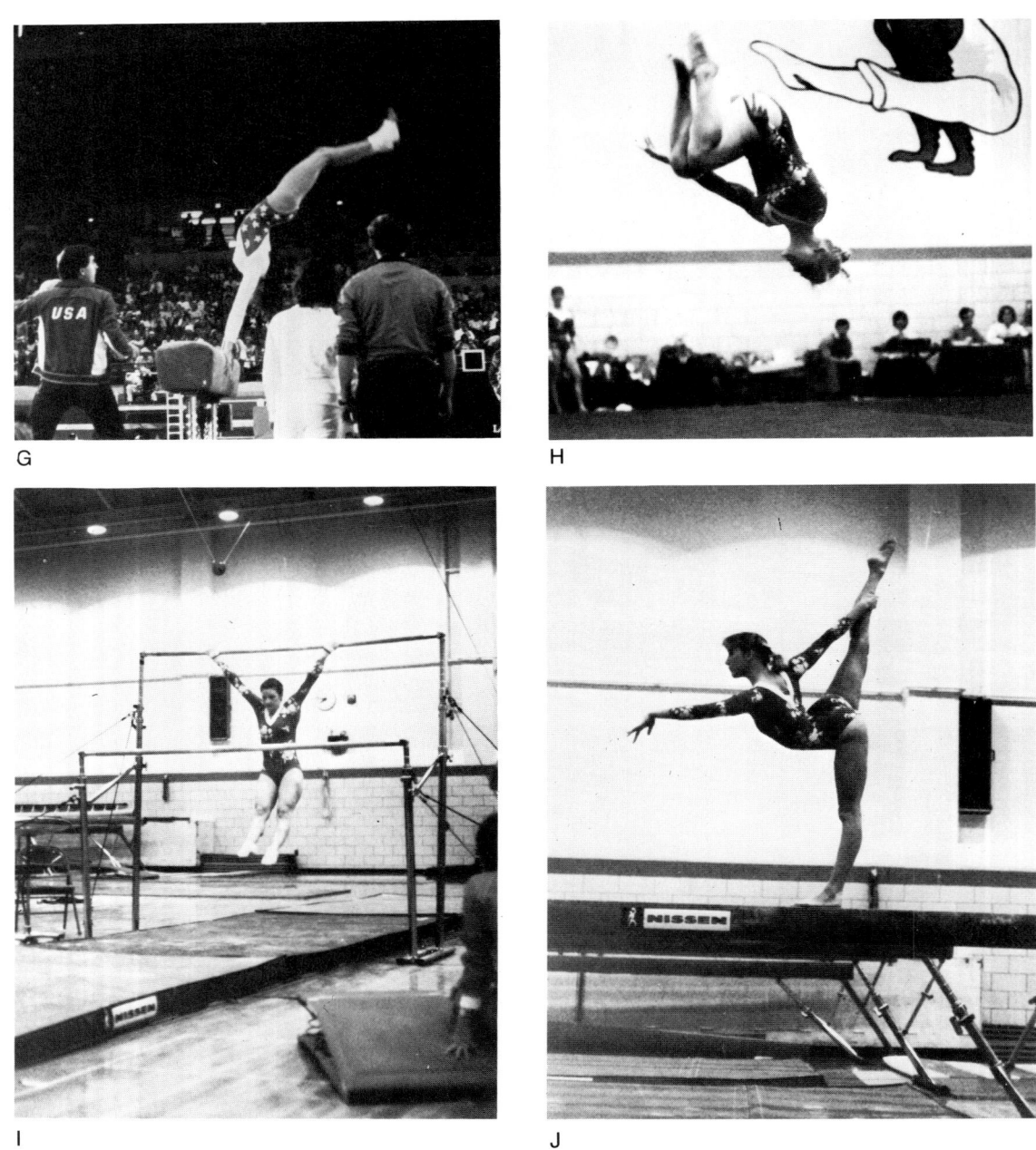

FIGURE 24–1. *Continued.*

NUTRITIONAL AND EATING DISORDERS

One of the most significant medical concerns in the young female gymnast is that of eating disorders and nutritional abnormalities. The age of menarche in a young growing adolescent gymnast is in fact delayed by almost 2 years.[10] The exact etiology may be related to the intensive exercise and training required by the sport as well as specific nutritional deficiencies. Eating disorders such as anorexia nervosa and bulimia are common in this population. The intensity and the obsession used to perfect one's gymnastic technique may also be manifested in the extreme parallel of an eating disorder. Loss of nutritional integrity, relative malnutrition, and loss of calories, protein, vitamins, and/or trace elements may result in incompetence of the musculoskeletal system. As in the dancer (Chapter 27), this relative malnutrition may compromise the ability of the gymnast's body to respond to physical stress, resulting in an increased incidence of overuse injuries. The physician must pay attention to the general condition of the intense young gymnast and frequently remind her of the relationship between adequate nutrition and optimal performance.

THE EPIDEMIOLOGY OF GYMNASTIC INJURIES

Several authors have evaluated the epidemiological aspects of orthopedic gymnastics injuries.[1,6,7,8,12,15] Snook, evaluating injury patterns in women gymnasts, concluded that this may be a "hazardous" sport for the competitor.[15] He found the incidence of injuries to be highest in the lower extremity, followed by the upper extremity and the trunk. Ankle sprains were the most common of all traumatic or overuse injuries. Garrick and Requa,[1] evaluating school, club, and collegiate gymnasts, concurred that the highest incidence of injuries was in the lower extremity, followed by the upper extremity, spine, and trunk. Once again, ankle sprains were the most common injury. Floor exercise was the event that had the highest association of injuries. In addition, sprains followed by strains qualitatively had the highest incidence in this study. Goldberg further defined and stressed the importance of overuse and developmental problems associated with gymnastic activities during the adolescent years.[2] He emphasized the need for the clinician to elicit the historic details of the athlete's training program and astutely analyze them to help prevent or minimize overuse and other orthopedic injuries. McAuley et al.,[8] in a survey of the girls gymnastics injury literature, noted that the incidence of injury increased dramatically as skill level increased.[1,7,16] They noted two possible reasons for this: first, that the difficulty of maneuvers increased with each skill level and, second, that the practice time and thus the exposure increased with each skill level. They also reported that floor exercise demonstrates the highest injury rate in women's gymnastics, followed by balance beam and uneven parallel bars, with vaulting a distant fourth.

Therefore, it appears that the sport of gymnastics, by virtue of the age of initiation, the type of risk inherent in complex routines and maneuvers, and the factor of human error, remains a challenge with respect to injury and prevention. Understanding the nuances of gymnastics and its coaching techniques will allow the physician to focus the preparticipation physical on appropriate details and facilitate the athlete's participation in the sport.

WRIST INJURIES

Wrist pain has become an increasing problem in this young, avidly participating athletic population.[9,11] The incidence in the young female gymnast is about 70 percent. Our studies in collegiate gymnasts indicate an incidence of 72 percent in the 21-year-old male athlete and 33 percent in his female counterpart.[10] This kind of pain causes a significant diminution in training, participation, and performance.

The etiological explanation for what appears to be a common and increasing problem has been obscure. One cause may be the increased utilization of "round-off" activities during training and competition in recent years. A round-off is a tumbling maneuver that requires a gymnast to pivot a half twist while weight bearing on the hands. Some elite and highly competitive coaches believe that these maneuvers have increased by two to three times. A consequence of the increase in the number of round-offs and upper extremity weight-bearing activity has been a concomitant increase in wrist pain. In general, the pathogenesis of wrist pain appears related to chronic repetitive upper extremity weight bearing during the growth and development years. Moreover, our study indicates that there is a direct correlation between wrist pain, the age of the gymnast, and the total hours of gymnastics. Based on these details, we have theorized that many of these wrist problems may be related to trauma to the distal radial physis during development.[14] Three separate studies using 11-, 16-, and 21-year-old gymnasts indicate that the relative length of the ulna with respect to the radius is significantly increased when compared with age-matched nongymnast con-

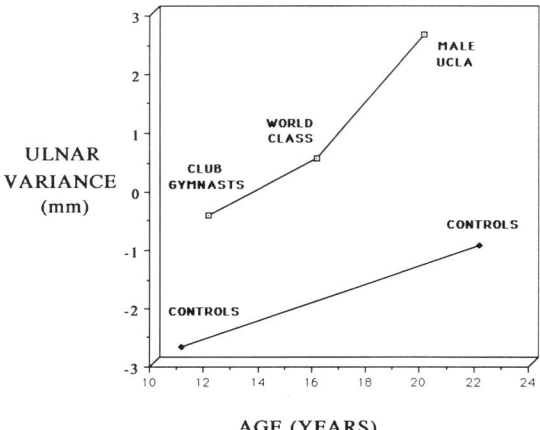

FIGURE 24–2. Graph depicting relationship of age to ulnar variance. The gymnastic curve is significantly different than the control population.

trols (Fig. 24–2). This increased incidence of positive ulnar variance can result in a myriad of pathoanatomical changes that most recently have been detected utilizing magnetic resonance imaging (MRI) and arthroscopy. Using these techniques, we can now define a spectrum of pathological entities including chondromalacia of the articular surfaces of the lunate, triquetrium, scaphoid, and the distal radius. Other problems that may be related to this pathogenetic progression include ganglion cysts of the tendon sheaths or of the wrist capsule.

In conclusion, it appears that the overuse or "overdose" of the biped wrist as compared with its quadruped progenitor has left the wrist unable to adapt to the additional loads during the years of growth and development. This then leaves us with several goals for the sports medicine physician caring for the gymnast with wrist pain: minimizing the morbidity associated with this problem, maximizing the performance of those gymnasts who have wrist pain, and lastly, preventing it in the younger new population of gymnasts.

EVALUATION AND MANAGEMENT

An algorithm has been developed for effective management of wrist pain in the gymnast (Fig. 24–3). The initial evaluation of wrist pain in the young gymnast should begin with an accurate history and physical examination. Important historical details include total number of hours of gymnastics relative to

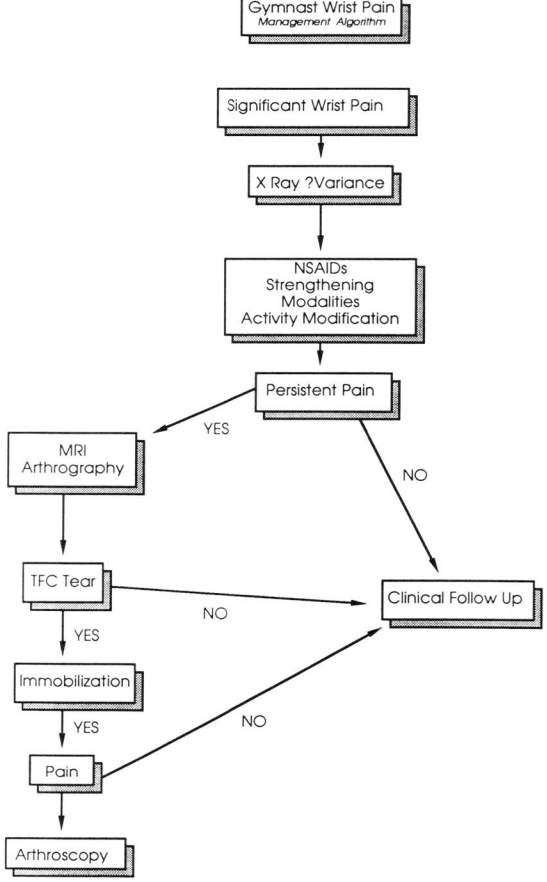

FIGURE 24–3. An algorithm for effective management of wrist pain in the gymnast.

the time spent in the gym and the qualitative progression of pain. Specific details regarding the overuse injuries to the bone or physis of the radius are heralded by a typical "crescendo" in the gymnast's pain: first pain during activity, followed by pain during and after activity, followed by pain before, during, and after activity. Physical examination should be performed with specific attention to muscle symmetry, points of maximal tenderness, and areas of pain in association with motion, loaded motion, and specific loaded motions with gymnastic activities.

Primary diagnostic tests include routine radiographs. It is essential to obtain reproducible examinations including anteroposterior (AP) and lateral projections. The AP projection should be performed with the shoulder at 90 degrees, the elbow at 90 degrees, and the wrist at neutral pronation. The following details should be evaluated: (1) ulnar variance, which can be measured with

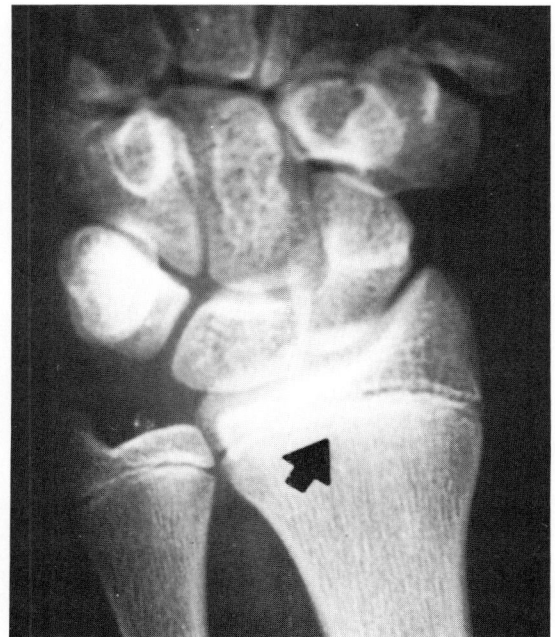 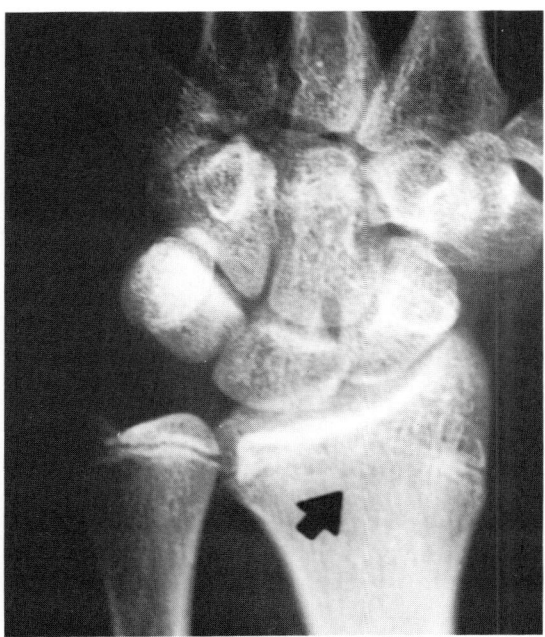

FIGURE 24–4. (A) Plain radiograph of a 13-year-old female gymnast who is asymptomatic demonstrating normally open distal radial and ulnar physis. (B) Plain radiograph in young gymnast showing premature distal radial physeal closure and consequent positive ulnar variance.

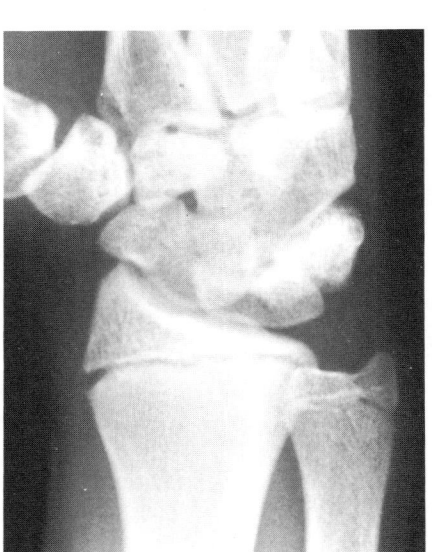 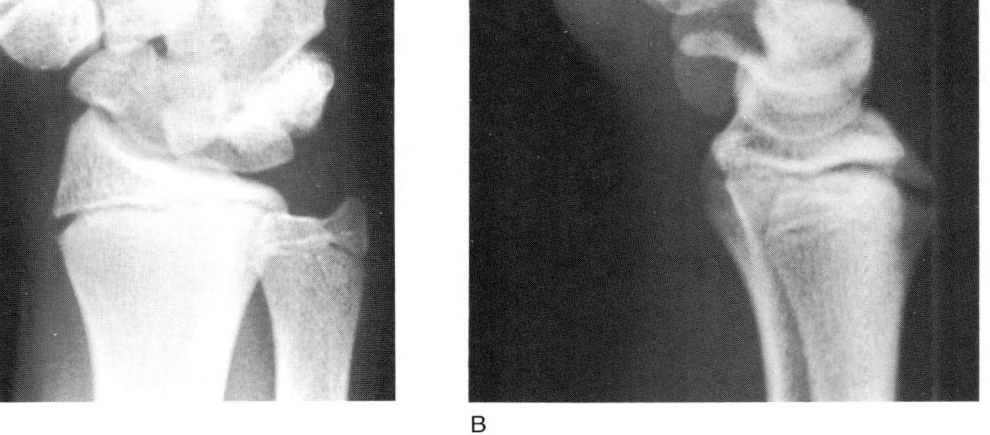

FIGURE 24–5. (A) Plain film in AP projection demonstrating widened distal radial physis. These changes are typical radiographic abnormalities seen in the young gymnast. (B) Lateral radiograph demonstrates metaphyseal beaking.

concentric circles (Fig. 24–4), and (2) specific changes in the distal radius or ulna physis including metaphyseal beaking, cysts, areas of hypersclerosis or new periosteal bone formation (Fig. 24–5), presence of fractures,[10] and ligamentous instabilities.[9]

Stress injuries should be treated with standard orthopedic techniques of rest, immobilization as necessary, and restorative rehabilitative protocols. Persistence of pain after an approximate 6- to 9- week period following this protocol should be evaluated by a second set of radiographs. Persistence of pain on the dorsal, ulnar, or middorsal portion of the wrist should be followed by arthrography and/or MRI, depending on accessibility (Fig. 24–6). At this juncture, ruling out intraarticular abnormalities such as triangular fibrocartilage tears, loose bodies, and/or ligamentous instabilities is essential. Prior to any other therapeutic intervention, a period of immobilization for 6 weeks once again is attempted.

ARTHROSCOPY

If pain persists in the face of a triangular fibrocartilage tear as defined by the imaging study of choice, wrist arthroscopy may ensue as a diagnostic and therapeutic endeavor. It is essential to maintain specific inclusion criteria for arthroscopy, which include the described immobilization period, trials of nonsteroidal antiinflammatories and/or aspirin, and a positive finding on the imaging studies. Partial tears in the triangular fibrocartilage can be specifically treated with partial debridement of the tear or rarely repair. Most overuse tears of the triangular fibrocartilage occur at the point of insertion at the sigmoid notch of the distal radius and respond well to debridement. Very few surgeons have significant experience with repair of the triangular fibrocartilage. We would only recommend repair in the case of an acute injury associated with a total and peripheral tear of the triangular fibrocartilage complex. The postarthroscopic rehabilitation protocol should be extremely gradual in terms of physical therapy and gradual upper extremity weight bearing (Table 24–1). It should always be stressed that after a long period of nonparticipation in upper extremity weight-bearing activities, an extended period of cyclically progressive training is required to reestablish the preinjury level of participation.

TABLE 24–1. Postoperative Rehabilitation Following Arthroscopic Debridement of the Triangular Fibrocartilage in the Gymnast

Phase I
First 10 days following surgery
The wrist is immobilized in the anatomical position of function with a bulky soft dressing and a volar splint

Phase II
10 days to 6 weeks postoperatively
Gentle range-of-motion exercises, at first without resistance but progressing to resistance with a small weight.

Phase III
6 weeks to 3 months postoperatively
Continue with range-of-motion and resistive exercises
Full painless range of motion should be achieved by the tenth week
By the twelfth week, mild push-ups and other gentle weight bearing activities should be done in a range of motion that prevents weight bearing in the fully extended position.

Phase IV
3 to 4 months postoperatively
The athlete gradually progresses to full loading of the wrist in hyperextension

Note: The rehabilitation process should progress in a cyclical manner; if the wrist becomes painful during the process, a period of rest with use of the splint may be necessary.

Thus, wrist pain in these athletes can be a difficult diagnostic and therapeutic dilemma, but a systematic approach must be made to restore the athlete to levels of participation and competition.

PREVENTION

The physician and coach can work together to benefit the largest number of gymnasts by implementing the following wrist injury prevention program. This may not only help prevent overuse injuries of the distal radial physis but may also reduce the incidence of secondary problems that occur later owing to the pathological positive ulnar variance. Specific steps that may help reduce wrist problems in gymnasts include the following:

1. Gymnasts should obtain biannual AP radiographs of the wrist to rule out widening of the epiphyseal plate and positive ulna variance (Figs. 24–4 and 24–5).

2. Avoid overloading of the wrists at an early age with gradually increased weight-bearing supports as the gymnast matures, es-

GYMNASTICS 423

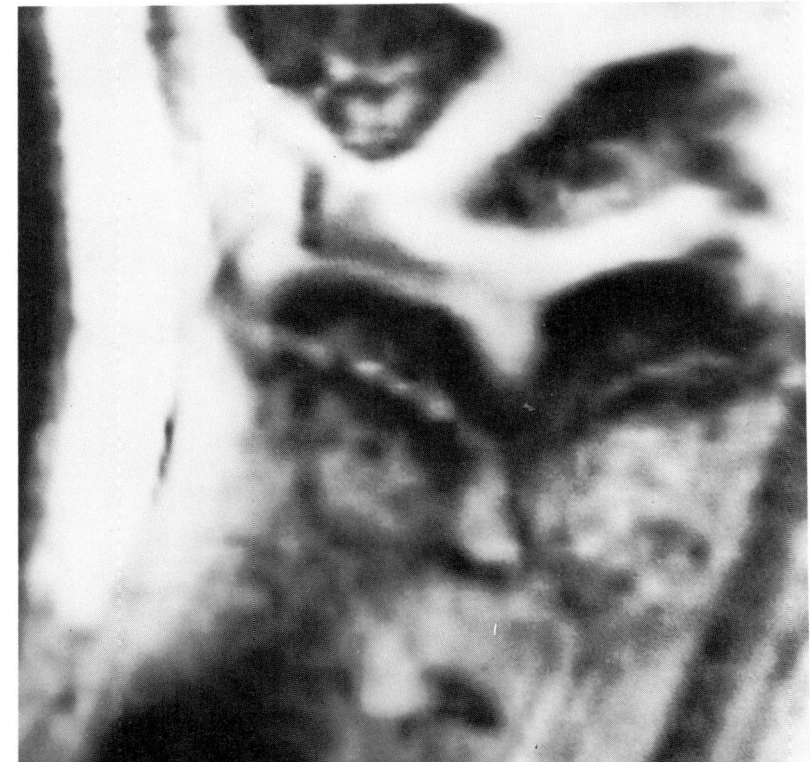

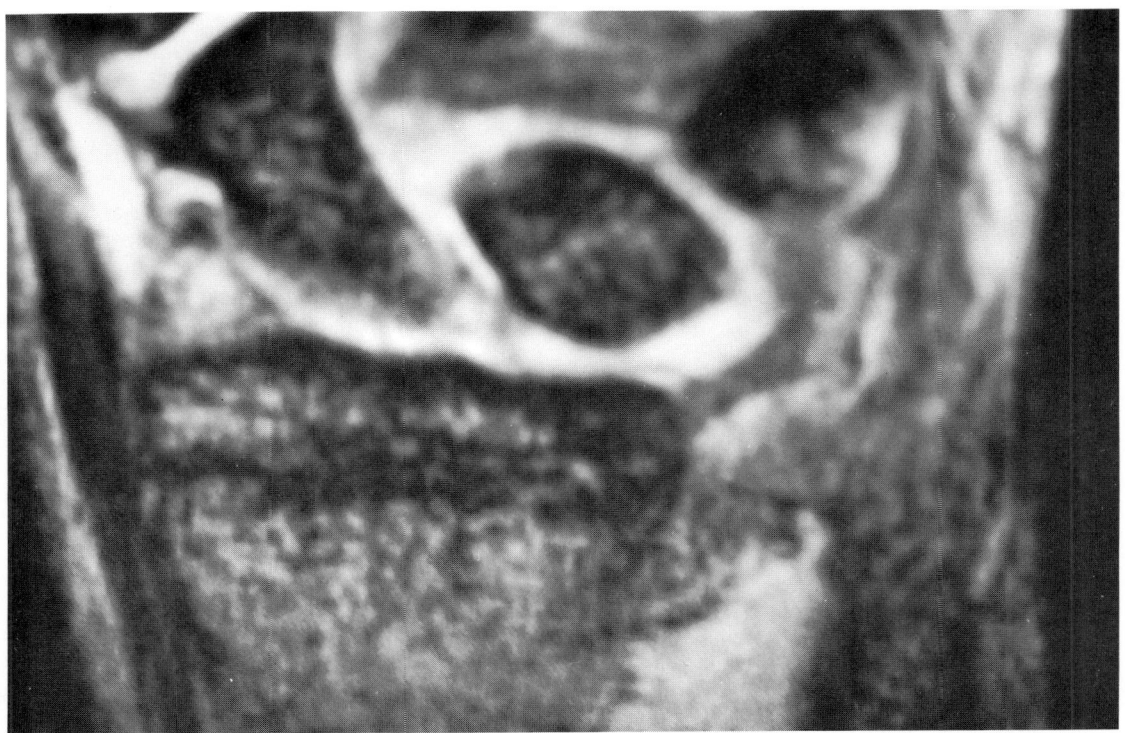

FIGURE 24–6. (*A*) Coronal MRI demonstrating triangular fibrocartilage showing insertion into sigmoid notch. (*B*) Coronal MRI depicting triangular fibrocartilage and insertion into distal radius.

pecially for boys on the pommel horse (Fig. 24–7).

3. Wrist strengthening and flexibility exercises should be performed before and after workout for all ages. The specific exercises should include isokinetics and isotonic free weights during motions of flexion/extension, radial/ulnar deviation, and pronation/supination. Attention should be placed on high repetition with low weight. Anecdotally, there appears to be a direct relationship between those individuals who have decreased flexibility and the overall incidence of wrist problems. Those individuals who have decreased flexibility should be specifically identified and treated with aggressive flexibility augmentation exercises.

4. Training should be done in a cyclically progressive manner so that the athlete is not increasing the dose of load bearing in a progressive stepwise fashion but rather in a cyclical manner so that every escalation is followed by a decrease in overall load for a week's time, followed by another increase, thereby allowing reparative time for connective tissue structures.

5. Swinging and support events should be alternated during workouts.

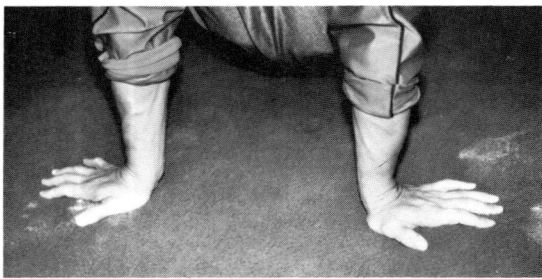

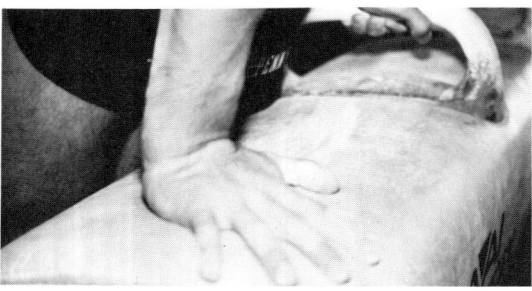

FIGURE 24–7. Gymnastics may produce large, complex loads on the flexed wrist. (*A*) Gymnast demonstrates "power" weight-bearing position. Note hyperflexion and slight radial deviation. (*B*) A strain gauge was built into this pommel to assess loads and forces during pommel horse maneuvers.

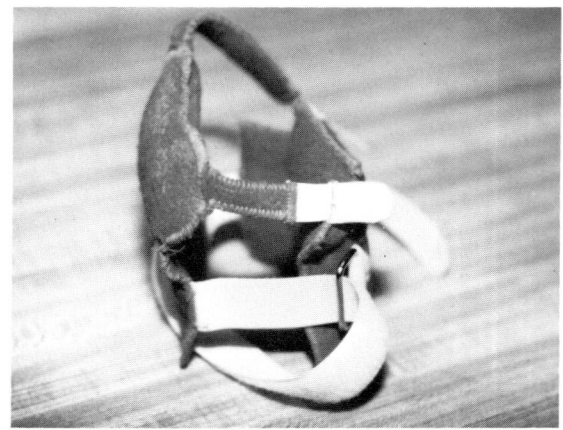

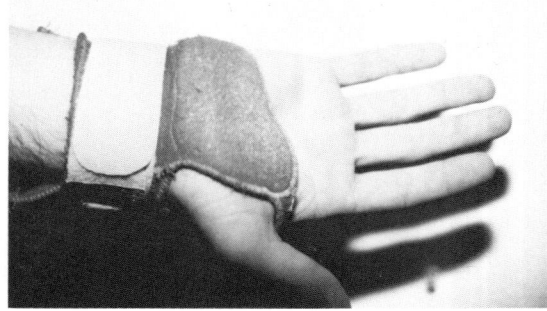

FIGURE 24–8. Ulnar variance brace. This device functions to distribute and transfer loads optimally and consequently precludes a painful wrist cycle.

6. The wrists should be turned neutrally during a round-off.

7. A foam pad should be used on the horse to absorb impact forces during the vault or the pommel horse.

8. A variance wrist brace should be worn to absorb some of the compression stresses and decrease the extension angle in support (Fig. 24–8). This brace is currently in its experimental stage. We envision that it ultimately will be utilized at all times as a therapeutic and prophylactic intervention.

OTHER UPPER EXTREMITY INJURIES

FOREARM

Other common problems in the upper extremity include acute injuries to the radius and ulna. One dramatic group of acute forearm injuries is related to malfunction of the

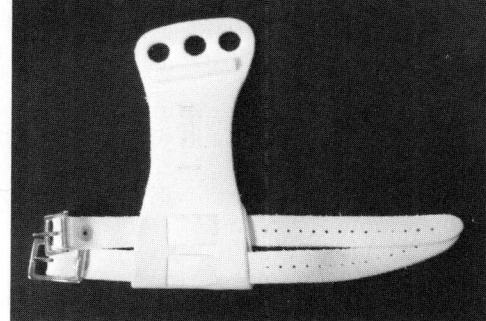

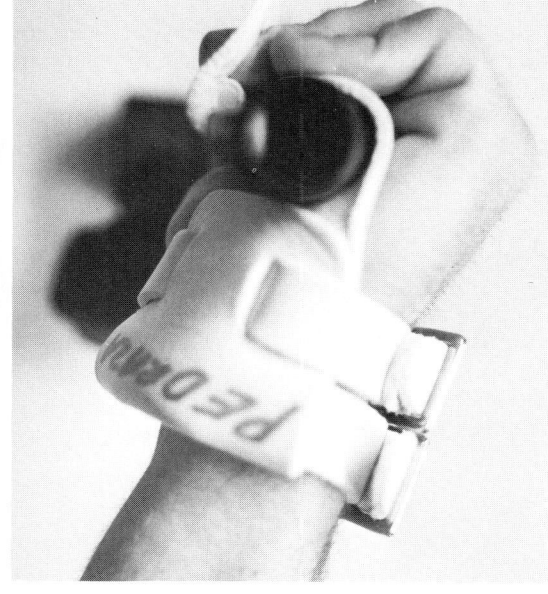

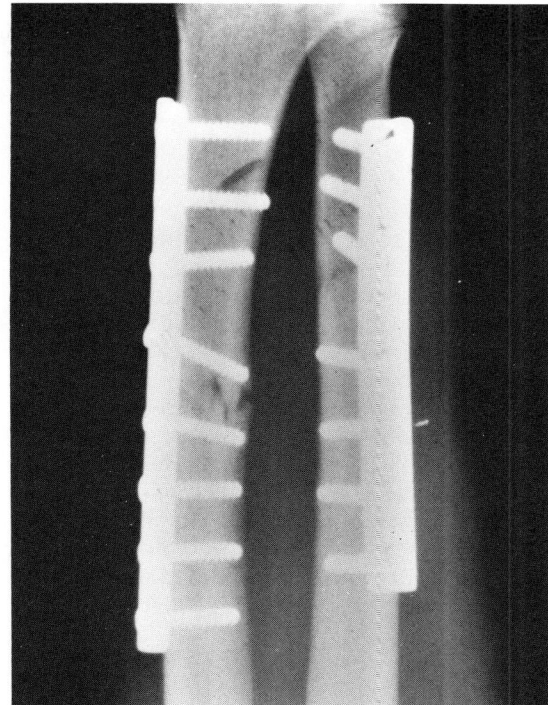

FIGURE 24-9. (*A*, *B*) Dowel grips, which allow the athlete to hold on to the high bar during high-speed maneuvers, may occasionally "freeze" on the bar, causing injury to the wrist or forearm. (*C*) This comminuted forearm fracture resulted from such a "grip lock" episode in a 16-year-old high school gymnast.

dowel grips used by male gymnasts on the high bar. These leather grips permit the athlete to hold on during the spectacular high-speed-trick swings that make contemporary high bar routines so thrilling to watch such as the one-armed giant (Fig. 24-9). If the grip "freezes" during its rotation around the bar, momentum will usually cause the athlete to continue to rotate until a both-bones forearm fracture or severe wrist sprain is produced. These should be treated with standard orthopedic management. One should be aware that in the gymnast use of open reduction and internal fixation with plate and screws has a significant disadvantage. Standard use of a plate and screws followed by removal at 1 year mandates the need for activity restriction in the gymnast as a result of stress risers and the decreased tensile strength of the radius. However, an optimal reduction is necessary to permit the return of complete forearm rotation, and this usually requires plates and screws. Thus, these injuries carry a significant morbidity for the young male gymnast. Although all the factors contributing to grip lock are not known, wearing of grips that are too large or have stretched out has been suggested as a possible cause. To minimize these injuries, young gymnasts should be carefully instructed in the use of dowel grips and taught to fit them carefully and examine them frequently for signs of wear.

ELBOW

Elbow dislocations occur most commonly in the female gymnast on the uneven parallel bars.[13] The mechanism is apparently hyperextension and results in injury to the capsule as well as the posterior and medial ligamentous structures. These athletes are effectively treated with functional rehabilitation including early mobilization and range-of-motion exercises as permitted by symptoms. Aggressive rehabilitation and conditioning should allow full restoration of gymnastics function within a 3-month period.

Gymnasts commonly present with medial epicondylitis and flexor tendon mass origin tendinitis. This results from the upper extremity weight bearing while maintaining a valgus carrying angle. Treatment includes appropriate restriction of activity level, strengthening of the involved muscle groups, and nonsteroidal antiinflammatory drugs. Attention to conditioning and strength programs is an essential step in preventing these problems.

SHOULDER

Gymnasts, by virtue of the sport's requirements for flexibility, tend to have increased ligamentous laxity, resulting in a spectrum of glenohumeral instability disorders. Subluxation and dislocation of the glenohumeral articulation and association labral abnormalities remain difficult entities to diagnose and effectively treat in this population.

Shoulder pain in the gymnast should be approached in a systematic fashion. After appropriate history and physical examination, it is essential to classify the problems as shoulder pain, instability, or instability plus pain. Furthermore, it is essential to differentiate the impingement syndromes with and without rotator cuff injuries. Since most gymnasts have a significant level of glenohumeral laxity, these differentiations can be difficult since they might have a degree of impingement in association with these relatively lax articulations. Therefore, a systematic approach should be initiated with definition of the degree of instability. For those individuals with recurrent subluxation or dislocation, initiation of an aggressive physical therapy program directed at augmenting rotational strength is essential. Failure in this management can be followed with a reconstructive procedure aimed at refixation of a Bankart lesion. The surgeon should be careful to avoid restricting shoulder range of motion.

Impingement syndromes are common in gymnasts and may be caused by supraspinatus and/or bicipital tendinitis. These should be initially treated with nonsteroidal antiinflammatories, icing, and rest. Constant rehabilitation and conditioning are essential to prevent these injuries. For those individuals who are not able to be effectively treated with conservative management, MRI has been an excellent diagnostic tool to define both labral and rotator cuff abnormalities. Arthroscopic evaluation and treatment of anterior and superior labral tears has been an effective mechanism of minimizing pain in this population. If there is a large rotator cuff tear in the face of significant impingement, acromial decompression and rotator cuff repair should be performed. This is a relatively rare but significantly debilitating problem.

Prevention of shoulder injuries should be approached early. Aggressive rehabilitation and conditioning programs should be instituted for those individuals with restricted shoulder motion and/or pain. At all times it is essential to ensure symmetrical strength and flexibility to prevent overuse and acute injury.

LOWER EXTREMITY INJURIES

ANKLE

Problems of the lower extremity are extremely common in this population. By virtue of the high energy of the dismount, athletes often land with the foot and ankle in a nonplantigrade position. This subjects the knee and ankle to torsional loading and results in complex ligamentous injuries.

As noted, ankle sprains have been shown to be the most common injury in gymnastics.[8,15] Most often this can lead to chronic recurrent sprains characterized by pain, functional instability, and weakness. In addition, as these athletes continue to have recurrent ankle sprains, they can eventually develop anteromedial or anterolateral impingement syndromes. The pathogenesis apparently is that of hypertrophic soft tissue fibrovascular invasion in the anterolateral gutter, resulting in soft tissue, cartilage, and/or bony impingement. Clinically, it is imperative to differentiate those ankles that are stable from those that are functionally unstable. Initial evaluation consists of plain and stress radiographs to make this differentiation. Those ankles that are determined to be stable are started with a period of rest, nonsteroidal antiinflammatories, and an aggressive physical therapy program. If pain persists after a 2-month period, an imaging study such as MRI is performed to rule out avascular necrosis and/or osteochondritis dissecans. Persistence of pain can be treated effectively with arthroscopic evaluation and debridement of the hypertrophic anterior tissue impingement. This can result in full restoration of function within a 2-month period.

Some debate remains in this country as to the best approach to acute ligamentous injuries in the athlete. To date, it is not well accepted to perform ligamentous repairs in the acute setting by virtue of the great number of athletes returning to full function with conservative management. Therefore, acute ligamentous repair is only performed in rare circumstances. Those individuals who have significant instability as documented by stress radiographs can be initially treated with aggressive rehabilitation and conditioning. If there is persistence of instability despite aggressive rehabilitation, we would proceed with a modification of the Chrisman-Snook or the Brostrom procedure. Our procedure is performed with a peroneus brevis graft sewn into the anterior fibulotalar ligament (AFTL), brought obliquely across the fibula, and then fixed to the calcaneus with a screw and ligamentous washer. These have had good success in restoring the athlete to full gymnastics function.

KNEE

Traumatic knee problems continue to be of significant importance during dismount mishaps[4,12] and floor exercise. Higher energy injury results in complex ligamentous injuries, meniscal tears, and fractures. These entities need to be acutely evaluated and appropriately treated. In the gymnast with open physes, anterior cruciate ligament (ACL) repair and/or reconstruction is not performed in the acute setting but delayed until the physis closes. Results with acute repairs in this group of athletes have been less than optimal. Therefore, acute ligamentous injuries in the young athlete are evaluated individually and treatment is based on the severity of each injury. Knee braces have been effectively utilized in the nonoperative management of ACL tears. Standard patellar tendon reconstruction of the ACL can be performed in these athletes after growth has been completed. For older teenagers who are full grown or within 1 year of physeal closure, arthroscopic patellar tendon reconstruction of the anterior cruciate ligament is recommended. We allow these athletes to return to the gym 8 weeks following surgery, gradually increasing activities, with a goal of full return to gymnastics 1 year postoperatively. Retrospectively, the majority of knee injuries can be attributed to premature attempts at new skills, poor mental and physical conditioning, and inadequate athlete or coaching preparation. The key in these situations is prevention through education, preparation, and methodical and systematic coaching progressions.

INJURIES TO THE SPINE

Problems of the spine continue to produce significant morbidity in the gymnast. This includes both acute trauma and overuse injuries. The acute injuries to the cervical, thoracic, and lumbar spine may have catastrophic consequences when associated with neurological compromise. These remain the most devastating sports medicine problems in the sport of gymnastics, leading to high degrees of morbidity and even mortality. They are the true emergencies of gymnastics, and all attempts must be made at preventing these rare but devastating mishaps. Keen attention to details such as level of participation, skill, fitness, adequate spotting, and coaching are all necessary to ensure safe participation with minimal risk to the spinal column.

Chronic overuse injuries of the spine have been a significant problem in the young gymnast. It is the chronic repetitive flexion, rotation, and extension of the spine during gymnastic activities that cause injuries to the spinal elements.[3] Common problems include damage to the pars intraarticularis with resultant spondylolysis and spondylolithesis,[5] discogenic pathology, and vertebral end plate abnormalities. As described in Chapter 10, evaluation of low back pain should be performed in a systematic fashion. The physician caring for gymnasts should be attuned to the characteristic clinical picture of spondylolysis. The time for its occurrence in the gymnast is between 9 and 13 years of age. Understanding the predilection in this population as well as the potential for progression to spondylolithesis is essential. Early treatment of the spondylolysis should be done with rest and possibly an orthotic. A gymnast may perform multiple substitute activities during effective rest and immobilization, including conditioning of the upper and lower extremities, swimming, and bicycling. If in fact the spondylolysis progresses to spondylolithesis, this is associated with higher morbidity and less potential for full restoration of function. There have been several cases of gymnasts who competed with grade II and III spondylolithesis without significant disability. In those instances where there is persistent pain in the face of grade II, III, and IV spondylolithesis, surgical intervention can be undertaken with a 50 percent chance of return to full function. There have been elite gymnasts who have returned to full competition after L5–S1 fusion.

CONCLUSION

Gymnastics has proven to be a tremendously demanding sport. The young athlete trains and performs at levels of physical and psychological stress that may result in a spectrum of medical, orthopedic, and overuse disorders. The health care professional should be aware of this spectrum and maintain the goals of prevention and minimization of morbidity while maximizing performance. The concept of titrating the "dose" of gymnastic stress to the "response" of the gymnast's body should be understood by the athlete, the coach, and the parents. The age of initiation, sport selectivity, progression of advancement, and technique should be individualized and reevaluated at various intervals. Adherence to specific recommendations is essential to ensure safe, enjoyable, and successful participation in the sport of gymnastics.

References

1. Garrick, J. G., Requa, R. K.: Epidemiology of women's gymnastics injuries. Am. J. Sports Med. 8:261, 1980.
2. Goldberg, M. J.: Gymnastics injuries. In Symposium on Sports Injuries. Orthop. Clin. North Am. 11:717, 1980.
3. Hall, S. J.: Mechanical contribution to lumbar stress injuries in female gymnastics. Med. Sci. Sports Exerc. 18:599–602, 1986.
4. Hunter, L. Y., Torgan, C.: Dismounts in gymnastics: should scoring be reevaluated? Am. J. Sports Med. 11:208–211, 1983.
5. Jackson, D. W., Wiltse, L. L., Cirincione, R. J.: Spondylolysis in the female gymnast. Clin. Orthop. 117:68, 1976.
6. Kirby, R. L., Simms, F. C., Symington, V. J., et al,: Flexibility and musculoskeletal symptomatology in female gymnasts and age-matched controls. Am. J. Sports Med. 9:160–164, 1981.
7. Lowry, C. B., Leveau, B. F.: A retrospective study of gymnastics injuries to competitors and noncompetitors in private clubs. Am. J. Sports Med. 10:237–239, 1982.
8. McAuley, E., Hudash, G., Shields, K., et al.: Injuries in women's gymnastics. Am. J. Sports Med. 15:558–565, 1987.
9. Mandelbaum, B. R., Bartolozzi, A. R., Davis, C. A., Teurlings, L., Bragolnier, B.: Wrist pain syndrome in the gymnast: pathogenetic, diagnostic and therapeutic considerations. Am. J. Sports Med. 17:(3):305–317, 1989.
10. Mandelbaum, B. R., Teurlings, L.: Wrist pain in the young gymnast. Am. J. Sports Med. In preparation.
11. Marizione, P.: Stress fracture of the scaphoid wrist. Am. J. Sports Med. 9:268–269, 1981.
12. Pettrone, F. A., Ricciardelli, E.: Gymnastic injuries: the Virginia experience 1982–1983. Am. J. Sports Med. 15:59–62, 1987.
13. Priest, J. D., Weiss, D. J.: Elbow injury in women's gymnastics. Am. J. Sports Med. 9:288, 1981.
14. Roy, S., Caine, D., Singer, K. M.: Stress changes of the distal radial epiphysis in young gymnasts. Am. J. Sports Med. 13:301–308, 1985.
15. Snook, G. A.: Injuries in women's gymnastics. A five year study. Am. J. Sports Med. 7:242, 1979.
16. Weiker, G. G.: Club gymnastics. Clin. Sports Med. 4:39–43, 1985.

25
SWIMMING

PETER J. FOWLER
M. SUSAN WEBSTER-BOGAERT

Swimming, both recreational and competitive, remains the most popular participatory sport in the United States.[13] As a recreational sport, swimming provides both upper and lower body strength training as well as cardiovascular fitness. Extreme dedication to the sport is required because rather minute differences in the swimmer's stroke, breathing, or attitude make the difference between the top-level swimmers. The majority of orthopedic complaints occur in swimmers of the competitive class.

In the 1972 Olympic games in Munich, the late Dr. J. C. Kennedy, chief medical officer of the Canadian team, noted a high incidence of orthopedic complaints among swimmers. Thirty-five swimmers registered 43 of a total of 127 consultations for a Canadian Olympic team of 296 total members. There were 1.23 complaints per swimmer versus 0.43 complaints per other athlete, a somewhat skewed distribution. A breakdown of orthopedic consultations for the Canadian Olympic swimming team was as follows: shoulder, 16, knee, 12, calf and foot, 8; and miscellaneous, 7.[15]

Later, in a survey of the major swimming clubs in Canada, Kennedy and Hawkins studied 2496 competitive swimmers who swam an average of 5000 yards per day.[14] Of 261 swimmers who had orthopedic complaints, 90 percent had shoulder, knee, calf, or foot problems. Eighty-one swimmers had shoulder conditions that resulted from the freestyle, the butterfly, and occasionally the backstroke. There were 85 calf and foot problems evenly divided among the four major swimming strokes. The 70 knee problems were all caused by the breaststroke.[15]

GENERAL STROKES AND TRAINING

STROKES

Competitive swimming has four different strokes: front crawl, backstroke, breaststroke, and butterfly. (Fig. 25–1). They are swum various distances alone or all four in combination. The biomechanics of the four strokes, with respect to the arm action, are deceptively similar. There are phases common to all strokes. The *reach* is the portion of the arm cycle where the arm reaches forward as it enters the water; the term *entry* is synonymous. The time the swimmer begins to scull or pull on the water is the *catch* phase of the swimming stroke. During the catch, which is similar for all competitive strokes, the elbow flexes to approximately 100 degrees and the shoulder begins to extend, horizontally abduct, and slightly medially rotate. The *pull* phase, although slightly different for every stroke, consists of the swimmer sculling, pulling, or pushing the water for the most efficient and forceful propulsion. In all strokes except the breaststroke, the arm starts at maximum elevation and ends in extension. The *recovery* phase finds the arm returning to start another pull. In all strokes except the breaststroke, this is performed in the air. Front crawl, butterfly, and backstroke all rely on the arms for the majority of the propulsion

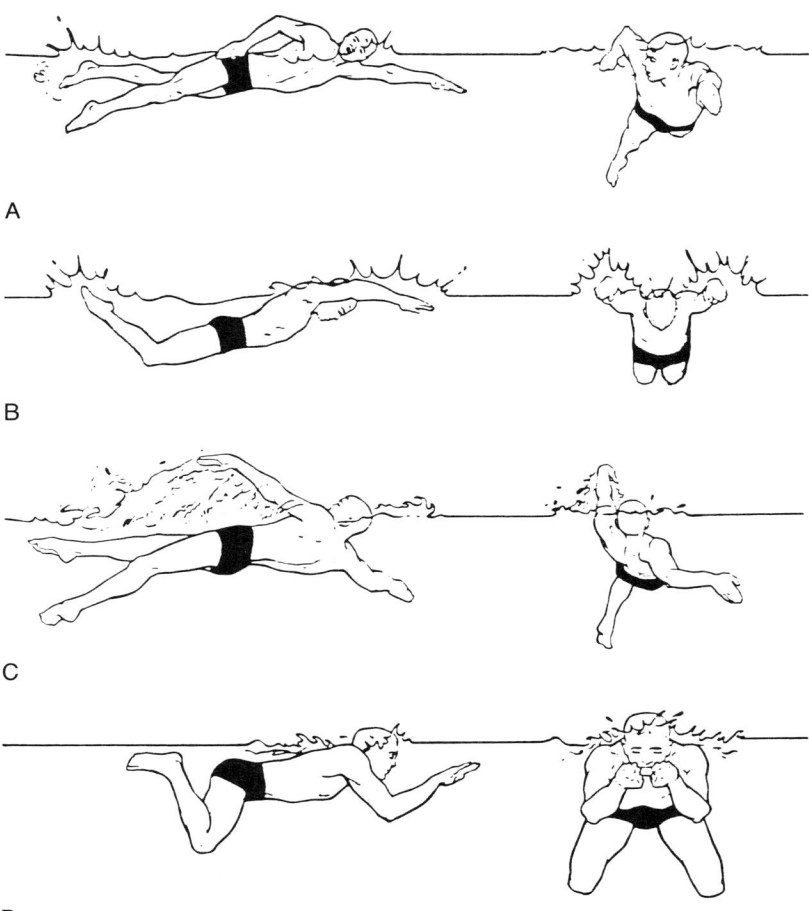

FIGURE 25–1. (A) Freestyle. (B) Butterfly. (C) Backstroke. (D) Breaststroke. (From Counsilman J. E.: The Science of Swimming. Englewood Cliffs, N.J. Prentice-Hall, Inc, 1968.)

forward (75 percent), whereas in the breaststroke the legs and arms contribute equally. In the freestyle event, the stroke performed is optional. Most competitors use the front crawl. In this chapter, we will use the term *freestyle* for the front crawl stroke, as is done in the swimming milieu.

Freestyle

The fastest stroke and the one most frequently used in practice is the freestyle. The standard racing distances for this stroke range from 50 to 1500 meters. The entry of the hand is usually a foot in front of the shoulder; the hand reaches ahead until the arm is fully flexed. The pull phase is initiated with a sculling motion. The torso is rolled about its longitudinal axis so the arm can be positioned deeper in the water. An S-shaped curving pull is produced under the torso, with the hand ending at the hip. The recovery of one arm occurs during the pull phase of the other arm. The recovery is synchronized with a body roll to enable the arm to be released from the water and sweep into the entry position again. The legs perform a flutter kick.

Butterfly

The butterfly is the second fastest stroke and in the evolution of competitive swimming the newest one. The underwater arm action is similar to the freestyle. The arms do not alternate but move in unison through the pull phase and the recovery. To relieve stress on the shoulder and to move faster through the water, a dolphin motion is produced with the whole body. The legs perform a dolphin kick, similar to the flutter kick except the legs move together.

Backstroke

The backstroke arm pull is very similar to the freestyle. The arm entry is performed with the shoulder in its fully elevated position. The arm is straight entering the water, but the body roll enables the arm to produce much the same S-shaped pulling pattern, only at the side. A flutter kick is used.

Breaststroke

The breaststroke is the oldest of the swimming strokes. The arms move together in the pull and recovery phases. Compared with the other strokes, the breaststroker is allowed only half a pull; the arms are not allowed to pull below the waistline. The recovery is under water. Variations in the kicking action continue to prevail. Counsilman described and assessed breaststroke kicks with respect to propulsion potential.[5] He concluded that the whip-style kick was superior in every respect, including speed and propulsion force. Initially, the legs are fully extended with the feet plantar flexed. The recovery begins with flexion at the hips and knees. At the end of the recovery, the foot dorsiflexes and external tibial rotation occurs. The angle between the trunk and thigh is 120 degrees. The foot is then pushed outward and backward as the knee extends. The dorsiflexed foot engages the water with the sole. Meanwhile, the thigh is driven upward toward the surface of the water by the hip extensors. The maximal force of the kick occurs as extension continues at the hip and knee while the legs are brought together. The knee is almost fully extended when the feet are a few inches apart. The kick is finished with the foot in plantar flexion. The kick does not invite natural musculoskeletal forces or motion at the knee joint.

TRAINING

Training for competitive swimming is rigorous. The typical age group or national caliber swimmer practices in the water twice per day a minimum of 5 days per week. These sessions are approximately 2 hours in length. Dry-land training is performed to increase strength and endurance. Although philosophies differ among coaches with regard to training distances, a normal range would be 4000 to 8000 meters per practice session. Time is spent in the water not only to improve conditioning but also to improve technique on strokes, turns, and starts. Once individual stroke and racing distance specialties have been established, swimmers are divided into groups to focus training.

THE SHOULDER

Injury to the shoulder is the most common problem facing competitive swimmers of all ages. The repeated demands made on the upper body stress the shoulder muscles and their tendons far in excess of normal usage and design. Anatomical features and biomechanical forces may combine in the swimmer to produce *swimmer's shoulder*. This term refers to tendinitis of the rotator cuff, usually the supraspinatus and/or the biceps tendon and was first used in the clinical literature by Kennedy and Hawkins in 1974.[14] They reported that 3 percent of the competitive swimmers surveyed had experienced shoulder pain. Recent papers have quoted a history of shoulder pain in 50 percent of swimmers. An increase in the intensity of training schedules, coupled with biomechanical factors, may be a causal factor in the increased incidence of swimmer's shoulder.

In 1981, Webster et al. circulated a questionnaire to age group swimmers in the province of Ontario.[28] Its aim was to formulate a profile of the athlete with tendinitis. Of the 155 responses, 48.4 percent reported present or past episodes of shoulder pain. Some 99 percent used the freestyle as their main practice stroke.

Understanding the factors involved in the occurrence of shoulder pain can assist swimmers and their coaches to plan training programs that reduce its incidence. An informed coach is the best ally a sports physician can have; prevention is easier than rehabilitation.

FUNCTIONAL ANATOMY OF THE SHOULDER MECHANISM

The shoulder joint is the most mobile joint in the human body and has little bony support or protection. It relies on its capsule, the surrounding ligaments, and rotator cuff muscles as well as larger muscles such as the pectoralis major and the serratus anterior for the stability that allows the arm to function with power and precision throughout its range of motion.

The four rotator cuff muscles work in a force couple combination with the deltoid and long head of biceps to contain the head of the humerus in the glenoid fossa. The supraspinatus muscle inserts on the uppermost facet of the greater tuberosity. It acts as a fulcrum for the deltoid during abduction and is active throughout that movement. It also assists the other rotator cuff muscles to resist any upward displacement of the humeral head in other arm actions. The infraspinatus and the teres minor are external rotators. In the horizontal plane, the infraspinatus abducts the humerus. The infraspinatus muscle also works in combination with the supraspinatus and the subscapularis to depress the humeral head.

A primary internal rotator of the shoulder is the subscapularis. It stabilizes the head of the humerus by resisting anterior or inferior displacement in the glenoid fossa and exerts a depressive force on the humeral head in combination with the supraspinatus and the infraspinatus.

In addition to activity during forward flexion of the shoulder, the long head of the biceps also has an important role in stabilizing the head of the humerus. Biceps function should not be overlooked in shoulder mechanics.

The scapular muscles—the serratus anterior, the rhomboids, and the trapezius—work constantly in the swimming arm action. If they fatigue, especially the serratus anterior, the scapula may have relative downward tilt, altering the mechanics of the glenohumeral joint. This in turn can increase subacromial stress as one forward flexes the arm.

TENDINITIS

Neer and Welsh have provided clinicians with a chronological framework for the progression of tendinitis.[22] Stage 1, edema and hemorrhage, is most often seen in athletes under 25 years. Stage 2, fibrosis and tendinitis, occurs in athletes between 25 and 40, whereas stage 3 most often develops in those over 40. Osteophytes form under the acromion, and tendon ruptures, either partial or complete, can occur. However, in the competitive athlete, these stages can occur at any age.

Overwork, subacromial loading, and hypovascularity are three main factors in contributing to impingement tendinitis in the competitive swimmer. Although the anatomical factors predispose some swimmers to tendinitis, changing training programs and modifying stroke technique can be used effectively both as a preventative measure to reduce its incidence and as a part of treatment to control its progress.

Overwork

The shoulder joint is least stable and therefore most vulnerable to injury in the overhead position. Swimming puts continuous repeated demands on the shoulder in this position. The muscles of the rotator cuff may work excessively hard to contain and stabilize the humeral head. The work load may overfatigue the muscles, starting a chronic condition. In addition, superior migration of the humeral head may occur with cuff fatigue, increasing the subacromial loading. This, in turn, may be a precipitating factor in the onset of tendinitis. Not only does the rotator cuff fatigue, but the scapular muscles fatigue as well. This may alter the mechanics of the whole shoulder complex.

Subacromial Loading

The supraspinatus and the biceps tendons anatomically are particularly susceptible to impingement. Their tendons insert on or across the humerus directly below the coracoacromial arch, formed by the coracoid process, the rigid coracoacromial ligament, and anterior acromion. When the arm is in abduction, forward flexion and internal rotation, the head of the humerus moves under the arch, and the tendons may be impinged.[21] This position is assumed in the catch phase of all competitive strokes. If the mechanics of the scapula have been altered, the tendons may be impinged against the arch, which may result in a mechanical irritation and an inflammatory response or tendinitis. The inflammation may further compromise the available space under the coracoacromial arch. If untreated, the inflammatory process can go on to include the subacromial bursa and the acromioclavicular ligament.

In 1986, Bigliani and his associates reported a study attempting to discover a correlation between acromial shape and full thickness rotator cuff tears.[1] They examined the acromions of 140 cadavers and classified them according to shape, angle of anterior slope, and the presence of spurs.

Three acromial shapes were identified: type I, flat; type II, curved; type III, hooked (Fig. 25–2). There were variations in the angle of the slope from 13.1 to 28.7 degrees. There were rotator cuff tears in 70 percent of the type III acromions, a disproportionate number. Bigliani's findings suggest an ana-

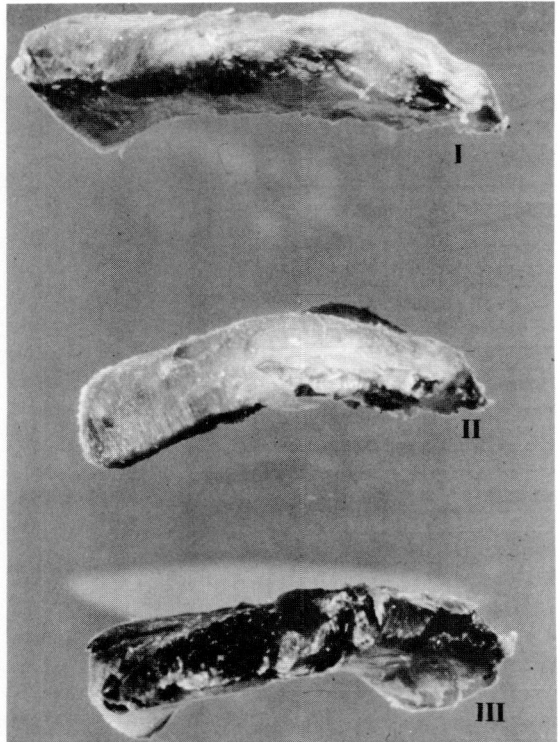

FIGURE 25–2. Bigliani's acromion shapes. (From Bigliani N. U., Morrison D. S., and April E. W.: The morphology of the acromion and its relationship to rotator cuff tears. Orthop Trans 10(2):216, 1986.)

tomical factor leading to a refractory tendinitis. A type III acromion in a competitive swimmer may precipitate impingement because the subacromial space is already compromised. A tendinitis would be more easily developed and more resistant to treatment. The type III slope described by Bigliani can be documented on X-ray using a lateral scapular view taken 10 degrees caudal. However, further studies are required to confirm its association with refractory tendinitis.

Wringing Out/Hypovascularity

Rathbun and Macnab's study of the functional relationship between arm position and blood supply to the supraspinatus and biceps tendon is well known.[25] In adduction and neutral rotation, the tendons are stretched tightly over the head of the humerus and their blood supply is compromised. In abduction, the vessels fill, restoring full circulation. This "wringing out" mechanism, or repeated hypovascularity, may contribute to early degenerative changes in the tendon. It occurs in the area of the tendon most vulnerable to impingement, compounding the potential for damage by repetitive stress.

Stroke Mechanics and Causal Factors

At entry and the first half of the pull phase, the shoulder is in forward flexion, abduction, and internal rotation. This forces the head of the humerus under the anterior acromion and coracoacromial ligament and may impinge the supraspinatus and biceps tendon, particularly in the fatigue situation.

Lateral impingement may be associated with the recovery phase of freestyle and butterfly strokes. To return to the entry position, the arm must abduct. If there is associated internal rotation and/or horizontal abduction, the head of the humerus comes up against the lateral border of the acromion.

During the end of the pull phase, the shoulder is in adduction and internal rotation, a position corresponding to the wringing out mechanism.

An analysis of the freestyle arm position at the time swimmers experienced pain seemed to correlate with the biomechanical factors implicated in tendinitis. Almost one half of the swimmers who had shoulder pain said it occurred during entry or the first half of the pull phase; 14 percent said they experienced pain during the second half of the pull phase, and 23 percent reported pain during the recovery; the remaining 17.8 percent had pain during the entire pull or the recovery phase, and some of these had pain throughout the entire stroke.[28]

TENDINITIS AND LAXITY

Overwork as a factor in tendinitis in competitive swimmers has already been described. However, if the athlete has loose or lax shoulders, the muscles of the rotator cuff may already be working hard merely to contain the humeral head. The added rigor of training makes additional demands on already fatigued or fatiguing muscles. Increased laxity should not be overlooked as a contributing factor in an athlete with resistant tendinitis.

In 1982, Fowler and Webster[6] evaluated 188 competitive swimmers between 13 and 26 years of age and compared them with a control group of 50 recreational athletes. Each subject was evaluated clinically both in regard to past history and any current signs of shoulder difficulty.

Anterior instability was tested using the "apprehension test." A positive response was recorded if the athlete displayed any sign of pain or anxiety. The sulcus sign indicated inferior instability. Posterior laxity was evaluated using the "load and shift" test conducted in two positions, sitting and supine. Posterior laxity was based on the excursion of the humeral head with respect to the glenoid fossa. Translation greater than 50 percent was considered excessive.

Fifty percent of the 188 swimmers had a history of shoulder pain. Almost 55 percent of the swimmers and 52 percent of the controls had some degree of posterior laxity in one or both shoulders. These results suggest that swimming does not predispose an athlete to increased posterior laxity. Twenty-five percent of the swimmers had a history of tendinitis and increased posterior laxity; the tendinitis was always in the lax shoulder. There does seem to be a relationship between tendinitis and increased laxity.

Many of these swimmers demonstrated weakness of the external rotators with gross manual testing. Forty athletes had gross weakness in one or both shoulders; 33 had both weakness and a history of tendinitis in that shoulder.

To delineate better rotation strength about the shoulder, 119 swimmers and 51 controls, all between 13 and 26 years of age, were tested on the Cybex II dynamometer. The controls were competitive athletes participating in sports that did not primarily require arm rotation strength.[7]

Internal and external rotation strength was measured in neutral, 90 degrees abduction, and 90 degrees flexion. There was a significant difference in the torque ratio between the two groups in abduction and neutral. The difference in the ratio was attributable to the swimmers' greater strength in internal rotation. There was no significant difference in external rotation strength between the two groups.[7]

This indicates that swimmers have an imbalance in rotation strength ratios when compared with other athletes. This is probably due to the emphasis in their training programs, both swimming and dry land, in strengthening the internal rotators and extensors to improve swimming speed and endurance.

Modifying training programs to include external rotation strengthening to restore and maintain the normal strength ratios should be a preventive measure against tendinitis. Evaluation of external rotation strength in swimmers with a resistant tendinitis can give the clinician added valuable information concerning the effectiveness of conservative management.

INSTABILITY ALONE

Pain as a result of shoulder instability alone is seldom seen in competitive swimmers. Anterior instability is often secondary to a traumatic incident in another sport. The arm is seldom in the provocative position in any swimming stroke as compared with the throwing mechanism. An exception is the conventional backstroke turn where the arm can be levered anteriorly. An alternative type of backstroke turn can biomechanically alleviate this problem.

In contrast to anterior instability, swimmers with frank posterior instability may have pain from being dislocated in the swimming stroke cycle. The "at-risk" position of forward flexion and internal rotation occurs in all strokes. Those with multidirectional instability, congenital or acquired, are susceptible to this. It is important that pain from instability alone be differentiated from those suffering from painful tendinitis and concomitant increased laxity.

PHYSICAL EXAMINATION

Palpation of the supraspinatus tendon medial to its insertion on the greater tuberosity will elicit tenderness if the tendon is inflamed (Fig. 25–3). If the long head of biceps

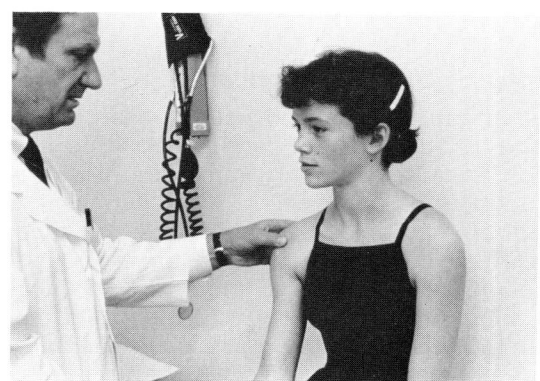

FIGURE 25–3. Palpation for supraspinatus tenderness.

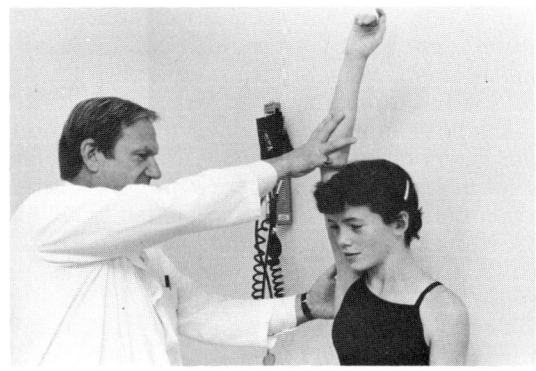

A

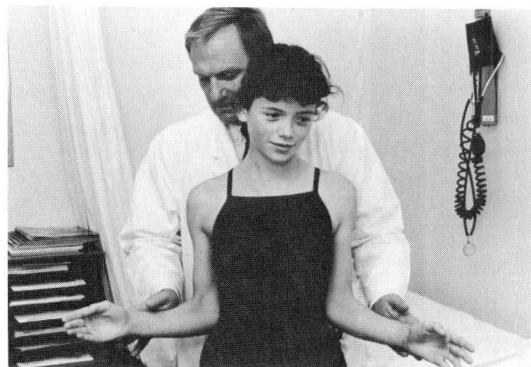

FIGURE 25-5. External rotation weakness.

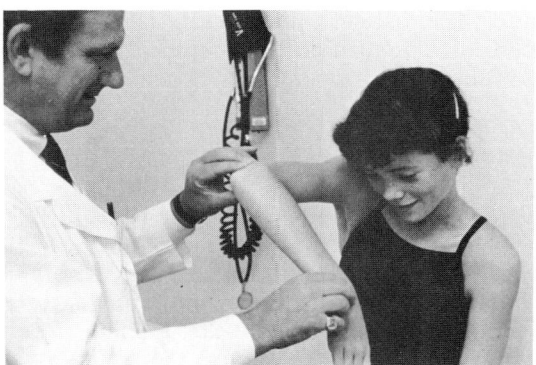

B

FIGURE 25-4. Impingement tests. (A) Hyperflexion test. (B) Internal rotation test.

is involved, there will be tenderness over the bicipital groove.

Those with supraspinatus tendinitis often demonstrate the classic "painful arc syndrome." There is pain with active abduction between 60 and 100 degrees. Symptoms of biceps tendinitis can be reproduced by resisting forward flexion of the straight arm while the forearm is supinated. The presence of a biceps tendinitis can be indicative of a refractory supraspinatus tendinitis. Clinical pain is often reproduced by placing the shoulder in the impingement aggravated position (Fig. 25-4).

Muscle weakness about the shoulder should be looked for, particularly in the external rotators (Fig. 25-5). Gross weakness will be readily apparent. This test is often accompanied by pain.

The generalized laxity of the swimmer is assessed particularly as it relates to the shoulder. Increased laxity or frank instability needs to be documented, as it contributes to a tendinitis progression or may in fact be the total cause of the pain. In anterior instability,

the apprehension test is very helpful (Fig. 25-6). A positive sign is obtained when the patient exhibits a feeling of anxiety, often with pain, or will not allow further external rotation. This feeling may be alleviated by applying posterior pressure on the upper arm, keeping the humeral head contained.

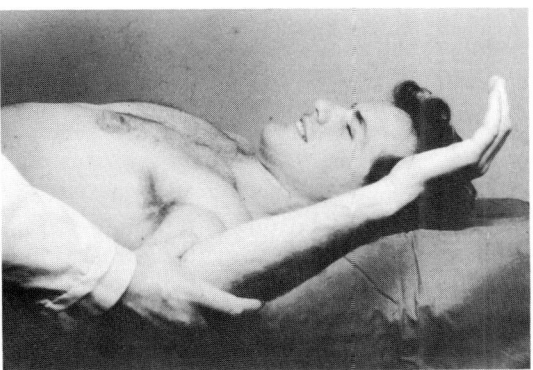

A

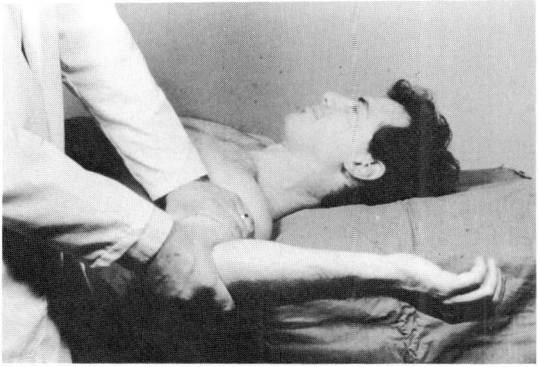

B

FIGURE 25-6. (A) Anterior apprehension. (B) Posterior pressure on the upper arm to contain the humeral head.

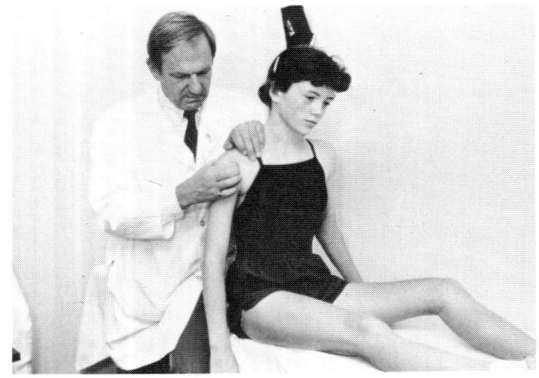

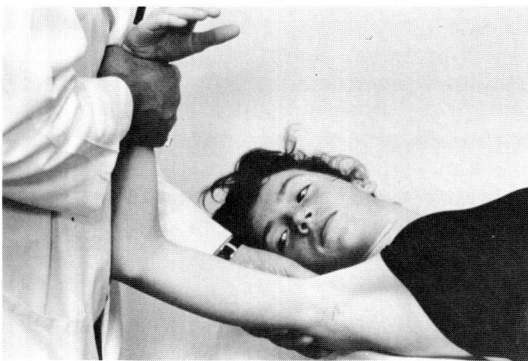

FIGURE 25-7. (A) Sitting posterior translation test. (B) Supine posterior translation test.

Posterior translation should be assessed (Fig. 25-7). Movement of the humeral head 50 percent of the glenoid width is considered normal, and motion greater than that—while not necessarily abnormal—would influence the mechanics of the shoulder by creating an increased work load to the rotator cuff. If the shoulder is unstable, applying an axial load may reproduce the symptoms the patient is having while swimming. This would be pain from the instability itself. In a second test, with the athlete sitting, the shoulder girdle is stabilized with one hand and forearm while the other hand translates the humerus posteriorly. The amount of movement is assessed. The presence of a sulcus with inferior traction indicates instability in this direction.

CLINICAL PICTURE

The progression of tendinitis is insidious. Pain becomes generalized about the shoulder and is often present at night or at rest. The athlete tends to avoid painful positions, and subtle changes in stroke mechanics are developed to minimize pain. In other activities as well, the athletes will modify all positions that aggravate the symptoms. Cuff tears are seldom seen in age group swimmers and are rare in all athletes under 25 years of age.

Clinical classification of tendinitis is based on Blazina's categories for jumper's knee.[2] In grade I tendinitis, the athlete has pain after the activity; in grade II, pain occurs during and after the sport but is not disabling. A grade III tendinitis describes disabling pain during and after activity, whereas a fourth and the most serious category is pain so severe that the athlete has pain with daily activities.

PREVENTION

Overuse syndromes about the shoulder are easier to prevent than to treat, and the principles for prevention should be incorporated into the athlete's training program early in his or her career (Table 25-1). The importance of an informed coach cannot be overemphasized. The coach can conduct an ongoing stroke analysis and guide the swimmer away from stroke errors that contribute to impingement tendinitis. The coach plans the

TABLE 25-1. Prevention of Swimmer's Shoulder

Training Regime
Gradually increase training distance
Gradually increase training severity
Place most rigorous sets at the beginning
Proper warm-up and warm-down
Warm-up after kicking sets

Strengthening
Include external rotators in dry-land program
External rotators strengthened more than three times per week
Include exercises for the muscles surrounding the scapula
Proper warm-up and warm-down after dry-land training
No pain involved

Stretching
Under 15 years of age, single stretching
Over 15 may stretch in pairs
Passive or PNF stretching only
No ballistic stretches
No pain involved

Stroke Mechanics
Proper mechanics used during fatigue situations
Proper body roll

training program and monitors the athlete's performance, preventing overwork and fatigue of the rotator cuff.

Training Regime

Overwork is one of the primary causes of tendinitis and is often the result of increased intensity of the training set. Putting athletes through rigorous training sessions before they are ready or through "extra-hard" practice at the beginning of training may do more than show swimmers how much work they need to do. Either of these can trigger the onset of tendinitis.

Training should gradually increase the demand on swimmers as the schedule progresses. Each training session can be designed so the difficult portion of the practice is earlier in the workout, before the swimmer begins to become overtired. Practice can continue with emphasis on stroke drills, alternating strokes with leg work, and start and turn technique to provide the swimmers with relative rest to the structures at risk. With proper instruction, swimmers can learn to guard against the damaging effects of fatigue using increased awareness and good stroke mechanics to minimize the potential for injury.

Strengthening

Imbalance in muscle strength about the shoulder results from emphasis on specific muscle groups during pool and dry-land training and contributes to overwork for the cuff muscles. A balanced exercise program that includes external rotation (Fig. 25-8) strengthening may reduce the incidence of tendinitis, particularly that associated with increased posterior laxity. The training program should not overlook exercises for the biceps and scapular muscles (Fig. 25-9). As in the swimming stroke, one should avoid painful subacromial loading positions when doing weight training. Using paddles while swimming is a method of increasing resistance. Paddles must be used with caution, as the increased leverage can overload the rotator cuff muscles.

Stretching

Stretching should be done regularly and well as part of the daily training warm-up. Three times weekly is insufficient. In 1985, Griep studied the relationship between shoulder flexibility and the incidence of tendinitis in swimmers.[8] He measured shoulder

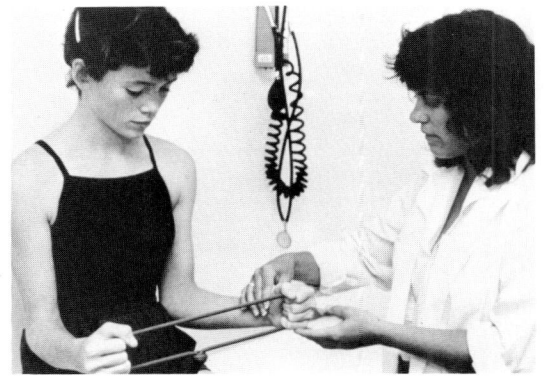

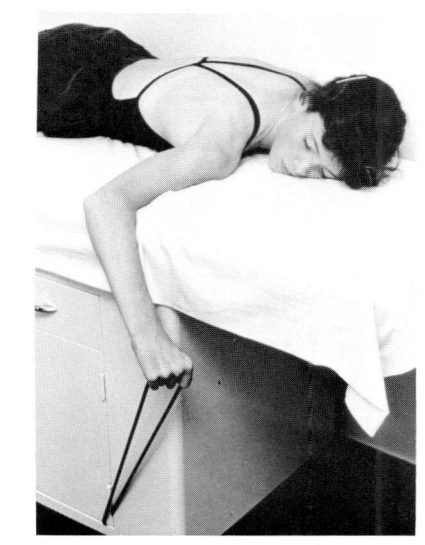

FIGURE 25-8. (A) Strengthening external rotators in neutral. (B) Strengthening external rotators in 90 degrees abduction.

flexibility in a group of 168 swimmers and recorded the information by gender and by stroke most frequently used. At the end of 6 months, Griep was able to predict with 93 percent accuracy which swimmers would develop tendinitis. Regardless of category, the swimmers with restricted flexibility were more likely to develop a tendinitis than those who maintained it with a stretching program.

Swimmers over age 15 should be sufficiently mature to stretch in pairs (Fig. 25-10). The stretching techniques can be either passive or proprioceptive neuromuscular facilitated (PNF). In passive type of stretching, the partner stretches very slowly to the limit of pain-free range and then holds the position. In PNF stretching, the swimmer

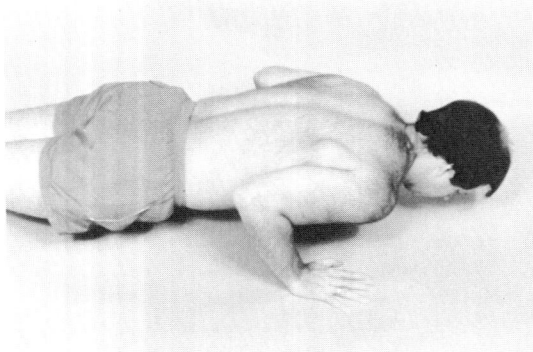

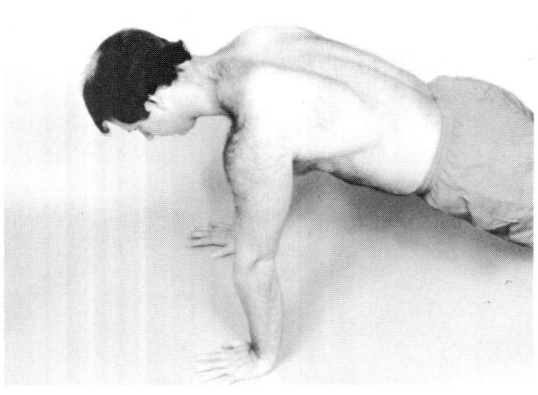

FIGURE 25–9. Muscle strengthening for the scapular muscles and biceps is important.

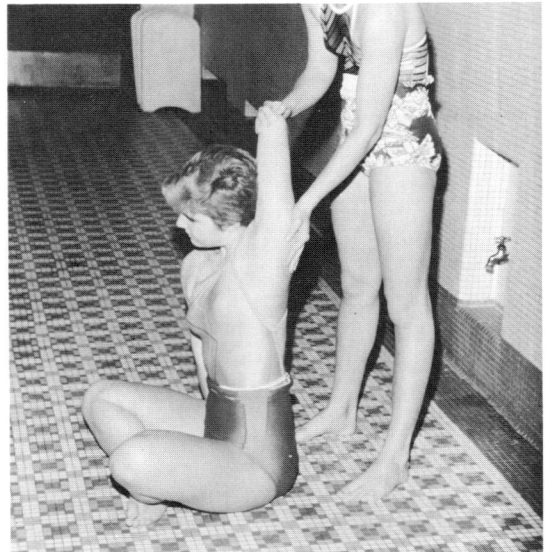

FIGURE 25–10. Pairs stretching.

to be stretched moves to the limit of range. The partner then maintains that position while the swimmer contracts against the partner's resistance.[9] This is then repeated a variable number of times. Partner stretching has to be done very carefully, as overstretching of the soft tissues can increase the irritation to the tendons of the rotator cuff.

Swimmers under the age of 15 are less likely to understand the pitfalls of pairs stretching. For safety reasons, they should be taught to stretch on an individual basis (Fig. 25–11).

Stroke Mechanics

Poor stroke mechanics can be a large factor in tendinitis production. Swimmers must be made aware that poor technique not only slows them down but also puts them at risk for injury. Analysis of changing stroke technique during fatigue situations is essential. Insufficient body roll in freestyle or backstroke can contribute to lateral shoulder impingement. In the freestyle, the swimmer may be told to attain a high elbow position during the recovery. The high elbow position must be achieved with body roll rather than muscle activity. Forcing the elbow into a higher position without body roll may induce subacromial humeral head impingement.

In the catch phase of all strokes, one is preparing for maximum propulsion. Overreach with excessive internal rotation may cause undue subacromial loading and excessive activity for the cuff muscles to contain the humeral head. Also, excessive internal rotation at the end of the stroke may intensify the wringing out phenomenon. Altering body roll, reach, and the degree of shoulder internal rotation can reduce both the frequency and the length of time the shoulder is in the precarious position.

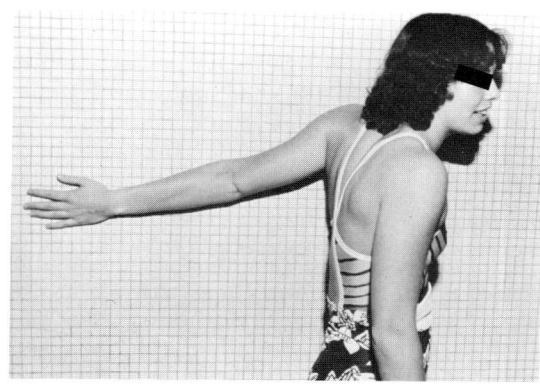

FIGURE 25–11. Single stretching.

There is contradictory evidence that breathing patterns affect the incidence of tendinitis. Breathing to alternate sides keeps the swimmer from leaning constantly on the same shoulder.

TREATMENT

Grade I Tendinitis

A grade I tendinitis (Blazina) responds well to management (Table 25–2). Swimmers are told to increase the time spent in both the prepractice stretch and in the pool warm-up. Stretches should pay attention to all structures including the anterior ones. Appropriate stretching can restore lost range of motion, increase the blood flow, and reduce the potential for further impingement injury. In the pool, warm-up should be prolonged, at a very slow pace and in pain-free strokes. Additional arm warm-up should be done after kicking sets. A swimming warm-down is recommended after the training session.

After the practice, the athlete should ice the sore shoulder for no more than 15 minutes to reduce pain and inflammation (Fig. 25–12). Ice cups are the simplest and most effective way to do this. If the swimmer has weakness of the external rotators, this should be corrected. The exercises should work the external rotators beginning in adduction and progressing to varying degrees of abduction. This improves the control of the glenohumeral joint, which in turn results in more efficient muscle work and a better perfor-

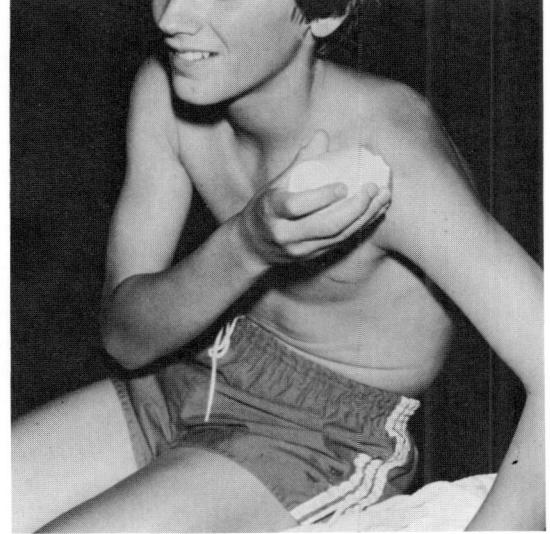

A

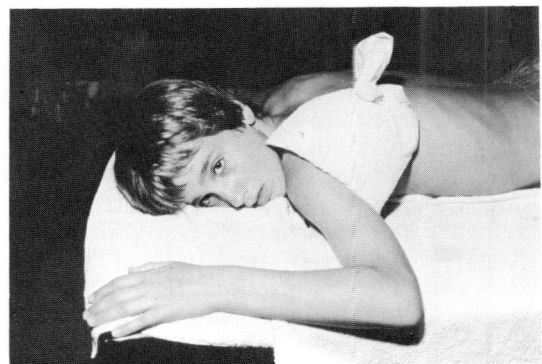

B

FIGURE 25–12. Techniques for icing after practice. (A) Ice cup. (B) Ice bags.

mance potential. The rotation exercises and swim practice should be as pain free as possible. If the swimmer has pain only when the work load is too heavy, the load must be reduced for a time and then gradually increased. If only one stroke causes symptoms, the athlete should discontinue it temporarily. Once the symptoms have subsided, the stroke, with any faults corrected, can be gradually introduced back into the training program.

Grade II Tendinitis

A grade II tendinitis requires rest and perhaps medication and physiotherapy in addition to the previous management. Rest does not mean total absence from the sport. One can work on strokes that do not elicit pain or

TABLE 25–2. Treatment of Swimmer's Shoulder

Grade I
Ice
Modification of stroke technique
Active rest
Extra Stretching
Strengthening of external rotators, no pain
Grade II
Above
More rest
Medication
Physiotherapy
Grade III
Above
Option for surgery
Option to change sport
Grade IV
Above

concentrate on leg work. In the latter case, kick boards should not be used, as they place the shoulder in the pain-provoking position. For aerobic training, running and cycling can supplement the shorter swim workout.

A short course of antiinflammatory medication in conjunction with these measures will help improve symptomatic relief.

At this stage or in the grade III tendinitis, the athlete may be referred for physiotherapy. The therapist will assess the athlete's shoulder to determine intensity and duration of pain, range limitations, and any loss of strength in the muscles of the arm and the shoulder girdle. Treatment is determined by the assessment findings and may include the use of modalities such as ultrasound, interferential therapy, or transcutaneous nerve stimulation (TENS). Loss of range is treated with passive mobilization techniques and range-of-motion exercises.

If there is an imbalance in muscle strength or significant weakness in any muscle group, the therapist will plan an appropriate strengthening program. Depending on the nature and presentation of the pain, joint range, and weakness, the exercises will be isometric, isotonic, or where possible, isokinetic. However, an effective treatment program can be developed using only free weights or rubber surgical tubing. The exercises should not reproduce pain. Often the pain is felt only in certain positions, and the exercises can be done around such positions. If, however, the exercise is painful throughout range, it should be discontinued or decreased in repetition or resistance to the level at which it is pain free.

If the treatment program is successful, the athlete gradually returns to full program, but is advised to continue with therapy until the preinjury level of activity is attained. If the tendinitis is not responding to treatment and there is still a painful response to the impingement aggravating test, a steroid injection into the subacromial space may be considered. Such injections should never be used routinely. If the situation merits its use, the athlete's swimming load should be decreased following the injection and gradually returned to former levels over 4 to 6 weeks.[16]

Grade III Tendinitis

In some cases, none of these measures is successful and the athlete progresses to a grade III stage or beyond, with the tendinitis becoming refractory. At this time, options available to the athlete include a change of sport or surgery. Unless a high-caliber career is possible at the national or international level, most young swimmers correctly select the former option and in most incidences should be so encouraged. Surgical options include resection of the diseased segment of tendon along with adjacent subacromial bursal tissue, if involved, and/or decompression of the same area.

Prior to selecting surgery as an option, it should be made clear to the athlete that the postoperative recovery period involves a serious personal commitment. During that time, rehabilitation will include a progressive exercise program to restore range of motion and balanced muscle strength. The athlete's cooperation and compliance with the program will directly affect its outcome. The return to the pool should begin with slow swimming progressing to interval training and guided stroke modification as well as an overlapped period from formal rehabilitation.

Grade IV Tendinitis

A grade IV clinical presentation—pain with all activity—is most often seen in the mature athlete. It may indicate a tear of the rotator cuff. Conservative treatment may not satisfactorily relieve these symptoms. Although the diagnosis may be made clinically, imaging techniques such as arthrography, ultrasonography, and magnetic resonance may give confirmation. Arthroscopy of the shoulder joint and the subacromial space can help identify such lesions as partial thickness tears and thickened subacromial bursae. Although not a frequent cause of pain, particularly in younger swimmers, superior quadrant labral tears, anterior or posterior, can cause pain in the swimmer and be successfully treated with arthroscopic excision.[19]

In younger athletes, bursectomy alone can provide relief, followed by appropriate rehabilitation. A more radical decompression to include resection of the anteroinferior acromion and a portion of the coracoacromial ligament is usually recommended. It is unlikely that the injured athlete will return to the preinjury level of participation, and this should be made clear preoperatively. Formal physiotherapy plays a significant role postoperatively, for range of motion is often lost and muscle strength, endurance, and power deteriorate. Classically, the abductors and the external rotators are the weakest groups postoperatively, but all muscle groups about the shoulder girdle must be included in the program.

Prevention/Treatment of Anterior Instability

Stroke modification and balanced strengthening exercises are the primary conservative treatments available to the swimmer with anterior instability. The turn in the backstroke brings on the symptoms reproducing the sensation that the joint is dislocating. The traditional turn can be modified by having the swimmer reach across the body to touch the pool wall (Fig. 25–13). This is followed by a somersault to come out of the turn. If symptoms do not subside, examination under anesthesia and/or arthroscopy can assist in diagnosing intraarticular lesions such as the Bankhart or Hill-Sachs. An anterior stabilizing procedure can provide relief and return the athlete to preinjury levels if he or she regains former motion and strength.

Prevention/Treatment of Posterior Instability

Persistence with a nonoperative program in this entity is suggested for prolonged periods. Stroke modification, correction of strength deficits, and alteration of training programs all designed to minimize the magnitude and incidence of abnormal motion can be used successfully in most cases. Surgical treatment possibilities include an inferior capsular shift, a "reefing procedure" to the posterior cuff and capsule, and a glenoid osteotomy. Such procedures should be considered only when nonoperative treatment has been completely exhausted. Restriction of motion by these procedures will undoubtedly terminate a competitive swimming career at a high competitive level. Such treatment can be realistically undertaken to provide symptomatic relief for daily activities and for participation in recreational swimming and other sports.

SUMMARY

Swimmer's shoulder is most commonly experienced from tendinitis. The etiology of this tendinitis in a competitive swimmer may be complex. It requires the combined effort and cooperation of the athlete, coach, therapist, and physician for successful prevention and management.

THE ELBOW

The arm pull in the butterfly stroke and breaststroke, and less frequently in the freestyle, is the main cause of stress syndromes about the elbow.[15] Most competitive swimmers use a form of "elbow up" pull in which the elbow is bent and held higher than the hand throughout the first part of the pull. This position permits maximal backward thrust of the hand by allowing the swimmer to push the water backward at the most efficient angle. The elbow then must bend as the arm is pulled under the body. This bend is about 100 degrees. Medial rotation of the upper arm occurs along with forearm pronation. With a high elbow position, the swimmer has a sensation of "reaching over a barrel." Lateral epicondylitis can ensue. A common fault in the swimmer's stroke pattern is "dropping" the elbow. This results in a less efficient angle to push the water backward, hence requiring more force in the common extensor muscles.

This disorder, frequently referred to as *tennis elbow*, is described in detail by Nirschl.[23,24] There is inflammation of the extensor carpi radialis brevis and extensor

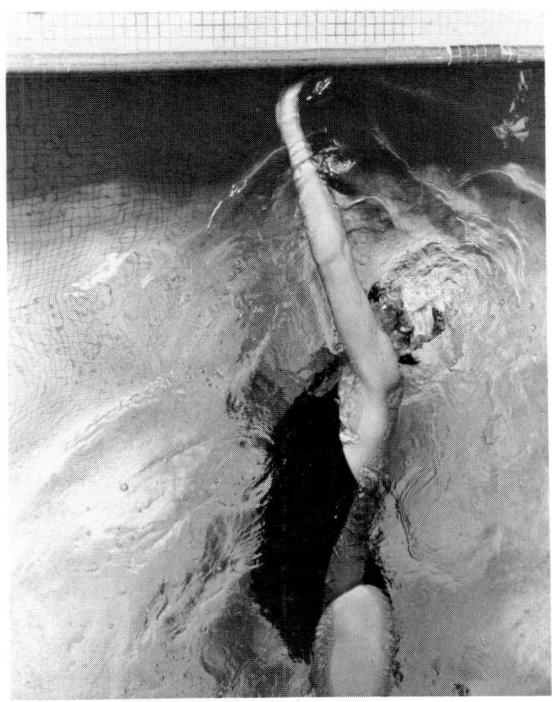

FIGURE 25–13. Modified backstroke turn.

communis aponeurosis at the lateral epicondyle of the humerus. The prime etiological factor in swimming appears to be overwhelming moments of force along with repetitions. This results in a combination of extrinsic overload in conjunction with excessive muscle contraction.

TREATMENT

The treatment of this condition includes relief of acute and chronic inflammation; increase in forearm extensor power, flexibility, and endurance; decrease in the moments of force placed against the elbow by stroke alteration; and very infrequently, surgery.

The forearm muscles are best strengthened by applying eccentric loads to aid in both flexibility and muscular strength and endurance. Relief of acute inflammation is aided by the application of ice, the judicious use of antiinflammatory medication, and physiotherapy modalities such as ultrasound. Stroke alteration in most cases is essential for management in the long term. In resistant cases, there is a place for steroid injection to the localized area. These injections should be performed cautiously, judiciously, and infrequently. There is evidence of collagen disorganization and weakening associated with such an injection for up to a 6-week period, as has been verified by Kennedy and Willis.[16]

Surgical treatment in refractory cases may include exposure and excision of the degenerative lesion most frequently found in the extensor carpi radialis brevis, as described by Nirschl. A slow, methodical return to swimming training must follow such a surgical treatment.

THE KNEE

The three most commonly sited causes of knee pain in the swimmer are medial collateral ligament stress syndrome, patellofemoral syndrome, and medial synovitis with or without pathological medial synovial plica.

Counsilman reports that few of his swimmers developed painful knees, and he attributes this to "proper" performance of the whip kick.[5] Stulberg et al., in their study of 23 breaststrokers, believed the condition to be found in young competitive swimmers with improper execution of the technique.[27] Kennedy and Hawkins believe that the elite class breaststroker swimmers are not immune, even with proper technique, because of the severity and number of repetitions of the kick.[13]

MEDIAL COLLATERAL LIGAMENT

Injury or strain to the medial collateral ligament (MCL) is the most common but not the only source of knee pain in the elite breaststroker. The problem is found in the superficial fibers of the medial collateral ligament, which arise from the adductor tubercle of the femur and extend downward and forward to their insertion 4 to 5 cm distal to the knee joint on the anteromedial surface of the tibia. Kennedy and Hawkins studied the pathomechanics of the problem using underwater photography and experimentally testing strain in cadaveric knees. Tension increased in the medial collateral ligament as the knee moved from flexion to extension, increased further with a valgus stress, and dramatically increased when external rotation forces were applied to the knee.[13]

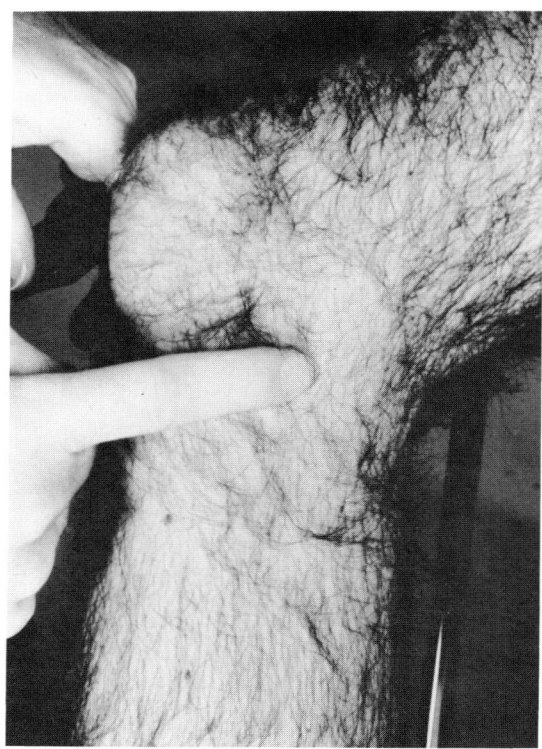

FIGURE 25–14. MCL point tenderness in "breaststroker's knee."

The diagnosis of medial collateral stress syndrome is suggested by the point tenderness along the course of the ligament (Fig. 25–14). Often this is located at its origin at the adductor tubercle of the femur, but just as frequently it is found where superficial fibers cross the upper tibial margin. Applying a valgus external rotation force to the knee flexed at 20 to 30 degrees will often reproduce the pain.

PATELLOFEMORAL PAIN

Stulberg et al., after examining 23 breaststroke swimmers with painful knees, noted that 18 had signs of a patellofemoral syndrome.[27] Five of these also had tenderness along the medial collateral ligament, with an additional five having medial collateral ligament tenderness as the only cause of the pain. They attributed the differing locations of pain to individual variations in whip kick technique.

The clinical findings of patellofemoral syndrome do not differ in the swimmer. Abnormal alignment of the lower extremity may be noted as well as hypermobility or frank instability of the patellofemoral joint. This may be associated with patella alta. Tenderness will be noted upon palpating the patellar facets or femoral condyles. Symptoms may be reproduced with the patellofemoral compression test or by laterally deviating the patella. In our experience, the more serious patellofemoral syndromes occur in the age group swimmers. This may be due to improper execution of the kick. In those whose patellofemoral joint demonstrates inherent instability, however, the forces generated by the whip kick will often preclude the swimmer from reaching elite levels of breaststroke swimming.

MEDIAL SHELF/PLICAE/SYNOVITIS

Keskinen et al. verified only the presence of medial synovitis in seven of nine breaststroke swimmers with knee pain submitted to arthroscopic examination.[17] They concluded that the combination of high angular velocities and excessive outward rotation might be the primary cause for this synovitis. Rovere and Nichols in 1985 reviewed 36 breaststrokers with knee pain.[26] They found a significant relationship between more frequent knee pain and increasing swimmer's age, increasing years of competitive swimming, increasing training distance, and decreasing warm-up distance. They found the most common site of knee pain to be the medial aspect and implicated the medial synovial plica syndrome because 47 percent of the subjects had tender thickened medial plicas. The extension phase of the breaststroke kick produced pain that was similar to pain reproduced by plica palpation. The medial synovial plica is a fold of synovium often described as the medial shelf.

Iino, cited by Jackson et al., described four types of such medial shelves in 1939.[11] According to Rovere and Nichols,[26] the pain is secondary to friction produced as the fold or plica snaps across the medial femoral condyle during repeated flexion and extension of the knee. With such friction, there is inflammation of this medial plica. This synovitis may be the same type noted by Keskinen et al. in their arthroscopic examination.[17] The diagnosis is made by eliciting local tenderness and palpating the thickened synovium as it crosses the medial femoral condyle.[20]

OTHER DIAGNOSES

One must consider other types of knee pathology found in this age group. Chronic ligamentous instability of the knee from an injury not related to swimming must be ruled out. A torn medial meniscus, uncommon in the stable knee in this age group, is still a possibility. Osteochondritis dissecans should be looked for radiologically, particularly if there is any chronicity to the complaints. Kennedy et al. conducted a retrospective study of swimming veterans.[12] They contacted 98 Canadian former world-class swimmers from the past 20 years competing in the Olympics, the Pan American Games, and the Commonwealth Games. Of those having knee problems during their competitive years, 46 percent continued with knee problems an average 15.5 years later. It would seem unusual for an inflamed ligament to persist in being irritable when its etiological stress has been removed. Hence, a multifactorial etiology may be present in many knee problems.

PREVENTION

As with other overstress syndromes, the ideal treatment of knee pain in the breaststroker is prevention. Kennedy and Hawkins suggest altering the training program for breaststroke swimmers so that much of their workout is devoted to swimming other strokes. They also suggest that breaststrokers, particularly among the class of elite competitive swimmers, have at least 2 months of total rest from swimming a year.[13]

Rovere and Nichols believe that an adequate warm-up period is an important preventive measure. They recommend a minimum of 1000 to 1500 meters of warm-up before hard breaststroke training begins. Increase in breaststroke training distance must be gradual to prevent acute knee pain.[26]

DIAGNOSIS/TREATMENT

Once the swimmer experiences pain, an early diagnosis is most helpful. Identifying the cause then becomes paramount in the long-term treatment. If the problem is technique, the knowledgeable coach may identify faulty whip kick technique.[18] Communication among coach, physician, and therapist is therefore essential.

Anatomical problems, such as significant patellofemoral or ligamentous instability, may be incompatible with the repetitive form of stress inherent in the whip kick. It behooves the physician to discuss this with coach and swimmer prior to embarking on a prolonged treatment program doomed to eventual failure.

The swimmer with knee pain can continue swimming training by swimming other strokes or breaststroke with arms only. Other therapeutic measures depend on the diagnosis. Antiinflammatory medications for those with inflamed medial collateral ligament or medial synovium may be of benefit. Ice and ultrasound also help control acute symptomatology. Strengthening muscle deficiencies in those with patellofemoral pain and the instruction in and maintenance of a stretching program for all the musculature about the lower extremity are mandatory. Steroid injections should not play a major role but have been noted by Rovere and Nichols to be effective in the treatment of the inflamed medial synovial plica.[26] When instituted, this injection should be into the inflamed pathological synovial tissue and should not be intraarticular.

After the treatment of the acute phase of the injury, there is a need for ongoing prevention and treatment programs. Breaststroke training should be reintroduced gradually and under a watchful eye to help prevent recurrence.

In the usual situation, knee pain in the elite breaststroker is a problem that is more easily controlled than severe shoulder pain in swimmers. As previously stated, those with anatomical instability, most frequently in the patellofemoral joint, may be forced into early retirement, at least from the breaststroke.

THE FOOT AND ANKLE

Foot and ankle pain are not unknown to swimmers, regardless of the stroke performed. The most common cause is tendinitis of the extensor tendons of the ankle and foot where they are firmly bound over the dorsum of the ankle by the extensor retinaculum.[15] In this area, these tendons enclosed in their sheaths are susceptible to irritation.

In both the flutter and dolphin kicks, the ankle and foot are carried into extreme plantar flexion and then back to neutral. There is little room for inflammation under the tight retinaculum. The diagnosis is frequently obvious. Crepitations may be felt and heard as the foot is passively brought from plantar flexion into dorsiflexion.

TREATMENT

Local therapeutic modalities including ice and ultrasound help in this situation. Antiinflammatory medication as well as wrapping of the foot and ankle are often of benefit. Preventive stretching of the extensor tendons should be carried out prior to practices. One can usually continue swimming with less vigor or no kicking. Return to swimming with normal kicking is achieved in a graduated program.

THE BACK

Recent and significant changes have occurred in the arm action of the breaststroke. From the glide position with the arms extended, many breaststroke swimmers now pull with an earlier elbow flexion and increased arm abduction. The "elbow up" position is prolonged by this, propelling the upper torso above the water. In most, this aggravates the already lordotic attitude of the lower back. With this stress, a variety of lower back problems may ensue, including stress fractures of the pars interarticularis or even frank spondylolisthesis. More often, accentuation of a mildly symptomatic spondylolisthesis or a mechanical low back pain from posterior facet irritation occurs and limits the competitive breaststroker's training. Such back complaints are not always confined to the breaststroke and have been encountered in the butterfly stroke. In the latter stroke, inefficient and improper mechanics are often the cause.

One should attempt to make an accurate and precise diagnosis. Most frequently, the main complaint is back pain with some radiation into the buttocks. Hamstring tightness may lead one toward a diagnosis of spondylolisthesis. Palpation of a step deformity at the spine of L5 and an abnormal gait with a backward tilt to the pelvis are frequent positive findings. The diagnosis is confirmed radiographically. If the X-rays are normal, a bone scan will help in the diagnosis of a pars stress fracture. If the diagnosis is a stress fracture of recent origin, a prolonged period of rest is paramount in the treatment program. The treatment of spondylolisthesis is symptomatic and dependent on the severity of the complaints. Following a period of temporary rest from training, a slow return using a carefully planned program is important. Hamstring stretching and abdominal strengthening exercises are of particular importance in the ongoing treatment.[4]

Mechanical low back pain will often respond to a similar program. The more resistant cases may require prolonged treatment with other modalities such as transcutaneous nerve stimulation or repeated mobilizations to the affected area. Occasionally, a steroid injection to the inflamed facet is necessary for relief.

Wilson and Lindseth coined the term "adolescent swimmer's back."[29] They described three adolescent swimmers with backache aggravated by swimming the butterfly stroke. These patients were all diagnosed as having Scheuermann kyphosis. The authors were not certain whether the forceful contraction of the chest and abdominal musculature during the power phase of the butterfly stroke caused the vertebral abnormalities or merely was an aggravating factor.[10] Two of three experienced dramatic relief by stopping the butterfly stroke. Such patients should be encouraged to continue with their swimming program but should confine their swimming to the backstroke and freestyle.[3]

CONCLUSION

The practitioner need not be an expert in swimming but should understand the rudiments of the strokes and training techniques to which patients are subjected. This will aid in proper identification and analysis of the problem. The solution may require the resources of a physician, therapist, coach, and parent as well as swimmer.

References

1. Bigliani N. U., Morrison D. S., and April E. W.: The morphology of the acromion and its relationship to rotator cuff tears. Orthop Trans 10(2):216, 1986.
2. Blazina M. E.: Jumper's knee. Orthop Clin North Am 4(3):65, 1980.
3. Blount W. P., and Moe J. H.: The Milwaukee Brace. Ed 2. Baltimore, Williams & Wilkins, 1980.
4. Boxall D., et al: Management of severe spondylolisthesis in children and adolescents. J Bone Joint Surg 61A:479, 1979.
5. Counsilman J. E.: The Science of Swimming. Englewood Cliffs, NJ, Prentice-Hall, Inc, 1968.
6. Fowler P. J., and Webster M. S.: Shoulder pain in highly competitive swimmers. Orthop Trans 7(1):170, 1983.
7. Fowler P. J., and Webster M. S.: Rotation strength about the shoulder: establishment of internal to external strength ratios. Presented at the American Orthopaedic Society for Sports Medicine Annual Meeting, Nashville, TN, July 1985.
8. Griep J. F.: Swimmer's shoulder: the influence of flexibility and weight training. Phys Sports Med 13(8):92, 1985.
9. Holt L. E.: Scientific Stretching for Sport. Halifax, Nova Scotia, Dalhousie University, privately published.
10. Ippoloto E., and Ponseti I. V.: Juvenile kyphosis—histological and histochemical studies. J Bone Joint Surg 63A:175, 1981.
11. Jackson R. W., Marshall D. J., and Fujisawa Y.: The pathologic medial shelf. Orthop Clin North Am 13:307, 1982.
12. Kennedy J. C., Craig A., and Schneider R. C.: Sports Injuries: Mechanics Prevention and Treatment. Baltimore, Williams & Wilkins, 1985.
13. Kennedy J. C., and Hawkins R. J.: Breaststroker's knee. Phys Sports Med 2:33, 1974.
14. Kennedy J. C., and Hawkins R. J.: Swimmer's shoulder. Phys Sports Med 2(4):35, 1974.
15. Kennedy J. C., Hawkins R. J., and Krissoff W. B.:

Orthopaedic manifestations of swimming. Am J Sports Med 6:309,1978.
16. Kennedy J. C., and Willis R. B.: The effects of local steroid injections on tendons: a biomechanical and microscopic correlative study. Am J Sports Med 4:11, 1976.
17. Keskinen K., Eriksson E., and Komi P.: Breaststroke swimmer's knee. Am J Sports Med 8(4):228, 1980.
18. McLean I. D.: Swimmer's injuries. Aust Fam Physician 13(7):499, 1984.
19. McMaster W. C.: Anterior glenoid labrum damage: a painful lesion in swimmers. Am J Sports Med 14(5):383, 1986.
20. Munzinger U., Ruckstuhl J., Hawkins R. J., et al: Internal derangement of the knee joint due to pathologic synovial folds: the mediopatellar plica syndrome. Clin Orthop 155:59, 1981.
21. Neer C. S.: Anterior acromioplasty for the chronic impingement syndrome in the shoulder. J Bone Joint Surg 54A:41, 1972.
22. Neer C. S., and Welsh R. P.: The shoulder in sports. Orthop Clin North Am 8:585, 1977.
23. Nirschl R. P.: Tennis elbow. Orthop Clin North Am 4:787, 1973.
24. Nirschl R. P., and Petrone F. S.: Tennis elbow. J Bone Joint Surg 61A:832, 1979.
25. Rathbun J. B., and Macnab I: The microvascular pattern of the rotator cuff. J Bone Joint Surg 52B(3):544, 1970
26. Rovere G. D., and Nichols A. W.: Frequency, associated factors and treatment of breaststroker's knee in competitive swimmers. Am J Sports Med 13(2):99, 1985.
27. Stulberg S. D., Shulman K., Stuart S., et al: Breaststroker's knee, pathology, etiology, and treatment. Am J Sports Med 8(3):164, 1980.
28. Webster M. S., Bishop P., and Fowler P. J.: Swimmer's shoulder. Undergraduate thesis, University of Waterloo, Waterloo, Ontario, 1981.
29. Wilson F. D., and Lindseth R. E.: The adolescent swimmer's back. Am J Sports Med. 10:174, 1982

26
BASEBALL

WILLIAM BRYAN

Baseball is different from many other popular American sports, stressing quickness and skill rather than strength or endurance. Unique in its emphasis on throwing, baseball produces a panoply of shoulder and elbow injuries not seen in other sports. The highest development of the throwing act is encompassed in the art of pitching. Unfortunately, this also subjects pitchers to the greatest risk of throwing injuries. Although throwing injuries certainly occur at other positions, they usually are less severe and create less disability; in fact, part of the treatment of pitching injuries may be to move the athlete to another position. This chapter will therefore concentrate on pitching injuries of the shoulder and elbow. Throwing injuries that occur to players at other positions may be treated with the same fundamental concepts. Injuries that occur in other parts of the body are generally not unique to baseball and may be treated with the methods described in Part II of this text.

This chapter will look at the unique demands placed on the adolescent's throwing arm, provide a rationale approach for keeping the throwing arm healthy, and present guidelines for diagnosing and treating common throwing injuries to the shoulder and elbow.

UNIQUE CHALLENGES FOR THE ADOLESCENT THROWER

Preadolescent throwing pains are common, but significant injuries in this age group are rare, as seen in a study by Gugenheim et al. that showed that in boys aged 9 to 12, 17 percent had a history of elbow symptoms, but only 1 percent had elbow symptoms that ever excluded them from pitching.[9] No X-ray changes were seen in this group, leading to the conclusion that the preadolescent may successfully play organized baseball without fear of developing permanent arm problems.

Adolescent baseball brings several new challenges to pitchers not seen in the preadolescent Little League group. The physical dimension of the playing field expands and the distance from the pitching mound to home plate increases from 45 to either 53 feet in Pony League or 60 feet in Little League's teenage Junior and Senior leagues. The hitters have more time to react to pitches thrown over these increased distances. Caring Little League mothers are now replaced by fathers determined to see adult performance from their suddenly adult-sized sons. Peer pressure reaches its zenith in this group in which success on the field may be perceived as essential to life. Fewer boys traditionally participate in adolescent baseball. Smaller rosters are thus common and place added expectations on available pitchers. Rules may be less stringent on innings pitched per week, as shown in Table 26–1. Outstanding pitchers may play on both high school teams and community-based teams, doubling their time on the mound.

Much bleacher discussion centers around growing pains and their relationship to adolescent endeavors. The disproportionate growth of bone over muscles and ligaments will give rise to occasional midarm muscle tenderness, but it is unacceptable to pass off

TABLE 26–1. Pitching Limits in Youth Baseball

Team	Age Group	Pitching Limits
Little League—Minors	10–12	Six innings per week; local restriction—four innings per night
Little League—Majors	11–12	Six innings per week
Little League—Juniors	13	Nine innings per week
Little League—Seniors	14–15	Nine innings per week
Pony League	13–14	Seven innings per week; no two adjacent nights
American Legion	16–18	No restrictions
Texas High School	—	No restrictions

"throwing pains as growing pains," and a more scientific basis for throwing dysfunction is advisable.

The biological uniqueness of the growing adolescent arm must be understood to appreciate many throwing injuries.[17] Longitudinal skeletal growth occurs throughout adolescence by addition of cells at primary epiphyseal growth centers. The complex shape of the bony structure around joints is provided by secondary growth centers. Metabolically active cartilage cells are dividing and being calcified to form mature bone at these sites. Biomechanically, these areas are weak compared with surrounding calcified tissue. Repetitive stress or a catastrophic event may result in growth plate injury.

The proximal humeral epiphysis is active throughout adolescence and closes at age 16. The distal humeral epiphysis closes at age 15 but is rarely involved in throwing injuries. The secondary growth centers about the dis-

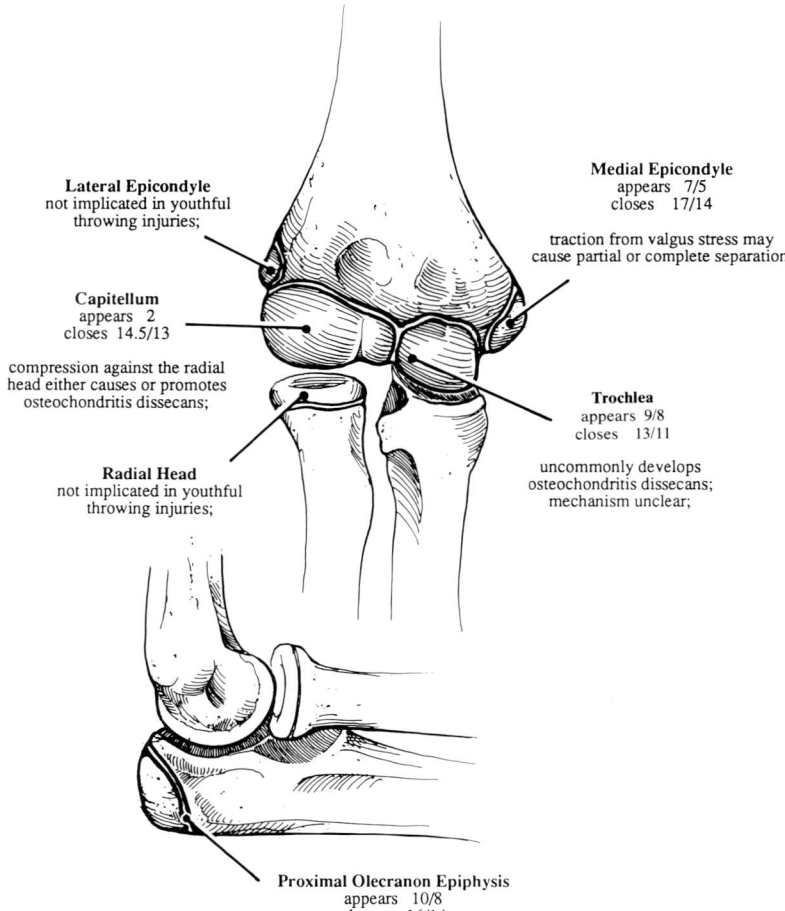

FIGURE 26–1. Epipyseal growth plates of the elbow.

tal humerus appear and close in a predictable fashion and are shown in Figure 26–1 along with appropriate clinical concerns.

The lateral elbow growth centers are subject to compression and repeated vascular insults, potentially leading to osteonecrosis from repetitive throwing. The capitellum appears at age 2 and fuses at age 14.5 in males and 13 in females. It is at risk for osteonecrosis in adolescents. The radial head appears at age 5 and fuses at 16 in males, 14 in females.

In contrast, the medial growth centers are injured by traction. These partial or complete avulsions primarily affect the medial epicondyle, to which the flexor-pronator group of the forearm is attached. This growth center appears at ages 7 and 5 in males and females, respectively, and closes at ages 17 and 14. The trochlea appears at ages 9 and 8, respectively, and fuses at 13 and 11.

Posteriorly, the olecranon process is vulnerable to both traction with violent triceps contraction and compression from elbow hyperextension. It appears at ages 10 and 8 and fuses at 16 and 14, males and females, respectively.

While growth centers usually appear and remain a single bony centrum, in some instances two or more foci of ossification may appear. When there is concern for osteochondrosis or other injury, always compare with contralateral radiographs and recall that variations in size and irregular density with fragmentation suggest pathology and not normal variation.

THE THROWING ACT

One needs only to watch a budding 9-year-old pitcher attempt to complete a baseball pitching delivery to realize that striking out batters is not a "natural act." Unlike the cricket bowler with his or her running windmill delivery, the baseball pitcher must start from a stationary position, occasionally watch opposing base runners, and be in command of several pitches. After release, he or she must suddenly become another defensive player. In response to these demands, the unique mechanics of the baseball delivery arose in the early 1800s and have been unchanged for the last 150 years.

It is convenient to separate the throwing act into four distinctive phases when teaching the art of pitching: windup, cocking, acceleration, and follow-through.[15, 22]

WINDUP

The windup takes between 0.5 and 1.3 seconds[18] (Fig. 26–2). It is a stage of physical and mental preparation in which the pitcher turns his or her body away from the batter, synchronizes his or her body parts, hides the ball from the batter, and concentrates on the pitch to be delivered. As the pitcher rotates the trunk, he or she balances on the hind foot and reaches the "gathering point" as the hands are lowered to the waist and the front hip is flexed to elevate the knee.

Balanced on the rear foot, the thrower is now ready to bring the baseball into maximal position for throwing. It is critical to reach this "flamingo balancing point," stabilizing the center of gravity before the arm is brought into action and the center of gravity is accelerated toward the target. Too often young pitchers rush this phase in order to start ball release, thereby losing all benefit from the power their legs and trunk can provide in delivering the baseball.

COCKING

Cocking (Fig. 26–3) takes place in 0.5 seconds as the ball is separated from the glove and the throwing arm brings the projectile behind the body and quickly over the head. The arm is simultaneously brought into 90 degrees of abduction and maximal external rotation as the catapult is placed under tension. Successful throwing demands at least 90 degrees of shoulder external rotation.[18] This is not normal motion and is achieved only by repetitive and progressively stronger tosses in the warm-up. Failure to warmup may result not only in unsatisfactory performance but in shoulder injury as well. Jobe et al.[14] have demonstrated considerable rotator cuff and deltoid contraction during the cocking phase, much related to the combination of shoulder external rotation and abduction. Subscapularis function is especially vigorous at the extremes of external rotation as the rapid transition to internal rotation is about to be made. The front foot contacts the ground midway through this phase, and the oblique and abdominal muscles are poised to initiate trunk rotation toward home plate.

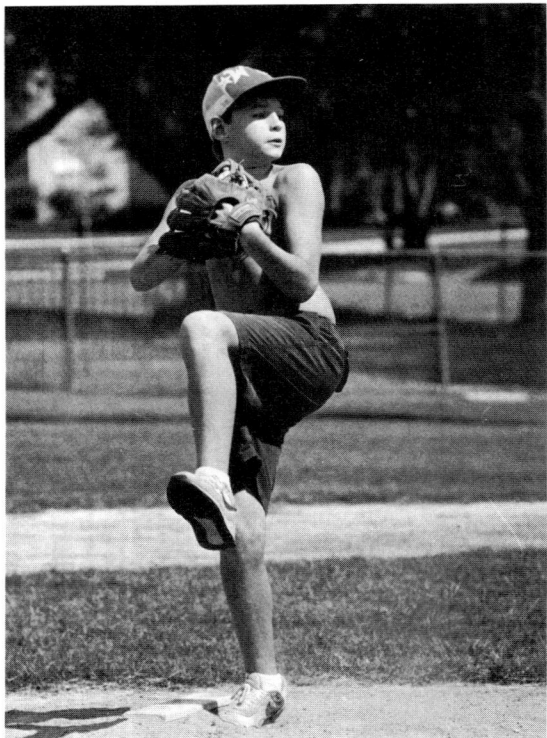 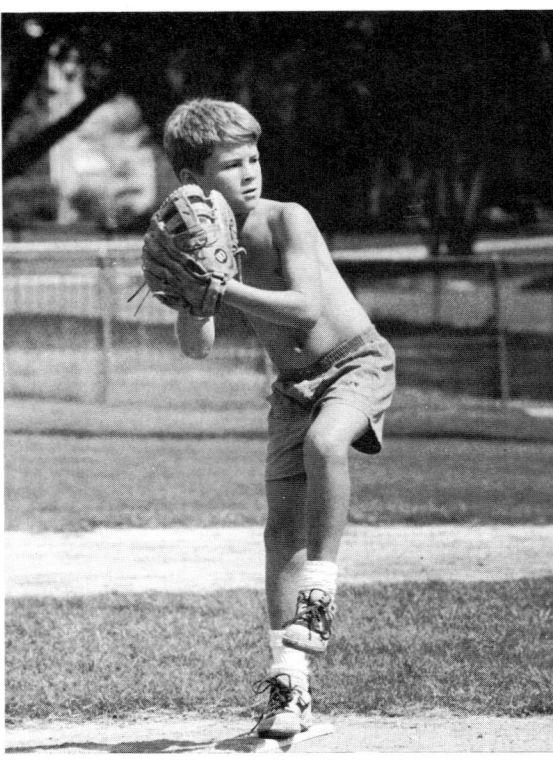

A B

FIGURE 26–2. Wind up. Getting to the "gathering point." The windup should culminate in one-legged balance with the trunk rotated as in the pitcher in *(a)*. The other pitcher *(b)* has not reached good balance, has inadequately elevated his left leg, and is likely to rush the delivery.

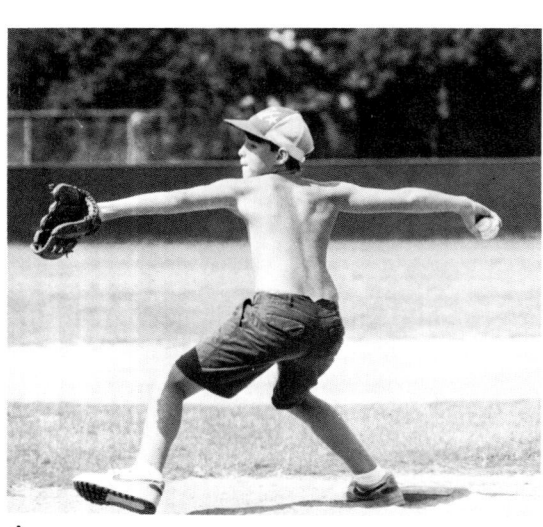 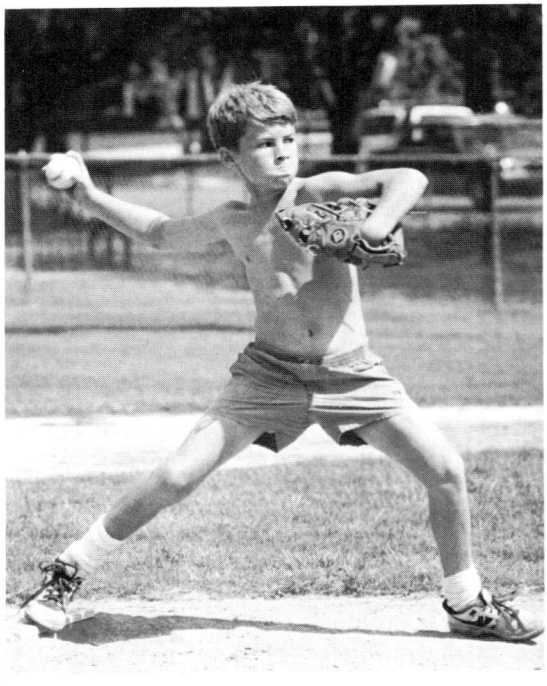

A B

FIGURE 26–3. Cocking. Maximal tension is applied to all the muscles that will accelerate the ball. The pitcher in *((A)* has his hand properly on top of the ball and is in better preparation for acceleration. The pitcher should concentrate on keeping the opposite shoulder pointing toward the batter to avoid "opening up too soon."

ACCELERATION

The third phase of delivery proceeds within 0.1 second as the pitching arm internally rotates and the ball is released (Fig. 26–4). Weight is shifted to the contralateral leg, and the trunk is sharply rotated toward the batter. The highly stretched anterior shoulder capsule and rotator cuff recoil like a spring. With the powerful muscle contracture of pectoralis major, serratus anterior, and latissimus dorsi, the shoulder is whipped into internal rotation at speeds reaching 6000 degrees per second.[18] It is critical that the pitcher keep the shoulder abducted to at least 90 degrees, as anything less may provoke elbow stress.

Wrist flexion begins early in this phase and provides some increased velocity at ball release. Overemphasis on wrist flexion or pronation/supination to throw breaking pitches is sure to produce elbow problems. Many clinicians and parents are concerned about the safety of throwing breaking pitches. The correct technique of throwing curves and sliders is by selective wrist position and finger pressure. If breaking pitches are thrown in this manner, there is not cause for concern. If, on the other hand, the pitcher relies on twisting forearm motion, he or she is likely to develop medial elbow problems.

The synchronous movement of trunk rotation and forward motion of the arm is critical. When the pitcher rotates the trunk before he or she accelerates the arm, the athlete is said to "open up too soon," placing unacceptable stress on the anterior shoulder. An attempt to get the ball to release properly now requires undue arm motion. The young thrower should be taught to keep the opposite shoulder tucked under the chin, thereby allowing arm motion to accelerate before trunk rotation. Rushing the delivery is the most common cause of opening up too soon. Other causes are a short stride, placing the front stride foot too far to the opposite of the midline, or failing to lift the knee high enough during windup.[20]

FOLLOW-THROUGH

Within 0.4 seconds, the pitching delivery is completed with follow-through (Fig. 26–5), a controlled deceleration maneuver that should be smooth and rhythmic. Studies have shown that arm deceleration forces are twice that of acceleration and act over a period twice as long.[18]

As the ball travels toward home plate, the rotator cuff and deltoid muscles are contracting violently to maintain the humerus within the glenoid cavity. The posterior shoulder structures are stretched as the humerus subluxes, and therefore the infraspinatus and

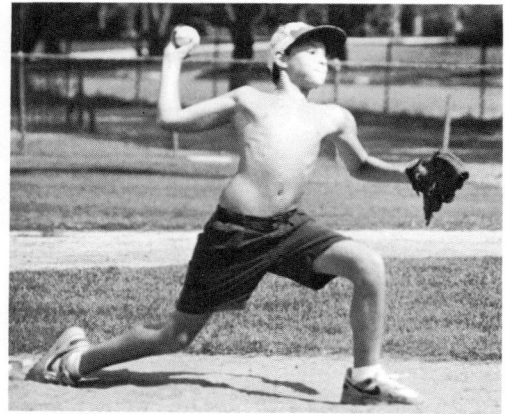
A

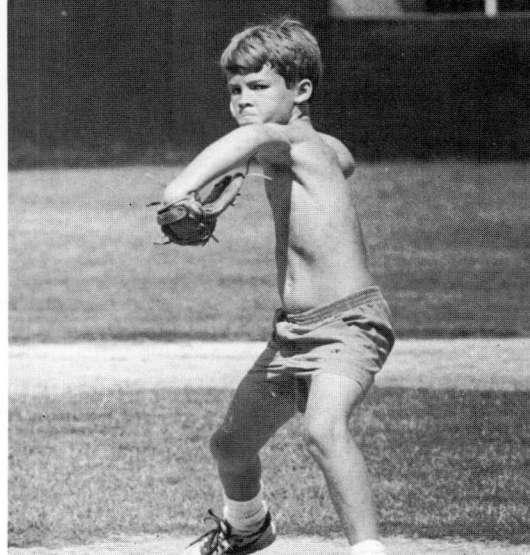
B

FIGURE 26–4. Acceleration. Energy is transferred from the body to the arm as the baseball is accelerated from zero to final velocity. Pitcher in *(A)* has improperly allowed his arm to fall behind trunk rotation. He has dropped his elbow and is "shortarming" the ball in an effort to complete the delivery.

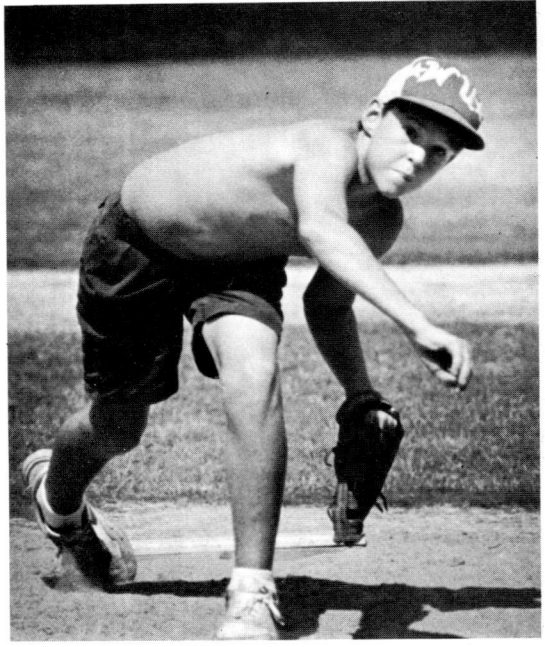 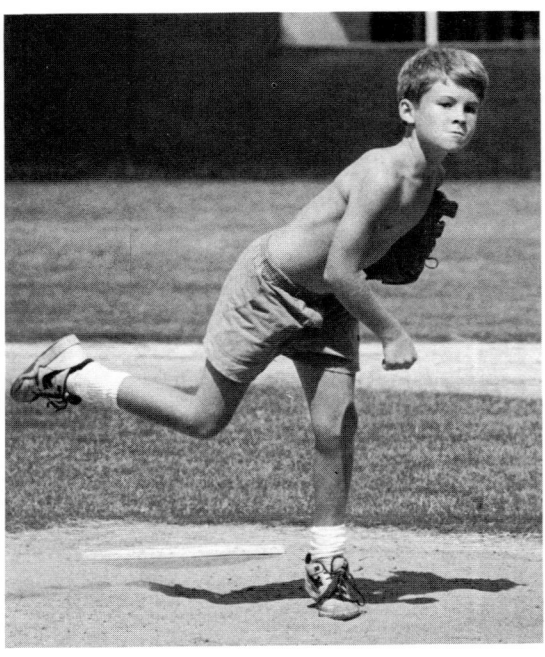

FIGURE 26–5. Release and follow-through. Great forces are developed to decelerate the shoulder and elbow after ball release. Pitcher in *(A)* is properly landing on a flexed knee with adequate trunk flexion. The pitcher in *(B)* is finishing too "upright" and on a stiff knee. This recoil may cause arm and back problems.

teres minor muscle groups are eccentrically contracting. This eccentric contraction may create problems that are discussed later in the chapter.

The trunk continues into flexion and rotation, and the planted leg with a flexed knee begins to absorb the shock. If the stride foot is placed short of the midline, the pelvis will not properly rotate. The body then loses its momentum, and the pitcher will "open up" late. This is called "pitching with the arm." The stride leg should have its knee slightly flexed to avoid a jarring landing. This would destroy the rhythmic nature of the delivery and might even "bull whip the shoulder" and possibly cause injury.

PITCHING DELIVERIES

The aforementioned phases of the pitching act are mandatory, but they may be completed in slightly different manners, giving rise to different pitching deliveries. Braatz and Gogias[2] have done an excellent job in reviewing the biomechanics of pitching, and Figure 26–6 demonstrates the kinematics of different deliveries.

OVERHEAD

In the overhead delivery (Fig. 26–6A), the trunk is bent sidewards during late cocking and acceleration so that the axis of motion passes through the left hip, transversing the pelvis and providing a larger moment arm for greater ball velocity. As the ball is released from a higher point, the trajectory is sloped and may prove very deceptive to the hitter. Overhand delivery may be extremely difficult to teach to young pitchers, as it requires supreme coordination of trunk and arm. If the synchrony of body movement is lost, the thrower will have control difficulties and may injure his or her shoulder from overuse.

THREE-QUARTER

The most popular delivery, the three-quarter delivery (Fig. 26–6B), is characterized by an erect trunk and a vertical forearm during the acceleration phase. The trunk rotates in its vertical axis throughout acceleration so that all arm motion will come from shoulder internal rotation. This delivery is easiest to teach despite the added demands

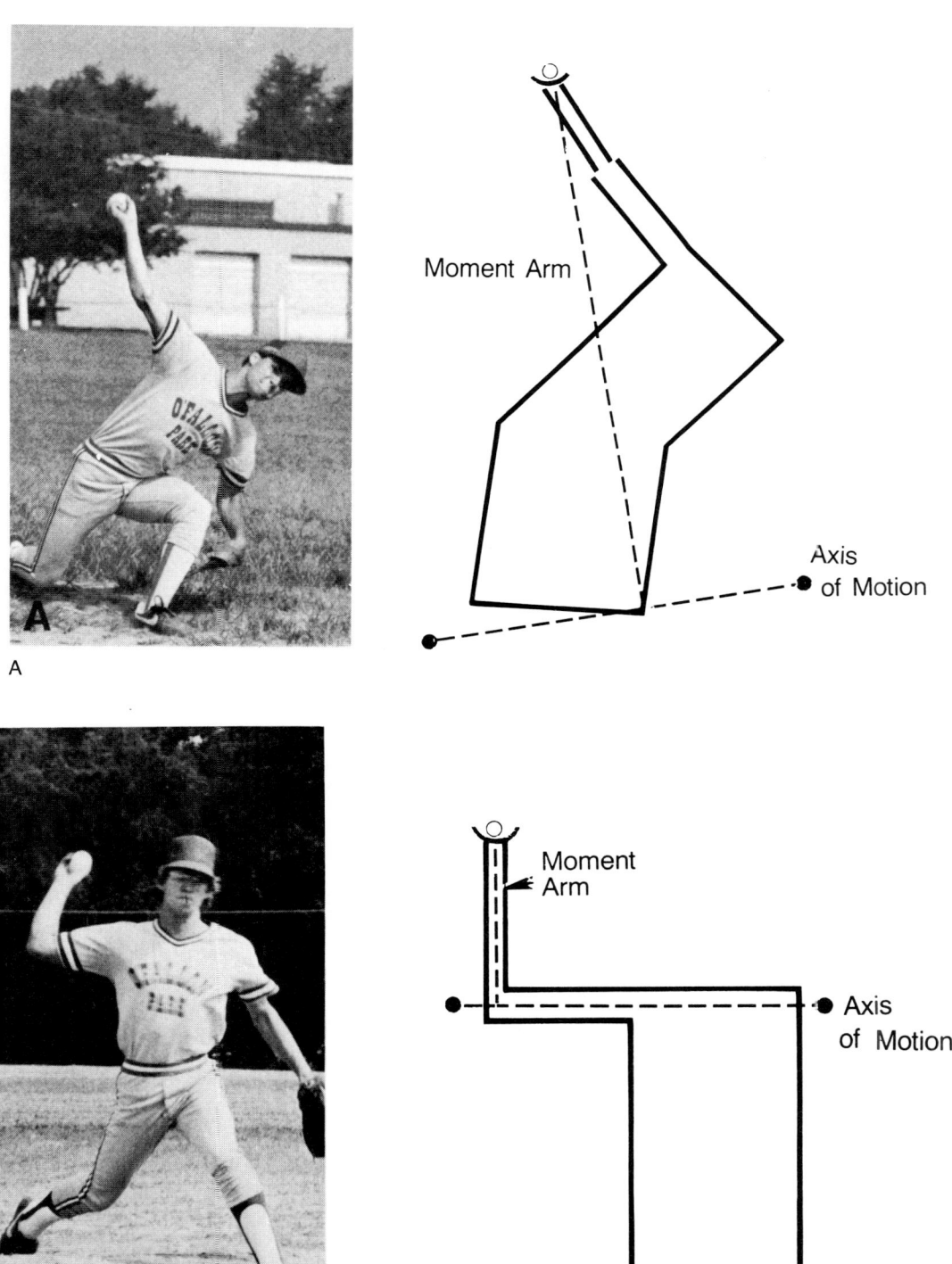

FIGURE 26-6. The one factor common to all these deliveries is 90 degrees of shoulder abduction. The three-quarter arm delivery is the most popular, as control is maximized by a stable trunk and easily reproduced arm position. *(A)* Overhand delivery. *A*, Ball in the overhand release arc; *B*, kinematics of the overhand delivery. *(B)* Three-quarter arm delivery. *A*, Three-quarter arm acceleration; *B*, kinematics of the three-quarter arm delivery.

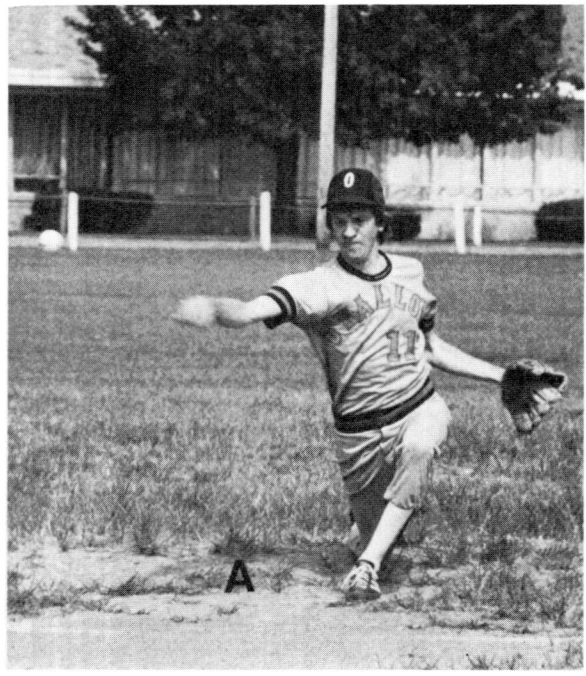
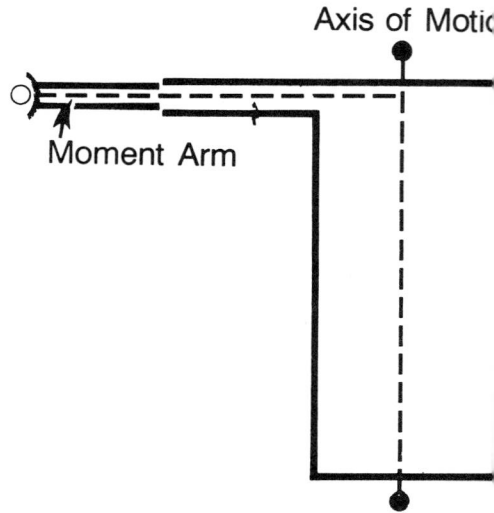

C

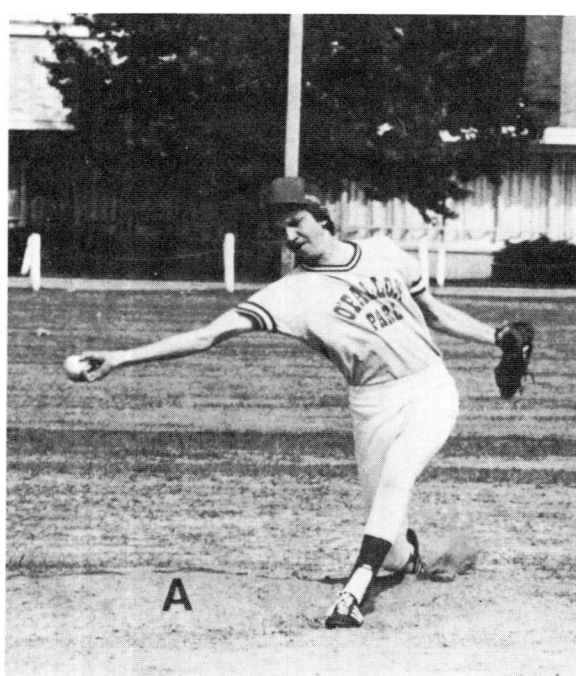
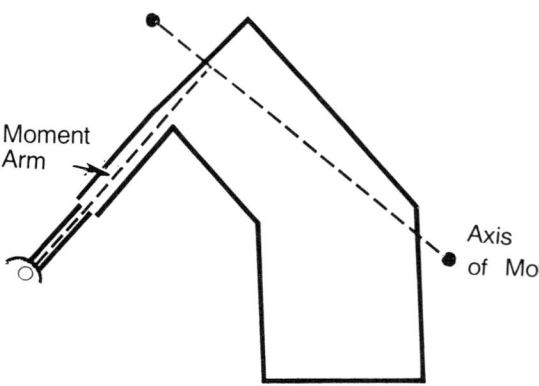

D

FIGURE 26–6. *Continued* (*C*) Sidearm delivery. *A*, Early arm follow-through from the sidearm motion; *B*, kinematics of the sidearm delivery. (*D*) Underhand delivery. *A*, Release point during an underhand pitch; *B*, kinematics of the underhand delivery. (From Braatz J. H., Gogias P. P.: The mechanics of pitching. J Orthop Sports Phys Ther 9(2):56–59, 1987.)

on shoulder function. Trunk motion is minimized, and balance is thus more stable. The disadvantage is that ball trajectory is flatter owing to a lower release point and velocity may be lower than with the overhead approach.

SIDEARM

In the sidearm delivery (Fig. 26–6C), the trunk remains erect as the pitcher extends the elbow early in the acceleration phase. The ball is held at a relatively long moment arm from the axis of trunk rotation, and good velocity may be generated. The shoulder is placed under considerable stress because of this long moment arm. This delivery demands precise coordination of trunk and arm motion to avoid opening up too soon. Its advantage lies with the ability to generate more velocity from this unusual release point. The flat plane of release makes it difficult, however, to throw breaking pitches and change speeds.

UNDERHAND

Many observers do not realize that the arm remains abducted to 90 degrees although the arm falls below the horizontal when a ball is thrown with the "submarine pitch" (Fig. 26–6D). This delivery is in no way akin to the underhand technique of softball. The trunk must be radically rotated toward the pitching arm and the shoulder thus tilted. All other aspects of the throwing act remain the same. The batter is easily confused by these pitches, which start low and stay low as they cross home plate. The submarine technique is difficult to master owing to its demands on balance and reproducibility of the throwing arc.

WHAT SEPARATES THE PROFESSIONAL FROM THE AMATEUR PITCHER?

The ability to throw a baseball 90 miles per hour with pinpoint accuracy has always stimulated the academic mind as coaches and parents seek to unlock those secrets for their young charges. Better understanding of this difference also seems valuable for preventing and treating throwing arm problems.

A recent study[8] sought to examine the electromyographic differences between professionals and amateurs and came to the conclusion that the only difference was greater activity of the latissimus dorsi and subscapularis muscles in professionals along

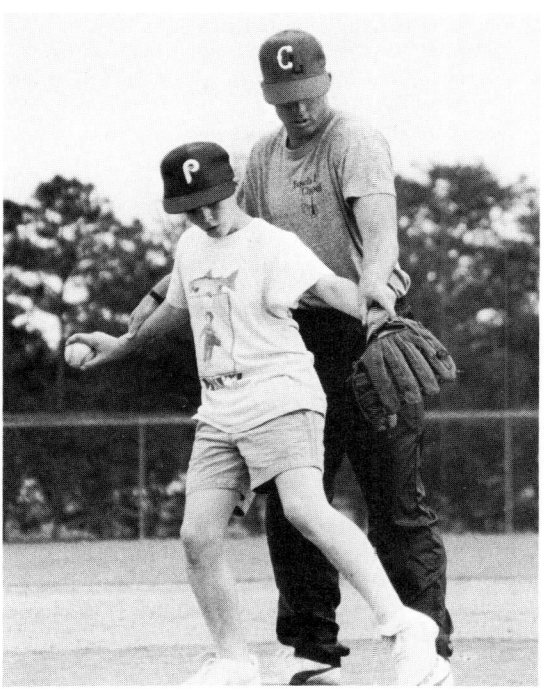

A

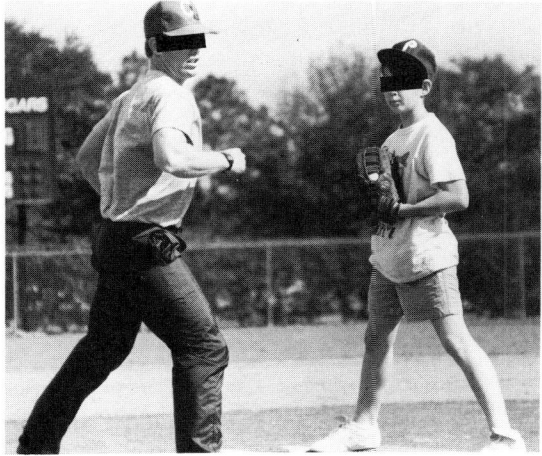

B

FIGURE 26–7. Baseball throwing is an unnatural act requiring expert teaching and constant evaluation of performances. Youth coaches such as Raynor Noble are indispensable in pitching success. Video cameras are also useful in allowing the young athlete to see himself or herself throwing.

TABLE 26–2. Raynor Noble's 10 Commandments for Proper Pitching

1. *Do not throw until your muscle temperature is elevated.* This will require stretching, calisthenics, and some light jogging.
2. *Proper arm action is crucial.* Break point must align with release point.
3. *Balance throughout the delivery is very important.* Do not start your pushing action toward the plate until the hand separates from the glove and the lead leg goes down.
4. *Stay closed with the hips and lead shoulder until the end of the pushing sequence.* This will maximize hip rotation toward the plate, resulting in added velocity and less strain on the shoulder and elbow.
5. *Use your legs and hips.* Pushing with the back leg and popping the hips add up to greater velocity and increased movement on your pitches.
6. *Follow through after releasing the pitch.* Proper follow-through will ensure that the throwing shoulder stays low, resulting in strikes in the lower portion of the strike zone.
7. *Take care of your arm.* Keep your entire arm covered when not pitching, especially in cooler climates. Never throw without a proper warm-up.
8. *Condition yourself physically to pitch.* This basically entails a daily running and stretching routine coupled with a light weight-lifting program suited for yourself. Note: Use light weights with greater repetitions on upper body, medium weights with average repetitions on the lower body. Don't forget about those sit-ups.
9. *Condition yourself mentally to pitch.* Imagine yourself pitching to good hitters. Put yourself in tough situations in a ball game and *imagine* yourself making good pitches to get out of the jam you are in. The more times you mentally, as well as physically, go through your delivery, the more you reinforce that action. Therefore, when you finally do get to that big game or get into that jam, you've already rehearsed how you are going to handle it.
10. *Be yourself.* Study your own body dynamics and pitching form. So many times I've seen pitchers try to emulate the form of their heroes, and it just was not good for themselves.

Source: From Raynor Noble, personal communication.

with shortened use of the rotator cuff muscles. Amateur pitchers used their cuff muscles throughout the throwing cycle, possibly increasing the chance for fatigue, overuse, and injury. In our experience, professional pitchers are extremely consistent in their deliveries and avoid overthrowing and risking injury. This dedication to consistency is the hallmark of every great pitcher.

Raynor Noble (Fig. 26–7), former professional baseball player and pitching coach at the University of Houston, has spent extensive time working with adolescent pitchers in his private clinics. Table 26–2 summarizes his "Ten Commandments" for teaching the art of pitching to youngsters.

CONDITIONING THE ADOLESCENT THROWING ARM: TOTAL BODY CONDITIONING IN AND OUT OF SEASON

It is difficult to impress upon young baseball players that it takes total body effort to throw effectively and without injury. Leg and trunk strength and endurance are critical to continued and ever-improved performance.

TABLE 26–3. The Nolan Ryan In-Season Running Program

Running is an essential but often neglected part of the total conditioning program for baseball. Players must run to improve endurance, speed, and power. Distance running will improve stamina so that performance will be maintained throughout the game. It will also facilitate recovery between pitches, innings, and games. Speed running (sprints) will improve speed and power.

For maximum results, players should run five to six times per week. A good approach is to do distance and sprint work on alternate days. Youth league players should run 1 to 1.5 miles. Sprints can be run on a track, in the outfield, or on the base paths. A good sprint routine using the base paths is as follows:

1. Five sprints from home to first base
2. Five sprints from first base to third base
3. Five sprints from home to second base
4. Five sprints from second base to home
5. Three sprints from home to third base
6. Two sprints from home to home
7. Five sprints backward from home to first base

Source: From Nolan Ryan, personal communication.

Sprints and middle distance running, bicycling against resistance, and trunk exercises are critical in and out of season. Nolan Ryan's running program (Table 26–3) and lower body calisthenics program (Fig. 26–8), along with bicycling, provide an excellent year-round training program without a lot of frills or specialized equipment.

Shoulder conditioning must strengthen the rotator cuff muscles, which are important in every phase of the baseball delivery.[12] Weights over 4 pounds have no place in adolescent rotator cuff strengthening. The 10-point program designed by Dr. Gene Coleman and Nolan Ryan (Fig. 26–9) will build considerable strength, as demonstrated in a recent high school study.[5]

Rex Jones, Houston Astros trainer, was asked to summarize advice for a high school–level pitcher. Table 26–4 provides his outline for off-season training. Table 26–5 sum-

TABLE 26–4. Rex Jones's Off-Season Training Program for Pitchers

Skill Development
Throwing during the off-season
   Three times per week throw off mound 10 to 15 minutes
     Proper throwing mechanics
     Keep location of pitches down
     Velocity and intensity 75 to 80 percent
     Every third outing finish 95 to 100 percent velocity
Pitchers' fielding practice (PFP)
   Pickup drills
   Cover first base
   Throws to second base
   Field bunts and throw first base and third base sides
   Throws to first inside of bag
Pickoff moves
   First base
   Second base
   Multiple runners on base
Bunting practice
   Once a week practice the following:
     Down first
     Down third
     Squeeze

Participation during the baseball off-season in other sports is very important in development of a well-rounded athlete. By participating in other sports, you will maintain and gain in muscle development, maintain and gain in cardiovascular development, and maintain and gain in flexibility.

Muscle Development*
Endurance
   Three times per week
   High repetitions (15 to 25)
   Three to five sets
   50 percent of maximum or less, depending on body part
Strength
   Two times per week
   Low repetitions (3 to 10)
   One to three sets
   60 to 75 percent of maximum

Cardiovascular Development
   Run minimum of 20 minutes, three to five times per week
   Or swim three to five times per week
   Or bike three to five times per week
   Minimum heartrate of 120 beats per minute

Flexibility
   Quadriceps and hamstring stretch
   Low back and abdominal stretch
   Shoulder stretch internal/external rotation

*Avoid bench press for baseball.
Source: From Rex Jones, personal communication.

TABLE 26–5. Rex Jones's In-Season Training Program for Pitchers

Day 1
Game day
   Overall body flexibility program; emphasis on legs and trunk
   Shoulder exercise program; one set 10 repetitions with 3-pound weight
   Shoulder stretching program
   Easy jog of 50 to 60 yards, five to seven times; sprints 70 percent at a distance of 60 to 90 feet
   Light tossing
   On-mound game preparation
   Game
   Milk down and/or ice throwing extremity
   Fluid replacement, primarily water
   Diet: restore energy supplies

Day 2
Day after game
   No throwing off mound; may long toss 5 to 10 minutes
   Overall body flexibility program
   Overall body strength program
   Long-distance running
   Shoulder exercise program: one set of 25 repetitions at regular workout weights of 3,5,8 pounds

Day 3
Throw on the side (bull pen)
   Shoulder flexibility program
   Easy jogging
   Light warm-up tossing
   On the mound work with pitching coach, 10 to 15 minutes
   Running program: distance and sprints
   Shoulder exercise routine: normal workout
   Milk down and/or ice

Day 4
Day before start
   Overall body flexibility program
   Overall body strength program
   Overall body conditioning program
   Shoulder exercise program: normal routine

Day 5
Game day, repeat Day 1

Source: From Rex Jones, personal communication.

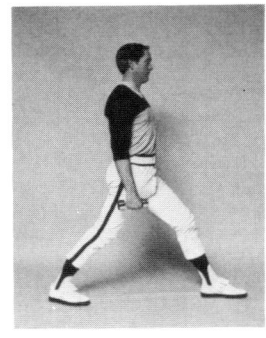 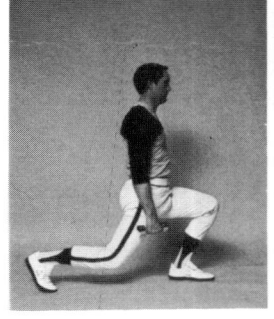

A　　　　　　　　B

LUNGES (A,B)

(1) Stand erect with one foot forward and the other foot back. (2) With weight in each hand, lower body by bending front leg. (3) Return to starting position and repeat with opposite foot forward.

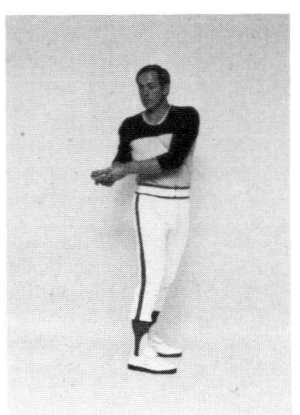

TRUNK TWIST (C)

(1) Place a mark on a wall at waist level. (2) Hold weight at waist level, stand at 10–12" away from mark with back to mark. (3) Turn to right and touch weight to mark. (4) Turn to left and touch weight to mark. (5) Repeat 10 times each direction.

FIGURE 26-8. Nolan Ryan's exercises for strengthening/stretching legs and trunk. (Courtesy of Dr. Gene Coleman and Nolan Ryan.)

C

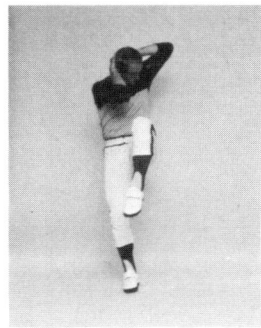

(D) KNEE LIFTS

(1) Stand erect with hands behind neck. (2) Bring left knee towards right shoulder. (3) Twist at waist and bring right elbow to left knee. (4) Repeat with right leg and left elbow. (5) Walk forward as you do this exercise. (6) Repeat 10 times each side.

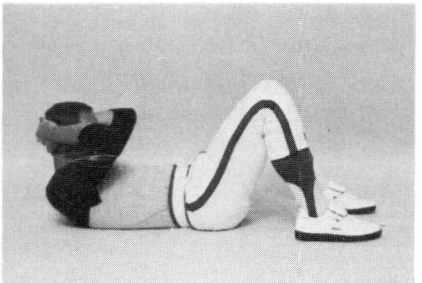

(E) CURL-UP

(1) Lie on back, knees bent, feet flat on floor and hands behind head. (2) Curl head and shoulders 6" off floor. (3) Keep chin to chest and hold for 6 seconds. (4) Return and repeat 10 times.

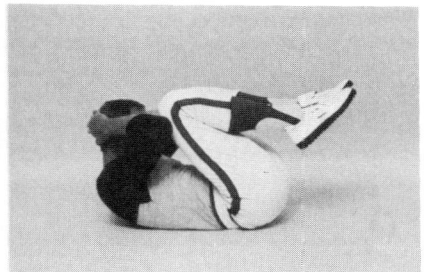

(F) V-UP

(1) Curl head and shoulder off floor and hold for 3 seconds. (2) Bring knees to chest and hold for 3 seconds. (3) Return and repeat 10 times.

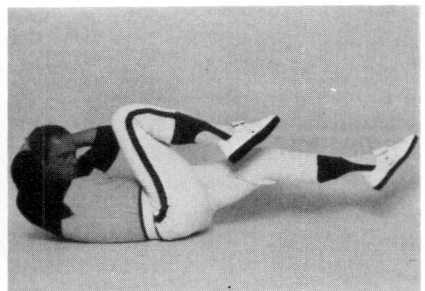

(G) PUMP SIT-UPS

(1) Curl head and shoulders off floor. (2) Bring right knee to chest. (3) Twist at hips and touch left elbow to right knee while extending left leg. (4) Alternate touching opposite elbow to opposite knee.

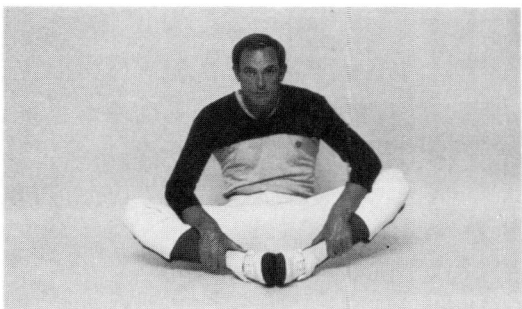

(H) GROIN STRETCH

(1) Sit erect, soles of feet together, elbows resting on knees. (2) Bend forward and grasp ankles. (3) Gently push down on knees with elbows. (4) Remove elbows from knees, bend forward and try to touch head to toes. (5) Hold 6-10 seconds. (6) Relax and repeat 3 times.

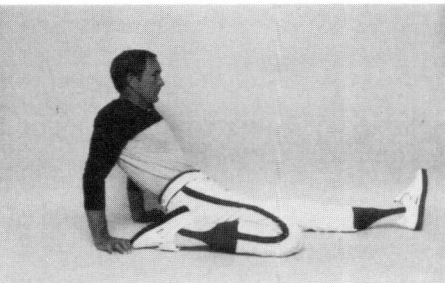

(I) QUAD STRETCH

(1) Sit with left leg straight and (2) right leg bent at knee, toes straight behind leg. (3) Lean backwards and hold 6-10 seconds. (4) Relax and repeat 3 times.

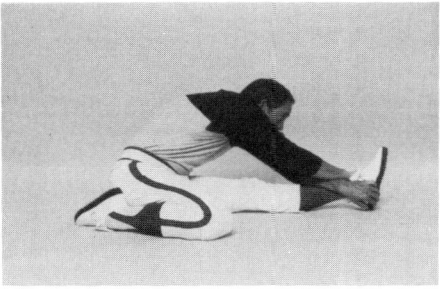

(J) HAMSTRING STRETCH

(1) Sit with left leg straight and (2) right leg bent at knee, toes straight behind leg. (3) Bend forward, grasp ankle and hold 6-10 seconds. (4) Relax and repeat 3 times.

FIGURE 26–8. *Continued*

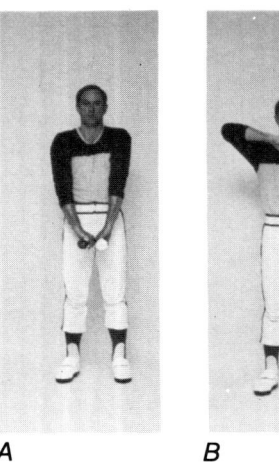 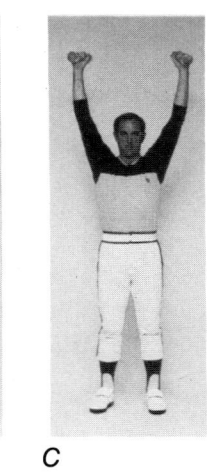 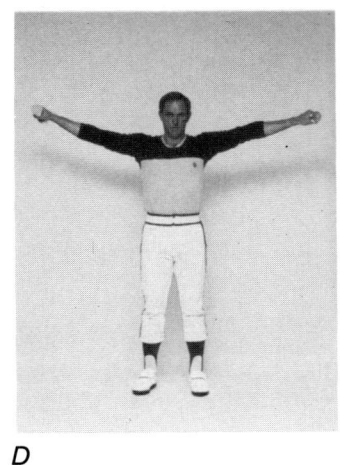 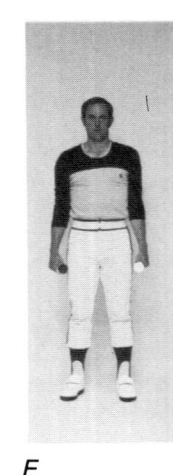

RAINBOW (A–E)

(1) Hold a pair of dumbells in front of body, elbows straight, arms inward rotated and knuckles together. (2) Slowly raise the dumbells to chin level, elbows above the head. (3) Continue to raise the dumbells over head until palms are together. palms outward and slowly lower the dumbells to the side ing elbows straight. (5) Return to starting position and

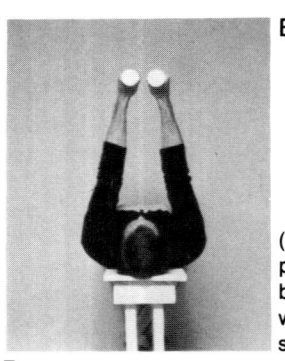

BUTTERFLY (F,G)

(1) Lie with back on bench, palms facing inward. (2) With elbows slightly bent, slowly lower weights to sides. (3) Return to starting position and repeat.

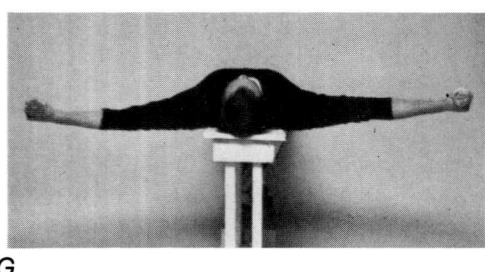

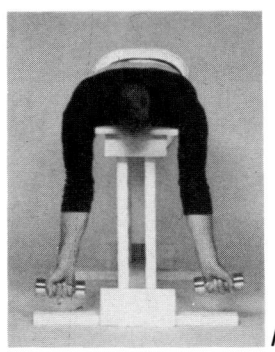

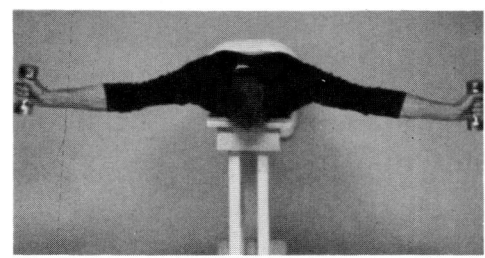

REVERSE BUTTERFLY (H,I)

(1) Lie with stomach on bench, arms straight and thumbs forward. (2) Raise weights until arms are straight and level with floor. (3) Return to starting position and repeat.

FIGURE 26-9. Nolan Ryan's rotator cuff strengthening exercises. (Courtesy of Dr. Gene Coleman and Nolan Ryan.)

BASEBALL   461

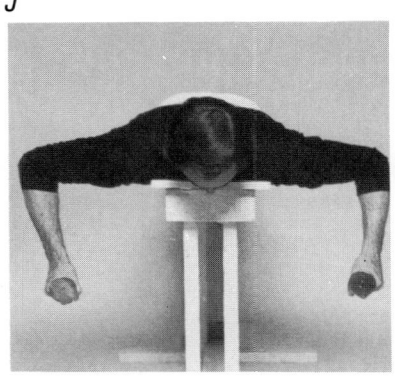
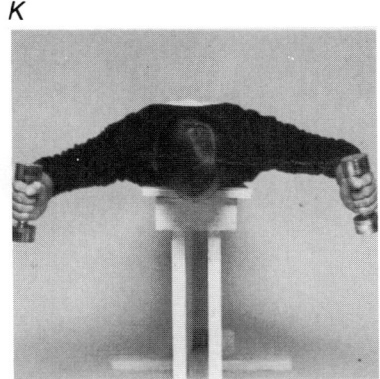

UPWARD ROTATION (J,K)
(1) Lie on stomach, arms raised to shoulder level, elbows at right angles and thumbs pointed forward. (2) Rotate weights upward until forearms are level with floor. (4) Return to starting position and repeat.

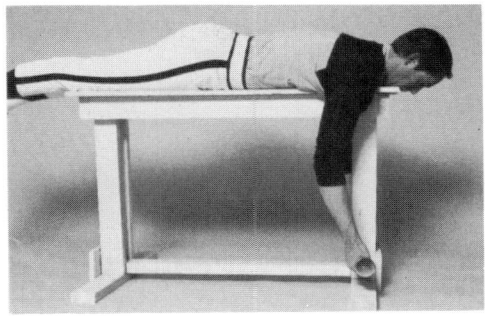
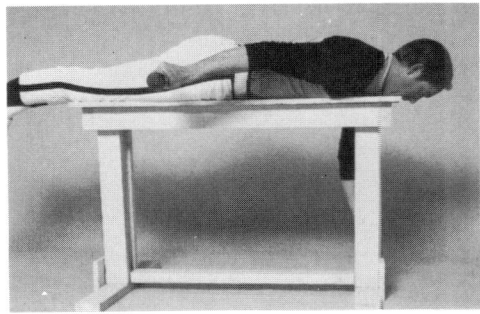

ROWING (L,M)
(1) Lie with stomach on bench, arm straight, weight pointed to floor, thumbs out. (2) Slowly pull one hand to top of bench and return to starting position. (3) Repeat with other arm.

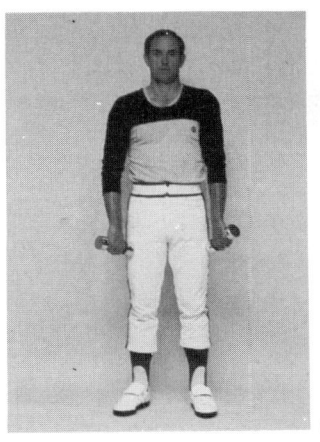
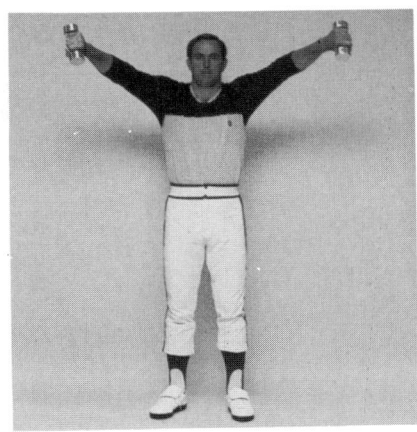

SUPRASPINATUS (N,O)
(1) Hold dumbells in front of body, elbows straight and thumbs toward floor. Slowly raise arms to shoulder level in a plane approximately 30 degrees forward. (2) Lower to starting position and repeat.

FIGURE 26–9. *Continued*   *Illustration continues on following page*

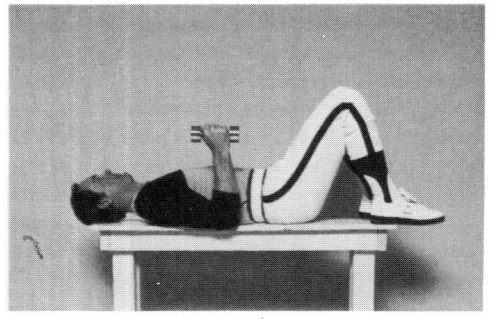 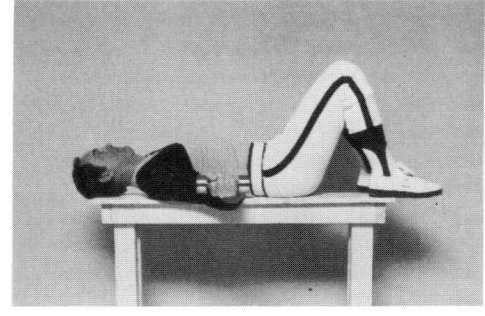

INTERNAL ROTATION (P,Q)

(1) Lie on back, right elbow against right side, weight pointed to ceiling. (2) Lower weight (outward rotate) away from side. (3) Raise weight (inward rotate) to starting position and repeat.

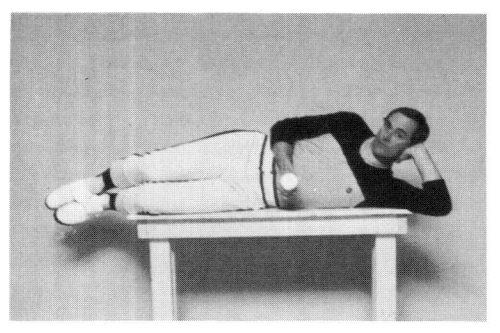 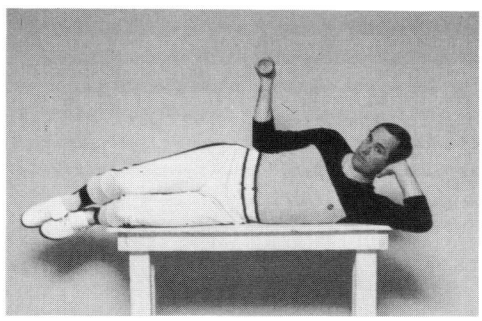

EXTERNAL ROTATIONS (R,S)

(1) Lie on left side, right elbow close to ribs, hand and dumbell across stomach with thumbs up. (2) Slowly raise weight until pointed at ceiling. (3) Lower to starting position and repeat.

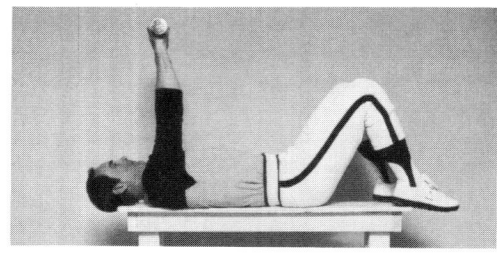

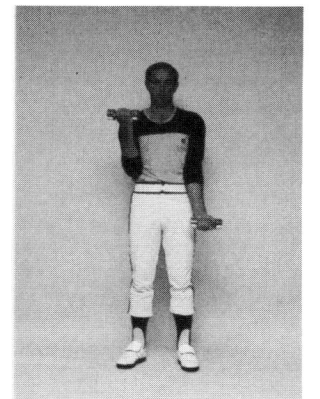 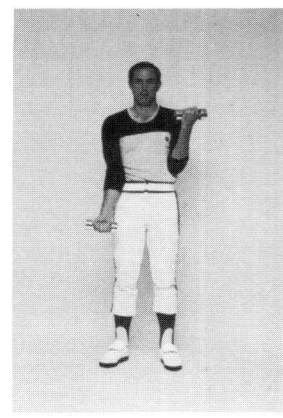

CURL (V,W)

(1) Hold a dumbell in each hand with both arms straight. (2) Flex the right elbow and curl the weight to the right shoulder. (3) Slowly lower the right arm as you flex (curl) the left arm. (4) Repeat alternating right and left arms.

PULLOVER (T,U)

(1) Lie on back, arms straight, palms facing forward. (2) With elbows straight, slowly lower weight behind head. (3) Return and repeat.

FIGURE 26–9. *Continued*

marizes his in-season program of maintenance. These programs are meant for healthy throwers. In the event of throwing shoulder injuries, a more individualized approach is warranted and will be discussed in subsequent sections.

This type of skill-oriented strength and conditioning program is much more relevant to baseball than the heavier weight training program that may be appropriate for other sports. It remains to be shown that heavy weight lifting exercises have any biological or physiological role in preparing or maintaining the preadolescent throwing arm. Children in latency are not endeared to such activity. Conversely, in adolescence, the drive to overtrain is a major problem for the treating physician as the forces of football-coaches-turned-baseball-managers, overzealous fathers, and the adolescent drive to get the "body beautiful" may conspire to overemphasize strength training.

Upper body strength has never been correlated with pitching velocity or ball control. Players who engage in heavy weight lifting off-season artificially increase body weight and bulk, arriving at spring practice with the misconception that they can overpower the opposition with increased arm strength. They have ignored total body conditioning and the fact that the baseball is thrown with a coordinated body effort. They are often stiff and never regain enough flexibility to avoid injury.

THROWING INJURIES TO THE SHOULDER

A detailed history that analyzes the events leading to the injury and a careful physical examination will allow the physician to determine the etiology of the pain and design a rational rehabilitation program.

HISTORY

Injured athletes seldom volunteer all the information necessary to evaluate a throwing injury adequately. "Kindly inquisition" may be necessary to make the correct diagnosis and set into motion corrective action. The following questions are essential in any throwing shoulder work-up:

1. Did the athlete start the season with a preexisting injury from baseball or other activities?
2. What physical preparation preceded the season?
3. How did the coach prepare the athlete in preseason? Was there a demand to throw hard in early practices?
4. Was the athlete asked to throw any new pitches?
5. How were his or her mechanics evaluated as the season progressed?
6. How heavy was the work load in the several games preceding the injury? This is best determined by asking how many hitters were faced or how many games he or she pitched.
7. Was weight training overemphasized?
8. Can the thrower correlate a specific pitch with the onset of injury?
9. Can the thrower correlate his or her pain with any specific phase of the throwing cycle?
10. Does it hurt with light tosses or full-velocity pitches?
11. Where exactly is the pain?
12. Does it hurt during throwing or after the game?
13. What treatment was started after injury? Did this include antiinflammatory medicines, cortisone shots, or heat or cold?
14. Did the athlete try to throw "hurt" or attempt weight-lifting as a cure?

The significance of these questions will become apparent as we discuss various injury situations.

PHYSICAL EXAMINATION OF THE THROWING SHOULDER

Stripped to the waist, the young athlete should now have both shoulders examined. It is extremely important to compare the injured shoulder with the opposite side. Palpate the sternoclavicular (SC) joints, as SC subluxation may occur primarily, often with a hard batting swing or indiscretion in the weight room. Secondary SC subluxation may occur where glenohumeral motion is restricted and increased stress is felt at the SC joint.

Palpate the acromioclavicular (AC) joint. Lingering problems from contact sports or weight lifting may have created AC dysfunction ranging from a torn AC cartilage to AC instability from chronic ligament insufficiency. Just lateral to the coracoid press, deep palpation will allow you to evaluate the anterior joint line. Injury to the anterior capsule-glenohumeral ligaments will create local tenderness here. Roll the biceps tendon in its groove to check for uncommon biceps tendinitis. Palpate the subacromial space and bring the arm into extension with the opposite hand to move the supraspinatus tendon anterior to the acromion for digital examination of the most frequently injured portion of the rotator cuff and the position of an often inflamed bursa.

Ask the athlete to abduct and externally rotate, observing for smooth, painless motion. Bring the arm passively into full abduction–external rotation and check for impingement symptoms. With the arms at 90 degrees of abduction, full internal rotation, and 30 degrees of flexion, the supraspinatus is isolated for manual strength testing. Ask the athlete to abduct further against resistance to see if this is a painful maneuver.

One of the most important observations is that of active and passive shoulder internal rotation. Ask the athlete to move his or her hand up the spine (Fig. 26–10) and compare it with the opposite arm. Any difference spells trouble and the potential for posterior shoulder problems. Feel the posterior shoulder joint line where there may be tenderness from acute or chronic strain on the posterior capsule and external rotators. Look for absence of the infraspinatus mass in throwers with chronic posterior pain (Fig. 11–10) and check for external rotator strength by asking for resistance against a flexed forearm.

SHOULDER INSTABILITY AS AN UNDERLYING CAUSE OF THROWING DYSFUNCTION

We have come to realize that most throwing shoulder pains are due to repetitive stress creating chronically inflamed support structures in a minimally unstable shoulder.[7] The examination for instability is therefore critical to pick up congenital laxity or acquired instability from the demands of throwing. Dr. Russell Warren has outlined an excellent approach, and the reader is referred to Chapter 11.

The alternating motion of shoulder abduction–external rotation in the cocking phase and adduction–internal rotation in the deceleration phase places unique stress on the rotator cuff and capsule, which together contain the humerus within the glenoid. Acute or chronic shoulder instability may create a number of clinical situations that result in shoulder pain, decreased velocity, and impaired control. Combinations of symptoms are common such as pain in the anterior joint line and impingement symptoms or complaints of anterior "clicking" and posterior discomfort.

It is our feeling that if many of these conditions are diagnosed early and treated with proper rest and rehabilitation, the stretched supporting shoulder structures will heal. If, on the other hand, the athlete has congenital laxity or has been allowed to throw over a long period of time with shoulder instability, there may be a serious threat to his or her pitching future.

For ease of discussion, we have described the pathoanatomy of distinct regions to help

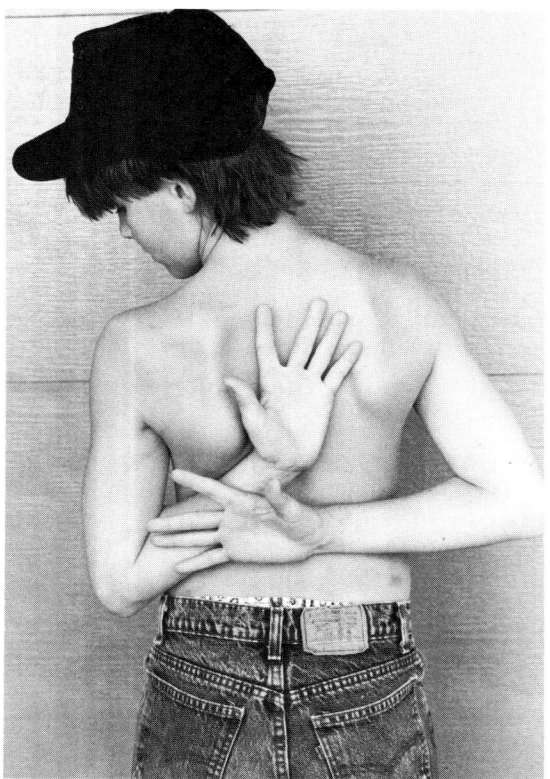

FIGURE 26–10. A lack of internal rotation often occurs in pitchers owing to repetitive eccentric strain on the posterior shoulder structures. Ask the athlete to move each hand up his or her spine and record the difference in vertebral level between dominant and nondominant sides. Note this right-handed pitcher with tight posterior shoulder structures creating a four vertebral level difference. Stretching exercises must be initiated lest he repetitively injure these taut external rotators.

the treating physician or trainer identify selected areas of concern and properly follow them with serial exams. Often the location of the pain is the primary key to the diagnosis of shoulder problems in pitchers.

ANTERIOR SHOULDER PAIN SYNDROMES

In the cocking phase, the anterior cuff (supraspinatus–subscapularis) along with the shoulder capsule and its thickened portions (called the middle and inferior glenohumeral ligaments) may be severely sprained with overthrowing or poor mechanics (opening up too soon, requiring the arm and not the body to accelerate the ball during middelivery). Anterior joint line pain results from this traction injury (Fig. 26–11), and many pitchers will be able to identify its occurrence during the late cocking–early acceleration phase. Secondarily, the anterior labrum may become torn from recurrent anterior shoulder subluxation and add to anterior discomfort. In many cases, the examiner will be able to

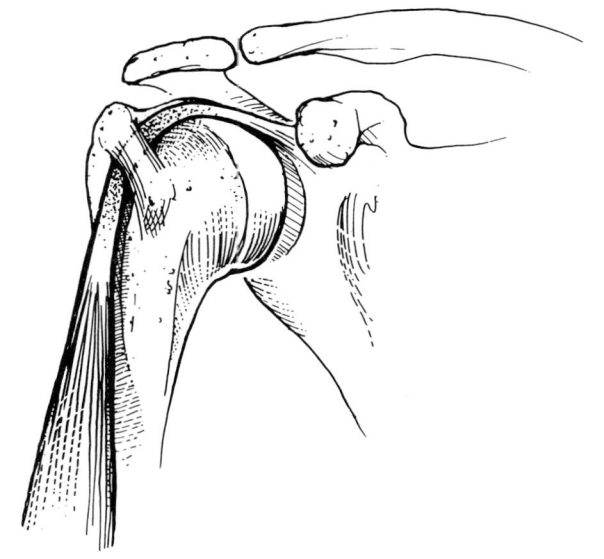

Long Head Biceps Tendonitis
Uncommon in throwers but often confused with anterior instability syndromes.

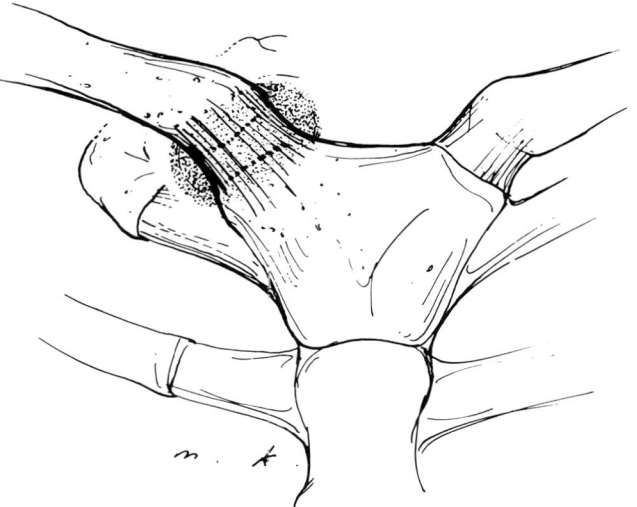

Sternoclavicular Sprain
Hard swings with a bat or a vigorous weight lifting program may loosen the ligaments connecting the clavicle to the sternum.

FIGURE 26–11. Anterior shoulder pain syndromes.

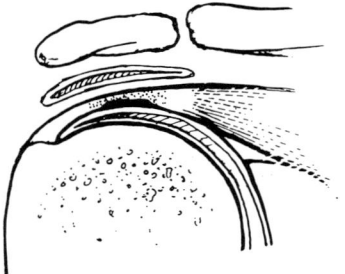

Rotator Cuff Dysfunction Syndromes
Traction tendonitis secondary to the repetetive stress of cocking-acceleration and anterior instability leads to subacromial pain. When symptoms are severe and performance is significantly impaired, consider the presence of a partial rotator cuff tear. Burning "at rest" pain may also indicate an inflammed bursa.

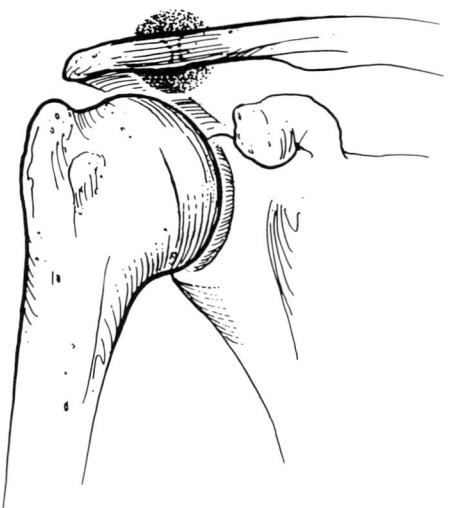

Acromioclavicular Dysfunction
Three different situations are encountered:
- gross instability from old separation
- popping or snapping from a torn AC cartilage
- distal clavicle osteolysis- pain over joint with X-rays demonstrating cysts in distal clavicle secondary to slight instability and/or chronic AC cartilage tear

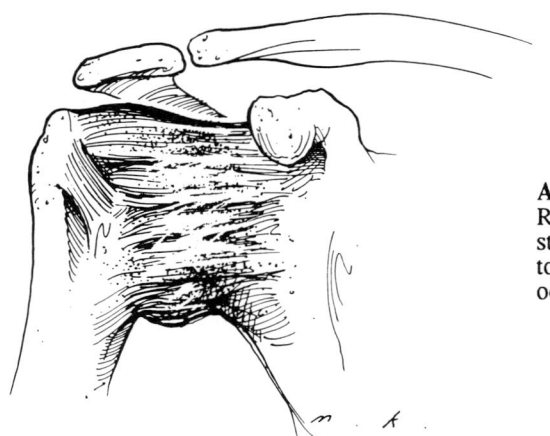

Anterior Capsule Ligament/capsule Sprain
Repetetive stretching in the cocking phase may stretch the anterior restraining structures leading to joint line pain; fraying of the labrum may occur but is of little clinical significance.

FIGURE 26–11. *Continued*

sublux the glenohumeral joint passively anteriorly.

History and physical examination alone should make this diagnosis, as anterior joint line tenderness is quite specific for this problem. Imaging tests may confirm the diagnosis but seem redundant and expensive and will have a questionable impact on the course of treatment.

Our approach in pitchers with painful, unstable shoulders is to suspend all throwing for several weeks, during which time we forbid all heavy weight lifting and start a general rotator cuff strengthening program. When return to play starts, it is essential for the pitcher to throw with proper mechanics and slowly increase the repetition and velocity of pitches. David Labossiere, the Astros head trainer, has outlined a program of rehabilitation for the pitcher attempting to come back from an unstable shoulder, shown in Table 26-6. These principles are not tied to any specific time frame but are adjusted as symptoms decrease and the athlete demonstrates sufficient progress.

Chronic shoulder instability will end many late-teenage pitching careers, and some thought has been given to reconstructive procedures. The anterior capsule may be tightened through a minimal incision without detaching the subscapularis. Jobe and Kvitne have described their approach in a recent publication.[11] The shoulder is first arthroscoped to evaluate the glenohumeral joint for labral tears, loose bodies, instability, and rotator cuff pathology. If the anterior supporting structures (anterior middle and inferior glenohumeral ligaments) are thought incompetent, the athlete will be brought back for a "subsequent anterior capsulolabral reconstruction." Through an anterior shoulder incision, the subscapularis is split in the direction of its fibers at the junction of the upper two thirds and lower one third. The capsule is incised in the same direction as the supscapularis, providing access to the glenohumeral joint. The anterior capsule is then secured to the glenoid rim by drill holes, thereby ablating the "baggy anterior capsule syndrome." A year of rest and rehabilitation

TABLE 26–6. Dave Labossiere's Rehabilitation for Rotator Cuff in Pitchers

	Phase I—Acute Phase
	This phase may vary from 2 days to 3 weeks or more.
Goal	Relief of symptoms
Plan	Rest, modalities if prescribed by physician
Program	Rest, no activities that aggravate the condition
	Modalities
	Ultrasound and muscle stimulation, preferably in combination
	Ice
	Oral antiinflammatory medicine
Notes	Our treatment regime is 10 minutes of ice, the ultrasound, and stimulation combination followed by 15 minutes of ice (BID). We maintain this till the symptoms have calmed down.
	Phase II—Range of Motion
	This phase often lasts for 4 weeks.
Goal	Increase ROM in internal-external rotation, shoulder abduction, shoulder horizontal abduction
Plan	Passive, active assistive, and active exercises
Program	Passive—wand and pulley used so it can be done at home
	Active—same program as passive except patient assists; we begin to use the Cybex at this time for ROM work in external rotation
Exercises	Wand (only to 90 degrees)
	Shoulder flexion
	Shoulder abduction
	Shoulder extension
	Shoulder internal-external rotation
	Shoulder horizontal abduction
	Cybex is done in cardinal plane with elbow flexed to 90 degrees; it is set at 300 degrees per second and it is stressed that ROM is the goal; advise the patient that minimal resistance and max ROM is the goal
	Pulley (full ROM)
	Shoulder flexion
	Shoulder abduction
Notes	We do the program four to five times per day. We encourage moving to active motion as soon as possible. We also begin doing functional motions as soon as possible because we believe that functional motion helps against muscle guarding. The therapist or trainer must work to achieve motion that is not guarded. If the patient has an unstable shoulder, we initially deemphasize external rotation ROM.

TABLE 26–6. *Continued*

Phase III—Strength

Phase III is continued for the second and third month after initiating the rehabilitation program.

Goal	Increase strength in all shoulder motions
Plan	Part A—selected motion work
	Part B—overall shoulder strength work
Program	Part A—specific rotator cuff exercises, some deltoid work
	Part B—large muscle work in addition to Part A
Exercises	Part A

    Unassisted ROM work becomes first strength program (weight of limb)
    Cuff routine begins unloaded and progresses to 25 reps with 5 pounds
    Stand (#1)—four-part deltoid only to 90 degrees (flexion, Jobe position, straight abduction, extension)
    Prone (#2)—90 degrees elbow flexion, 90 degrees shoulder abduction, wrist supinated and externally rotated
    Prone (#3)—arm hanging to floor, shoulder externally rotated, lift arms straight out from side
    Prone (#4)—arm hanging to floor, shoulder externally rotated, lift arms straight out along side
    Standing (#5)—shoulders flexed to 90 degrees, move arms together from side to side without moving trunk
    Supine (#6)—hold other end of tube in hand and externally rotate shoulder (90–90 position); extend leg to increase resistance, lower into internal rotation slowly (an eccentric contraction of external rotators)

Notes	We continue the motions mentioned in the ROM phase, but these become strength work because they are active motion. Cybex is now used as a strength tool. We use a velocity spectrum regime 10 reps at each setting. The settings are 300, 270, 240, 240, 270, and 300 degrees per second.
	Part B

    Large muscle exercises are begun
        Butterflies
        Rowing
        Military press
        Chest press (light weights at all times)
        Lateral raises

Note	These exercises are done three sets of 8 to 12 reps.

Phase IV—Return to Function

Begins 3 to 5 months after injury and only if the athlete is symptom free.

Goal	Return to activity
Plan	Ease into activity using controlled situations
Program	We use the following activities for return:

    Cybex setting at 90–90 position, 300 degrees per second
    Sleeve toss
    Long toss
    Throwing on side
    Simulated games

Exercise	We try to ease them into throwing by:

    Simulating the motion (Cybex)
    Throw in a special sleeve in training room
    Long toss on field (time or number restricted)
    Throwing on mound (noncompetitive situation)
    Simulated games (throwing to hitters but not in game situation)
    Restrict the number of pitches on return to game speed

Final Notes

The throwing athlete needs extreme external rotation, so this ROM must be worked diligently, but do not neglect internal rotation ROM, which also needs work.

Be sure to isolate the glenohumeral movements from the scapulothoracic movements when stretching internal-external rotation.

It is extremely important that the athlete be given an opportunity to ease into activity.

BID = Twice a day
ROM = Range of motion
Source: From Dave Labossiere, personal communication.

is started. The long-term results of such surgery are still unknown.

Anterior instability syndromes may occur easily in congenitally lax shoulders. In those individuals, it may be the best advice to suggest playing a different position. No amount of rest or physical therapy will be effective in returning these hyperlax individuals to successful pitching.

SHOULDER IMPINGEMENT SYNDROMES

Often the young pitcher has a combination of anterosubacromial or subacromial pain experienced during the late cocking–acceleration phase. Subacromial pain is the summation of a traction injury to the supraspinatus tendon with resulting inflammation, bursa formation, and secondary impingement symptoms. Often they have anterior joint line tenderness from concomitant stretched, inflamed anterior structures. In many cases, a partial rotator cuff tear may be seen on arthrogram (Fig. 26–12).

In throwers with impingement symptoms, rest for several weeks may be in order, especially if complaints of loss of velocity or control are elicited. Suspicion for an inflamed bursa is seen when extreme pain under the acromial arch is elicited by palpation or forced abduction–external rotation. A single steroid injection is warranted to decrease pain with simple activities of daily living. All throwing activities are ceased, but general conditioning may continue. We start a simple rotator cuff strength program in which all resistive exercises above the horizontal are forbidden, lest they recreate impingement symptoms. The rehabilitation program outlined in Table 26–6 is begun. If the arthrogram or arthroscopy reveals a partially torn rotator cuff, the athlete, trainers, and coaches may expect several months of rest to be necessary before throwing can be resumed.

Arthroscopy is reserved for those cases where a suspected labrum tear may be causing glenohumeral impingement or where other pathology such as a loose body is suspected. Shaving the partially torn rotator cuff makes little biological sense and may further threaten its integrity. Acromioplasties, open or arthroscopic, are contraindicated in throwers with impingement symptoms, as they will not address the stretched rotator cuff.

LATERAL SHOULDER PAIN

Most lateral shoulder pain represents rotator cuff tendinitis in the posterior supraspinatus and anterior infraspinatus regions. In these cases, the treatment is similar to that described above for impingement syndrome. If the tenderness is on the tip of the acromion,

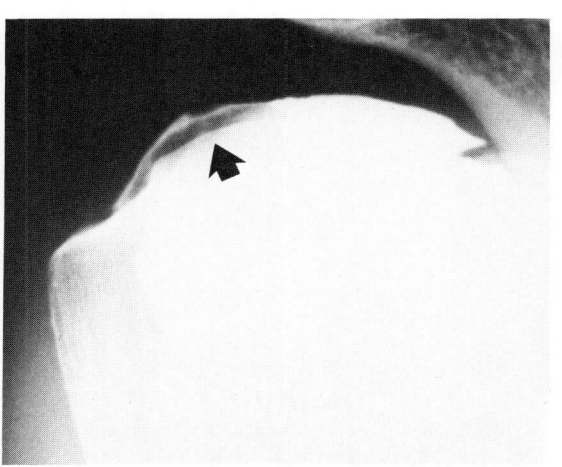
A

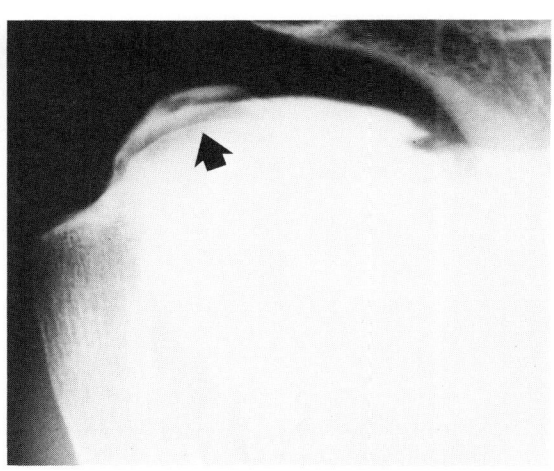
B

FIGURE 26–12. Shoulder arthrogram demonstrating partial rotator cuff tear. *(A)* Slight irregularity of the dye column over the greater tuberosity signifies possible rotator cuff pathology in this 19-year-old pitcher with impingement syndromes. *(B)* After 2 minutes of exercise with the arthrographic dye in place, a partial tear is clearly demonstrated.

it may, however, be considered deltoid tendinitis. In this latter case, rest for several days is appropriate.

POSTERIOR SHOULDER PAIN

Deceleration places significant stresses on the posterior capsule and infraspinatus muscle-tendon complex as the arm is twisted violently into adduction–internal rotation (Fig. 26–13). If anterior instability is present, the humerus will sublux anteriorly and place further traction on the already sprained tissues. Unlike the anterior structures that become loosened, the posterior structures lose their elasticity and tighten with greater resistance to repetitive stress. Physical exam will often demonstrate an internal rotation contracture in cases where repetitive injury has

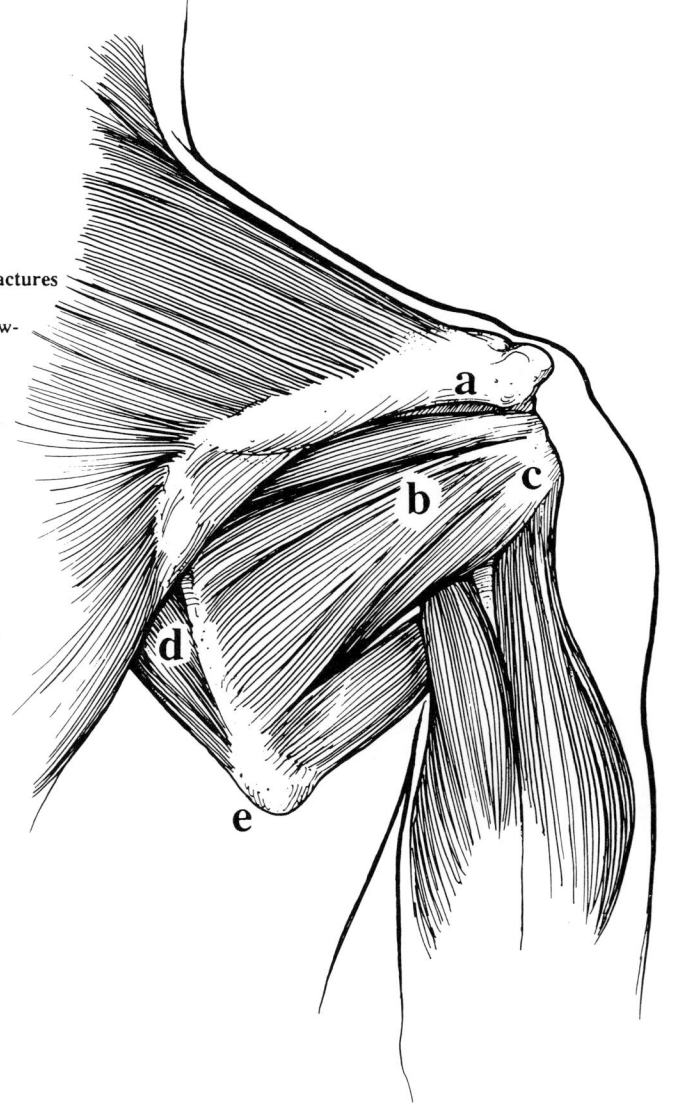

a. Infraspinatus Traction Tendonitis

Pain under the posterior acromial arch is not likely due to traction tendonitis on the posterior rotator cuff tendons

b. Infraspinatus Fibrosis and Internal Rotation Contractures

Repeated infraspinatus microtears may occur during follow-through, leading to muscle fibrosis. A secondary internal rotation contracture will develop

c. Posterior Capsule Sprain

Follow-through stretches the posterior capsule, leading to joint line tenderness and pain on instability testing.

d. Rhomboid Strain

Any of the periscapular muscles may be strained from the forces of follow-through.

e. Periscapular Bursitis

Deep burning pain beneath the scapula may be due to a scapulothoracic bursa.

FIGURE 26–13. Posterior shoulder pain syndromes. *a,* Infraspinatus traction tendonitis. Pain under the posterior acromial arch is not likely owing to traction tendonitis on the posterior rotator cuff tendons. *b,* Infraspinatus fibrosis and internal rotation contractures. Repeated infraspinatus microtears may occur during follow-through, leading to muscle fibrosis. A secondary internal rotation contracture will develop. *c,* Posterior capsule sprain. Follow-through stretches the posterior capsule, leading to joint line tenderness and pain on instability testing. *d,* Rhomboid strain. Any of the periscapular muscles may be strained from the forces of follow-through. *e,* Periscapular bursitis. Deep burning pain beneath the scapula may be due to a scapulothoracic bursa.

occurred (Fig. 26–10). In rare cases, one will see frank atrophy of the infraspinatus from either entrapment–traction of the inferior branch of the suprascapular nerve or actual nerve avulsion.[4]

The combination of anterior joint line tenderness and anterior subluxation with posterior joint line tenderness and internal rotation contracture has led us to the concept of the "loose-in-the-front-and-tight-in-the-back" syndrome. It is one of the most common problems in late adolescent and adult pitching shoulders. The imbalance of soft tissue tension further propagates itself with throwing. When untreated, this may lead to prolonged disability of career-threatening proportions.

Treatment consists of immediate rest. When there has been prolonged disability or severe symptoms, an arthrogram is ordered to document the presence or absence of partial rotator cuff tear, the presumption being that its presence will require a longer rest period. The athlete should be prepared to stop pitching for several weeks as he or she progresses through a rehabilitation program.

Astros trainer Dave Labossiere has designed a series of trainer-athlete interactive exercises to build cautiously anterior cuff strength while stretching the contracted posterior tissues (Fig. 26–14). We use these during the several weeks of rest imposed on adolescent throwers with the shoulder "loose-in-the-front-and-tight-in-the-back" syndrome. We suggest that it also be used in-season to maintain flexibility in pitchers with a propensity to develop posterior tightness.

PROXIMAL HUMERAL EPIPHYSIOLYSIS

A rare but important cause of deep global shoulder pain is due to a traction injury to the proximal humeral epiphysis.[1] Seen in young adolescent pitchers who pitch excessively or with overpowering effort, this condition leads to deep, throbbing shoulder pain reproduced by palpating the humeral neck region. Radiographs show a widened epiphyseal plate when compared with the opposite shoulder (Fig. 26–15). Rest for several weeks and gradual return to throwing are in order. Often several months must pass before it is comfortable to throw.

INJURIES TO THE THROWING ELBOW

HISTORY AND PHYSICAL EXAMINATION

The same concerns discussed under shoulder problems should be addressed when working up a young athlete with elbow problems. The classic questions of "What, where, when, and how" are to be asked under the guidelines previously presented.

The elbow is but one link in a kinetic chain of several joints and must be considered in context, particularly with regard to any shoulder problem. Limitation of shoulder motion or focal shoulder pain implies that the elbow may have sustained added stress while the athlete was throwing with a compromised shoulder.

Flexion and extension should be compared with the opposite side and recorded in degrees. Similarly, pronation and supination restrictions should be measured.

Palpation should be carried out in an orderly fashion, concentrating on several critical areas. Careful palpation can usually identify the injured structure responsible for the pain. Thorough knowledge of the ligamentous and bony anatomy (Chapter 13) is essential in obtaining the maximum amount of information from this examination.

Anterior

Anterior elbow pain is often seen in conjunction with elbow flexion contractures, which are discussed below. Ascertain whether the entire anterior elbow capsule is inflamed or whether the tenderness is confined to the attachment of the lateral or medial muscle groups.

Lateral

Lateral epicondylitis is uncommon in throwers yet may be present from other activities (such as hitting with a fungo bat) and may compromise overall elbow function. Anterolateral tenderness, along with decreased pronation and supination, suggests the diagnosis of radiocapitellar incongruity from osteochondrosis. Bulging beneath the anconeus muscle indicates an elbow effusion or hemarthrosis. Aspiration with a needle and syringe is warranted to decrease pain and determine the nature of the intraarticular fluid.

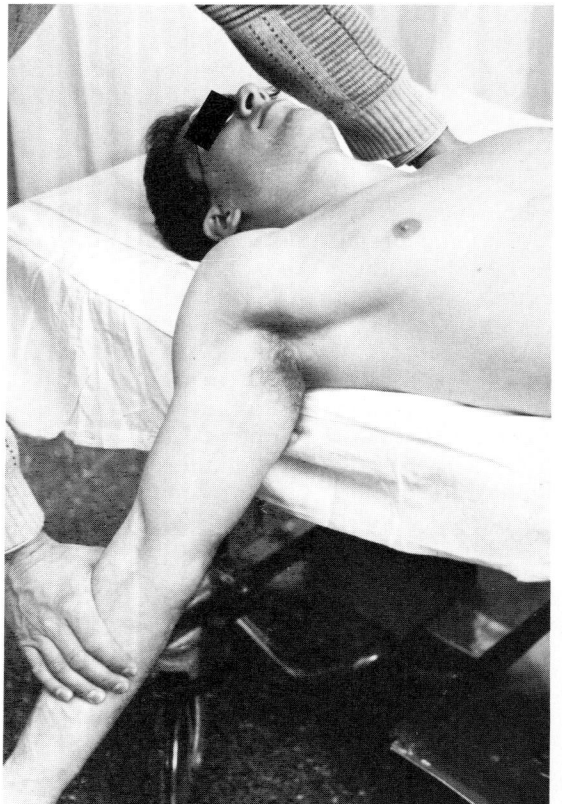 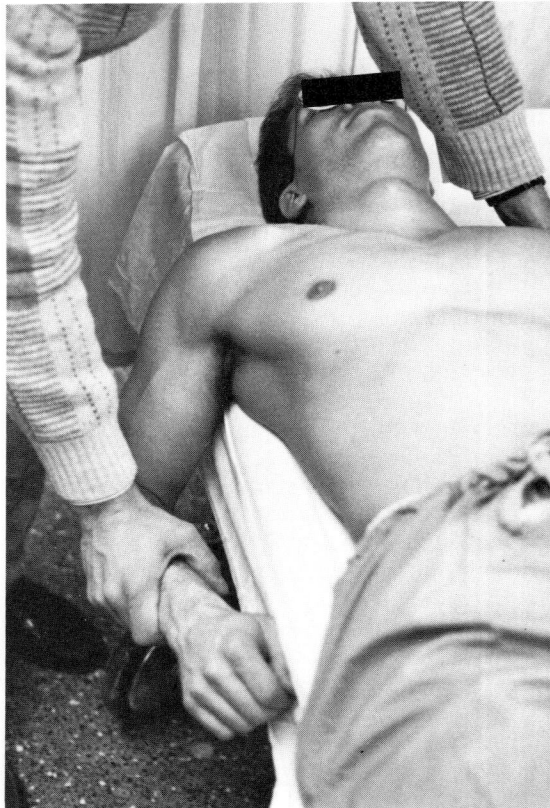

FIGURE 26–14. Manual shoulder flexibility program. The following program is a program of shoulder flexibility exercises used by the Houston Astros baseball team for the maintenance and rehabilitation of shoulder injuries. It is designed for therapists and trainers who are interested in keeping their throwing athletes flexible enough for the rigors of their sport. It should not be used by people who have no experience in active assistive flexibility techniques. All the positions may be used with proprioceptive neuromuscular facilitated (PNF) techniques such as contract–relax or hold–relax. We generally use between 5 and 10 repetitions of each position. There are several positions that are alike except for the blocking of the scapula and/or humeral head. Please note when the figures show the blocking techniques, as these are essential to stretching the shoulder and surrounding structures fully. One positioning term that will be used throughout this program is 90–90, which refers to the position of 90 degrees of shoulder abduction and 90 degrees of elbow flexion. *Shoulder extension.* We use two exercises for stretching of the anterior portion of the shoulder. One is done with the elbow extended, the other is done with the elbow flexed. *Exercise #1 (A).* The patient is supine with the arm and elbow in extension. The operator pushes the shoulder into extension and mild scapula horizontal adduction. This stretches anterior structures such as anterior capsule, long head of biceps, and anterior deltoid. *Exercise #2(B).* Same positioning as above except the elbow is flexed as the operator pushes shoulder into extension. This once again stretches the anterior structures but negates stretch on the long head of the biceps. *Shoulder external rotation (C).* You are stretching the internal rotators. The patient is supine and in the 90–90 position. The operator moves the arm into external rotation while maintaining the 90–90 position. *Shoulder internal rotation.* We are moving into internal rotation, which stretches the external rotators. The patient is supine again in the 90–90 position. *Exercise #1(D).* The operator supports the elbow and pushes into internal rotation, allowing the glenohumeral joint to roll forward off the table while maintaining the position of 90–90. This method stretches external rotators as well as the scapula adductors. *Exercise #2(E).* The positioning is the same, but the operator blocks the glenohumeral joint from rolling forward while pushing into internal rotation. This must be done *carefully!!* This stretches only the external rotators, particularly the supraspinatus, infraspinatus, and teres minor. *Shoulder internal rotation. Exercise #3(F,G).* The patient is supine with hand behind back (in lumbar area). The operator blocks the glenohumeral joint and lifts the elbow upward. This is done in two positions—first, with hand just covered by back (F), then with hand well behind the back (G). This should also be done *carefully!! Shoulder horizontal abduction.* We will stretch the scapula horizontal adductors in two positions. One is done with the scapula blocked, and the other is done unblocked. *Exercise #1 (H).* The patient is supine with the arm across the chest. The operator pushes the arm (held

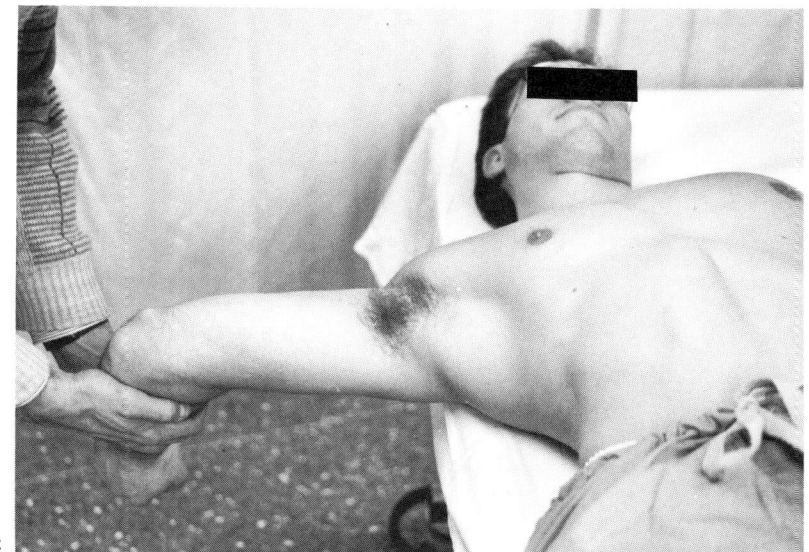

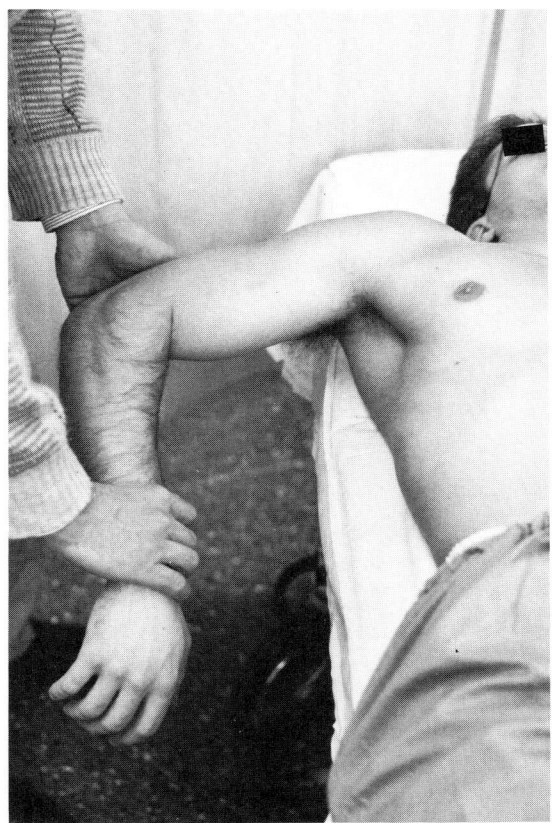

above the elbow) across the chest. This is done at three angles: directly across the chest, just under the chin, and just above the hip. This stretches the rhomboids and trapezius. Exercise #2 (*I*). Same position as #1. The operator blocks the lateral border of the scapula with the heel of his or her hand. The patient then reaches with the other hand and grabs his or her arm just above the elbow and pulls it cross chest. The operator must prevent the scapula from normal scapular excursion. This stretches the posterior scapulohumeral muscles such as infraspinatus and teres minor. (From Labossiere, D.: Manual shoulder flexibility program (unpublished).)

Illustration continues on following page

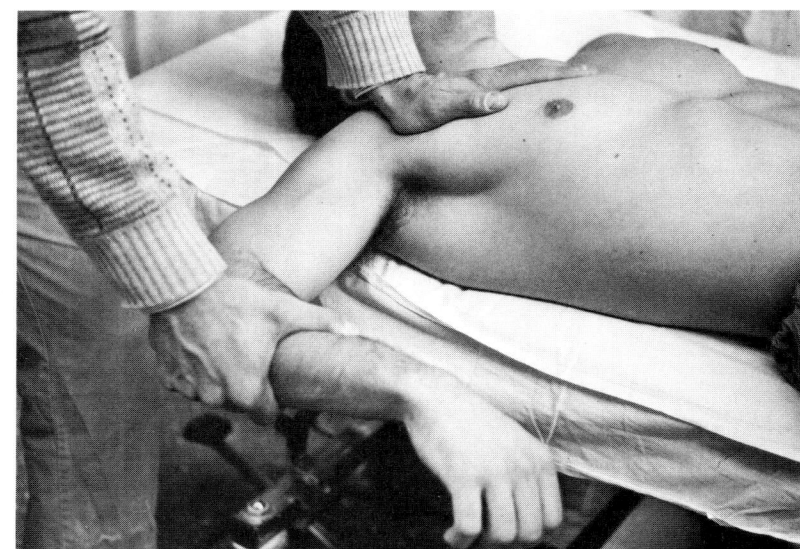

E

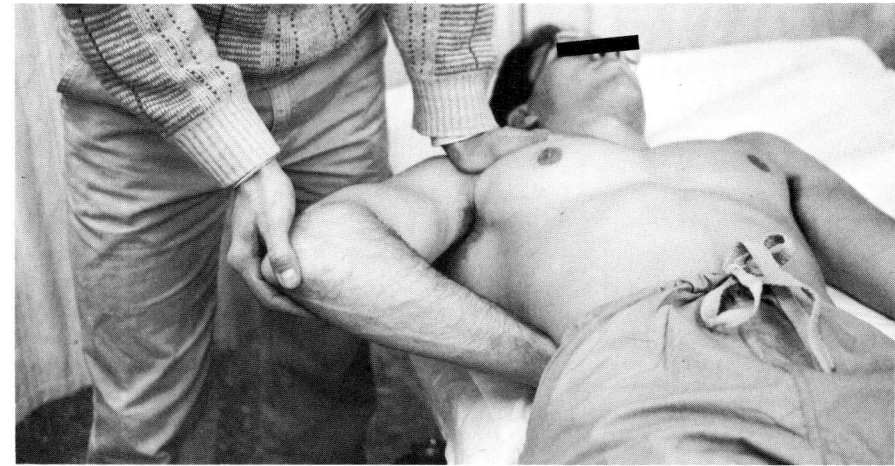

F

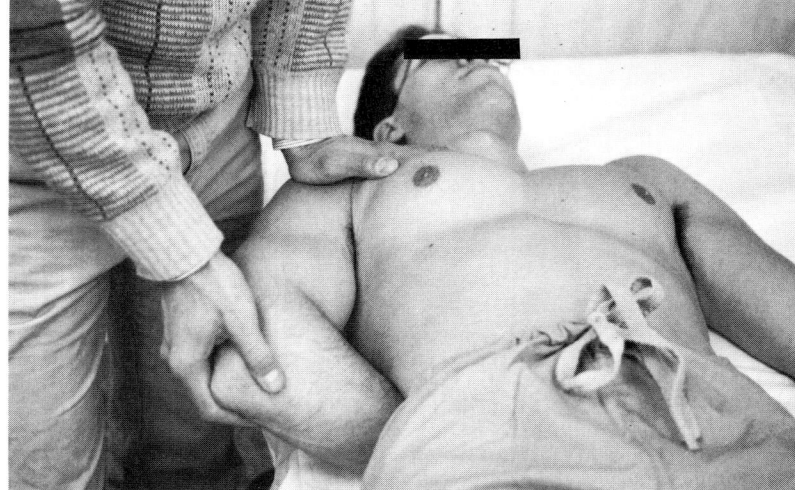

G

FIGURE 26–14. *Continued*

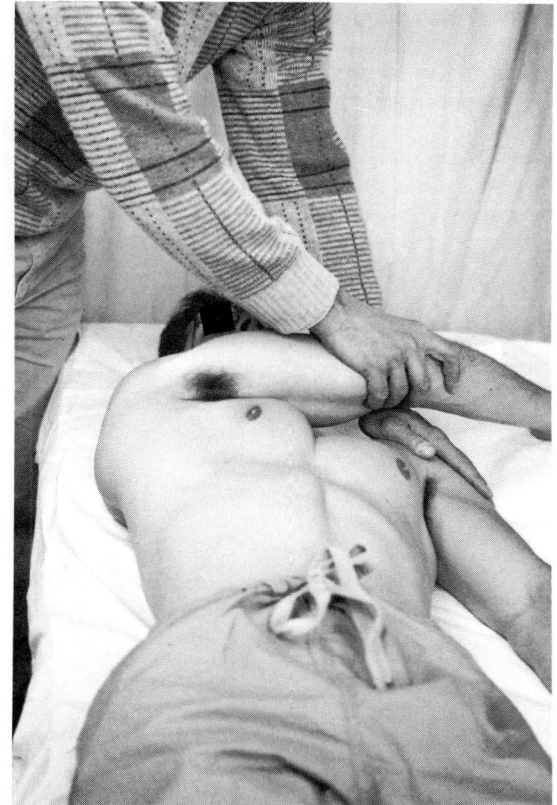
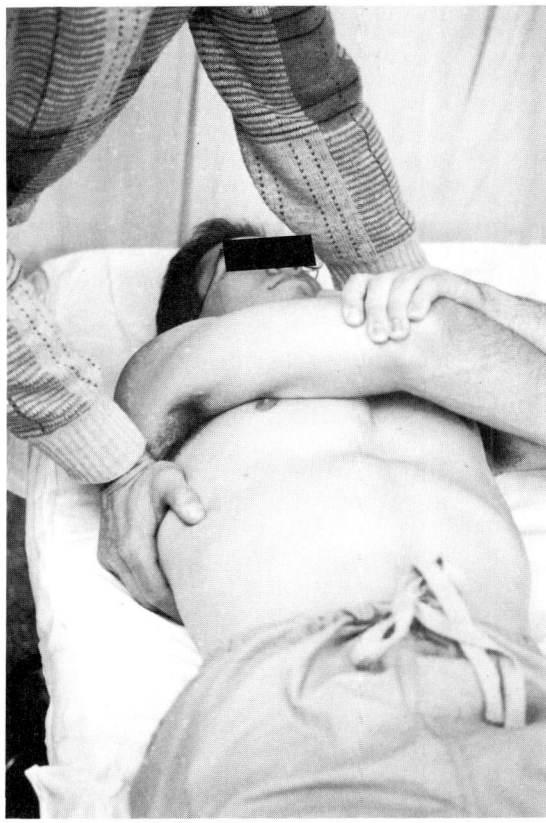

H   I

FIGURE 26–14. *Continued*

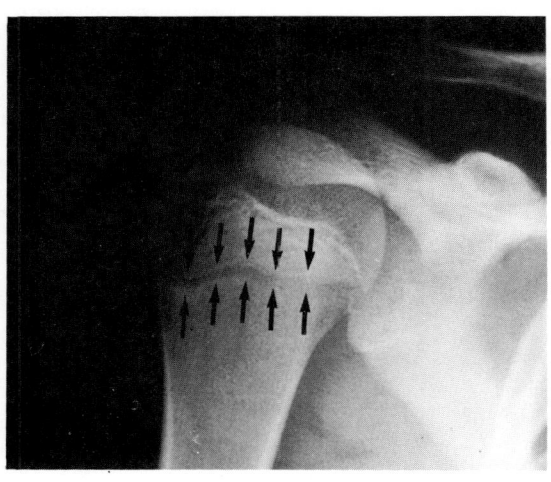
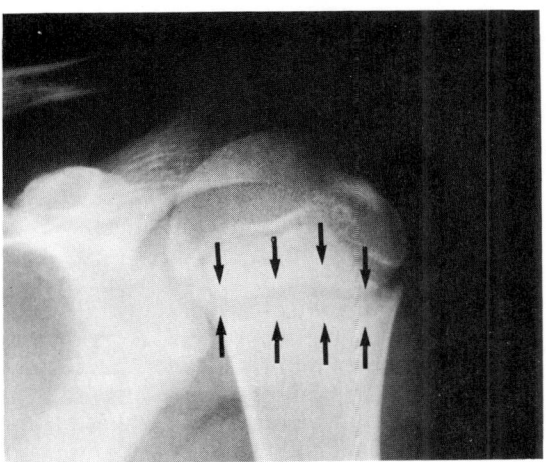

A   B

FIGURE 26–15. (*A*) A narrow epiphyseal plate is seen in this nondominant right shoulder of a 13-year-old pitcher. (*B*) A widened but nonfragmented epiphyseal plate is seen in this 13-year-old pitcher with persistent deep shoulder pain. Widening is enough to make a diagnosis of epiphysiolysis. Fragmentation is rare.

Posterior

Carefully feel the distal triceps tendon for localized tenderness and in the adolescent thrower exert pressure over the proximal olecranon process, as traction injury to the olecranon apophysis may have occurred. The medial olecranon area is often tender from extension compaction chondromalacia. Tenderness here should easily be distinguished from medial collateral ligament problems.

Medial

The examiner should be prepared to separate the areas of flexor-pronator tendinitis, medial collateral ligament sprains, and ulnar nerve irritation by digital exploration and valgus stress testing, the latter designed to bring out severe cases of medial instability. To test for abnormal valgus laxity, flex the elbow 30 degrees in order to unlock the olecranon from the humeral fossa and apply abduction stress to the elbow while stabilizing the humerus.

OSTEOCHONDRITIS DISSECANS OF THE CAPITELLUM

Capitellar osteochondritis dissecans may lead to symptoms of tightness, stiffness, swelling, clicking, grinding, or pain.[3] The average age of these patients is 12, and most have been pitching baseball for several years. Gradual onset of pain is the most common presentation and accounts for the fact that many of these diagnoses are made on a delayed basis.

Pain over the lateral and anterior elbow is made evident with deep palpation or pronation-supination maneuvers. Restricted pronation-supination is the rule, and a flexion contracture is common.

X-rays will show ill-defined, patchy decalcification and cysts in the capitellar area (Fig. 26–16). Comparisons with the opposite elbow are invaluable. X-rays may also show loose bodies, products of exfoliated articular cartilage from the diseased area. Arthrograms are often ordered but must be interpreted with caution, as reactive synovitis may be so pronounced that filling defects from the synovium will be misinterpreted as "loose bodies." Magnetic resonance imaging (MRI) and computerized tomography (CT) scans may confirm necrotic changes but offer little in guiding the physician's treatment plan.

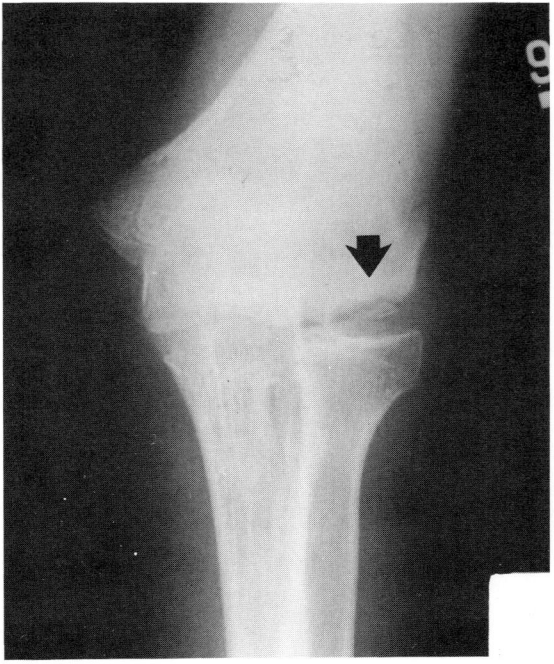

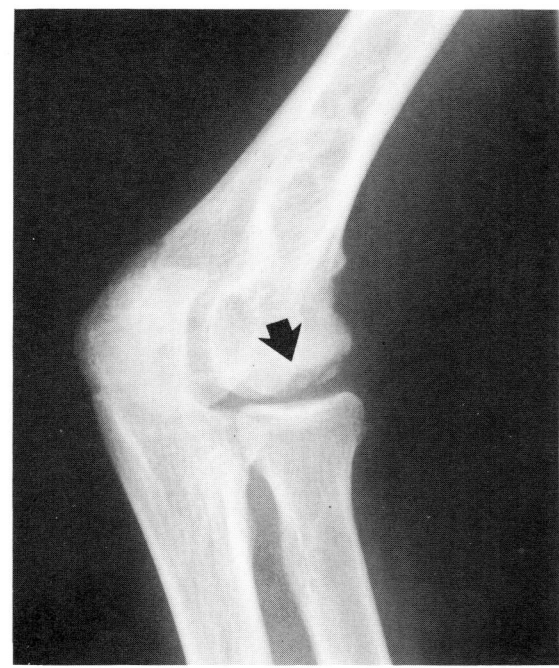

FIGURE 26–16. An anteroposterior (A) and oblique view (B) demonstrate osteochondritis dissecans in this 14-year-old shortstop with a 25 degree elbow flexion contracture. No loose bodies were found at arthroscopy.

When the diagnosis of osteochondritis dissecans is made, complete rest from pitching is instituted. The thrower is asked to start gentle passive stretching exercises to maintain as much flexion–extension and pronation–supination as possible. We feel it is safe to continue playing baseball but preferably at first base or right field.

All identified osteochondritis dissecans need not be operated on. Surgery is indicated when:

1. The osteochondral defect is large as demonstrated on plain X rays and the young athlete complains of grinding and catching from roughened articular surface or an unstable flap of osteochondral tissue.
2. A loose body has formed and is causing mechanical problems.

The arthroscope has proved attractive for exploring the anterior compartment but may not allow proper debridement of roughened surface or removal of large loose fragments. A small anterolateral arthrotomy will suffice in most cases and may be completed in day surgery with same-day discharge.

ELBOW FLEXION CONRACTURES

Lack of full elbow extension may occur suddenly or progress slowly with months and years of throwing in the absence of osteochondritis dissecans. These chronic contractures cause little functional disability and should not raise clinical concern. Acute lack of extension is often associated with pain and is thought due to chondromalacia of articular surfaces with secondary reactive synovitis and joint motion guarding. Other cases are due to hyperextension that may occur during contact with another player or during base sliding.

It is extremely important to diagnose the cause before embarking on treatment of restricted motion. No adolescent with a painful flexion contracture should be allowed to return to throwing until the pain has been relieved and preinjury motion restored.

Treatment begins with nonsteroidal antiinflammatories to decrease symptoms during activities of daily living. We prefer to rest the athlete from throwing and weight lifting, during which time the individual is asked to passively stretch the contracted joint gently with the opposite arm. Within a few weeks, more vigorous stretching with free weights may be started. We have not found other physiotherapy modalities or extension braces to be helpful in these cases.

MEDIAL ELBOW PAIN

The very nature of the throwing act places great demands on the medial elbow structures (Fig. 26–17). Several forces are at play in creating medial elbow pain, including the valgus stress during acceleration and forceful wrist flexion at ball release.

Flexor-Pronator Tendinitis

Sisto et al.[23] performed electromyelographic studies on the forearm musculature and arrived at the conclusion that breaking pitches demand no excessive work from the wrist flexors and forearm pronators. This is what one would expect from highly trained pitchers, but in the adolescent and preadolescent group, many breaking pitches are not thrown with subtle wrist position or differential finger pressure but rather violent pronation before ball release. This often gives rise to strain on the flexor-pronator origin at the medial elbow. It may prove difficult to implicate breaking pitches in many cases, as often these are the same youngsters who are also throwing their fast balls excessively hard.

Flexor-pronator tendinitis is easily identified by tenderness over the muscle mass just distal to its origin from the medial epicondyle. Discomfort is reproduced by wrist flexion against resistance. In a college player, we have observed the equivalent of a compartment syndrome that responded to a fascial release, but this is rare. As with any muscle strain, 10 days of rest from throwing and a gradual return are usually effective. The athlete should be observed and corrected for excessive pronation or wrist flexion, especially on breaking pitches.

Pain over the medial epicondyle, especially in the ages 10 to 14, should arouse concern for a traction injury to the secondary growth plate in this area.[26] Such an injury demands radiographic evaluation to rule out the unusual complete avulsion of the medial epicondyle, which would require open reduction and internal fixation with a screw (as smooth pins have proven inadequate). More often, comparison radiographs will show a widened space between the epicondyle and underlying humerus, indicating a chronic traction injury. Pitchers with this injury should be rested for 4 to 6 weeks and then allowed to throw if the commonly associated flexion contracture has resolved. During this time, they may bat but should avoid weight lifting or any resistive arm exercises for the first month. A light resistive program may then be instituted.

Medial Collateral Ligament Sprains

Numerous studies[16] have confirmed the all-important role played by the medial collateral ligament (MCL) in providing medial support and preventing anterior ulnar sub-

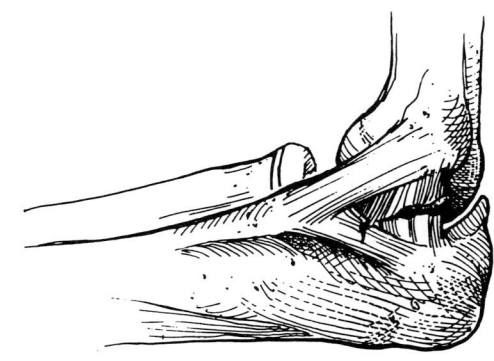

Medial Collateral Ligament Sprain
The valgus stress of throwing stretches the MCL with each toss. Poor mechanics or a single catastrophic injury from over-throwing will partially or completely tear this critical ligament. Frank valgus instability is uncommon unless the ligament is completely disrupted.

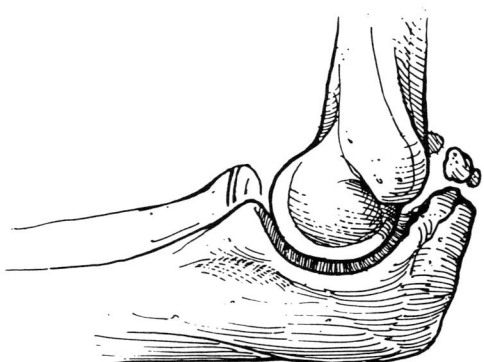

Posteromedial Impingement
Tenderness over the medial olecranon is due to impingement against the humeral fossa, leading to chondromalacia. Repetitive injury will lead to exfoliation of osteocartilagenous fragments and loose bodies.

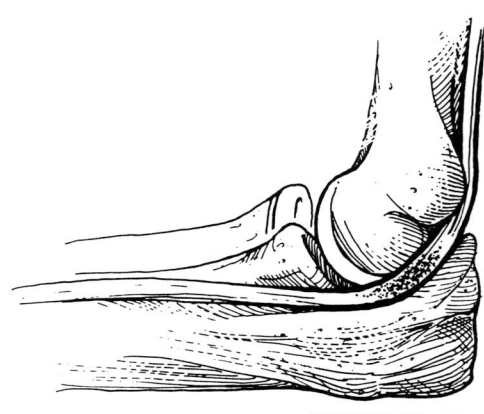

Ulnar Neuritis
The ulnar nerve sits in a shallow groove behind the medial epicondyle. The nerve maybe irritated from repeated throwing. If medial instability is present the nerve is stretched with each toss. Ulnar neuritis must not be considered an isolated condition in such a situation.

FIGURE 26–17. Medial elbow pain.

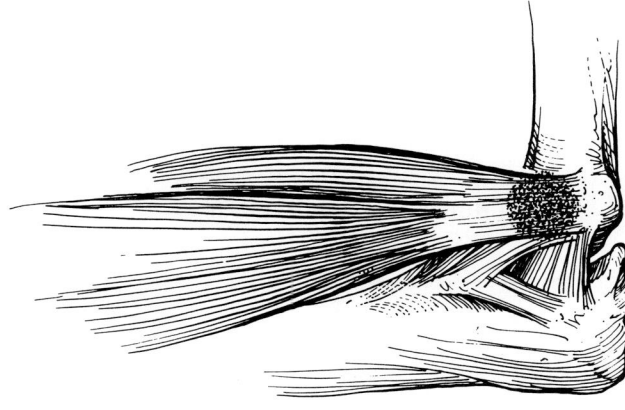

Flexor-Pronator Tendonitis
Sudden or repetitive stress upon the flexor muscle-tendon will cause local tenderness. Symptoms are reproduced by resistance against wrist flexion.

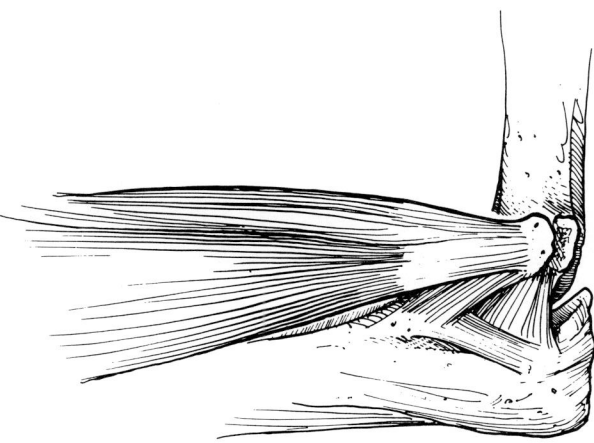

Medial Epcondylar Fracture
Traction overload on this open epiphysis may cause local pain directly over the medial epicondyle. Catastrophic failure will result in separation and an avulsed medial epicondyle.

FIGURE 26–17. *Continued*

luxation with the elbow in flexion.[21] Most of the throwers with MCL sprains have overstressed their elbows by either opening up too soon or by dropping the elbow below the horizontal.[24] This latter technical error tends to arise late in the game as the shoulder becomes fatigued.

MCL sprain pain is localized to the area just beneath the medial epicondyle and flexor-pronator mass. The proper diagnosis may be made by careful palpation of the ligament. Discomfort produced by valgus stress testing at 30 degrees of elbow flexion is a less reliable sign unless there is significant MCL disruption. Radiographs are normal unless there has been an avulsion fracture in a young teenager and should not be used to make determinations about the presence or absence of medial collateral pathology.

Uncommonly, the athlete may hear a loud pop, experience immediate medial elbow pain, and come out of the game with a complete rupture of the medial collateral ligament. Valgus stress testing will produce pain and "a jog of instability."

Medial collateral ligament sprains are often ignored or treated with ice and cortisone injections under the belief that some "sports medicine magic" will hasten recovery. Yet this is a ligamentous structure, and like any other ligament sprain, an elbow medial collateral ligament injury deserves considerable rest and concern as to the cause of its injury. Throwing should be prohibited for several weeks in acute cases and several months in chronic cases, which characteristically involve repeated injuries. Throwing should progressively resume with attention to mechanics and a strong rotator cuff group to prevent shoulder fatigue and secondary elbow stress. If the thrower returns without correction of faulty mechanics, reinjury will recur no matter how long rest was carried out.

Surgical repair of significant *acute* medial collateral ligament tears has never been shown to hasten recovery or prevent recurrent instability. Just as knee medial collateral ligament tears heal successfully with rest, we have found that acute elbow medial collateral ligament sprains will heal without surgical repair. A customized thermoplastic cast–brace with Velcro straps should be worn during waking hours for 6 weeks after

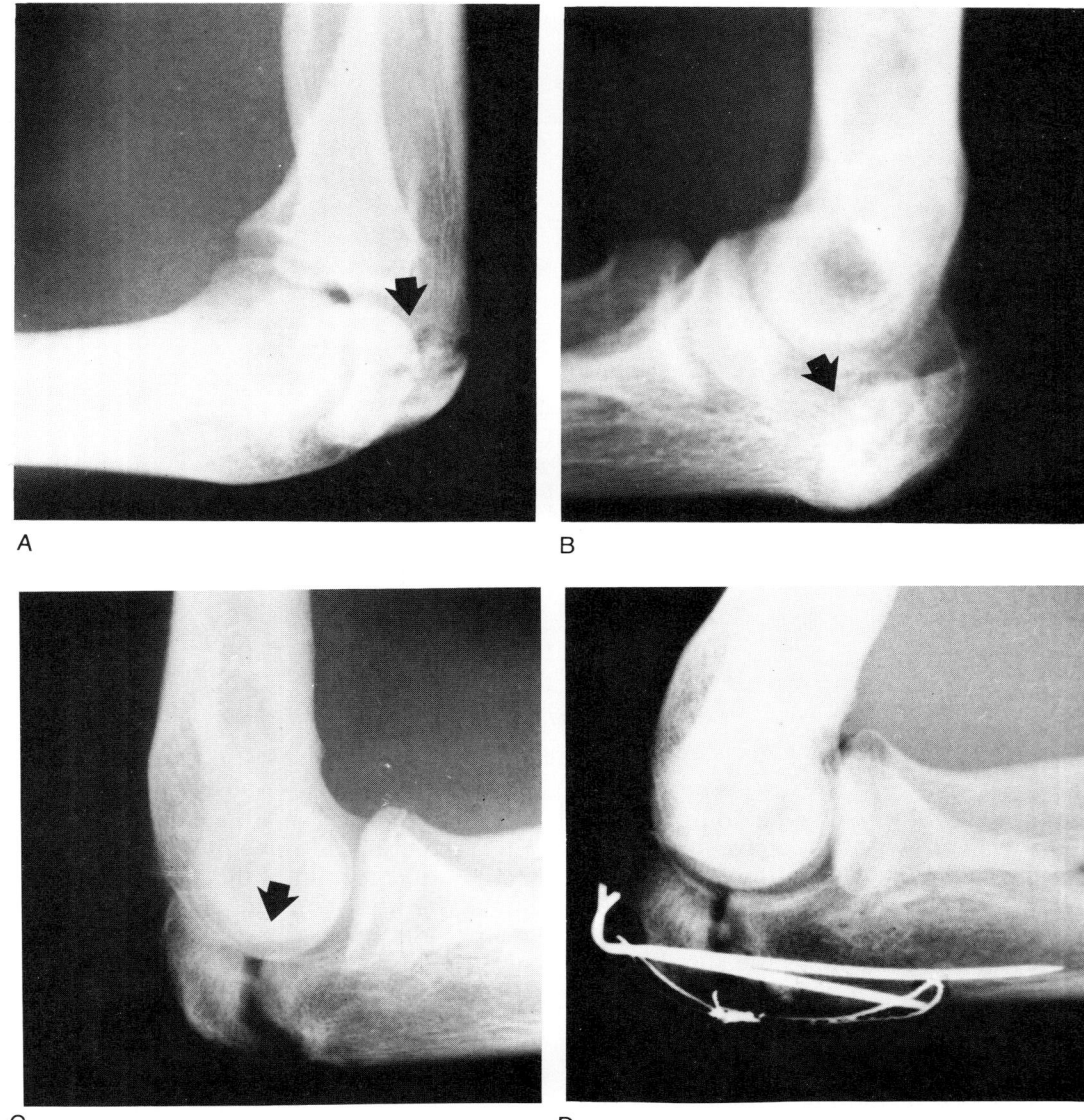

FIGURE 26–18. Proximal olecranon epiphysiolysis is thought to occur from repetitive traction, but impingement from hyperextension may also play a role. (*A*) Posterior elbow pain and fragmentation of the olecranon epiphysis as seen in a 15-year old pitcher. Rest at this point led to spontaneous recovery. (*B*) The lateral elbow X ray of an 18-year-old pitcher shows he had proximal olecranon epiphysiolysis that healed with hypertrophied bone and persistent symptoms. No surgery was warranted. (*C,D*) This 16-year-old pitcher and quarterback threw for 2 years with pain and a progressive elbow flexion contracture. At surgery a frank pseudoarthrosis was discovered. Bone graft and tension band wiring were successful. Three years later he is throwing without restriction.

injury. Full flexion–extension is encouraged.

Chronic recurring medial collateral ligament sprains are often seen in adult pitchers with mechanical problems and may prove to be career-ending such that some enthusiasm exists for reconstructive procedures.[13] It is my opinion that if teenagers develop such problems at an early stage of their throwing careers, it is a less-than-subtle sign that they might not have the "right stuff." I therefore discourage young players from having reconstructive elbow ligament surgery of any sort for fear of recurrent problems from faulty mechanics.

Ulnar Neuritis

Ulnar neuritis may occur in three[6] different situations: (1) hypermobile nerve with anterior subluxation,[25] (2) ulnar nerve traction from valgus instability, or (3) cubital tunnel irritation without elbow instability.

Some athletes have the disadvantage of a hypermobile ulnar nerve, which may sublux out of the cubital tunnel with rapid elbow flexion and extension. This may prove to be a serious deterrent to pitching, as permanent nerve transfer is not without risk.

Most players with persistent ulnar neuritis have accompanying medial collateral ligament instability, accounting for the increased traction on the tethered nerve. The swollen, inflamed tissues surrounding the injured medial collateral ligament also contribute to nerve compromise by direct compression. This may have come from too many pitches on a weak and fatigued shoulder or faulty pitching mechanics. When instability and ulnar neuritis are encountered together, we suggest several months of rest with a complete overhaul of throwing techniques.

Nerve transfer has been carried out in skeletally mature athletes,[6] but there is limited success owing to the combined factors of persistent instability, nerve entrapment in the anterior position, and the inability of the athlete to change mechanics when he or she returns to play. In youthful players, conservative treatment with prolonged rest is prudent.

Ulnar neuritis without medial collateral ligament injury is unusual and carries a better prognosis. Often these are pitchers who may remember a single pitch where we presume the nerve was momentarily stretched. Return to pitching is allowed when light tossing produces no symptoms.

POSTERIOR ELBOW PAIN

Proximal Olecranon Traction Injury

The proximal olecranon growth center appears at age 9 and closes at age 15. During this period, it is subject to traction from violent and repeated triceps contraction such as occurs in late ball release and early deceleration.[10, 19] Tenderness over the olecranon should lead to lateral radiographs of both elbows, looking for a widened epiphyseal line. Most players will be successfully treated by moving them to a position other than third base or shortstop for several months. We have had one case where a pseudoarthrosis developed in the epiphyseal plate, necessitating open reduction and internal fixation with a tension band (Fig. 26–18).

Posteromedial Impingement

The olecranon was designed to fit snugly within the olecranon fossa with full elbow extension. Posteromedial impingement may occur with or without medial instability, giving rise to chondromalacia and in late situations osteophytes that may break off, forming loose bodies[24] (Fig. 26–19). Rest and a single steroid injection are acceptable in the older teenage throwers, but once the local tissues

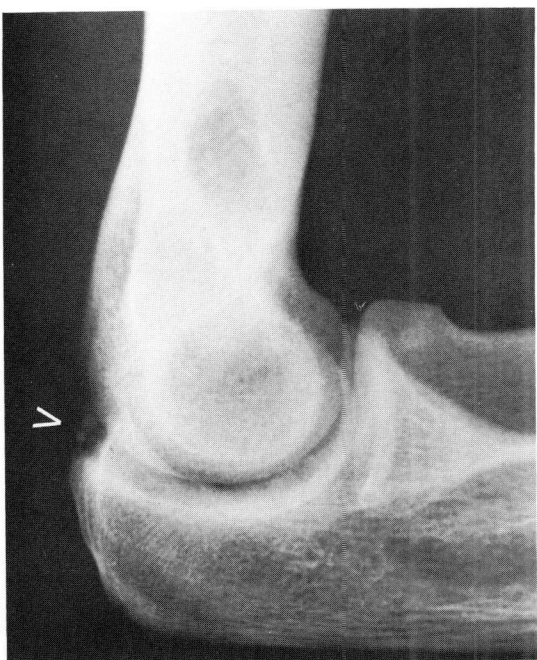

FIGURE 26–19. Posteromedial impingement may be associated with osteophyte formation around the tip of the olecranon.

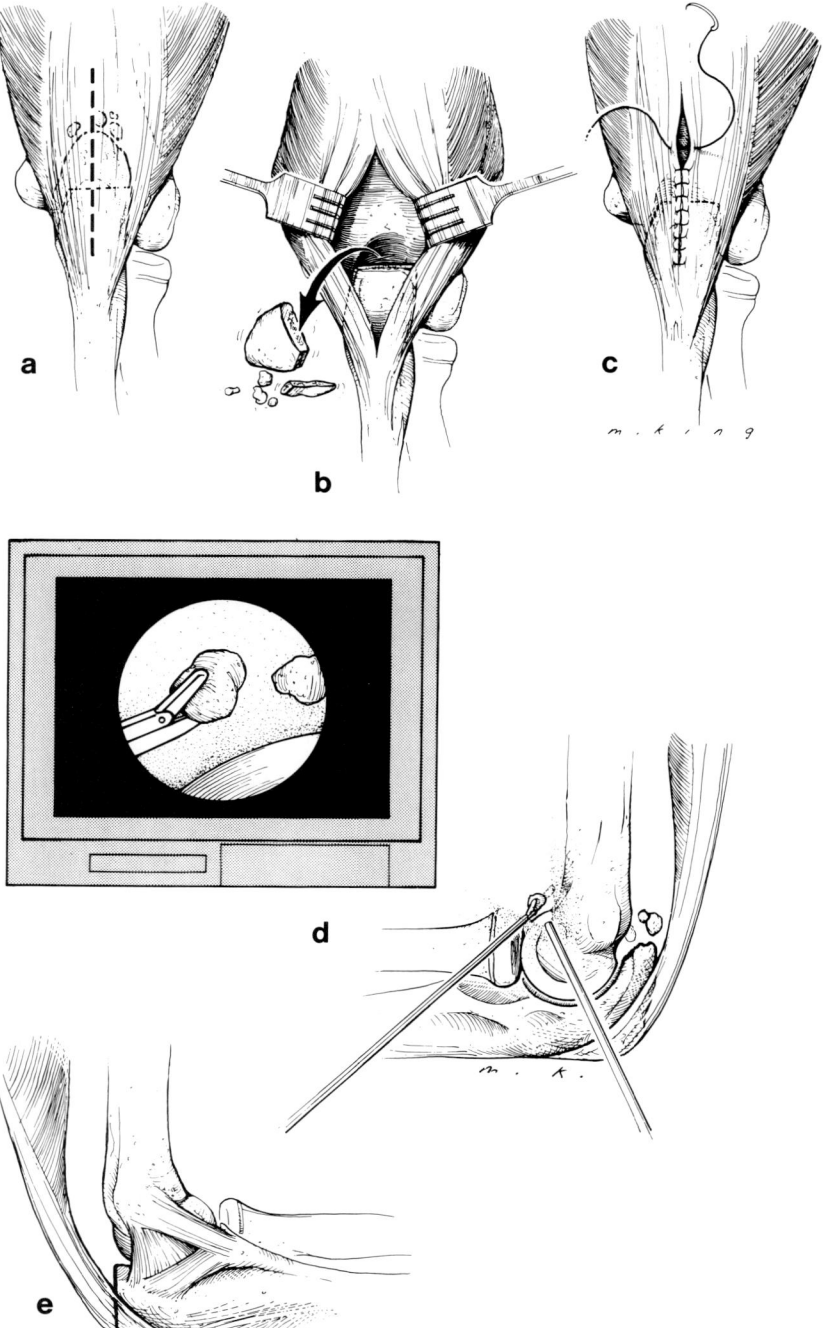

FIGURE 26–20. Proximal medial olecranonectomy. (*a*) A straight five centimeter posteromedial incision is created over the proximal olecranon and distal triceps. This incision will allow the posterior compartment to be cleaned of any loose bodies and for an appropriate amount of proximal impinging olecranon to be removed. (*b*) The medial 1/3 triceps is reflected to expose the proximal-medial olecranon. The ulnar nerve is safely protected and needs no formal exposure. (*c*) An osteotome removes the proximal centimeter of olecranon with a transverse cut. A slightly angled cut removes the medial olecranon. The triceps is sewn side-to-side and the skin closed with subcuticular sutures. (*d*) Elbow arthroscopy is indicated if there is suspicion of anterior loose bodies. The loose bodies may be removed arthroscopically or through a small lateral wound anterior to the radial head. (*e*) Summary: A proper proximal olecranonectomy will not violate the triceps attachment. Nor will it have removed enough olecranon to sacrifice any ulnar attachment of the medial collateral ligament.

enlarge from repeated contact and inflammation, the only solution may be off-season resection of the posteromedial olecranon.

A triceps-splitting incision (Fig. 26–20) is carried out in day surgery under either general anesthesia or a regional block. The posterior compartment may harbor cartilaginous loose bodies, and these should be flushed from the joint. A generous proximal olecranonectomy may be carried out without triceps detachment. A small portion of the medial olecranon should also be removed, but care should be exercised in avoiding more than 2 mm of removal, lest the attachment of the medial collateral ligament be violated. Often significant chondromalacia on the olecranon fossa is seen but will recover once contact from the olecranon is relieved. The athelete is sent home the same day in a resting splint; 2 days later, vigorous active and passive motion is started; 6 weeks after surgery, a light tossing program is started, and at 10 weeks, full pitching is reinstated.

Beware the pitcher with concurrent medial instability, for such a procedure will not correct the underlying cause of excessive ulnar motion against the humerus. Teenagers who develop this combination of problems (medial collateral insufficiency with posteromedial impingement and loose bodies) are faced with a difficult task to return to pitching under any circumstances.

References

1. Barnett L. S.: Little League shoulder syndrome: proximal humeral epiphysiolysis in adolescent baseball pitchers. J Bone Joint Surg 67A:495–496, 1985.
2. Braatz, J. H., Gogias P. P.: The mechanics of pitching. J Orthop Sports Phys Ther 9 (2):56–59, 1987.
3. Brown R., Blazina M. E., Kerlan R. K., et al: Osteochondritis of the capitellum. Am J Sports Med 2:27–46, 1974.
4. Bryan W. J., Wild J. J.: Isolated infraspinatus atrophy. A common cause of posterior shoulder pain and weakness in throwing athletes? Am J Sports Med 17:130–131, 1989.
5. Coleman, E.: Personal communication regarding Clear Creek High School shoulder strength study, 1986.
6. Del Pizzo W., Jobe F. W., Norwood L.: Ulnar nerve entrapment syndrome in baseball players. Am J Sports Med 5:182–185, 1977.
7. Glousman R.: Dynamic EMG analysis of the throwing shoulder with glenohumeral instability. J Bone Joint Surg 70A:220–226, 1988.
8. Gowan I. D., Jobe J. W., Tobone J. E., Perry J., Moynes D. R.: A comparative electromyographic analysis of the shoulder during pitching. Professional versus amateur pitchers. Am J Sports Med 15: 586–590, 1987.
9. Gugenheim J. J., Stanley R. A., Woods G. W., Tullos H. S.: Little League survey: the Houston study. Am J Sports Med 11:3–11, 1983.
10. Hunter L. Y., O'Connor G. A.: Traction apophysitis of the olecranon. A case report. Am J Sports Med 8:51–52, 1980.
11. Jobe F. W., Kvitne R. S.: Shoulder pain in the overhand or throwing athlete: the relationship of anterior instability and rotator cuff impingement. Orthop Rev 18:963–975, 1989.
12. Jobe F. W., Moynes D. R., Tibone J. E., Perry J.: An EMG analysis of the shoulder in pitching: a second report. Am J Sports Med 12:218–220, 1984.
13. Jobe F. W., Stark H., Lombardo S. J.: Reconstruction of the ulnar collateral ligament in athletes. J Bone Joint Surg 68A:1158–1163, 1986.
14. Jobe F. W., Tibone J. E., Perry J., Moynes D.: An EMG analysis of the shoulder in pitching: a preliminary report. Am J Sports Med 11:3–11, 1983.
15. King J., Brelsford H. J., Tullos H. S.: Analysis of the pitching arm of the professional baseball pitcher. Clin. Orthop. Rel. Res. 67: 116–123, 1969.
16. Morrey B. F., An K. N.: Articular and ligamentous contributions to the stability of the elbow joint. Am J Sports Med 11:315–319, 1983.
17. Pappas A. M.: Elbow problems associated with baseball during childhood and adolescence. Clin. Orthop. Rel. Res. 164:30–42, 1982.
18. Pappas A. M., Zawacki R. M., Sullivan J. J.: Biomechanics of baseball pitching: a preliminary report. Am J Sports Med 13:216–222, 1985.
19. Pavlov H., Torg J. S., Jacobs B., et al: Nonunion of olecranon epiphysis: two cases in adolescent baseball pitchers. AJR 136:819–820, 1981.
20. Sain J., Andrews J. R.: Proper pitching techniques. In Zarins B., Andrews J. R., Carson W. G. (eds): Injuries to the Throwing Arm Philadelphia: WB Saunders Co, pp 30–37, 1985.
21. Schwab G. H., Bennett J. B., Woods G. W., et al: Biomechanics of elbow instability: the role of the medial collateral ligament. Clin. Orthop. Rel. Res. 146:42–52, 1980.
22. Seaver T.: The Art of Pitching. Ed 1. New York: Hearst Books, 1984.
23. Sisto D. J., Jobe F. W., Moynes D. R., Antonelli D. J.: An electromyographic analysis of the elbow in pitching. Am J Sports Med 15:260–263, 1987.
24. Wilson F. D., Andrews J. R., Blackburn T. A., et al: Valgus extension overload in the pitching elbow. Am J Sports Med 11:83–88, 1983.
25. Wojtys E. M., Smith P. A., Hankin F. M.: A cause of ulnar neuropathy in a baseball pitcher: a case report. Am J Sports Med 14:413–424, 1986.
26. Woods G. W., Tullos H. S.: Elbow instability and medial epicondyle fractures. Am J Sports Med 5:23–30, 1977.

27
BALLET

WILLIAM G. HAMILTON

There has been a "dance explosion" in America in the last 10 years. As the number of young dancers increases rapidly, the number of children and adolescents seeking medical attention for dance-related disorders likewise will grow. Frequently, overuse injuries in the young dancer are the result of poor training, but they may also be a warning that the dancer's body is unable to withstand the demands of the art form.

A BRIEF PRIMER ON DANCE FOR THE NONDANCER

Ballet is considered the queen of dance. It had its origins in Renaissance Italy, and was brought to France by Catherine de Médicis (1519–1589) when she married Henry II. It flourished in the courts of the French kings in the seventeenth and eighteenth centuries, reaching its pinnacle under Louis XIV at Versailles. Ballet was the natural outgrowth of the arts of the Renaissance gentleman as practiced at court. These included court dancing, classical fencing (the five positions of the feet in ballet were supposedly derived from positions used in fencing), and classical horsemanship. All positions of the feet and poses of the body were codified by Pierre Beauchamps circa 1680, Louis XIV's ballet master, and these same positions and French names continue to be used today. The five positions of the feet are fundamental. In all positions, the feet are turned out 180 degrees so that the audience sees a maximum profile or "line." The dancers dance on the balls of their feet on *demi-pointe* in soft ("ballet") shoes or on *full pointe* (females only) in toe-shoes that contain a hardened cardboard toe-box. Certain positions (Fig. 27–1) and movements are basic:

- First position. The heels are together and the feet are turned out 90 degrees from the saggital plane (Fig. 27–1*A*).
- Second position. The feet are shoulder width apart and turned out (Fig. 27–1*B*).
- Third position. The feet are turned out and overlapped by 50 percent so that the heel of one foot is next to the instep of the other foot (rarely used in ballet today) (Fig. 27–1*C*).
- Fourth position. The feet are turned out but apart from front to back by about a foot (Fig. 26–1*D*).
- Fifth position. The feet are turned out and completely overlapped so that the heel of one foot is next to the toe of the other foot. This is the position that is most commonly used and is also the most difficult to achieve when a dancer has a poor turnout. The dancer who cannot externally rotate her feet enough to bring them snugly against each other in this position is said to be unable to "close in fifth" (Fig. 27–1*E*).
- *Relevé*. The movement from foot flat to the ball of the foot (*demi-pointe*) or onto full toe (*full pointe*) (Fig. 27–2).
- *Plié*. The ballet dancer's knee bend. The heel is left on the floor in the *demi-plié* but comes off the floor in the deep knee bend, or *grand plié* (Fig. 27–3).
- *Tendu*. A stretching out of the foot, either forward, sideways or backward, usually from first or fifth position. As the foot moves, the toes are kept close to the floor (Fig. 27–4).

This chapter copyright © 1991 by William G. Hamilton.

BALLET 485

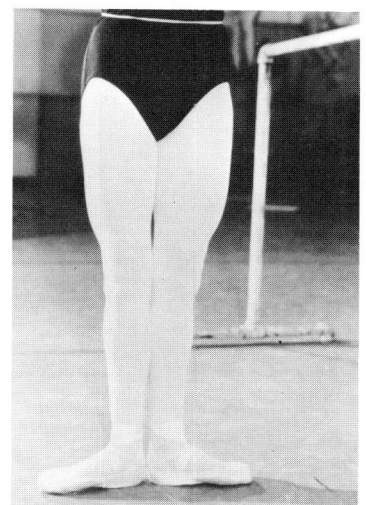
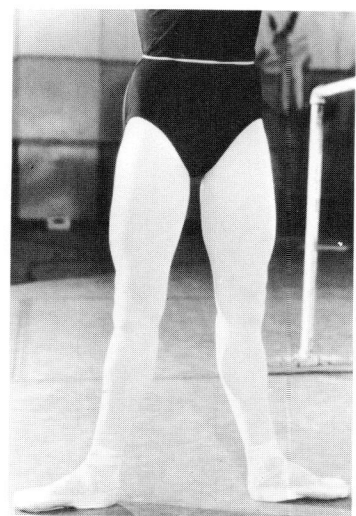
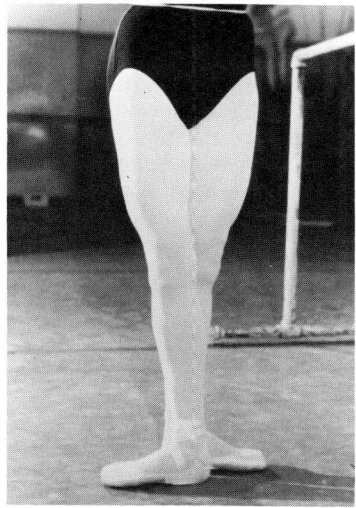
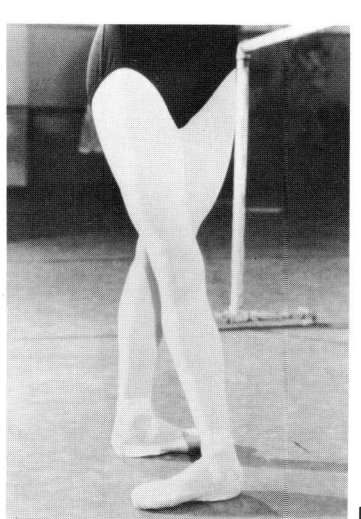
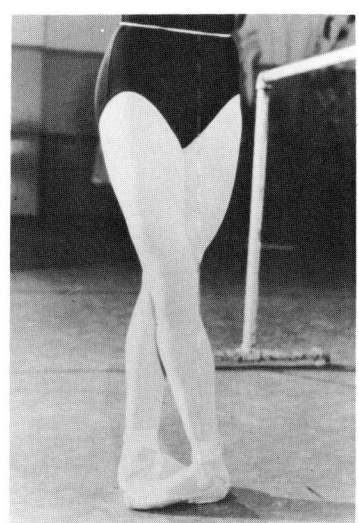

FIGURE 27–1. The five positions of the feet.

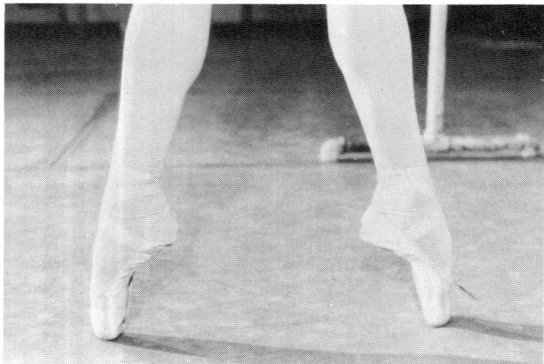

FIGURE 27–2. The *relevé*.

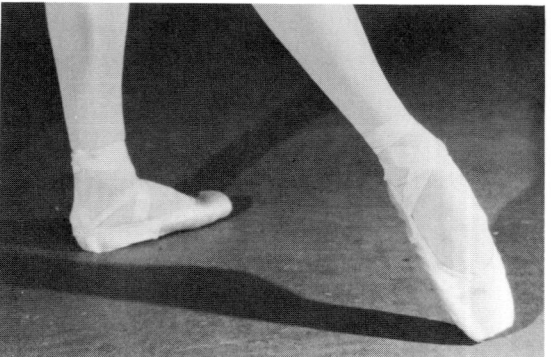

FIGURE 27–4. The *tendu*.

- *Passé.* One foot is moved upward along the inner border of the opposite leg to the level of the knee. The hip remains in the turned-out position (Fig. 27–5).
- *Developé.* From the *passé* position, the leg is then extended either forward, backward or sideways.
- *Rond de jambes, en l'air, en terre.* The foot is moved so that it traces a circle in the air or on the ground.
- *Battement.* A throwing of the leg into the air with the knee in extension.
- *Arabesque.* A pose on one leg while the other leg is extended backward with the knee straight (Fig. 27–6).
- *Attitude.* A position similar to the *arabesque*, but the knee of the leg behind is bent 90 degrees (Fig. 27–7).
- *Jeté.* A leap forward.
- *Entrechat six.* The dancer jumps off the ground from fifth position and, while in the air, changes the position of the feet from front to back six times (three times with each foot). Many sprained ankles in females occur during this step, especially if the dancer is tired and is only able to execute five and half changes while in the air.
- *Double saut de Basque.* A flamboyant jump done by male dancers in the style of the Basques. It is a turning step in the air with the leg in the *passé* position and is a frequent cause of sprained ankles in male dancers.

In proper ballet technique, the knee should remain over the foot when the foot is in the turned-out position and should not move inside of it. This causes excessive rotation in the knee and pronation in the foot (*rolling in*) (Fig. 27–8).

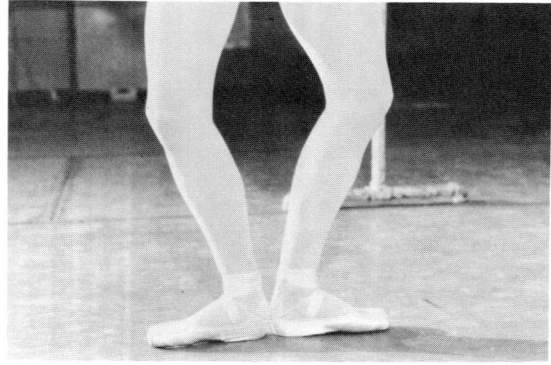

FIGURE 27–3. The *demi-plié*.

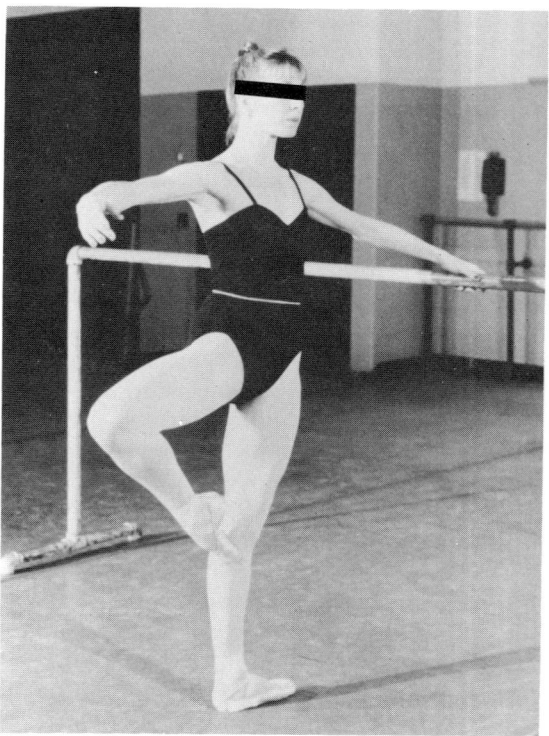

FIGURE 27–5. The *passé*.

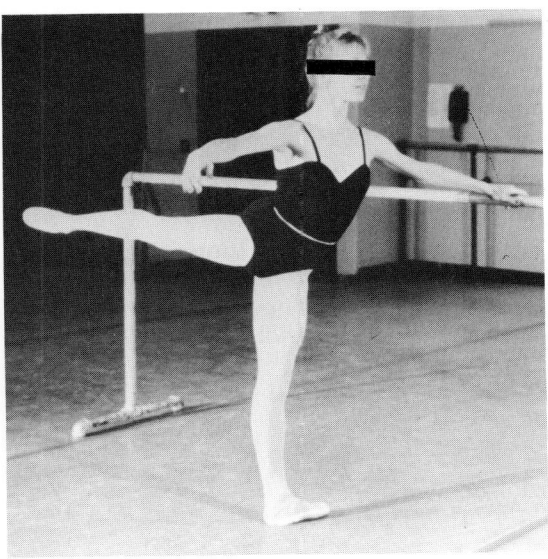

FIGURE 27-6. The *arabesque*.

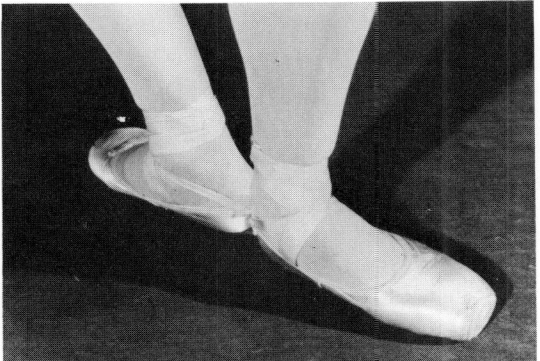

FIGURE 27-8. Rolling in.

NATURAL SELECTION AND BODY TYPES

One cannot overemphasize the role that selectivity plays in problems that dancers have with their bodies.[24] Dance, especially ballet, is a highly selective art form. Only the astronaut in our society is a more selected individual than the professional ballet dancer. In a study by Nicholas in 1975,[37] 61 common sports were evaluated and rated for difficulty. Only professional football was found to be more demanding in this study than professional ballet. Beginning with the first ballet class, there is a constant natural selection process at work, weeding out the dancers with the wrong bodies and those who lack the talent or tenacity to persevere. This "Darwinism" begins early and continues throughout a dancer's career, eventually eliminating everyone from the system for one reason or another (Fig. 27-9).

When treating injured dancers, one must always consider what role this selectivity may be playing in their problem. The vast majority of the problems that are seen in amateur dancers are the result of trying to do things with their bodies that they are poorly suited to do. This situation is not as common among professional dancers, as they usually have survived the weeding-out process and have the proper "equipment" or they would not have made it to the professional level.

Of course, an absolutely perfect body for dancing is a very rare thing, so even professionals can develop problems on the basis of imperfections in some part of the body. If you push any biomechanical system long enough and hard enough, you will eventually find its weak link. Injury patterns in professionals tend to be more subtle and related to the background and training of the dancer, the type of choreography performed, and the touring schedule, including types of stages and patterns and lengths of layoffs.

What are the prerequisites for a professional caliber dancer?[20] The most important

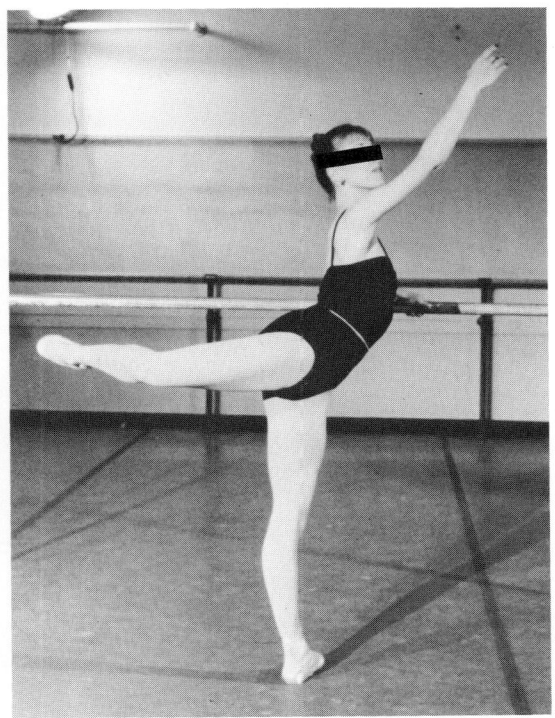

FIGURE 27-7. The *attitude*.

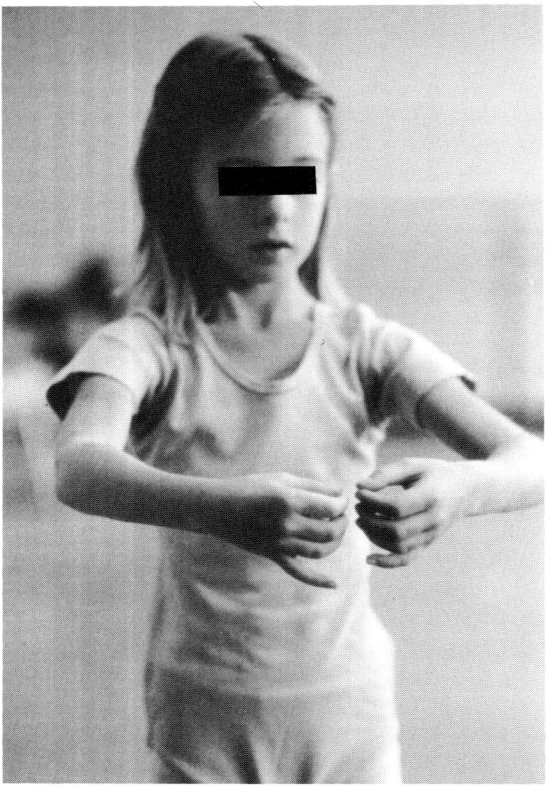

FIGURE 27–9. A young dancer.

and most elusive factor is *talent*—whatever talent is! A dancer with talent can overcome incredible physical shortcomings, but a dancer with a perfect body and no talent is useless. Besides the physical attributes, a dancer needs a sense of musicality, rhythm and timing, self-discipline, maturity, and a large dose of perfectionism. Dancers should always be regarded as artists and not athletes, although there are athletic aspects to their injuries. In addition to talent, certain physical attributes are desirable.

PROPORTIONS

A dancer should have proper proportions for her size. She should be thin and attractive but not emaciated. Generally accepted as unaesthetic for dancing are combinations of long trunks, short legs, big buttocks, swayback, round shoulders, spinal curves, big heads, and short necks. Overall size is also a factor. Some ballet companies, such as the English Royal Ballet, stress uniform height, especially in the corps de ballet. Others, like the New York City Ballet, find use for short as well as tall dancers. Height has its limitations; 5 foot 9 inches is considered the maximum height for a female ballet dancer. This does not hold true for modern dance, where many females over 6 feet tall have had successful careers. Taller girls may have difficulty in finding male partners with which to dance, as most male dancers are about 6 feet tall. They also take longer to mature in their dance training. Balanchine felt that short girls were mature at 18, but many of his tall dancers were still weak and in need of training as late as age 21.[2]

LIGAMENTOUS LAXITY

Being loose jointed is one of the fundamental requirements of dance. Children tend to be naturally loose jointed, so it is uncertain whether dancing selects loose-jointed individuals or simply maintains the suppleness natural to youth. Tight dancers, like tight athletes, are prone to muscle pulls and tendon strains. Exceptionally loose dancers are prone to sprains, dislocations, and impingement syndromes. Flexible joints require muscles that have enough strength to control the excessive motion.

TURNOUT OF THE HIPS

Turnout is the single most fundamental physical attribute in ballet. Proper turnout of the hip is the cornerstone of correct ballet technique. (Turnout is not confined to the hip but is the sum total of the turnout of the entire leg, hip plus knee, tibia, ankle, and foot.) Without it, the dancer must constantly compensate, forcing the turnout from the floor up rather than from the hip down. This compensation stresses the leg below the hip and essentially increases the Q angle at the knee, contributing to patellar malalignment and many other problems. If the foot is planted in more external rotation than is present at the hip, the additional turnout will be forced at the knee joint. The knee is a modified hinge joint and is not designed to rotate more than a few degrees. Unphysiological rotatory motion in the knee is an excellent way to develop internal derangement.

How much the hip turns out is determined

primarily by the bony architecture of the hip joint itself, by the torsion or "version" present in the upper femur. Most babies are anteverted at birth and slowly change as they grow, reaching 15 degrees of normal anteversion around age 6. Pigeon-toed people are common in the general population. These people have increased torsion in the hip and are anteverted. Others are born "duck footed" or turned out. These children are born to ballet and will have natural turnout of the hip.

Whether turnout comes from femoral retroversion, anterior capsular stretch, or a combination of the two is not known. Miller et al.[35] measured anteversion in Cincinnati Ballet dancers and found it to be normal, but these were regional dancers. A study of ballerinas in the New York City (NYC) Ballet and American Ballet Theater has shown that the external rotation of the hip gained for turnout is matched by an equal loss of internal rotation, so that the total range of motion is normal but is oriented in external rotation.[27] This would imply that a torsional deformity exists in the upper femur. Perhaps this controversy will be resolved by magnetic resonance imaging (MRI) studies in the future. Can turnout be increased to any significant degree by early ballet training? This also is not known. A study presently under way at the School of American Ballet in NYC will measure the range of motion in the hips of young dancers and see if it changes from age 8 to 16. The orthopedic literature suggests that anteversion is genetically predetermined and cannot be easily altered to any great degree. It is also probable that turnout is almost formed by age 11.[41] If this is true, it means that turnout probably can be improved to some extent by early training, perhaps by stretching the capsular tissues around the joint. However, a child who has poor turnout from the beginning will probably never have adequate turnout and can set herself up for all kinds of problems later, both physical and emotional, by trying to get too serious about a career. This does not mean that only children with perfect bodies should take ballet class. There are many beneficial aspects of ballet for children, even if they have poor bodies: poise, posture, balance, body image, self-discipline, and the like. These students must, however, work within their limitations and not become too serious about choosing it as a career.

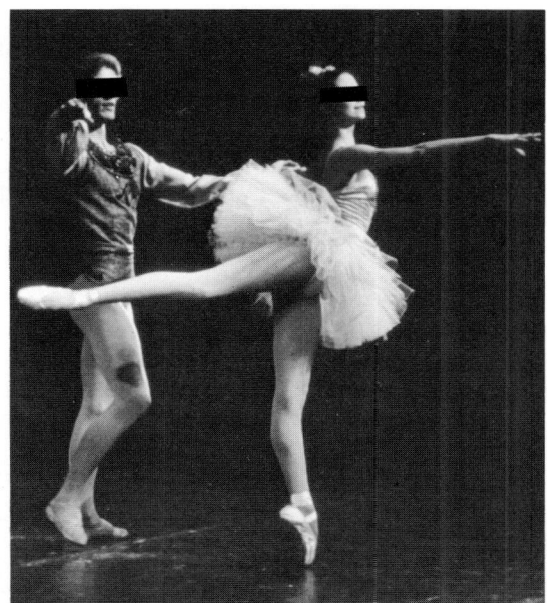

FIGURE 27–10. The "S-curve" of the ballerina's leg on *pointe*.

HYPEREXTENSION OF THE KNEE

Some degree of hyperextension of the knee is desirable for several reasons. It results in a more pleasing line on *pointe* and better placement of the upper body. The desired line of the leg on *pointe* is a gentle "S" curve, not a straight line, and hyperextension places the center of gravity forward of the knee and gives a pleasing forward and upward appearance to the trunk and upper body (Fig. 27–10). Mild hyperextension is a reflection of laxity of the ligaments and allows some "forgiveness" in the knee for rotatory or torsional forces. It is fine in theory to say that sufficient hip turnout eliminates the need for rotatory forces in the knee, but in practice those rotatory forces cannot be avoided. A dancer whose knee hyperextends must develop enough strength and technique to control the knee and prevent injury.

ALIGNMENT OF THE LEG

Axial alignment of the leg is important for dancers, both aesthetically and practically. Most good dancers are slightly bowlegged, as are most good athletes. The hyperextension usually present in the knee tends to exaggerate the genu varum. Genu valgum is undesirable (Balanchine[2] hated it). There are several problems resulting from a knocked-knee deformity: It does not look good, it makes closing in fifth position and doing beats and changements difficult, and it subjects the knee to forces that can cause patellar and meniscus problems.

EXTERNAL TIBIAL TORSION

If one examines dancers' turnout carefully, many different patterns are found, and one leg may differ considerably from the other in the same individual. Normally, about 60 percent of the turnout comes from above the knee and 40 percent from below.[27] The turnout in the hips may be lost, or augmented, by that below the knee. Some dancers have good external rotation in the hip but have internal tibial torsion below, resulting in mediocre or poor total turnout. Others have the opposite—poor turnout in the hip—and their turnout comes from external tibial torsion. The best get their turnout both above and below the knee.

ANKLE–INSTEP FLEXIBILITY

All alignment is interrelated. If the foot on *pointe* is to be in a vertical position, there must be enough plantar flexion in the foot and ankle not only to move the foot all the way down but also to compensate for the hyperextension in the knee above. This plantar flexion is the result of the combined motion of three joints: the ankle joint, the subtalar joint, and the midtarsal joints. The ability to *relevé* completely up necessitates more than 90 degrees of combined motion in these joints. An effective way to evaluate this combined motion is to look at the feet when the dancer is on *relevé* in the second position. Ideally, the feet should be the prolongation of the line of the anterior tibia (Fig. 27–11).

Unfortunately, generalized ligamentous laxity does not always include the instep. People who are otherwise loose may have tight, relatively inflexible insteps ("spoons"), so the feet must be evaluated separately from the rest of the body. There are several factors that can limit motion in these joints: the presence of an os trigonum, poor subtalar motion due to fibrous coalitions, and general

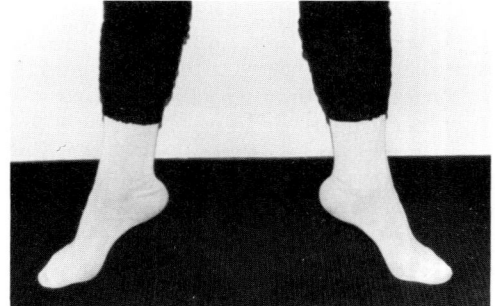

FIGURE 27–11. A poor *relevé*. The anterior tibia as a gauge of the *relevé*.

stiffness of the midfoot—often a problem in a dancer who started late and was not able to develop flexibility while the bones were growing. A flat foot is the worst foot that a dancer can have, but the opposite cavus foot is a mixed blessing; it has a beautiful *relevé* but little or no *plié*. It is rigid, absorbs energy poorly, and is prone to stress fractures and ankle sprains.

THE FOOT

Considering the amount of punishment that a dancer's foot must absorb, it had better be well suited for it. A dancer is best off with a broad, square foot so that the forces are shared equally by all the metatarsals running down to the ball of the foot (Fig. 27–12). Several types of feet are undesirable—though not impossible to work with. The "Grecian" or Morton's foot, with its shortened first and fifth rays, is prone to soft corns and fractures at the base of the second metatarsal. The splayfoot or simian foot has metatarsus pri-

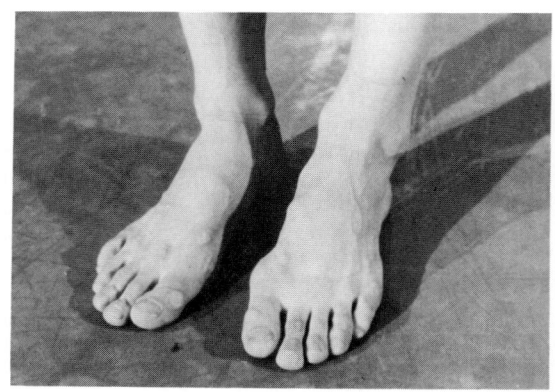

FIGURE 27–12. A dancer's foot.

mus varus, usually with a hypermobile first ray. This foot has a tendency to pronate or roll in and is often a precursor to hallux valgus, bunions and bunionettes.

THE TOES

The normal range of motion in the first metatarsophalangeal (MTP) joint is listed as 63 degrees of dorsiflexion and 37 degrees of plantar flexion.[1] Dancers must routinely have 80 to 90 degrees of dorsiflexion to allow a full relevé onto demi-pointe (Fig. 27–13). This motion is usually obtained by dancing as the musculoskeletal system is forming so the joints can be molded. Unfortunately, there are some young dancers who never develop adequate motion in this important joint. These individuals will have a very difficult time dancing ballet or modern dance and are better off studying jazz or tap.

There are few if any absolute contraindications to dancing. Very poor turnout of the hips or acetabular dysplasia usually preclude a career in ballet. Artistry and talent override the physical ideals described above, and every dancer has his or her shortcomings. Most of all, it is important for dancers to realize their limitations and to work within them.

THE STAGES IN A YOUNG DANCER'S TRAINING

The phases in a young dancer's training are:

- The beginning, ages 8 to 12, the pre-pointe years
- The middle, ages 12 to 16, the development years

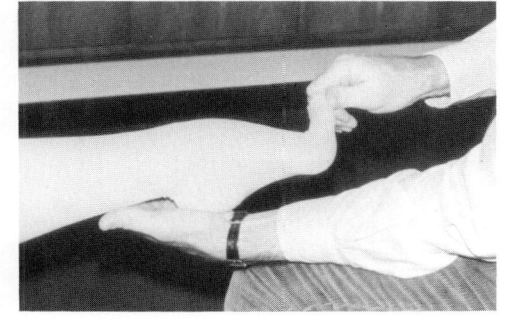

FIGURE 27–13. The dorsiflexion necessary in the first MTP joint.

- The apprentice, ages 16 to 20, the start of a career

Each of these has its particular set of problems, for there is a correlation between a dancer's age, skeletal maturation, and stage in dance training.

THE BEGINNING

There are few injuries in the pre-pointe age group. The body at ages 8 to 12 is very forgiving, and the demands placed on it are minimal. Problems seen are mainly the result of early selectivity: body proportions, flexibility, turnout, good relevé (i.e., full plantar flexion of the foot-ankle complex), musicality, and ability to learn.

Scoliosis can be found at the end of this phase, and when it is, it is usually ominous. Curves beginning this early have a long time to progress before spinal maturity is reached.

When to Start Pointe Work

In any discussion of ballet training, the question of the proper age to begin working on full pointe always arises. It has been traditionally held that young dancers could injure their feet by dancing on full pointe while the bones were still growing; so full pointe work has been started when the bones of the feet were near maturity—age 12 to 13 for girls. In fact, there is little evidence that dancing on pointe at an early age can damage the feet. In South America, children are allowed to dance on full toe as early as age 5 or 6 without evidence of injury, and dancing on demi-pointe places as much stress on the feet, other than the toes, as dancing on full pointe. There is no evidence that Freiberg's disease is more common in dancers who go on pointe "too early." More germane, however, is what George Balanchine had to say about the controversy.[2] He felt that there was no reason to get a young dancer up on full pointe if she could not do anything when she got up there! He believed that it took 4 years of serious ballet training before students were strong enough and trained enough to do anything when they went on full toe. Serious training in ballet usually begins around age 8, so 4 years of training works out to ages 11 to 13 anyway.

A problem can arise when a dancer takes up dancing late, for example, at 14 or 15. An excited, enthusiastic teenager will not be willing at this late age to wait 4 years. She wants to get onto *pointe* as soon as possible, and this can lead to problems.

One of the many advantages in starting ballet early is that training, ability, body weight, strength, and musculoskeletal development can proceed in concert. This is especially so in the feet. When training begins early, the *demi-pointe* and *full pointe* work put relatively small forces into the feet because the young dancer does not weigh very much. As the dancer grows, the feet are subjected to increasing stresses in a slow, steady manner as body weight increases, allowing the bones of the feet to respond to the extra stress by building up greater strength according to Wolff's law. This means that at age 16 when the dancer weighs 100 to 115 pounds, the bones in the feet will be strong enough to sustain the forces produced in *pointe* work at that age. The dancer starting late (especially if she has a delayed menarche or is amenorrheic)[48] may not have sufficient body strength, and stress fractures of the metatarsal bones can occur. Unless she has sufficient muscle strength, there is also a real risk of sprained feet and ankles.

A background in gymnastics can provide the necessary preparation for dancing. Most successful ballerinas who started late had their early training in this field.

THE MIDDLE

The development years, ages 12 to 16, constitute a period of rapid growth and progressive acceleration in the training demands placed on the dancers and their musculoskeletal system.

The Demands for Thinness in Ballet

Ballet dancers reflect, to an extreme degree, the obsession with thinness that is so common in our society.[15] Thinness in ballet can be traced to the romantic period when choreographers created mystical roles that required dancers of extraordinary thinness and grace such as nymphs, fairies, and sylphs who appeared to float across the stage. George Balanchine introduced the ultrathin look to ballet in the 1920s with his neoclassicism, intensifying the desire for leanness. Most national ballet companies today have rigid standards for height, body shape, and body composition. For the young ballet dancer auditioning for the corps de ballet, physical composition is extremely important. Without the proper body, even the most technically adept dancer may not be accepted into a company because of her body size or an anatomical variation that does not project the right look. Consequently, constant concern about minimizing calories to maintain thinness has become an everyday part of a dancer's life. These patterns are picked up by adolescents early and can be the source of many problems.

Dancers are considerably thinner than average females their age (15 to 18 percent below their ideal weight)[7] and are more likely to have a delayed menarche when compared with population norms. Studies of menstrual patterns in dancers suggest that a delay in menarche may influence long bone growth.[47,48] Dancers with delayed menarche were observed to have a decreased upper-to-lower-body ratio and a significantly increased arm span compared with the nondancer female members of their families. If a long, linear body is associated with a delay in menarche, it is possible that the delay seen in dancers may be the result of preselection for this somatotype. It would seem that the thin body typical of a ballet dancer is achieved through a complex interplay of selection and behavior—selection, in that girls with linear builds are favored; behavior, in that a combination of nutritional restrictions, aberrant eating patterns, and exercise are used to maintain an acceptable form.

Delayed Menarche

In our society, the average age of menarche is age 12.5.[3] In dancers, this is usually delayed 2 years, occurring around age 15—but sometimes as late as age 19. In a survey of adult ballet dancers, all of whom were members of national ballet companies, 70 percent reported a delay in menarche.[8] This delay is caused by many factors and has far-reaching implications, both mental and physical.

It is felt that menstruation in young females cannot begin until they acquire a critical amount of adipose tissue, thought to be about 20 percent of body weight.[11] With increasing age, even girls who have not reached these body weights begin menstruating, implying that other factors are involved in initiating puberty. A high level of exercise during the adolescent years is thought to impose an energy drain on the reproductive function of dancers and athletes that can affect the menstrual cycle. A process of adaptation to increased metabolic demands may then ensue, resulting in a natural form of fertility control that reverses with the cessation of exercise. In fact, in one study, 15 ballet dancers, aged 13 to 15, were followed over a 4-year period. The progression of sexual development and menarche correlated in 10 of 15 subjects with a decrease in exercise and/or injury, causing forced rest of at least 2 months' duration. During this interval, weight gain was minimal or absent, with no significant change in body composition.[47] The progression of puberty was also more evident in the leaner girls when activity decreased. Thus, ballet exercise during adolescence may prolong the prepubital state and induce primary amenorrhea.

Adolescent dancers with delayed menarche are 10 pounds lighter than those with normal menarche,[7] suggesting that a low weight is associated with this delay. Delayed menarche is also found in other groups that have weight standards for their sport, such as gymnasts and ice skaters. Girls for whom low weights are not required, such as swimmers, are less likely to have pubertal delays.[5] For some, delayed menarche is due to a combination of genetic and environmental factors.[16]

Secondary amenorrhea also appears to be related to the low weight maintained by dancers. In one series, 78 percent of the adult dancers and over 50 percent of the adolescent dancers surveyed reported prolonged amenorrhea.[7,8] These dancers were thinner and were also more likely to have eating problems. It is likely that the synergistic effects of intense exercise and thinness are more likely to result in amenorrhea than either factor separately.

Skeletal Growth

Prolonged hypoestrogenism secondary to amenorrhea can be associated with a higher incidence of scoliosis and stress fractures.[48] A survey of 75 female dancers from four national ballet companies revealed a 24 percent incidence of scoliosis. This is significantly higher than the 3.9 percent found in the general population of young women.[49] In addition, 83 percent of the scoliotic dancers had an age of menarche of 14 years or later, and the incidence of scoliosis increased with increasing menarcheal age.[15] The scoliotic dancers also had higher scores on a questionnaire measuring anorectic behavior than the non-scoliotic dancers, suggesting that nutritional factors may be important in the pathogenesis of this deformity and may also play a role in the development of menstrual abnormalities. The incidence of stress fractures in this same group was 45 percent and rose with increasing menarcheal age. These dancers also had an incidence of secondary amenorrhea twice as high and of longer duration than dancers without stress fractures. Ballet training begins at a young age and much of it takes place during adolescence. Since dieting to achieve a low body weight is common, it seems that ballet dancers as a group are likely to experience the effects of delayed sexual maturation on the growing skeleton. In fact, it is not unusual to see a dancer of 19 or 20 years old with an iliac apophysis still ununited on X ray.

There is evidence that ballet training may mold the young skeleton as it is growing to obtain turnout and the extreme range of motion in the joints of the lower extremity. This is especially true of the hip and ankle.

Nutritional Intake

To maintain thinness and minimize their caloric intake, dancers often do not eat well. In nutritional surveys, dancers have been found to be undernourished compared with other women of similar age, weight, and height.[9,14] More than one half of the dancers were consuming less than 85 percent of the recommended daily allowance (RDA) of calories, in spite of the fact that they were dancing 3 to 4 hours per day.[14] Four of the dancers fell below 66 percent of the RDA, and two took in less than 50 percent of the RDA for calories. Their diets were also poor in nutritional density, with the majority taking in less than the RDA of calcium, iron, and niacin. Many of the dancers showed poor knowledge of sound nutrition. They did not know the four basic food groups or that carbohydrates were the best energy source. Most believed that vitamin supplements could be used as a source of energy for exercise.[9]

Dancers should be cautioned regarding poor eating habits because the physical requirements of ballet are considerable.[15] Poor nutrition and excessive dieting can lead to a dangerous loss of energy. To a great extent, normal energy comes from the glycogen stored in the muscles of the body. The highest glycogen storage is provided by carbohydrates, which should compose approximately 60 percent of a dancer's diet. Depletion of muscle glycogen stores by poor nutrition is associated with exhaustion. A lack of education about sound nutrition is often responsible for dancers omitting carbohydrates from their diets because they are falsely considered to be high in calories. For the dancer who is dieting aggressively and achieving a rapid weight loss, 50 percent of that weight lost is lean muscle mass; the rest is fat and fluids. Because it is typical to gain weight back, and because the muscle gain is slow, the dancer may very well gain the weight back as fat, making this kind of dieting particularly fruitless.

Eating Problems

Not only is nutrition restricted, but dancers score higher on tests designed to detect eating disorders. Eating problems seem to be more common in dancers than in other female athletes. In one study, adolescents were compared who were engaged in three sports that varied in two dimensions: energy expenditure and weight demands.[6] Dancing requires a low weight but has a low energy expenditure; figure skating requires a low weight and has a high energy expenditure; and swimming does not require a particular weight and has a high caloric expenditure. Menarche was delayed and weight for height was lower in dancers and figure skaters than in swimmers. In addition, dancers engaged in more dieting behavior to maintain their low weight than did figure skaters, owing to the low energy expenditure of dancing.

Eating Disorders (Anorexia Nervosa, Bulimia, and Purging)

An even greater consequence for dancers than becoming compulsive dieters is the potential for the development of serious eating disorders. Dance students have a sevenfold increased chance of developing anorexia nervosa (AN) than their high school peers.[12] This incidence is related to the level of competition. Dancers from more competitive settings have double the incidence of AN—7.6 percent versus 3.5 percent—than dancers from less competitive settings. This higher incidence is attributed to the greater performance expectations and higher demands of the more competitive schools. Professional dancers are at an even higher risk for developing eating disorders than are adolescent dance students.

It appears that dancers who are not naturally thin are most vulnerable to the development of eating disorders.[16] This is probably due to the fact that these women are fighting their genetic "setpoint" by excessive dieting to achieve a dancer's low weight. The primary emphasis in ballet is a long, lean, and linear body. Certain national companies choose their dancers from company schools where extremely rigid standards for weight, shape, and technique have been consistently met throughout pubertal development. Typically, only 5 percent of the girls who begin their training at these selective schools survive the weeding out process and graduate 9 years later.[10] Other companies select their dancers from large general auditions that are open to students from any background. Dancers who have been through this less stringent process of early selection have significantly more eating problems (anorexia nervosa, bulimia, and purging) than those selected from company schools. In addition, the less selected dancers have an incidence of familial obesity that is similar to that found in the general population but eight times higher than that reported by the more highly selected dancers. Because family-line resemblances in fatness can run as high as 80 percent, and dieting in general is not very effective in reducing weight, it appears that the less selected dancers may often achieve an appropriately low weight by practicing deviant eating behaviors. That the less selected dancers report significantly more eating problems, while exhibiting a higher incidence of familial obesity, supports this theory.

The fact that ballet is a discipline that involves both physical and artistic considerations without sharing the high energy expenditure of many other athletic endeavors is a major dilemma for the professional dancer. Studies of the exercise characteristics of ballet have shown that the physiological profiles of professional dancers are above those of unconditioned athletes but not on the level of endurance athletes.[37,42] Ballet dancing requires only brief periods of low- to high-level activity that are usually spaced far enough apart to limit an intervening training effect. Because of this, ballet is basically not an aerobic activity; women in a 1-hour ballet class typically expend only 200 calories. Swimming is an excellent way for a dancer to achieve the additional calorie expenditure needed to maintain a steady weight without resorting to deviant eating behaviors. In terms of a darwinesque selection of the fittest, ballet favors the naturally thin female.

Specific Problems

The Forefoot. Genetically, there are several kinds of feet, some good and some not so good for dancing. Having the wrong foot does not preclude a career in dancing, but it does predispose a dancer to certain foot problems related to their profession. The *Grecian*, or *Morton's, foot* is the most common foot type in dancers and in the general population. It has a short first toe and a long second toe, sometimes to an extreme degree. The difference in toe length is really due to shortening of the first ray, especially the first metatarsal (MT). If the foot is examined carefully, the fifth ray is also shortened. The inequality of the toe lengths predisposes this dancer to soft corns in the fourth and first web spaces. The shortened first ray transfers load into the second metatarsal, requiring extra strength in this bone. One can see cortical hypertrophy of the second metatarsal on the X ray with this type of foot. This process takes time and is one of many reasons why females must start their training early while their skeleton is adaptable. Figure 27–14 shows a teenage dancer who began her training at age 15, trying madly to catch up with her peers. Notice the lack of cortical hypertrophy in the metatarsals and the stress fracture in the third MT. Interestingly, the second MT is usually the longest, but in this dancer the third is the longest and it is the one that has fractured. The treatment for this injury is simply "modified activities"—that is, "Don't do what hurts until it doesn't hurt to do it anymore"—and swimming to stay in shape. The average healing time is 4 to 6 weeks.

The *Egyptian foot* is the opposite of the Grecian foot. It has a long first toe and a relatively short second toe. Because of the added stress on the first ray, it tends to have trouble with the hallux: derangement of the MTP joint and the interphalangeal (IP) joint.

The *model's foot* is a thin foot with a relatively long first ray and a short fifth ray. This tapered configuration bears weight unevenly in the *relevé*. It is a foot that is pleasing to the eye, but it does not work very well and tends to be hypersensitive and painful. It is not a good foot for a dancer.

The *Simian foot*, or splayfoot, has an atavistic first ray that is hypermobile and deviates toward the midline—metatarsus primus varus. This is the "bunion-prone" foot that, if put into a narrow shoe, will develop a bunion and often a bunionette.

The *peasant's foot* is a broad, square foot with a uniform metatarsal length. It provides a stable base on which to *relevé*. This is the ideal foot for the ballet dancer.

The necessity for 90 to 100 degrees of dorsiflexion in the first MTP joint has been noted. People are rarely born with this much motion in this joint, so it must be obtained by some molding of the growing epiphysis. This can result in an epiphysitis of the proximal phalangeal epiphysis, presenting with tenderness, inflammation, and pain with activity relieved by rest. The condition tends to recur but disappears when the epiphysis fuses at maturity. This condition in many ways resembles Osgood-Schlatter disease so commonly seen in the adolescent's knee, and is known as *Osgood-Schlatter disease of the foot* (Fig. 27–15). Treatment consists of modified activities for 4 to 5 weeks until the symptoms subside and then gradual resumption of normal routines as tolerated.

The *adolescent bunion* has been mentioned above. Spacers placed between the first and second toes will usually make it more functional, as this alignment maintains maximum motion in the MTP joint (Fig. 27–16). The young female dancer with this

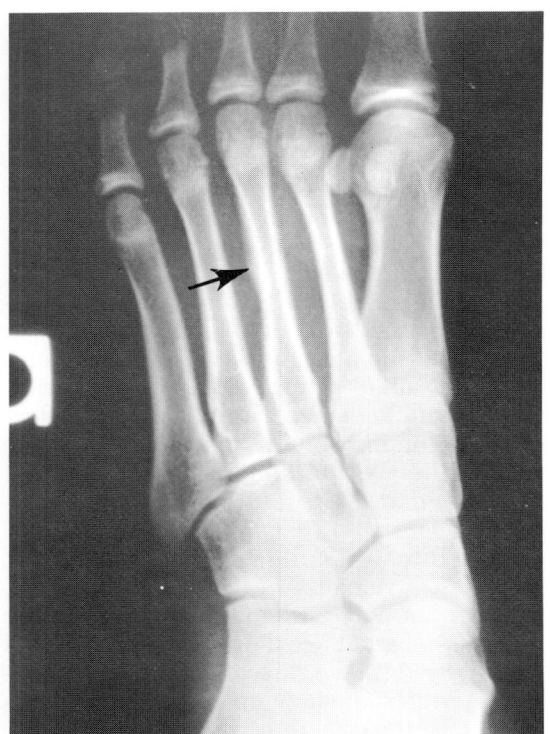

FIGURE 27–14. A stress fracture of the third metatarsal. Note the lack of cortical hypertrophy.

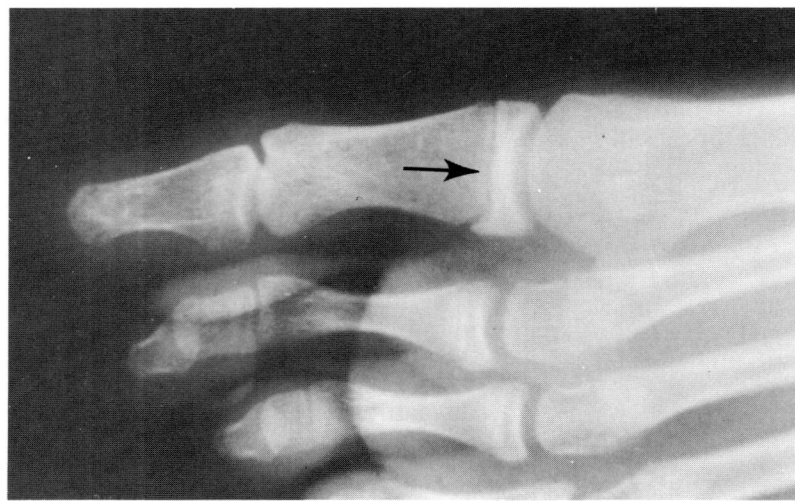

FIGURE 27-15. "Osgood-Schlatter disease" of the first MTP joint.

problem should be encouraged to wear wide shoes (i.e., boys' sneakers) and to resize their toeshoes often—at least yearly and every 6 to 8 months if they are in a "growth spurt." Bunions should *never* be operated on in a serious dancer because the operation, no matter how carefully performed, will usually limit the motion in the first MTP joint. Ideally, 90 to 100 degrees of dorsiflexion is needed in this joint for normal ballet function (Fig. 27-13). It is impossible to preserve this motion after surgery, and once it is lost, it cannot be reclaimed. Many careers in dancing have been terminated by well-meaning foot surgeons performing bunion surgery on aspiring ballerinas.

The Midfoot. The *hypermobile first ray* can be a source of problems. The most common is "rolling in", excessive pronation when attempting to gain a full 180 degrees of turnout. Good dance teachers should recognize this fault in technique and correct it before it becomes a habit.

An *accessory navicular*, as any orthopedist knows, can be a frustrating problem in a teenager. I usually try to postpone surgery on this condition until age 16 or 17 because many that are painful in the early teens will stop hurting with skeletal maturity. Arch supports are usually prescribed for this condition, but I am not convinced that they make a difference. If surgery is necessary, I have found that simply shelling out the medial fragment works as well as the rerouting of the posterior tibial tendon as described by Kidner and requires much less dissection. Following surgery, a short leg cast is worn for 6 weeks. The acutely tender accessory navicular may require cast immobilization until the symptoms subside.

The Hindfoot and Subtalar Joint. Forefoot pronation and heel valgus "unlock" or loosen the subtalar joint, giving added equinus to the ankle-subtalar complex. It is desirable in dancing to have as much plantar flexion and dorsiflexion of the ankle as possible for a full *relevé* and *plié*. Examination of the X ray of a dancer on *pointe* will show considerable opening of the subtalar joint, demonstrating its contribution to ankle motion (Fig. 27-17). Conversely, any condition that limits subtalar motion will markedly limit these motions in a dancer. For this reason, tarsal coalitions, either bony, cartilaginous or fibrous, will often show up early in a dancer's career. These stiff, inflexible, and immobile feet in the dance world are known as "spoons" and are most undesirable. It is diffi-

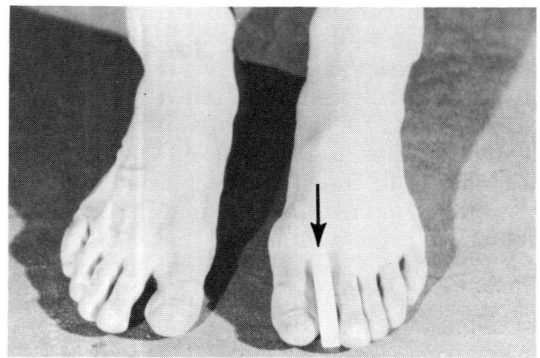

FIGURE 27-16. Spacers.

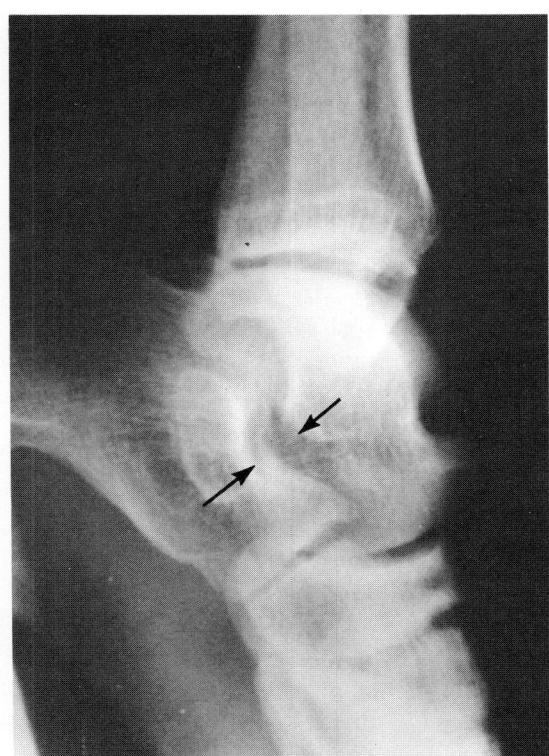

FIGURE 27–17. Opening of the subtalar joint in the *relevé*.

cult for an adolsecent with this condition to pursue a career in dancing. In my limited experience with resection of the tarsal coalition, I have not found the operation able to restore enough motion to allow ballet dancing in a female; the requirements for the male dancer, however, are much more lenient.

The Ankle. Two things separate ballet from other forms of dancing: (1) the 180 degrees of turnout at the hips and (2) the ballerina dancing on *full pointe* in a toeshoe. Thus, the full equinus position is essential for proper ballet technique, especially in females. Not only should there be at least 90 degrees of plantar flexion in the foot/ankle complex (see subtalar motion) but preferably 10 to 15 degrees more than that to compensate for the recurvatum usually present at the knee.

The shape of the dome of the talus can vary considerably from one individual to another. Some are round like an oil drum and have excellent motion, both in plantar flexion and dorsiflexion. Others are congenitally flat and have very limited motion. It is possible that this, too, can be molded and improved to some degree by beginning training at an early age, but a stiff, flat foot and flat domed talus will never achieve the desired amount of motion, and this dancer is far better off choosing a career in some form of dancing other than ballet.

Early training usually produces a notch in the neck of the talus to accept the anterior lip of the tibia and allow a deep *plié* (Fig. 27–18). Conversely, some posterior molding may be necessary, especially if there is an os trigonum or trigonal process present. The topic of posterior impingement is discussed in some detail later. In this younger age group, posterior ankle pain is frequently seen when an

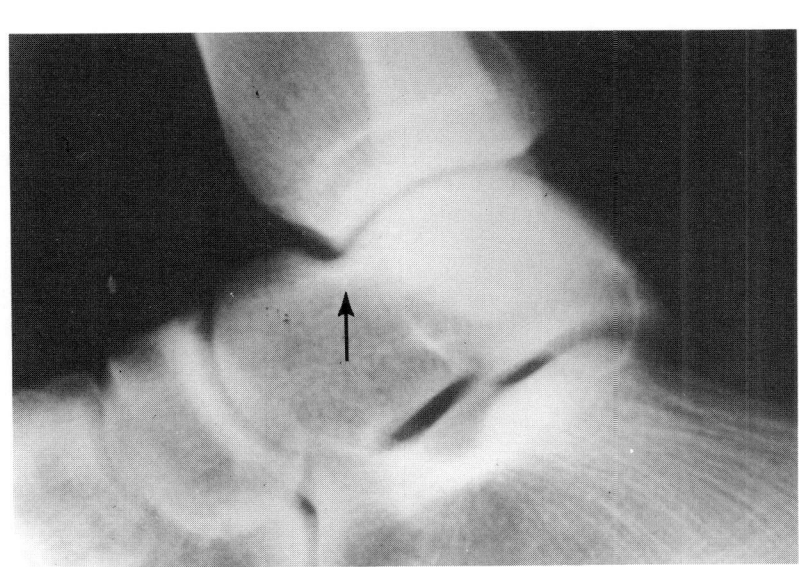

FIGURE 27–18. The notch in the neck of the talus.

os trigonum is present and full plantar flexion is restricted, especially if the other ankle is normal. The symptoms in this situation are usually due to the machinations that the young dancer is going through to force the "bad" ankle to go down as far as the "good" one. These include hooking the toes underneath the piano and levering the forefoot into equinus, sitting on the heels with the foot in full plantar flexion or having one of their friends do this, and so on. The diagnosis should be made and the problem explained to the dancer and her family. The symptoms will usually subside when she stops forcing the ankle after she realizes that the lack of motion is due to a bony block and that the ankle cannot go any further, no matter how hard she pushes.

The Knees. With proper ballet technique, the turnout should come from the hip down and not from the floor up. If there is insufficient turnout in the hip and the dancer gets it by turning out the foot on the floor, the knee is caught in between the turned-in hip above and the turned-out foot below (Fig. 27–19). Some rotatory motion is present in the knee, especially when it is flexed, so the young dancer learns early that she can get more turnout by flexing her knees in a *plié*, turning out to 180 degrees, then straightening the leg with the feet turned out. This has been called "screwing the knee." Almost all young dancers do it, but it should be discouraged. It can result in chondral damage or meniscal damage and can contribute to patellar malalignment.

Osgood-Schatter disease is just as common in young dancers as it is in young athletes. The treatment is the same: modified activities until the pain subsides. Older dancers who had this disease when they were young sometimes have problems later with the prominent tibial tubercles, especially if there are ossicles in the attachment of the patellar tendon. These areas often become tender when doing floor work on the knees in modern dance or "turns to the knee" in ballet. Removal of the ossicles may sometimes be necessary.

Excessive recurvatum is often found in this group with generalized ligamentous laxity. It is usually not a problem if the dancer learns early how to control the condition and not to work too far back into the knee. If they do not, then they can occasionally develop signs of anterior impingement and posterior capsular stretching. The excessive recurvatum can make the dancer appear to have more genu varum than they actually have ("pseudo–genu varum"). As the knees go past the neutral position into hyperextension, they separate, giving the appearance of more varus than is actually present. If the dancer is examined on a flat surface that limits recurvatum, the axial alignment of the leg and thigh can be more accurately assessed.

Patellar malalignment, subluxation, and *dislocation,* problems so often seen in loose-jointed females, can be particularly frustrating in dancers. The full-blown syndrome of patellar dislocation usually precludes a serious career in ballet. Malalignment and subluxation are exacerbated by lack of turnout in the hips because the turnout must then be obtained by external rotation of the tibia below the knee. This external rotation of the tibia markedly increases the Q angle at the knee, compounding the malalignment problems. Management involves the usual progressive constellation: quadriceps strengthening, arthroscopic lateral release, and proximal patellar realignment. Dancers cannot wear patellar stabilizing braces on a regular basis but may do so for class. The unstable patella is a potentially serious condition. The most serious injury seen in the professional dancer is the total "wipeout" of the knee that occurs landing from a jump when the patella dislocates and the rest of the medial knee and both cruciates are torn.

Osteochondritis dissecans is usually seen in this age group and should be suspected when a young dancer has unexplained swelling and discomfort in the knee. It can best be seen on the "tunnel view" X ray of the knee and can usually be managed arthro-

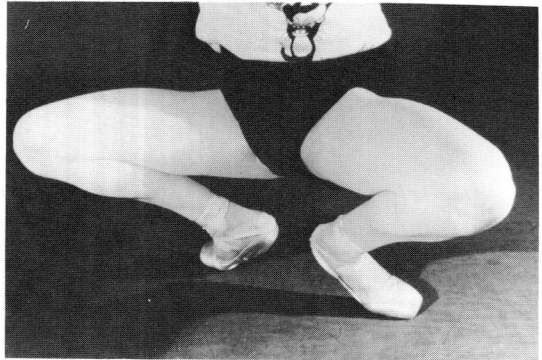

FIGURE 27–19. Turning out below the knee and "rolling in."

scopically (see Chapter 15). It should be noted that like all the osteochondritis conditions, the symptoms can precede the X-ray findings by as long as 6 months; so if the condition is strongly suspected but not seen on X ray, a bone scan or MRI study may pick it up.

The *discoid lateral meniscus* often appears in this age group and should be suspected when there is loud repetitive popping in the knee with the *plié*. It usually can be accurately diagnosed with an MRI study. This anomaly can often be treated conservatively. If surgery is required (see Chapter 16), the chances of returning to dance are good.

The Hips. External rotation of the hip is absolutely essential for a professional career in ballet; at least 45 degrees, but 60 to 70 degrees is even better. Trying to pursue a serious career in ballet with poor turnout can set the young dancer up for a lifetime of ailments in one form or another followed ultimately by disappointment.

The *snapping hip*, usually seen in young girls, is rare in ballet dancers because in the turned-out position the greater trochanter is rotated posterior to the iliotibial band. Instead, a medial snapping hip in the groin is seen. This is almost always the iliopsoas tendon snapping over the anterior hip capsule. It can be palpated when the dancer performs a *passé*. The condition is not serious but tends to be self-perpetuating; that is, the more it snaps, the easier it is to snap. The dancer usually knows what position will cause the hip to snap. The treatment is to avoid that position until the problem resolves.

Subclinical slipped femoral epiphysis in young male dancers fortunately is rare, but it should be considered if hip or knee pain is present. As the epiphysis slips posteriorly and inferiorly, the turnout in the hip will increase. Dancers have been seen with this condition when they develop degenerative joint disease in their hips at a later age—having gone into ballet because they had good turnout. Unfortunately, they also contained the seeds of their own destruction.

The Spine. Proper ballet technique demands an extreme range of motion in all segments of the spine. Fortunately, serious spine problems and injuries are rare, compared with football and other contact sports, but some spine conditions do occur.

Scheuermann's disease (adolescent kyphosis) is common in young males and can be painful and produce stiffness and round-back deformity. It should be treated symptomatically. It is rare that the patient has to give up dancing completely.

Young dancers learn early that they can gain extra turnout in the hips by increasing their lumbar *lordosis* (swayback) and can develop a habit of working this way. This technique is unsightly and potentially damaging to the lower spine. Most dance teachers are aware of the problem and will correct it early on. However, some dancers will continue to work this way, especially if their turnout is suboptimal and they have to struggle to close the feet in fifth position. The swayback posture can lead to spondylolytic stress fractures of the lumbosacral spine.

Scoliosis is extremely common in adolescent female ballet dancers, especially those with a delayed menarche.[48] Adolescent dancers with scoliosis do not require any special restrictions. The cornerstone of the modern treatment of scoliosis is the early diagnosis and aggressive early treatment (with bracing) of curves that are progressing beyond 20 to 25 degrees.

Anyone involved in the care or teaching of young dancers should remember Dr. John Moe's postulates:[51]

1. It occurs in families and is hereditary.
2. Small flexible curves may be present throughout growth without progression.
3. Other curves are progressive and become structural (fixed).
4. There is no way to predict which course these curves will follow.
5. All curves must be watched carefully. All structural curves that show progression should be treated.

If a curve is going to progress, neither manipulation, physical therapy, nor exercises against the curve will control the progression.

THE APPRENTICE

General Problems

In the 17 to 19 age group, high-level stresses begin to take place on a not-quite-mature skeletal system, since a delay in menarche and skeletal maturation are common in dancers.[48] An apprentice will be dancing a minimum of 6 hours per day, 6 days a week. The traditional rules of thumb used in orthopedics may not apply. Examples of this are seen in girls with scoliosis whose iliac apophyses have not fused at age 20. Also, it is not uncommon to see strains and partial avulsions of the anterior wing of the ilium at the insertion of the oblique abdominals in dancers 19 to 21 years of age. The treating orthopedist should keep in mind the high incidence of stress fractures associated with amenorrhea and delayed menarche.

Specific Problems

The Feet. *Corns* and *calluses* are the necessary result of the interaction between the foot and the toeshoe. Just as they are necessary on the sole of the foot for comfortable walking, they are necessary on the toes for comfortable toe dancing. They are really "Wolff's law of the soft tissues." The calluses can be troublesome when they build up excessively, cause blisters, or become infected. Dancers often use various over-the-counter dental remedies containing local anesthetic preparations to allow them to dance with toe pain.

Soft corns are commonly seen in dancers in this age group, especially in those with a Grecian, or Morton's, foot. Normally, there is a "fit" between adjacent phalanges so that the condylar prominences on the phalanges of one toe fit into the recess of the diaphyseal portion of the phalanx of the other toe. With this arrangement, there is no concentration of pressure on the skin in the web space. When the metatarsals are shortened, the prominences can line up with each other, and a soft corn may form. Treatment consists of debridement of excess callus if it forms and lamb's wool or spacers to keep the toes apart. If the problem is chronic, condylectomy or partial phalangectomy is usually indicated. In Europe, webbing of the fourth web space is done for this problem, but this is not a popular procedure in this country.

Modern dancers work in bare feet and have problems related to calluses on the sole of the foot. They should be extra careful regarding their foot hygiene but rarely are. They are prone to splinters and cracks on the sole of the foot in the margins of the large calluses that form there. These can get infected and, if neglected, can require surgical drainage and intravenous antibiotic therapy.

The usual *nail problems* are seen in these dancers. *Subungual hematomas* are common under the great toenail. When this happens, I encourage dancers to leave the dead nail on as long as possible, even if they have to tape it in place, to protect the new nail and allow them to dance while it is forming. Square trimming of the nail will prevent *paronychias*. If the paronychia becomes recurrent, the nail can be partially excised without problems later with dancing. Some dancers will have trouble with sensitivity of the fifth toenails where they rest against the toebox. If this is recurrent, they can be safely excised permanently (the Thompson-Terwillinger[45] procedure).

Interestingly, dancers are said to have ugly feet. This is mostly due to the calluses formed to allow toe dancing. They will hardly ever have claw toes or hammer toes because their feet are "intrinsic plus" and their proximal interphalangeal (PIP) joints are straight. Claw toes form in the "intrinsic minus" foot, which is rarely seen in the dancer.

Sesamoiditis and *sesamoid fractures* can be an annoying problem because they heal so slowly. Sesamoiditis has many causes:

- *Contusion.* This will respond to conservative therapy but often heals slowly.
- *Sprain* of a bipartite sesamoid. The injury X ray compared with an old film will sometimes show widening of the distance between the two fragments.
- *Stress fracture.* The bone scan will be positive.
- *Fracture.* It will usually heal either by bony or fibrous union.
- *Avulsion fracture* of the proximal pole.
- *Osteonecrosis.*[40] This condition occurs often in the lateral sesamoid, occasionally in the medial, and on rare occasions in both. The cause is unknown and the prognosis is often poor because the bone may fragment as it heals and pain may persist. In some patients, healing will occur, but the process is slow and uncertain (Fig. 27–20).
- *Osteoarthritis* with loss of the cartilage space and spur formation seen on the X-ray sesamoid view. This is a problem usually seen in adults.
- *Entrapment neuropathies,* especially adjacent to the medial sesamoid, can mimic sesamoiditis or be part of the problem. In this condition, a Tinel's sign will usually be present.

There is an old expression in foot surgery: "Don't mess around with the sesamoids!" This admonition is based on the unpredictable results and complications seen following sesamoidectomy. This operation is usually not necessary in a dancer because the pain will almost always eventually subside with conservative therapy alone. It is often

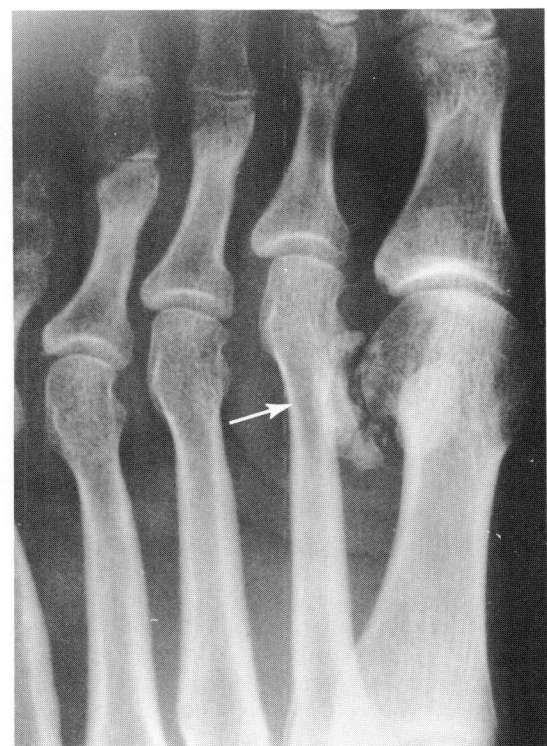

FIGURE 27–20. Osteonecrosis of the lateral sesamoid.

difficult to get the dancer to be patient, but the pain will usually go away if one can just wait long enough. The exception to this rule is osteonecrosis.[32] This has a poor prognosis and a long healing time. Almost all the sesamoids that I have removed in dancers have been for this problem.

Conservative therapy of sesamoid problems may take 6 to 12 months. During this period, pads may be used to unweight the sesamoids, and *demi-pointe* work should be minimized. If the dancer is still having disabling symptoms after 1 year of conservative treatment, sesamoidectomy may be considered. Because of the poorer prognosis, the period of conservative treatment may be shortened to 6 months in osteonecrosis. Both sesamoids should never be removed.

Metatarsalgia is not common in dancers in spite of the beating that the metatarsals take. When it is seen, it should arouse suspicion that there may be something else going on, such as a subluxing joint or Freiberg's disease.

The collateral ligaments of the lesser MTP joints can be torn by a dorsiflexion sprain or, in an older dancer, can be stretched out, slowly leading to instability in the joint and resulting in MTP joint subluxation. When the dancer does a *relevé* onto the ball of the foot, the base of the phalanx subluxes onto the dorsum of the head of the metatarsal, forcing it downward (the "dropped metatarsal"), causing metartarsalgia (Fig. 27–21). When the dancer comes back down to the floor, the phalanx relocates and appears to be normal. The regular set of X rays will also be normal. To pick this condition up on physical exam, you must do a *Lachman test* on the MTP joints similar to that done on the knee.[44] When tested in this manner, the affected toe will easily dislocate and then relocate, making the diagnosis apparent. Conservative management is difficult; once the ligaments

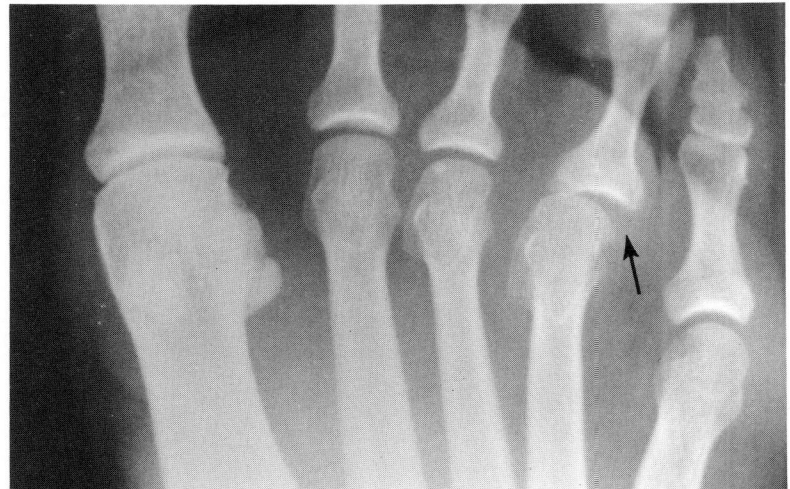

FIGURE 27–21. Subluxation of the MTP joint in the *relevé*.

are loose, they cannot be tightened other than by surgery. Sometimes flexion exercises and a toe retainer with padding under the metatarsal head will at least make the problem workable. If surgery is necessary, the flexor-to-extensor transfer, which as a rule works well in athletes, will often not work in dancers because, in order to control the instability, the joint must be tightened so much that the patient loses the 80 to 90 degrees of dorsiflexion necessary for a full *relevé*. The best solution to this problem usually is a resection arthroplasty (Keller) procedure, but only if conservative measures have failed. This should not be necessary in the adolescent.

Freiberg's disease[44] is no more common in dancers than nondancers, but it can be a problem because it occurs in young adults and can be symptomatic for as long as 6 months before the diagnosis is made on X ray (Fig. 27–22). When the avascular necrosis occurs, several things may happen, leading to a classification based on the degree of the pathology and method of treatment:

- *Type I.* The metatarsal head heals by "creeping substitution" with minimal deformity and loss of motion. No further treatment is necessary.
- *Type II.* The head heals with the articular surface intact but with a ring of marginal osteophytes around the dorsum of the joint that limit dorsiflexion. This can often be corrected by a generous cheilectomy that will restore most of the normal motion.
- *Type III.* There is extensive destruction of the metatarsal head, and the joint surface is loose within the joint "like an orange peel." This type will require a resection arthroplasty with debridement of the MT head. (You need to take more out than you think when you do this procedure or you will not get as much motion as you hoped for.)
- *Type IV.* There is multiple head involvement. This type is rare and probably represents a form of epiphyseal dysplasia. It is a difficult problem but usually not the end of a career.

Freiberg's disease usually presents with pain, stiffness, and swelling at the MTP joint. A bone scan should be done if radiographs are normal and the condition does not improve with rest. Restricted dancing, including avoidance of *relevés*, will be necessary for 6 to 8 months to allow spontaneous healing.

Stress fractures of all the metatarsals occur, but by far the most common one in a dancer is the *base of the second MT*. The bones of the midfoot are solidly connected like the stones of a Roman arch, with the middle cuneiform as the keystone. The base of the second metatarsal is countersunk into the arch at this point and firmly fixed in position to anchor the second ray as the most rigid in the foot. This creates a natural stress riser just distal to the base of the second metatarsal where the bone tends to fracture. As with many stress fractures, it is often difficult actually to see the fracture on the X ray, especially within a week or so of the onset of the symptoms. Persistent tenderness in the proximal first web space or around the base of the second metatarsal in a dancer means a stress fracture until proven otherwise! This is usually an

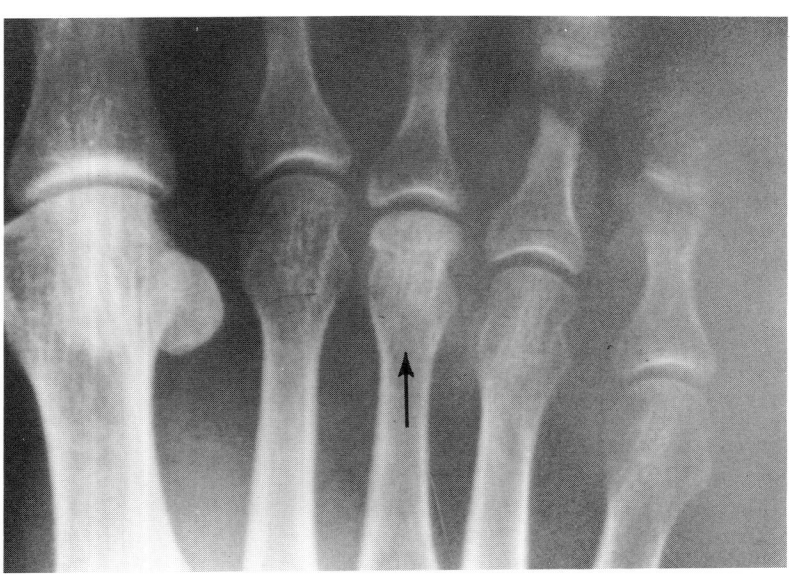

FIGURE 27–22. Early Frieberg's disease. The symptoms may precede the X-ray appearance. The third metatarsal head is involved.

indication for a bone scan, unless the dancer is very young, in which case she is simply taken off jumping and *grand pliés* until the pain and tenderness are gone. This fracture does not normally have to be put in a plaster cast. Activity modification ("Don't do what hurts") for 6 to 8 weeks is usually sufficient for the fracture to heal, providing they have not been working on it for a prolonged period of time while it was hurting. If they have, I usually warn them that it will probably take as long to heal as they have been working on it while it was hurting. Predisposing factors to fracture of the second MT include:

- Amenorrhea and anorexia nervosa
- A Grecian (Morton's) foot with a short first ray and a transfer lesion onto the second MT
- A cavus foot with a rigid, high arch that absorbs energy poorly
- An anterior impingement in the ankle that drives the metatarsals downward (often seen in combination with a cavus foot)

The "*dancer's fracture*," the most common acute fracture seen in dancers other than insignificant toe fractures, is the spiral fracture of the distal one third of the fifth metatarsal (Fig. 27–23). It is analogous to the fracture of

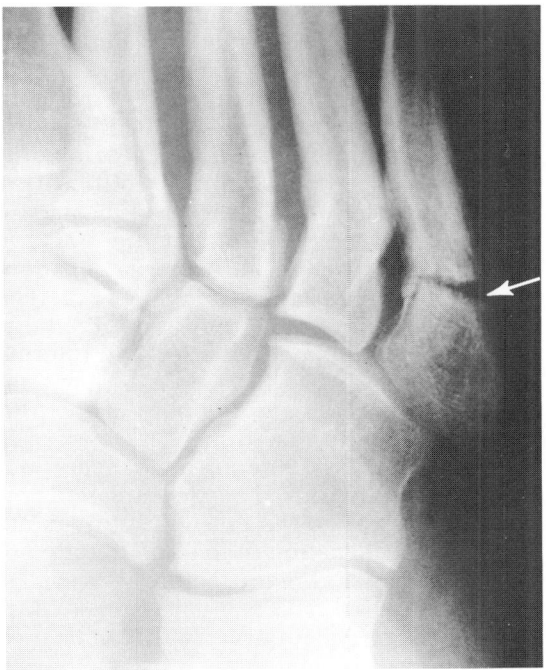

FIGURE 27–24. The Jones fracture of the fifth metatarsal.

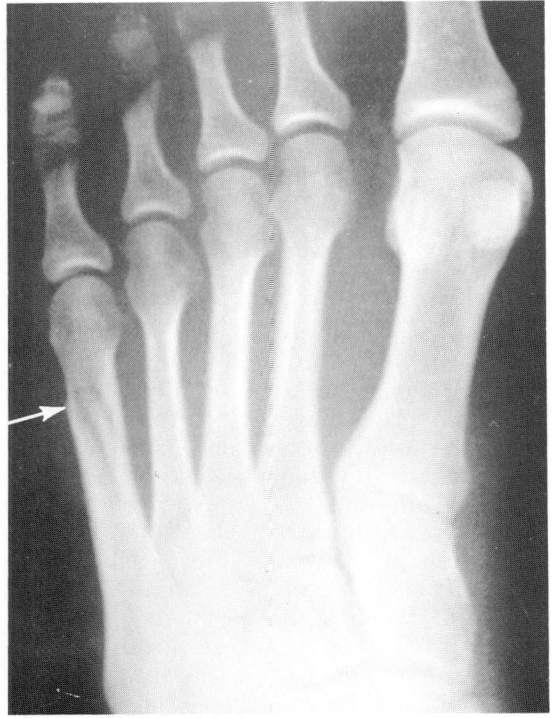

FIGURE 27–23. The "Dancer's fracture" of the fifth metatarsal.

the tubercle at the base of the fifth metatarsal seen in athletes. Dancers sustain this fracture when they lose their balance while on *demi-pointe* and roll over the outer border of the foot. If the fracture is displaced, it may be necessary to put the dancer in a walking cast for 4 to 6 weeks while it heals. (A considerable amount of displacement can be accepted with this fracture.) In fractures that are minimally displaced, it is often sufficient to treat them in a comfortable running shoe with restricted activities until healed. This will allow them to swim and stay in shape while they are waiting to dance again.

Occasionally, a markedly displaced and comminuted fracture will be seen and reduction and internal fixation will be necessary.

In 17 years of treating dance injuries, I have never seen this fracture fail to unite. I have seen two irreducible fractured fifth metatarsals due to muscle interposition. These required open reduction and internal fixation, but they both healed.

The *Jones fracture of the proximal shaft of the fifth metatarsal*[30] (Fig. 27–24), so commonly seen in basketball players, is rare in dancers, especially ballet dancers, because they spend so little time in the plantigrade position. When seen, it is usually in a

Broadway dancer. Care must be taken to recognize this injury for what it is and not to mistake it for the benign fractures seen in the distal shaft and proximal tubercle. Treatment must be aggressive because of the high incidence of nonunion. Undisplaced fractures should be treated in a non–weight-bearing short leg cast for 6 to 8 weeks until healed on X ray. Displaced fractures should undergo anatomical reduction and internal fixation, usually with a lag screw through the tubercle. Delayed and nonunions will require a bone graft along with open reduction and internal fixation.

Avulsion fractures of the base of the fifth metatarsal at the insertion of the peroneus brevis tendon are common in dancers, but they are usually caused by stepping in a pothole on the way to the theater, not by dancing. They occur while in the plantigrade position and are a benign fracture that can be treated by supportive bandage and a loose running shoe. This injury should not be mistaken for an os vesalianum, an accessory ossicle sometimes found at the base of the fifth metatarsal. It is not usually necessary to put the patient in a plaster cast for this injury.

Plantar flexion sprain of the first MTP joint is a painful injury that is slow to heal. It is caused by the toe of the ballet shoe catching on the floor and forcing the toe into plantar flexion. It should be given whatever time it takes to heal because tampering with it can result in osteophyte formation on the dorsum of the first MT head where the capsule has been avulsed. Later on, this spurring can result in a hallux limitus.

Lisfranc sprains are very rare in young dancers. They are usually seen in adult performers. When it does occur, this injury is a serious and career-threatening event. Recognition and treatment are essential. Normal anatomy must be restored by closed or open means.

The *subluxing cuboid*[33,36] is a common but poorly recognized condition that presents as lateral midfoot pain and an inability to "work through" the foot, that is, to go smoothly from foot flat to *relevé*. This may present as an acute sprain or an insidious overuse injury. The dancer is unable to run, cut, jump, or dance without a marked increase in discomfort or a feeling of weakness and lack of intrinsic support in the foot. Pressing on the plantar surface of the cuboid in a dorsal direction is painful. The normal dorsal/plantar joint play is reduced or absent when compared with the uninjured side. Severely subluxed cuboids leave a shallow but definite depression on the dorsal, and a palpable fullness on the plantar aspect of the cuboid. Treatment usually involves a manual reduction, the "cuboid whip," by a therapist familiar with the condition and may need to be repeated. The most important thing about the subluxed cuboid is to be aware of its existence and to recognize it when it is present.

The Ankle. The flat foot is a poor foot for a dancer. It is prone to develop posterior impingement. The cavus foot is a desirable foot for the dancer but is prone to anterior impingements, ankle sprains, and Achilles tendinitis at its insertion in the os calcis.

Osteochondritis dissecans of the talus is a disorder common in males in this age group. It may be posttraumatic or spontaneous and should be considered when a young man presents with painless unexplained swelling in the ankle. Often it heals spontaneously (Fig. 27–25). Treatment depends on whether the dissected fragment is loose or still in place. As long as it is in place, there is potential for revascularization and healing. If the fragment is loose and there is joint fluid beneath or around it, it cannot heal and should be arthroscopically debrided.

The *anterior impingement syndrome of the ankle*[31,38] is common in both athletes and dancers. It is the result of years of "hitting bottom" in the *plié* in dancers who dance the "bravura" technique of big jumps and grandiose lifts, who have an exceptionally high arch and thus a shallow *plié* to begin with, or who have loose lateral ligaments due to old ankle sprains (Fig. 27–26). Surgery for this condition is hardly ever indicated in a young dancer. The person needing surgery is usually an older male dancer with osteophytes. If the symptoms are disabling, an anterior debridement either through a small anterior medial incision or arthroscopically may be indicated. The diagnosis is important because the condition is often mistaken by the dancer and the dance teacher for "tight Achilles tendons." Obviously, there is no point in working on Achilles stretching if the restriction in motion is due to a bony impingement in the front of the ankle. A second reason to diagnose this problem in a young dancer is to correct his technique to avoid the irritation that may lead to osteophyte formation later.

There are other conditions that can mimic the anterior impingement syndrome: de-

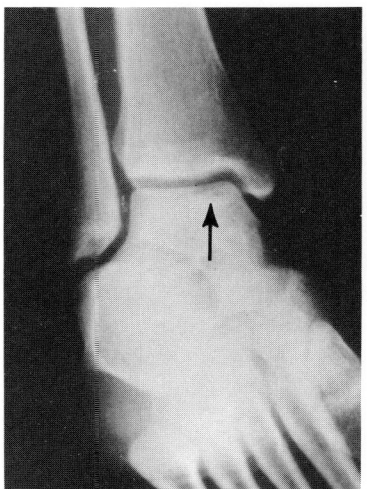 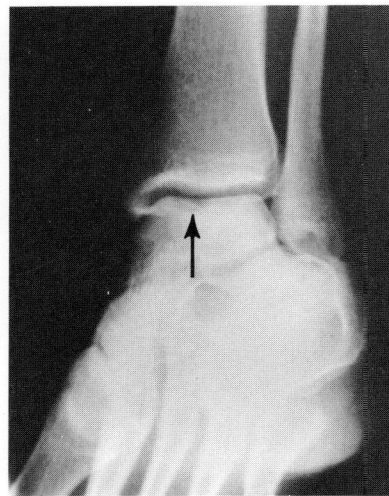

FIGURE 27–25. Bilateral asymptomatic osteochondritis dissecans of the talus.

generative joint disease of the tibiotalar or talonavicular joints, especially in the early phases when the X-ray findings are subtle; and an *osteoid osteoma* in the tarsal navicular (Fig. 27–27). Both of these conditions will give a characteristic picture on the bone scan.

The *posterior impingement syndrome of the ankle* (Fig. 27–28), or talar compression syndrome,[22,29,39] is the natural result of full weight bearing in maximum plantar flexion of the ankle in the *demi-pointe* or *full pointe* position, especially if an os trigonum or trigonal process is present. It presents as posterior lateral pain in the back of the ankle when the os calcis closes against the posterior lip of the tibia as in the *tendu*, the *frappé*, the *relevé*, or leaving the ground in a jump (Table 27–1). It can be confirmed on physical exam by tenderness behind the lateral malleolus (often mistaken for peroneal tendinitis) and by pain with forced passive plantar flexion of the ankle—the *"plantar flexion sign."* It is commonly seen in 15- to 16-year-old female dancers with an os trigonum, who are trying to force their foot to go down as far as the one that does not have an os trigonum. A lateral radiograph in the *full pointe* position will also be helpful. In this particular group, it is

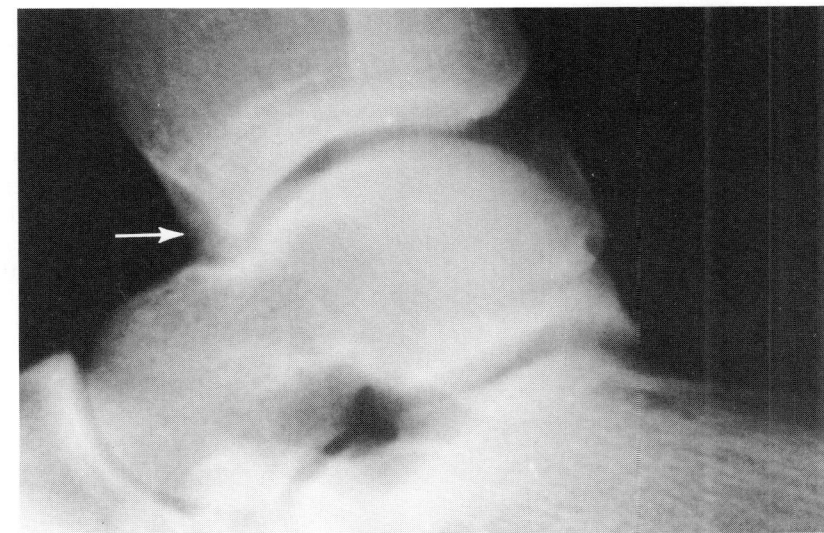

FIGURE 27–26. Anterior impingement of the ankle.

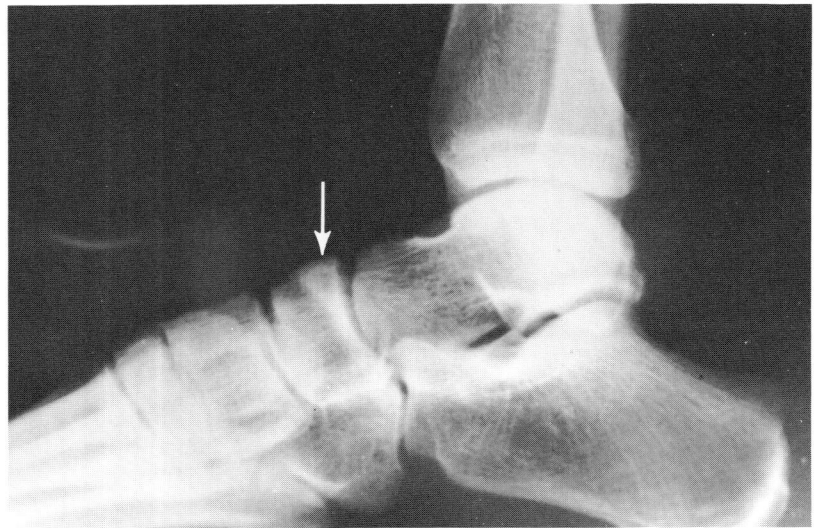

FIGURE 27–27. Osteoid osteoma of the tarsal navicular.

often sufficient to tell them what the problem is, have them accept a mild limitation to the plantar flexion in the ankle, and work with what they have. They should be told that the pain comes from trying to force the foot further down than it has the ability to go and that the pain will subside when they stop forcing the plantar flexion.

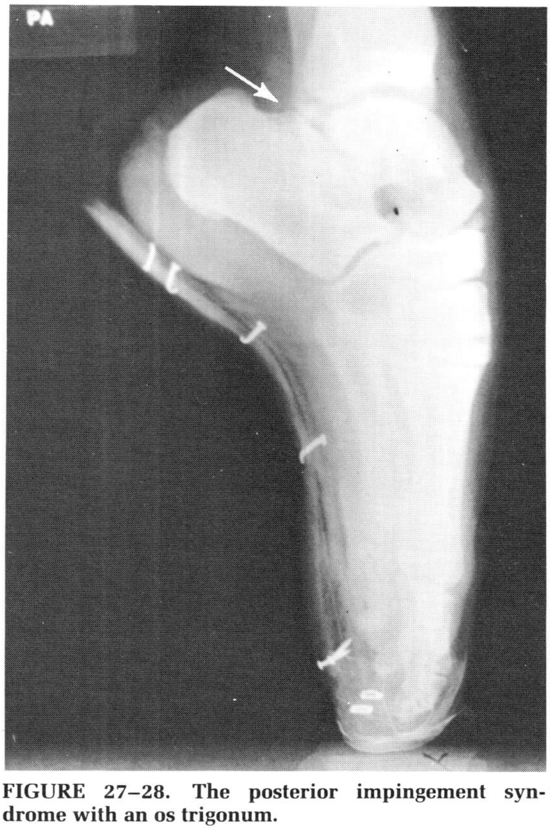

The syndrome is often, but not always, associated with an os trigonum (OT) or trigonal process on the back of the ankle. The posterior aspect of the talus normally has two tubercles, the medial tubercle and the lateral tubercle. Between the two tubercles lies the fibroosseus tunnel of the flexor hallucis longus (FHL) tendon. The os trigonum is the ununited lateral tubercle on the posterior aspect of the talus. It is present in 7 to 10 percent of people and has a 50 percent incidence of bilaterality. Most people who have an os trigonum are not aware of its presence, and the posterior impingement syndrome is rare in athletes. In dancers, it may or may not be symptomatic, and the degree of the symptomatology is not always related to the size of the OT. Large ones can be minimally symptomatic and small ones are sometimes disabling. Usually, the symptoms are mild, and on the whole, the OT is more often asymptomatic than symptomatic. Many world-famous ballerinas have asymptomatic OTs, and they work with them without any trouble. It is important to stress this fact to the patient and her mother when discussing this condition because there is often a tendency for the problem to get blown out of proportion, sometimes owing to the dramatic appearance of the bone on the X ray. It is best seen on a lateral view of the ankle on *pointe* or in full plantar flexion. The diagnosis can be confirmed if necessary by injecting 0.5 cc of Xylocaine into the posterior soft tissues behind the peroneal tendons.

FIGURE 27–28. The posterior impingement syndrome with an os trigonum.

TABLE 27–1. Posterior Pain Syndromes of the Ankle in Dancers: FHL Tendinitis versus Posterior Impingement

FHL Tendinitis	Posterior Impingement (Os Trigonum Syndrome)
Posteromedial	Posterolateral
Tenderness over FHL tendon	Tenderness behind fibula
Pain with motion of hallux	Pain with forced plantar flexion of the ankle (the "plantar flexion sign")
Tomasen sign[46] positive	Tomasen sign negative
Mistaken for posterior tibial tendinitis	Mistaken for peroneal tendinitis

Treatment of the posterior impingement syndrome should be graded. The first approach, similar to tendinitis, is modification of activities ("Don't do what hurts"); nonsteroidal antiinflammatory drugs (NSAIDS) if the dancer is over age 16; and physical therapy. Patients should be told that it will take a few weeks for the pain to subside—usually as long as they have been dancing with the condition before they began treatment; that is, if they have been working with the pain for a month, then it will often take a month of treatment and reduced activities before they can resume normal activities without discomfort. In cases where this approach has failed, or the symptoms recur, and the patient is 16 years or older, an injection of 0.5 cc of a mixture of long- and short-acting corticosteroid can often give dramatic and permanent relief of symptoms. Before injecting the steroid preparation, the diagnosis should be confirmed with Novocain. If the Novocain does not relieve the symptoms, there is no point in injecting the steroids. It should be stressed that the os trigonum is not usually a surgical problem; most dancers with an os trigonum do not need to have it removed surgically.

Occasionally, the os trigonum does cause enough disability to warrant surgical excision. As with most elective surgery, it is only indicated after the failure of conservative therapy in a dancer at least 16 years old. If the problem is an isolated OT with no medial symptoms, then it can be approached posterolaterally (protect the sural nerve). Not infrequently, there may be a combined problem of FHL tendinitis and os trigonum syndrome. In these patients, it is best to go in posteromedially so that the neurovascular bundle can be isolated and protected. A tenolysis of the FHL and removal of the adjacent OT can then be performed safely.

As mentioned under ankle sprains, a previously asymptomatic OT may become persistently symptomatic following an ankle sprain, sometimes owing to disruption of its ligamentous connections and a subtle shift in position. A posterior impingement may also follow ankle sprains that cause loose lateral ligaments that cannot hold the talus under the tibia in the *relevé*.[25] As the talus slips forward, the posterior lip of the tibia comes to rest on the os calcis. This is difficult to differentiate clinically from other cases of posterior impingement, but the subluxation may be seen on a lateral weight-bearing radiograph taken during *relevé* (Fig. 27–29). The

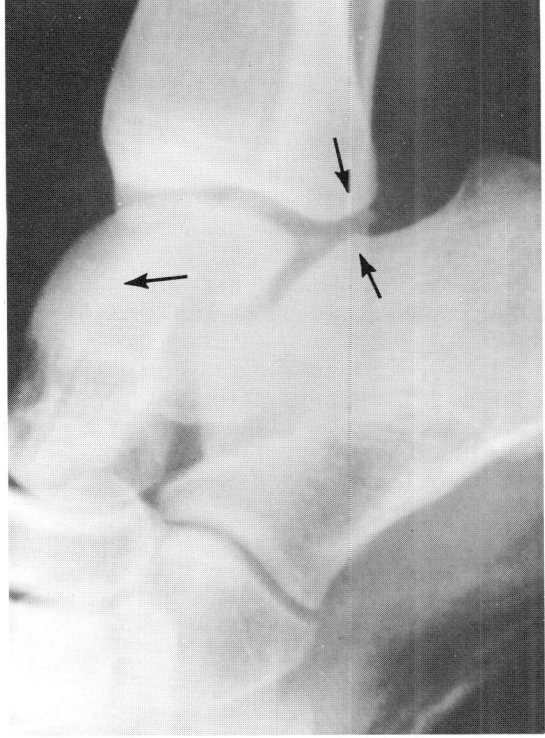

FIGURE 27–29. The posterior impingement syndrome secondary to loose lateral ligaments.

treatment for this type of posterior impingement is to tighten the lateral ankle ligaments. If the drawer sign can be corrected, the posterior impingement will usually disappear.

There also can be a *pseudomeniscus* or plica in the posterior ankle,[21,22] with or without an os trigonum. It can cause the posterior impingement syndrome without an OT or loose ligaments and can cause locking and other mechanical symptoms more often seen in the knee than the ankle. Because this plica cannot be differentiated clinically, it should be looked for during surgical exploration for posterior impingement.

Tendinitis of the FHL tendon behind the medial malleolus of the ankle is so common that it is known as *dancer's tendinitis* (Table 27–1).[18,22,25] It is often misdiagnosed as posterior tibial or Achilles tendinitis, but careful examination will usually reveal the true diagnosis. The FHL is the "Achilles tendon of the foot" for the dancer. It passes through a fibroosseus tunnel behind the talus like a rope through a pulley. Where it passes through this pulley, it is easily strained. When strained, rather than moving smoothly in the pulley, it begins to bind. This binding causes irritation and swelling, which in turn causes further binding, irritation, and swelling—setting up the familiar cycle: Because it is swollen and irritated, it binds; and because it binds, it is swollen and irritated. If a nodule or partial tear is present, triggering of the big toe may occur—*hallux saltans* (Fig. 27–30)—or the tendon may become completely frozen in the sheath, causing a *pseudo–hallux rigidus*. This tendinitis typically responds to the usual conservative measures. Rest is an important component of the therapy so that the chronic cycle described above can be broken. NSAIDs can help, but they should only be used as part of an overall treatment program and not as medicine to kill the pain so that the dancer can continue dancing and ignore the symptoms. As with other tendon problems, steroid injections should be avoided. On some occasions, FHL tendinitis may be recurrent and disabling. In these cases, operative tenolysis may be indicated but only after failure of at least a year of conservative therapy in the young dancer or 6 months in a professional.

FHL tendinitis will usually occur behind the medial malleolus, but it can occasionally be found at Henry's knot under the base of the first metatarsal where the flexor digitorum longus (FDL) crosses over the FHL and under

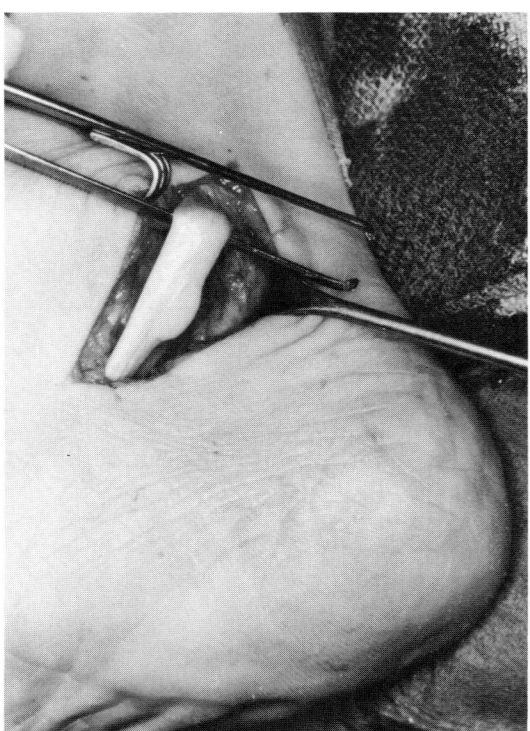

FIGURE 27–30. Nodule on the FHL tendon causing triggering of the big toe—hallux saltans.

the head of the first metatarsal where it passes between the sesamoids. Occasionally, a fibrous subtalar coalition may be present in the posteromedial ankle mimicking FHL tendinitis or the tarsal tunnel syndrome. This condition should be suspected when there is less than normal subtalar motion on physical exam.

The *tarsal tunnel syndrome* is extremely rare in dancers. What appears to be tarsal tunnel syndrome is usually either FHL tendinitis or posterior impingement. The only true cases of the tarsal tunnel syndrome that I have seen in dancers have been due to abnormal structures, such as ganglions arising from the subtalar joint, lying within the tarsal tunnel.

The most common acute skeletal injury in the dancer, other than the stubbed toe, is the *inversion sprain* of the ankle.[21] Sprains may occur in any ligament in the foot or ankle, but the most common ones involve the lateral ligament complex (the anterior talofibular, the calcaneofibular, and the posterior talofibular ligaments), the anterior tibiofibular ligament, the lateral talocalcaneal ligament,

TABLE 27-2. Working Classification of Acute Ankle Sprains

	Anatomical Injury	Physical Exam	X-ray Findings
Grade I	Partial tear; ATF or CF	Negative or 1+ drawer sign	Negative drawer sign; negative talar tilt
Grade II	Torn ATF; intact CF	2+ Drawer sign	Positive drawer sign; negative talar tilt
Grade III	Torn ATF; torn CF	3+ Drawer sign	Positive drawer sign; positive talar tilt

ATF = Anterior talofibular ligament
CF = Calcaneofibular ligament
Note: Drawer sign (4 to 5 mm): 1+, slightly greater than normal side; 2+, definitely greater than normal; 3+, grossly positive (greater than 15°).

and occasionally, the deltoid ligament (see Table 27–2).

Other conditions, however, can closely resemble the classical sprained ankle, and the physician is well advised to examine the patient carefully for the following injuries that can simulate or accompany a simple sprain:

- A complete tear of the lateral collateral ligaments (really, a medial dislocation of the talus that has spontaneously reduced)
- An injury to the anterior inferior tibiofibular ligament
- A complete tear of both the distal anterior and posterior tibiofibular ligaments (the syndemosis) and the interosseous membrane without fracture of the malleoli but with diastasis of the ankle mortise and, occasionally, fracture of the proximal isthmus of the fibula—the "Maisonneuve fracture"
- A sprain of the subtalar joint with disruption of the lateral talocalcaneal ligament
- A fracture of the base of the fifth metatarsal
- An undisplaced fracture of the lateral malleolus, or malleolar epiphysis, in a young dancer
- A fracture of the "beak" of the os calcis in the sinus tarsi[28] (Fig. 27–31)
- Subluxation of the cuboid[33,36]
- A fracture of the posterior lip of the distal tibia or fracture of a trigonal process behind the talus (Shepherd's fracture)
- A fracture of the medial malleolus or sustentaculum tali
- A lateral sprain of the tarsometatarsal (Lisfranc) joints
- A rupture of the Achilles tendon
- A lateral process fracture of the talus

Ankle sprains are usually graded as I, II, or III, depending on the extent of the injury.[21,26] Grade I sprains are partial tears, usually of the anterior talofibular ligament or occasionally the anterior tibiofibular ligament (the "high" ankle sprain) with little or no resultant instability. On physical exam, the

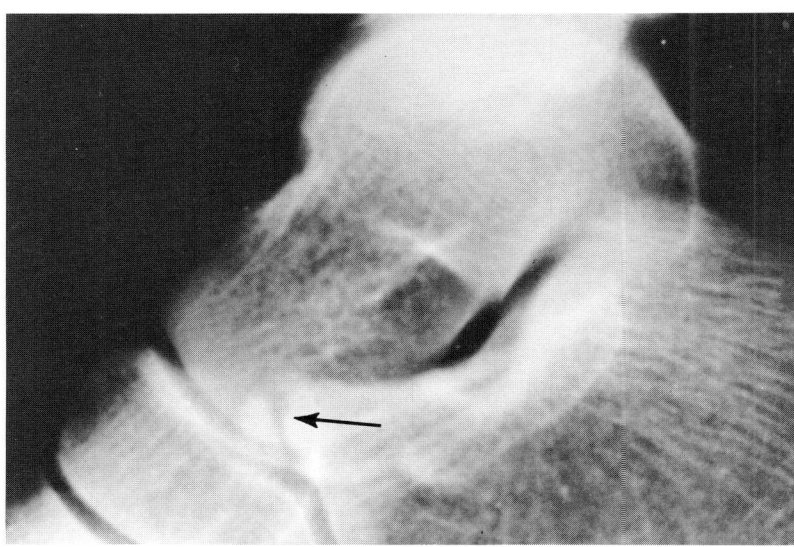

FIGURE 27–31. Fractured "beak" of the os calcis.

drawer sign and the stress films are normal. After the initial 48 hours of rest, ice, compression, and elevation, the patient should begin early active use of the limb with a compression bandage, taping, or an "air splint."

Grade II sprains are complete tears of the anterior talofibular ligament, with minimal damage to the calcanealfibular ligament. They produce a moderately positive drawer sign but a normal or minimal talar tilt on the stress film. They often result in some residual instability, but this can usually be controlled by good peroneal strength. Treatment consists of some type of support—either taping, air splint, or a walking plaster cast for 3 to 6 weeks followed by aggressive peroneal rehabilitation.

This is the type of ankle sprain most commonly seen in dancers. It usually occurs when they are on *demi-pointe*. In this position, the anterior talofibular ligament is almost vertical, in the position normally taken by the calcanealfibular ligament when the foot is plantigrade, and it is easily torn when an adduction-inversion force is applied. In this position, the calcanealfibular ligament is almost parallel to the floor; it is out of harm's way and is rarely injured.

The *grade III* sprain is fortunately a rare injury, for it represents a complete rupture of the lateral ligament complex and results in gross instability. It is actually a spontaneously reduced medial dislocation of the talus. The drawer sign and stress films are grossly positive on physical exam and X ray (Fig. 27–32). The healing time, 3 to 4 months, is long and uncertain, and the likelihood of significant permanent laxity of the ligaments is high. Curiously enough, dancers with residual laxity of the lateral ankle ligaments from this injury usually complain more of rotatory instability than of varus instability; that is, they develop anterolateral rotatory instability of the ankle analogous to ligament injuries of the knee. They can feel the talus rotate within the mortise when they do "inside" turns, that is, turning to the right on the right foot. For this reason, many orthopedists, including myself, feel that (grade III) lateral ankle sprains in professional athletes and dancers should be repaired surgically, within 7 to 10 days of the acute injury.

The repair described by Gould et al.[13] is a simple procedure done under regional anesthesia with a small incision over the distal fibula. The ligaments are easily identified, as they are within the capsule itself. They are usually avulsed from the fibula rather than torn in their midsubstance, making them easy to reattach to their anatomical origin on the fibula. Occasionally, the calcaneofibular ligament is avulsed from the calcaneus rather than the fibula, making the repair somewhat more difficult. Postoperative immobilization in a short leg walking cast for 4 weeks is followed by protection in an air splint and early rehabilitation. Here again, complete restoration of peroneal strength is critically important.

Regardless of the method of treatment, adequate physical therapy and proper rehabilitation are necessary to restore normal use fol-

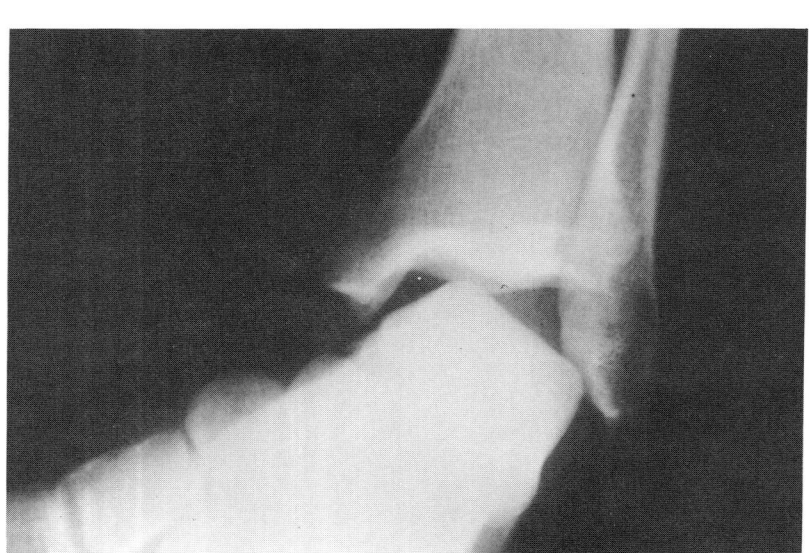

FIGURE 27–32. A grade III sprain of the ankle.

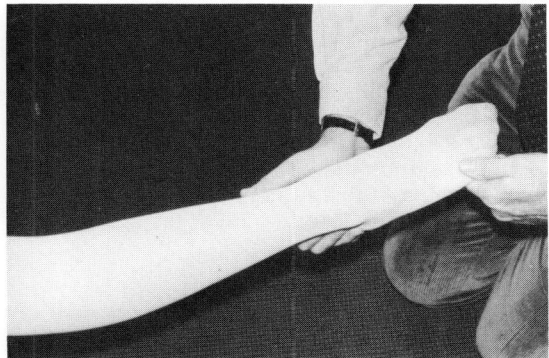

FIGURE 27–33. Testing peroneal strength.

lowing injury. Full peroneal strength is essential. My preferred method is progressive resistive exercises (PREs) in the fully plantar-flexed position. Residual peroneal weakness is a commonly unrecognized condition in dancers[19] and can cause a myriad of obscure symptoms such as unexplained swelling and discomfort or poor timing with "beats." Any dancer complaining of these symptoms should be checked for weak peroneals. This is done by having them place their foot in the *tendu* position of full plantar flexion and neutral abduction-adduction and asking them to hold this position against varus and then valgus stress (Fig. 27–33). A well-conditioned dancer should be able to resist as much force as you can manually apply to the foot in this position. The uninjured side can be checked for comparison if necessary. The most common fault is that the dancer either has not been adequately rehabilitated or she has been exercising in the neutral position rather than full plantar flexion. Exercise machines are not very good for ankle rehab, as they cannot be placed in full equinus. I use a home exercise program over

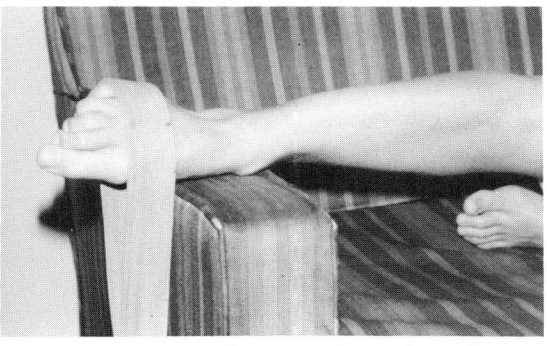

FIGURE 27–34. The peroneal exercise regimen.

the end of a sofa or couch with the dancer on her side using a weight bag in full plantar flexion (Fig. 27–34). Abduction exercises are performed with the ankle supported so that it can only move upward in valgus and the patient can relax the ankle in between lifts. They lift 3 pounds, 25 times slowly, morning and evening, increasing the weight in the bag by 3 pounds each week to a total of 15 pounds. When they can lift 15 pounds slowly 25 times, they are adequately rehabilitated. I have never seen this method fail to restore normal peroneal strength. The symptoms do not always disappear, and if they do not, the clinician should suspect that one of the other conditions mentioned above or below may be mimicking or complicating the ankle sprain.

Secondary or delayed ankle ligament reconstruction is occasionally necessary in a dancer, but it should only be considered after full peroneal strength has been obtained (see above) and the dancer is still unable to dance. Often, as previously mentioned, the problem is rotatory instability rather than varus instability. It must be emphasized that reconstruction should be done only for functional difficulties and not simply on the basis of a drawer sign or a positive stress X ray. There are many professional dancers working quite well with loose ankles that are not symptomatic enough to warrant surgical repair.

I feel strongly that the peroneus brevis tendon should not be used for ankle reconstruction in a professional dancer for two reasons. First, the peroneus brevis is too important as a support tendon for dancing on *full pointe* to be sacrificed. Second, it is not necessary to use it: I have had excellent results using the Brostrom repair as described by Gould et al.[13,26] The procedure is simply a reefing of the anterior talofibular and calcaneofibular ligaments with reattachment to their proper locations on the fibula, then sewing the lateral extensor retinaculum over the tip of the fibula in a "pants over vest" manner to limit inversion. (The stability of the subtalar joint should be checked at the time of exploration because some of the ankle instability is often coming from this joint. If unstable, it may be necessary to reef the lateral talocalcaneal ligament as well.) The patient is placed in a short leg walking cast for 1 month, then taken out for rehab and swimming and protected in a removable air splint for another 2 to 3 weeks. In 18 professional dancers, this technique has not failed to give an excellent result, with full range of motion and strength.

Miscellaneous problems following ankle sprains are not uncommon:

- A *trigonal process may be fractured* at the time of the sprain and may continue to be symptomatic after the sprain heals—Shepherd's fracture. A bone scan will detect this when there is clinical uncertainty.
- Dancers will often develop an FHL *tendinitis* and/or *posterior impingement syndrome* following an ankle sprain, occasionally involving an os trigonum that had previously been asymptomatic.[25] These complications are not always related to the severity of the sprain.
- A unique type of posterior impingement may follow grade III sprains with residual laxity. In this condition, the loose anterior talofibular ligament cannot hold the talus under the tibial plafond in the full *relevé* position, and the talus slips forward, allowing the posterior lip of the tibia to settle down on the os calcis (Fig. 27–25).
- If there is lateral ligament laxity in the ankle, an *anterior impingement* may follow with osteophyte formation in the anterior tibiotalar joint, secondary to rotatory instability, often opposite the tip of the medial malleolus. This problem is insidious and presents years after the original injury. It is diagnosed and treated the same as other anterior impingements. It does not develop in all dancers with laxity; therefore, it is not, by itself, an indication for ligament repair.
- Problems around the *tip of the fibula* may persist after the sprain heals:
  Soft tissue entrapment (the *"meniscoid"* of the ankle).[50] This condition can be diagnosed and corrected by arthroscopy.
  An *avulsion fracture* of the tip of the fibula.
  A previously *asymptomatic accessory ossicle* (the os subfibulare) that becomes symptomatic.
  An unrecognized *fracture of the beak of the os calcis*. This fracture is an avulsion fracture of the extensor digitorum brevis origin (often best seen on the oblique X ray of the foot).[28] Excision of the fragment may be necessary if conservative therapy fails to control the symptoms (Fig. 27–27).
  An unrecognized fracture of the talus (Fig. 27–35).
  The sinus tarsi syndrome.[4,43]

When a tendon is strained, the surface, rather than being smooth and shiny, becomes roughened and appears frayed like an old rope. Rather than moving smoothly, it now will bind as it moves in its sheath, causing pain, swelling, tenderness, and crepitus. Certain tendons in dancers are particularly prone to *tendinitis*. Tendinitis of the FHL, or dancer's Tendinitis has been already discussed.

The *Achilles tendon* is the largest tendon in the body. It connects the triceps surae (medial and lateral gastrocnemius and soleus muscles) to the os calcis and transmits the forces necessary to propel the body in walking, running, and jumping. These forces range from two to three times body weight in walking to four to six times body weight in running and jumping.[23] Their magnitude makes the Achilles tendon a common site for tendinitis secondary to repetitive overload or faults in technique in dancers, such as "roll-

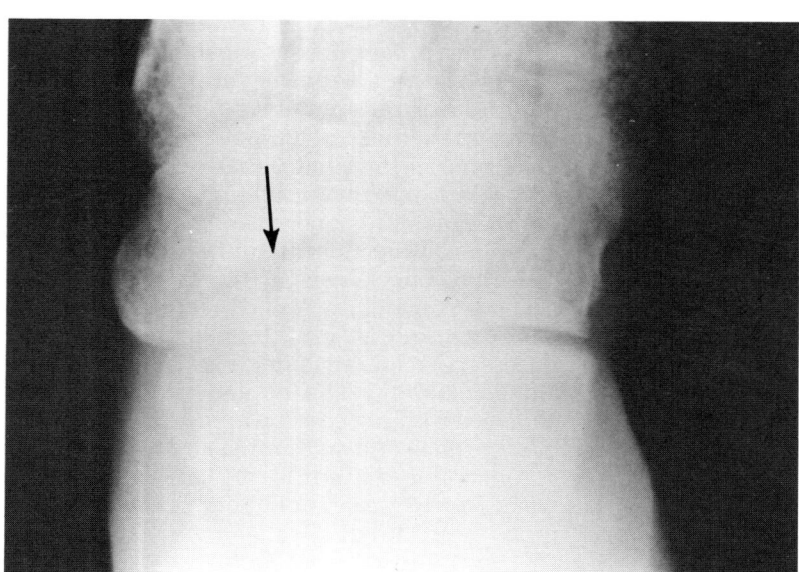

FIGURE 27–35. An unrecognized fracture of the talus.

ing in" (pronation) and landing hard on the heels.

Achilles tendinitis is rarely seen before the age of 16, probably because of the low body weight of the young dancer. It is relatively rare until the dancer is in her twenties. Similar to other forms of tendinitis, it is an inflammatory response surrounding the tendon triggered by microscopic tearing of the collagen fibers secondary to overload. The tearing may be on the surface or in the substance of the tendon (interstitial); thus, clinically there are types and gradations of severity. The simplest type results in pain, tenderness, swelling, and thickening of the pseudosheath surrounding the tendon, usually at its isthmus or narrowest point. There may also be crepitus present on active motion. If the condition is chronic, nodules usually form around the tendon or on its surface. These may result in adhesions between the tendon and its sheath. A more severe strain results in a localized, fusiform swelling of the tendon itself, "like a snake that has swallowed a pig." This latter injury is slow to heal and has a guarded prognosis.

Certain factors can contribute to the development of Achilles tendinitis:

- *Heel cord tightness* is the most common cause of Achilles strain in the recreational athlete and dancer.
- The *size* of the tendon varies considerably from person to person and from one side to the other and is not always related to body size. People with small tendons are prone to strains and overloads.
- *Pronation,* usually called "rolling in" in dancers, subjects dancers to increased risk of developing Achilles tendinitis.
- A *"ribbon burn"* at the place where the toeshoe ribbons encircle the tendon above the ankle can result in Achilles tendinitis. This is usually caused by wearing the ribbons too tight and can be relieved by sewing a segment of elastic in the ribbons at this location (Fig. 27–37).
- A *cavus foot* with prominence of the posterior superior os calcis often causes *chronic retrocalcaneal bursitis* ("pump bumps") and tendinitis of the Achilles overlying the bursa. Occasionally, this condition can result in a *partial tear of the Achilles tendon* just above its insertion, causing chronic pain and swelling. This condition is not uncommon in dancers, as they are selected for having cavus feet. Exploration, debridement of the bursa, partial excision of the os calcis, and repair of the tendon may be necessary if the condition does not respond to conservative therapy. The retrocalcaneal bursa is a dangerous place to inject steroids; such an injection in dancers can weaken the Achilles insertion and cause the tendon to pull loose. I have seen this happen in two major professional dancers.

Treatment of Achilles tendinitis, like so many other sports-related injuries, should be two phased: First, the injured tendon must be allowed to heal. Rest, antiinflammatory medicines, and physical therapy modalities such as ice, contrast baths, and ultrasound will promote healing. Second, rehabilitation with a trainer or therapist is necessary to restore both strength and flexibility. Any faults in technique should be corrected prior to resumption of full activities. "Injured athletes should not try to play themselves back into shape but should get into shape and then play."

In the NYC Ballet and American Ballet Theater, we have reduced the incidence of Achilles tendinitis in half by the use of the "stretch box," a wedge-shaped box that is kept in the wings during the season so that the dancers can stand on it to stretch their Achilles tendons while they are waiting backstage during performances and rehearsals (Fig. 27–36).

Rupture of the Achilles tendon can occur without warning but is usually preceded by tendinitis or degeneration. Fortunately, it is extremely rare in adolescents. If the tendon is accidentally lacerated, it should be surgically repaired. A detailed discussion of the surgical repair of the Achilles tendon is beyond the scope of this chapter; however, a few comments are in order. It used to be said that a ruptured Achilles tendon was automatically the end of a dancer's career. This need

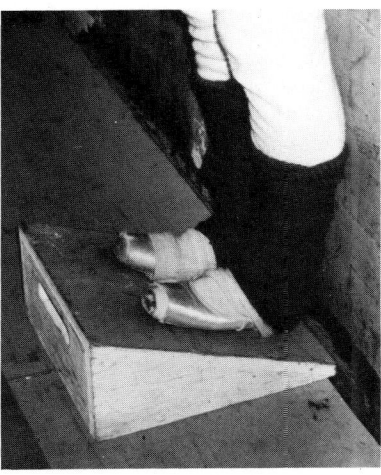

FIGURE 27–36. The stretch box.

not be the case. If the tendon can be restored to its original length, and if the dancer is willing to devote the time and effort (1 full year) necessary for the postoperative rehabilitation, he or she can dance again. The type of repair used is not as important as the concept of the restoration of physiological length.[25] My preferred method is to use the plantaris tendon as an autogenous "figure-of-eight" suture to approximate the ends of the tendon under proper tension. This tension is best determined by having the uninjured leg prepped in the field so that the resting length of the contralateral Achilles is available for comparison when the tension is set in the repair. By sighting across both ankles, the tension can be adjusted to place the injured and uninjured ankles in the same resting position relative to one another. An incision placed on the medial rather than the posterior aspect of the leg will minimize postop skin problems, and splitting the Achilles sheath anteriorly prior to the repair will allow a layered closure of the wound at the end of the procedure. Postoperatively, the patient is placed in a short leg walking cast in neutral for 8 weeks and then rehabilitation is begun.

Peroneal tendinitis and *posterior tibial tendinitis* do occur, but they are not nearly as common in dancers as they are in athletes. More often than not, "peroneal tendinitis" is really the posterior impingement syndrome and "posterior tibial tendinitis" is usually FHL tendinitis. Tendinitis of the peroneus longus does occasionally occur where it passes around the cuboid into the sole of the foot.

Fortunately, *Peroneal subluxation* and dislocation is not common in dancers, because it has a poor prognosis without surgery. Acute primary subluxations should be treated by cast immobilization for 6 weeks, followed by a vigorous rehabilitation program emphasizing peroneal strengthening. The patient should not return to dancing for a total of 8 weeks. Unfortunately, this often does not prevent the condition from becoming chronic. There is no need for cast immobilization in the chronic subluxators; I treat them in an air splint similar to an ankle sprain. The condition can be repaired surgically in a manner similar to the delayed repair of the lateral ligaments of the ankle. The retinaculum can be reefed and then sewn into its original location in the fibula in a small trough created with a thin osteotome. The Achilles tendon should *not* be used for this repair because of the stiffness that usually follows this method of treatment.

The Leg. Many dance problems are seen in the leg. The fibula has a proximal and a distal isthmus, and *stress fractures* occur in both these locations, especially distally. This is the area where the toeshoe ribbons encircle the distal leg. If they are worn too tightly and if the fibula happens to be very thin in this area, as it often is, a stress fracture can occur. This fracture can rarely be seen on the regular X ray, so a bone scan is needed to confirm the diagnosis. I usually make the diagnosis on the basis of the physical exam alone because the localized tenderness at this location is so characteristic of the fracture. Treatment involves restricted activities and no *pointe* work until the tenderness is gone. This normally takes 4 to 6 weeks. When the dancer returns to the *pointe* shoe, she should sew elastics in the toe ribbons to relieve the tightness that caused the fracture (Fig. 27-37).

The most common problem in the leg is the differential diagnosis between *shin splints*, *tibial stress fractures*, and *compartment syndromes*. Shin splints in dancers occur mainly along the posterior border of the tibia along the soleus and flexor digitorum longus origins (not the posterior tibial origin, which lies on the posterior lateral border of the tibia along the interosseous membrane). Shin splints commonly occur in September after a summer layoff, not in midseason, and give a

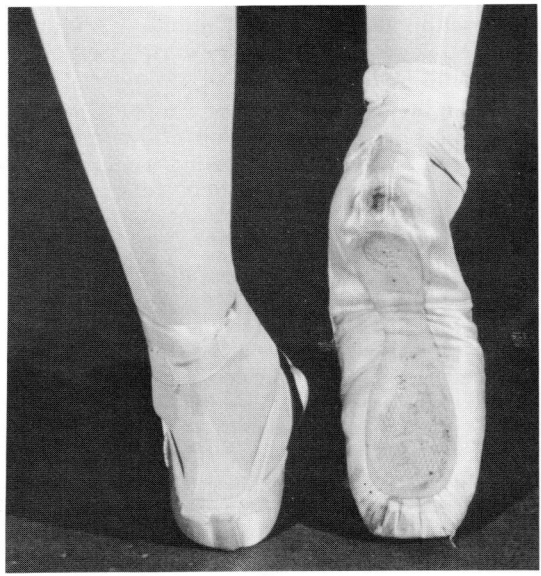

FIGURE 27-37. Toeshoe ribbons with elastics.

characteristic pattern on the bone scan, a diffuse uptake over several centimeters. Tibial stress fractures occur in midseason, and the symptoms and bone scan are quite localized. In dancers, they are almost always on the anterior border of the middle third of the tibia. If the stress fracture has become chronic, there will usually be a tender, palpable excrescence on the surface of the tibia at the site of the fracture. Compartment syndromes are very rare in dancers because their exercise patterns are intermittent. Compartment pressures can be measured if this condition is suspected. The *soleus syndrome*[34] is seen in dancers. It is a pain syndrome resembling a posterior shin splint, but it occurs on the posterior border of the tibia just above the medial malleolus. It is caused by an abnormally distal origin of a leash of the soleus muscle. Surgical release of this leash may be necessary in recalcitrant cases. The treatment of these conditions in the adolescent dancer is the same as most overuse syndromes—reduced activities until the problem heals. Swimming is used during the rest period to stay in shape. If the dancers are apprenticed to a company or are dancing professionally, then I recommend ice, physical therapy (iontophoresis), technique modification, and in the case of stress fractures, a bone stimulator, although there is no hard evidence as yet that these make a stress fracture heal faster.

The time a tibial stress fracture takes to heal is highly variable. It depends mainly on how early the condition is diagnosed and treatment is begun and on how compliant the dancer is with the treatment regimen. If they have been "working through" the pain, I warn them that it will take at least as long to heal as they have been working with the pain.

The Knee. By far the most common knee problem in dancers is the *painful patella syndrome*. This condition, so common in athletes, is exacerbated in dancers if they are turned in at the hip and are getting their turnout from the knee, thus increasing their Q angle. The differential diagnosis includes:

- Patellar malalignment and subluxation
- Chondromalacia patellae
- The plica syndrome
- The bipartite patella
- Quadriceps tendinitis
- Infrapatellar tendinitis
- Osteochondritis dissecans

A careful history and physical exam will usually reveal which of these conditions is causing the pain. If the diagnosis is not apparent, I have found small (0.5 cc) injections of a local anesthetic with a tuberculin syringe into various anatomical sites to be helpful in locating the problem. An accurate diagnosis is desirable in the treatment of these conditions. The presence of several different problems at the same time often makes the treatment of these disorders difficult. Frequently, the diagnosis is infrapatellar tendinitis, the *jumper's knee*. This can be a frustrating and difficult condition to treat. It heals slowly and tends to recur. Treatment involves modified activities, friction massage, ice, and eccentric quadriceps strengthening. Unrecognized eccentric quad weakness is felt to be a predisposing factor in this condition. The dancer must avoid jumps and *grand pliés* as much as possible. In older dancers, this condition may need to be "scraped" under local anesthesia to induce healing.

Torn knee ligaments constitute the most serious dance injury. Often they follow on the heels of a patellar dislocation. There may be partial tears, complete tears, or isolated tears—usually of the anterior cruciate ligament (ACL), medial collateral ligament (MCL), and menisci. Early, accurate diagnosis and treatment are essential if optimum function is to be obtained following this injury. An MRI study and diagnostic arthroscopy are usually indicated to assess the damage and determine whether or not the ACL is partially torn, avulsed, or surgically repairable (usually it is not). Surgical repair of completely torn collateral ligaments may be necessary. Unfortunately, a knee with torn ligaments is never completely normal afterward, regardless of treatment.

Perhaps because of the normal hyperextension present in the dancer's knee, isolated tears of the ACL do occur. If the MCL is intact, sufficient stability may occur in external rotation of the tibia, in the turned-out position used in ballet, to allow the dancer to continue her career without reconstruction. There is often a striking difference between the stability present in the turned-out position and the stability present in the parallel, or turned-in, position. This makes the prognosis somewhat better in the ballet dancer than the modern dancer who does not turn out and thus stabilize her knee. I recommend conservative treatment of 1+ and 2+ laxities but favor primary repair or reconstruction of 3+ ("loose as a goose") laxities. The others can be reconstructed later if the knee is symptomatic in spite of rehabilitation. If reconstruction is necessary, the infrapatellar tendon with bone blocks is the method of choice.

Meniscal and *coronary ligament problems* in teenage dancers are very rare, and when they occur, it is usually due to an accident that occurs outside dancing. The advent of the MRI study for diagnosis and operative arthroscopy for treatment have been a tremendous boon to the dancer as well as the athlete. Currently, meniscorrhaphy is preferred to meniscectomy whenever possible. Arthrotomy of the knee should be avoided if at all possible in dancers. As with all high-level athletes, postoperative management and rehabilitation are as important as the surgery itself.

The Hip. *Tendinitis* about the hip in dancers is relatively common, especially if they are forcing their turnout. It can be found in the sartorius, rectus femoris, iliopsoas, pectineus, and posteriorly, in the tensor fascia lata and the pyriformis (the "turnout tendon"). Diagnosis is based on the physical exam. The clinician should try to pinpoint the exact location of the tenderness and define which motions are painful when resisted. The most common sites are the sartorius and iliopsoas anteriorly and the pyriformis posteriorly. Treatment includes modified activities and physical therapy until the pain subsides. The recovery time is related to the patient's age and the duration of the symptoms.

Tendon avulsions, either gross or microscopic, are seen fairly often in the early teens before the apophyses have fused. It should be remembered that dancers often have a delayed menarche and skeletal development, leaving the iliac apophyses open at a later skeletal age than might be expected. Avulsions occur in the rectus origin on the anterior inferior iliac spine, the oblique abdominal insertion on the anterior iliac wing, the iliopsoas insertion on the lesser trochanter, and the hamstring origin on the ischial tuberosity. These avulsions heal slowly and may be difficult to diagnose because they are not always apparent on the radiographs. The diagnosis is based on the physical exam. Treatment consists of modified activities until the symptoms and tenderness subside.

Stress fractures of the femoral neck, a cause of hip pain in runners, are rare in dancers.

Finally, some of these young women have hip pain associated with a shallow acetabulum. These dancers with *acetabular dysplasia* usually have excellent turnout because of the shallow socket but ironically contain the seeds of their own destruction. They present initially with recurrent strains and muscle pulls around the hip. The characteristic groin pains usually come later. Any adolescent with recurrent hip or groin pains should be X-rayed to look for this condition. The findings on X ray are subtle (Fig. 27–38). Young dancers with this condition who are persistently symptomatic should not pursue a career in ballet. This condition may be responsible for the high incidence of arthritis of the hip in older ballet dancers.

The Spine. *Scoliosis* was discussed in the younger age group. As well, dancers need also be concerned with several *congenital anomalies*. Conditions such as *bilateral sacralization* of the lower lumbar spine prevent the fifth lumbar segment from functioning normally. The dancer with this condition has to do with four lumbar vertebrae what other dancers do with five. *Hemisacralization of L5*

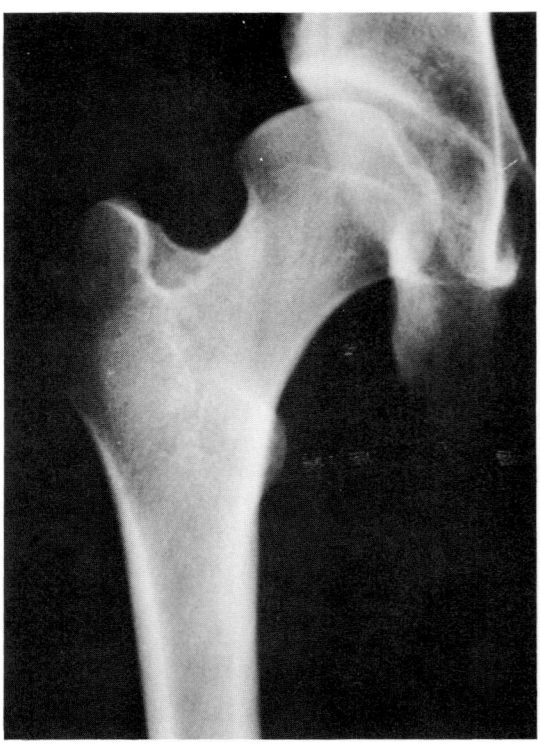

FIGURE 27–38. Acetabular dysplasia.

is even worse because it is as stiff as the bilateral condition but is often more painful and traditionally causes disk disease at the level above on the opposite side.

Segmental fusions or *"block" vertebrae* and *cervical ribs* can become symptomatic in female dancers as they whip the head around when doing pirouettes or turns. The dancer will usually pick out a light or spot in the auditorium to focus on when turning, thus their expression "spotting." Fortunately, this condition is something that they can usually work with.

Lordosis and the need for an extreme range of motion may predispose the teenage dancer to a stress fracture of the pars interarticularis of the lower lumbar spine, resulting in *spondylolysis*. If recognized, diagnosed, and treated, these stress fractures can heal. If unrecognized, they will usually go on to a fibrous union and a permanent condition. The 15- to 18-year-old dancer with recurrent unilateral lumbosacral pain and pain with the *arabesque* on that side has a spondylolysis until proven otherwise. The lesion may be seen on the oblique X ray of the lumbar spine, but like many stress fractures, it may not appear on the film for some time. A bone scan will usually confirm the diagnosis (Fig. 27–39). My clinical impression is that the incidence is about equal between females and males. If the condition is diagnosed early before a diastasis is seen on the radiographs, I recommend a Boston-type brace and no athletics other than swimming for 3 to 6 months. The exact time of enforced rest depends on evidence of healing on subsequent radiographs. If diastasis or a fibrous union is already present at the time of diagnosis, I treat them symptomatically. Occasionally, the back pain can be due to an osteoid osteoma. This benign bone tumor can cause many different pain patterns in the back and can be difficult to diagnose. Fortunately, it is easily seen on a bone scan.

Many ballet schools do not pay enough attention to the upper body strength of their young male dancers. Often there is no preparation for partnering: One day they just begin to lift the girls. This may be appropriate for boys who have good natural development of their upper bodies, but it leaves some underdeveloped. They often fear the appearance of being "muscle-bound." Most young male dancers, especially if they have a history of back problems, should be put on a routine exercise program for the upper extremity and

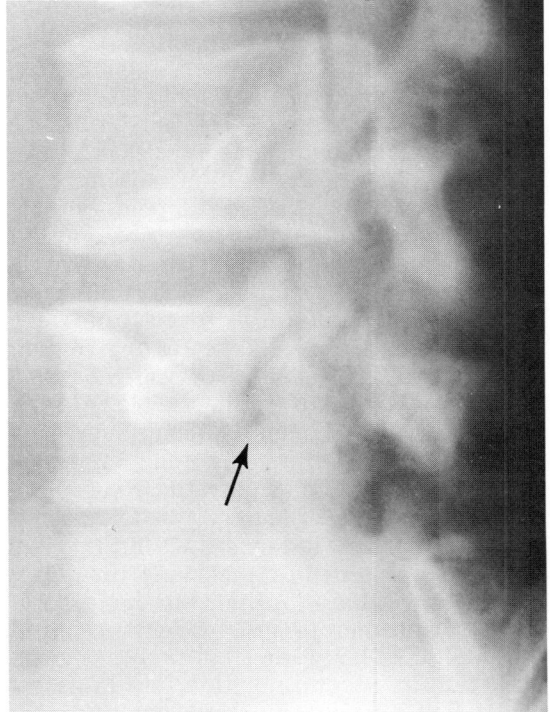

FIGURE 27–39. Spondylolysis.

abdominal muscles. I tell these dancers to do push-ups, pull-ups, and sit-ups with the knees bent as part of their daily bar exercises. Of course, they should be cautioned not to do these exercises when their back is hurting.

If a spondylolysis is present bilaterally, it can allow the spine to slip forward on the vertebra below, resulting in a *spondylolisthesis*. This condition is very common in ballet dancers and gymnasts. It may cause some occasional discomfort, but not to the degree that it does in the general population—perhaps because of the thinness, flexibility, and strength that dancers have. It is usually a small slippage (grade I) and is not a contraindication to a career in dancing.

The problems associated with *disk herniation* and *sciatica* are fortunately rare in young dancers.

REHABILITATION OF THE INJURED DANCER

This topic is far too extensive to be discussed in great detail and is covered in other chapters of this volume, but some principles should be noted. With dance injuries, there are three phases of recovery: the healing phase, the rehabilitation phase, and the return-to-dancing phase. The rehab phase itself has four stages that must be passed through sequentially: motion, strength, endurance, and timing. Each depends on the successful completion of the prior one. Because dancers as a group are directed toward performing regular exercise, it is counterproductive to ask them simply to rest, unless it is *absolutely* necessary. It is better to give them something else to do while they are healing. I have found swimming to be the best alternative to dancing. I usually recommend that they do 25 to 50 laps in a pool, depending on how well they swim, followed by stretching on the side of the pool afterward. The stretching is important because swimming alone tends to tighten the dancer. As the injury heals, I have them do their bar exercises in the pool and then progress from there out of the pool to a "baby bar" that includes *grand pliés* only in second position (not in first or fifth), half turnout in third position, and *relevés* on two feet only. When they are returning to their dancing, I favor a graduated program in stages. For example, when they are ready to do jumps, I tell them to do changements first and, when they are comfortable, jumps on two feet facing the bar, just as they did in children's first division. When that is comfortable, they do jumps on one foot at the bar, then on two feet in center, and finally on one foot in center.

With dancers, one should always look for contributing or predisposing factors that may have played a part in the injury. These may involve an unrecognized weakness or tightness from a prior injury, environmental factors, defects in technique, as well as psychological factors. In a recent study of elite dancers, overachievers were found to have a significantly higher incidence of stress-related injuries. Thus, the very qualities that are necessary in the dancer's continual drive toward physical perfection can also lead to injuries if carried too far.[17] The *team approach* to dance injuries cannot be overemphasized. This team ideally should involve the orthopedist, the physical therapist or trainer, the dance teacher, technique coach or ballet mistress, and occasionally, the psychologist, when emotional factors are involved.

CONCLUSION

Dancing is not a dangerous activity. Serious injuries are rare, and its many benefits, both physical and emotional, far outweigh the few risks involved. It is necessary, however, that dancers recognize their limitations and learn to do the best they can with what they have to work with. Not everyone is going to have the perfect physique, and many physical problems in dancers are the result of trying to get perfect technique from an imperfect body. As the television commercial says: "It's not nice to fool Mother Nature."

References

1. American Academy of Orthopedic Surgeons: Joint Motion: Method of Measuring and Recording. Chicago, IL, 1965.
2. Balanchine G.: Personal communication.
3. Bean J. A., Leeper J. D., Wallace R. B., et al: Variations in the reporting of menstrual histories. Am J Epidemiol 109: 181–185, 1979.
4. Bernstein R. H., Bartolomei F. J., McCarthy D. J.: The sinus tarsi syndrome: anatomical, clinical and surgical considerations. J Am Podiatry Assoc 75(9):475–480, 1985.
5. Brooks-Gunn J.: Antecedents and consequences of variations in girls' maturational timing. J Adolescent Health Care 9:365–373, 1988.
6. Brooks-Gunn J., Burrow C., Warren M. P.: Attitudes toward eating and body weight in different groups of female adolescent athletes. In J Eating Dis 7:749–758, 1988.
7. Brooks-Gunn J. Warren M. P.: The effects of delayed menarche in different contexts: dance and nondance students. J Youth Adolescence 14:285–300, 1985.
8. Brooks-Gunn J., Warren M. P., Hamilton L. H.: The relationship of eating problems to amenorrhea in ballet dancers. Med Sci Sports Exerc 9:41–44, 1987.
9. Calabrese L. H., Kirkendall D. T.: Nutritional and medical considerations in dancers. Clin Sports Med 2:539–548, 1983.
10. Dunning J.: But First a School: The First Fifty Years of the School of American Ballet. New York, Viking Press, 1985.
11. Frish R. E., Wyshak G., Vincent L.: Delayed menarche and amenorrhea in ballet dancers. New Engl J Med 303:17–18, 1980.
12. Garner D. M., Garfunkel P. E.: Socio-cultural factors in the development of anorexia nervosa. Psychol Med 10:646–656, 1980.
13. Gould N., Seligson D., Gassman J.: Early and late repair of the lateral ligament of the ankle. Foot Ankle 4:84–89, 1980.
14. Hamilton L. H., Brooks-Gunn J., Warren M. P.: Nutritional intake of female ballet dancers: a reflection of eating problems. Int J Eating Dis 5:109–118, 1986.
15. Hamilton L. H., Brooks-Gunn J., Warren M. P., Hamilton W. G.: The impact of thinness and

dieting on the professional ballet dancer. J Med Prob Perf Artists, pp 117–122, Dec 1987.
16. Hamilton L. H., Brooks-Gunn J., Warren M. P., Hamilton W. G.: The role of selectivity in the pathogenesis of eating problems in ballet dancers. Med Sci Sports Exerc 20 (6):560–565, 1988.
17. Hamilton L. H., Hamilton W. H., Meltzer J. D., Marshall P, Molnar M.: Personality, stress, and injuries in professional ballet dancers. Am J Sports Med 17(2):263–267, 1989.
18. Hamilton W. G.: Tendinitis about the ankle joint in classical ballet dancers; "dancer's tendinitis." J Sports Med 5:84, 1977.
19. Hamilton W. G.: Post traumatic peroneal tendon weakness in classical ballet dancers. Am Orthop Soc Sports Med, Lake Placid, NY, July 1978.
20. Hamilton W. G.: The best body for ballet. Dance Mag, 82–83, Oct 1982.
21. Hamilton W. G.: Sprained ankles in ballet dancers. Foot Ankle 3(2):99–102, 1982.
22. Hamilton W. G.: Stenosing tenosynovitis of the flexor hallucis longus tendon and posterior impingement upon the os trigonum in ballet dancers. Foot Ankle 3(2):74–80, 1982.
23. Hamilton W. G.: Surgical anatomy of the foot and ankle. CIBA Clin Symp 37 (3), 1985.
24. Hamilton W. G.: Physical prerequisites for ballet dancers. J Musculoskel Med 13: 61–66, 1986.
25. Hamilton W. G.: Foot and ankle injuries in dancers. In Yokum L (ed): Sports Clinics of North America, Philadelphia, Williams & Wilkins, 1988.
26. Hamilton W. G., Thompson F. M.: The Brostrom/Gould repair for lateral ankle instability. Presented at the American Academy of Orthopedic Surgeons, Las Vegas, NV, 1989. (Submitted to Foot and Ankle for publication)
27. Hamilton W. G., Marshall D., Molnar M.: A profile of the musculoskeletal characteristics of elite professional ballet dancers. (Submitted to Am J Sports Med).
28. Harburn T., Ross H.: Avulsion fracture of the anterior calcaneal process. Phys Sports Med 15(4): pp, 1987.
29. Howse J. A. G.: Posterior block of the ankle joint in dancers. Foot Ankle 3(2):31–84, 1982.
30. Jones R: Fractures of the fifth metatarsal bone. Liverpool Med Surg J 42:103, 1902.
31. Klieger B.: Anterior tibiotalar impingement syndromes in dancers. Foot Ankle 3(2):69–73, 1982.
32. Kliman M., Gross A., Pritzker P., Greyson D.: Osteochondritis of the hallux sesamoid bones. Foot Ankle 3(4):220–223, 1983.
33. Marshall P. M., Hamilton W. G.: Subluxation of the cuboid in professional ballet dancers. (Submitted)
34. Michael R. H., Holder L. E.: The soleus syndrome: a cause of medial tibial stress. Am J Sports Med 13(2):87–94, 1985.
35. Miller E. H., Schneider H. J., Bronson J. L.: A new consideration in athletic injuries—the classical ballet dancer. Clin Orthop 111:181, 1975.
36. Newell S., Woodie A.: Cuboid syndrome. Phys Sports Med 9(4):71–76, 1981.
37. Nicholas J. A.: Risk factors, sports medicine and the orthopedic system: an overview. J Sports Med 3:243–258, 1976.
38. Parkes J. C., Hamilton W. G., Patterson A. H., Rawles, J. G.: The anterior impingement syndrome of the ankle. J Trauma 20(40):895–898, 1980.
39. Quirk R.: The talar compression syndrome in dancers. Foot Ankle 3(2):65–68, 1982.
40. Richardson G.: Injuries to the hallucal sesamoids in the athlete. Foot Ankle 7(4):229–244, 1987.
41. Sammarco J.: The dancer's hip. Clin Sports Med 2(3):385–398, 1983.
42. Schantz P. G., Astrand P.: Physiological characteristics of classical ballet. Med Sci Sports Exerc 16:472–476, 1984.
43. Taillard W., Meyer J. M., Garcia J., Blanco V.: The sinus tarsi syndrome. Int Orthop 5(2): 117–130, 1981.
44. Thompson F. M., Hamilton W. G.: Problem of the second metatarsophalangeal joint. Orthopedics 10(1):83–89, 1987.
45. Thompson T. C., Terwilliger C.: The terminal Syme operation for ingrown toenail. Surg Clin North Am 31:575, 1951.
46. Tomasen E.: Diseases and Injuries of Ballet Dancers. Denmark, Universitetsforlaget D Arhus, 1982.
47. Warren M. P.: The effects of exercise on pubertal progression and reproductive function in girls. J Clin Endocrinol 51:115–157, 1980.
48. Warren M. P., Brooks-Gunn J., Hamilton L. H., Warren F., Hamilton W. G.: Scoliosis and fractures in young ballet dancers: relationship to delayed menarcheal age and amenorrhea. New Engl J Med 314:1338–1353, 1986.
49. Winter R. B.: Adolescent idiopathic scoliosis. New Engl J Med 314:1370–1380, 1986.
50. Wolin T., Glassman F., Sideman S., Leventhal D.: Internal derangement of the talofibular component of the ankle. Surg Gynecol Obstet 91:193–200, 1950.
51. Moe J.: Personal communication, 1969.

28
WRESTLING

RANDALL R. WROBLE
JAMES T. HOEGH
JOHN P. ALBRIGHT

Wrestling is one of the most ancient of sports. Artifacts recovered from a 5000-year-old Sumerian temple depicted wrestlers in action. In an ancient Egyptian wall painting from 1850 BC, a "manual of wrestling" documented the course of a match and demonstrated knowledge of many holds still used today. In the *Iliad*, Homer gives a detailed description of a wrestling match. Later in classical Greece, wrestling was one of the sports contested in the Olympics and was an important part of the physical training of every young man. In addition, early roots of wrestling are found in central Asia, Japan, and China.

The modern sport of amateur wrestling emerged in the 1870s and 1880s from club tournaments in the New York area and was termed *American folkstyle*. The first college teams were at Yale, Columbia, Penn, and Princeton, with the first college championships held in 1905 in Philadelphia. Weight classes were established, and early matches consisted of three 10-minute periods. The United States sent its first wrestling team to the Olympics in 1904. The sport grew steadily as evidenced that by 1924, 3000 athletes competed for spots on the U.S. Olympic team.[34]

Currently, wrestling remains a popular youth, high school, and college sport. An important element in its popularity relates to the opportunity for participation by men and boys of all sizes. In 1981, the National Federation of High Schools listed wrestling as the fifth most popular sport for boys, involving 300,000 to 400,000 participants annually.[44] Thousands of wrestlers from several hundred institutions compete at the college level each year.

In virtually all reports examining injury rates in sports, the number of injuries in wrestling is significantly high, often second only to football. Why this high injury rate? First, wrestling is a contact sport, and unlike many other similarly designated sports, contact in wrestling occurs virtually 100 percent of the time. There is no question that this increases the at-risk period. Second, wrestling is also a collision sport. Collisions occur when one wrestler "shoots" or attempts a takedown. Injuries occur during takedowns because of the explosive nature of these moves. We have clearly demonstrated that the takedown is indeed the truly highest risk situation in wrestling.[67]

Wrestling rules ban certain holds or moves that obviously exert potentially injurious torque or force to the extremities or spine.[1, 32] These fall into two categories. The first includes the full nelson (Fig. 28–1); choke holds; hammerlocks with elbow flexion past 90 degrees (Fig. 28–2); twisting of the flexed knee out of the sagittal plane (Fig. 28–3); twisting or hyperextension of individual fingers; forceful "slamming" of an opponent to the mat; headlocks without an arm included (Fig. 28–4); head scissors (Fig. 28–5); any hold over the mouth, eyes, or the anterior throat; holds that bend, twist, or force the

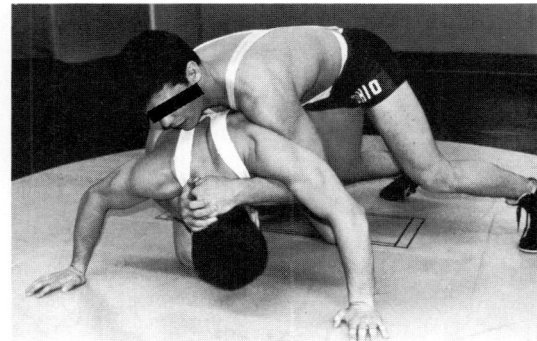

FIGURE 28–1. Full nelson.

head or extremities beyond their normal range of motion; or any hold administered for punishment alone. Should these situations arise, the referee stops the action and calls an "illegal hold." The opponent of the offending wrestler is given one point for the first time this occurs in a match. The second violation called for an illegal hold also results in a one-point penalty. The third violation mandates a two-point award, and the fourth, disqualification. Should an opponent injured by application of an illegal hold be unable to continue, the aggressor forfeits the match.

A second group of holds are deemed "potentially dangerous."[1,32] These are legal holds that when applied with excessive force may cause injury. Examples of potentially dangerous holds are the double wristlock, hyper–plantarflexion of the ankle (note that this is an illegal hold in high school) (Fig. 28–6), the chicken wing or arm bar when turned into a twisting hammerlock (Fig. 28–7), and hyperextension–abduction of the shoulder (Fig. 28–8). When the referee makes this call, the match is stopped and restarted as if the wrestlers had gone out of bounds. No penalty points are assessed.

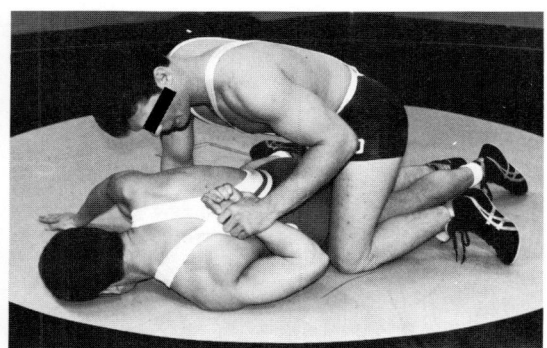

FIGURE 28–2. Hammerlock. The elbow is flexed past 90 degrees.

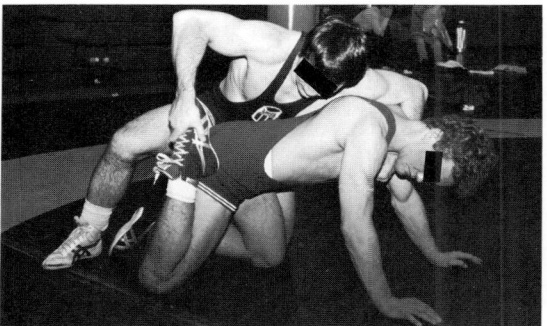

FIGURE 28–3. Valgus force applied to the flexed knee. (From Wroble, R. R., Mysnyk, M. C., Foster, D. T., and Albright, J. P.: Patterns of Knee Injuries in Wrestling at the University of Iowa—A Six Year Study. Am J Sports Med, 14:55–66, American Orthopaedic Society for Sports Medicine, 1986.)

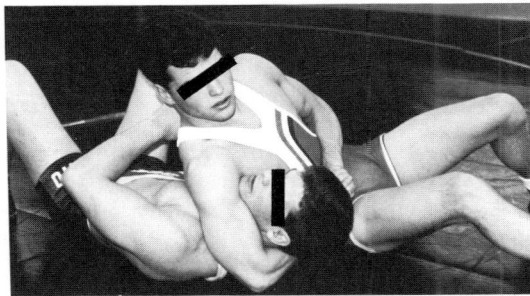

FIGURE 28–4. Headlock applied without an arm included.

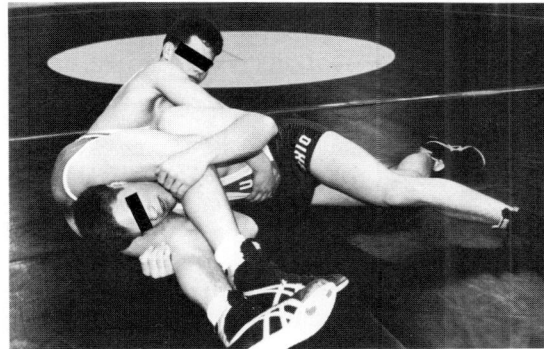

FIGURE 28–5. Head scissors.

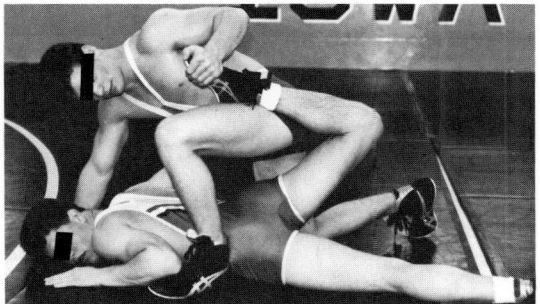

FIGURE 28–6. Ankle hyper–plantarflexion.

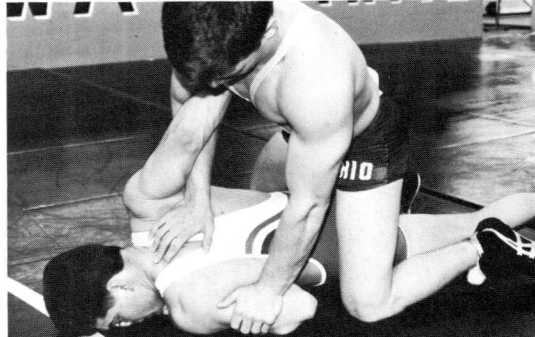

FIGURE 28–7. Arm bar used as a twisting hammerlock.

Rules such as these have substantially reduced the number of injuries in wrestling and have certainly discouraged the use of dangerous practices by wrestlers.

It is also clear, however, that while the injury rate is much higher in matches, most wrestling injuries occur during practice, reflecting the vast amount of time the average wrestler spends in preparation for a match. Wrestlers are also at higher risk for injury early in the season or if they have sustained a previous injury to a given body part.[65,67] Tournaments carry greater risk than dual meets. Tournaments entail wrestling three to six times per day, often with only a 1-hour rest between matches. Because there are so many matches, a minor injury that would go unnoticed in a dual meet can easily progress to a significant injury when five more matches have to be wrestled within that same day, with resulting potential for aggravation. For these reasons, we recommend that a qualified athletic trainer or team physician be present at all wrestling practices and matches.

When covering a wrestling match or tournament, the physician or trainer must realize that several other rules of wrestling come into play. If an injury occurs during a match and time is called, the referee instructs the scorer to start an injury time clock. Once the clock starts, the wrestler has limited time—only 2 minutes (90 seconds in college)—to resume wrestling or to default the match. This time is cumulative throughout the match but does not include time taken for control of bleeding. During that 2 minutes, the health care professional must make a decision regarding participation. In a tournament setting with multiple matches on the same or consecutive days, defeat due to injury default does not eliminate an athlete from further wrestling in the tournament. However, the tournament medical personnel are responsible for determining his ability to compete.

Once a wrestler has been injured and a plan for treatment is being developed, one must take into consideration an additional factor—noncompliance. An endemic problem among wrestlers, we have found a relationship between this and increased rate of injury recurrence. In the group of wrestlers we studied at the University of Iowa, only about half were considered compliant. Additionally, we use the term *compliance* in a relative sense. Using a strict definition, probably none of our wrestlers would have been called compliant. The noncompliant group's injury recurrence rate was over twice that of our compliant group's.[67] While our impression is that compliance is better in the school-age wrestler, noncompliance and its

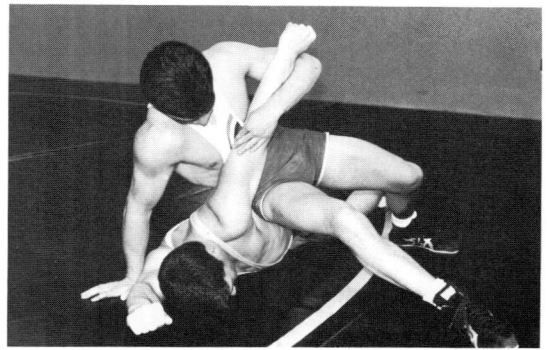

FIGURE 28–8. Shoulder hyperextension–abduction.

TABLE 28–1. Percentage of Injuries by Anatomical Region, University of Iowa, 1976–1977 to 1983–1984

	Percentage of Total
Head, neck, face	31.0
Head	3.0
Neck	12.0
Ear	5.5
Face	8.0
Teeth	2.5
Upper extremity	22.0
Shoulder	12.0
Arm, elbow, forearm	5.0
Wrist, hand	5.0
Trunk and lower back	10.0
Lower extremity	37.0
Hip, thigh	4.0
Knee	24.0
Leg, ankle	8.0
Foot	1.0

effect on reinjury must be considered in treating these athletes as well.

In our 7-year review of wrestling injuries at the University of Iowa, we found that the most commonly injured anatomical regions were the knee; the head, neck, and face; the shoulder; the trunk and back; and the ankle (Table 28–1).[65] We will go into detail about some of the more common injuries we have encountered. Particular attention will be paid to mechanism of injury and to treatment methods where they are specific to the sport of wrestling.

HEAD, NECK, AND FACE INJURIES

Injuries to these areas make up about 30 percent of the total of all wrestling injuries.

CONCUSSION

Concussion[8,13,14] is a reversible pathophysiological condition of the brain occurring without identifiable structural damage to the brain itself. Clinically characterized by immediate but transient impairment in the level of consciousness, it is usually associated with blurred vision and loss of equilibrium and memory.

We have typically seen three or four per year out of a group of 30 to 35 college wrestlers, most often mild but occasionally moderate in severity. The most common mechanism is head-head or head-knee collision during takedowns. Less commonly, concussions are produced by contact with a wrestling mat. The padding of the mat and the proscription of slamming an opponent to the mat make serious head injury less likely via this mechanism.

Clinically, concussion has been divided into three categories. Mild or *grade 1 concussion* applies to a patient with slight disorientation without loss of consciousness. Dizziness without loss of equilibrium or memory may occur. The patient is slow to get up, feels fatigued, or is somewhat confused. Headache may or may not be present.

Moderate or *grade 2 concussion* is defined as loss of consciousness for 3 to 5 minutes, then subsequent disorientation and presence of retrograde amnesia (loss of memory for events immediately preceding the injury) lasting up to 24 hours.

Severe or *grade 3 concussion* consists of loss of consciousness for greater than 5 minutes or posttraumatic amnesia lasting more than 24 hours. These patients are at risk for developing intracranial hemorrhage.

The unconscious wrestler should be assumed to have a concomitant cervical injury and should be treated as such. Priorities also include maintenance of ventilation by ensuring patency of the nasopharynx (clear of secretions and/or vomitus).

In the most common cases, the wrestler is responsive—that is, mild to moderate concussion—and initial exam[8] assesses the level of consciousness and the status of the cervical spine. Items to be included are:

1. *Evidence of cervical spine injury.* Can the wrestler localize the pain in his neck? Is he numb anywhere? Can he move all four extremities?
2. *Level of unconsciousness.* Was the wrestler unconscious briefly? How long did he remain that way? Could he get up initially? If so, was he very unsteady?
3. *Balance and dizziness.* Is the wrestler able to stand up and walk unaided in a straight line? Can he close his eyes and maintain his balance?
4. *Vision.* Does bright light hurt his eyes? Can he see the examiner clearly? Are there any visual field defects? Are his pupils equal?
5. *Occult evidence of skull fracture.* Is there any discharge from the ears or nose or signs of contusions or lacerations about the face or head that would indicate a more serious head injury than the level of consciousness would lead one to believe? Are there any contusions or lacerations about the face or head that would indicate possible skull fracture? Are there any areas of ecchymosis, bogginess, crepitus, or tenderness any place on the skull, particularly behind the earlobes or the temporal regions and anterior and superior to the ears? These signs would indicate a skull fracture.
6. *Orientation.* Is the wrestler oriented to time (What day is it? What period is it? How much time is left in the match? What is the score?); place (Who are we wrestling? What town is this?); person (Who am I? What is the coach's name?).
7. *Retrograde memory.* What street clothes did you wear to the match today? What is your team's won and loss record this year?

TABLE 28–2. Concussion—Return to Competition Criteria

Fully alert
No dizziness, headache, anisocoria
Absence of amnesia and impaired concentration
History of less than two previous concussions

Give strong consideration to neurosurgical consultation in wrestlers with moderate or grade 2 concussion. Unconsciousness for greater than 5 minutes (grade 3), progressively worsening headache, or presence of any focal neurological deficit dictates immediate transport to a hospital for further evaluation.

Criteria for return to action are somewhat less well defined[8,14] (Table 28–2). Because of the limited amount of injury time, when a concussion occurs during a match, decisions need to be made promptly. Wrestlers with mild concussion may return to a match or to practice without known risk of sequelae only if they first become fully alert, without dizziness, headache, anisocoria, persistent retrograde amnesia, or impaired concentration. With more severe concussions, care should be taken to ensure that the completely asymptomatic, preinjury neurological state has been reached before return to competition. This may frequently take 1 to 2 weeks for moderate concussions and 1 month for severe concussions.

In about 10 percent of severe concussions, a decrease in ability to process information occurs. This impairment is greater and lasts longer with repeated concussions, suggesting a cumulative effect.[8,14] It is generally felt, therefore, that three concussions in a given sport are sufficient to give consideration to terminating participation in that sport at least for one season, if not permanently.

NOSEBLEEDS AND LACERATIONS

Lacerations occur commonly to the eyebrow region and to the lips. The former occurs when the supraorbital ridge impacts against the opponent's head or knee, resulting in a crushing, tearing type wound. The latter results when the lip is violently struck against the teeth, again commonly on contact with the opponent's head or knee. In this case, the wound is made by the teeth cutting the lip. As with concussions, these situations usually arise during takedowns.

If a laceration occurs during a match, the referee will call time-out promptly should bleeding be any more than minimal. In order for the match to continue, the blood flow must be stopped. Time does not permit suturing the wound (but note that the 90-second injury time limit does not apply for bleeding). We have found several treatment techniques to be effective. First, a brief period of compression is attempted. If the bleeding stops, this is followed merely by application of a small amount of bacitracin ointment. If it is apparent that this treatment will be ineffective, one of two options is available. Pressure dressings offer the advantage of keeping the wound clean but must be applied properly or they are apt to fall off. They must be applied to a (relatively) dry, sticky surface. To achieve this in a profusely sweating wrestler requires the use of collodion or an adhesive spray to the forehead. The dressing is applied circumferentially below the greatest diameter of the skull (i.e., below the occiput and frontal prominence). It must be put on extremely tightly to prevent slipping. It may even cause a headache when needed tension is used. The ears and supraorbital ridge help prevent downward migration of the bandage. Alternatively, we employ adhesive spray, followed by Steristrips or butterfly strips. This provides the best apposition of skin edges but is more difficult because of the sweating of the skin in the area.

Primary suture, the obvious treatment of choice for all but the smallest lacerations, is performed as soon as practical after completion of the match. Facial lacerations can be safely closed up to 24 hours postinjury. We generally use a 6/0 nonabsorbable monofilament suture that is not black (this simplifies suture removal from the eyebrows by eliminating confusion between hair and suture). In wrestling, lacerations rarely involve layers deeper than the skin, but should the galea be involved, it should be closed in a separate layer with absorbable sutures.

The lip consists of three layers: the mucosa, subcutaneous tissue, and muscle (orbicularis oris), from superficial to deep. Involvement of the deep layers is reasonably common. Best results are achieved by closure in layers after adequate anesthesia is obtained by infiltration with 1 percent lidocaine with epinephrine. Muscle is closed with 3/0 chromic suture, whereas the subcutaneous tissue and skin are closed with 4/0 chromic suture. With large, deep lacerations within the mouth, Penicillin V, 500 mg, four times a day, is given orally for 1 week.

Nosebleeds occur commonly owing to a combination of trauma and drying of the nasal mucosa secondary to relative dehydration and generally low ambient relative humidity in gyms and wrestling rooms. Most occur in the anterior region of the nose.[56] Digital compression is initially employed, followed by introducing a cotton plug (a cut-down tampon is effective) soaked in 1 percent phenylephrine (Neo-Synephrine) into the nose. After 1 or 2 minutes, when ready to resume wrestling, the nostril is packed with a cylindrical gauze plug or cut-down tampon covered with Vaseline.

AURICULAR HEMATOMA

An all-too-common wrestling injury, auricular hematoma (Fig. 28–9) results from direct trauma to the ear, either on direct impact with another wrestler's head or knee, causing it to be smashed against the mastoid process, or by abrasive, friction-causing forces as when wrestlers "tie up" while standing. A small amount of blood then accumulates beneath the perichondrium of the external ear. It is very important to recognize that while most often hematomas result when wrestling headgear is not being worn, hematomas can and do happen with headgear on![51] Once the wrestler begins to sweat, the headgear can slide and *cause* the hematoma itself by abrading the external ear. Several design features contribute to this—shallow depth of the ear piece, an inadequate number of straps for fixation, and construction with slick plastic materials that allow sliding of the headgear.

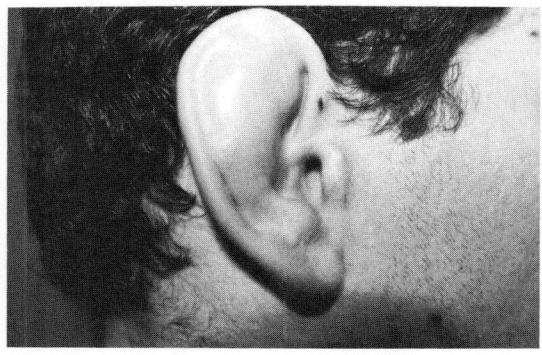

FIGURE 28–9. An inadequately treated or untreated auricular hematoma can evolve into this deformity—the cauliflower ear.

We currently recommend headgear with four straps (chin, forehead, crown, and occiput) and with deep ear pieces. We often add a $\frac{1}{4}$-inch to $\frac{1}{2}$-inch Plastizote "donut" around the ear piece to increase its depth further (Fig. 28–10). Headgear is required during all matches. We also recommend that it be worn by all wrestlers at all practices.

Historically, treatment has been apparently ineffective for several reasons. First, and most unfortunate, is that some wrestlers regard the "cauliflower ear" as a mark of distinction that identifies them immediately as a wrestler. Education is the answer to this sort of abhorrent thinking. Second, treatment *is* painful and may be avoided on that basis. Third, a wrestler may shy away from treatment because of fear of being told he needs to take time off.

The acute hematoma requires prompt needle aspiration by or under direct supervision of a physician. We must emphasize the strict use of aseptic techniques. Should an infection arise in the subperichondrial space, cartilage necrosis with loss of a great portion of the external ear may ensue. Approximately 2 to 3 cc of blood can be aspirated from the typical acute hematoma and is routinely sent for aerobic and anaerobic culture and sensitivity. A 1-inch 19-gauge *short bevel, thin wall* needle works well and is our preference. It provides a large inner diameter that seems less apt to clog and allows removal of more viscous fluid. Following aspiration, we have used two types of pressure dressings. Our preference is the collodion cast (Fig. 28–11). It is applied in the following manner: Apply digital pressure until post-aspiration bleeding in the ear stops, dry the ear thoroughly, then pour about 1 ounce of collodion into a cut-down paper cup and assemble ten to twelve 1- to 1$\frac{1}{2}$-inch strips of $\frac{1}{2}$-inch Nu-Gauze.

Place a Q-tip in the external meatus so that the collodion does not run down into the auditory canal. Saturate each strip of Nu-Gauze with collodion and then wring them out with the gloved fingertips. Use the Q-tips to get good "total" apposition of the collodion-soaked strips onto the ear. The strips begin at the top of the ear well above the start of the lesion. Each strip starts over the back of the ear and then runs down over the helix and antihelix. Use the Q-tips to push the gauze down against the ear in all places. Lay on strips continuously, overlapping by about one-half of the width of the strip. Carry the

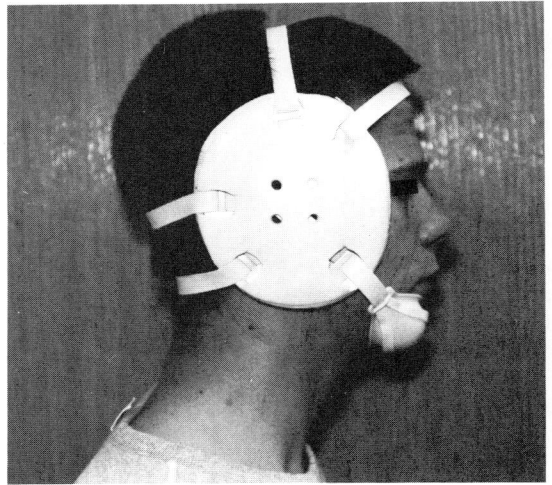
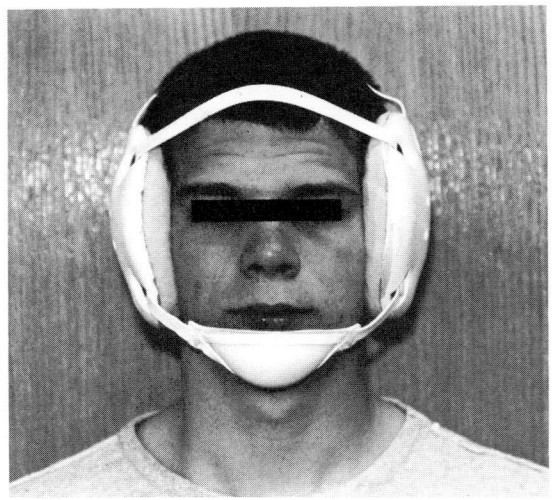
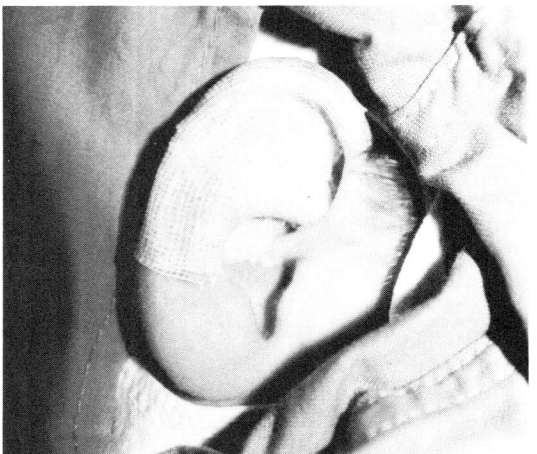

FIGURE 28–10. Headgear that we recommend. Note the location and position of the four straps and the depth of the ear pieces. (A) Side and (B) front views. (C) With the headgear removed, the additional Plastizote around each ear piece is apparent.

FIGURE 28–11. Close-up view of a newly applied collodion cast.

strips down the entire length of the ear. After completing this first layer, apply a second identical layer over the first. Paint the entire cast thoroughly with additional collodion to get a very slick-looking appearance. A hair dryer may be used to dry the cast faster. Intermittent pressure must be kept on the cast during the procedure if the ear is actively bleeding.

Advise the patient that he may not practice wrestling for 24 hours and that he should not sleep on the newly formed cast. Inform him that the cast should be hard in 30 minutes but that it should not get wet that night. He may practice the next day.

Warn each wrestler in a collodion cast of the consequences of infection. They should follow up in 2 days by phone. If there is re-

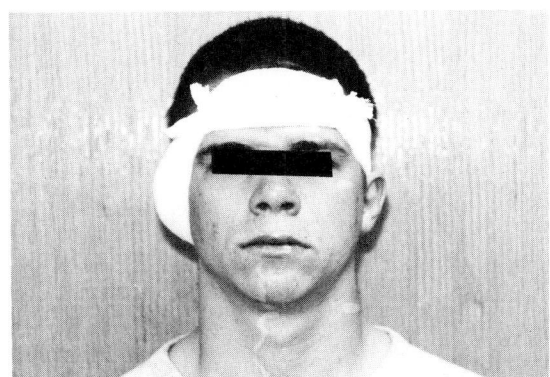

FIGURE 28–12. A standard mastoid dressing.

currence in the cast, reaspiration and recasting are appropriate. Total duration of casting is 5 to 7 days. We estimate that there is a 25 percent chance of recurrence if the wrestler returns to participation on the next day. There is a 10 percent recurrence rate if the wrestler stays out until cast removal.

Remove collodion casts by soaking for 10 minutes with rubbing alcohol placed on by four-by-fours. After this, the cast is cut along the edge of the helix and pulled off very gently, as the hairs in the ear make it painful to do otherwise.

Our second choice consists of wet cotton molded to the shape of the ear, followed by a standard mastoid dressing (Fig. 28–12). This is changed daily with concomitant reaspiration if fluid has reaccumulated. If fluid continues to accumulate after 3 days, we recommend referral to an otolaryngologist. This technique allows serial observation of the ear, but it makes competing or practicing difficult. (If used, it is best—but not absolutely required—that the wrestler sit out 2 to 3 days.) Our success rate with both these methods has been very high when we get wrestlers to come in acutely and to comply with instructions.

NECK[65]

Amateur wrestling at the high school and collegiate levels very rarely results in a fatality or paralysis from head or neck injury.[46] Noncatastrophic injuries to the neck, however, are common despite generally superior neck muscle strength among wrestlers. The cumulative effects of neck injuries are seen in some wrestlers as evidenced by an increasing incidence of degenerative changes on radiographs, by the incidence of days lost from acute injuries among collegiate and club wrestlers, and by long-term symptoms reported by ex-wrestlers.

The incidence of neck injury at the grade school and high school levels is low, but the patterns of injury are basically the same as at the college level. The maneuver of bulling the neck into hyperextended position while attempting, or blocking, a takedown appears to be associated with the greatest number of neck injuries (Fig. 28–13).

The majority of legal claims for severe neck injuries in athletics focus not on faulty equipment but on the techniques for the initial treatment and transportation of the athlete. Thus, health care professionals must be thoroughly familiar with the guidelines of safe on-the-mat care and must be certain that their medical staff is well drilled in the techniques involved.

In wrestling, the most common presentation of neck injury is acute neck pain with or without radiation. The first responsibility of the health care professional is to determine the nature and severity of the injury and make a correct decision regarding continuance of participation despite extrinsic pressures of the moment.

ON-THE-MAT ASSESSMENT OF ACUTE NECK INJURIES

The on-the-mat exam consists of the following: The minimum historical information requires determining the location of pain; the

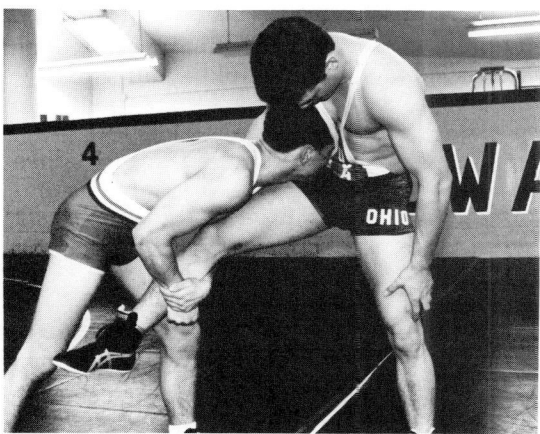

FIGURE 28–13. During a takedown, the neck is extended while the wrestler forcefully drives straight forward, producing hyperextension plus axial load.

detailed mechanism of the injury with particular attention paid to the position of the head and neck at the time of injury; aggravating and relieving factors (such as coughing, sneezing, or traction); presence, location, and duration of any neurological symptoms; and history of previous neck injury.

In addition to the neurological findings of motor weakness, deep tendon reflex changes, and sensory loss, the most reliable clinical tests involve the identification of the site of maximal tenderness, the position that produces the most pain, and finally, range-of-motion (ROM) testing.

The wrestler must be asked to remain supine. He is informed that his cooperation in relaxing muscles at critical points will help to determine the nature of his injury. Palpation is performed to identify the site of maximum tenderness. Cases of neurologic deficit or in which pain or localized tenderness suggest even a slight possibility of cervical instability are immobilized and transported to a hospital for full evaluation.

Wrestlers with apparently minor injuries are examined for active and finally gentle passive range of motion (Fig. 28–14). The examiner should move the head slowly through the entire range of motion. The position producing the most pain is noted. Whether the pain is more severe with flexion or extension is of help in the differential diagnosis. For example, increased pain with flexion suggests extensor strain, distraction injury to the posterior elements, or acute cervical disk herniation. Conversely, increased pain with extension suggests posterior element compression fracture, facet joint sprain, or traumatic compression neuritis. When discomfort is noticed, slight traction should be placed on the head in the same position to see if distraction will bring relief. This maneuver lowers intervertebral pressure and widens the neural foramina and so potentially decreases pressure on nerve roots, lessening concomitant pain.

The next step is to determine the effect of axial compression of the spine against the examiner's hand or leg. Isometric contraction of the cervical musculature, applied by creating slight pressure against the examiner's hand during repeat palpation of the tender spot, is then checked to assess possible instability.

On the mat, it is not important to establish the difference between brachial plexus and nerve root injury. Since neurological involvement with motor or sensory loss determines whether an athlete should continue wrestling, be held out for observation, or referred for consultation, direct the neurological exam toward those areas. Although impairment can be determined by testing for sensation, motor function, and deep tendon reflexes (DTRs), systematically evaluating each nerve root level, sensory testing takes the most time and is the least reliable test in an acutely injured athlete. By far the best and most obvious impairment estimate on the mat can be obtained by spending time establishing the presence or absence of muscular weakness.

In general, when dealing with athletes, as opposed to the rest of the population, it is best to gain the maximum mechanical advantage possible in order to develop the most sensitivity in picking up even minor weaknesses (Fig. 28–15). The first sign to appear (and the last to leave) is early fatigability of the muscle. Prolonged recovery time is also characteristic of an injured motor unit. Therefore, motor testing should always be repeated three to four times for each muscle in question. On the mat, time constraints may dictate checking each group only once. We recommend testing the cervical spine flexors and extensors, deltoid (C5), biceps and wrist extensors (C6), triceps (C7), finger flexors (C8), and finger abductors (T1).

The degree of weakness should if possible be recorded as percentage of the normal opposite side. This sort of "percentage of normal" information proves valuable in the recovery phase in assessing the wrestler's readiness to return to action.

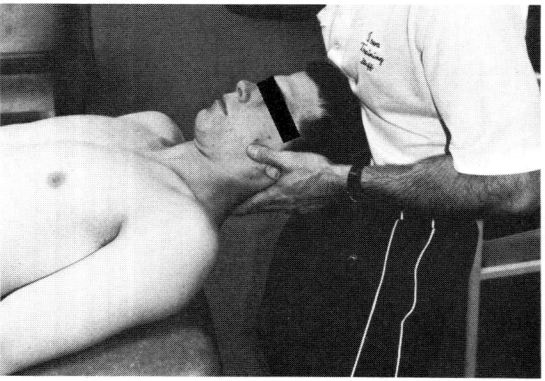

FIGURE 28–14. The ideal position for examining the cervical spine. The athlete is supine with his head and neck supported over the table's end.

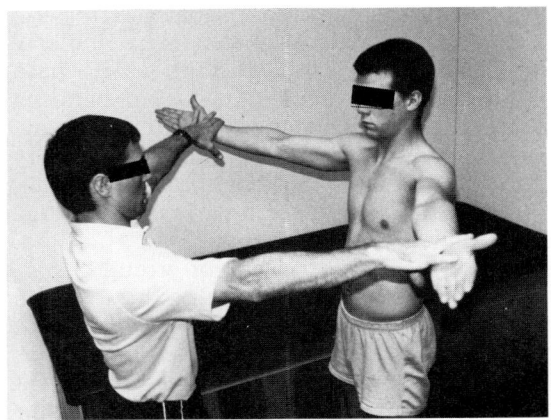

FIGURE 28–15. Test of deltoid strength. The more distal the examiner places his or her hands, the greater the mechanical advantage and thus the sensitivity of the test.

It is obvious that treatment is determined by the severity of the findings on examination. In no instance should a wrestler return to action until a full, pain-free range of motion has returned, neurological symptoms have disappeared, strength has normalized, and the axial compression test is negative. Suggestion of significant ligamentous sprain or presence of a transient radiculopathy requires at least a period of observation before deciding on a final disposition. If any doubt remains in the examiner's mind as to the risk of further injury on immediate return to action, the wrestler should be held out. Any suspicion of fracture or ligamentous injury sufficient to create clinical instability requires immediate splinting and transfer to an emergency room for radiographs and more definitive diagnosis. Any wrestler who must be held out for the remainder of a match or misses more than 1 day of practice or one match should have radiographic evaluation. We have noted, however, that radiographic differentiation of old from new injury is very difficult owing to the frequent presence of radiographic changes in even the youngest collegians.

When referral to an emergency room facility is indicated, it is essential that information about mechanism and progression of injury be relayed to the responsible consulting physician or that a member of the primary care team stays with the wrestler until the need for consultation is determined.

ACUTE CERVICAL STRAIN

A cervical strain is a tear of one of the musculotendinous units in the neck. The muscles most commonly involved include the trapezius, the sternocleidomastoids, the erector spinae, the scalenes, levator scapulae, and the rhomboids. The spectrum of injury ranges from mild to moderate, with rupture being extremely rare. These injuries all result from mechanical overloading with forces too great for the extensor mechanism to withstand. Sprain injuries to ligaments and capsular structures of the cervical spine itself are frequently seen with concomitant muscle strain syndromes, thus often making it difficult to differentiate between the two. The usual mechanism for sprains is a hyperextension twisting injury.

The course of the injury is usually fairly characteristic. At first, there is localized pain and tenderness with localized inhibition of voluntary muscle contraction. With a sprain, pain tends to be less localized but, nonetheless, is confined to the neck and interscapular area and possibly the upper arm in a nonradicular pattern. Initially, even the most severe injury can appear quite benign. After the first few minutes, the immediate pain of the injury will subside and range of motion will remain full. Often, the only sign is weakness demonstrated through an inability to resist the examiner's hand. Muscle soreness and swelling with limitation of motion do not appear to reach a maximum until several hours after the competition is over. With mild strains, the discomfort may not be noticed until awakening the next morning. With a pure strain injury, bending of the neck to the contralateral side produces pain. In contrast, with sprains, extension and ipsilateral bending are the most painful. In addition with strains, distraction may cause discomfort because of stretching the injured muscle. With sprains, axial compression, particularly in extension, produces pain by causing periarticular tissue to impinge on nerve roots. The degree of limitation of motion, soft tissue swelling, and discomfort at 24 to 48 hours after the injury serve as prognostic signs. There are no neurological deficits (except motor weakness secondary to pain) and no radicular symptoms. Radiographs are normal.

Most of the acute injuries in this category can be treated symptomatically, with occasional brief immobilization in a hard cervical

TABLE 28–3. Acute Neck Injury—Return to Competition Criteria

Full, pain-free range of motion
No neurological symptoms
Normal strength
Negative axial compression test
No tenderness

---

collar, nonsteroidal antiinflammatory drugs (NSAIDS), and cold modalities until the range of motion has returned to near normal. Isometric exercises must begin as soon as tolerated because return of normal muscle strength is also necessary to return to action. Symptoms are usually transient and do not result in permanent disability. Return to competition is predicated upon achieving a near-normal pain-free range of motion. Additionally, a test of axial compression must be assessed. Positive axial compression indicates that swelling and inflammation around the sprained joint remain to such a degree that nerve root impingement is possible even under the low load conditions of the test. Therefore, this test must be tolerated in all positions of the head before the athlete resumes wrestling (Table 28–3).

NEUROGENIC PAIN SYNDROMES — "STINGERS"

Most commonly due to traumatic stretching or pinching of the brachial plexus or nerve roots, neurogenic injuries occur almost exclusively during takedowns. The most common mechanism is forced hyperextension and ipsilateral flexion that occurs when a wrestler "shoots" a takedown with his neck bulled, striking his opponent's chest or thigh with his forehead. The vast majority of these are neuropraxic lesions.

The clinical picture of the typical injury is characteristic. Severe electric shocklike pain occurs at the time of impact and extends from shoulder to fingertips. These momentary dysesthesias are replaced by a dull ache and numbness and weakness of the arm and hand, lasting from a few seconds to a few minutes (usually 5 minutes or less).

On physical examination, the wrestler is noted to have the arm hanging limply at his side. Often, the wrestler shakes the wrist and rubs the affected arm. Tenderness is noted in the ipsilateral paraspinous muscles and trapezius. Range of motion tends to be decreased in all planes, and guarding occurs. Changes in range of motion, particularly lateral bending, are persistent.[15] The pain is reproduced by ipsilateral side bending and extension coupled with axial loading. Neurological deficits are most commonly found in the upper brachial plexus distribution (C5–C6), but in contrast to other sports, low brachial plexus lesions (C7–T1) are not uncommon. Deficits in motor strength, particularly of the biceps, deltoid, and external rotators of the shoulder, are the rule, but these usually normalize within 5 minutes. Occasionally, weakness persists for an extended period of time and less often becomes chronic with noticeable muscle atrophy. Persistence of mild weakness is common. Changes in sensation and deep tendon reflexes are also noted only transiently.

If complete recovery without symptoms occurs within 1 to 2 minutes, immediate return to action is permitted.[61] If any neurological abnormality exists after that time, the wrestler is restricted from action.

Acute treatment involves ice to reduce spasm and bleeding and for analgesia for the first 24 to 48 hours (Table 28–4). A Philadelphia collar is used if symptoms are severe. Its use is confined to a short time. Transcutaneous electrical nerve stimulation (TENS) has also been employed acutely. A course of a nonsteroidal antiinflammatory agent (typically naproxen, 500 mg, two times a day, or sulindac, 200 mg, two times a day) is used for the first 5 to 7 days. A dexamethasone burst can be used for the first 72 hours (12 mg, twice a day; 8 mg, twice a day; and then 4 mg, twice a day) but is rarely indicated in the school-age athlete. Exceptional circumstances, such as injury close to postseason championship tournaments (particularly in high school seniors) may dictate their use, but only after a thorough explanation of risks and side effects to the wrestler and his par-

TABLE 28–4. "Stingers" — Treatment Recommendations

Ice
NSAIDs
Early range of motion
Isometric strengthening
Optional
    Hard cervical collar (less than 48 hours)
    Corticosteroid burst
    TENS

NSAIDs = Nonsteroidal antiinflammatory drugs
TENS = Transcutaneous electrical nerve stimulation

ents. Approximately 48 hours after injury, range of motion is begun. Hot packs and ultrasound (with or without hydrocortisone phonophoresis) are also employed.

Rehabilitation begins after pain and stiffness have diminished. Initially, passive ROM and isometric exercises are used. When near-normal motion is attained, manual resistance exercise is done with a partner (the athletic trainer). Use of a neck machine or Nautilus training comes next and continues as part of the wrestler's routine workout.

Return-to-action criteria are (1) minimal or no tenderness, (2) full, active range of motion, (3) normal neck strength without pain, (4) normal neurological examination, and (5) absence of neurological symptoms.

If the wrestler returns to action before pain, tenderness, and range of motion have returned to normal, the likelihood of a recurrence is extremely high.[6, 8] Reinjuries appear to occur with less severe trauma but in terms of time loss are not necessarily more severe.[6,15,65] Repetitive acute injuries in the same season will often lead to persistent rather than just transient weakness.[8] Individuals beginning a new season with residual symptoms are also at high risk of reinjury.[6,8] However, individuals who return to a new season without symptoms or radiographic changes have no obvious increased risk over their teammates.[6, 8]

The more severe the changes to the neurological structure and the longer the period of recuperation, the less advisable it is for the wrestler to return to the sport for fear of increased vulnerability to permanent injury. Repeated trauma, mostly minor compression/hyperextension injury, appears to cause osteophyte formation with further foraminal narrowing.[43,65] We have several wrestlers with permanent neurological loss and severe X-ray changes on this basis (Fig. 28–16).[65] Despite stopping the repetitive trauma of wrestling, 28 percent of ex-wrestlers with history of neck injury continue to have symptoms.[37] While no absolute guidelines exist, the wrestler and his parents should be informed of the evidence so that individual decisions regarding participation can be made.

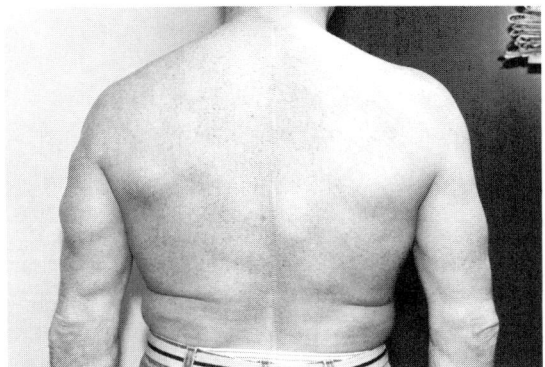
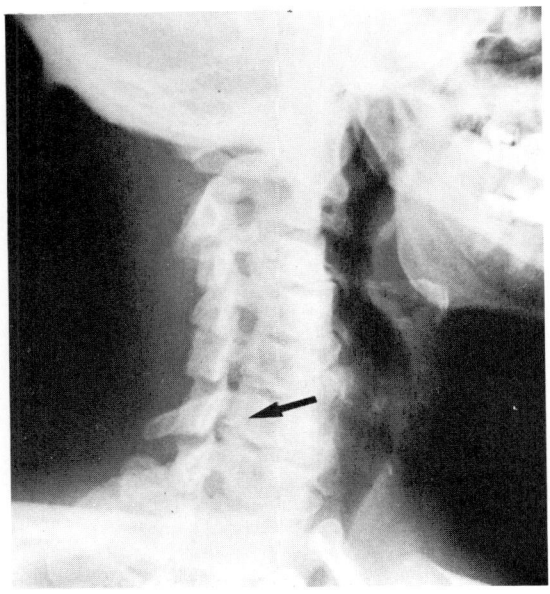

FIGURE 28–16. A former college and international wrestler with permanent neurological loss with a history of multiple neck injuries. (A) Obvious triceps and supraspinatus wasting. (B) Degenerative changes at multiple levels with large foraminal osteophytes seen on an oblique radiograph. (From Wroble, R. R., and Albright, J. P.: Neck and low back injuries in wrestling. Clin Sports Med, 5:295–325, W. B. Saunders Co., 1986.)

NECK INJURY PREVENTION

Prevention of cervical spine injuries is facilitated by rules in amateur wrestling that declare illegal all holds that result in a wrestler being thrown to the mat "out of control," specifically with "spearing" of the head and shoulders to the mat. If a wrestler is injured during such a move and is unable to continue, his opponent is disqualified and the injured wrestler's team receives the maximum of six team points.

Preseason examination is very important.[7] At the time of entry into high school or upon starting in a new program, radiographs of the cervical spine should be obtained on those individuals who have either positive history or physical examination for previous neck injury. A positive history consists of neck pain severe enough to have caused the wrestler to miss at least one practice or match. A positive physical examination includes limited range of motion, cervical tenderness, or pain with axial compression. A history of neck injury requires thorough investigation of the wrestler's medical records and a special effort to contact the treating physician.

Supervision by physicians and trainers can certainly play a great role in the reduction of both catastrophic and the more common mild-to-moderate neck injuries by establishing and enforcing strict criteria for return to action. Furthermore, the establishment of proper lines of responsibility for medical care of acute injuries is extremely important. Administrators of school systems should be convinced to hire full-time certified athletic trainers, or at the least, all the coaches in contact sports should be required to earn continuing education credit through instructional courses or clinics sponsored by the National Athletic Trainers Association.

Proper management of neck injuries obvi-

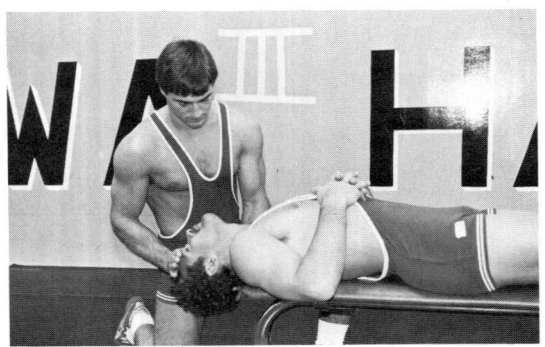
A

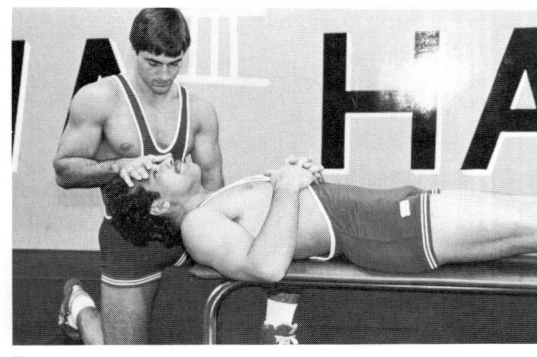
B

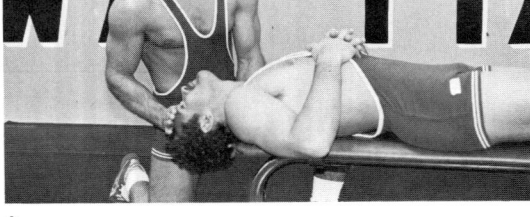
C

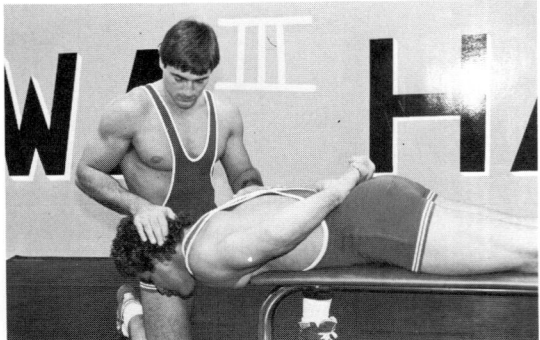
D

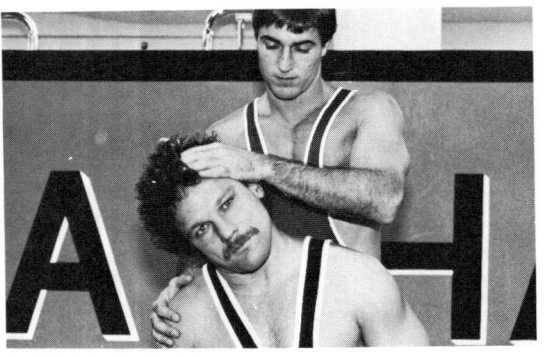
E

FIGURE 28–17. (*A, B*) Neck strengthening series. Exercise 1: Neck flexion against manual resistance is accomplished from extension (*A*) to flexion (*B*). (*C, D*) Exercise 2: Neck extension is accomplished against manual resistance from a fully flexed position (*C*) to maximal extension (*D*). (*E*) Exercise 3: Left lateral flexion is accomplished in a sitting position against manual resistance from a position of maximal right lateral flexion moving toward the left shoulder. This is repeated in the opposite direction. (From Wroble, R. R., and Albright, J. P.: Neck and low back injuries in wrestling. Clin Sports Med, 5:295–325, W. B. Saunders Co., 1986.)

ously should be a thoroughly familiar procedure to all medical personnel involved in the care of participants in high-risk sports. This includes cardiopulmonary resuscitation training as well as the acute care of head and neck injuries. Not only should the lines of responsibility be well worked out in advance, but the routine should be practiced by the primary care team on a regular basis.

Education of the coaching staff is also very important. It should be the responsibility of the trainer or the physician, or both, to make the coach aware of the occurrence of minor head and neck injuries as well as those athletes known to be at high risk. The coach should also be taught the importance of preseason neck strength conditioning, the relationship between the hours of contact and the incidence of such injuries, and the signs and symptoms that are important to recognize in the injured wrestler.

No scientifically sound studies have been done to demonstrate the protective factor of strength and endurance of neck musculature in the well-conditioned athlete. However, it is our impression that strength, endurance, and flexibility are important elements in decreasing the frequency of neck injuries. A simple neck exercise program requiring no equipment should therefore be incorporated into each team's conditioning program (Fig. 28–17).

UPPER EXTREMITY

Upper extremity injuries account for about 20 percent of all wrestling injuries.

SHOULDER

The shoulder region is one of the more commonly injured areas in wrestling. These injuries come about via two principal mechanisms. When being thrown to the mat from a standing position, a wrestler may attempt to brace his fall with his extended arm. This may then impart force to the shoulder girdle severe enough to cause injury. If he is unable to extend his arm, the fall may be taken directly on the shoulder, causing damage in this way.

The most common problem that we have found is recurrent anterior glenohumeral subluxation, whereas frank dislocations rarely occur. In the typical case, the initial subluxation appears to occur early in a wrestler's career, as many of our entering college freshmen are already affected. In some, generalized ligamentous laxity exists (with concomitant bilateral shoulder laxity). In most, however, this is not present. Most commonly, the wrestler cannot identify a single inciting event. All wrestlers, nevertheless, are subject to forces that tend to stress or stretch the anterior structures of the shoulder: the half nelson, arm bars, landing on a "posted" arm (Fig. 28–18)—all activities that place the shoulder in abduction and external rotation.

Wrestlers differ in some important clinical aspects from other athletes with shoulder subluxation. First, their subluxations occur anteriorly almost exclusively. Second, almost all are aware that their shoulders "slip in and out." Presentation with pain and weakness *alone* is rare. Third, two groups are distinguishable. One, characterized by awareness of the subluxation but no associated symptoms such as pain or weakness, occurs more commonly in those with generalized laxity. The other group notes awareness of subluxation but *is* symptomatic, particularly with respect to weakness. Previously asymptomatic wrestlers may move into the symptomatic group after repeated trauma. We presume this to be on the basis of damage to the glenoid labrum either acutely or with accumulation of repetitive trauma chronically.[64]

Pain, when present, occurs anteriorly or posteriorly, or both. Posteriorly, it results

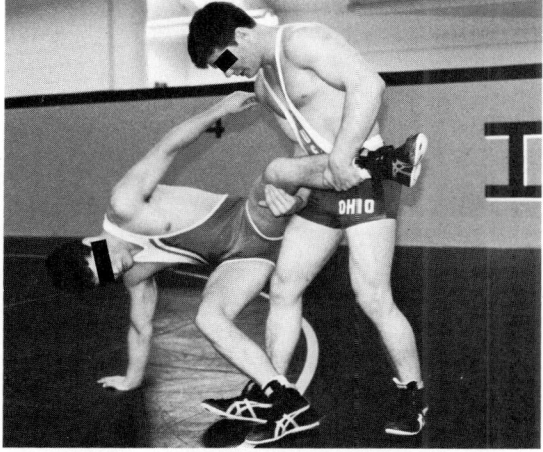

FIGURE 28–18. The wrestler's right arm is posted. Landing in this way can stress the anterior shoulder capsule.

from irritation subsequent to traction on posterior structures during the subluxations. Anteriorly, it is due to impingement produced by the increased excursion of the humeral head.[64]

On physical examination, tenderness may appear anteriorly or posteriorly. Range of motion is often decreased, particularly external rotation (this is tested both with the arm at the side and with the arm abducted to 90 degrees). Stability examination, while always abnormal, only rarely reveals a markedly positive apprehension test. The wrestler is tested supine with the shoulder at the exam table's edge. Since instability is obliterated by active contraction of the rotator cuff muscles, which act to compress the humeral head against the glenoid, relaxation is extremely important. All planes of instability are evaluated. Inferior subluxation is tested by axial traction with the arm at the side or by an inferiorly directed force on the abducted proximal humerus (Fig. 28–19). Translation detected by the examiner's opposite hand in the axilla or over the glenohumeral joint anteriorly, a "clunk" felt as the head passes over the labrum, or a sulcus visualized beneath the acromion indicates inferior instability. Anterior instability is tested in external rotation with differing combinations of flexion/extension (from slight flexion to slight extension) and abduction from 45 to 135 degrees (Fig. 28–20). Anterior pressure is applied to the posterior humeral shaft while the humeral head is palpated anteriorly. Anterior translation, a "clunk," or an indication from the patient that a particular maneuver reproduces his symptoms indicates a positive test. Posterior instability is assessed by applying an axial load to the flexed, slightly adducted shoulder, again feeling for translation or a clunk (Fig. 28–21). Positional weakness is also sought. Both upper extremities are placed in the position found to be "positive" on stability examination or that which the wrestler describes as being the vulnerable one. Internal rotation and extension versus resistance is then checked. At the subluxed position, a dramatic decrease in strength on the affected side occurs (Fig. 28–22).

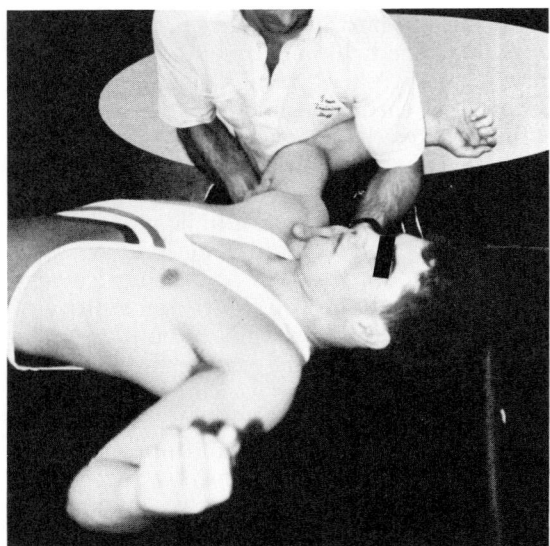

FIGURE 28–20. Anterior shoulder stability is checked in this position.

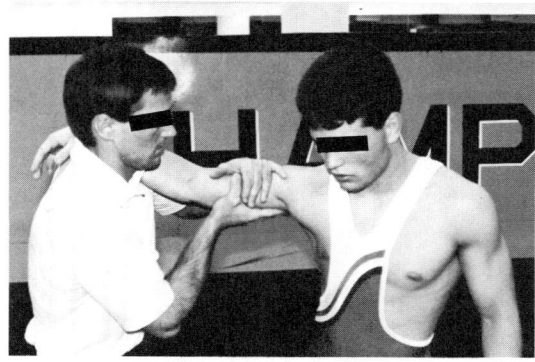

FIGURE 28–19. The position for testing inferior shoulder subluxation.

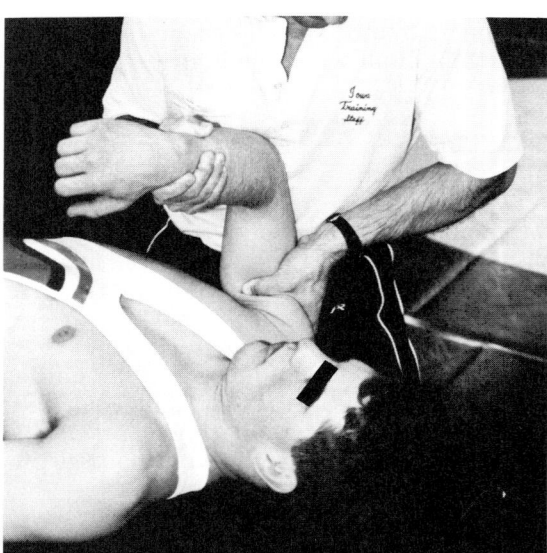

FIGURE 28–21. Check posterior shoulder stability in this position.

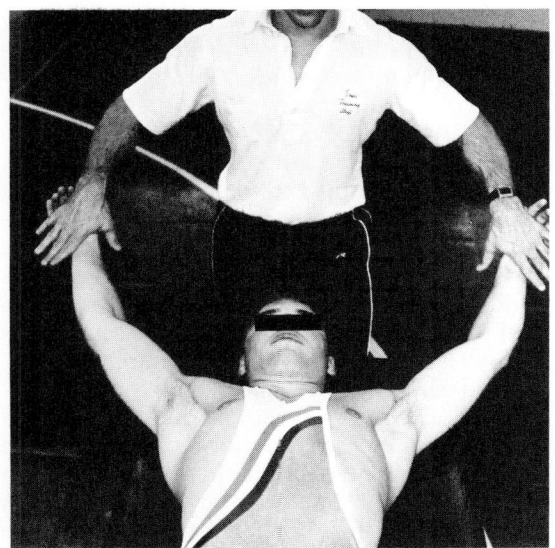

FIGURE 28–22. Positional weakness is demonstrated by pushing up against the examiner's hands.

In the case where a wrestler has a clear-cut inciting event, treatment of an acute first-time subluxation consists of immobilization for 2 to 3 weeks in a sling and swathe (removed for bathing, elbow ROM exercises, and pendulum exercises), followed by gradually increasing ROM and strengthening exercises. Strengthening of the internal and external rotators constitutes the mainstay of treatment.

The asymptomatic group generally needs no further treatment. For the symptomatic group, that is, those with positional weakness that affects their wrestling, we add other modalities. Concomitant tendinitis or other inflammatory processes dictate usage of NSAIDs. Most important though, we employ a series of exercises called "shoulder shifts." Based on the principles of proprioceptive neuromuscular facilitation (PNF), they consist of the following steps:

1. The wrestler identifies the subluxed and reduced position of the shoulder and what maneuvers produce these.
2. The position of weakness (i.e., the subluxation position) is established.
3. Manual resistance exercise (with the therapist as a partner) is performed positioning the shoulder about, but not at, the position of weakness.
4. The range of strengthening is gradually brought toward the position of weakness.
5. Once near-normal strength is achieved, "fanning" exercises are begun, first fanning toward, then through, the position of weakness, gradually increasing in speed (Fig. 28–23).

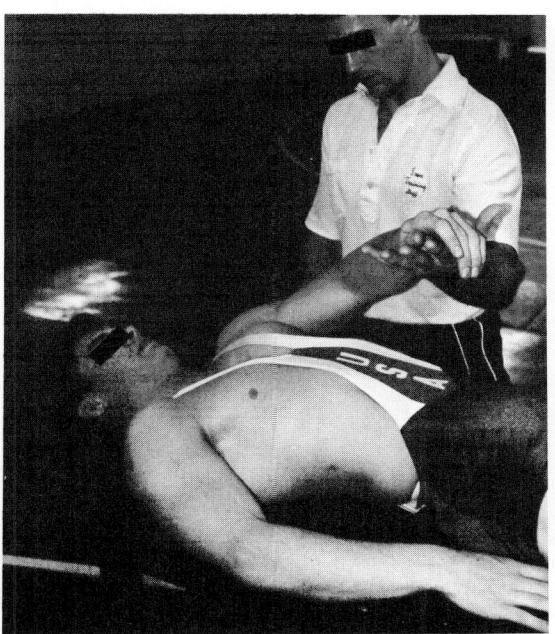 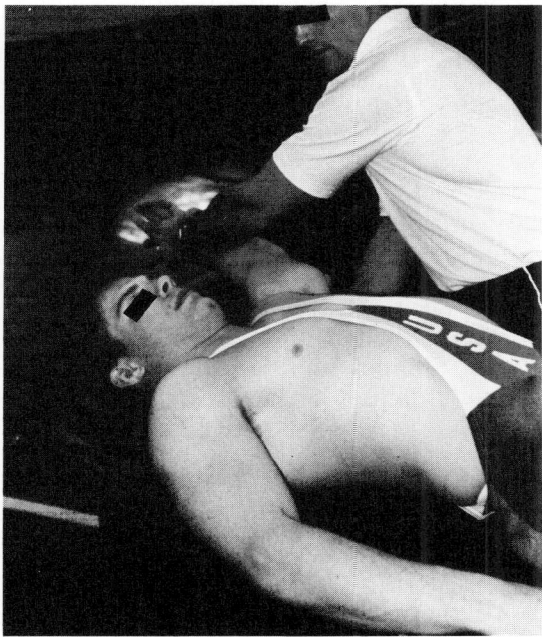

FIGURE 28–23. The shoulder shift program for treatment of anterior shoulder subluxation involves "fanning" the shoulder through a range of motion against manual resistance.

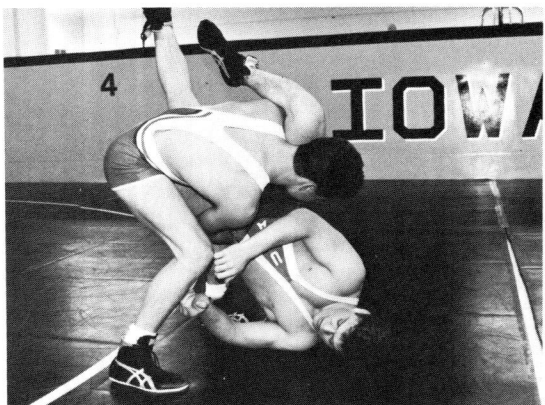

FIGURE 28–24. The defensive wrestler is taken to the mat, landing directly on his shoulder. This is the classic mechanism of an AC joint injury.

In our hands, this has been extremely successful; we have had no wrestlers who have required surgical intervention for this problem. Surgical options, however, consist of arthroscopy with labral debridement and open or arthroscopic anterior repair. Based on a limited number of cases, it appears that after full rehabilitation, an athlete may safely return to wrestling without undue risk of recurrence of instability (whether a subluxation or dislocation). We have generally not found taping or bracing to limit abduction to be useful or necessary.

Acromioclavicular (AC) sprains happen nearly as commonly as anterior instability. Together these account for the majority of shoulder injuries in wrestling. The mechanism for their occurrence consists almost exclusively of a fall on the unprotected shoulder. This happens when a wrestler, taken down by his opponent, is brought to the mat with his arm trapped (Fig. 28–24). In this way, the downward force on the acromion drives the scapula and clavicle inferiorly until the clavicle strikes the first rib.[22] Continued force then causes sprain of the AC ligaments. Similarly, with a force imparted more laterally rather than superiorly to the shoulder, damage occurs mainly to the intraarticular structures. In the former mechanism, trapezius strain occurs at its insertion onto the acromion and distal clavicle. Occasionally, the force is transmitted medially along the clavicle, and simultaneous (but less severe) sprains of the ipsilateral sternoclavicular joint occur. Rarely, a fall on the outstretched hand with resultant upward force may cause AC injury.

Almost all AC injuries are type I or very mild type II. These are differentiated by severity of pain and tenderness, slight prominence of the outer clavicle, and sensation of instability on palpation in the type II injury.

Should an AC sprain occur during a match, the wrestler is allowed to continue wrestling as long as he can tolerate the pain. An exception is the type III sprain; with this, the wrestler must withdraw. We use various modalities with success in treating the typical AC sprain including ice, analgesics (NSAIDs), TENS, and neuroprobe. Early return to competition is the goal, but the probability of repetitive direct trauma and also of aggravation by direct traction on the affected arm makes this problematic at times. With a type I injury, the wrestler returns as his symptoms permit. With the type II injury, we have occasionally used slings for comfort. Return after these injuries is based on the following: (1) no clinically detectable laxity and (2) manual muscle testing of the deltoid and the external rotators returned to 90 percent of the opposite side. In the mild type II injuries we typically see, this averages 2 to 3 weeks. In the more severe type II and all type III injuries, we accept the deformity, immobilize for a short period in a sling, allow early range of motion (as soon as tolerated), and emphasize scapular and shoulder rotational strengthening.[25] Return criteria include (1) no tenderness, (2) 90 percent strength of deltoids and external rotators, and (3) no pain with downward traction on the adducted arm. Time to return averages 3 to 6 weeks. Laxity and deformity will persist in many of these patients. To prevent aggra-

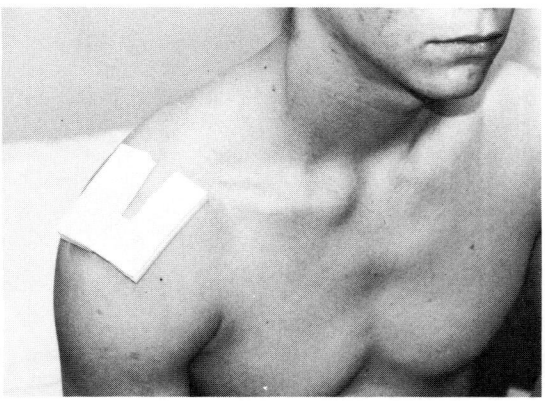

FIGURE 28–25. A thick foam rubber horseshoe applied to protect the healing AC joint.

TABLE 28–5. AC Sprains—Return to Competition Criteria

Type I and mild type II
  No laxity
  Deltoid and external rotators equal to or greater than 90 percent strentgh versus contralateral side
Severe type II and type III
  No tenderness
  Ninety percent deltoid and external rotator strength
  No pain with stress testing

vation by direct trauma during the period when the wrestler first returns to the mat, we do employ padding. A foam rubber horseshoe relieved over the AC joint is taped on with heavy elasticized tape during practice and matches (Fig. 28–25). We occasionally see a wrestler with posttraumatic osteolysis of the distal clavicle, which can cause nagging, persistent pain. Table 28–5 summarizes the criteria for return to wrestling following AC sprains.

HAND

Relatively commonplace, injuries to the hand are almost always of a minor variety. Fractures or dislocations occur uncommonly. Nearly all happen in the same way. The thumb or fingers come in contact with the mat such that sufficient torque is generated to produce injury. This typically happens in a takedown when a wrestler is being thrown to the mat. With his opponent in control, he lands, putting out his hand in an effort to break the fall. Wrestling rules dictate that prying back of individual digits is illegal. Performing such an act will result in a wrestler's opponent being awarded a penalty point. Thus, injuries due to this type mechanism rarely happen.

By far the most common injuries are metacarpophalangeal (MP) and proximal interphalangeal (PIP) sprains along with thumb MP ulnar collateral ligament sprains (gamekeeper's thumb). The bulk of these are first or second degree. Third-degree injuries rarely occur. Mallet fingers occasionally occur. We maintain a very low threshold for obtaining radiographs in hand injuries, particularly with a gamekeeper's thumb. Undisplaced fractures need proper care to avoid their conversion to more serious, debilitating displaced fractures. Radiographs allow differentiation between bone and soft tissue injury and between bone injuries requiring casting (e.g., a large, minimally displaced avulsion fracture at the attachment of the ulnar collateral ligament of the thumb MP joint), those requiring only splinting or taping (small volar plate avulsions), and those requiring surgery (flexor digitorum profundus avulsion).

The most significant problem we have identified with hand injuries in wrestlers is recurrence. Wrestlers are never willing to miss working out because of hand injuries, but there is no way to avoid repetition of stresses at the affected joints. This presents somewhat of a challenge.

The primary treatment methods of hand problems consist of splinting and taping. Although up to the referee of each match, in general no splint is allowed that has sharp, unprotected edges or that has the potential for causing injury itself. Bearing this in mind, we have been pleased with our success in using a small dorsal hood splint for gamekeeper's thumb. Made of orthoplast, the splint covers the dorsum of the thumb MP joint. It also encircles the base of the proximal phalanx (Fig. 28–26). Secured by tape, it is lightweight, comfortable, and effective. In contrast, we find taping alone to be ineffective unless the thumb is held adducted. Wrestlers find this objectionable and thus will not tolerate it. For MP and PIP sprains, however, buddy taping seems adequate in most cases. We do not splint the MPs, as we feel this increases the injury rate at the PIP joint of the splinted digit. We have used dorsal PIP splints made of orthoplast, but it is unusual to need them.

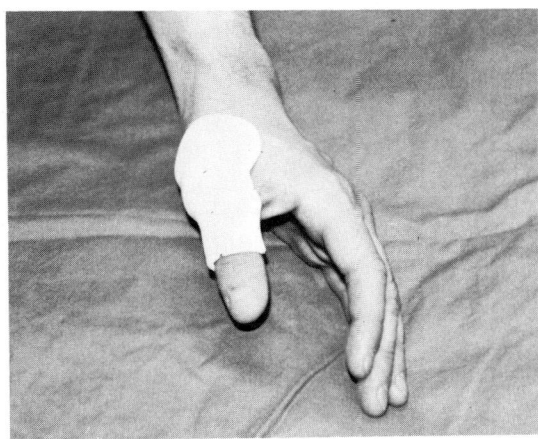

FIGURE 28–26. Orthoplast splint used for thumb MP joint injuries.

TRUNK AND LOW BACK

Truck and low back injuries make up about 10 percent of all wrestling injuries.

RIB CAGE

Injuries to the rib cage result primarily from direct trauma during takedowns. Thus, the head or shoulder of the opponent strikes the anterior chest with considerable force (Fig. 28–27). A less common mechanism of injury occurs when direct pressure is applied during a bear hug or gut wrench (Fig. 28–28). When the opponent lifts or throws the wrestler while in this position, the force generated by the opponent's hand can be enough to cause chest wall injury. Rib contusions and rarely rib fractures occur, but a reasonably common injury is to the costochondral articulations. These range in severity from contusion to sprain to dislocation. The injuries are located at the anterior margin of the ribs about three to four fingerbreadths lateral to the sternum. There the ribs articulate with the costal cartilages, which in turn articulate with the sternum.

Clinically, the wrestler complains of anterior chest pain worse with coughing, sneezing, and—because the anterior abdominal muscles also attach at the lower costochondral junctions—twisting motions. Physical findings include localized tenderness and swelling lateral to the sternum. Pain occurs with direct pressure over the injured area, with pressure over the same rib laterally (in the axillary line), and with sternal pressure. With subluxation or dislocation, a step-off may be felt or a click may be elicited by palpation. Symptoms, of course, worsen with increasing severity of injury. In general, this

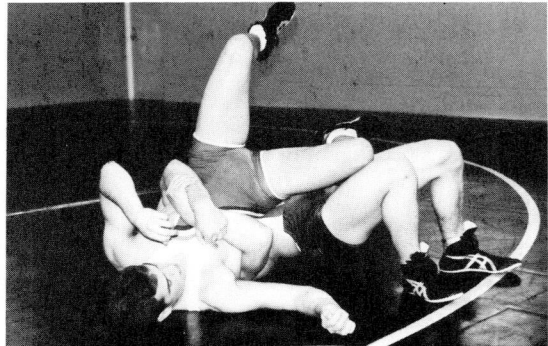

FIGURE 28–28. Tremendous pressure is exerted on the ribs during a gut wrench.

is quite a painful injury. Radiographs provide no help, as the injured area rarely can be visualized.[36, 40]

Treatment is symptomatic with ice and TENS used for pain control. The wrestler stays out of action until symptoms permit return—rarely more than 7 to 10 days and more commonly 2 to 3 days. Initially on return, we pad the affected area with a thick adhesive foam. We have not had occasion to employ injections of local anesthetics or steroids. Occasionally, this injury is complicated by the late development of calcifications of the injured costochrondral junction. This produces a painless mass at the area; it is usually only a cosmetic problem (Fig. 28–29).

LOW BACK[65]

Low back injuries in wrestling are much less common and are not as severe as those in

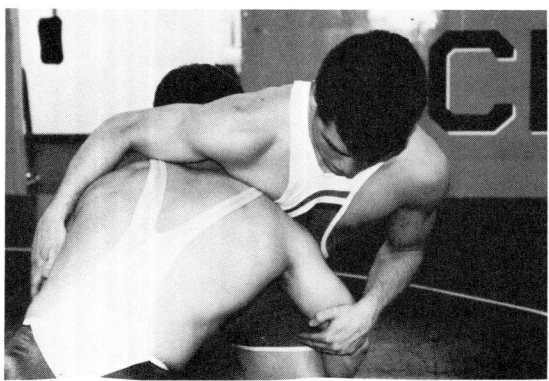

FIGURE 28–27. The shoulder is driven into the rib cage with considerable force during a takedown.

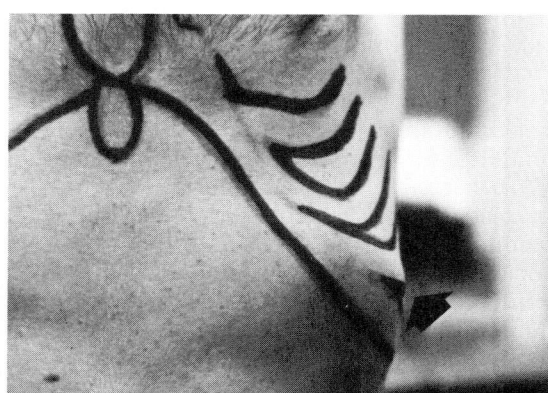

FIGURE 28–29. A former high school and collegiate wrestler with a history of a costochondral separation. Note the rib cage deformity and its typical location.

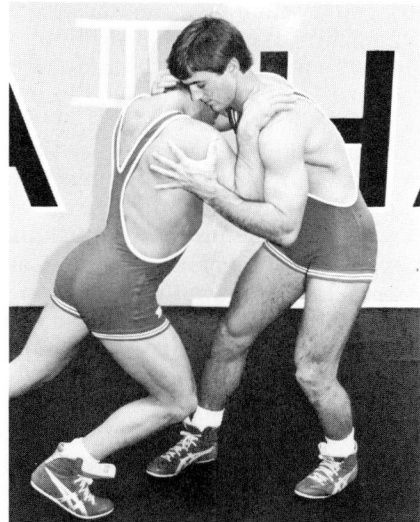

FIGURE 28–30. Wrestlers sparring. Note the hyperextension of the lumbar spine. (From Wroble, R. R., and Albright, J. P.: Neck and low back injuries in wrestling. Clin Sports Med, 5:295–325, W. B. Saunders Co., 1986.)

the neck. The most frequent injuries are sprains and strains. More serious injuries, such as herniated disk or fracture, have a very low incidence. Chronic low back pain with or without radiographic degenerative changes occurs uncommonly.

Most low back injuries take place during takedowns. During sparring, wrestlers pull and push against one another with the lumbar spine in mild hyperextension, much like linemen in football (Fig. 28–30).[24] This extension, coupled with twisting, results in injuries. Extension against resistance, as in lifting an opponent off the mat when "deep" in on his legs (Fig. 28–31), and hyperflexion, as when rolling (Fig. 28–32), are also mechanisms for low back sprain or strain. On the other hand, low back injury may result not only from a single episode but also from repeated microtrauma, that is, overuse.[33]

Furthermore, on interviewing our wrestlers we have found that many low back injuries resolve in 1 to 2 weeks and because wrestling is continued, medical care is never sought. Nevertheless, many wrestlers who presented to us with low back complaints had symptoms for months.

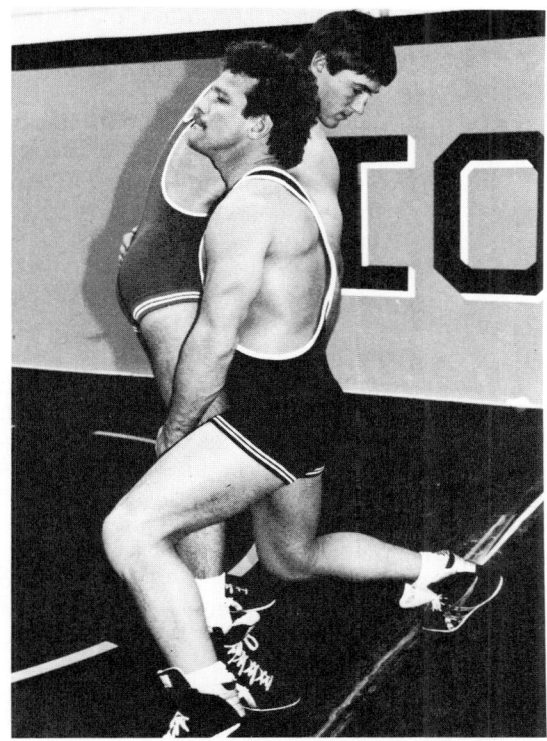

FIGURE 28–31. A wrestler lifting his opponent off the mat, demonstrating extension of the lumbar spine against resistance. (From Wroble, R. R., and Albright, J. P.: Neck and low back injuries in wrestling. Clin Sports Med, 5:295–325, W. B. Saunders Co., 1986.)

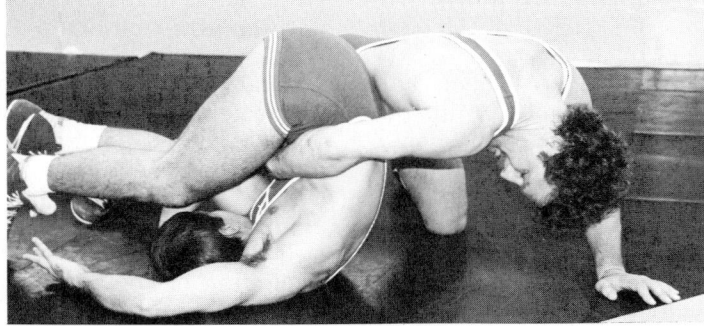

FIGURE 28–32. Hyperflexion of the lumbar spine occurs when a wrestler is caught in a roll. (From Wroble, R. R., and Albright, J. P.: Neck and low back injuries in wrestling. Clin Sports Med, 5:295–325, W. B. Saunders Co., 1986.)

Athletes describe a sensation of "something twisting" or their back "going out." Pain may be unilateral or bilateral and is usually localized to a muscle belly or its insertion. Typically, the pain reaches a maximum 24 to 48 hours after the injury. Exam reveals decreased range of motion in the lumbar spine, normal neurological examination, and negative tension signs.

With posterior element pathology, such as pars stress lesions or spondylolysis, the pain has an insidious onset. Usually confined to the lumbar spine without radiation, it tends to localize unilaterally and is worse with twisting or hyperextension activities. On exam, neurological findings are absent, tension signs are negative, and pain is reproduced with extension in the standing or prone position. Bending to the affected side accentuates the pain.

The examination of the low back is done sequentially with the patient in five different positions. Clothing covering the entire area to be examined is removed. The patient is first examined standing erect with the arms hanging at the sides and is viewed from all sides. Posture, gait, presence of a list, scoliosis or kyphosis, and lumbar lordosis are noted. The heights of the iliac crests are observed. A "forward bend" test for structural scoliosis is performed. The spine is hyperextended to elicit pain from the posterior elements. This pain is often more easily elicited when the hyperextension maneuver is performed with the athlete standing on one leg. The spinous processes, paraspinous muscles, iliac crests, sarcroiliac joints, glutei, sciatic notches, and symphysis are palpated, noting any tenderness or muscle spasm. Viewing from the back and side, the range and pattern of motion are observed and measured. Strength testing of the quadriceps (L4) and gastrocnemius (S1), tested by repetitive one-leg squats and repetitive one-leg toe raises, respectively, is also best done standing.

Next, the patient kneels on a chair and flexes over the examination table. In this position, the Achilles reflex is tested.

Perform manual muscle testing of the hip flexors (L2), hip adductors (L3), anterior tibialis and extensor hallucis longus (L5), and peronei (S1) with the patient sitting on the examination table. Sensory examination is performed using light touch and pinprick in all lower extremity dermatomes. The patellar tendon and posterior tibialis reflexes are checked.

With the patient supine, assess sciatic nerve tension signs: Bilateral straight leg raising and increased pain with ankle dorsiflexion (Lasègue test) or pressure in the popliteal fossa (bowstring test) are noted. Thigh and calf circumferences measured at fixed distances above and below the knee joint line allow quantitation of atrophy. Assess the sacroiliac joint by compression of the iliac crest, by the fabere test, and by the Gaenslen test. A rectal examination is rarely performed—only in those cases of acute injury with neurological deficit and history and physical consistent with possible sacral nerve root involvement.

Finally, turn the patient prone with a pillow beneath the abdomen to flatten the lumbar lordosis. Have the athlete hyperextend the spine by lifting his chest off the table with his arms. This causes pain in those with posterior element problems. Repeat palpation and assess femoral nerve tension by hyperextension of the hip with the knee in moderate flexion. Larson's test of instability is performed by first locating the level of maximal tenderness, then applying pressure to this area initially with the paravertebral muscles relaxed, followed by palpation of the same area with the extensors tense (the patient lifts his chest off the exam table without using his hands, thus arching his back). Elimination of tenderness with muscle contraction, a positive test, indicates instability at the involved level.

Unlike the nonathletic population, we have found little use for attempting to elicit Waddell's nonorganic physical signs in our highly motivated athletes.[63] Anterior-posterior (AP) and lateral radiographs of the lumbosacral spine are routinely obtained if symptoms are severe enough to bring the wrestler into the clinic. Oblique views show pars lesions best and are obtained if low back pain is persistent despite treatment. A bone scan appears useful if plain radiographs are normal and a high index of suspicion exists for posterior element pathology.

An essential concept in the treatment of back injuries in athletes is prevention. Conditioning and stretching comprise the key elements in preventing back injuries. A stretching program should include not only stretching of the low back but also of the hamstrings and hips.

Treatment of the acute low back injury is divided into three general areas: rest, reduction of pain and spasm, and patient educa-

TABLE 28–6. Acute Low Back Injury—Treatment Recommendations

Activity reduction
Pain control—ice, massage, TENS, corset or brace (occasionally)
Reduction of muscle spasm
Allow conditioning and strengthening
No overhead weight lifting
Flexibility/stretching exercise
Extensor and flexor strengthening

TENS = Transcutaneous electrical nerve stimulation

tion.[29] In most wrestlers, absolute bed rest is an unlikely, and probably undesirable, goal. Therefore, we prescribe relative rest in which we allow the conditioning and strengthening portions of the wrestler's routine. We eliminate weight training exercises in which a significant load is transferred through the lumbar spine (military press, for example). Actual wrestling is curtailed for a short period (Table 28–6).

Modalities used for pain control include ice, massage, ultrasound, TENS, NSAIDS, mobilization, and epidural steroid injections (if radicular symptoms are present). A corset or antilordotic back brace may be helpful in controlling pain during the period of activity modification. These are not practical once the wrestler returns to competition. As the acute phase of the injury resolves, we add heat, flexion and stretching exercises, and review of activities of daily living.

We spend a great deal of time with the wrestler discussing the nature of low back pain, its implications, and prognosis. This tends to reduce the anxiety associated with these injuries and the stigma attached to them.

Most injuries are self-limited, with return based on criteria of full range of motion and strength. Although we have had cases of chronic recurrent low back injury, all wrestlers have returned to full competition. Athletes with back pain have a better prognosis than nonathletes because athletes have more localized pathology, less psychological overlay, and fewer secondary gains from prolonged disability.[29] We have noted very few long-term sequelae of back injuries in wrestlers.

LOWER EXTREMITY

Lower extremity injuries make up 40 percent of all wrestling injuries, with knee injuries constituting the majority of the total.

KNEE[67]

The knee is the single most commonly injured anatomical region. In addition, knee injuries make up an even larger proportion of serious time loss injuries (more than 7 days lost). As with most other injuries in wrestling, the risk of sustaining a knee injury in a match greatly exceeds that of sustaining one in practice. In fact, on a per-minute basis, we calculated this risk to be 40 times greater in a match.[67] Early season matches carry particularly high risk. Tournaments represent an increased risk compared with dual meets. Based on an average squad size of 35, we extrapolated a rate of one knee injury for every 12 practices, every 10 dual meets, or every two tournaments.[67]

Multiple injuries are frequent, with noncompliance contributing to a higher reinjury rate. A wrestler with a previous knee injury is about twice as susceptible to a second injury as he was to sustaining the initial injury.[67]

Takedowns are involved in the majority of knee injuries of all types. Usually the wrestler on the defense sustains the injury. The lead leg is in general more frequently injured. We have been unable to discern any trend toward more frequent injury in a given period of a match or during a given time period within a practice. There is no apparent relationship between knee injury rate and years of wrestling experience. We have found that reserves (i.e., second- and third-string wrestlers) lose more time from competition than varsity wrestlers for an equivalent injury. They do not tend to get more severe injuries.

The overall knee injury rate in wrestling is high, but the severity of injury is not as great as in football. For example, we found a very low incidence of anterior cruciate ligament (ACL) and other catastrophic knee injuries. Nonetheless, we are aware of two knee dislocations occurring in wrestling matches. The most common injuries are prepatellar bursitis, medial and lateral sprains, and medial and lateral meniscus tears (Table 28–7). Lateral mensical tears are proportionately more common in wrestling than in any other sport.[9]

On-the-Mat Assessment of Acute Knee Injuries

When a knee injury occurs in a match and time is called, the team physician or trainer must decide within the allotted 2 minutes of

TABLE 28–7. Knee Injuries by Diagnosis

Diagnosis	Percentage of All Knee Injuries
Prepatellar bursitis	21.0
Lateral sprains	12.5
Medial meniscus tears	10.0
Lateral meniscus tears	10.0
First degree MCL sprains	8.0
Second degree MCL sprains	8.0
ACL sprains	3.0

MCL = Medial collateral ligament
ACL = Anterior cruciate ligament

injury time whether to allow a wrestler to continue. First, with the wrestler supine on the mat, we palpate to determine the location of maximal tenderness. We then assess stability of the tibiofemoral and patellofemoral joints. Patellar apprehension testing is followed by varus-valgus stress testing at 0 and 30 degrees flexion. Anterior and posterior Lachman tests are done. We have found it advantageous to perform the stabilized Lachman test, which is done in the following manner (Fig. 28–33).[66] With the wrestler supine on the mat, to examine the left knee the examiner kneels on the wrestler's left side perpendicular to and just opposite the knee. With his right knee hyperflexed and his right hip internally rotated, the examiner places his or her knee beneath the wrestler's distal thigh. The thigh is further stabilized by placing the right hand firmly on its anterior aspect. Anterior and posterior loads are then sequentially applied to the proximal tibia in the usual fashion with the left hand. This technique decreases femoral rotation during testing and allows the examiner to quantitate tibial translation more easily and reproducibly. Laxity is compared with the contralateral side if necessary. If there is no instability found, the wrestler attempts short arc quadriceps contractions, then short arc hamstring contractions against resistance. These are done to rule out reflex inhibition of muscle firing secondary to pain and to quantitate roughly any weakness. After executing these successfully, we ask the wrestler sequentially to stand, to squat, and then to shadow wrestle. If the wrestler meets the following criteria, he may continue: (1) no ligament sprains greater than first degree (i.e., no clinically detectable instability), (2) full range of motion, (3) quadriceps and hamstring strength 90 percent or greater, and (4) satisfactory performance of functional tests without pain (Table 28–8).

Prepatellar Bursitis[39,67]

Not only the most common knee injury, prepatellar bursitis is associated with the largest number of recurrences, often ultimately requires surgery, and accounts for the most time lost of any knee injury. Prepatellar bursitis can be caused by a single traumatic event—that is, forceful impact of the knee to the mat—or by chronic repeated trauma. In both, takedowns are frequently implicated.

Diagnosis of prepatellar bursitis usually is not difficult. There is usually a history of trauma even though the exact inciting incident is often unknown. Swelling, essential for the diagnosis, occurs superficial to the patella (Fig. 28–34). Bursal effusion, generally not present early in the course, may or may not occur at all. The posterior aspect of the knee is normal and the knee range of motion relatively painless (even in cases of sepsis) except with maximum flexion. Septic bursitis, of which we have had but one case per year, may present with the typical local evidence of infection but is often bereft of these signs. *Staphylococcus aureus* is the most common offending organism. Most cases are believed to result from direct pene-

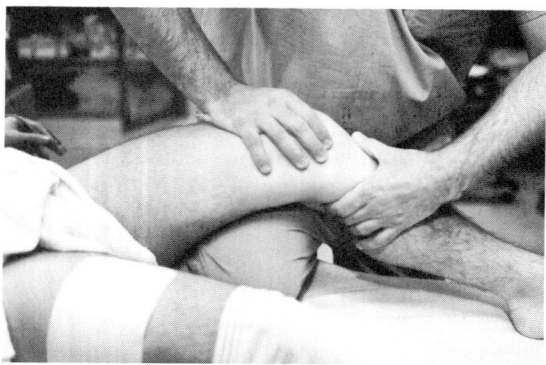

FIGURE 28–33. Performing the stabilized Lachman test decreases femoral motion during testing.

TABLE 28–8. Acute Knee Injuries—Return to Competition Criteria

On the mat
  No instability
  Full range of motion
  No substantial quadriceps or hamstring strength deficit
  Able to squat and shadow wrestle comfortably

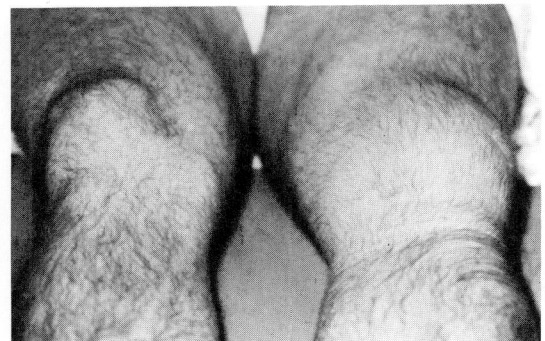

FIGURE 28-34. This case typifies the superficial swelling seen in prepatellar bursitis.

tration through the skin even though a wound is rarely seen. Knee trauma and minor mat burns, extremely common in wrestling, may allow bacterial seeding and ultimately infection to occur.

Bear in mind that conservative treatment is difficult since wrestlers are often noncompliant and repeated irritation is inherent to the sport. Nonetheless, if diagnosed and treated early enough so that fluid has not accumulated, we have had a high success rate with the following treatment protocol. When a wrestler presents to the training staff with typical symptoms and signs of prepatellar bursitis but no effusion, we start phonophoresis with 5 percent hydrocortisone, along with aspirin or an NSAID. Wrestling is rarely curtailed: We send them back on the mat with a neoprene knee sleeve with extra neoprene anteriorly (Fig. 28-35). We apply petrolatum to the anterior aspect of the knee before the sleeve is put on. This decreases friction between the skin and the sleeve, thereby decreasing irritation of the prepatellar bursa. Most cases respond to this routine with resolution of symptoms.

We encourage all our wrestlers but particularly those with a history of prepatellar bursitis to wear knee pads (those shown in Fig. 28-35). We have not made their use mandatory, and indeed less than one half of our athletes are using them. Our retrospective study on wrestling knee injuries failed to show any relationship between wearing knee pads and occurrence of prepatellar bursitis.[39,67] It is our impression, however, that the knee pad we presently use is of benefit in this regard.

Our current treatment for the initial episode of prepatellar bursitis with effusion consists of aspiration (sending fluid for culture and sensitivity, and Gram stain), compressive wrap, NSAIDS, and decreased activity for approximately 1 week. Following this, the wrestler may return to full workouts with a knee pad. If there is a recurrence, we repeat the same procedure, often increasing the rest period. If a second recurrence arises and the season is not at a point where a month off will jeopardize tournament participation, we recommend bursectomy. Because most wrestlers are highly motivated and also often noncompliant with conservative treatment, surgery with the second recurrence appears to provide the best means of getting the wrestler back in action as soon as possible. We did not find any effect on recurrence rate or time lost with intrabursal corticosteroid injections and thus do not use them[39] (Table 28-9).

Surgical Techniques for Prepatellar Bursectomy. Since the bursa is typically grossly enlarged, a transverse incision centered over the proximal one half of the patella gives the best exposure. It is usually easiest to identify the bursal border medially or laterally, and this is where to start dissection. Staying in the correct tissue plane is facili-

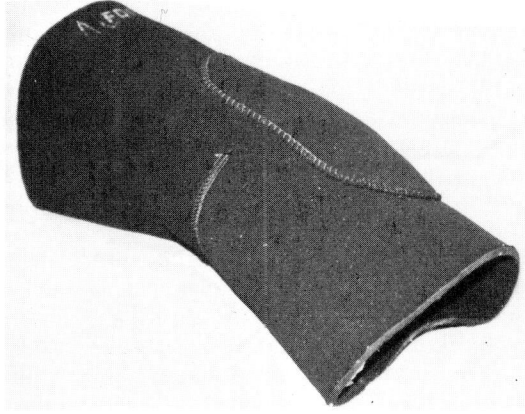

FIGURE 28-35. The knee pad we use has reinforcement anteriorly over the patella.

TABLE 28-9. Prepatellar Bursitis—Treatment recommendations

No effusion
  Neoprene knee sleeve with petrolatum
  NSAIDs
  Five percent hydrocortisone phonophoresis
With effusion
  Aspiration—send culture and Gram stain
  NSAIDs
  Decrease activity
  Third episode—bursectomy

NSAIDs = Nonsteroidal antiinflammatory drugs

tated by maintaining tension on the intact bursa. Distally, the bursa may be stuck down to the tibia or the patella tendon, and proximally the fascia of the quadriceps may easily be entered by mistake if care is not taken to avoid this. Hemostasis is important, and if there is any question, use a drain.

Return to wrestling after bursectomy is based on (1) absence of swelling and effusion, (2) lack of tenderness, and (3) full, pain-free range of motion. This averages about 6 to 8 weeks.

Because systemic or even local symptoms are often lacking, early septic bursitis is often more difficult to diagnose than septic arthritis. However, since the prepatellar bursa is ordinarily a closed space not communicating with the joint, complications of septic bursitis are rare, especially when compared with those of septic arthritis. Still, it has been demonstrated that the duration of necessary antibiotic treatment is prolonged if initiation of treatment is delayed. Aspiration, Gram stain, and cultures should initially be done on all cases of bursitis, whether they appear infected or not. Once the diagnosis is established, and even before if clinical suspicion is high, antibiotics, preferably a first-generation cephalosporin or a penicillinase-resistant penicillin should be started.

Antibiotics may be given orally if the infection is not severe and the patient can be trusted to rest his knee. The athlete may need to be admitted for parenteral treatment if the infection is severe, if oral treatment fails, or if compliance problems make it necessary. Incision and drainage with irrigation using local anesthesia are necessary only if the bursa appears loculated and clinical improvement does not occur with aspirations. One week of oral antibiotics after apparent clinical "cure" will be sufficient in most cases. In cases not responsive to the above regimen, or with any second recurrence, we recommend surgery.

Meniscus Injuries

Meniscus injuries are the most common leading to surgery. A higher ratio of lateral to medial meniscus tears occurs in wrestling than in any other sport.[9] In our experience, the ratio is 1:1 versus 1:4 in all other sports.

We have seen a variety of mechanisms for both medial and lateral tears. Most have one thing in common: They occur during takedowns and most often to the lead leg. A commonly implicated mechanism for a medial tear is depicted in Figure 28–36: a twisting

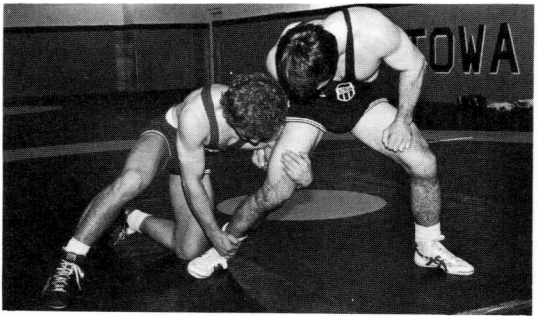

FIGURE 28–36. Medial meniscal tears can occur in situations where valgus stress is exerted on a weight-bearing leg. (From Wroble, R. R., Mysnyk, M. C., Foster, D. T., and Albright, J. P.: Patterns of Knee Injuries in Wrestling at the University of Iowa—A Six Year Study. Am J Sports Med, 14:55–66, American Orthopaedic Society for Sports Medicine, 1986.)

valgus stress on a weight-bearing leg. Lateral tears reportedly occur as in Figure 28–3, with hyperflexion, twisting, and valgus. We feel this latter mechanism is quite uncommon, as this is an illegal hold.

We noted several cases in which the meniscus injury resulted from a seemingly trivial stress or during noncontact activities in which the wrestler went through actions performed literally thousands of times previously without apparent consequences. We could relate these types of injuries to two pathophysiological explanations. Several of the injuries were horizontal cleavage tears of the "degenerative type." We suggest that the knees of these young wrestlers have undergone stresses that occur in nonwrestlers over a much longer time period. Thus, they suffer degenerative tears at at early age. A second explanation is that in some cases meniscal injury had already occurred but was not reported unless swelling, locking, or disability was present. For example, the injury may have been first reported only when a previously undisplaced bucket handle tear became displaced with concomitant locking.

The clinician should be aware that the torn meniscus may present atypically in wrestlers. It occurs more frequently on the lateral side of the knee, not uncommonly in situations associated with minimal trauma. Although the wrestler may give a history of locking in the past, a rather benign knee examination may be found simply because these highly motivated athletes have continued to practice and compete despite the pain of the acutely injured knee.

Surgical treatment involves either arthroscopic partial excision of small radial or complex degenerative tears or arthroscopic meniscal repair for large radial or peripheral tears. With a wrestler who works very hard after meniscectomy, it is not unreasonable to return to the mat in 2½ to 3 weeks, given that they have achieved a full range of motion, greater than 80 percent quadriceps strength, have resolved any effusion, and have no tenderness. After meniscal repair, the time course of meniscal healing dictates a slower return. Swimming, cycling, cross-country ski machines, and stair machines as well as swimming pool running are started at 8 weeks. We institute a progressive running protocol at 12 weeks. Return to wrestling is slow and gradual, averaging about 6 months.

Ligament Injuries

Taken together, ligament sprains constitute the most common knee injury in wrestling. The overwhelming majority of injuries, however, occur to the medial and lateral collateral ligaments with relative sparing of the cruciates,[53] a situation quite in contrast to that seen in football. Once again, a relatively high number of lateral injuries is seen. Third-degree sprains, as well as "triad" or other catastrophic knee injuries, rarely happen. Injuries tend to be divided evenly between first- and second-degree.

Not surprisingly, most injuries occur during takedowns with the defensive wrestler being injured almost exclusively.[67] A specific form of mat wrestling, the "leg ride," accounts for occasional medial and lateral sprains (Fig. 28–37). The lateral injury typically results from the defensive wrestler grabbing the offensive wrestler's foot and applying a varus stress to the knee (Fig. 28–38). This occasionally occurs abruptly but usually is a more controlled maneuver, and the alert referee is often able to stop this before an injury occurs. Medial collateral ligament (MCL) injuries occur with a much more explosive move. In instances in which this injury occurred, the top wrestler had "laced" his foot around his opponent's leg, essentially anchoring his foot and toes. When his opponent (on bottom) snapped his knee into extension to free his leg, it caused a valgus–external rotation stress on the opponent's knee (Fig. 28–39).

A few aspects of the treatment of ligament injuries deserve mention. First- and second-degree MCL and lateral collateral ligament (LCL) sprains receive nonoperative treatment. We employ an aggressive rehabilita-

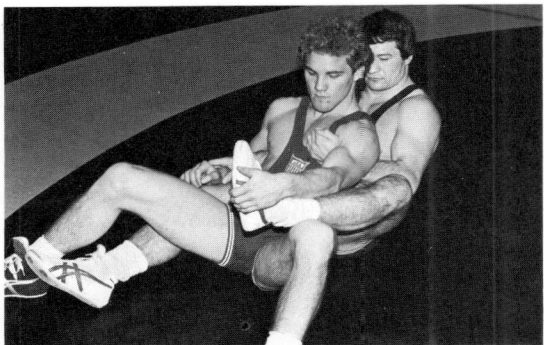

FIGURE 28–38. The defensive wrestler counters the leg ride by rolling to a sitting position and grabbing his opponent's foot, pulling it toward his head, resulting in a varus stress at the knee. (From Wroble, R. R., Mysnyk, M. C., Foster, D. T., and Albright, J. P.: Patterns of Knee Injuries in Wrestling at the University of Iowa—A Six Year Study. Am J Sports Med, 14:55–66, American Orthopaedic Society for Sports Medicine, 1986.)

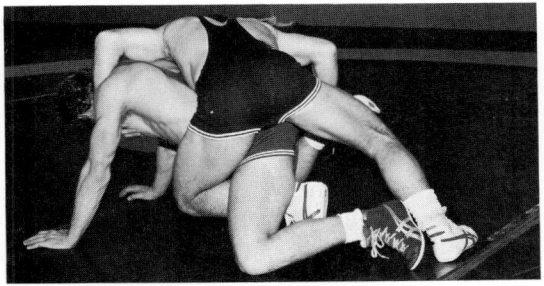

FIGURE 28–37. In this ride, the top wrestler has his left leg hooked over his opponent's left leg. (From Wroble, R. R., Mysnyk, M. C., Foster, D. T., and Albright, J. P.: Patterns of Knee Injuries in Wrestling at the University of Iowa—A Six Year Study. Am J Sports Med, 14:55–66, American Orthopaedic Society for Sports Medicine, 1986.)

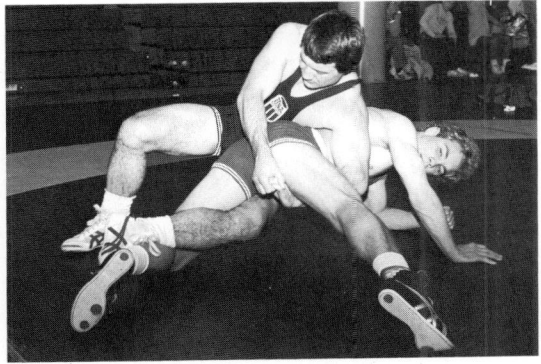

FIGURE 28–39. In this counter, the defensive wrestler rapidly extends his knee, causing a valgus–external rotation stress on his opponent's knee. (From Wroble, R. R., Mysnyk, M. C., Foster, D. T., and Albright, J. P.: Patterns of Knee Injuries in Wrestling at the University of Iowa—A Six Year Study. Am J Sports Med, 14:55–66, American Orthopaedic Society for Sports Medicine, 1986.)

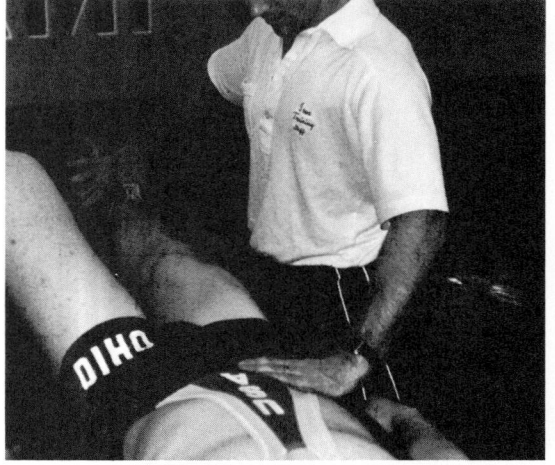
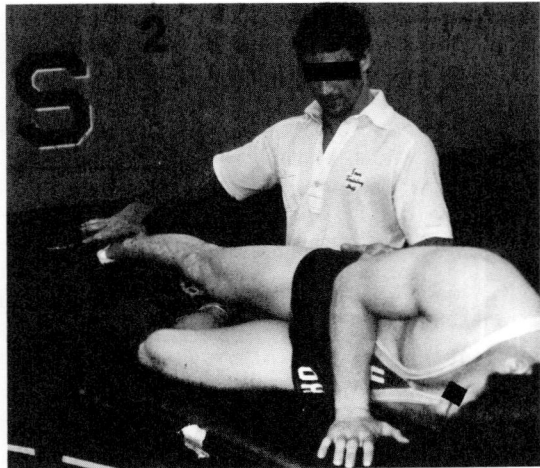
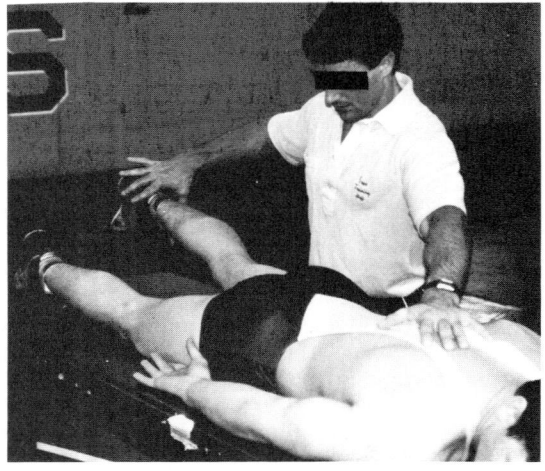

FIGURE 28–40. After a second-degree MCL sprain, straight leg raising against resistance is done supine (*A*), lateral decubitus (uninvolved side down) (*B*), and prone (*C*).

tion program that emphasizes gradual phasing in of more and more strenuous wrestling activities (Fig. 28–40).

Controlled return to the mat occurs when there is (1) no point tenderness, (2) no pain with stress, (3) near-normal laxity compared with the opposite knee, (4) virtually full range of motion and (5) 60 to 70 percent of normal quad and hamstring strength. Initially, all that is allowed on the mat is shadow (solo) wrestling and wrestling with a training dummy. Jump rope and exercise bicycling are also introduced.

Approximately 4 to 5 days later, provided symptoms do not recur, we introduce running and unlimited strength training. When strength has returned to 80 to 90 percent of normal, we permit full wrestling.

Cruciate ligament injuries present another set of problems. Some wrestlers may function reasonably well in the short term with cruciate-deficient knees because the demands of the sport are such that the knee is uncommonly in a position where tibial subluxation could occur. There is no jumping and essentially no cutting. Acceleration and deceleration occur primarily with the wrestler moving straight ahead or straight back. During virtually all actual wrestling, the knee is flexed greater than 30 degrees. At this degree of knee flexion, the iliotibial band acts to prevent anterior tibial subluxation, that is, the pivot shift. Nonetheless, as with other populations, most wrestlers will not have satisfactory function in their sport, and the vast majority of athletes with ACL-deficient knees will go on to have long-term problems. We therefore generally recommend ACL reconstruction with return to wrestling at about 9 to 12 months. For those who elect not to have surgery, we employ an aggressive program emphasizing hamstring strengthening and a pivot-shift control regimen.[23]

Taping of the knee has not been generally employed during rehabilitation or as a prophylactic measure in wrestlers with previous knee injuries. We are skeptical that this affords any protection, and more important, the decrease in flexibility it causes is probably more harmful to the wrestler. Psychologically, it seems to cause a big disadvantage. The wrestler is more aware of his own "disability." He also knows that his opponent is aware of it and may try to exploit it. Indeed, more often than not, he is correct!

We have a similar view regarding knee braces in wrestlers. Prophylactic braces are of the same questionable value as taping and offer identical, serious disadvantages. We do not recommend them. We also do not recommend functional braces for wrestlers with cruciate-deficient knees. On the other hand, we never discourage a wrestler who wishes to wear a brace from doing so. Those who do use them must have them taped and padded for matches and practice. Wrestling rules dictate that any device used must be protected so that it cannot cause injury to the opponent by sharp corners, exposed metal, and the like. The rules also state that braces may not limit motion. The referee makes a determination regarding any brace worn immediately prior to a wrestling meet and uses the above two criteria for acceptability. The 5- to 10-degree extension block hinges on most functional braces as a rule pass this referee's inspection without difficulty.

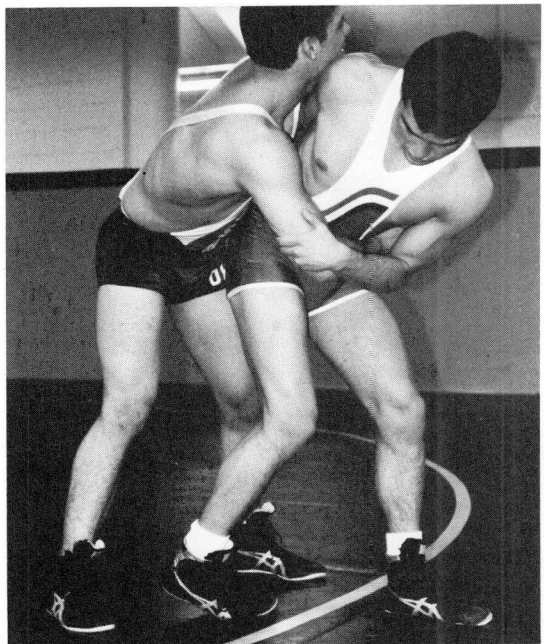

FIGURE 28–41. The wrestler in control inverts his ankle as he attempts to throw his opponent to the mat.

ANKLE

Moderately frequent (approximately five per year at the University of Iowa), the ankle injury to look for is the lateral ligament sprain. These almost always occur during takedowns. We have identified two specific mechanisms. First, when a wrestler attempts to throw his opponent, and so rises onto his toes and twists, a momentary loss of balance may cause him to "roll over" his ankle into a hyperinverted position (Fig. 28–41). The second occurs to the defensive man during a takedown. In this, the opponent controls one of the wrestler's legs with all weight then on the other leg. As his opponent attempts to bring him to the mat by various combinations of rapid changes in direction or trips, inversion stress can occur (Fig. 28–42).

The design of the standard wrestling shoe affords little protection to the ankle. They

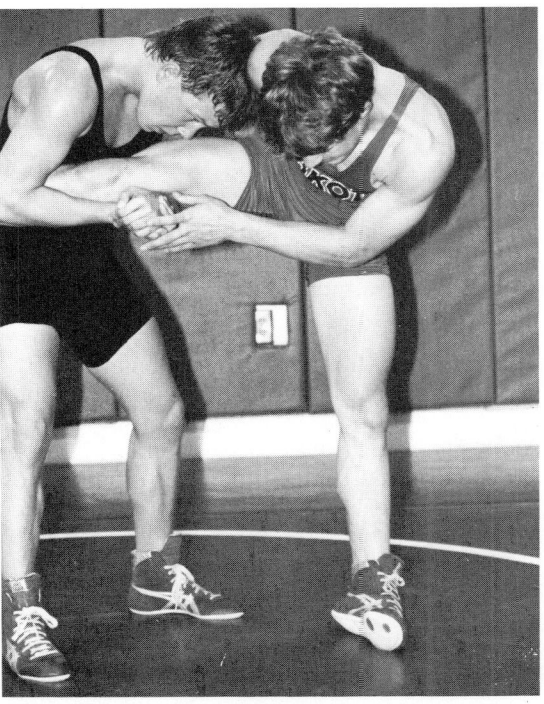

FIGURE 28–42. With one leg up in the air, an ankle sprain results when the wrestler's supporting leg is tripped or when his opponent initiates rapid change in direction.

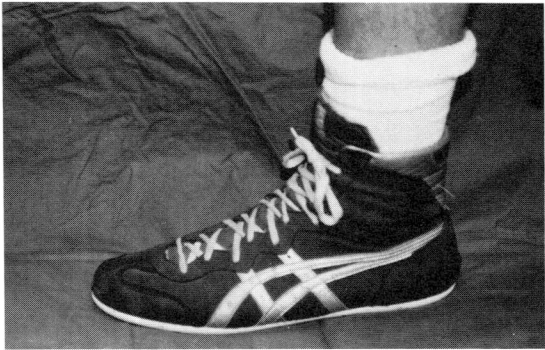

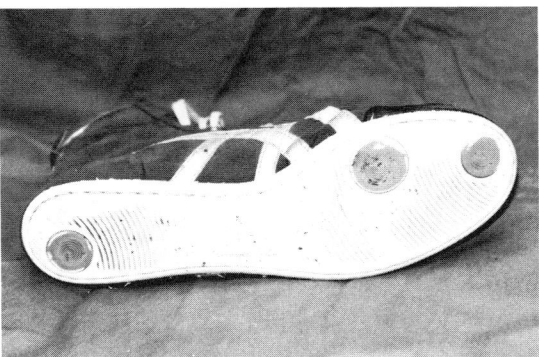

FIGURE 28–43. A commonly used wrestling shoe. Note the high-friction rubber sole and the soft, flexible nylon uppers.

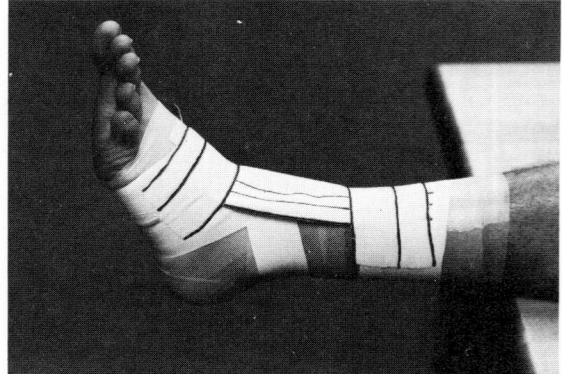

FIGURE 28–45. An example of "front support" taping. Note that the dorsum of the foot is reinforced.

have a rubber sole that has very high friction with the mat, allowing virtually no "give." Although they extend above the ankle, the uppers consist of nylon or soft leather and offer little support (Fig. 28–43).

Most often, these sprains are first-degree, and thus no laxity results. Accompanying strains of the peronei or toe extensors occur reasonably commonly. Physical findings are point tenderness over the anterior talofibular ligament (ATFL) and pain with stretch of the involved tendons.

Treatment, basically symptomatic, begins with ice, then is followed by ultrasound or hydrocortisone phonophoresis after 48 hours. Usually 1 day of rest is all that is required. Thereafter, we employ taping and splinting, both on and off the mat as needed. We use "outside" taping (Fig. 28–44), limiting inversion for wrestlers in whom the ATFL causes the most symptoms; "front support" taping (Fig. 28–45) limiting plantar flexion is used for those with prominent symptoms of extensor strain. Unlike most other athletes, wrestlers do not feel handicapped by limited plantar flexion. Full plantar flexion is rarely required in any wrestling move, and therefore wrestlers tolerate front support taping. Likewise, we have used posterior orthoplast splints (Fig. 28–46) with good results. These are taped on and worn

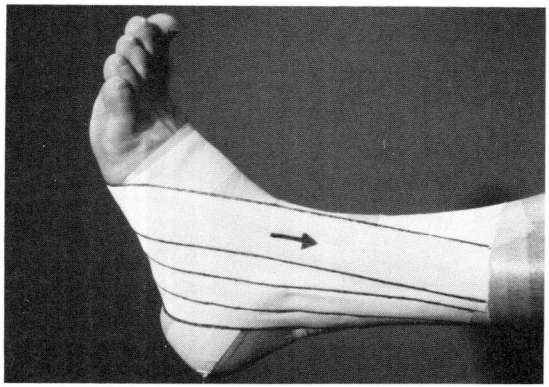

FIGURE 28–44. An example of "outside" taping. Note the extra tape strips on the lateral aspect of the ankle.

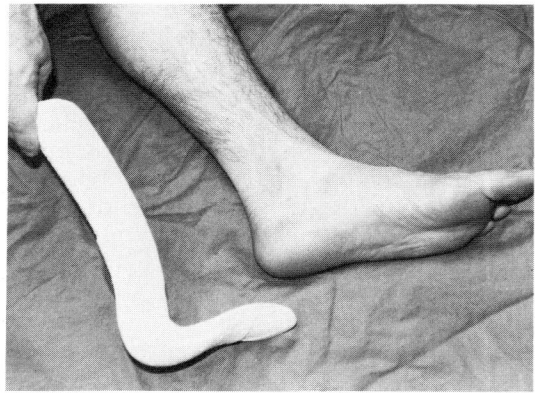

FIGURE 28–46. Orthoplast splint used in wrestlers with ankle problems.

inside the wrestling or street shoe. Used at practice or in matches, they do not appear to compromise performance.

At 5 to 7 days after injury, we begin ankle strengthening work. We have used the multiaxial ankle exerciser (MAAE). Compliance is a problem, but we feel employing a daily exercise regimen provides some modicum of prevention.

ISSUES IN WEIGHT LOSS AND NUTRITION

BODY FAT

In a weight-matched competition where the goal is to maximize power, quickness, and endurance for every pound of weight, excess noncontributing fat is a disadvantage. Minimal percentage of body fat is estimated to be 5 percent for most wrestlers and 7 percent for those who are still growing.[41,59] Common body fat measurement techniques include underwater weighing, anthropometric measurements, and skinfold thicknesses. Reliability of these measurements depends in large part on the experience of the examiner and the techniques used. The Tcheng-Tipton equation, based on six skinfold sites, was developed to compute an estimated percentage of body fat in wrestlers.[41] Knowing the athlete's current body weight and estimated percentage body fat, a minimum recommended wrestling weight can be determined for a body fat percentage between 5 and 7 percent. Calculations should be made at the beginning of the school year to allow for a gradual weight loss of 1 to 3 pounds per week. To monitor progress of fat reduction, both skinfolds and weight should be evaluated on a monthly basis. The athlete should be instructed by a qualified health professional on how to create effectively the required negative energy balance necessary to lose fat. Weight loss may be accomplished by moderate reduction in food intake in combination with increased energy expenditure.[52] Dietary records may be kept during this time to evaluate nutrient and calorie adequacy.

DEHYDRATION AND WEIGHT LOSS METHODS

Wrestlers often lose large amounts of weight in a short period of time. Fluctuations in weight may occur frequently throughout the season.[28, 45, 54, 57, 60] Studies in weight loss practices among high school and college wrestlers indicate that from 3 to 20 percent of the preseason body weight is lost prior to certification or competition. Most of this weight loss occurs in the final days or day before the official weigh-in, with team members who are youngest or lightest, or both, losing the highest percentage of their body weight.

In order to lose weight, many wrestlers use a combination of food and fluid restriction. Dehydration unfortunately appears to be the most commonly used method for acute weight loss and is typically induced by fluid restriction and exercise at elevated temperatures. Methods such as use of rubber suits and sauna are common, although they are ruled illegal at the high school level. Of special concern is reliance upon induced vomiting, laxatives, and diuretics to make weight.[28, 39, 54, 55, 57, 58, 60] The effects of acute and prolonged dehydration are significant reductions in blood plasma volume, performance, and muscular strength.[12, 18, 21, 27, 49, 50, 62] When fluid loss exceeds 2 percent of normal stable body weight, significant changes occur during submaximal work that include elevated heart rate, reduced stroke volume, and lowered cardiac output. These changes in cardiovascular function are potentially dangerous, especially in combination with elevated core temperature, altered electrolyte balance, and possible renal changes.[68,69] Current rules call for weigh-ins to take place within a maximum of 1 hour and a minimum of 1/2 hour before the scheduled start time of a dual meet. But even when 5 hours is allowed between weigh-in and the match, this time is not sufficient for restoration of electrolyte balance and replenishing muscle glycogen concentration.[27, 68, 69] The practice of fluid deprivation has been discouraged by both the American College of Sports Medicine (ACSM)[5] and the American Medical Association (AMA),[2] as well as the National Collegiate Athletic Association (NCAA) Wrestling Committee.[1] We strongly recommend that school-age wrestlers limit weight loss in the hours before weigh-in to 2 percent of normal body weight.

Only one study documents the long-term effects of repetitive weight loss. Mysnyk et al. studied 336 former wrestlers, all over the age of 30, and a control group of 224 normal males. Both groups underwent measurement of pulse, blood pressure, urine protein and creatinine, and serum creatinine.[38] The investigators found no significant differences between the wrestlers and nonwrestlers for any of these parameters. Additionally, they found no correlation between the values of these parameters and the estimated amount of weight lost per week. The authors concluded that repetitive weight loss and dehydration did not cause detrimental renal effects.

FLUID REPLACEMENT

The most critical nutrient for any athlete during training and competition is water. Dehydration compromises optimal performance and, if allowed to become severe, may be life threatening. Because thirst is an unreliable mechanism for determining fluid replacement and hypohydration, athletes need to drink beyond satisfying thirst to rehydrate.[30] Fluids should be taken before, during, and after exercise. While cold water appears to be the best fluid replacement, carbohydrate-electrolyte drinks can also be used effectively. When choosing a replacement fluid other than water, the most important factor to consider is promotion of rapid gastric emptying. Gastric emptying is affected by volume, temperature, and caloric content. Increasing fluid volume (up to 500 ml) and decreasing fluid temperature will increase gastric emptying.[20] Increasing caloric content, the most important factor, decreases the gastric emptying rate. During exercise, however, dilute glucose solutions are emptied as quickly as water.[35] Although fluid is absorbed preferentially in the small intestine rather than the stomach, and is enhanced by glucose and sodium, the gastric emptying rate is slower than the intestinal absorption rate. Thus, the limiting step remains how fast the fluid leaves the stomach. Athletes may find it uncomfortable to exercise after a large volume of liquid is consumed and may therefore prefer smaller amounts taken every 10 to 15 minutes. Ideally, the drink should contain a glucose concentration less than 2.5 grams per 100 ml of water, as higher levels of glucose will significantly slow gastric emptying. Low levels of potassium and chloride ions should be present but only become vital with extreme, prolonged exercise. All fluids should be taken cold.[4] Most commercial fluid replacement drinks have higher than optimal electrolyte or carbohydrate content or both, so dilution may be used to enhance emptying and absorption. Palatability is improved with carbohydrate-electrolyte drinks compared with water, and this may enhance fluid consumption so that desired replacement volumes are reached. Some investigators have shown that carbohydrate feedings may actually enhance prolonged exercise performance.[35] We recommend that cold water be readily available and frequently taken by wrestlers during practices and tournaments. If commerical drinks are used, we suggest dilution to half strength (Table 28–10).

TABLE 28–10. Fluid Replacement—Ideal Characteristics

Cold
Small volumes
Taken during and after exercise every 15 to 20 minutes
Good taste
Water or dilute glucose solutions

NUTRITION

Wrestlers, like many athletes, are prone to believe common food fallacies and frequently lack a good understanding of basic nutrition.[55, 60] Too often nutrition information is received from peers or other unreliable sources. Because weight control is an important aspect of wrestling, it would be helpful for wrestlers to understand the basic principles of nutrition. Information provided by a qualified professional can minimize misinformation.

It has been estimated that calorie expenditure for wrestling is 14.2 kilocalories per minute.[3] In general, daily calorie consumption should not fall below 2000 kilocalories to ensure that the nutrient needs of training and growth are met.[52] Wrestlers who are in negative calorie balance compromise their ability to synthesize glycogen, the fuel used by muscle during athletic activity. An adequate carbohydrate intake is essential for maintenance and repletion of glycogen stores. It has been recommended that carbohydrate intake for the wrestler contribute 55 to 60 percent of total caloric intake.[30] While protein is essential for synthesis and repair of muscle, protein intake above 15 percent of total calories does not benefit the athlete.[26, 30]

Once protein needs are met, excess is either utilized for energy or converted to and stored as fat. Muscle size, while independent of protein intake, depends on genetic potential and training regimen.[26,30] Fat, though a valuable source of energy for muscle activity, should not exceed 30 percent of total calories.[30]

Adequate intake of vitamins is essential for a variety of physiological functions related to exercise, including energy metabolism (B complex) and tissue repair (vitamin C). However, no evidence exists that hard exercise in a hot environment increases the requirement for any vitamins above the recommended dietary allowances (RDAs).[16] Excessive intake of fat soluble vitamins (A,D,E,K) can be toxic as a result of their increased storage in the body. Although excess water soluble vitamins are generally excreted and not stored, complications have been reported for megadoses (in excess of 10 times RDA) for niacin, vitamin C, and B_6.[30] The use of a multivitamin that supplies 100 percent RDA, not more, is considered safe and may be indicated for the wrestler who has unusual dietary habits or is on a strict weight loss regimen.[26] Significant losses of sodium, potassium, magnesium, and chloride in sweat have been reported.[11,17] In general, these losses can be replaced by a balanced daily diet. However, if an athlete loses 4 to 6 percent of body weight from dehydration on a daily basis, some electrolyte replacement may be considered. Salt tablets should be avoided, as they irritate the stomach lining, delay water absorption, and further promote intracellular dehydration if taken with inadequate amounts of water.

PRE-EVENT MEAL

While allowing for personal preferences and psychological factors, the pre-event meal should be high in carbohydrate, nongreasy, and readily digested. For wrestlers who may be in a dehydrated state, protein intake should be minimal prior to a match. Fat intake should also be minimized, as fat slows gastric emptying time. Other foods that should be limited prior to competition include bulky, high-fiber foods; foods high in sodium; and those that are spicy or gas-producing. The pre-event meal should be consumed 3 to 4 hours prior to competition to allow for digestion and for plasma insulin

TABLE 28–11. Pre-event Meal—Ideal Characteristics

High carbohydrate
Adequate fluids
Timing—3 to 4 hours before a match
Avoid bulky, high-fiber, spicy, or gas-producing foods
Avoid high salt, high fat, high protein

and glucose to return to basal levels. Examples of carbohydrate-rich, easily digested foods include pasta, baked potatoes (without butter and sour cream!), pancakes, muffins, and cereals.

The wrestler may not want to eat prior to a match owing to nausea, nervousness, or difficulty in digesting food after prolonged restriction. A liquid replacement meal may solve this problem. These products provide adequate carbohydrates, contribute to hydration, and are digested rapidly and completely, leaving little residue.[48]

Ingestion of carbohydrate $1\frac{1}{2}$ to 2 hours or less before competition begins is not recommended, as this will result in an increased concentration of circulating insulin, which promotes glucose uptake from the blood and suppresses mobilization of free fatty acids from adipose tissue.[19] The net result can be a rapid decline in blood glucose, resulting in hypoglycemia and premature utilization of glycogen stores, leading to a reduced exercise capacity.[19] Consequently, it is recommended that a high school wrestler consume only water if there is only 1 hour allocated between weigh-in and match (Table 28–11).

DERMATOLOGICAL PROBLEMS

Owing to the extensive physical contact inherent to wrestling, participants are exposed to transmissible diseases, especially those of the skin. This requires early recognition of common dermatological problems so that prompt and appropriate treatment may be administered. Proper management of these cases may not only hasten the course of the skin lesion but also serves to protect teammates and opponents from exposure to the infectious agent.

Skin diseases have become such a significant problem that the NCAA wrestling rules committee recommends that a physician be present at weigh-ins to examine contestants for communicable diseases in all tournaments and meets. Referees may serve this function when physicians are not available. Disqualification of an individual from competition may occur if, in the opinion of the examining physician, there is the presence of a communicable disease that makes participation inadvisable.[1]

STAPHYLOCOCCAL INFECTIONS (FOLLICULITIS, FURUNCULOSIS)

The skin is always populated with large numbers of harmless strains of bacteria. Pathogenic staphylococci are present periodically or constantly on the skin, especially in proximity to the mucous membranes. Environmental factors are important in the colonization of the skin by pathogenic staphylococci. In particular, moisture promotes the growth of staphylococci. Predisposing factors, then, include warm, moist climates; occlusive clothing and footwear; closely opposed skin surfaces; and constant exposure to water. Skin constantly moistened by sweat is vulnerable to the growth of pathogenic microorganisms, and for this reason, keeping the skin dry is the most important mechanism to prevent bacterial overpopulation. While prevention may largely be dependent on proper skin hygiene, it is advisable to change workout clothing daily. Wrestling mats and equipment should be cleansed daily with an effective germicidal product. Soap and water may serve as the most effective means of "cleansing" the skin, as soaps containing antibacterial agents offer uncertain advantages and may be associated with contact allergy (Table 28–12).

Staphylococcal infections generally originate in the hair follicles. *Folliculitis*, characterized by a purulent lesion at the base of the hair follicle, is a superficial infection (Fig. 28–47). In wrestlers, these lesions are most commonly seen on the thighs and in the popliteal area, possibly owing in part to knee pad irritation and in part owing to the skin con-

TABLE 28–12. Skin Diseases— Recommendations for Prevention

Good skin hygiene—"soap and water"
Daily washing of workout clothes
Adequate drying of skin (particularly in flexural areas)
Hold out infected wrestlers
Occlusive coverage of isolated lesions (not applicable to *Staphylococcus aureus*, impetigo, or herpes infections)
Mats cleaned daily

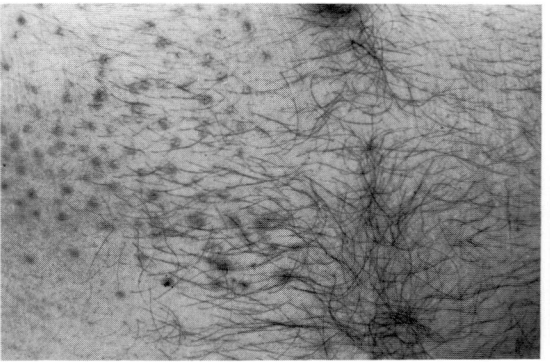

FIGURE 28–47. Folliculitis.

tact occurring with knee hyperflexion—a common position for wrestlers.

Folliculitis may be bacterial or traumatic. Bacterial folliculitis is generally caused by *Staphylococcus aureus*. If this organism is isolated from a lesion, the wrestler should be held out from participation involving contact with other wrestlers. If no organism is isolated, then it is not necessary to hold a wrestler out. This traumatic folliculitis is indeed found in many cases among wrestlers. Most folliculitis may be effectively managed through reduction in follicular irritation and improvement in skin care. Hibiclens scrub used two to three times daily is generally effective in controlling the majority of these problems.

A *furuncle* is characterized by acute inflammation arising deep in the hair follicle. It presents as a fluctuant local area of tenderness and with erythema surrounding a central pustule (Fig. 28–48). There may be associated lymphadenitis and, in advanced cases, identifiable lymphangitis. When exudate is obtainable, culturing is advisable to identify

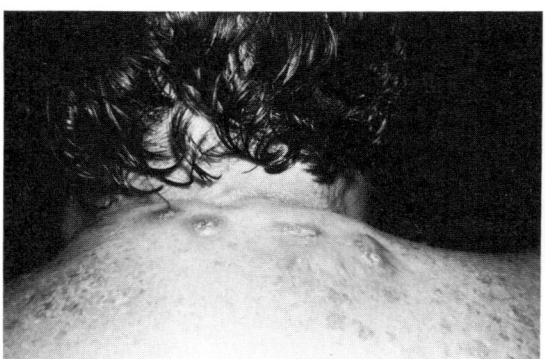

FIGURE 28–48. Furunculosis. Multiple adjacent furuncles showing erythema around central pustules.

the organism and its antibiotics sensitivities. Treatment includes systemic antibiotics and multiple daily application of hot, moist compresses. In many circumstances, particularly when there is secondary lymphangitis and active drainage, the wrestler is held from activity. This helps minimize progression of the inflammatory process and also protects teammates from contacting the infection. If there is no associated lymphangitis, conditioning alone is generally permitted. In circumstances of a mild infection without associated lymphangitis, it may be determined that the athlete can resume contact or individual conditioning if the lesion can be effectively covered and protected. In all cases where *Staphylococcus aureus* is identified, the wrestler is held from contact until the infection has been treated.

STREPTOCOCCAL INFECTIONS (IMPETIGO)

Impetigo, usually caused by beta-hemolytic streptococci, may be secondarily infected by staphylococci. While rare among college wrestlers, it is common among the younger high school athletes. Although impetigo may present on previously healthy skin, it is generally preceded by an abrasion or similar injury to the skin barrier. The initial lesion is a subcorneal bulla that is rarely intact because of its superficial position. The remnants of the blister are seen at the edge of the lesion as a shriveled epithelial remnant. The lesion may be solitary but also may consist of multiple scattered lesions. The characteristic finding is the presence of a superficial, honeycombed, amber-colored crust (Fig. 28–49). In some cases, the lesions may progress to deeper erosion with little surface spread (ecthyma). In school-age wrestlers, the face is the most common site but, unlike in nonwrestlers, may be localized to the arms and legs. Systemic antibiotics must be given, as acute glomerulonephritis may follow certain cases of streptococcal impetigo. The crusts should be removed with warm water soaks prior to application of topical antibiotics two to three times daily. Daily change of bedding and items such as towels is also recommended. The athlete must be withheld from all wrestling contact and must refrain from common usage exercise equipment until lesions are gone. Preventive measures are as for staphylococcal infections.

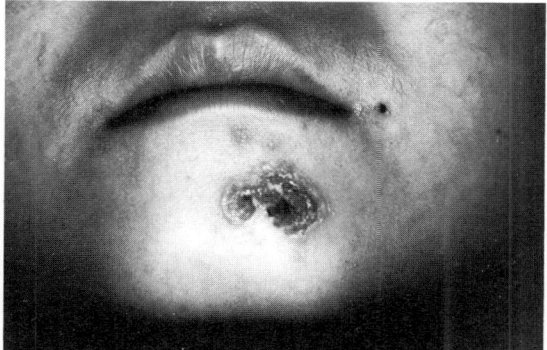

FIGURE 28–49. Impetigo. A large facial lesion with typical amber-colored crust.

VIRAL INFECTIONS

Herpes simplex type I, referred to as herpes gladiatorum in this population, is the most common cutaneous infectious disease of wrestlers.[10] In one study, 19 percent of a group of college wrestlers had a history of herpes in a single season.[10] Owing to its highly contagious nature, caution should be exercised when dealing with infected wrestlers or other contact sport athletes.

The typical clinical presentation is an acute onset of a cluster of tense, serous-filled vesicles (Fig. 28–50). Prodromal symptoms include tingling or burning of the skin prior to eruption. The infection site commonly covers an area less than 1 cm in diameter, but in some cases of primary infection, it may cover large and perhaps multiple areas of skin. There is associated discomfort and possible local swelling with lymphadenitis. Sys-

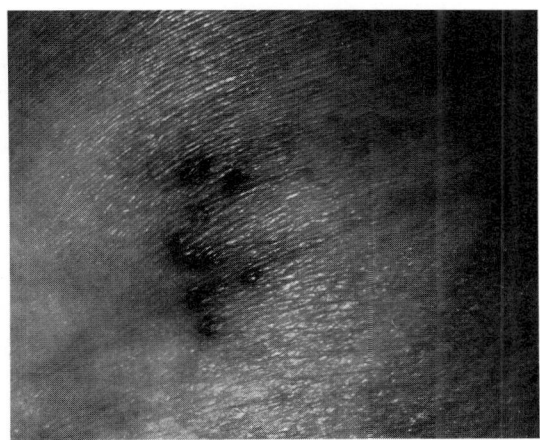

FIGURE 28–50. Herpes simplex type I. Note the vesicular appearance.

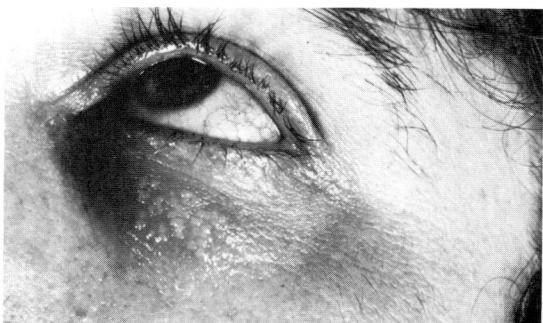

FIGURE 28–51. Herpetic lesion bordering the eye. Potentially blinding keratoconjunctivitis can result.

temic illness is often present at the onset of a primary infection. Lesions may present on any part of the skin surface, with a common site being the periphery of the lip and adjacent facial tissue. Recurrence is common and frequently presents at the same anatomical location. The vesicles, situated in the epidermis, readily burst and may become secondarily infected. Herpes lesions near the eye (Fig. 28–51) are of special concern, as involvement of the conjunctiva or surrounding skin may have serious implications for vision.[47] Ophthalmologic consultation is strongly advised in these instances.

Herpes virus tends to persist in a latent state for a person's entire life. Reactivation with resultant observable lesions may follow a known or an unrecognized triggering event.[31] Most commonly, lesions appear with an upper respiratory infection or sunlight exposure, but some individuals regularly develop herpes simplex during periods of stress or exhaustion or on exposure to cold temperatures. Some athletes may therefore have a tendency to develop the infection prior to or during stressful times of the season, such as key matches and tournaments. This is an important consideration for, as the NCAA rules committee outlines, confirmed herpes virus infection may be considered a disqualifying condition.[1, 32]

Prevention may be aided by identification and avoidance of specific precipitating factors. While no satisfactory treatment of herpes simplex exists, several drugs can inhibit replication of herpes virus in laboratory models.[31] Oral acyclovir, 200 mg, five times a day for 2 weeks, *may* serve to reduce viral shedding and shorten healing time and can be used for both primary and recurrent infections. Use of acyclovir for chronic suppressive therapy (i.e., prophylaxis) has not been reported for herpes gladiatorum but has been used for up to 6 months for genital herpes.[10] Nausea or vomiting, headache, and diarrhea are the most common side effects with long courses of acyclovir. But, in addition to this, unanswered questions remain about the potential for reproductive system toxicity and mutagenicity, so the drug cannot be used with complete impunity. Frequent application of 70 percent ethanol may also serve to reduce symptoms and assist in drying of the lesions. Ethanol may also serve to reduce the local bacterial population, thereby reducing the risk of secondary infection.[42, 47] Most affected wrestlers report at least one match against an opponent with cold sores or vesiculopapular rash;[10] so no contact with teammates should be permitted until lesions reach a dry, crusted (noninfectious) state. Although in some rare cases the infectious process will persist for as long as 2 weeks, the lesions usually dry and form a flat crust in 3 to 7 days, at which time return to participation may be allowed.

SUPERFICIAL FUNGUS INFECTIONS

Tinea infections, especially of the feet and groin area, are common among wrestlers but only in rare advanced cases necessitate removal from participation. Moisture and sweat contribute to the development of infection. The inflammation associated with superficial fungal infections varies from slight scaling and fissuring to more extensive dry, reddish scaling and to acute vesicular and bullous flare-ups. Although the diagnosis is almost always made clinically, definitive diagnosis, as for all fungus skin disorders, is by microscopic examination of scraped scale or bulla.[47]

Tinea pedis (Fig. 28–52) presents with scaling and varying degrees of maceration of the skin between the toes, commonly between the fourth and fifth toes. There also may be heavy scaling, vesicles, and pustules on the soles. The nails may also be involved with thickening and dystrophic changes.

Tinea corporis (Fig. 28–53), involving areas of the trunk, limbs, and face, is the least common of the fungal infections among wrestlers. It presents as scaling, erythematous areas with activity primarily at the margins and central clearing, thereby producing

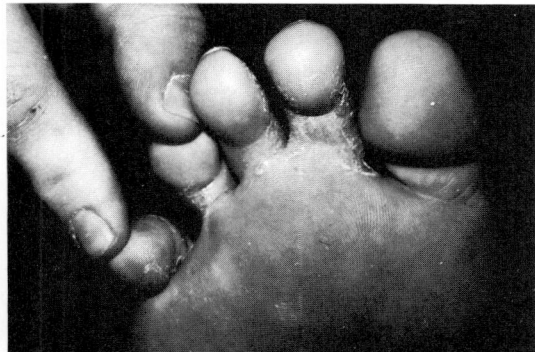

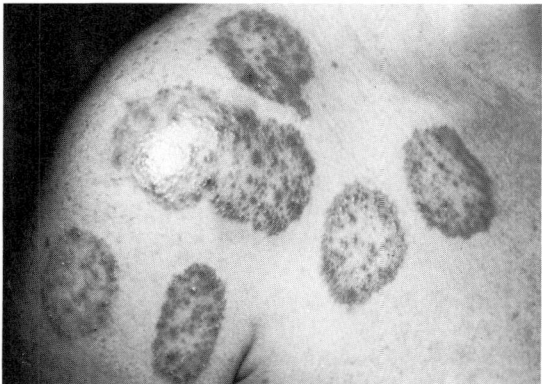

FIGURE 28–53. Tinea corporis. Note the annular appearance of the lesions.

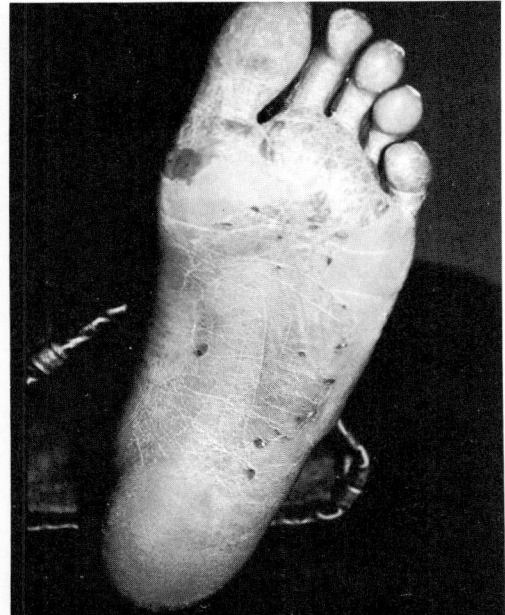

FIGURE 28–52. Tinea pedis. (A) Scaling, fissuring, and erythema between the toes. (B) More extensive involvement of the soles.

an annular appearance. The lesions are of various sizes and number.

Tinea cruris is localized in the groin. As with other types of fungal infections, poor hygiene, heat, and humidity contribute to wider dissemination.

Treatment and prevention involves foot and skin hygiene; the wearing of clean, well-ventilated shoes and clothing; frequent change of socks; medicated topical ointments (tolnaftate or miconazole); and in rare cases, oral griseofulvin for 4 weeks. Nonmedicated dusting powders and creams may also be of value as a preventive measure.

Tinea versicolor (Fig. 28–54) most frequently affects the upper trunk and abdomen. Typical lesions appear as multiple sharply demarcated macular patches of varying sizes and shapes, ranging in color from whitish to tan to brown. Scaling is not prominent. It responds readily to overnight application of selenium sulfide 2.5 percent suspension (Selsun), but relapses are frequent.

DERMATITIS (CONTACT DERMATITIS, ATOPIC DERMATITIS)

Dermatitis is a clinical term used to describe a wide variety of inflammatory skin conditions. There are many different etiological agents and pathogenic mechanisms involved in different types of dermatitis. Although the occurrence of dermatitis among wrestlers is relatively uncommon, two disorders deserve special mention: contact dermatitis and atopic dermatitis.

Contact dermatitis may be due either to the direct irritative nature of the contact or to a

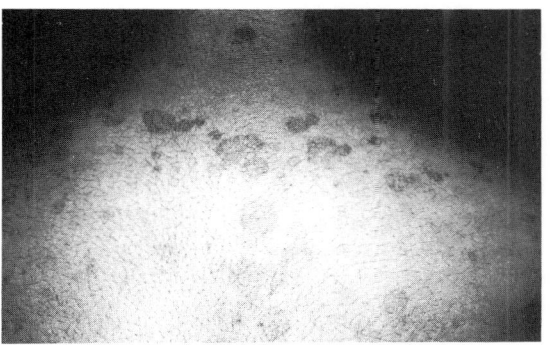

FIGURE 28–54. Tinea versicolor.

delayed hypersensitivity reaction to various chemical agents. The best example of the latter is poison ivy. In wrestlers, reactions to tape are probably most common. Contact dermatitis varies from a mild eczematous disease to a severe bullous erythematous eruption. Itching is a frequent feature, and therefore secondary bacterial infections are a risk owing to violation of the protective skin barrier. The location and configuration of the skin eruption often provide important clues to the causative agent since the reaction appears at the site of exposure to the offending agent. Reactions to primary irritants generally appear within 12 to 24 hours, whereas allergic reactions may require 48 hours or more to appear. If the causative allergen can be identified, removal from exposure cures the eruption. If exposure to the offending substance is continued, further exacerbations can occur.

A mild contact dermatitis can frequently be effectively treated with wet, cool compresses and topical application of 1 percent hydrocortisone cream. The size of large bullae may be reduced by puncturing them and allowing the serous exudate to drain, but removal of the protective roof of the blister should be avoided unless there is secondary infection. Occlusive dressings are generally not advised. Careful observation for secondary bacterial infections is necessary, and if it occurs, systemic antibiotics should be used.

In most instances of mild contact dermatitis, it is not necessary to withhold the athlete from participation. In more severe cases with large bullae formation, it is recommended that the wrestler refrain from contact until there is no longer exudation.

Atopic dermatitis is a type of dermatitis that occurs in patients with a personal or family history of an atopic diathesis (hay fever, allergic rhinitis, etc.). The etiology of the dermatitis is not fully elucidated, but affected individuals have dry skin and demonstrate a low tolerance to irritants, which often increase the dryness. Frequent bathing also tends to increase the dryness. The patients have eczematous lesions with thickening of the skin, most commonly in the flexural areas but also occurring on the face and the dorsum of the hands. Fissuring of the skin is common. Severe itching may develop with characteristic involvement of the trunk and extremities.

Management[31, 42, 47] of the disorder includes first minimizing contributing factors.

Therapy should attempt to mitigate itching, thereby reducing scratching and resultant dermatitis. Dryness benefits from the frequent use of emollients, which often are combined with 1 percent hydrocortisone applied two or three times daily. Only advanced cases necessitate withholding a wrestler from activity. Table 28–12 summarizes measures for prevention of skin diseases in wrestlers.

References

1. Adams D. H. (ed.): 1987 NCAA Wrestling Rules and Interpretations. Shawnee Mission, KS, NCAA Publications 1987.
2. AMA Committee on the Medical Aspects of Sports: Wrestling and weight control. JAMA, 214:1269, 1970.
3. American Alliance for Health, Physical Education and Recreation: Nutrition for Athletes. A Handbook for Coaches. Washington, DC, AAHPER, 1971.
4. American College of Sports Medicine position paper. Med Sci Sports Exerc, 7:1, 1975.
5. American College of Sports Medicine position stand on weight loss in wrestlers. Med Sci Sports Exerc, 8:xi–xiii, 1976.
6. Albrigh, J. P., McAuley E., Martin R. K., Crowley E. T., and Foster D. T.: Head and neck injuries in college football: an eight-year analysis. Am J Sports Med, 13:147–152, 1985.
7. Albright J. P., Moses J. M., Feldick H. G., Dolan K. D., and Burmeister L. D.: Nonfatal cervical spine injuries in interscholastic football. JAMA, 236:1243, 1976.
8. Albright J. P., Van Gilder J., El-Khoury G. Y., Crowley E., and Foster D.: Head and neck injuries in sports. In Scott W. M., Nisonson B., and Nicholas J. A. (eds): Principles of Sports Medicine. Baltimore, Williams & Wilkins, 1984.
9. Baker B. D., Peckham A. C., Pupparo F., and Sanborn J. C.: Review of meniscal injury and associated sports. Am J Sports Med, 13:1, 1985.
10. Becker T. M., Kodsi R., Bailey P., Lee F., Levandowski R., and Nahmias A. J.: Grappling with herpes: Herpes gladiatorum. Am J Sports Med, 16:665, 1988.
11. Beller G. A., Maher J. T., Hartley L. H., et al: Changes in serum and sweat magnesium levels during work in the heat. Aviat Space Environ Med, 46:709, 1975.
12. Bosco J. S., Terjung R. L., and Greenleaf J. E.: Effects of progressive hypohydration on maximal isometric muscular strength. J Sportsmed Phys Fit, 8:81, 1968.
13. Bruce D. A., Schut L., and Sutton L. N.: Brain & cervical spine injuries occurring during organized sports activities in children and adolescents. Clin Sports Med, 1:495, 1982.
14. Cantu R. C.: Guidelines for return to contact sports after a cerebral concussion. Phys Sports Med, 14:75, 1986.
15. Chrisman O. D., Snook G. A., Stanitis J. M., and Keedy V. A.: Lateral-flexion neck injuries in athletic competition. JAMA, 192:117, 1965.

16. Consolazio C. F.: Nutrition and performance. Progress in Food and Nutrition Science, 7:1, 1983.
17. Consolazio C. F., Nelson R. A., Matoush L. O., Harding R. S., and Canham J. E.: Excretion of sodium, potassium, magnesium and iron in human sweat and the relation of each to balance and requirements. J Nutrition, 79:407, 1963.
18. Costill D. L., Cole R., Miller E., and Wynder S.: Water and electrolyte replacement during repeated days of work in the heat. Aviat Space Environ Med, 46:795, 1975.
19. Costill D. L., and Miller J. M.: Nutrition for endurance sport: carbohydrate and fluid balance. Int J Sports Med, 1:2, 1980.
20. Costill D. L., and Saltin B.: Factors limiting gastric emptying during rest and exercise. J Appl Physiol, 37:679, 1974.
21. Costill D. L., and Sparks K. E.: Rapid fluid replacement following thermal dehydration. J Appl Physiol, 34:229, 1973.
22. DePalma A. F.: Surgery of the Shoulder. Philadelphia, JB Lippincott Co, 1983.
23. Eldridge V. L.: Development of pivot shift control. Phys Ther, 64:751, 1984.
24. Ferguson F. J., McMaster J. H., and Stanitski L. L.: Low back pain in college football linemen. Am J Sports Med, 2:63, 1974.
25. Galpin R. D., Hawkins R. J., and Grainger R. W.: A comparative analysis of operative versus nonoperative treatment of grade III acromioclavicular separations. Clin Orthop, 193:150, 1985.
26. Hecker A. L.: Nutritional conditioning for athletic competition. Clin Sportsmed, 3:567, 1984.
27. Houston M. E., Marvin D. A., Green J. H., and Thomson J. A.: The effects of rapid weight loss on physiological functions in wrestlers. Phys Sportsmed, 9:73, 1981.
28. Hursh L. M.: Food and water restriction in the wrestler. JAMA, 241:915, 1979.
29. Jackson D. W., and Mannarino F.: Lumbar spine injuries in athletes. In Scott W. N., Nisonson B., and Nicholas J. A. (eds): Principles of Sports Medicine. Baltimore, Williams & Wilkins, 1984.
30. Katch F. I., and McArdle W. D.: Nutrition, Weight Control and Exercise. Philadelphia, Lea & Febiger, 1983.
31. Krupp M. A., and Chatton M. J.: Current Medical Diagnosis and Treatment. Los Altos, CA, Lange Medical Publications, 1983.
32. McGinness F. L.: Official High School Wrestling Rules. Kansas City, Mo, National Federation Publication. 1987.
33. Micheli L. J.: Back injuries in gymnastics. Clin Sports Med, 4:85, 1985.
34. Morton G. W., and O'Brien G. M.: Wrestling to Rasslin: Ancient Sport to American Spectacle. Bowling Green, OH, Bowling Green State University Popular Press, 1985.
35. Murray R.: The effects of carbohydrate-electrolyte beverages on gastric emptying and fluid absorption during and following exercise. Sports Med, 4:322, 1987.
36. Mustalish A. C., and Quash E. T.: Sports injuries to the chest and abdomen. In Scott W. N., Nisonson B., and Nicholas J. A. (eds): Principles of Sports Medicine. Baltimore, Williams & Wilkins, 1984.
37. Mysnyk M. C., and Albright J. P.: Relative risk and long-term impact of injuries from amateur football and wrestling competition. Unpublished abstract, 1989.
38. Mysnyk M. C., Freeman R. M., Albright J. P., Yesalis C. E., and Oppliger R. A.: Long term effects of weight reduction on blood pressure and renal function in former wrestlers. Submitted for publication, JAMA, 1990.
39. Mysnyk M. C., Wroble R. R., Foster D. T., and Albright J. P.: Prepatellar bursitis in wrestlers. Am J Sports Med, 14:46, 1986.
40. O'Donoghue D. G.: Treatment of Injuries to Athletes. Philadelphia, WB Saunders Co, 1962.
41. Oppliger R. A., and Tipton C. M.: Weight prediction equation tested and available. Iowa Med, p 449, 1985.
42. Pillsbury D. M., and Heaton C. L.: A Manual of Dermatology. Philadelphia, WB Saunders Co, 1980.
43. Reid S. E., and Reid S. E. Jr.: Head and Neck Injuries in Sports. Springfield, IL, Charles C Thomas, Publisher, 1984.
44. Requa R., and Garrick J. G.: Injuries in interscholastic wrestling. Phys Sports Med, 9:44, 1981.
45. Ribisl P. M.: Rapid weight reduction in wrestling. J Sports Med, 3:55, 1975.
46. Rontoyannis G. P., Pahtas G., Dinis D., and Pournaras N.: Sudden death of a young wrestler during competition. Int J Sports Med, 9:353, 1988.
47. Rorsman H., Dermatology. Chicago, Year Book Medical Publishers, Inc, 1976
48. Rose R. D., Schneider P. J., and Sullivan G. F.: A liquid pregame meal for athletes: report on a field trial. JAMA, 178:30, 1961.
49. Saltin B.: Aerobic and anaerobic work capacity after dehydration. J Appl Physiol, 19:1114, 1964.
50. Saltin B.: Circulatory response to submaximal and maximal exercise after thermal dehydration. J Appl Physiol, 19:1125, 1964.
51. Schuller D. E., Strauss R. M., and Dankle S. K.: Auricular injuries and the use of headgear in wrestlers. Med Sci Sports Exerc, 20:524, 1988.
52. Smith N.: Weight control in the athlete. Clin Sportsmed, 3:693, 1984.
53. Stanish W. D., Rubinovich M., Armason T., and Lapenskie G.: Posterior cruciate ligament tears in wrestlers. Can J Appl Sport Sci, 11:173, 1986.
54. Steen S. N., and Brownell K. B.: Weight loss in college wrestlers. Abstract. Presented at annual meeting of the American Diabetic Association, 1986.
55. Steen S. N., and McKinney S.: Nutritional assessment of college wrestlers. Phys Sportsmed, 14:100, 1986.
56. Stevens H.: Epistaxis in the athlete. Phys Sportsmed, 18:31, 1988.
57. Tcheng T. K., and Tipton C. M.: Iowa wrestling study: anthropometric measurements and the prediction of a "minimal" body weight for high school wrestlers. Med Sci Sports, 5:1, 1973.
58. Tipton C. M.: Physiologic problems associated with the "making of weight." Am J Sports Med, 8:449, 1980.
59. Tipton C. M., and Oppliger R. A.: The Iowa wrestling study: lessons for physicians. Iowa Med, 74:381,1974.
60. Tipton C. M., and Tcheng T. K.: Iowa wrestling study. Weight loss in high school students. J Am Med Assoc, 214:1269, 1970.
61. Torg J. S.: Athletic injuries to the cervical spine and brachial plexus. Contemp Orthop, 9:65, 1984.
62. Torranin C., Smith D. P., and Byrd R. J.: The effect of actual thermal dehydration and rapid

rehydration on isometric and isotonic endurance. J Sports Med Phys Fit, 19:1, 1979.
63. Waddell G., McCulloch J. A., Kummel E., and Venner R. M.: Nonorganic physical signs in low back pain. Spine, 5:117, 1980.
64. Warren R. F.: Subluxation of the shoulder in athletes. Clin Sports Med, 2:339, 1983.
65. Wroble R. R., and Albright J. P.: Neck and low back injuries in wrestling. Clin Sports Med, 5:295, 1986.
66. Wroble R. R., and Lindenfeld T. N.: The stabilized Lachman test. Clin Orthop Rel Res, 237:209, 1988.
67. Wroble R. R., Mysnyk M. C., Foster D. T., and Albright J. P.: Patterns of knee injuries in wrestling at the University of Iowa—a six-year study. Am J Sports Med, 14:55, 1986.
68. Zambraski E. J., Foster D. T., Gross P. M., and Tipton C. M.: Iowa wrestling study: weight loss and urinary profiles of collegiate wrestlers. Med Sci Sports, 8:105, 1976.
69. Zambraski E. J., Tipton C. M., Tcheng T. K., Jordan H. R., Vailas A. C., and Callahan A. K.: Iowa wrestling study: changes in the urinary profiles of wrestlers prior to and after competition. Med Sci Sports, 7:217, 1975.

29

FOOTBALL

BRUCE REIDER
ROBERT BELNIAK
DARRYL W. MILLER

The care of football injuries occupies a unique place in sports medicine in the United States. The prominent social and economic role of football in American life and the large number of participants on club, scholastic, and collegiate football squads give the care of football players a special importance. The relatively small number of games in each season and the potential for college scholarships and later rewards can put even greater pressure on the physician to return the athlete to competition than in other sports. As the most widely practiced collision sport, football commonly produces impact injuries that are unusual in other sports, although some of the worst "football injuries" may be noncontact ones. Football's large number of specialized positions require a wide variety of skills: throwing, catching, running, blocking, and tackling. It is almost a collection of sports, with each position requiring its own somatype, athletic skills, and training regimen and even predisposing players to different types of injury that may have different requirements for rehabilitation and return to play.

The physician caring for football players must always keep this specialization in mind. A grade II ulnar collateral ligament sprain of the thumb may be devastating to a quarterback but inconsequential to a lineman; a restrictive shoulder harness may be tolerable to the same lineman but disabling to a wide receiver. In youth and high school football, this specialization is often less rigid. The physician may take advantage of this fact by suggesting that a player temporarily or even permanently be reassigned to a new position to reduce the impact of a particular injury. The better a physician knows the details of football and the requirements of each position, the better he or she will be able to care for each individual player.

The origins of football are usually traced to the game between Princeton and Rutgers universities in 1869. Its popularity quickly spread across college campuses in the East and Midwest. Organized blocking began with the introduction of the "flying wedge" in 1884. In 1885, referees entered the game, soon followed by the first penalty, 5 yards for delay of game. The early pioneers such as Amos Alonzo Stagg, Walter Camp, Pop Warner, John Heisman, and Felding H. Yost began introducing innovations and formations that were rapidly employed.

However, as the popularity of the game began to grow, the number of injuries (and even deaths) increased as well. Interest in safety began to emerge. The first team physician is generally recognized to be Dr. William Conant of Harvard in 1890. Helmets were first worn in 1896. Nevertheless, it became evident that stricter control of rules and regulations was necessary to control the violence and promote safety. President Theodore Roosevelt in 1905 thus proposed the formation of a guiding institution, the Intercollegiate Athletic Association, which was founded in 1906 and in 1910 became the

National Collegiate Athletic Association (NCAA). Rule changes, such as elimination of the flying wedge, were adopted to increase safety. Regulation of play, the use of protective equipment, and proper injury treatment have continued to be the keys to player safety at all levels of competition.

EPIDEMIOLOGY AND INJURY PREVENTION

Although it is methodologically difficult to compare injury rates in different sports, football is generally agreed to have one of the highest injury rates among high school sports. Garrick and Requa in 1978[32] reported an injury rate of 0.81 per player for football players over two seasons, followed by wrestling (0.75), girls' softball (0.44), and girls' gymnastics (0.40). Of course, many of these injuries are mild; three different studies have estimated the percentage of injuries resulting in less than 1 week of lost participation to be 14 percent,[68] 50 percent,[38] and 75 percent.[74]

In 1987, Thompson et al.[90] critically reviewed prior studies of football injuries. They cited data published in 1974, which estimated that 1.5 million young males were participating in organized football in the United States. Calculating with exposure rates that varied from 11 percent[68] to 81 percent[33] depending on the study, they estimated that "a minimum of 165,000 and more likely 200,000 to 1,215,000" preadolescent and adolescent males sustain football injuries in the United States each year. Thompson et al. noted that methodological problems called into question some of the details of each study. For example, the risk of injury was found to increase with age by Robey et al.[79] and Goldberg et al.[38] and was found to be increased in players who had been injured the previous year by Robey et al.[79] and Mueller.[61] However, Thompson et al. pointed out that older athletes and those who had been injured the previous year (and therefore had played the previous year) were more likely to see playing time and therefore might have increased exposure to injury.

With injuries so common, the impetus to predict or prevent them has been strong. The clearest benefit in this regard has come from rule changes and improvement in coaching techniques. Most notable has been the decrease in cervical spine injuries as a result of the prohibition of "spearing" or head-butting tackling techniques. Increased awareness of the potentially catastrophic nature of injuries sustained by players utilizing these techniques has been the result of the implementation of the National Football Head and Neck Injury Registry, inspired by the work of Torg et al.[95] The elimination of the "crackback block"[71,72] has also been responsible for decreases in major knee injuries, although the violent nature of the game continues to expose competitors to trauma to the knee ligaments.

Another approach to injury prevention that appears to make sense is detection and rehabilitation of unrehabilitated injuries and preseason conditioning for all athletes. Cahill and Griffith[14] found that the rate of knee and ankle injuries in a conference of eight Illinois high schools that had a preseason conditioning program (4.1 percent) during the years from 1973 to 1976 was significantly lower than the rate during previous years (1969 to 1972) when no such program was in place (6.8 percent). Thompson et al. pointed out that the historical comparison design is a weakness of this study, since other changes during the period of the study, such as the elimination of blocking below the waist in 1973, may have also contributed to the drop in injury rates. In a randomized study of soccer players, which may also have relevance for football, Ekstrand et al.[27] noted that a seven-point prophylactic program, including: (1) correction of training, (2) provision of optimum equipment, (3) prophylactic ankle taping of players with prior injuries, (4) controlled rehabilitation of lower extremity injuries, (5) exclusion of players with grave knee instability, (6) information at training camps about the importance of disciplined play and the increased risk of injury, and (7) correction and supervision by doctor(s) and physiotherapist(s), resulted in a 75 percent decrease in injuries. Although the efficacy of each point is difficult to prove, principles such as proper conditioning, proper equipment fitting, and proper detection and rehabilitation of injuries would appear to be a sound basis for injury prevention.

The benefit of other types of screening is less obvious. The report of Nicholas[65] that increased ligamentous laxity predisposed football players to knee injuries prompted a spate of similar studies. However, subsequent investigators have failed to confirm the ability of general laxity tests to predict an increased risk of knee injury.[35, 40, 51, 52, 60] In 1974, Klein[54] stated that an isokinetic muscle imbalance of greater than 10 percent between the hamstrings and quadriceps predisposed to knee injuries, an idea also espoused by others. However, Grace et al.'s 1984 well-controlled study of 206 New Mexico high school football players failed to confirm such a relationship.[39]

The effects of shoe design and playing surface on the incidence of injuries have received considerable attention. In the late 1960s and early 1970s, a number of innovators sought to reduce the incidence of knee and ankle injuries with original cleat modifications. At the time, conventional football shoes had seven $\frac{3}{4}$- or $\frac{1}{2}$-inch cleats. Designs included a heel disk[42] and a metallic forefoot turntable.[15] Torg and others[24] championed the "soccer-style" shoe with many shorter cleats. Torg et al. showed in laboratory studies[94] that such shoes had a lower "release coefficient" than the conventional shoe. Torg and Quedenfeld's clinical studies[92, 93] corroborated the laboratory investigations, documenting a marked decrease in severe knee injuries among high school football players wearing soccer-style shoes with molded soles containing fourteen $\frac{3}{8}$-inch cleats compared with players wearing conventional shoes with seven $\frac{3}{4}$-inch cleats. Torg recommended that football shoes should meet the following specifications: (1) synthetic molded sole, (2) a minimum of 14 cleats, (3) cleat diameter at least $\frac{1}{2}$ inch, and (4) maximum cleat length of $\frac{3}{8}$ inch.

Torg's laboratory studies emphasized that the shoe and the playing surface must be considered together, demonstrating that the release coefficient varies with the type of surface, natural or artificial, wet or dry, as well as the number, length, and diameter of the cleats. Since the first such artificial surface, Astroturf, made its debut at the Houston Astro Dome in 1966, players, coaches, and physicians have wondered whether they predispose to injury. Stanitsky et al.[88] in 1974 showed that player speed was increased on artificial turf compared with grass, a factor that might predispose to injury. They also noted that Astroturf absorbed 5 to 10 percent less energy than grass, and Bowers and Martin noted that its ability to absorb impact decreased with time.[10] A decreased ability to absorb impact has been felt to increase the chance of injuries from direct contact. Larson and Osternig[55] noted an increased incidence of prepatellar and olecranon bursitis and Keene et al.[53] a higher incidence of scrapes on synthetic turf.

An important question is whether synthetic surfaces predispose to serious injuries, such as knee injuries requiring surgery. Unfortunately, conclusions from comparative studies have been limited because of differences in equipment, field conditions, personnel, and the precise type of synthetic surface. It has often been pointed out that "natural grass" can vary tremendously according to location, maintenance, and weather.

In 1972, Bramwell and Garrick,[12] in a study of high school football players, reported an increase in the incidence of serious injuries on artificial turf. Conversely, Keene et al.[53] found more serious injuries on grass, although the two surfaces were studied consecutively and not concurrently. A more recent study by Powell[73] of professional teams found increased injury rates on artificial turf that would cause each team to have one more major (causing 21 days loss from play) knee injury every 20 games and one more surgical knee injury every 50 games. These differences were not analyzed using traditional statistical tests for significance.

It thus appears that the definitive epidemiological study on artificial turf has yet to be written. Artificial turf remains a popular option where durability of the playing surfaces under intense use is important. When playing on such surfaces, appropriate shoes and protection from contusions, scrapes, and other impact injuries are clearly essential.

Overall, interscholastic football injuries remain an annual autumn epidemic. Coaches, trainers, and team physicians each play a critical role in the prevention, detection, and rehabilitation of these injuries.

THE HEAD AND NECK

Most interscholastic football players experience an injury of varying severity to their nervous system during their competitive careers. Many of these injuries go unreported to medical personnel, since most players expect to occasionally "get their bell rung" or experience a "stinger" or "burner." Adherence to some basic guidelines in the sideline management of these injuries will protect these athletes from further injury and protect the team physician from unnecessary liability. It must also be emphasized that physicians and trainers must work with coaches to instruct young athletes in proper tackling techniques to minimize the occurrence of more severe head and neck trauma.

Concussions can be graded according to the presence of amnesia and its severity as well as by the presence of loss of consciousness. The complete loss of consciousness often associated with the term *concussion* is relatively unusual in football. Alterations in mentation, sometimes very transient or subtle, are much more common. Players may refer to this as "seeing stars" or "having your bell rung." The physician, trainer, coaches, and teammates must be alert for players whose mildly aberrant or confused behavior may signal a mild concussion, since these athletes often neglect to report their symptoms and may even be unaware of their own condition. As detailed in Chapter 9, transient episodes of confusion and incoordination without amnesia and with full recovery are characteristic of a grade I concussion. After repeat screening examinations, a player suffering a grade I concussion can usually be allowed to return to competition. A grade II concussion is marked by posttraumatic amnesia. Athletes with this symptom should be kept out of competition for the day and may be prone to develop postconcussive symptoms of headache, dizziness, and lack of concentration. Players with these symptoms should be screened with computerized tomography (CT) or magnetic resonance imaging (MRI) for a chronic subdural hematoma and withheld from competition until all symptoms clear. Postconcussive syndrome can be a frustrating condition for the athlete and the physician, because it may take weeks to resolve and little can be done to speed its resolution. Allowing a player to return to contact before all symptoms are gone will usually lead to their recurrence. Retrograde amnesia is the hallmark of a grade III concussion, whereas loss of consciousness characterizes a grade IV concussion. Athletes with either of these symptoms should be withheld from competition, with repeated neurological evaluation for signs of increased intracranial pressure. Transfer to a hospital by ambulance for further observation is mandatory if any such signs are present. Evaluation and treatment of severe head injuries are covered in detail in Chapter 9.

The work of Torg et al.[91, 95] has served to make most orthopedic surgeons aware of the potential catastrophic nature of football injuries to the neck. The mechanism of axial compression associated with incorrect tackling techniques or "spearing" has been well shown by the analysis of game films of numerous injuries, and resulting rule changes have decreased the incidence of fatal and catastrophic neck injuries. Players should now be instructed to tackle with their "heads up" instead of with the tops of their helmets. This reduces the chance of dangerous axial loads across the cervical spine. Nonetheless, cervical fractures do occur and are discussed in Chapter 9. In general, the sideline physician is obligated to investigate further any suspicion of injury to the cervical spine with hospital transfer for radiographic evaluation. Although unstable cervical spine injuries are thankfully rare, they are potentially so devastating that the physician should always evaluate and transport the athlete as if the cervical spine were unstable if there is any suggestion of such an injury. Although it is difficult to set down any rules that would cover all possible circumstances, certainly any unconscious athlete or any player who is down on the field and complains of significant neck pain, especially when accompanied by any localized cervical tenderness or even transient neurological symptoms, warrants such cautious management. Helmet removal at the field is inappropriate if cervical injury is suspected and should be delayed until baseline radiographs are completed. If airway management is an issue, the face mask can be removed, and a screwdriver and bolt cutters for that purpose should be available.

Frequently, the team physician is confronted with a player who has experienced a "burner," an injury named for the burning, dysesthetic pain that usually radiates down the upper extremity. Transient paresthesias and motor weakness in the upper extremities, often without neck pain, are the most common clinical presentations of such an injury.[18] Grade I injuries are those that recover sensation and strength rapidly. The most common motor manifestation of these injuries is deltoid weakness, so the athlete should be tested for symmetrical shoulder abduction strength (Fig. 29–1). These probably represent a neuropraxia of the brachial plexus, and the player may return to the game when symptoms resolve. In a grade II injury, weakness may persist for several weeks or more, and prolonged rehabilitation may be necessary for full return of muscle strength.

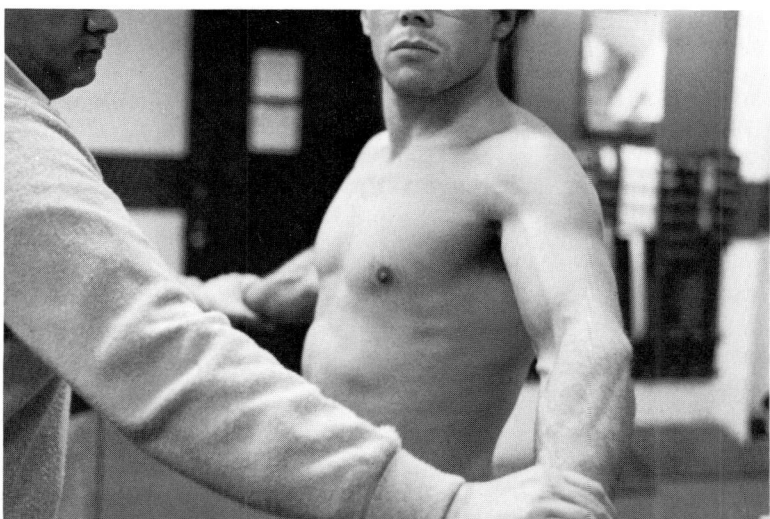

FIGURE 29–1. The most common motor deficit in a "burner" is deltoid weakness, so shoulder abduction strength should be checked after each episode.

These athletes will usually exhibit severe deltoid weakness and a milder decrease in biceps strength. The athlete should be withheld from competition until this has resolved. The rare grade III injuries have deficits that persist for a year or more. Because the mechanism of burners is felt frequently to involve lateral bending of the neck toward the contralateral shoulder, a wide variety of neck rolls and collars have been developed to help the player who has recurrent grade I burner episodes (Fig. 29–2). They may help decrease the frequency or severity of these episodes, although we know of no controlled studies that prove they do so. Off-season neck strengthening and flexibility exercises are also traditional for the player with a tendency to develop burners. Sometimes recurrent grade I burners may become so distressing to the athlete that it is wise to withhold him from contact for a week or more, even when no motor deficit is present.

Torg et al.[95] have helped to elucidate a syndrome of transient quadriplegia in football players, which can often be associated with congenital, degenerative, or posttraumatic stenosis of the cervical spinal canal (Chapter 9). Continued participation in football following an episode of transient quadriplegia can often be a vexing decision for the young athlete, his parents, and his physician. Although it has not been shown that an episode of spinal cord neuropraxia predisposes the athlete to permanent quadriplegia, the physician may be reluctant to assume the liability of returning such an athlete to play.

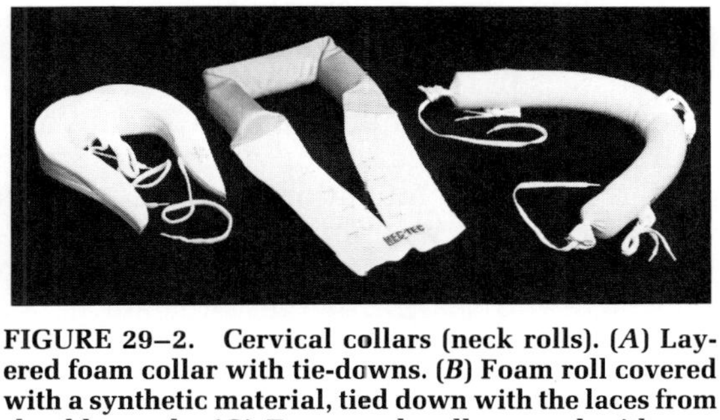

THE LUMBAR SPINE

Low back pain is a common problem in football players. McCarroll et al. reported an incidence of 21 percent among players at Indiana University.[57] Spondylolysis appears to be the most common cause of recalcitrant low back pain in football players. Saal, a physiatrist specializing in spine problems, stated that among football-related spine problems referred to him after the failure of 6 weeks of "nonspecific care," 70 percent involved the posterior elements and 25 percent involved the intervertebral disk.[85]

Interior linemen have been classically identified as susceptible to developing spon-

FIGURE 29–2. Cervical collars (neck rolls). (A) Layered foam collar with tie-downs. (B) Foam roll covered with a synthetic material, tied down with the laces from shoulder pads. (C) Foam neck roll covered with surgical stockinet and tie-downs.

dylolysis, but players at any position may develop it. In McCarroll et al.'s study, 74 percent of the cases occurred in nonlinemen, suggesting that other factors such as weight training errors or congenital predisposition may contribute. However, an incidence of spondylolysis of 15 percent compared with 6 percent in the general population implies that football may predispose to this condition, although their sample only contained 145 players.

Eighty-six percent of the Indiana University players with spondylolysis arrived at college with abnormal radiographs, a fact that suggests that they had developed the condition in high school or earlier. Because of this, the team physician must carefully evaluate each young football player with low back pain. Any athlete with moderate to severe or recalcitrant pain should have plain radiographs, and those with normal radiographs but persistent pain should be studied with bone scans. Pain with extension of the lumbar spine is typical of spondylolysis and should signal a close investigation. Players with normal radiographs and bone scans but severe or radicular pain may have intervertebral disk pathology and should be treated and evaluated accordingly.

Because there is evidence that the patient with normal radiographs but increased activity on bone scan may achieve bony healing, we hold such players from contact and fit them with a custom-molded lumbar orthosis. (Fig. 10–6). If spondylolysis is clearly evident on radiographs, we feel that the prospect for bony healing is small and treat such patients symptomatically with a course of nonsteroidal antiinflammatory drugs (NSAIDS) and a temporary reduction in activity level. Some occasionally require a prefabricated lumbar support. Spondylolisthesis, when present, is rarely greater than grade I. Since there is no evidence that such patients are predisposed to traumatic paraplegia, we allow these athletes to play according to pain tolerance unless they show signs of a radiculopathy or progression of spondylolisthesis (Fig. 10–2). McCarroll et al. found that all their patients with spondylolysis were able to complete their college football careers; this is generally true of high school football players, although younger ones may have to be excluded if they show signs of progression of spondylolisthesis or may themselves choose to change to a less traumatic sport.

THE SHOULDER

Instability of the shoulder, trauma to the proximal humerus, and injuries of the shaft and articulations of the clavicle are frequently seen in the scholastic football player. Precise anatomical diagnosis may often be difficult, particularly in the case of instability and rotator cuff tendinitis, two entities whose interrelation is only beginning to be elucidated.

Recurrent episodes of shoulder instability may be caused by constitutional factors such as ligamentous laxity or may be posttraumatic. History and physical examination may often serve to help the clinician differentiate between these patterns. This is discussed in more detail in Chapter 11. One dilemma that frequently presents itself is the case of an athlete who sustains a primary shoulder dislocation in early or midseason. Although there is a consensus that the frequency of recurrence in school-age athletes is high regardless of the treatment, it is still controversial whether immobilization after the primary episode can reduce the risk of recurrence.[4, 47, 48, 82, 86] We generally recommend 3 weeks of immobilization but explain to the parents and athlete that uncertainty exists regarding its prophylactic efficacy. This allows the family to make an informed judgment, should they wish to choose immediate rehabilitation and early return to play for social reasons such as a college scholarship. In the future, the ability to predict with arthroscopy or MRI which shoulders are prone to recurrence may allow us to distinguish which are unlikely to benefit from immobilization. Recurrent anteroinferior dislocations and subluxation in the young athlete are often resistant to rehabilitation programs owing to the presence of injury to the labral-ligamentous complex. A player with recurrent anterior instability may elect to finish the season after a program of strengthening exercises, although surgical stabilization in the off-season is usually advisable if the athlete wishes to continue to participate in football. In the absence of convincing evidence that recurrent subluxations or dislocations predispose the glenohumeral joint to degenerative changes, we will allow a player to complete the season in these instances, always with a supervised rehabilitation program and with a harness if his position allows it. For the surgical repair in these young athletes, we prefer anatomical procedures

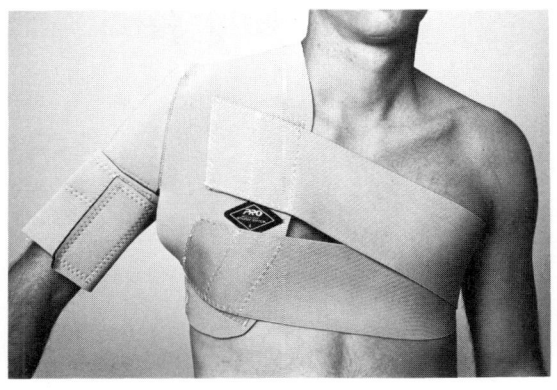 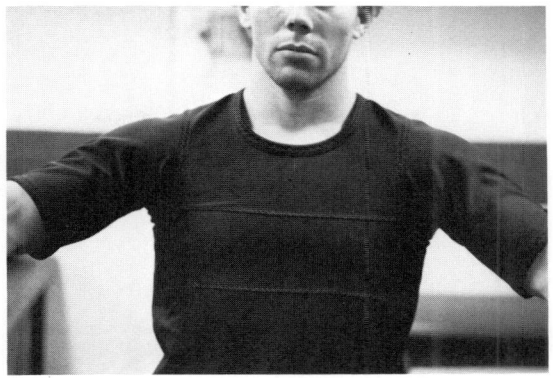

FIGURE 29–3. (A) This brace is constructed of elastic and neoprene rubber with Velcro fasteners to restrict abduction, external rotation, and elevation beyond 90 degrees. Indications are recurrent anterior subluxation and/or dislocation of the glenohumeral structure. (B) A stiffly-knit, snug-fitting "bench press" shirt made for power lifters may provide some security for an athlete who cannot wear a more restrictive device. Another style of restraint is depicted in Figure 30–8.

that leave no internal fixation such as the Bankart procedure[81] or one of its modifications[77] or a capsular shift if multidirectional instability exists.[64]

Various restraining devices may help reduce the chance of recurrence while the athlete is awaiting surgery. (Fig. 29–3A). Since these attempt to prevent anterior dislocation by restricting the shoulder from the abducted–externally rotated position, they will not be acceptable for players whose positions require full overhead motion, such as receivers or defensive backs, and will not be effective in players whose shoulders dislocate in less extreme positions. The stiffly knit, snug-fitting "bench press" shirts designed for power lifters may give some additional stability or feeling of security to athletes who cannot wear a more restrictive device (Fig. 29–3B).

Trauma to the proximal humerus produces characteristic fracture patterns. The Salter Harris type II (physeal-metaphyseal) injury is commonly seen in adolescents. Fortunately, remodeling potential in these cases is great, and the inherent mobility of the shoulder girdle compensates for residual deformity. Therefore, all but the most severely displaced or angulated fractures can be managed by closed, conservative means. Abduction splints are awkward but may be necessary to achieve satisfactory closed reduction (Fig. 29–4). The lightweight ones manufactured for rotator cuff surgery are usually effective and more tolerable than a shoulder spica cast. Lack of fracture pain and tenderness as well as return of shoulder motion and strength are the guidelines for returning to competition after such an injury. Similarly, fractures of the shaft of the clavicle are nearly universally treated conservatively with gradual return to activity as tolerated and produce no long-term disability.

Treatment of dislocations of the ends of the clavicle have caused a great deal of controversy in the orthopedic literature. Their classification and treatment are covered in Chapter 12. A peculiar feature of acromioclavicular dislocations in the immature skeleton is the tendency of the distal clavicle to "squirt" out of its periosteal sleeve, giving the clinical and radiographic picture of a grade III injury despite the presence of intact acromioclavicular and coracoclavicular ligaments. Consequently, we favor symptomatic treatment of almost all acromioclavicular dislocations in the young athlete. Grade III dislocations in the older population can be treated in a similar fashion.

Football players are particularly prone to acromioclavicular injuries owing to the frequency of tackling or falls on the shoulder. Even well-fitting shoulder pads cannot completely eliminate these injuries. Modifications to the shoulder pads, such as "risers" or "lifters," can easily be made to protect previously injured joints once the athlete returns to play. (Figs. 29–5 and 29–15).

The diagnosis of sternoclavicular dislocation requires a high degree of suspicion. Many anterior dislocations can be managed nonoperatively, often with closed reduction.

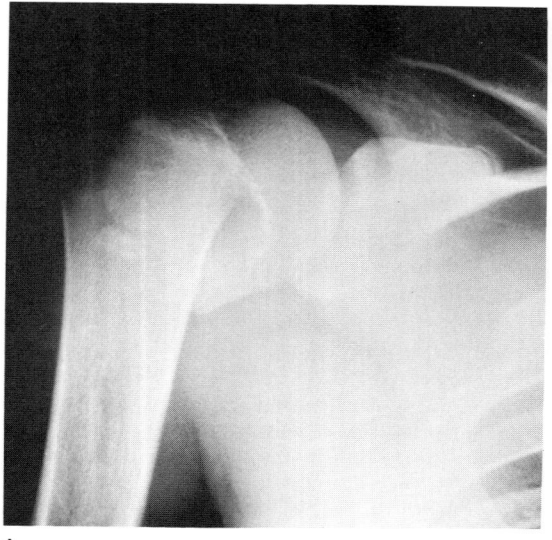 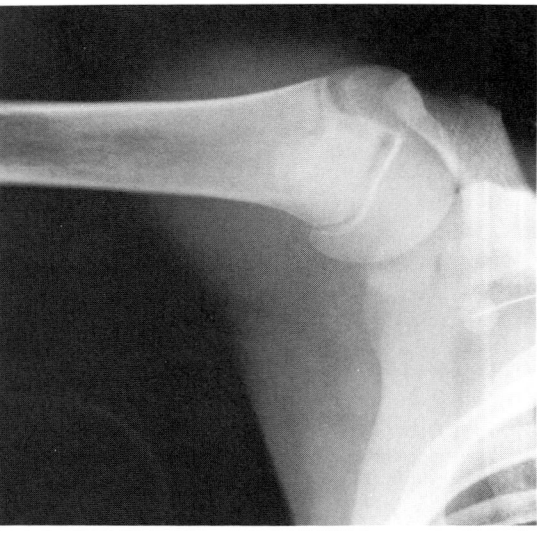

FIGURE 29–4. (A) This physeal fracture in a 15-year-old football player was treated with closed reduction and (B) immobilization in an abduction splint for 1 month.

A potentially more devastating injury, although fortunately rarer, is the posterior sternoclavicular dislocation. Prompt reduction and observation for the complications related to intrathoracic penetration are mandatory (see Chapter 12).

Injuries to the wrist and hand are common in football. Chapter 14 discusses their treatment in detail. Metacarpal and finger fractures tend to heal rapidly in school-age youngsters. Many injuries will be stable in 3 weeks time; a reliable athlete can then be allowed full mobilization during daily activities while being protected with a playing cast or splint during football. In the case of some injuries, such as flexor profundus tendon avulsion, optimal treatment may not be compatible with early return to football. In these cases, the parents and players must decide whether the potential benefit of continued participation justifies accepting the deformity or disability of a compromised result.

The use of "soft" playing splints or casts may allow a player to return to participation while a fracture or ligament injury is still healing. They are particularly useful for metacarpal fractures and thumb injuries. Bergfeld et al. reported the use of such splints in 32 wrist fractures, including 11 scaphoid injuries, with no apparent ill effects;[8] of the 6 acute scaphoid injuries, 5 healed primarily, and 1 was lost to follow-up. Some injuries can be treated immediately with a "soft cast" while others should be initially immobilized in a conventional cast and then changed to a soft cast after two to four weeks. In each case, of course, the physician should make an individual assessment of the stability of the injury and the suitability of treatment in a "soft" playing splint or cast.

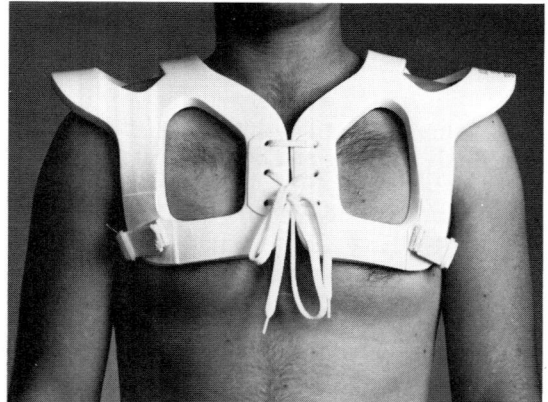

FIGURE 29–5. Lifter (modified shoulder pad). Lifters provide additional support by absorbing shock from impact and dispersing the forces from impact via the cutout over each acromioclavicular joint.

HIP AND PELVIS

Fortunately, major hip and pelvic fractures and dislocations are infrequent in contact sports. The vast majority of injuries encountered on the football field are either direct contusions or muscular avulsions. The physis of the immature skeleton is the "weakest link" in the muscle origin complex, predisposing the pelvic ring to avulsion injuries at any one of its numerous muscle attachment sites.

The most common sites of avulsion fractures in the immature pelvis are the anterior superior iliac spine (sartorius origin), the ischial tuberosity (hamstrings), the lesser trochanter (iliopsoas), the anterior inferior iliac spine (rectus femoris), and the iliac crest (external oblique and hip abductors). Generally, all these injuries can be conservatively managed according to the guidelines set out by Metzmaker and Pappas.[59] Initially, a period of rest with positioning to relax the involved muscle group is prescribed. Once pain and spasm have resolved, the patient may gradually be allowed to increase the range of motion of the affected muscle and joint. Resistive exercises are withheld until full motion is achieved. Return to sport-specific practice activities can be initiated as strength returns, and competition may be allowed once the athlete has recovered full strength.

Chronic nonunion of these avulsions has been reported[34] and may be painful. In these unusual cases, excision of the ununited fragment may be indicated.

The iliac crest is particularly vulnerable to trauma in football players, and contusions to this area of the pelvis, or "hip pointers," can be the source of considerable disability for the athlete. Aspiration of large iliac crest hematomas may occasionally give symptomatic relief, but generally these injuries can be managed with the acute application of ice and compressive dressings and NSAIDS. Tenderness and lameness may persist for days or weeks following this injury. We generally allow these athletes to return to contact with special padding when the pain is tolerable and any limp has disappeared (Fig. 29–15). Injecting the acute hematoma with a small amount of steroid has been successful in preventing most of the morbidity of these injuries in college and professional players, but we do not advocate the routine use of this technique in the school-age athlete.

True fractures and dislocations of the hip joint are fairly rare in football. Clinicians caring for adolescent athletes with hip or knee pain need to be constantly vigilant of the possibility of slipped femoral capital epiphysis, which may also present with referred pain in the knee. Legg-Calvé-Perthes disease, bone infections, and tumors are other nontraumatic causes of hip, thigh, and knee pain to which school-age football players are not immune.

MUSCLE CONTUSIONS AND MYOSITIS OSSIFICANS

Direct blows to the muscle masses of the thigh or arm can produce significant contusions and large intramuscular hematomas. Severe quadriceps contusions may be associated with a knee effusion in the absence of a specific knee injury. Jackson and Feagin's study of 65 quadriceps contusions in West Point cadets[50] outlines the basic management strategy for these injuries and for the prevention of their complications. The hospitalization that they recommended for severely injured cadets does not seem to be necessary for the school-age athlete with a supportive family. The severity of the injury can usually be graded by the consequent loss of knee motion. Ice and rest are the mainstays of acute treatment, with the goal of minimizing hemorrhage. After the first 48 hours, gentle quadriceps stretching and strengthening exercises are implemented, with care taken to avoid overzealous passive stretching. Upper extremity lesions, which usually occur in the biceps or brachialis, may be treated similarly. The athlete may return to competition once full range of motion and 90 percent of contralateral strength are regained, but protective thigh pads are important to avoid reinjury (Fig. 29–12).

Occasionally, for reasons poorly understood, the more severe of these contusions may evolve into myositis ossificans, where heterotopic ossification occurs in the substance of the affected muscle. The prediction of myositis ossificans can often be made when the initial swelling persists or enlarges and the muscle becomes very warm and tender. Radiographic changes may occur 3 to 4 weeks postinjury. The unsuspecting clinician may mistake these changes for those of osteogenic sarcoma, and haphazard biopsy may yield a diagnosis consistent with malignancy. Jackson and Feagin emphasized that this condition is very different from the disabling myositis ossificans that may develop around joints in neurologically impaired patients or following surgery. They noted that myositis ossificans tended to form in patients with more severe degrees of injury but that it did not correlate with the duration of disability and none of these patients had permanent disability. We therefore do not treat these patients differently from other patients with muscle contusions but allow them to return to contact with padding when they meet the criteria of full joint motion and nearly normal strength. Surgical resection of myositis ossificans is rarely indicated, as these lesions will regress with time.

THE KNEE

A knee injury is the most common reason for a football player to seek medical evaluation by a sports medicine specialist. In 1982, Pritchett[75] calculated that knee injuries accounted for 12.7 percent of high school football injuries reported to an insurance company and 31.8 percent of all medical costs paid by the company. Specific knee injuries are covered separately in the text, and the reader is referred to these chapters for detailed management of these clinical entities. A discussion of these injuries as they relate to football and the controversies regarding knee brace wear will be considered here.

ANTERIOR CRUCIATE LIGAMENT INJURIES

With more media attention focused on athletes and their injuries, well-informed competitors may fear an injury to their anterior cruciate ligament (ACL) as signaling the end of their football careers. Certainly, rupture of the anterior cruciate ligament is a potential cause of extensive secondary morbidity in a school-age athlete. Not long ago, we commonly encountered young athletes who underwent prolonged treatment, endured multiple giving-out episodes, and had one or both menisci removed before an underlying anterior cruciate ligament tear was diagnosed. An increased awareness of the common nature of anterior cruciate ligament tears in football and many other sports is leading to earlier diagnosis and treatment for these athletes.

The details of decision-making in the treatment of the young athlete with an acute or chronic ACL tear are explained in Chapter 18. In general, the prognosis for playing football with an anterior cruciate–deficient knee is not good. The experience of Hawkins et al.[45] and others is that teenage athletes as a group do poorly following ACL tears. Studies such as that of Giove et al.[34] that are relatively optimistic regarding return to sports following nonoperative treatment of an ACL tear tend to include an older patient population that does not wish to return to sports as stressful as football: "Sports requiring quick turns, sudden stopping, jumping, or lateral movements (such as football, volleyball, basketball, and racquetball) showed the lowest levels of return to participation."[34] Since the demands of the different positions vary, it may be more feasible for some players such as linemen to play successfully without ACL reconstruction than others such as linebackers or backs.

The athlete and his family should be presented with all this information, including the details and risks of surgery, and allowed to make their own decision. Some will choose to stop playing football; many will request surgical reconstruction. The prognosis for postoperative return to football, if desired, appears to be good with contemporary reconstruction techniques. In some cases, surgery may have to be postponed until skeletal maturity. Those electing nonoperative treatment must be well educated about their condition so that they will seek further care before they have destroyed their knees with repeated episodes of giving way.

The efficacy of functional knee bracing as part of the nonoperative treatment of ACL tears is under continued investigation. Clinical studies show that they reduce the incidence of giving-out episodes in many unstable knees, although biomechanical studies seriously question the proposition that they do so by physically stabilizing the knee. For example, in a clinical study, Colville et al.[23] found that 69 percent of braced patients experienced a significant reduction in giving-way episodes and improved athletic performance, although they were unable to show by instrumented testing that the brace reduced anterior subluxation of the tibia.

The two major styles of functional knee braces are the (1) hinge, post, and strap (Fig. 29–6A) and (2) the hinge, post, and shell (Fig. 29–6C). In an in vitro study, Beck et al.[7] found that the hinge, post, and shell braces tend to work better as a group, although the effectiveness of all braces in controlling anterior tibial displacement decreases as the

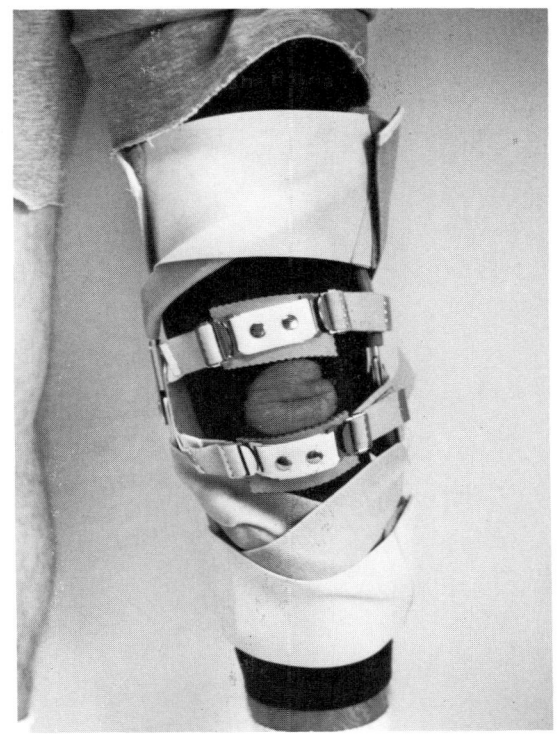
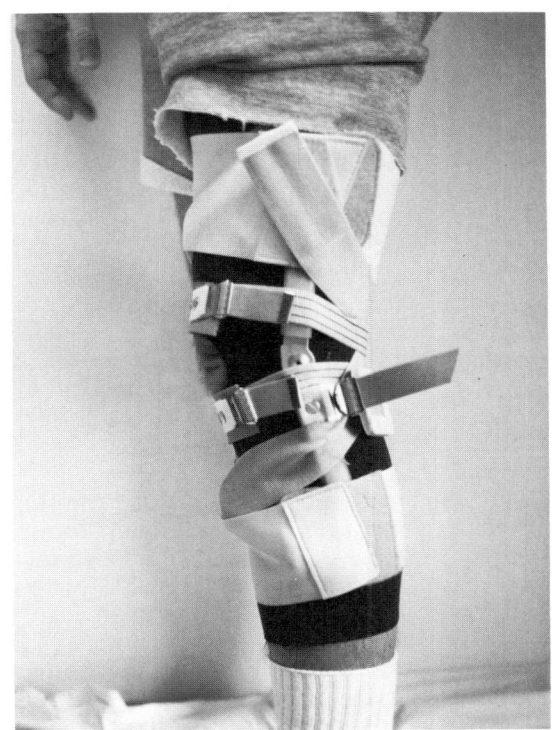
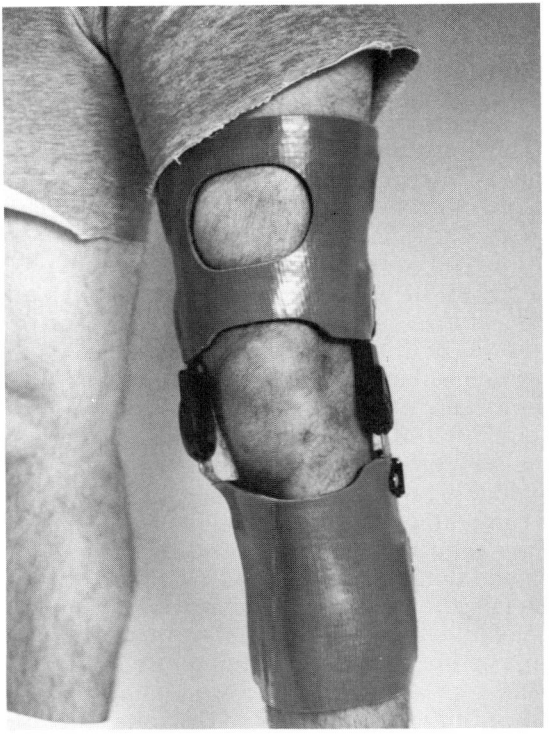
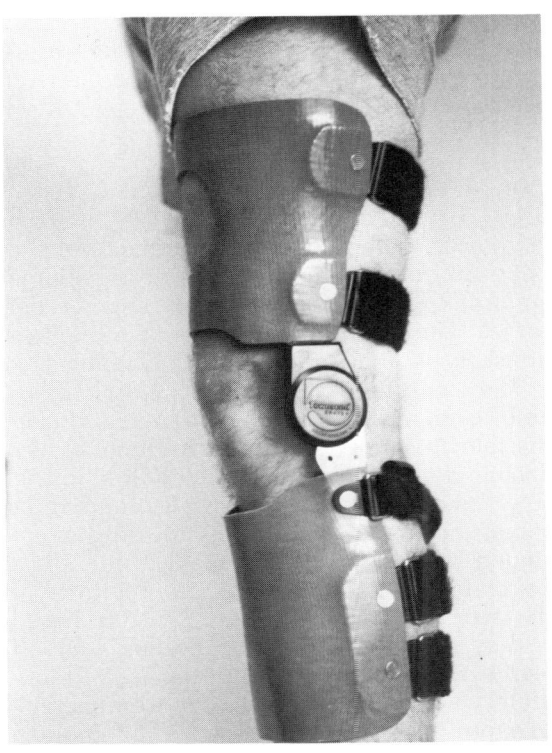

FIGURE 29–6. The two major styles of functional knee braces are the hinge, post, and strap (*A, Front; B, lateral*) and hinge, post, and shell (*C, Front; D, lateral*).

applied force increases. We currently favor the new generation of hinge, post, and shell braces with complex hinges that try to mimic the rolling, gliding mechanism of the knee (Fig. 29–6B). Although there is no evidence that such braces are more effective than other types, they are less prone to the annoying tendency of braces with simpler hinges to "piston" up or down the leg. They thus tend to be better tolerated. Whatever brace is chosen, it should be emphasized to the patient that brace wear is not an absolute safeguard against further episodes of instability.

POSTERIOR CRUCIATE INJURIES

The diagnosis and treatment of posterior cruciate ligament (PCL) tears are detailed in Chapter 19. Most PCL tears in football players are isolated injuries and can be treated with functional rehabilitation with an excellent prospect of return to competition.[29, 69] If the PCL is torn in combination with other ligaments, surgery is more likely to be indicated. The potential for vascular damage should always be kept in mind when treating these "blow-out" injuries, and the integrity of the limb should not be risked to repair the ligaments. In the most severe ligament injuries, return to football may not be a realistic goal.

COLLATERAL INJURIES

Injuries to the collateral ligaments of the knee are frequent in football, causing a large amount of temporary disability and missed games. Their treatment is almost exclusively nonsurgical and is discussed in Chapter 17.

The common occurrence of medial collateral ligament (MCL) sprains in football led to the fabrication of prophylactic hinge braces designed to prevent or attenuate this injury[2] (Fig. 29–7). These braces have lateral or sometimes medial and lateral hinges designed to absorb valgus impact to the knee. Favorable initial anecdotal impressions of these braces caused them to be purchased widely by high school and college football teams. Subsequent epidemiological and laboratory studies have questioned their effectiveness. The study by Hansen et al.[43] found a decrease in ligament and meniscal repairs in braced players, but Hewson et al.'s[46] study the following year showed little difference

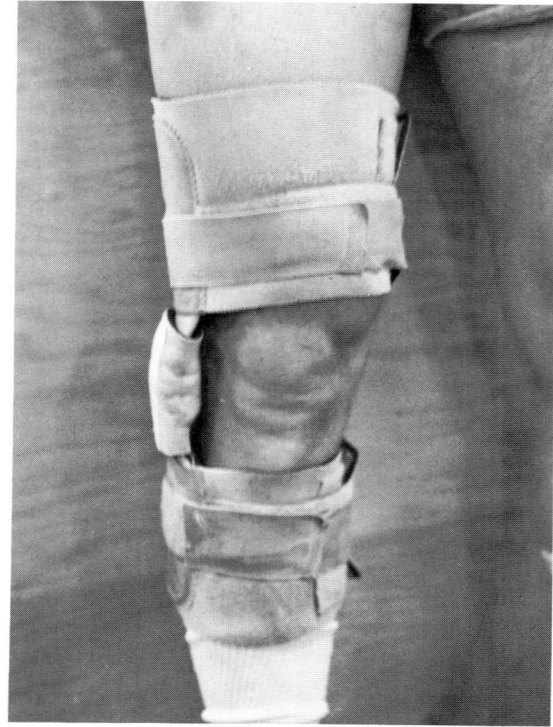

FIGURE 29–7. Prophylactic braces such as this were introduced to decrease the incidence of knee injury but have not been shown to achieve this goal.

between braced and unbraced players. Studies by Rovere et al.[80] and Teitz et al.[89] actually showed increased injury frequency in players wearing braces and raised the possibility that the braces might increase the chance of MCL injury by preloading it. The study by Teitz et al. included 6307 college football players in 1984 and 5445 in 1985. Grace et al.[99] confirmed these findings and also showed an increase in foot and ankle injuries in the braced players. Reviews of the available data by Garrick and Requa[31] and the American Academy of Orthopaedic Surgeons in 1987[1] have concluded that there is no evidence to support the use of currently available knee braces.

Laboratory studies by Paulos et al.,[70] France et al.,[30] and Baker et al.[6] have confirmed that the first generation of prophylactic knee braces is not capable of resisting the level of valgus stress that is probably involved in producing a clinical MCL sprain. France et al. and Paulos et al. showed that brace-induced MCL preload was negated by joint compression forces.

France et al. postulated that the "ideal" brace should decrease the lateral force at

MCL injury by 80 percent. Hopefully, future designs will achieve this goal and offer some protection against injury. For the moment, there is no convincing evidence that prophylactic braces decrease the frequency of injuries to the medial collateral ligament, and their routine use is not recommended. We have, however, found them very useful for providing gentle support during the rehabilitation of MCL sprains (Chapter 17).

FOOT AND ANKLE INJURIES

The athletic footwear industry has become increasingly visible recently, as consumers spend more dollars each year on sports shoes. Although many recreational athletes make footwear choices based more on current style than on biomechanical considerations, changes in playing surfaces and more vigorous training regimens have caused an increase in the number of foot and ankle injuries evaluated by the sports medicine physician. In one study at Rice University, ankle and foot injuries ranked just behind knee injuries as the most common cause of time loss from sports.[19]

The frequency of ankle sprains in football and other sports has prompted many attempts to prevent such injuries with some form of stabilization. The most commonly used method is that of ankle taping, although the cost of this technique in terms of materials and time has led to the use of reusable strapping or supports as an alternative (Fig. 29–8).

Studies of these techniques have attempted to determine (1) if they actually restrict excessive ankle motion and (2) if they reduce the risk of injury. In 1962, Rarick et al. published a study[76] in which they measured the passive excursion of the ankle to an inversion–plantar flexion test. They found that taping did indeed restrict this motion but that 10 minutes of exercise reduced the net support strength of the taping by 40 percent. In 1980, Laughman et al.[56] published their study that used an electrogoniometer system to measure restriction of motion associated with an inversion ankle sprain both before and after 15 minutes of zigzag running. They

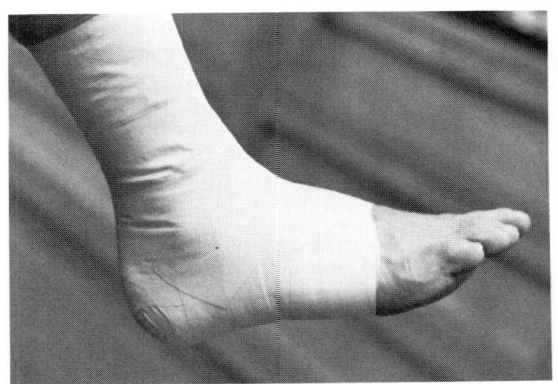

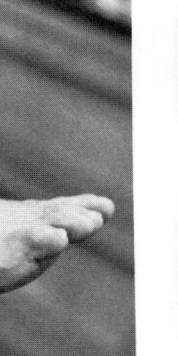

A

B

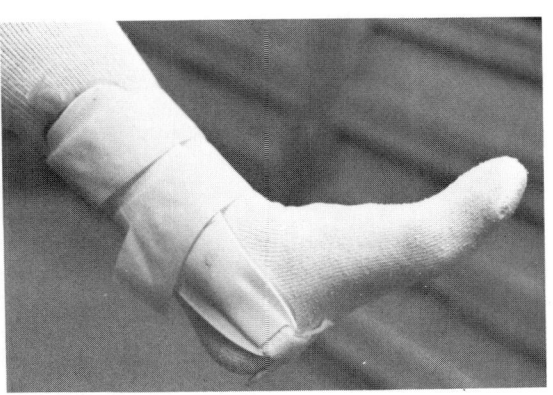

FIGURE 29–8. Techniques for externally supporting the ankle include (*A*) taping, (*B*) reusable canvas brace, and (*C*) the air splint, a plastic stirrup with an inflatable lining.

C

found that taping did restrict these motions an average of 27 percent, compared with the untaped control. Although exercise reduced this restriction by 12 percent, the effect remained significant. Taping thus appears to have the potential to protect against inversion sprains, but its effectiveness decreases during use. A 1983 study by Hughes and Stitts[49] showed a thermoplastic splint to offer restriction of motion similar to taping, indicating that less expensive reusable devices may also be helpful.

Garrick and Requa concluded in 1973 in a clinical study[31] that taping did indeed decrease the risk of ankle sprain. In a 1985 prospective study, Tropp et al. compared the incidence of ankle sprain among a control group of soccer players with those protected with a special brace and those given a coordination training program on an "ankle disk" for 10 weeks.[96] Among athletes who had a history of prior ankle injury, the incidence of sprain was 2 percent in the brace group and 3 percent in the disk-trained group compared with 25 percent in the controls. Among the athletes with no history of ankle injury, neither the brace nor training appeared to reduce the risk of injury. Based on these studies, it thus appears advisable to rehabilitate ankle sprains using a method that is designed to restore strength and proprioception and to protect these athletes with taping or bracing.

In the foot, the injury to the first metatarsophalangeal (MTP) joint whimsically called "turf toe" can be a vexing problem in football players. The great toe carries more than twice the load seen by the other toes, and 40 to 60 percent of body weight may act across its metatarsophalangeal joint. These large forces are reflected by the well-developed capsuloligamentous complex protecting this joint. Injuries to this complex can be graded according to their severity. Grade I injuries are marked by local tenderness without swelling or ecchymosis. Grade II injuries have swelling and ecchymosis, and tenderness may be less well localized. Grade III sprains have more marked tenderness, primarily dorsally, and probably represent a spontaneously reduced MTP dislocation.

In reported series of injuries to the great toe MTP joint, authors have noted a fairly consistent mechanism of joint hyperextension as well as a predisposition to this injury in football players competing on artificial surfaces. Traditional cleated football shoes have rigid forefoot components to allow for attachment of the cleats. Lightweight, noncleated, flexible shoes often preferred by players for use on synthetic surfaces are much more flexible in the forefoot, allowing the great toe to dorsiflex forcefully, causing the turf toe syndrome of MTP injury and resultant synovitis. In a study from Rice University,[19] 51 out of 53 reported injuries to the MTP joint of the great toe were seen in football players, all of whom were wearing flexible, lightweight shoes while performing on artificial (Astroturf) surfaces.

Treatment of these injuries has been fairly standard, with ice, compression, rest, and nonsteroidal antiinflammatory agents. Corticosteroid injections have generally worked poorly in these injuries and should be avoided.[19] Loss of playing time ranged from 0 to 56 days in one series. Several authors have stressed the possibility of prevention of turf toe by the use of shoes with stiffer forefoot components or shoe stiffening orthotic devices.[19, 21, 26] No definitive follow-up is currently available regarding these shoe modifications.

STRESS FRACTURES

Stress fractures are unusual but not unknown in football. The ones that we have seen have manifested themselves very early in the season and appear to be related to overly intensive running by the athlete during his preseason conditioning program. It is important to be alert to the possibility of such fractures, since some of them, such as fractures of the femur, navicular (Fig. 22–28), and medial malleolus (Fig. 22–29), may have serious consequences if undetected.

HEAT ILLNESS

No sport other than football is played in such a wide variety of weather conditions. Although heat illness is a concern in many other sports, it is a particular problem in football because of the large amount of protective equipment worn regardless of the ambient temperature. An ever-lengthening season and higher competitive demands make preseason practice sessions begin earlier, when summer heat and humidity can take an excessive physiological toll on fully padded players. Awareness of the signs of heat illness and active prophylaxis of the problem have decreased its incidence over the last 20 years. Nevertheless, there were 11 documented heat stroke deaths in American football between 1981 and 1988.[62] The spectrum of heat illness is a continuum, ranging from mild cramps to full-blown heat exhaustion. *Heat cramps* often occur in the calf muscles and can usually be treated symptomatically with oral hydration, ice, and rest. Similarly, *heat syncope* is manifested by fatigue, dizziness, and a weak, rapid pulse and can usually be managed by cessation of activity, cooling of the patient, and replenishment of lost fluids in the form of water. *Heat exhaustion* often requires more aggressive therapy. The patient is often delirious, complaining of thirst and fatigue, with an elevated body temperature and moist, sweating skin. This patient may often require hospitalization, with electrolyte replacement. The most serious form of heat illness, *heat stroke*, can be fatal if not promptly recognized and treated. A patient with heat stroke presents with a body temperature of 104° F or greater, with a strong, rapid pulse and hot, dry skin. Management of this patient involves rapid cooling and fluid replacement, as well as observation for coagulation abnormalities, renal failure, and hemorrhage in other viscera.

Prophylaxis of heat illness in terms of activity modification and fluid replacement is most important. Most experts recommend the use of a sling psychrometer to monitor wet bulb temperatures, a measure of both temperature and relative humidity. As wet bulb readings rise to a range of 68° to 73° F, all players should be required to drink water as a preventive measure. Between 74° and 79°, practice routines should be adjusted and any individuals known to be susceptible to heat illness should not be allowed to practice. If wet bulb readings rise above 80°, practice should either be postponed or conducted without pads.

The prevention of heat illness, then, primarily involves keeping the athlete well hydrated. Required daily weigh-ins are an easy way to detect the player who may be becoming progressively dehydrated before clinical heat illness has a chance to develop. Since sweat is hypotonic, players competing in hot and humid conditions will experience a total body water deficit. Salt tablets, soft drinks, and many commercially available solutions for athletes are hypertonic and therefore inappropriate for maintenance of correct fluid balance in the active athlete. Unlimited water should be available, and its use should be encouraged by coaches and trainers. In warm weather, trainers and physicians should keep an eye out for any player who may be sweating profusely and encourage him to drink water before any specific manifestations of heat illness develop. The sweaty player who is sitting on the bench "catching his breath" may be in the early, easily reversible stages of heat illness. Such players should be rehydrated orally and rested until profuse sweating has stopped and their resting pulse is normal.

SIDELINE DECISIONS

When he or she assumes the role of team physician, a doctor is given a wonderful opportunity to serve the community, not only through the care of injured athletes but by becoming a friend and role model to many healthy youngsters. In the United States, community and high school football teams provide the most common setting for a practitioner to serve as a team physician. One reason for this is the cultural importance of football to the typical American community, but another important reason is the very real medical benefit of having a physician available who knows the players and can be called on when injuries occur during practices and to provide sideline assistance during games. Although team physicians are most commonly identified with football, this concept is certainly applicable to most other team sports.

To function optimally as a team physician, the practitioner must establish a friendly rapport with the players when they are healthy. The physician should make it clear to the players that he or she is present for their benefit, to maximize their participation and enjoyment and prevent excessive time lost due to injury. It is important for the players to realize that the physician is neither an adversarial spoilsport dedicated to preventing their participation in football nor an extension of the athletic establishment, dedicated to returning them to play at any cost. If players come to regard the physician as a trusted friend, they will feel free to discuss their injuries with him or her instead of hiding them.

Having a standard series of functional tests for deciding the ability of players to return to the game will be a great help to the physician in making sideline decisions. Although each decision must be made on an individual basis, such guidelines will remove much of the subjectivity from these decisions and emphasize to the player that it is the injury, not the physician, that is keeping him off the field. Failing such simple functional tests will usually make it clear to the player that he is unable to return to play.

The presence of a physician on the football sideline has two principal purposes. The first is to detect and treat conditions that are serious or life-threatening and that require immediate attention. This includes evaluation and treatment of injury to the central nervous system, spine, or major internal organs or metabolic and medical problems such as heat illness, diabetic crisis, or asthmatic attack. The second purpose is to evaluate injuries that are less serious but may still produce a temporary or permanent functional disability. In such cases, the physician must decide whether continued participation following the injury will expose the player to a significantly greater risk of permanent disability or an unacceptable level of pain. In general, any significant increase in the risk of permanent disability is an indication for withholding the athlete from continued participation. Pain, however, is a more subjective matter. The desire or ability to play with pain varies from one athlete to another and often involves a personal choice.

Most sideline decisions can be guided by normal common sense. Any athlete who is visibly limping is not only at risk for secondary injury but is probably not functioning effectively and should not continue to play. In the case of injuries that are painful but do not appear to carry the risk of permanent disability, the physician should be responsive to the desires of the athlete and his family. Particularly when dealing with the school-age athlete, the physician should be sensitive to signs that the athlete is frightened or in severe pain and should advise such athletes not to return to competition. Sometimes the fear of being labeled a coward will prevent the athlete from verbalizing his desire not to play; the physician must sense when this is the case and relieve the youth of this responsibility. Since most school-age athletes are minors, parents should always be consulted in any case in which the decision is not clearcut. Especially in the absence of parental consent, the physician should always err on the side of protecting the athlete. It is important for the physician to remain slightly detached from the athletic establishment, so that he or she does not get swept up with enthusiasm during the pitch of competition. In general, when caring for school-age athletes who may be in a vulnerable stage of development as well as legally minors, it is important for the physician to be more conservative in sideline decisions than he or she might be with a college or professional team. At the same time, it is important for the physician to be aware of the importance of athletic participation to the athletes and their parents, not withholding an athlete who wishes to return to competition and whose risk is minimal.

It is important that the team physician have the complete backing of the coaching staff, so that it is clear to the players that the physician, and not the coaches, is responsible for deciding when an athlete is fit to return to competition following an injury. Not infrequently, the physician will encounter an enthusiastic athlete who challenges the decision to withhold him from competition. Giving such an athlete functional tests to perform will usually allow him to see the light of reason: A player with a sprained ankle who limps during sprinting and cutting tests will usually realize that he is not going to be an asset to his team on the field. Emphasizing that missing part of a game immediately following the injury may help an athlete avoid missing several successive games will also often influence him to cooperate with the physician's decision.

An important principle for the proper functioning of the team physician during a football game is that of sideline vigilance. The physician should get a feeling for the normal sideline behavior of football players; the athlete who is noted to be sitting quietly by himself on the bench is often trying to recover from a concussion, heat illness, or other injury. Players should also be warned to alert the physician to teammates who may be acting inappropriately owing to subtle forms of concussion.

Injuries to the abdominal viscera may have a surprisingly benign presentation. We have seen players with splenic contusions and renal hematomas complete a game before they inform the physician or training staff that they had a painful "rib injury." Any football player with significant localized abdominal or flank tenderness should be evaluated in a hospital setting. It is important to remember that conditioned athletes frequently have a resting pulse in the sixties, so that a pulse that remains in the nineties after the athlete has had a chance to "catch his breath" may signify hypovolemia from blood loss.

When a physician is called to see an athlete who is "down on the field," he will often find that player in an emotional and agitated state. After checking the athlete's vital signs and doing an appropriate abbreviated exam to verify that no urgent condition exists, the physician should allow the athlete to calm down in order to obtain a more accurate assessment of the location and magnitude of the injury. The management of potentially serious head and neck injuries in this situation has already been discussed. When the physician has enough information to conclude that it is safe to ambulate or transport the patient, the player should be taken to the sidelines where the evaluation may be completed in a relaxed, unpressured fashion.

Joint injuries should be examined for deformity and instability. If neither of these is present and the injury appears minor, the athlete should still be required to pass functional tests prior to being allowed to reenter the game.

Knee injuries are easiest to evaluate for abnormal laxity a few minutes following the injury, after the pain of the acute injury has eased but before swelling develops. Any abnormal laxity is a contraindication to returning to competition. Tenderness along a sprained collateral ligament may take 15 to 30 minutes to develop, and a hemarthrosis from a cruciate ligament tear, patellar dislocation, or osteochondral fracture may take even longer to manifest itself. Meniscal tears may be hard to diagnose acutely, as tenderness and swelling may take hours to develop. Athletes who demonstrate no abnormal laxity or deformity and who wish to return to play must complete a functional testing program. The players should be required to do a number of sprints along the sideline, followed by a zigzag run with sharp cuts. Side-to-side maneuvers such as cariocas may supplement these tests. To return to play, an athlete should be able to perform all these maneuvers without any limp or difficulty.

Injured ankles should be evaluated for abnormal anterior or varus laxity, deformity, or bony tenderness. The presence of any of these should be a contraindication to returning to play unless the laxity was preexisting and known to the physician. If these findings are absent, the player must be able to hop on the toes of the affected foot and perform the sprints and functional tests described for the knee without limp or difficulty before returning to play.

The shoulder should be examined for any deformity in the glenohumeral, acromioclavicular, or sternoclaviclar joints indicative of dislocation or subluxation. Significant localized tenderness on the clavicle or elsewhere should alert the physician to the possibility of a fracture. Although functional tests for the shoulder are less well established, a player should certainly have full active range of motion in the shoulder and normal strength of all major muscle groups prior to being returned to play. Since the upper brachial plexus is usually involved in the common "burner injury," the deltoid should be carefully evaluated for any loss of strength.

Common finger dislocations are traditionally reduced on the sidelines. If the joint can then be put through a full, active range of motion without crepitus and appears stable, the athlete may usually be allowed to return to play with the finger buddy taped to the adjacent digit. Nondisplaced fractures of the metacarpals or wrist may be difficult to diagnose clinically. Point tenderness over the suspected fracture site is usually present but is not specific, since it will also be present with a local contusion or hematoma. Pain generated at the suspected fracture site by the application of torque or pressure elsewhere in the bone is highly suspicious for a fracture. The physician must use his or her own judgment regarding the possibility of a displaceable nondisplaced fracture and should withhold the athlete if the physician believes that the chance of aggravating such an injury is significant.

The physician should never assume that all players wish to return to the game or that all parents wish them to do so. Even when the athlete passes all tests, behavioral cues from the player or his parents may indicate that the best decision is to withhold the athlete from competition.

PROTECTIVE EQUIPMENT FOR FOOTBALL

Although the physician will rarely be involved in the fitting of football equipment, he or she may be called on by scholastic authorities for advice in equipment selection. A knowledge of the nature and limitations of routine protective equipment will also help the physician know when to recommend supplemental protective padding.

Proper selection, fit, maintenance, inspection, and reconditioning of protective equipment are essential in any sport; however, with heavy collision sports such as football, these are of paramount importance to promote the safety of the participant. With increasing litigation related to sports equipment throughout the nation's high schools, the purchaser and user must have a solid understanding of the correct use and potential risks inherent in the misuse of that equipment.

Contact by the athlete with either an opposing player, teammate, or the playing surface may result in a sustained injury. Through the use of protective equipment over known vulnerable areas of the body, the number and degree of these injuries can be minimized. Thus, the two principles behind the use of protective equipment are created around the goals of injury prevention and reduction.

Within the last 15 years, two organizations have made major contributions to the improvement, standardization, and testing of protective sports equipment.[20, 28, 97] They are:

- The National Operating Committee on Standards for Athletic Equipment (NOCSAE)
- The American Society for Testing and Materials (ASTM) Committee on Sports Equipment and Facilities

Through close association with equipment manufacturers, these organizations have established recommendations for equipment usage, maintenance, and reconditioning. These recommendations are considered essential guidelines with which to ensure safe usage by the athlete. As an example, today *all* football helmets must have the following label (recommended warning) from the NOCSAE, visibly placed on the exterior shell of the helmet by the manufacturer or reconditioner:[22, 44, 97]

> Do not use this helmet to butt, ram or spear an opposing player. This is in violation of football rules, and can result in severe head, brain, neck injury, paralysis or death to you and possible injury to your opponent. There is a risk these injuries may also occur as a result of accidental contact without intent to butt, ram or spear. No helmet can prevent all such injuries.

Furthermore, the NOCSAE seal indicates the helmet has met all the requirements of football helmet tests, as established by the NOCSAE.

SELECTION AND FIT OF STANDARD FOOTBALL EQUIPMENT

The proper selection and fit of protective equipment are predicated on a basic level of knowledge, awareness, and expertise in the following areas:[3, 16]

- Materials and construction of equipment
- Fabrication—proper fit
- Inspection and maintenance
- Design styles and manufacturers
- Safety and inherent risks
- Rules and regulations
- Warranty (to include reconditioning and recertification procedures)
- Athlete education
- Cost

The individual who has taken time to develop a clear understanding in each of these areas has a distinct advantage in the prevention and management of athletic injuries. This knowledge and background can be considered an important first step in protecting the athlete from unnecessary injury.

The Helmet

Principally, football helmets on the market today can be differentiated by their type of internal suspension and the material properties of the outer shell. The internal system suspends and supports the head within the helmet in a favorable position to absorb safely forces experienced during impact to the outer shell. Today, football helmets are generally classified into three categories based on the type of suspension within the shell[3, 16, 28, 83] (Fig. 29–9). They include:

1. Padded
2. Air- and fluid-filled cells
3. Combination of air and padded suspension

The shell of all football helmets is constructed of a hard, resilient plastic. There is a distinction of shell construction, however, between youth and high school. The shell of high school football helmets (ninth grade and above) is constructed of a polycarbonate alloyed polymer plastic. A common reference to this material is the "Kralite II," manufactured by Ridell, Inc. The youth helmet shell

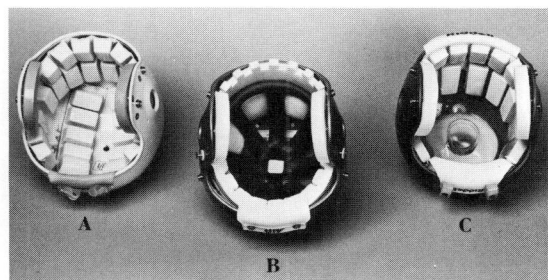

FIGURE 29-9. Football helmets may be (A) padded, (B) lined with fluid or air-filled cells, or (C) fitted with a combination of pads and air cells.

is constructed of ABS (acrylonitrile butadiene styrene) plastic. Both shell composites are strong and absorb energy well from impact; however, the youth ABS plastic shell is more susceptible to abrasion and less expensive. The ABS plastic shell is acceptable for youth (junior high level and below), based on the level of play generally found in junior high and younger athletes. Typically, there is a lesser degree of impact force owing to a lesser amount of strength, weight, and speed of the younger athlete compared with the high school athlete.

Internal suspension systems consist of a plastic vinyl liner, individual vinyl air cushions, and layers of energy-absorbing foams.

General Fitting Standards and Procedures. After the selection of manufacturer and model for the appropriate level of participation, proper fitting of the football helmet should be regarded as the most important way to maximize its potential for injury prevention and protection. The fitting procedures are outlined below. Additionally, one should always refer to each manufacturer's guidelines for the specific instructions of fitting each model or brand.[3, 16, 28, 44, 83]

1. Prior to fitting, visually inspect and manually stress the shell for cracks, defects, and/or deterioration. Repeat this same procedure when inspecting the internal suspension (i.e., air, liquid cell, and/or foam inserts). Check air cells for correct inflation levels as recommended by the manufacturer. Check foam inserts for cracking and discoloring. Inspect attachment sites (i.e., screws, grommets, rivets, and Velcro) for deterioration and looseness. Check chin strap and buckles for excessive wear and looseness. Face masks that have become distorted may alter the shape of the helmet and should be replaced.

2. Hair length can affect the fit, so the athlete should wet his hair to simulate a practice or game situation prior to fitting. Hair should remain approximately the same length throughout the season. Changes in hair length may require readjustment of the helmet.

3. Helmet size is determined by the following factors: head circumference (Measurement is taken 1 inch above the eyebrow with a cloth or steel measuring tape or calipers designed to measure head circumference and head shape. Determine any obvious variations such as large occipital bone, slanting forehead, and/or long oval head).

The above information will be helpful in determining approximate helmet size as specified by the manufacturer's sizing chart.

Helmet Fitting Adjustments. First, to insert the head into the helmet, the athlete should spread the ear flaps with the thumbs in the ear holes and rotate the helmet downward until firmly in place. Many inexperienced athletes will attempt to pull the helmet straight down, potentially causing much discomfort over the ears.

Next, fasten the chin straps and check to ensure that equal tension is felt on either side of the chin cup. Also, make certain the chin cup is centered over the chin to keep the jaw stabilized. Chin straps have either two or four snaps, with the four-snap strap stabilizing the helmet by limiting posterior and anterior rocking. The four-snap strap has become the strap of choice of the majority of coaches owing to the limitation of forward and backward movement. A properly adjusted chin strap will act as a safety device and release when excessive stress or pressure occurs[3, 28, 44] (Fig. 29–10A).

There are several other areas to check once the helmet is on properly. They are:

1. Crown adjustments
   a. The anterior rim or front of the helmet should rest approximately $\frac{3}{4}$ inch to two finger widths above the eyebrows. To ensure proper helmet height, adjust the thickness of the crown insert or inflate or deflate the air cells to raise or lower helmet (Fig. 29–10B).
   b. The posterior rim and pads placed at the back of the helmet should cover the base of the skull (occipital bone) but not impinge on the back of the

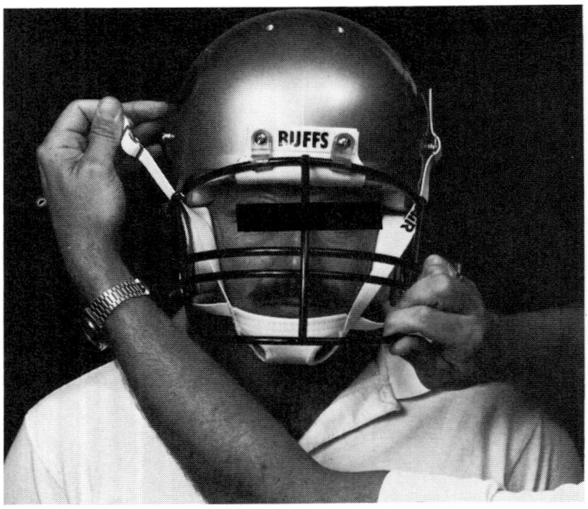

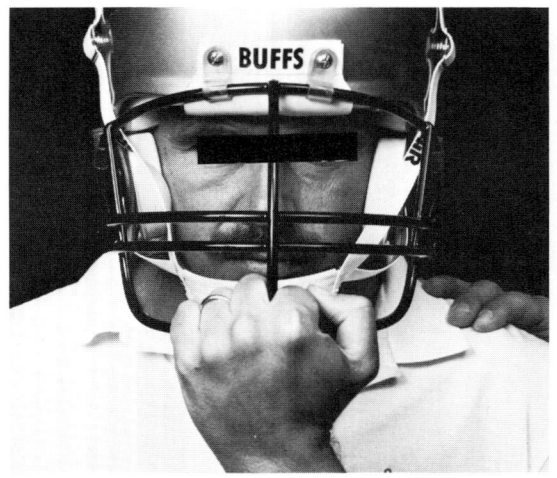
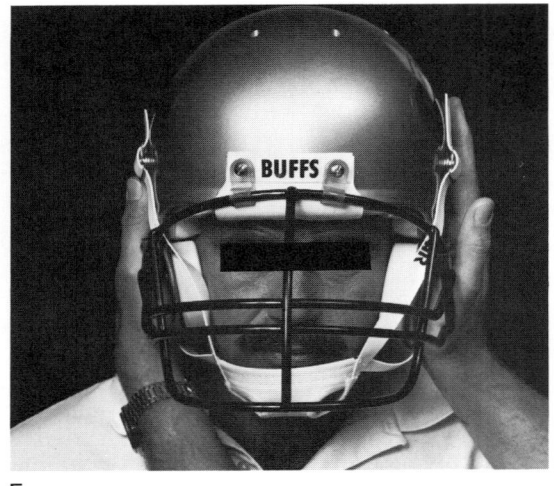

FIGURE 29–10. Helmet fitting technique. (*A*) Fasten chin straps and check to ensure equal tension is felt on either side and chin cup is centered. (*B*) Anterior rim/front of helmet should rest approximately $\frac{3}{4}$ inch to two finger widths above the eyebrow. (*C*) Posterior rim and pads at back of helmet should cover base of skull but not impinge on back of neck. (*D*) Cheek pads should fit snugly to prevent lateral rocking. (*E*) Grasp face mask and attempt to move in a forward/backward motion. (*F,G*) Turn helmet from side to side and in a lateral direction. (*H*) Apply downward pressure on top of helmet. There should be a minimal amount of give.

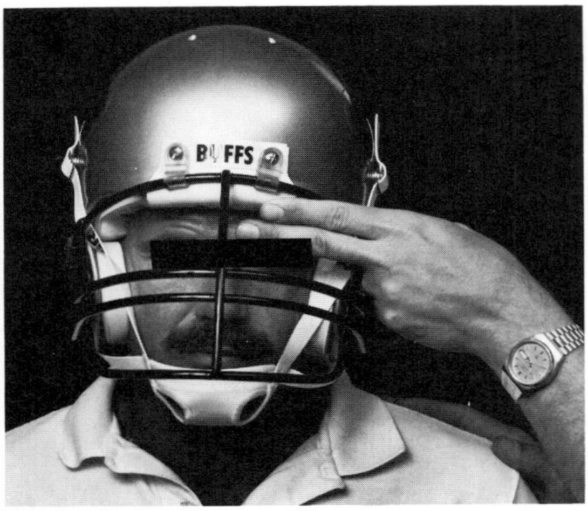

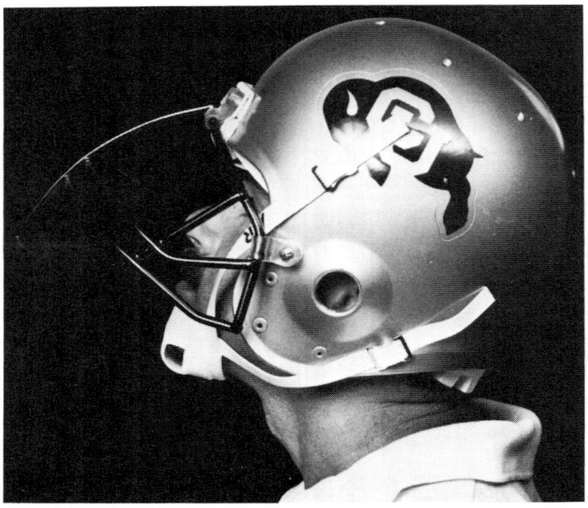

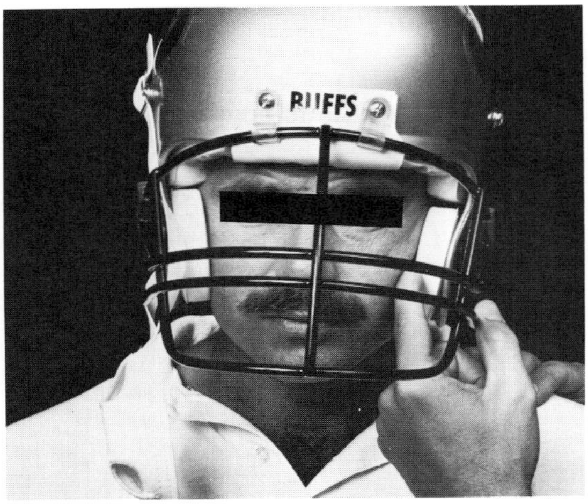

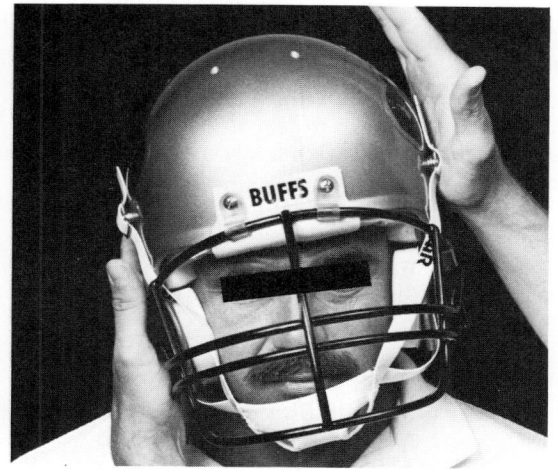 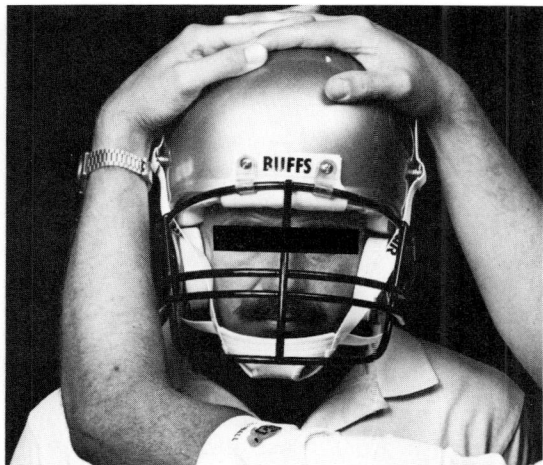

FIGURE 29–10. *Continued*

neck when the athlete is in full neck extension (Fig. 29–10C).
  c. Forehead clearance should be checked with the examiner firmly securing the back of the athlete's helmet with both hands and at the same time having the athlete press backward into the examiner's hands. Clearance from the forehead pad by the forehead should lessen but not produce a gap. Correct fit may be achieved by adjusting the back spaces or forehead pad.
2. Final checks
  a. Ear holes of the helmet should match the ear openings. Jaw or cheek pads should fit snugly to prevent lateral rocking (Fig. 29–10D).
  b. The face mask should match according to the athlete's position and the manufacturer's specifications. The face bar should be approximately 2 inches to no greater than three finger widths from nose and chin. The athlete should have a complete field of vision.
  c. With the helmet firmly in place, have the athlete resist your motions as you go through the following sequence:
    1. Grasp face mask and attempt to move helmet in a forward/backward motion (Fig. 29–10E).
    2. Turn helmet from side to side and in a lateral direction (Figs. 29–10F and 29–10G).
    3. Apply downward pressure onto the top of helmet (Fig. 29–10H).

The above sequences should elicit only a very slight or minimal amount of "give" when helmet is properly fitted. When the examiner tries to shift the helmet, there should be no movement without a simultaneous movement of the head. The athlete should be informed that the fit may seem tight, but within several days, he should be accustomed to the helmet.

Daily and weekly inspection and maintenance tasks should be carried out by the athlete and/or trained maintenance personnel. These tasks include:

- Cleaning and drying
- Visually checking shell for stress fractures and defects (especially around predrilled holes)
- Checking helmet padding for deterioration and wear; pads constantly exposed to oil or hair spray from hair will deteriorate much faster than when hair is dry and clean
- Checking air and fluid cells for leaks and proper inflation.
- Inspecting all inserts and attachments for wear and looseness
- Checking face mask for distortion and/or cracks
- Checking chin straps and buckles for wear

When traveling to areas where altitude is considerably greater or less than your usual location, the air cells must be checked routinely for proper inflation.

Football Shoulder Pads

The shoulder girdle, like the helmet, sustains great collision forces during football contests; thus, the same importance of fit and inspection given to the football helmet must be applied to the shoulder pads.

Shoulder pads are basically of two types, the flat pad and the cantilevered type (Fig. 29–11). The flat pad is worn by the quarterback, wide receiver, and kicker, who require less bulk and more mobility. Much improvement has been realized in the design and construction of shoulder pads. The objective behind this ongoing effort is to maximize the ability of the shoulder pads to absorb and disperse the great forces encountered during contact to protect the bony and muscular structure of the shoulder girdle. This has been achieved by the following features observed on today's shoulder pads:[3, 16, 28, 83]

1. The shoulder or deltoid cap is designed to protect the deltoid muscle and prevent any object from being lodged underneath the pad from the side.
2. Shoulder epaulets are placed over the deltoid cap, coupling and extending to the main body of the pad. Their purpose is to protect the top of the shoulder from direct impact.
3. The neck cutout or clavicle-channel is cushioned and constructed of leather. (Vinyl coverings will eventually crack owing to wear and moisture and may become abrasive.) The clavicle-channel combines with the cantilevered design to perform the most important function of the shoulder pad, diverting the pressure away from the clavicle to the surrounding torso.
4. Front and rear panels of shoulder pads have been extended along with the cantilever to increase the protection of the acromioclavicular joint by evenly absorbing the forces taken from the top of the shoulder.
5. Dense foam padding covered by a hard resilient plastic is used. Foam should be covered by nylon to decrease wear and drying time.
6. Underarm straps are of an elastic material and often cushioned by a rectangular pad.

Shoulder Pad Fitting.

1. Shoulder pad size is determined by measuring the width of the shoulders.
2. The shape of the shoulder pad must fit the chest, with inside padding extending over the ends of the shoulders.
3. The neck opening or clavicle-channel should provide enough coverage to protect the base of the neck and surrounding areas and allow for liberal movement of the arms but not permit sliding back and forth.
4. Shoulder caps should cover the deltoids with shoulder epaulets riding directly over the shoulder caps.
5. Underarm straps must be snug but not constrictive and should prevent the shoulder pads from shifting.
6. Front and back body arches should meet evenly with medial portion of neck opening close to the neck.
7. A tight-fitting porous jersey will provide sufficient pressure to keep pads in place and prevent the pads from being pulled out.

Shoulder pads that are properly fitted by the above guidelines will maximize the shoulder pads' ability to distribute and absorb the shock delivered to the shoulder complex and surrounding thoracic area evenly.

Hip and Tailbone Pads

Hip padding is designed to protect the iliac crest and the greater trochanter from direct trauma, whereas the tailbone or buttocks pad protects the sacrum and coccyx. These pads are generally thin and made of a dense foam covered with a hard plastic. When sold commercially, pads may come in the form of a meshed girdle style with pads inserted into pockets or a belt style with pads fastened by a snap. As a rule, the athlete should not be permitted to play without one. Thigh pads help to protect the quadriceps from contusions (Fig. 29–12).

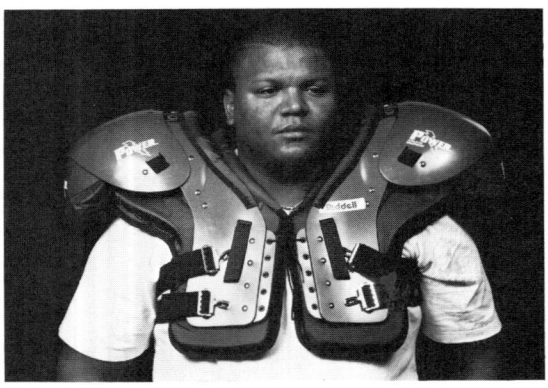

FIGURE 29–11. Cantilevered style shoulder pads with extended cantilever, front and rear panel and epaulets to increase protection of the acromioclavicular joint.

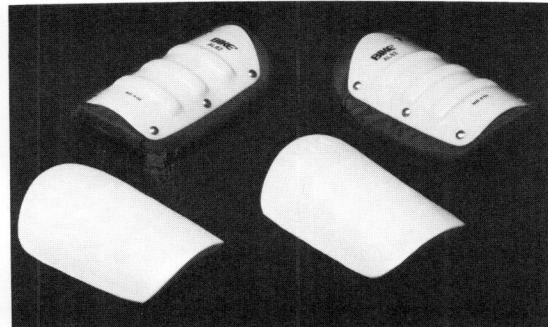

FIGURE 29-12. Thigh pads. Top pads are constructed of a closed-cell foam enclosed by nylon with a hard, unyielding polymer plastic shell. Bottom pads are a ½-inch thick closed-cell foam.

Mouth Guard

A correctly fitted intraoral mouth guard serves two purposes: to reduce and prevent dental injuries and to absorb the shock from a direct blow to the chin, thus decreasing the chance of possible concussion.[17, 37]

Mouth guards are constructed of a polymeric or polymer thermoplastic material. The physical properties of this material may change slightly depending on the additive fillers and plasticizers used. Research has shown the variance among mouth guard materials does not alter the protectability, durability, or stability against trauma to the head, neck, or teeth.[3, 17, 37] There are generally three types:

1. The ready-made type.
2. The commercially made piece that is individually fitted by boiling the hard resilient rubber in water and then molding the piece to the contour of the athlete's teeth.
3. The custom-fabricated style that is made from a plaster mold or impression taken from the athlete's maxillary arch.

A properly fitted mouth guard should be tight and stable around the teeth, not bite into gums, and allow for unrestricted air flow and speech. Maximum protection is achieved when the mouth guard is fitted to the upper jaw.

In the majority of high school today, mouth guards are required at all times during participation whether in practice or competition. During competition games, officials will enforce the use of mouth guards to the point of penalizing the team for their absence.

Footwear

Socks are often overlooked as an important component to proper footwear. Too often, a poorly fitting sock or worn sock is one of the major causes of blisters. In general, socks that fit properly should provide ample toe room, have a well-padded sole, fit snugly without wrinkles, and feel comfortable. Sock material should be a cotton or cotton blend (i.e., cotton, polyester, and/or nylon) for optimum dissipation of moisture away from the skin and lasting wear. The "tube sock" has become popular over the last decade as one size generally fits all. Another consideration is advising the athlete to wear two pairs of socks. This will reduce friction and prevent hot spots that may become blisters. The inner sock, as a rule, is usually thinner and lighter than the outer pair. Lastly, clean socks are a must in warding off fungus growth and maintaining the overall health of the athlete's feet.

Shoes

Proper selection and correct fit of shoes will return major dividends by keeping the athlete out of the training room and doctor's office. An ill-fitted or worn-out shoe can be the root of many problems (i.e., blisters, calluses, postural imbalance, and soft tissue and joint disturbances).[3]

Shoe Fit. Ensuring correct shoe size and fit requires several important factors:

- Shoes should not be purchased with the thought that the next larger size will allow the athlete to grow into them. The exact size is most important.
- When trying on shoes, the athlete should use the style of socks that will be worn in practice and competition.
- Both feet should be measured for possible size differences between feet.
- Correct shoe length is achieved when the great toe is approximately $\frac{1}{4}$ to $\frac{1}{2}$ inch from the tip or end of the shoe while the athlete is standing. Allowing for this room will provide the extra space needed for the foot to move forward when the athlete comes to a stop or is braking.
- Proper shoe width should permit full extension, flexion, and spreading of toes. Wearing the correct sock is important to guarantee proper fit. The eyelets of the shoes should be between $\frac{1}{2}$- and 1-inch distance from each when shoe is laced.
- The shoe should bend at the distal end of the metatarsal and/or the widest part of the shoe box.

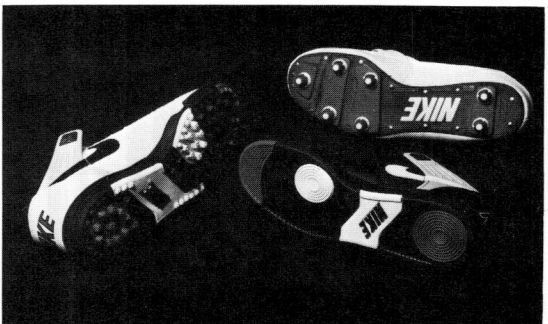

FIGURE 29–13. Three styles of shoes for different surfaces. *Left* to *right*: rubber molded cleat (wet artificial surface), flat sole (dry artificial surface), and screw-in cleat (natural grass).

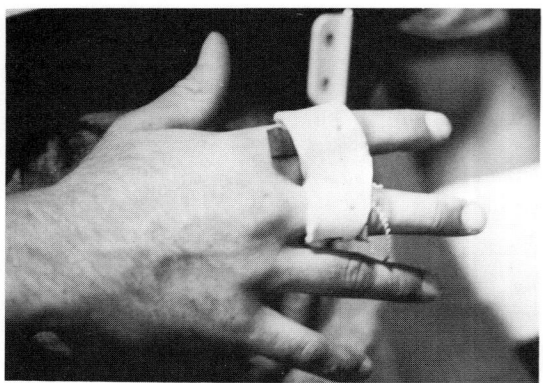

FIGURE 29–14. This quarterback sprained the ulnar collateral ligament of his index metacarpophalangeal joint. Buddy taping to the long finger, the standard method of protection, would not allow him to grasp a football. This custom splint was molded to his hand while he was holding a football.

- The heel counter must surround and encompass the heel and provide good rigidity.
- The shoe interior should contain an adequate arch support with a smooth, even insole.

When an athlete's foot is excessively narrow at the heel while the remaining shoe fits correctly, a strip of moleskin or thick, dense foam rubber secured to the inside of the heel will often resolve the problem.

Shoe selection should be based on the surface played on (whether grass or artificial turf) and the support needed. These factors will determine the rigidity of the shoe, the style of the sole, and the shoe height (low cut or high cut for added ankle support)[22] (Fig. 29–13).

SPECIAL PADDING AND SPLINTING TECHNIQUES

In conjunction with the use of supportive and preventive adhesive strapping, and various bandages used for support, there are a variety of materials employed today in the formation of custom protective devices. Special padding and splinting techniques can augment the protective qualities of football equipment (i.e., helmets, shoulder, hip, and thigh pads) and are essential in further limiting athletic injuries. The team physician should be aware of the various splinting and padding materials available and the regulations governing their use. Familiarity with these materials will help the physician or trainer develop creative solutions to unusual padding or bracing situations[3, 5, 16] (Fig. 29–14).

Prior to constructing a protective pad or orthotic, several questions should be asked:

For what protective purpose is the device to be used? What are the basic properties of the available materials? What are the location and severity of the injury?

The following additional questions should be asked:

1. Is there an available commercial device that will offer at a reasonable cost the same protection and durability as a customized splint or brace (e.g., commercial foam rubber pads and sleeves, elastic wraps and sleeves, and Velcro and canvas straps)? Commercial protective equipment such as pads and braces should in no way be altered from their original state or intended purpose. Changing the design or structure of the device will void the manufacturer's warranty and could result in potential litigation claiming negligence and wrongdoing.

2. Is the purpose of the custom supportive device to permit nearly complete or complete freedom of movement or activity with mild to moderate protection via soft, flexible, resilient, shock-absorbing materials? This would include foam rubber materials with various degrees of thickness, moldability, recovery, and energy absorption used as thumb splints, acromioclavicular pads, and hip pointer pads (Fig. 29–15).

3. Is the purpose of the custom supportive device to restrict or limit active joint range of motion while offering support via a reinforced elastic or rubber composite material (e.g., shoulder braces for the chronic subluxing or dislocating shoulder that act as a restraining apparatus to restrict the shoulder

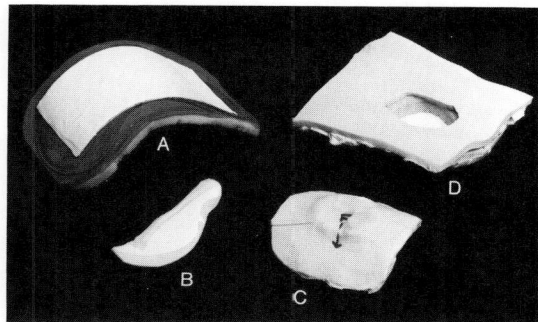

FIGURE 29–15. Custom-clinic-made pads. (*A*) Hip pointer or acromioclavicular pad. Pad is made from open- and closed-cell foam covered by a hard thermo-moldable plastic. (*B*) Thumb splint constructed from Orthoplast and lined with moleskin. (*C*) Acromioclavicular pad. Pad is open-cell foam covered by molded Orthoplast and moleskin. (*D*) Thigh contusion pad constructed with layers of closed-cell foam covered by Orthoplast to form rigid shell. Note donut cutout for placement directly over injury and Orthoplast shell to absorb and disperse forces from impact.

from excessive abduction, external rotation, or elevation beyond 90 degrees)?

4. Is the purpose of the custom supportive device to provide a rigid, nonyielding support to protect anatomically the injured area by dispersing the forces generated from high impact (e.g., a rigid nasal splint to protect an injured nose or a rigid splint to protect a healing fracture)?

The NCAA Football Rules (1979), Section 4, Article 5, requires there be

> no hard or unyielding substances on the hand, wrist, forearm, or elbow of any player, no matter how well covered or padded. No hard or unyielding substance in thigh guards, shin guards, knee or leg braces unless such an article is covered on both sides and all of its edges are overlapped with closed-cell slow-recovery foam padding no less than one-half inch thick or an alternate material of the same minimum thickness having similar physical properties.[63]

Regulations for school-age players vary from state to state but are similar in nature.

The severity, location, and restriction of the injury will dictate the physical properties and style of the materials needed (i.e., foam versus plastic; soft, flexible, and compressible versus rigid and unyielding; slow-recovery versus quick-recovery foam; open-cell versus closed-cell foam; donut versus bubble or bridge design).

The properly fabricated and fitted protective device should protect both the user and opposing player. Athlete education should focus on the safe use, maintenance, and limitations of the protective device. An improperly placed and secured device can reinjure or predispose the athlete to further injury.[5]

Custom Pad Construction Materials

Soft Materials. A large selection of soft material products is available through many manufacturers of sports medicine products. As stated at the beginning of this section, it is important to stay current with the many improvements made annually in protective equipment. The following examples represent a sampling of the more commonly used soft materials found in pad fabrication (Fig. 29–16).

FOAM. The properties and variety of foams used in protective padding have expanded and changed to keep pace with the great demand in custom-made pads for protective support in athletics. Foams offer many desired qualities. They provide a wide range of "shock absorption" and recovery properties. They come in several thicknesses ($\frac{1}{8}$ to $\frac{5}{8}$ inch), densities, and colors. Many of the foam products can be purchased with adhesive backing. Foams are generally classified as closed- or open-cell construction.[3, 5, 28, 67, 83]

Closed-cell foams are the most widely used primarily owing to two qualities: They resume their original contour after compression (some are thermomoldable and thus are easily molded), and they do not absorb perspiration, bacteria, or odors. Plastizote is one example of a thermomoldable closed-cell foam that is commonly used in training rooms to form various pads and splints.[3, 66, 67, 83]

Open-cell foams are generally less resilient than those of closed-cell construction. They are moisture and abrasion resistant and are

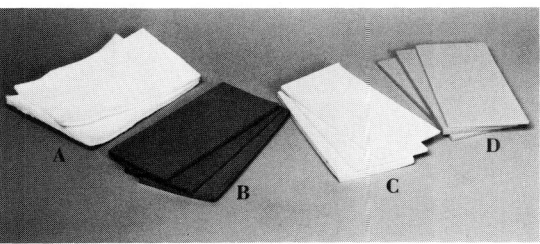

FIGURE 29–16. Soft material assortment. (*A*) Felt $\frac{1}{4}$- and $\frac{3}{8}$-inch thick. (*B*) Closed-cell foam $\frac{1}{8}$, $\frac{1}{4}$, and $\frac{1}{2}$-inch thick. (*C*) Thermomoldable foam (Plastizote) $\frac{1}{8}$-, $\frac{1}{4}$-, and $\frac{1}{2}$-inch thick. (*D*) Open-cell foam $\frac{1}{8}$-, $\frac{1}{4}$-, and $\frac{1}{2}$-inch thick.

generally used for lining splints and for protecting blisters and wounds. Rolyan contour foam is one type of open-cell foam with slow-recovery properties, unlike other open-cell foams, and has the ability to mold to the body after several minutes' exposure to the body's natural heat.[3, 20, 67, 83]

Foams with high-density and energy-absorbing qualities are being used in the orthotic industry to prevent blisters and chronic overuse syndromes such as stress fractures. Examples are Viscolas, Sorbathane, and energy impact foam (Fig. 29–17).

FELT. Felt is composed of compressed wool fibers and comes in varying thicknesses from $\frac{1}{4}$ to 1 inch. It is used in many orthotic applications and is also commonly used as a horseshoe-shaped cut-out support for an acutely sprained ankle. Felt must be replaced frequently when exposed to the body, as it absorbs perspiration and odors.

MOLESKIN. Moleskin is a material that is used for lining pads and splints and for the prevention of blisters. Moleskin is generally $\frac{1}{8}$-inch thick and comes with a self-adhesive backing.

Hard Materials.

PLASTICS. Plastics fall into the rigid, unyielding material classification and offer excellent bracing and splinting protection. Many of the plastics used in athletic training are of the thermomoldable or heat-forming type that lend themselves well to being accurately and directly molded to a body part. These materials come in both solid and porous sheets 24 by 36 inches and range from $\frac{1}{8}$- to $\frac{3}{8}$-inch thick. A common type of plastic used in training rooms is called Orthoplast. Many trainers combine Orthoplast and other materials such as the foam material Plastizote

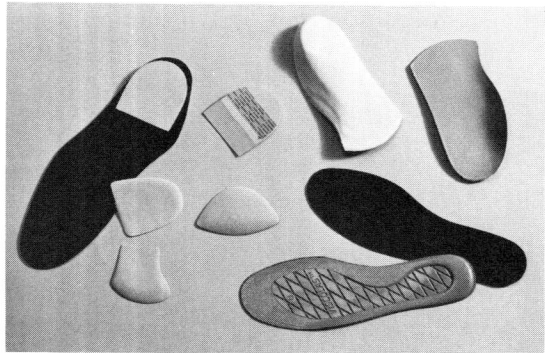

FIGURE 29–17. Commercial orthotic devices. Assortment of viscoelastic full-length shoe inserts, half-sole inserts, and heel and arch pads.

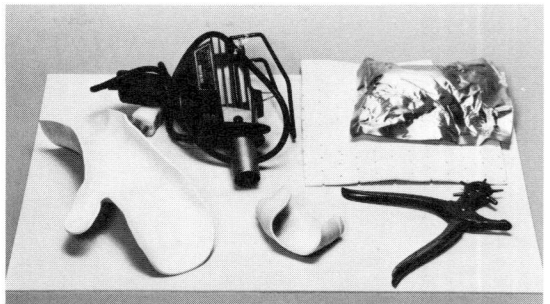

FIGURE 29–18. Hard materials and tools. *Left:* molded Orthoplast hand/wrist splint and heat gun. *Right:* porous sheet of Orthoplast, fiberglass, and rivet apparatus for making straps and perforating solid sheets of Orthoplast to increase moldability.

to improve further the safety, comfort, and support of the body part being protected[3, 5, 66, 67, 83] (Fig. 29–18).

CASTING MATERIALS. Plaster and synthetic casting material are the two common mediums used in applying casts to injured body parts. Synthetic casting material has become increasingly popular among trainers for fabricating hard shells for protective pads and splints. It comes in rolls of $1\frac{1}{2}$- to 6-inch widths of various colors. This material is heat activated by submersion in warm water for approximately 30 seconds and then can be molded. The material hardens within a few minutes and can be trimmed to shape with scissors or cast saw, depending on thickness.[3, 5, 66, 67, 83]

Hard casts will usually require softer external padding and may be totally forbidden by many referees. "Soft" casting materials have been developed for fabricating protective casts or splints that do not present a significant additional hazard to opponents. These have been used primarily for wrist and hand injuries.

Layering silicone rubber, gauze, and foam has been a popular technique for making these playing splints. Bergfeld et al.[8] showed that playing splints made from these materials approximated the hardness of six layers of adhesive tape and thus did not present an excessive hazard to opponents. These splints have two principal disadvantages. First, their fabrication is a rather lengthy and involved process. Second, they do not "breathe." If they are left on the body for long periods of time, the athlete's skin will become macerated. They must therefore be made removable and another cast or splint made to protect the athlete off the field. Not only is this expensive, but an unreliable patient may be tempted to remove such splints on his own.

A recent development that seems promising is "soft" synthetic casting material (e.g., Scotch Wrap). Its appearance is indistinguishable from conventional hard synthetic casting material, but it is relatively soft and resilient. Depending on the number of layers used, it can be made into casts or splints that are quite supportive, although we know of no objective studies comparing its supportive capabilities to hard casts. Casts or splints made with this material are acceptable in most venues. They are as easy to fabricate as a conventional cast and may be left in place for days or weeks because they are porous.

Commercial Pads

There are many commercially manufactured supportive devices available for the athlete. Prefabricated items offer several conveniences. One is their availability for immediate use. Another is the ability to select style, color, and quality from more than one manufacturer. Mass-produced products are often less expensive and will carry some type of warranty and liability statement. The disadvantages of stock items can be lack of availability due to demand, cost, sizing, and quality control. The descriptions of commercial items to follow are only a small sampling of the many common supportive devices used in sports.

Cervical Collar (Neck Roll). Neck rolls (Fig. 29–2) used in football are designed to limit or restrict cervical spine motion, thus avoiding a potentially serious neck or brachial plexus (burner/stinger) injury. An important factor to ensure maximum protection is securing firmly the tie-downs of the neck roll to the front or chest portion of the shoulder pads. Attaching the neck roll to the top of the shoulder pads alone does not provide the maximum fixation necessary.[20]

Ankle Supports. Ankle braces (Fig. 29–8) are designed to either provide protective or preventive support for the noninjured or weak ankle and/or are used following an acute ankle injury (e.g., sprain). Commercial ankle supports, as with other stock braces, come in a variety of styles. The main differences are in the type of material and configuration of that material in supporting the anatomical structures of the ankle. We are not aware of any well-controlled studies comparing the effectiveness of the different styles available. The air splint is used to provide support following an acute ankle injury.

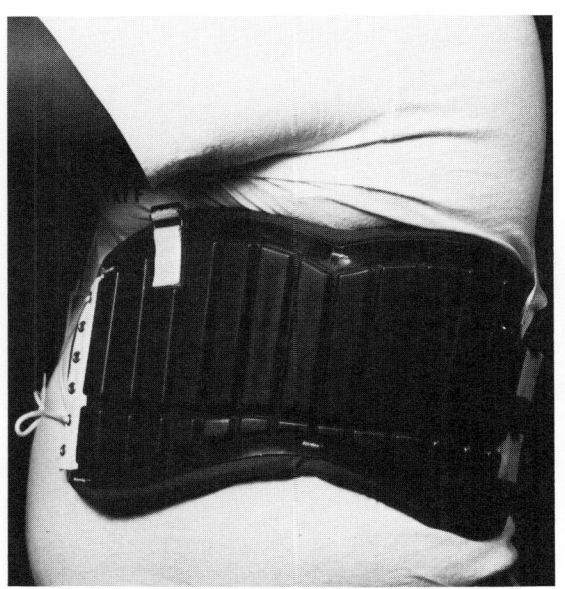 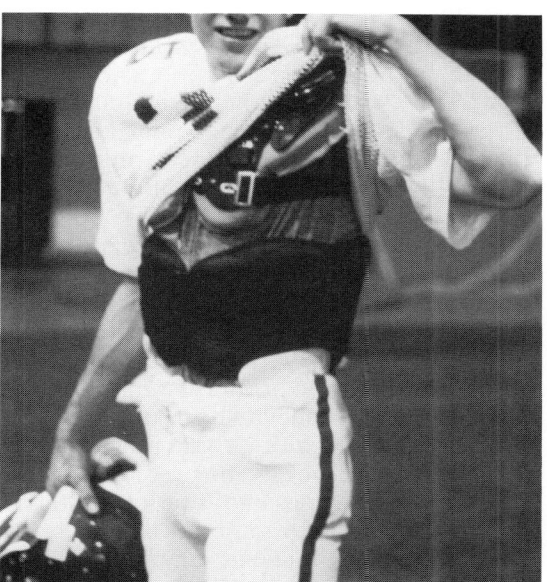

A B

FIGURE 29–19. Flak jacket (rib cage protector). (*A*) This rib protector is constructed of dense foam enclosed in nylon with a hard, rigid, variegated shell over the top. Note the nylon straps for adjustment to accommodate size variances among athletes. Rib belts fitted properly should protect the thorax and rib cage. (*B*) This player who has a history of a renal contusion is wearing a flak jacket for extra kidney protection.

Preinflated and adjustable air cells line the interior and are easily inflated or deflated to compress and accommodate the contour of the swollen tissue as needed. Additionally, inversion and eversion are restricted, whereas normal plantar and dorsiflexion are only minimally limited.[3, 5, 67, 83]

Lifters (Modified Shoulder Pads). Lifters (Fig. 29–5) perform two primary functions. First, they provide additional shock-absorbing support to the shoulder structure in conjunction with the shoulder pad. Second, they lessen the pressure around the acromioclavicular joints by dispersing the forces from impact via the cutout over each joint.

Flak Jacket (Thoracic/Rib Cage Protector). Rib belts have become the choice in protective wear for the protection of the rib cage. Today, the majority of quarterbacks whether injured or for prevention will don this piece of protective gear prior to competition. As seen in Figure 29–19, the rigid outside shell covering a dense foam offers considerable protection over the rib cage from high-impact forces. The adjustable straps accommodate for different-sized athletes and allow freedom of movement. There are a variety of rib belts available, with varying shell and foam materials.

Shoulder Harness. The shoulder brace (Fig. 29–3) is used to limit the motion of abduction, external rotation, and/or elevation above 90 degrees of the glenohumeral joint. This restriction of movement around the chest and upper arm is designed to reduce the occurrence of anterior subluxation and/or dislocation of the shoulder. Several styles of shoulder harnesses are available. The one in Figure 29–3A is made of an elastic rubber composite, whereas others use canvas strapping and linked chain to restrict motion.

Neoprene Sleeves. The use of neoprene sleeves (Fig. 29–20) has become popular among athletes. The primary functions of the neoprene rubber sleeve are to provide compression, heat retention, and prevention of abrasions. Their ability to protect the knee from shock (i.e., excessive anterior, posterior, valgus, varus, and rotational stress) is extremely limited; however, many companies are constructing various-shaped felt and foam buttresses that are sewn in or inserted into the sleeve for additional support. As there are no objective studies comparing these devices, selection is based primarily on the athlete's and physician's preferences.

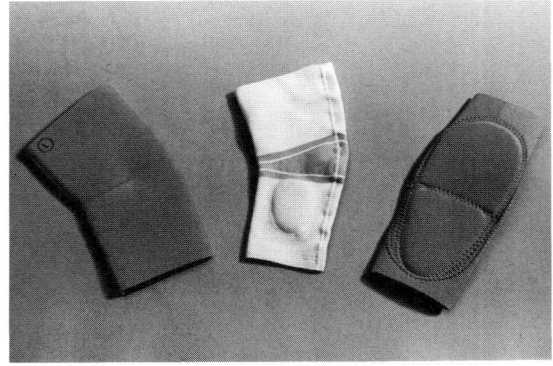

A

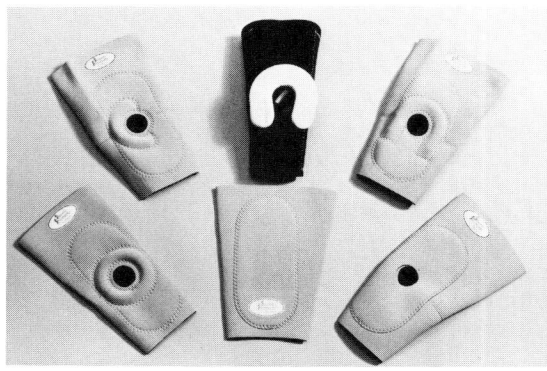

B

FIGURE 29–20. Protective neoprene sleeves. (*A*) Elbow sleeves. (*B*) Knee sleeves. Some of these have patellar cutouts or pads that may be useful in players with patellar pain or instability.

Summary

The design, fabrication, and application of custom- or commercially made pads, braces, or splints are important in providing optimum protection and safety for both the user and opponent. Athlete education and supervision are crucial to ensuring proper and safe use of the protective device.

References

1. American Academy of Orthopaedic Surgeons: A position statement. The use of knee braces. October 1987.
2. Anderson, G., Zeman, S. C., and Rosenfeld, R. T.: The Anderson knee stabilizer. Phys. Sportsmed. 7:125–127, 1979.
3. Arnheim, D.: Modern Principles of Athletic Training. 7th ed. Times Mirror/Mosby College Publishing, St. Louis, MO, 5:138–169, 1989.
4. Aronen, J. G., and Regan, K.: Decreasing the incidence of recurrence of first time anterior shoul-

der dislocations with rehabilitation. Am. J. Sports Med. 12:283–291, 1984.
5. Athletic Training and Sports Medicine. American Academy of Orthopaedic Surgeons, Chicago, IL, pp. 101–109, 1984.
6. Baker, B. E., Van Hanswyk, E., Bogosian, S., et al.: A biomechanical study of the static stabilizing effect of knee braces on medial stability. Am. J. Sports Med. 15:566–570, 1987.
7. Beck, C., Drez, D., Young, J., et al.: Instrumented testing of functional knee braces. Am. J. Sports Med. 14:253–256, 1986.
8. Bergfeld, J. A., et al.: Soft playing splint for protectin of significant hand and wrist injuries in sports. Am. J. Sports Med. 10(5):293–296, 1982.
9. Blyth, C. S.: Football injury survey. Part III. Injury rates vary with coaching. Phys. Sports Med. 2:45, 1974.
10. Bowers, D. K., and Martin, R. B.: Impact absorption, new and old Astroturf at West Virginia University. Med. Sci. Sports 6:217–221, 1974.
11. Bowers, K. D., Jr., and Martin, R. B.: Turf toe: a shoe-surface related football injury. Med. Sci. Sports 8(2):81–83, 1976.
12. Bramwell, S. T., Requa, R. K., and Garrick, J. G.: High school football injuries: a pilot comparison of playing surfaces. Med. Sci. Sports 4:166–169, 1972.
13. Bruno, L. A., Gennarelli, T. A., and Torg, J. S.: Management guidelines for head injuries in athletics. Clin. Sports Med. 6(1):17–30, 1987.
14. Cahill, B. R., and Griffith, E. H.: Effect of preseason conditioning on the incidence and severity of high school knee injuries. Am. J. Sports Med. 6:180–184, 1978.
15. Cameron, B. M., and Davis, O.: The swivel football shoe: a controlled study. J. Sports Med. 1:16–27, 1973.
16. Carey, R., et al.: Athletic Training—A Program Instructional Text. Cramer Products, Inc., Gardner, KS, F:143–155, 1986.
17. Chapman, P.: Player's attitudes to mouthguards and prevalence of orofacial injuries in the 1987 U.S. rugby football team. Am. J. Sports Med. 17(5):690–691, 1989.
18. Clancy, W. G., Brand, R. L., and Bergfeld, J. A.: Upper trunk brachial plexus injuries in contact sports. Am. J. Sports Med. 5:209, 1977.
19. Clanton, T. O., Butler, J. E., and Eggert, A.: Injuries to the metatarsophalangeal joints in athletes. Foot Ankle 7:162–176, 1986.
20. Clinics in Sports Medicine, Injuries to the Spine. W. B. Saunders Co., Philadelphia, 5:217–220, April 1986.
21. Coker, T. P., Arnold, J. A., and Weber, D. L.: Traumatic lesions of the metatarsophalangeal joint of the great toe in athletes. Am. J. Sports Med. 6:326–334, 1978.
22. College Athletic Management. College Athletic Administrator Inc., Ithaca, NY, 1(5), October 1989.
23. Colville, M. R., Lee, C. L., and Ciullo, J. V.: The Lenox Hill brace. An evaluation of effectiveness in treating knee instability. Am. J. Sports Med. 14:257–261, 1986.
24. Culpepper, M. I. and Nieman, K. M.: An investigation of the shoe-turf interface using different types of Poly-Turf and Astro-Turf: torque and release coefficients. Ala. J. Med. Sci. 2:387–390, 1983.
25. Dagiau, R. F.: Relationship between exposure time and injury in football. Am. J. Sports Med. 8:257–260, 1980.
26. Doller, J., and Strother, S.: Turf toe: an acute inflammatory response to athletic activity on artificial playing surfaces. J. Am. Podiatry Assoc. 68:512–514, 1978.
27. Ekstrand, J., Gillquist, J., and Liljedahl, S.: Prevention of soccer injuries: supervision by doctor and physiotherapist. Am. J. Sports Med. 2:116–120, 1983.
28. Fahey, T. D.: Athletic Training. Principles and Practices. Mayfield Publishing Company, Palo Alto, CA, pp. 45–50, 1986.
29. Fowler, P. J., and Messieh, S. S.: Isolated posterior cruciate ligament injuries in athletes. Am. J. Sports Med. 15:553–557, 1987.
30. France, E. P., Paulos, L. E., Jayaraman, G., et al.: The biomechanics of lateral knee bracing. Part II. Impact response of the braced knee. Am. J. Sports Med. 15:430–438, 1987.
31. Garrick, J. G., and Requa, R. K.: Role of external support in the prevention of ankle injuries. Med. Sci. Sports 5:200–203, 1973.
32. Garrick, J. G., and Requa, R. K.: Injuries in high school sports. Pediatrics 61:465–469, 1978.
33. Garrick, J. G., and Requa, R. K.: Epidemiology of foot and ankle injuries in sports. Clin. Sports Med. 7(1):29–36, 1988.
34. Giove, T. P., Sayers, J. M., Kent, B. E., Sanford, T. L., and Garrick, J. G.: Nonoperative treatment of the torn anterior cruciate ligament. J. Bone Joint Surg. 65A:184, 1983.
35. Godshall, R. W.: The predictability of athletic injuries: an eight year study. Am. J. Sports Med. 3:50–54, 1975.
36. Godshall, R. W., and Hansen, C. A.: Incomplete avulsion of a portion of the iliac epiphysis. J. Bone Joint Surg. 55A:1301–1302, 1973.
37. Going, E., et al.: Mouthguard materials; their physical and mechanical properties. JADA 89:132–138, 1974.
38. Goldberg, B., Rosenthal, P. P., and Nicholas, J. A.: Injuries in youth football. Phys. Sports Med. 12(8):122–130, 1984.
39. Grace, T. G., Sweetser, E. R., Nelson, M. A., et al.: Isokinetic muscle imbalance and knee joint injuries. J. Bone Joint Surg. 66A:734–740, 1984.
40. Grana, W. A., and Moretz, J. A.: Ligamentous laxity in secondary school athletes. JAMA 240(18): 1975–1976, 1978.
41. Hammer, D.: Artificial playing surfaces. Athletic Training 16(4):240–242, 1981.
42. Hanley, D. F.: Controllable external factors in lower extremity injuries. Presented at the Medical Society of the State of New York Symposium on Medical Aspects of Sports, 1969.
43. Hansen, B. L., Ward, J. C., and Diehl, R. C.: The preventive use of the Anderson knee stabler in football. Phys. Sportsmed. 13:75–81, 1985.
44. Harris, D., and Hawley, E.: Charlotte-Mecklenburg Schools Athletic Training Manual. Charlotte, NC, pp. 148–157.
45. Hawkins, R. J., Misamore, G. W., and Merrite, T. R.: Follow-up of the acute nonoperated isolated anterior cruciate ligament tear. Am. J. Sports Med. 14:205–210, 1986.
46. Hewson, G. F., Mendini, R. A., and Wang, J. B.: Prophylactic knee bracing in college football. Am. J. Sports Med. 14:262–266 1986.

47. Hovelius, L.: Anterior dislocation of the shoulder in teenagers and young adults. Five year prognosis. J. Bone Joint Surg. 69A:393–399, 1987.
48. Hovelius, L., Ericksson, K., Fedin, H., Hagberg, G., Hussenius, A., Lind, B., Thorling, J., and Weckstrom, J.: Recurrences after initial dislocation of the shoulder. Results of a prospective study of treatment. J. Bone Joint Surg. 65A:343–349, 1983.
49. Hughes, L. H., and Stitts, D. M.: A comparison of ankle taping and a semirigid support. Phys. Sports Med. 11:99–103, 1983.
50. Jackson, D., and Feagin, J.: Quadriceps contusions in young athletes. J. Bone Joint Surg. 55A:95–105, 1973.
51. Jackson, D. W., Jarrett, H., Bailey, D., Kausek, J., Sanson, J., Powell, J.: Injury prediction in the young athlete: a preliminary report. Am. J. Sports Med. 6:6–14, 1978.
52. Kalenak, A., and Morehouse, C. A.: Knee stability and knee ligament injuries. JAMA 234 (11):1143–1145, 1975.
53. Keene, J. S., Narechanta, R. G., Sachtjen, K. M., and Clancy, W. G.: Tartan Turf on trial. A comparison of intercollegiate football injuries occurring on natural grass and Tartan Turf. Am. J. Sports Med. 8:43–47, 1980.
54. Klein, K. K.: Muscular strength in the knee. Phys. Sports Med. 2:29–31, 1974.
55. Larson, R. L., and Osternig, L. R.: Traumatic bursitis and artificial turf. J. Sports Med. 2:183–188, 1974.
56. Laughman, R. K., Carr, T. A., Chao, E. Y., et al.: Three dimensional kinematics of the taped ankle before and after exercise. Am. J. Sports Med. 8:425–431, 1980.
57. McCarroll, J. R., Miller, J. M., and Ritter, M. A.: Lumbar spondylolysis and spondylolisthesis in college football players. Am. J. Sports Med. 14:404, 1986.
58. McCarthy, P.: Prophylactic knee braces: where do they stand? Phys. Sports Med. 12:102–115, 1988.
59. Metzmaker, J., and Pappas, A.: Avulsion fractures of the pelvis. Am. J. Sports Med. 13:349–358, 1985.
60. Moretz, A., Walters, R., and Smith, L.: Flexibility as a predictor of knee injuries in college football players. Phys. Sports Med. 10(7):93–97, 1982.
61. Mueller, F. U.: North Carolina High School Football Injury Study: equipment and prevention. Am. J. Sports Med. 2:1, 1974.
62. Murphy, R. V.: Heat illness in the athlete. Am. J. Sports Med. 12:258–261, 1984.
63. National Collegiate Athletic Association: NCAA Football Rules. NCAA, Shawnee Mission, KS, 1979.
64. Neer, C. S., and Foster, C. R.: Interior capsular shift for involuntary inferior and multidirectional instability of the shoulder. J. Bone Joint Surg. 62A:897, 1980.
65. Nicholas, J. A.: Injuries to knee ligaments. Relationship to looseness and tightness in football players. JAMA 212:2236–2239, 1970.
66. Nicholas, J. A., and Hershman, E. B.: The Lower Extremity and Spine in Sports Medicine. C. V. Mosby Co., St. Louis, 1:339–368, 1986.
67. Nicholas, J. A., and Hershman, E. B.: The Lower Extremity and Spine in Sports Medicine. Vol 2. C. V. Mosby Co., St. Louis, Chaps. 9, 44, 45, 1986.
68. Olson, O. C.: The Spokane Study: high school football injuries. Phys. Sportsmed. 7(12):75–82, 1979.
69. Parolie, J. M., and Bergfeld, J. A.: Long term results of nonoperative treatment of isolated posterior cruciate ligament injuries in the athlete. Am. J. Sports Med. 17:275–277, 1986.
70. Paulos, L. E., France, E. P., Rosenberg, T. D., et al.: The biomechanics of lateral knee bracing. Part I. Response of the valgus restraints to loading. Am. J. Sports Med. 15:419–429, 1987.
71. Peterson, T. R.: The cross body block, the major cause of knee injuries. JAMA 211:449, 1970.
72. Peterson, T. R.: Blocking at the knee, dangerous and unnecessary. Phys. Sportsmed. 1:47, 1973.
73. Powell, J. W.: Incidence of injury associated with playing surfaces in the national football league 1980–1985. Athletic Training 22:202–206, 1987.
74. Powell, J.: 636,000 Injuries annually in high school football. Athletic Training 22:19–22, 1987.
75. Pritchett, J. W.: A statistical study of knee injuries due to football in high school athletes. J. Bone Joint Surg. 64A:240–241, 1982.
76. Rarick, G. L., Bigley, G., Karst, R., et al.: The measurable support of the ankle joint by conventional methods of taping. J. Bone Joint Surg. 44A:1183–1190, 1962.
77. Reider, B., and Inglis, A.: The Bankart procedure modified by the use of Prolene pull-out sutures. J. Bone Joint Surg. 64A:628–629, 1982.
78. Robertson, W. C., Eichman, P. L., and Clancy, W. G.: Upper trunk brachial plexopathy in football players. JAMA 241:1480–1482, 1979.
79. Robey, J. M., Blyth, C. S., and Mueller, F. O.: Athletic injuries: application of epidemiologic methods. JAMA 217:184–189, 1971.
80. Rovere, G. D., Haupt, H. A., and Yates, C. S.: Prophylactic knee bracing in college football. Am. J. Sports Med. 15:111–116, 1987.
81. Rowe, C. R., Patel, D., and Souhmayo, W. W.: The Bankart procedure. J. Bone Joint Surg. 60A:1, 1978.
82. Rowe, C. R., and Sakllarides, H. T.: Factors related to recurrences of anterior dislocation of the shoulder. Clin. Orthop. 20:40–48, 1961.
83. Roy, S., and Irvin, R.: Sports Medicine, Prevention, Evaluation, Management, and Rehabilitation. Prentice-Hall, Inc., Englewood Cliffs, NJ, 4:45–51, 1983.
84. Rudner, M.: Football players who wear knee braces show fewer incidents of serious injury. Big Ten Conference News Service Bureau 2(6), 1988.
85. Saal, J. A.: Rehabilitation of football players with lumbar spine injury (part 1 or 2). Phys. Sports Med. 16:61–67, 1988.
86. Simonet, W. T., and Cofield, R. H.: Prognosis in anterior shoulder dislocation. Am. J. Sports Med. 12:19–24, 1984.
87. Smith, R. W., and Reischl, S. F.: Metatarsophalangeal joint synovitis in athletes. Clin. Sports Med. 7:75–78, 1988.
88. Stanitski, C. L., McMaster, J. H., and Ferguson, R. J.: Synthetic turf and grass. A comparative study. J. Sports Med. 2:22–26, 1974.
89. Teitz, C. C., Hermanson, B. K., Kronmal, R. A., et al.: Evaluation of the use of braces to prevent injury to the knee in collegiate football players. J. Bone Joint Surg. 70A:422–427, 1988.
90. Thompson, N., Halpern, B., Curl, W., Andrews,

J. R., Hunter, S. C., and McLeod, W. D.: High school football injuries: evaluation. Am. J. Sports Med. 15:117–124, 1987.
91. Torg, J. S., Pavlov, H., Genvario, S. E., Sennett, B., Wisneski, R. J., Robie, B. H., and Jahre, C.: Neuropraxia of the cervical spinal cord with transient quadriplegia. J. Bone Joint Surg. 68A:1355–1370, 1986.
92. Torg, J., and Quedenfeld, T.: The effect of shoe type and cleat length on incidence and severity of knee injuries among high school football players. Res. Q. 42:203–211, 1971.
93. Torg, J. S., and Quedenfeld, T.: Knee and ankle injuries traced to shoes and cleats. Phys. Sportsmed. 1:39–43, 1973.
94. Torg, J. S., Quedenfeld, T. C., and Landau, S.: The shoe surface interface and its relationship to football knee injuries. Am. J. Sports Med. 21:261–269, 1974.
95. Torg, J. S., Vegso, J. J., Sennett, B., and Das, M.: The National Football Head and Neck Injury Registry. 14 Year report on cervical quadriplegia 1971 through 1984. JAMA 254:3439–3443, 1985.
96. Tropp, H., Akling, C., and Gillquist, J.: Prevention of ankle sprains. Am. J. Sports Med. 13:259–262, 1985.
97. Warning Labels Now Required on Outside of Football Helmets. The First Aider. Cramer Products, Inc., Gardner, KS, 1986.
98. Yarnell, P. R., and Lynch, S.: The "ding" amnestic states in football trauma. Neurology 23:196, 1983.
99. Grace, T. G., Skipper, B. J., Newberry, J. C., et al: Prophylactic knee braces and injury to the lower extremity. J. Bone Joint Surg. 70A:422–427, 1988.

30
HOCKEY

ROBERT HUNTER

Skating is an ancient sport, having been described as early as the Stone Age when skates were made from animal bones. In the fourteenth century, metal replaced bone as the blade material, improving the durability and performance. By the late Middle Ages, skating had become quite a popular pastime in the Netherlands, with early evidence of both figure skating and hockey.[6] The first recorded skating injury was reported in *The Lives of the Saints* by Bergmann in 1498.

Full metallic skates were introduced into the United States in 1850 and in Europe in the following decade.[6] Skating competition followed shortly thereafter, with the first reported hockey game recorded in 1894 between two competing American colleges.[17] However, it was not until 1917 that professional hockey was initiated. Since that time, hockey has grown steadily in popularity and participation. At present, it is estimated that the American Hockey Association has 300,000 youth players and 12,000 teams.[17] In 1983, it was estimated that there were 24,000 high school hockey players, 20 percent of whom were in Minnesota.[3]

With the increased participation in hockey has come an increasing number of injuries. Hockey is by nature a collision sport, with a certain number of injuries expected and, to a certain extent, unavoidable. Sutherland has divided the causes of injuries into two broad groups: (1) the high-speed, low mass injuries and (2) the low-speed, high mass injuries.[18] The former are injuries caused by a puck or stick and result in contusions, lacerations, and concussions. The latter injuries, caused by collisions with bodies or boards, frequently result in fracture and sprain.

Contact, whether with the stick, puck, boards, fellow player, goal post, or the ice, accounts for the vast majority of injuries seen in hockey and has been reported to be responsible for as much as 82 percent of the injuries sustained.[4, 6]

The early interest in hockey injuries was precipitated in part by the devastating eye injuries sustained as a result of poor or no face protection. Pashby, writing in the *Canadian Medical Association Journal*, reported 257 eye injuries in Canadian hockey in the 1974–1975 season. These injuries occurred at an average age of 14 years, with 19 percent resulting in legal blindness.[13] As a direct result of this study and others, helmets and face masks became mandatory equipment in the Canadian Amateur Hockey Association. They are now required by the American Amateur Hockey Association as well as all collegiate and high school hockey teams. The effectiveness of helmets was suggested by an early study done by Kraus and coworkers in 1969. When helmets were added as a mandatory piece of equipment to a collegiate intramural hockey league, head injuries dropped from 8.3 injuries per 100 games to a level of 3.8 head injuries per 100 games. At the same time, lacerations were reduced from 51 to 36 percent.[9] Despite the encouraging data regarding the reduction in head and catastrophic eye injury, periodic reports of massive spinal injuries continue to be reported to the Committee on the Prevention of Spinal Injuries due to Hockey. Tator and Edmonds, writing in the *Canadian Medical Association Journal* in 1984 reported 42 such injuries between the years of 1976 and 1983.[19] The average age was 17 years. Seventeen of these injuries went on to complete paralysis as a result of the neck being struck from behind and forced into the boards; 39 of the 42 injuries involved the cervical spine, and 22 out of the 42 resulted in wheelchair confinement. The authors concluded that rule changes to reduce the incidence of boarding, cross checking, and checking from behind still required attention. In addition, they suggested muscle conditioning to increase neck strength, recommended against small ice rinks, and recommended in favor of better-fitting helmets.

Epidemiological studies have been attempted, looking at hockey injuries in a variety of settings and in a variety of countries. A cross comparison of these studies is made difficult by virtue of the fact that definition of injury is not consistent. The population at risk is often poorly identified and ranges from peewee to professional. Injury identification varies, data collection varies, and statistical analysis frequently varies. Despite these differences, trends can be seen. Hornof and Napravnik reviewed injuries sustained in Czechoslovakia between the years 1967 and 1968.[6] They found an overall injury rate of 29.6 injuries per 1000 players per year. Forty-five percent were the result of practice and 55 percent the result of games. The puck or stick was responsible for 53.9 percent of injuries; the boards, 16.6 percent; and contact with another player, 15.6 percent. Falling on the ice accounted for an additional 9 percent. The head was involved in 36.7 percent and the lower extremity in 35.7 percent.

Sutherland reported injury incidence in four different age groups over 1 year.[18] Between ages 11 and 14, an injury incidence rate of one per 100 hours of playing time was recorded, with 59 percent of the injuries to the face and scalp. Ages 15 to 18 years had an injury rate of one per 16 hours of play time, with 68 percent involving the face and scalp. Ages 18 to 21 years sustained injuries at a rate of one per 11 hours of play, with 26 percent involving face and scalp. Professionals, by contrast, had an injury rate of one per 7 hours of play, with 66 percent involving face and scalp. The author concluded that injury rate showed progressive increase with age. Sutherland also found that the injury rate in games was much greater than in practice, and early season injuries seemed to be more prevalent than late season.[18]

Müller and Biener reported a 5-year study of injuries sustained in Swiss hockey.[12] They found that 25 percent were caused by the stick, 5 percent by skates, 17 percent by the puck, 17 percent by collision, and the remainder by falls on the ice, body checking, crashing against the boards, and so on. Forty-two percent of the injuries involved the head and face; 21 percent, legs; 11 percent, feet; 11 percent, arms; 7 percent, hands; and 8 percent, trunk. Seventy percent of all injuries were sustained during the game and 30 percent a result of practice. In total, 2680 accidents were reported. In 1987, Gerberich et al. reviewed the injuries sustained by 12 Minnesota high school teams in the 1982–1983 season.[3] An injury rate of 75 per 100 players per year was recorded, with the head and neck accounting for 22 percent. Sixteen percent of injuries involved the shoulder; 13 percent, arm and hand; 12 percent, trunk; 11 percent, leg and foot; and 10 percent, knee. Fifty-four percent of these injuries were felt to be mild; 28 percent, moderate; and 18 percent, severe. The mechanism of injury was a collision with a player in 34.8 percent, collision with the boards in 19.8 percent, collision with the goal in 19.8 percent, falls to the ice in 8 percent, and contact with the puck in an additional 7.5 percent. In 4.8 percent, no contact was involved, and 14.9 percent were unknown. The vast majority of injuries sustained in this study were a result of competition.

Jorgensen and Schmidt-Olsen reviewed the injury pattern in the Danish Elite Hockey Program.[8] The ages ranged from 16 to 34, with an average age of 22.7. The injury incidence was found to be 4.7 per player per 100 hours. Game-related injuries occurred 25 percent more frequently than practice injuries. The head was involved in 28 percent, the lower extremity in 27 percent, the upper extremity in 19 percent, and the back in an additional 7 percent.

Sim and Chao[17] compared and contrasted several of these epidemiological studies including a work done by Hayes in 1972[5,10] Table 30–1 reviews the distribution of injury sites. The head had a uniformly high injury percentage, as did the shoulder, thigh, and knee regions. Table 30–2 reviews the distribution of injury mechanism. Although the skate would be expected to cause frequent lacerations because of its razor-sharp edge, in fact it is a fairly infrequent cause of injury and certainly much less important than the stick, puck, and collisions. The majority of injuries sustained are of the contusion and

TABLE 30–1. Distribution of Sites of Ice Hockey Injuries (in percent)

Site	Sutherland	Müller et al.	Hornof et al.	Hayes
Head	7.0	42	37.1	45.1
Scalp and face	45.9	—	—	—
Eye	2.6	—	—	—
Shoulder	8.6	18	21.9	9.2
Hand	2.1	—	—	7.9
Thigh (groin)	18.4	21	35.7	8.8
Knee	11.6	—	—	10.4
Trunk	—	—	—	8.9
Miscellaneous (back, ribs, foot, ankle)	3.8	19	5.3	9.7

Source: From Sim, F. H., Simonet, W. T., Melton, L. J., Lehn, T. A.: Ice hockey injuries. Am J. Sports Med 15(1): 30–40, 1987. Reprinted with permission.

TABLE 30–2. Distribution of Mechanism of Ice Hockey Injuries (in percent)

Mechanism	Mathe	Handzo et al.	Müller et al.	Hayes
Stick	8	18	25	29.1
Puck	16	20	17	15.2
Skate	5	6	5	3.5
Collision	33	14	17	38.3
Miscellaneous	38	42	36	13.9

Source: From Sim, F. H., Simonet, W. T., Melton, L. J., Lehn, T. A.: Ice hockey injuries. Am J Sports Med 15(1): 30–40, 1987. Reprinted with permission.

laceration variety, as demonstrated in Table 30–3.[17]

Although these studies give us insights into the frequency and type of injury patterns sustained in hockey, they were performed at a time before helmets and masks were uniformly used and before the improvement in shoulder pads. These equipment changes, in association with rule changes, have undoubtedly changed the pattern of hockey injury in 1990.

TABLE 30–3. Distribution of Types of Ice Hockey Injuries (in percent)

Type	Hayes	NEISS	Hornof et al.
Contusion	47.6	25	37.0 (skin)
Laceration	28.4	49.7	33.9 (joints)
Fracture	4.6	10	15.2 (bones)
Dislocation	2.7	1	7.9 (muscles)
Other	4.6	4	2.9 (nervous system)
Muscle or ligament strain	12.1	10.3	3.1 (other)

NEISS = National Electronic Injury Surveillance System, 1974
Source: From Sim, F. H., Simonet, W. T., Melton, L. J., Lehn, T. A.: Ice hockey injuries. Am J. Sports Med 15(1): 30–40, 1987. Reprinted with permission.

HOCKEY INJURIES

Hockey, by its nature, results in a large number and variety of injuries and injury patterns. However, the chapter will concentrate on those injuries that are endemic to hockey and certain others for which measures for injury prevention, treatment, or rehabilitation are specific to hockey.

"HOCKEY ANKLE"

Ankle sprains are a ubiquitous part of sports injuries. However, in hockey the common ankle sprain caused by a plantar flexion, inversion, internal rotation mechanism is a relatively rare occurrence because of the protection afforded by the modern stiff skating boot and because there is relatively little jumping and landing, which is a frequent cause of inversion injuries. More frequent and much more troublesome in skating is the dorsiflexion, eversion, external rotation ankle sprain. There are two principal etiologies for this sprain. The first and most common is the catching of the support blade in an ice rut, causing the skate to follow the rut, forcefully externally rotating and everting the ankle. The second etiology is a fall over the front of the skates, with the foot being caught in an externally rotated, dorsiflexed position under the body (Fig. 30–1).

Signs and Symptoms

This sprain mechanism results in immediate pain, which localizes in two distinct areas, the medial aspect of the ankle over the deltoid ligament and the anterolateral aspect of the ankle over the anterior tibiofibular ligament and distal interosseous ligament. The pain is increased with eversion, external ro-

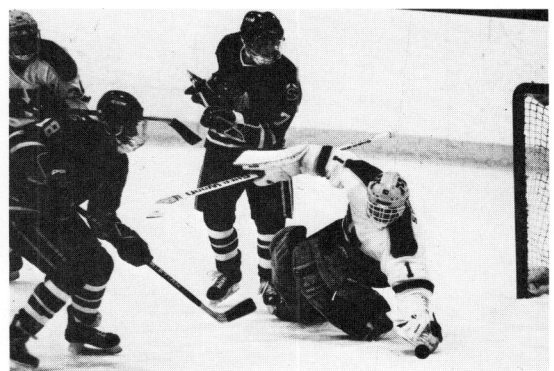

FIGURE 30–1. The goal tender's left foot shows a dorsiflexion, external rotation, eversion force being applied to the left ankle as a result of catching the skate blade in the ice rather than sliding smoothly.

tation stress of the dorsiflexed ankle. Inversion, internal rotation of the plantar-flexed ankle is relatively painless. When the mechanism of injury and clinical exam are consistent with an eversion sprain, stress X-rays should be initially performed to rule out a diastasis of the ankle syndesmosis. I routinely include the entire tibia and fibula on the film to avoid missing a proximal fibular fracture.

Treatment

The immediate treatment for this injury should be prompt compression, ice, and elevation, as the degree of swelling predicts the amount of ankle pain and the length of recovery time expected. When radiographic evidence of mortice widening or instability is evident, I favor open fixation with a syndesmodic screw to reduce and hold the ankle anatomically. Postoperative management includes non–weight bearing in a short leg cast for 6 weeks and full weight bearing in a short leg cast for an additional 6 weeks. The screw is removed 12 weeks postoperatively, and skating is resumed along with an ankle rehab program. Use of an air cast allows for daily removal for ankle range of motion. This reduces ankle stiffness and calf atrophy and will accelerate the postcast rehabilitation and return to function. An alternative treatment proposed is prolonged cast immobilization and non–weight bearing, provided a closed reduction is possible. If stress X-rays are negative for diastasis, crutches and compression dressing are continued until the initial injury pain subsides. At that point, weight bearing is allowed as tolerated. Early rehabilitation is designed to maintain cardiovascular fitness and allow plantar-flexion-dorsiflexion motion of the ankle as tolerated. The exercise bicycle and an ankle board are invaluable in this early phase (Fig. 30–2). Inversion-eversion strengthening is advanced as the tenderness over the anterior tib-fib ligament and interosseous space begin to subside. When biking, full weight bearing, and ankle strengthening are tolerated well, we advance to straight-ahead running on a treadmill or outdoors as the weather permits. The final, most difficult phase of the rehabilitation is return to skating because of the inherent external rotation, eversion forces placed across the ankle with normal skating stride. To help protect the ankle against excessive stress in this period, a "Roman sandal" compression taping is applied (Fig. 30–3). The purpose of the tape is to provide compression of the innerosseous space, to limit dorsiflexion, plantarflexion motion and to limit eversion, external rotation stress.

Prognosis

The ultimate prognosis for this injury is excellent, with no residual disability to the ankle, provided there has been no formal diastasis of the syndesmosis of the ankle. However, time for return to skating and hockey is prolonged relative to a standard ankle sprain. In my experience, 3 to 6 weeks

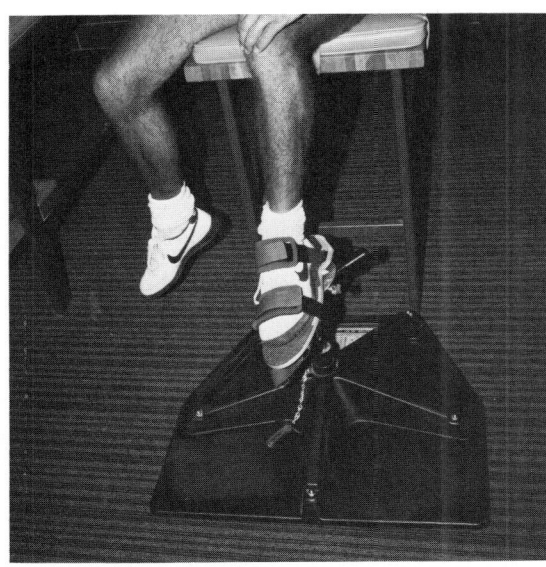

FIGURE 30–2. Inversion and eversion range of motion and strengthening can be progressed as pain allows. Both motion and resistance can be adjusted to accommodate each athlete.

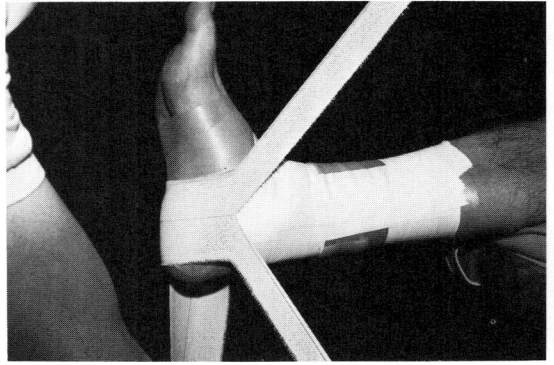
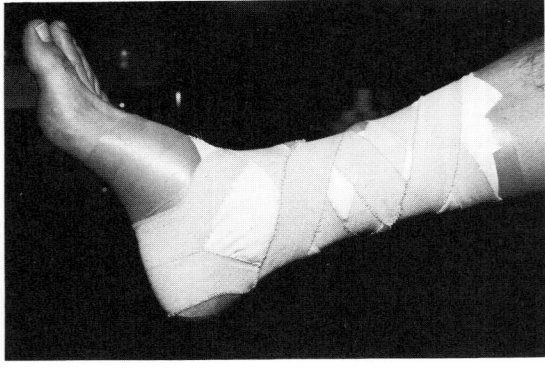
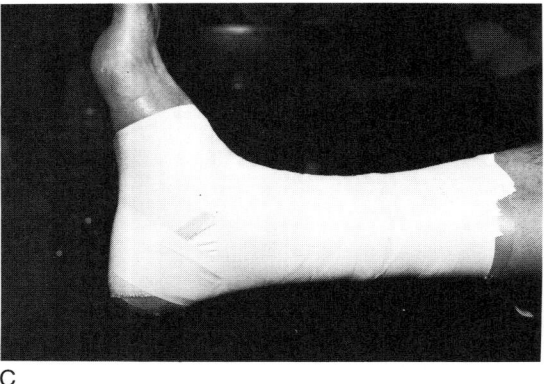

FIGURE 30–3. "Roman Sandal" taping after pretape preparation, the stirrup straps are placed. Four-inch Elastikon is split to the distal border of the malleolus, as shown in (A). Each arm of the elasticized tape is woven up the ankle from the medial and lateral sides, as shown in (B). A final layer of lateral and medial heel locks and figure-of-eight taping is placed over the top of the "Roman sandal" for further stability, as shown in (C).

is required before the ankle has rehabilitated to the point where skating can be performed effectively.

HIP ADDUCTOR STRAIN

Sim and Chao presented biomechanical data demonstrating the large forces placed across the hip and leg at the time of push-off during a skating maneuver. They hypothesized that these large forces could result in the adductor strain patterns seen commonly in skaters.[16] Merrifield and Cowan tested a series of high school athletes, looking specifically at leg adductor strength.[11] They compared the injury rate to preseason test results and found that all players suffering an adductor strain injured the weaker leg and further that all players who sustained an injury had an imbalance of greater than or equal to 25 percent on preseason strength testing. They recommended a strengthening and stretching program as prophylaxis against this injury pattern. Adductor strains continue to be a problem in hockey and, once present, plague the hockey player and skater for the duration of the season. Rather than presenting as an acute injury, adductor strain is generally an overuse injury, particularly related to push-off and rapid acceleration.

Signs and Symptoms

The presenting symptom is one of pain in the adductors, generally perceived in the muscle-tendon unit just distal to the origin on the pelvis. This pain is increased with resisted adduction and at times with resisted hip flexion. Rarely is there ecchymosis associated with this injury.

Treatment

The best treatment for this injury is avoidance. The author feels that part of the off-season strengthening program should include a hip abduction/adduction strength station as well as a hip stretching program (Fig. 30–4). Since initiating such a strengthening effort in the off-season, the incidence of adductor strains in the hockey players for whom the author has responsibility has dropped precipitously.

Once present, treatment is symptomatic. A hip spica wrap can be effective in maintain-

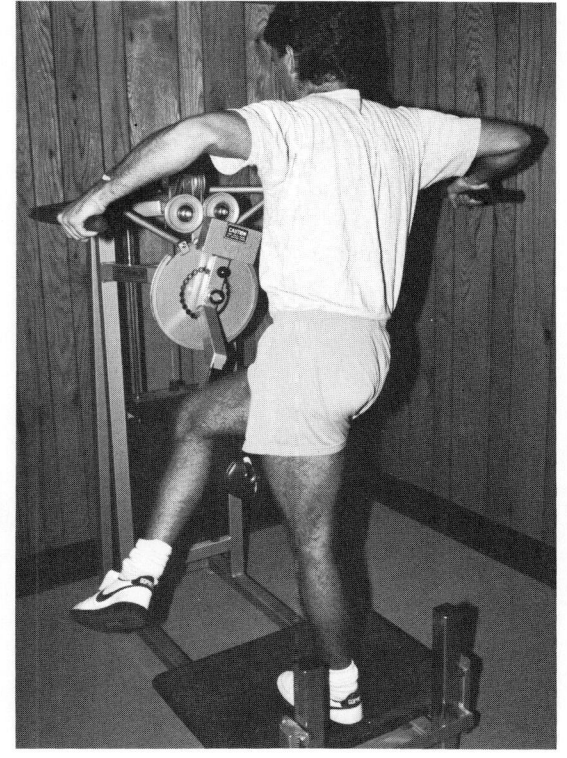
A

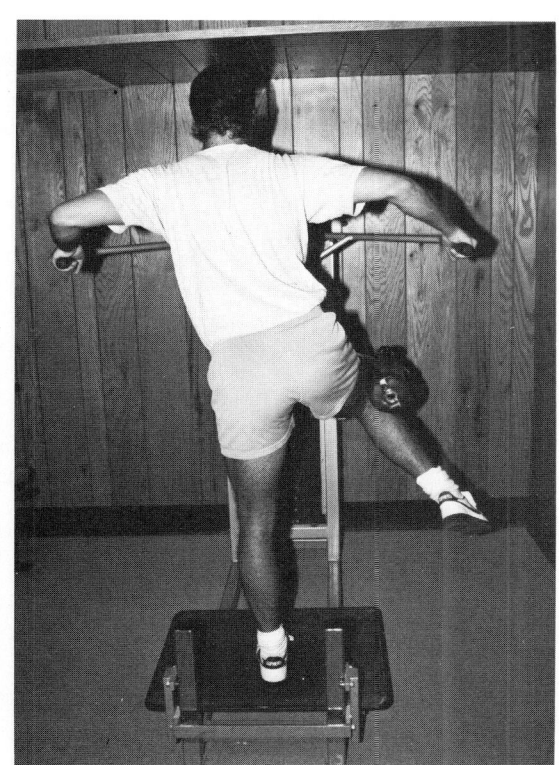
B

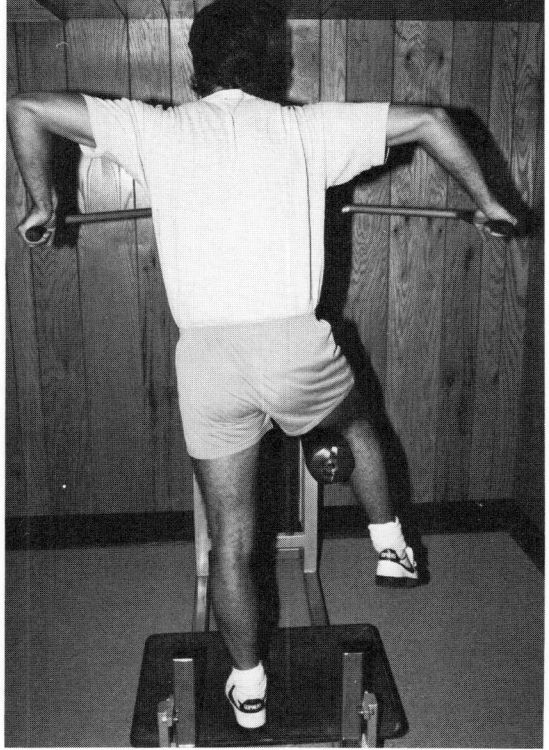
C

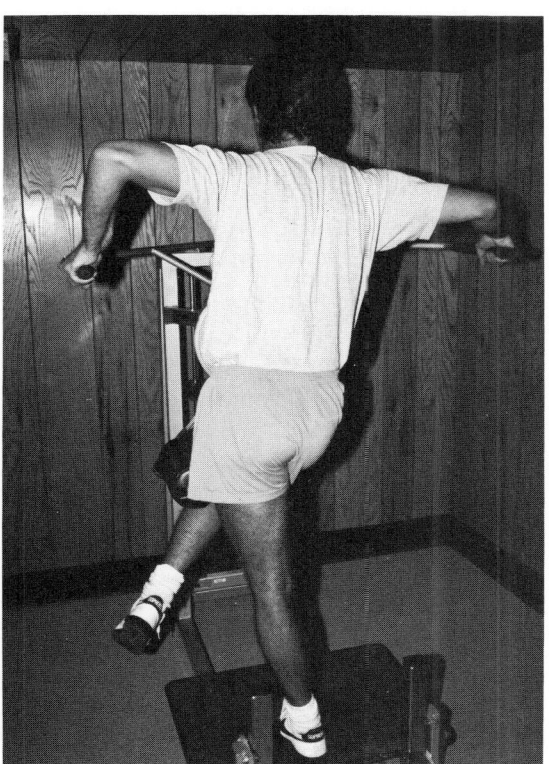
D

FIGURE 30–4. (*A*) and (*B*) show the starting and finishing positions for hip abduction strengthening. (*C*) and (*D*) demonstrate starting and stopping positions for hip adduction strengthening. (*E*) and (*F*) demonstrate the start and stop position for hip extension stretching.

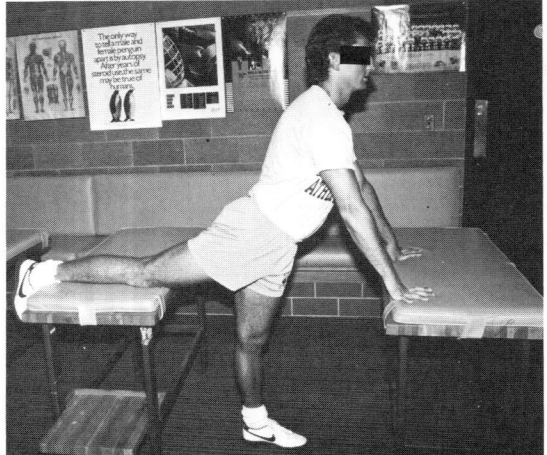 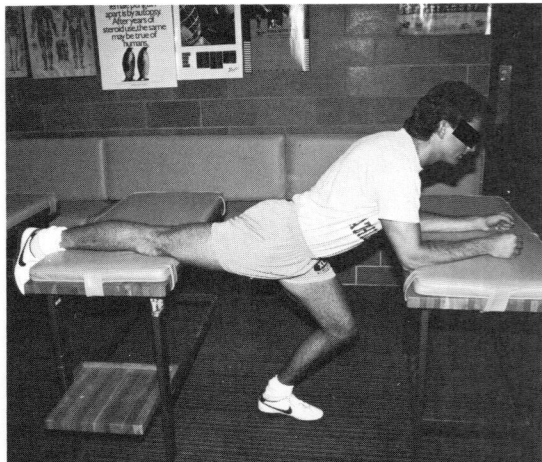

E F

FIGURE 30-4. *Continued*

ing slight pressure and heat in the area (Fig. 30–5). A hip adductor stretching program and gentle adductor strengthening have also been effective in season, minimizing the symptoms and allowing competition. All strengthening exercises should be done on a high repetition, low weight protocol to avoid reinjury to the irritated musculature.

Prognosis

The prognosis for complete recovery from adductor strains is excellent. However, once

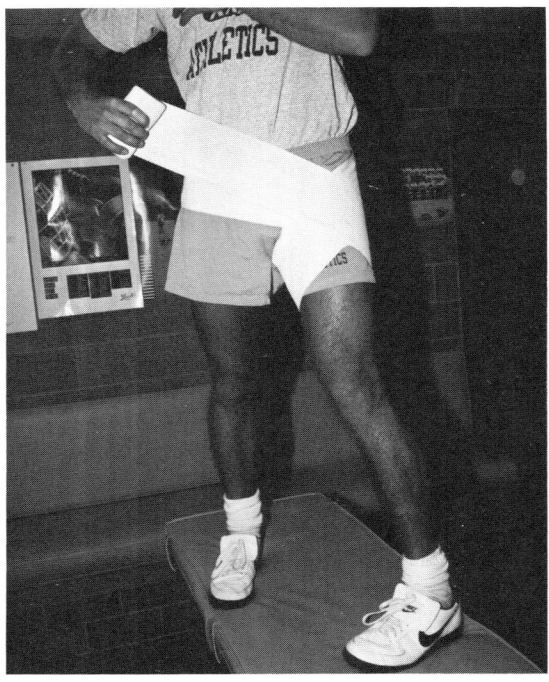 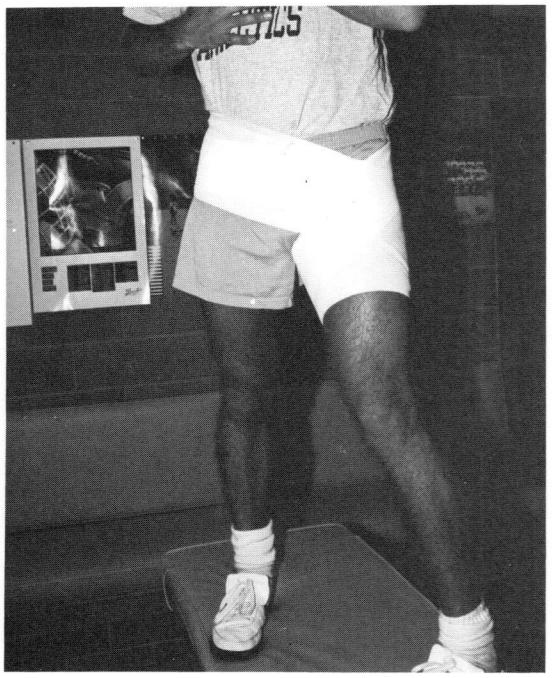

A B

FIGURE 30-5. The hip spica wrap for adduction strain is applied with the affected leg slightly abducted and internally rotated. The wrap is preformed with an extra long Ace bandage, encouraging further internal rotation (*A*). The bandage is locked in place with athletic tape, discouraging excessive abduction, as shown in (*B*).

present, it can be anticipated that the symptoms will persist for the duration of the season. For the most part, return to competition has been possible after the resolution of acute symptoms, lasting 5 to 7 days.

SHOULDER INJURIES

The shoulder is particularly vulnerable because of the frequency of falls on the outstretched arm, because of collisions with other players, and in particular, because of checking against the boards, where a player's shoulder is compressed between an opponent and a nonyielding side wall. Three specific shoulder injuries are most frequent and troublesome: the acromicolavicular (AC) joint sprain, anterior shoulder dislocation, and clavical fracture.

Acromioclavicular Sprain

Relatively little information is available concerning AC separations in children. Eidman et al. reviewed 25 cases of AC injuries treated surgically.[1] They found no cases of true AC dislocation in children under the age of 13 but rather distal clavical fractures. Their recommendations were for closed management of all AC dislocations under the age of 13 and operative repair in children over the age of 13.

The mechanism of injury is a fall directly on the tip of the shoulder or acute compression of the shoulder, driving the acromion down forcibly. This latter mechanism is very common with checking against the boards.

Signs and Symptoms. The principal symptom is pain, located over the AC joint. Grade I and II injuries have relatively few signs other than direct tenderness. A grade III separation will show elevation of the distal clavicle or, if palpated under a shoulder pad, will reveal gross motion between the clavicle and the acromion as longitudinal traction is placed on the humerus.

Treatment. The author has treated all acute shoulder separations nonoperatively in the adolescent. Treatment consists of a sling used for comfort, generally from 2 to 4 weeks. Motion is allowed as tolerated, with strengthening added to motion as motion progresses. Return to competition is allowed when motion is full, strength has returned to its preinjury level, and tenderness is minimal. A grade I sprain is usually able to return to hockey within 1 to 2 weeks. A grade III injury

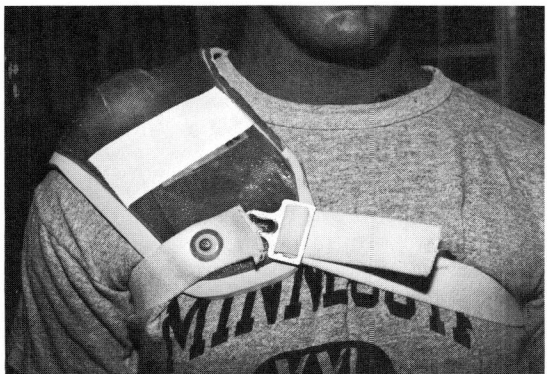

FIGURE 30–6. The AC splint can be effective in dissipating forces across the AC joint after a separation. When taking the mold, the AC joint is padded with felt or foam, creating a bump as shown in the photo. When the foam is removed, a pocket is created over the AC joint, which results in the dissipation of forces away from that location to the soft tissues of the chest and back.

will generally require 3 to 4 weeks before pain has subsided and motion and strength are restored to the point where competition is possible. On return to competition, a protective fiberglass pad is fabricated, which fits underneath the shoulder pad and dissipates forces to the soft tissues around the AC joint when direct contact is made in this area (Fig. 30–6). I have not seen a type IV or V lesion in this population but would treat it as recommended by Rockwood et al.[14]

Prognosis. The prognosis for complete symptomatic recovery from a shoulder separation in this population is excellent. A type III disruption can at times lead to a prominent distal clavicle, but rarely is this a symptomatic issue. I suspect that the improved prognosis in these injuries is the result of the protective periosteal tube that maintains continuity of the coracoclavicular ligaments and the inferior acromioclavicular ligaments, allowing for enhanced healing and restoration of stability.[2]

Shoulder Dislocations

Shoulder dislocations occur with much less frequency than AC separations. There is relatively little information available regarding dislocations in the adolescent population to offer advice in these demanding cases. Rowe, in 1963, felt that prognosis was most directly associated with the age of the patient at the time of initial dislocation and recorded a recurrence rate of 94 percent in patients between the ages of 11 and 20.[15] Hovelius reviewed his experience with shoulder dislocations in Swedish hockey. All patients were under the age of 30. The author found that the length of immobilization did not change the recurrence rate, which in his study was 76 percent. Like Rowe, he felt that the age of first dislocation was most important in prognosticating recurrence. In those patients under the age of 20, the recurrence rate was 90 percent, as opposed to 50 percent for those patients over the age of 25.[7] There are two potential mechanisms for anterior shoulder dislocation seen in hockey: an indirect force from a fall on an outstretched arm or a direct blow to the posterior aspect of the shoulder at the time of body contact (Fig. 30–7).

Signs and Symptoms. At the time of dislocation, the athlete will immediately support the involved forearm with the uninvolved hand, with the shoulder held in slight external rotation. Palpation will reveal a fullness in the anterior aspect of the shoulder and a depressed area lateral to the acromion process where the humeral head provides shoulder contour.

Treatment. After reduction, the author recommends placing the arm in a shoulder immobilizer with the involved upper extremity held in full adduction and internal rotation for a period of 3 weeks. I believe that this offers the maximum potential for anterior capsule healing, which may reduce recurrence rate. Immobilization is followed by an aggressive rehabilitation program, emphasizing internal and external rotation strengthening, in an effort to restore secondary stability, particularly of the internal rotators. When

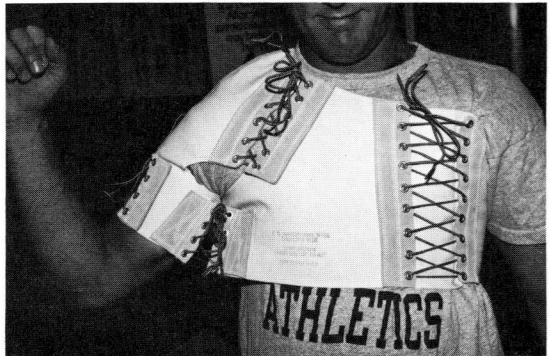

FIGURE 30–8. After anterior shoulder subluxation or dislocation, a shoulder harness can be used to discourage arm abduction and external rotation, thus avoiding the most vulnerable position for recurrent instability episodes.

range of motion has been restored and strength training can be accomplished without pain or shoulder tenderness, I allow return to competition. This occurs by 6 to 8 weeks following dislocation. On return to contact, the shoulder is protected with a shoulder harness that blocks motion and thus restricts the abduction, external rotation position, which might place the shoulder at risk of recurrent subluxation (Fig. 30–8). This brace is well tolerated by hockey players and does not seem to interfere with performance. We recommend that the harness be worn for a period of 6 months after the dislocation but have found a number of competitors who prefer to wear it for extended periods beyond the 6-month time limit because of the feeling of security that it offers.

Clavicle Fractures

Clavicle fractures are becoming less common in hockey as shoulder pads improve. Old-style shoulder pads provided little protection against axial load from a blow to the tip of the shoulder and also provided very little protection against a direct blow to the clavicle as a result of a high stick. New pads offer protection against both mechanisms (Fig. 30–9).

Signs and Symptoms. The principal symptoms are pain with a palpable defect in the shaft of the clavicle and gross motion at the fracture site. When the fracture is more distal, it can be very difficult to differentiate between a fracture and an AC joint separation. In the young patient, under the age of 13, it may be impossible to make this differentiation, short of open exploration.

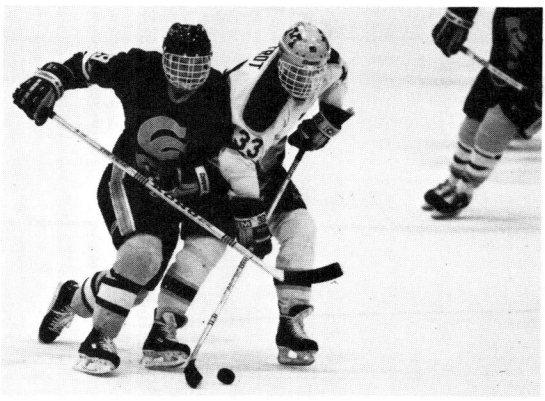

FIGURE 30–7. A direct blow to the posterior aspect of the shoulder, as shown in this game photo, can result in anterior translational forces causing subluxation or dislocation of the glenohumeral joint.

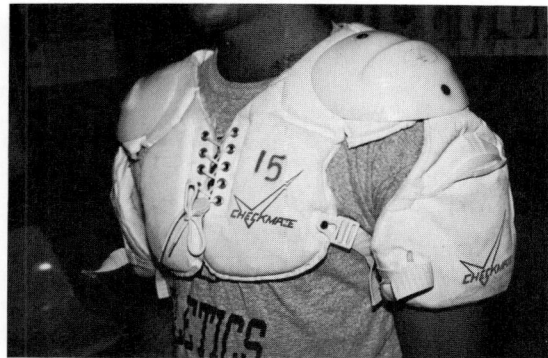

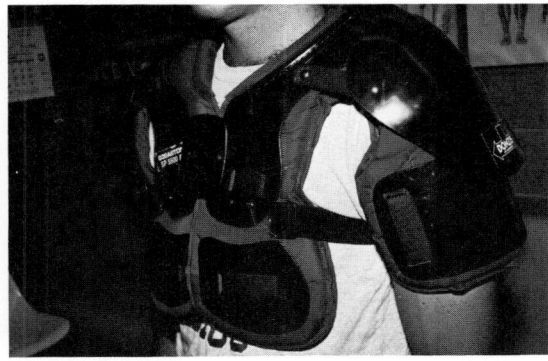

FIGURE 30–9. (A) demonstrates an old form of shoulder pad, which has minimal protection over the clavicle as well as the AC joint. By contrast, the newer, more protective pads (B) have extended protection over the clavicle as well as enhanced protection over the AC joint, shoulder, and proximal arm.

Treatment. Once the diagnosis has been made, the author treats all clavicle fractures in this population conservatively, using a figure-of-eight-styled harness to encourage shoulder extension. A harness is worn full-time for 2 to 3 weeks and then is removed for bathing and at night for an additional 2 to 3 weeks. In the younger child, abundant callus will be seen at the fracture site within 2 to 3 weeks of injury, with complete clinical union by 4 weeks, resulting in a fracture that is nontender and stable. In the older child, the healing progresses somewhat slower and can take 6 to 8 weeks.

Prognosis. The prognosis for complete recovery is excellent. However, there is a tendency to return these competitors to competition when their pain has subsided and motion has been restored. Clearly, the fracture is not firmly united at this point and places the athlete at risk for refracture or reinjury. Because of that, we discourage return to competition after a clavicle fracture for 12 weeks. We allow return to skating and noncontact practice at 6 weeks but protect the clavicle with a fiberglass molded cuff in an effort to dissipate forces to the surrounding soft tissues.

SUMMARY

Hockey injuries can never be eliminated because of the nature of the sport and because of the environment in which the sport is played. Skates, pucks, and sticks will always be sources of injury, as will collisions with competitors, with goals, and with boards. Nevertheless, great strides have been made, reducing injury incidence and reducing injury severity because of aggressive research that has resulted in rule changes and equipment improvement. Further progress can be expected if we continue to pursue proper athletic training, good and consistent coaching that begins at an early age, and officiating that provides maximum protection to all participants. With continuous review of rules and improvement in athlete protection, hockey can be made safer without adversely affecting the thrill or enjoyment of this wonderful sport.

References

1. Eidman, D. K., Sherwin, J. S., Tullos, H. S.: Acromioclavicular lesions in children. Am. J. Sports Med. 9:150–154, 1981.
2. Falstie-Jensen, S., Mikkelsen, P.: Pseudodislocation of the acromioclavicular joint. J. Bone Joint Surg. 64B:368–369, 1982.
3. Gerberich, S. G., Finke, R., Madden, M., Priest, J. D., Aamoth, G., Murray, K.: An epidemiological study of high school ice hockey injuries. Child's Nervous System 3:59–64, 1987.
4. Handzo, P., Novosad, S., Krivosudsky A.: Urazova zabrana pri ladovom hokeji. Teor Praxe tel Vych 8:125–132, 1960.
5. Hayes, D.: The nature, incidence, location and causes of injury in intercollegiate ice hockey. Thesis, University of Waterloo, Ontario, Canada, 1972.
6. Hornof, Z., Napravnik, C.: Analysis of various accident rate factors in ice hockey. Med. Sci. Sports 5(4):283–286, 1973.
7. Hovelius, L.: Shoulder dislocation in Swedish ice hockey players. Am. J. Sports Med. 6(6):373–377, 1978.
8. Jorgensen, U., Schmidt-Olsen, S.: The epidemiology of ice hockey injuries. Br. J. Sports Med. 20(1):7–9, 1986.
9. Kraus, J. F., Anderson, B. D., Mueller, C. E.: The effectiveness of a special ice hockey helmet to

reduce head injuries in college intramural hockey. Med. Sci. Sports 2(3):162–164, 1970.
10. Mathe, E.: The nature and occurrence of injuries in ice hockey. Presented at the Conference on Winter Sports Injuries, Madison, WI, 1967.
11. Merrifield, H. H., Cowan, R. F. J.: Groin strian injuries in ice hockey. J. Sports Med. pp 41–24, January/February 1973.
12. Müller, P., Biener, K.: Accidenti da hockey su ghiaccio. Minerva Med. 66:1352–1355, 1975.
13. Pashby, T.: Eye injuries in Canadian amateur hockey. Can. J. Ophthalmol. 20(1):2–4, 1985.
14. Rockwood, C. A., Wilkins, K. E., King, R. E. (eds): Fractures in Children. Vol 3. JB Lippincott Co, Philadephia, 1984.
15. Rowe, C. R.: Anterior dislocation of the shoulder: prognosis and treatment. Surg. Clin. North Am. 43:1609–1614, 1963.
16. Sim, F. H., Chao, E. Y.: Injury potential in modern ice hockey. Am. J. Sports Med. 6(6):378–384, 1978.
17. Sim, F. H., Simonet, W. T., Melton, L. J., Lehn, T. A.: Ice hockey injuries. Am. J. Sports Med. 15(1):30–40, 1987.
18. Sutherland, G. W.: Fire on ice. Am. J. Sports Med. 4(6):264–269, 1976.
19. Tator, C. H., Edmonds, V. E.: National survey of spinal injuries in hockey players. Can. Med. Assoc. J. 130:875–880, 1984.

31

BASKETBALL AND VOLLEYBALL

JAMES MICHAEL RAY
WALTER McCOMBS
ROY A. STERNES

Basketball and volleyball have become two major team sports and are being played more and more by adolescent athletes. Although basketball results in much more incidental body contact, they share many activity and injury patterns. Activities common to these sports are vertical jumping, run and jumping, pivoting, jump stopping, shooting, blocking, and occasionally diving to the floor. These activities put ankles, knees, and fingers at variable risk for injury. The injuries sustained may result from acute trauma or chronic overuse. The purpose of this chapter is to identify the injuries that are most common to these athletes and recommend preventive and treatment regimens to aid in safe and enjoyable participation. Basketball is more widely played than volleyball, and its injury patterns are better known; much of the knowledge gained from the care of basketball injuries may help the clinician care for volleyball players as well.

Basketball was invented by Dr. James A. Naismith in 1891. The game has evolved into one of the most enjoyable of participant and spectator sports. The teams are composed of five players each. The court is a rectangle that is 50 by 84 feet for high school and 50 by 94 feet for college and professional games. The purpose of the game is to score points by shooting the basketball through the opponents' basket.

The actual playing is divided into offensive and defensive strategies. Offensively, techniques that are used include dribbling, passing, and shooting. These activities require hand-eye coordination as well as running abilities. Defensively, running is also needed as well as fast footwork and leaping ability for shot blocking. Jumping is the one activity needed for performance on defense as well as offense.

Volleyball is also played on a rectangular court that measures 29 feet 6 inches by 59 feet from endline to endline. The teams consist of six players on each side. Scoring is done from the offensive side only. Serving and volleying are done from hand-ball contact. The purpose is to block the ball back into the opponents' court. The skills required also can be divided into offense and defense. Vertical jumping, run-jump, shot blocking, and footwork are necessary on the defensive side, whereas offense requires these skills plus the special eye-hand coordination necessary for serving.

The equipment necessary to participate in either of these two sports is very minimal. The basketball is an orange sphere made of leather panels cemented to an inner airtight rubber lining. A boys' basketball measures 29 to 30 inches in circumference and weighs 20 to 22 ounces, whereas the girls' ball measures 28 to 29 inches and weighs 18 to 20 ounces.

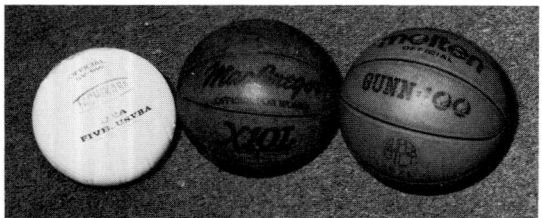

FIGURE 31–1. Volleyball, girls' basketball, and boys' basketball.

The volleyball is a smaller and lighter white sphere measuring 25 to 27 inches in circumference and weighing only 9 to 10 ounces (Fig. 31–1).

The basket is an 18-inch round rim, suspended from which is a net. The basket is placed approximately 10 feet from the floor. In volleyball, a net is suspended between two supports with its upper level approximately 7 feet ⅝ from the floor. The net serves to divide the court into two halves. The indoor courts usually have wood or tartan surfaces. Outdoor facilities may vary from cement to grass or sand. The playing surfaces contribute to injuries and must be taken into account when discussing variables.

The players' uniforms should accommodate the climate in which the game is being played. They usually consist of a shirt and short outfit; in volleyball, a one-piece uniform may be worn. Shoes are a very important part of the uniform because of the various running and jumping activities that must be performed. Shoes must be in good repair to give the athlete a good foot foundation on which to participate and to aid in the reduction of lower extremity injuries (Fig. 31–2).

EPIDEMIOLOGY OF BASKETBALL AND VOLLEYBALL INJURIES

The epidemiological literature on youth basketball injuries is not voluminous, and information on volleyball is even sparser. Some of the basketball studies suggest that girls are more likely to be injured than boys[18, 49, 100, 149, 152] In a 1978 survey of high school sports injuries, Garrick and Requa noted an injury rate of 0.31 per player for boys' basketball and 0.25 for girls'. The injury rate in volleyball was 0.10. They did not differentiate between major and minor injuries.[49]

In a small study of high school basketball players also published in 1978, Moretz and Grana found a startling difference in injury rates between the sexes—0.72 injuries per player for girls and 0.16 in boys. They attributed this difference to a perceived lack of preseason conditioning in girls.[100]

In 1985, Chandy and Grana published a much larger comparison of injury rates in several paired sports in 130 Oklahoma secondary schools over a 3-year period.[18] Again, they found that the female players had a significantly higher injury rate, 35.9 per 1000 athletes compared with 26.3 per 1000 athletes for the boys. Both sexes had similar types of injuries, but the girls had more severe injuries and more knee surgeries.

In a 1982 comparison study of a men's and a women's professional basketball team, Zelisko et al. also found an increased incidence of injuries among female players. Although the actual number of players was small, the authors found that the women's injury rate, expressed as injuries per 1000 player exposures, was 60 percent higher than the men's.[152]

A survey on high school basketball injuries was conducted by our University of Kentucky Sports Medicine staff for the 1987–1988 and 1988–1989 girls' and boys' basketball season (Fig. 31–3). The most common injury sustained was the sprained ankle, accounting for 55 percent (651 total) of the injuries in boys' basketball and 54 percent (311 total) of the injuries in girls' basketball.

Knee injuries accounted for 12 and 20 percent (140 and 118 total), respectively, followed by hand and wrist injuries at 9 and 7 percent (103 and 40 total). Sixty-six percent

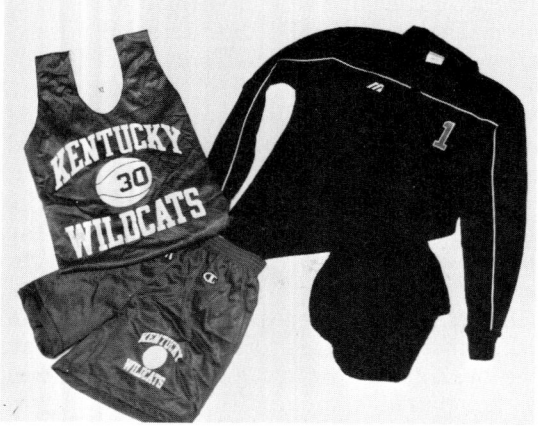

FIGURE 31–2. Basketball and volleyball uniforms should consist of a jersey and short set made of appropriate cloth for climate control. Shoes should be in good repair.

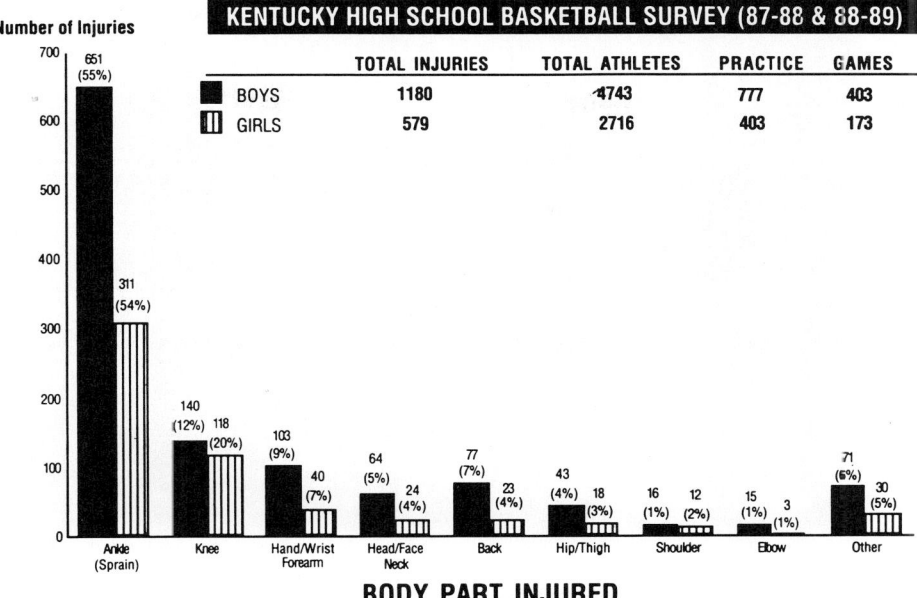

FIGURE 31-3. Kentucky High School Basketball Survey, 1987–1988 and 1988–1989.

of the boys' injuries and 70 percent of the girls' injuries occurred during practice. Only 33 percent of the boys' injuries and 30 percent of the girls' injuries occurred during the game activities. This distribution reflects the increased exposure time in practice. The Kentucky data situations are similar to other reports in the literature on injury statistics.[5, 12, 17, 34, 56, 95, 96, 101, 114, 146, 150, 151] Injuries occurring in volleyball show a similar anatomical injury distribution.

This chapter concentrates on the treatment of lower extremity injuries in basketball and volleyball. The treatment of hand and wrist injuries is not unique to these sports and follows the principles detailed in Chapter 14.

KNEE INJURIES

PATELLAR TENDINITIS

Overuse injuries of the tendinous portions of the extensor mechanism are so common in basketball and volleyball that they are often collectively called "jumper's knee."[9, 40, 41, 121] Tendinitis may occur at the junction of the patellar tendon and the patella, the patellar tendon and the tibial tubercle, or the quadriceps tendon and the patella.[73, 77, 84, 87] As in Achilles tendinitis, eccentric overloading of the tendon while landing from jumps is thought to cause microfailure in the tendon. Local inflammation at the area of the bone-tendon junction as well as within the tendon substance itself may cause symptoms during and possibly after athletic activities. If sporting activities are allowed to continue, the symptoms will persist.

Pain and tenderness near the junction of the patellar tendon and patella are typical of patellar tendinitis. Tenderness at the superior pole of the patella suggests insertional quadriceps tendinitis. Hamstring and quadriceps flexibility may also be limited in these conditions.

Radiographic examination of the knee should include AP, lateral, tunnel, and skyline views. The lateral view may demonstrate calcification at the inferior pole of the patella characteristic of Sinding-Larsen–Johansson disease.[126] Calcification within the tendon tissue itself or soft tissue swelling may also be noted.

Ultrasonography of the patella tendon is a noninvasive method of documenting edema, hemorrhage, partial rupture, or calcification within the tendon tissue that may not be visible on routine radiographs.[43, 45] Tendon thickness at the inferior pole of the patella has been calculated in normal individuals to be less than 5 mm. Hemorrhage and edema in the area of the proximal patella tendon increase this thickness to greater than 10 mm.

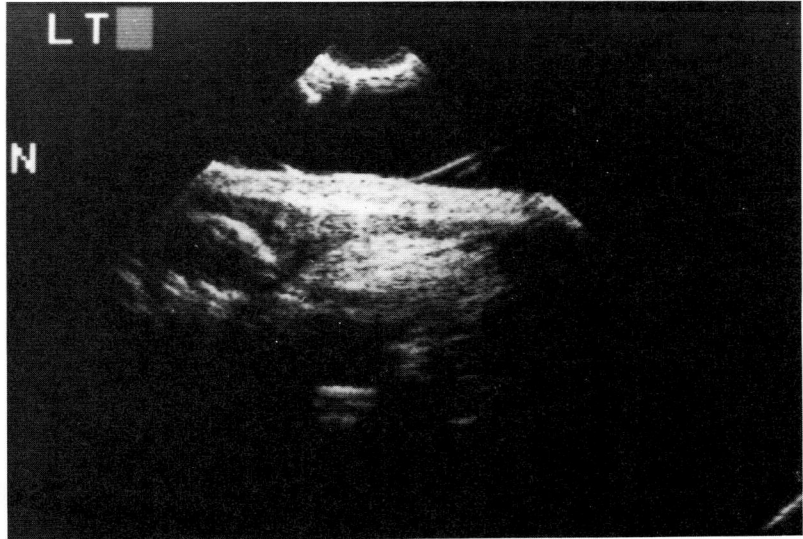

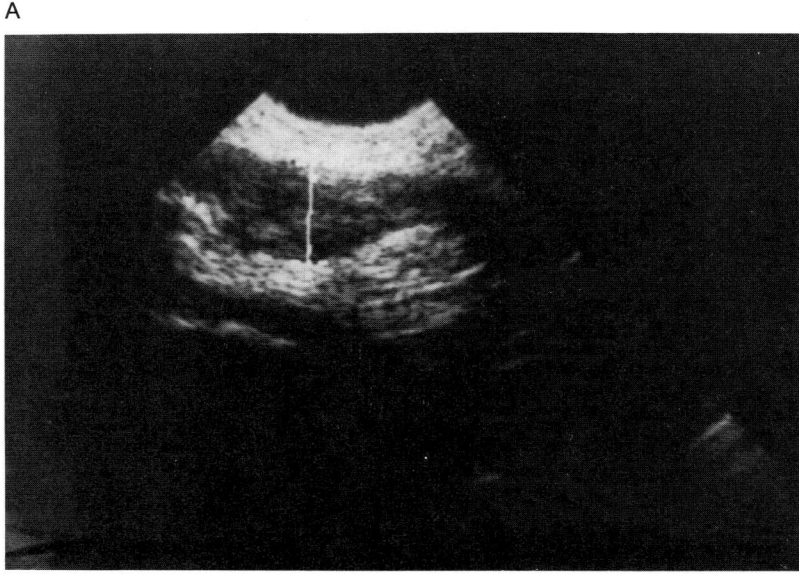

FIGURE 31–4. Sonograms of (*A*) normal patella tendon and (*B*) abnormal patella tendon showing calcification and hemorrhage.

Generalized edema and tendon thickening can be calculated with ultrasonography from the inferior pole of the patella to the tibia tubercle (Fig. 31–4).

Bone scans have also been utilized in the workup and evaluation of jumper's knee.[59, 60, 61] The radioactive tracer is noted to highlight the inferior pole of the patella in patellar tendinitis or the superior pole in quadriceps tendinitis (Fig. 31–5). Uptake of the tracer at the bone-tendon interface suggests an ongoing microfailure-reparative process.

Bone scanning and ultrasonography are useful together in evaluating chronic cases of patellar tendinitis that may require surgery. Athletes who present with the signs and symptoms of patellar tendinitis and who have a negative bone scan and a normal sonogram may respond to conservative management. Athletes with a positive bone scan and an abnormal sonogram most likely have a history of long-standing disease that has been refractory to conservative treatment regimens. These athletes will often require sur-

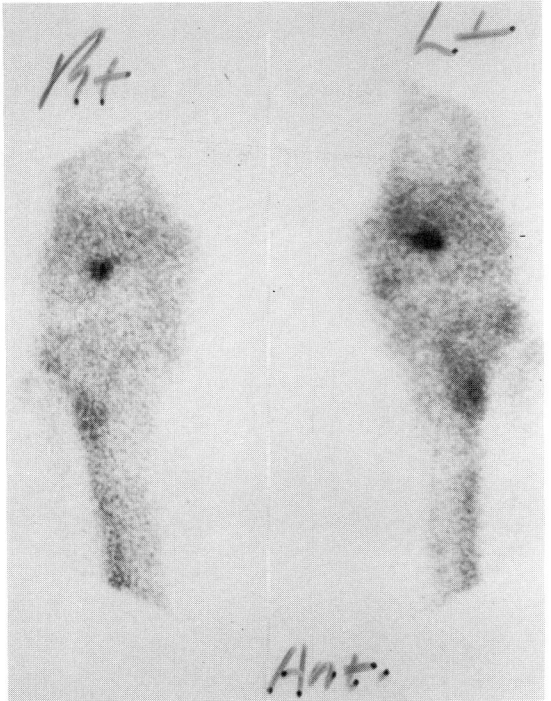

FIGURE 31-5. Bone scan of patient with bilateral patella tendinitis showing increased uptake at the inferior pole of the patella.

Cast treatment should be avoided. Analgesics are rarely indicated, and local steroid injections are contraindicated because of the risk of tendon rupture.[65, 74] The athlete and parents should be informed of the severity of the disease and its potentially serious implications. If the athlete is unable to compete despite extensive conservative treatment, then ultrasonography and bone scanning or MRI may be performed to document the severity of the disease.

Surgery for chronic patellar tendinitis involves exploration of the diseased portion of the patellar tendon as well as removal of the inferior pole with drilling of the patella.[87, 111] Arthroscopy of the knee to document articular surface chondromalacia of the patella is helpful in prescribing postop rehabilitation protocols. Debridement of the fat pad near the inferior pole of the patella as well as the patella tendon on its undersurface near the bone-tendon junction may result in tendon healing. Arthroscopic burring and drilling of the inferior pole of the patella may limit the surgical morbidity associated with open tendon exploration (Fig. 31-6).

Postoperatively, the knee is wrapped in a compressive dressing, not a cast, and early

gery. Athletes with either a positive bone scan and a normal sonogram or a normal bone scan and an abnormal sonogram may be placed on a conservative program but may come to surgery if this fails.

More recently, MRI has improved the documentation of bone disease, bone-tendon junction disease, and isolated tendon disease.[66] MRI is noninvasive, involves no radiation, and may be repeated to document disease progression or healing or results of surgical intervention. The use of MRI has added a new dimension to the evaluation of tendon disease but is currently limited owing to cost and availability.

The athlete with patellar tendinitis may continue to compete in the face of the inflammation and discomfort. Hamstring and quadriceps flexibility should be assessed and stretching exercises prescribed. A neoprene knee sleeve or a tendon strap may reduce symptoms by local compression of the tendon or from retention of body heat. Efforts aimed at reducing local pain and tissue reaction may include a 2-week course of oral nonsteroidal antiinflammatories, phonophoresis, ultrasound, or moist heat prior to exercise and ice applications after exercise.

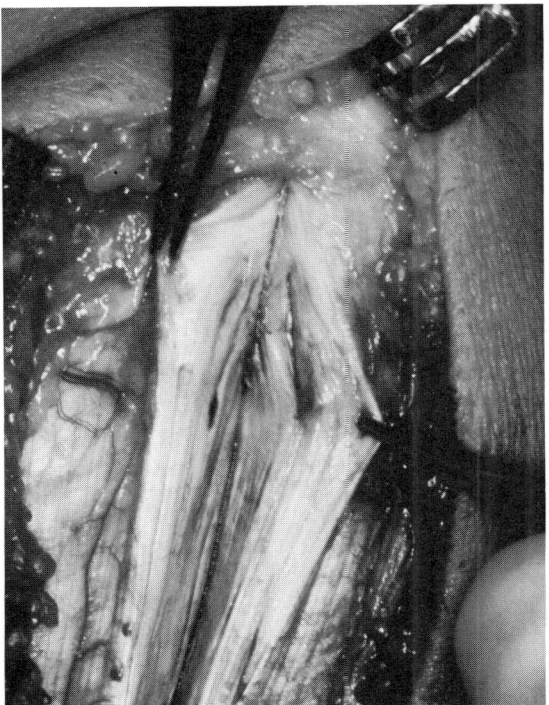

FIGURE 31-6. Surgical exploration of the patella tendon showing chronic degenerative change of the patella tendon.

range of motion is instituted. Resistive exercises through a full range of motion are not begun until tendon healing and symptoms of surgical pain have subsided. This takes 4 to 6 weeks. Terminal extension exercises may aggravate patellar tendon pain if instituted too soon. Alternative training may help to maintain conditioning during this period. Avoidance of jumping and sprinting is necessary until symptoms subside.

Advanced conditioning and training may be instituted once comfort and strength have returned to the knee. Resistive exercises with elastic bands or weights, sliding boards for lateral movement, and plymometrics concentrating on landing patterns and eccentric quadriceps activity are helpful prior to the athlete's return to the basketball or volleyball court.

OSGOOD-SCHLATTER DISEASE

Traction apophysitis, marked by pain, swelling, inflammation, and fragmentation at the tibial tubercle, is common in the younger adolescent basketball or volleyball player.[99, 108] The onset of this pain is usually coincident with or after the onset of rapid growth. Hamstring and quadriceps flexibility are decreased. Pain with exertion and at rest leads to a decreased level of athletic participation. Males are affected more than females. The prominence of the tibial tubercle makes it vulnerable to blunt trauma.

Radiographic examination may demonstrate swelling, fragmentation, and ossicle formation of the tibial tubercle. These changes are best seen on the lateral radiographs. Ultrasonography usually does not demonstrate tendon disease, and MRI studies are not indicated. Bone scanning shows an increased uptake of the radioactive tracer due to the fragmentation of the tibial tubercle as well as the open epiphysis and so lends very little to the diagnosis and treatment of the disease.

Treatment of Osgood-Schlatter disease should include hamstring and quadriceps flexibility exercises. Icing after athletic participation is helpful in controlling inflammation and pain. Reduction or elimination of running and jumping activities may be necessary when the athlete is symptomatic. Protective volleyball or basketball knee sleeves that provide a thick pad over the tibial tubercle may protect it from blunt trauma

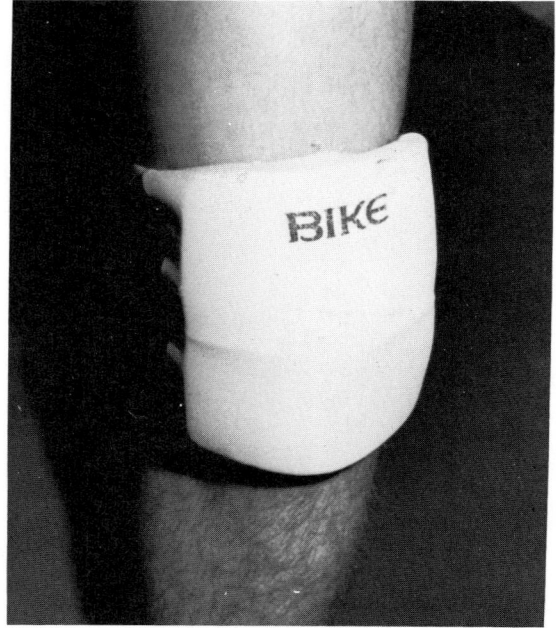

A

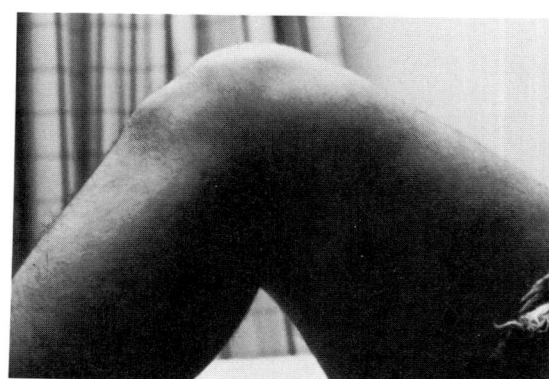

B

FIGURE 31–7. (A) Volleyball or basketball knee pads for soft tissue protection. (B) Lateral view of the knee demonstrating Osgood-Schlatter disease.

(Fig. 31–7). Casting of the knee has been discarded in favor of a more functional rehabilitation program. Oral antiinflammatory medication may be helpful during periods of severe symptoms. This disease is self-limiting and resolves with skeletal maturity. Surgical intervention is rarely indicated in the athlete with an immature skeleton.[109] Ossicles in the tendon will occasionally continue to be symptomatic after skeletal maturity and require surgical excision (Fig. 31–8). Rupture of the patellar tendon or avulsion of the tibial tubercle apophysis is rare in Osgood-Schlatter disease.[11]

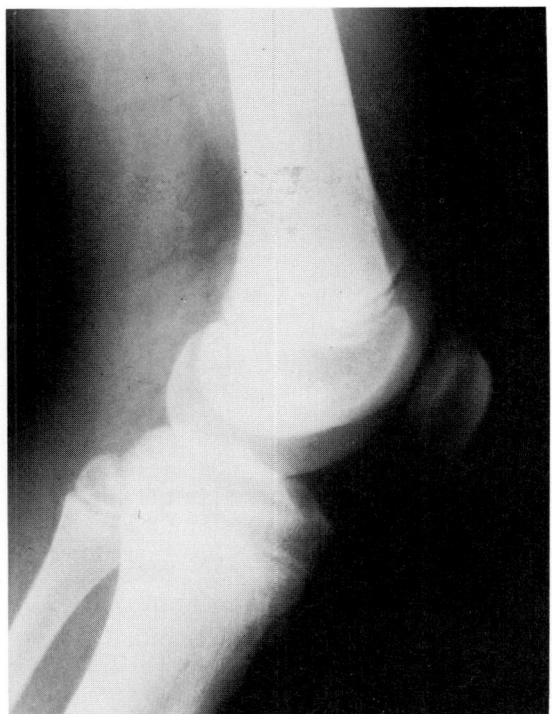

FIGURE 31–8. Lateral X ray of the knee showing radiographic changes of Osgood-Schlatter disease.

FRACTURES ABOUT THE KNEE

Fractures may occur through the physis of the distal femur or the proximal physis of the tibia.[88] The mechanism of injury for the distal femoral physis fracture is either hyperextension while landing from a jump or deceleration from a run. A valgus force directed at the flexed knee in the skeletally immature skeleton may also cause failure through the epiphyseal plate instead of a sprained medial collateral ligament (MCL). Intense pain, immediate swelling, and the inability to bear weight on the affected extremity cause the athlete to seek medical help on an emergent basis. Clinical examination localizes the pain and swelling to the distal femur. An injury to the MCL must be ruled out. If the routine radiograph does not reveal an obvious epiphyseal injury, valgus stress X rays will reveal the fracture (Fig. 31–9). Most epiphyseal injuries are Salter type II fractures and may be treated with closed reduction and casting. Salter type III or IV fractures require anatomical reduction and internal fixation with postoperative immobilization for satisfactory healing.[139]

Fractures through the proximal tibial epiphysis may involve the tibial tubercle apophysis.[103] The mechanism of injury may be related to hyperextension of the knee following landing from a lay-up or jump. A violent contraction of the quadriceps muscle during deceleration, leading to knee extension and compression, is also a cause of the injury. The athlete experiences an immediate onset of pain, swelling, and inability to extend the knee actively. Weight bearing is usually impossible, and emergent medical treatment is sought. Radiographic examination is diagnostic and dictates surgical treatment.[88] These fractures may be extraarticular or intraarticular. Intraarticular fractures demand anatomical reduction with internal fixation (Fig. 31–10). Because of involvement of the patellar tendon attachment, postoperative knee motion must be restricted to allow satisfactory bone healing. The anterior cruciate ligament is spared, as it is attached to the displaced tibial fragment. The anterior horn of the lateral meniscus may be torn at its peripheral attachment and thus require surgical repair. Once the tibial fragment is reduced and fixed, the knee becomes stable (Fig. 31–11).

Fractures of the patella may also occur in the adolescent basketball or volleyball player as a result of direct trauma. A fall on the

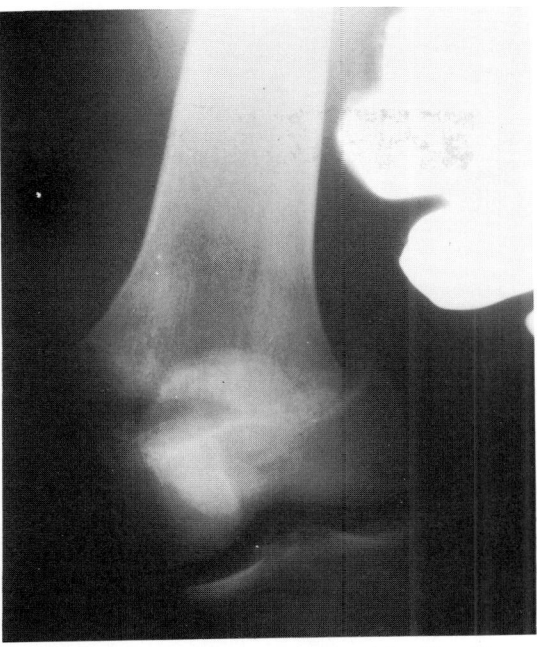

FIGURE 31–9. AP roentgenogram of the distal femur showing epiphyseal fracture.

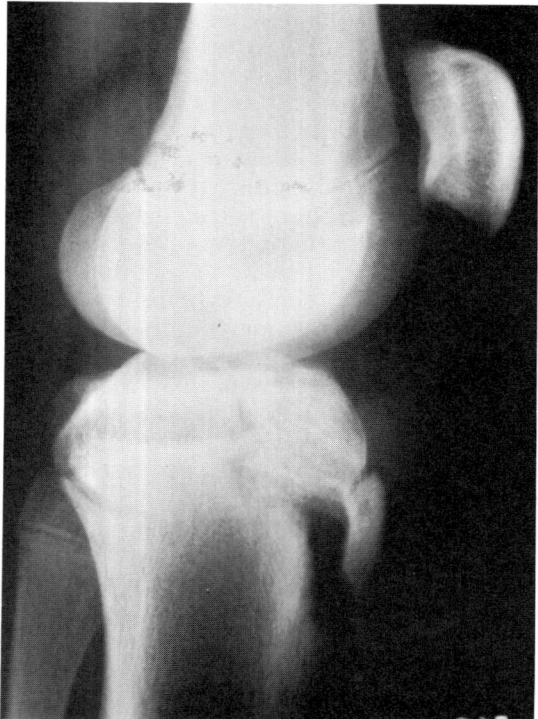

FIGURE 31-10. Lateral X-ray of the tibia showing fracture of the tibial epiphysis.

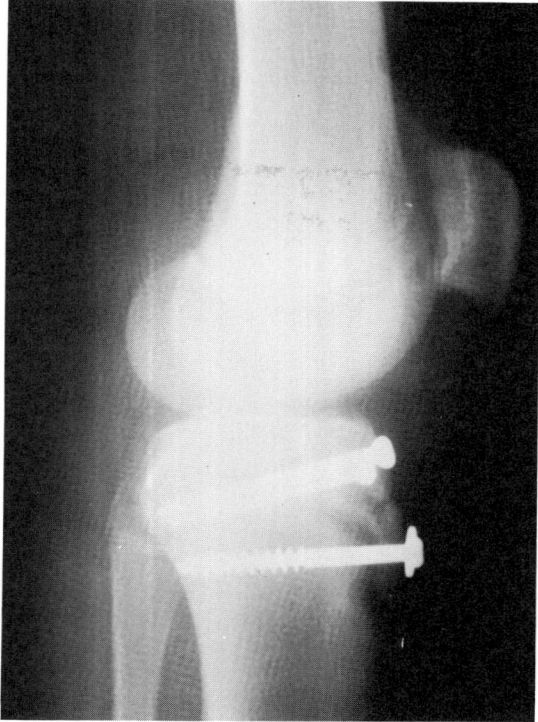

FIGURE 31-11. Lateral X-ray of the tibia showing postoperative internal fixation of tibial fracture.

flexed knee with the foot in a dorsiflexed position makes the patella prominent and vulnerable. In the immature skeleton, the patella is composed mainly of cartilage.[108] A fracture pattern unique to this age group is the sleeve fracture. The inferior pole of the patella is avulsed with a sleeve of articular cartilage (Fig. 31-12). This fracture requires surgical repair and anatomical reduction. One mechanism of sleeve fracture production is the placement of the basketball goal flush to the gym wall, since this does not allow sufficient floor space for deceleration and stopping after a lay-up (Fig. 31-13). The player contacts the wall with the patella of the flexed knee of the swing leg. In more skeletally mature athletes, transverse fractures and longitudinal fracture patterns similar to those of adults are seen. Stellate fractures are rare owing to the relatively low magnitude of the force applied to the patella.

Dislocation or subluxation of the patella is not rare in the adolescent basketball or volleyball player. The mechanism of injury is usually a violent quadriceps contraction with the knee flexed.[31] Predisposing factors may be vastus medialis dysplasia, increased Q angle, genu valgum, and developmental anomalies of the patellofemoral joint.

The athlete experiences an immediate onset of pain as well as a sensation of the knee shifting, giving way, or abnormal lateral movement of the patella. Swelling is immediate and restricts athletic participation and knee motion. Clinical examination demonstrates tenderness proximal to the femoral attachment of the medial collateral ligament where the vastus medialis obliquus (VMO) attachment has torn, allowing the patella to dislocate laterally. The inferior medial pole of the patella and the lateral border of the lateral femoral condyle may be tender. Radiographs should be examined carefully for osteochondral fragments from the medial patella or lateral femoral trochlea.[55]

Initial treatment for patellar dislocation is rest, compression, ice, and restricted knee motion and participation. Once the swelling and discomfort have subsided, a functional rehabilitation program can be instituted including range-of-motion exercises and hamstring and quadriceps strengthening emphasizing the vastus medialis obliquus. Running, cutting, and jumping are allowed once strength and comfort have returned. Return to basketball activity may require a neoprene patellar tracking sleeve or brace

BASKETBALL AND VOLLEYBALL 609

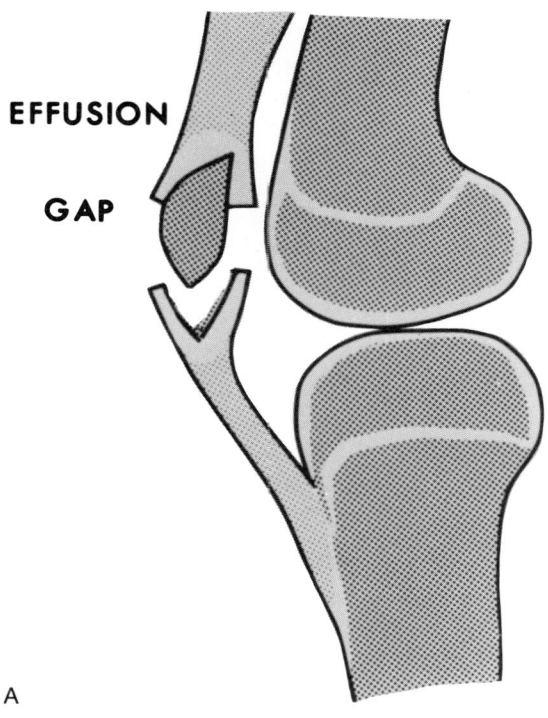

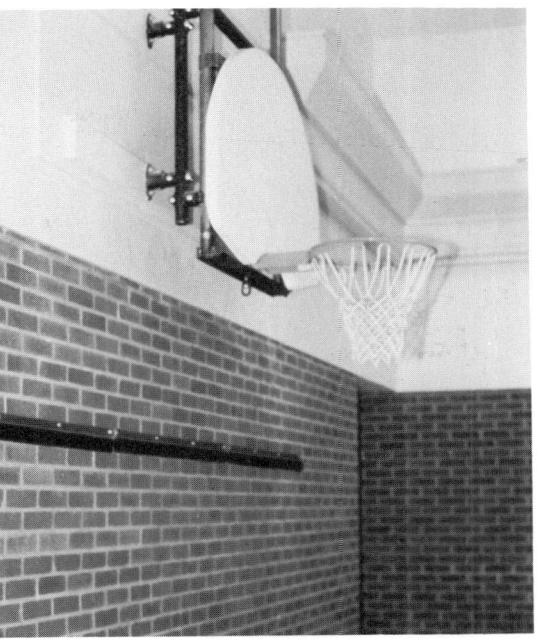

FIGURE 31–13. The basketball goal is too close to the wall, a cause of patella fractures.

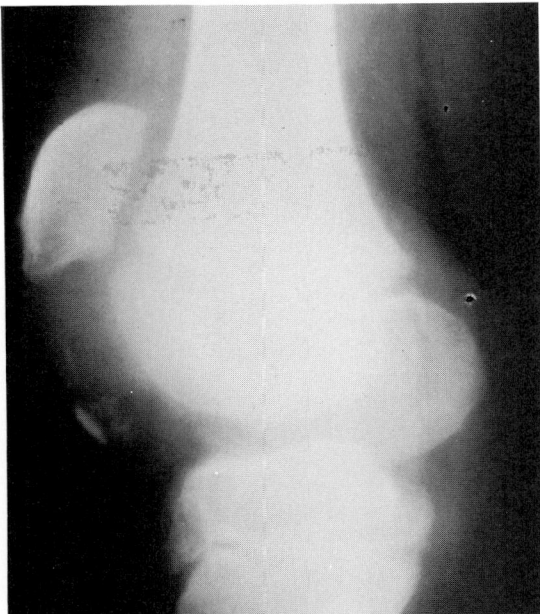

FIGURE 31–12. (A) Diagrammatic example of the sleeve fracture of the patella. (B) Lateral X ray of the knee showing a sleeve fracture of the patella.

for prophylaxis. Arthroscopic intervention is indicated if osteochondral fragments are noted on radiographs. The management of recurrent patellar instability is detailed in Chapter 20.

Stress fractures of the patella usually involve the inferior pole and may be seen in those athletes who have a history of chronic patellar tendinitis. The athelete presents with a history of chronic pain at the inferior pole of the patella. Minimal swelling is present, but tenderness is notable. Active knee extension will be possible but painful. The athlete will point to the area of the patella that is symptomatic (Fig. 31–14). Lateral

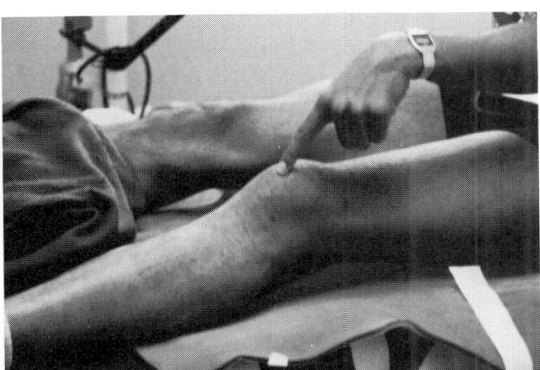

FIGURE 31–14. Athlete is pointing to the inferior pole of the fracture, denoting a stress fracture of the patella.

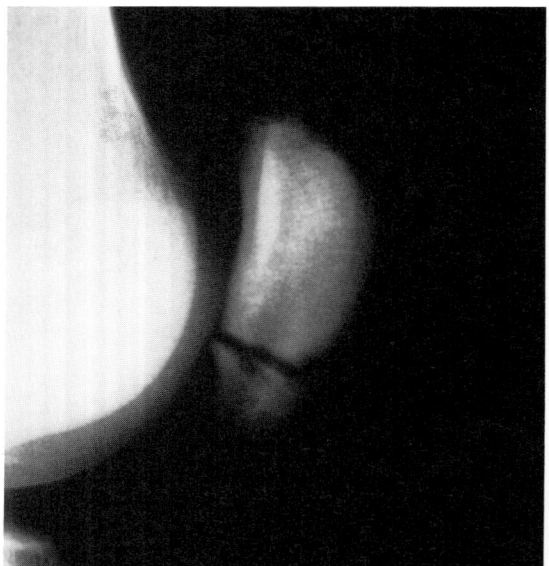

FIGURE 31–15. A lateral radiograph of the patella showing a stress fracture of the inferior pole of the patella.

radiographs demonstrate a fracture line that is sclerotic in chronic cases (Fig. 31–15). The extensor retinaculum is intact, and there is no displacement of the fracture fragments. Surgical intervention is rarely indicated. Rest from jumping, running, and weight lifting activities until symptoms subside, usually 3 to 6 weeks, is necessary. Alternative training to maintain conditioning is instituted. Antiinflammatory medication, ice, and neoprene knee sleeves are helpful in treating the symptoms. Stretching of the quadriceps and hamstring muscles is necessary to maintain flexibility. Return to competition is dependent on comfort, strength, and flexibility. Radiographic bone union is not a requirement for a player's return.

Stress fractures of the proximal tibial metaphysis, medial tibial diaphysis, or distal femoral metaphysis may also be seen in these athletes.[6, 36, 89, 90, 125, 131, 144] The use of crutches for protective weight bearing may be necessary only if there is impending failure of the integrity of the tibia or femoral cortices. The presenting complaints are that of pain with exertion and also at rest. The athlete can point to the exact spot of the discomfort. Radiographs may be normal if the symptoms are less than 3 weeks old. Clinical examination can usually make the diagnosis in these cases, but a bone scan may be obtained if

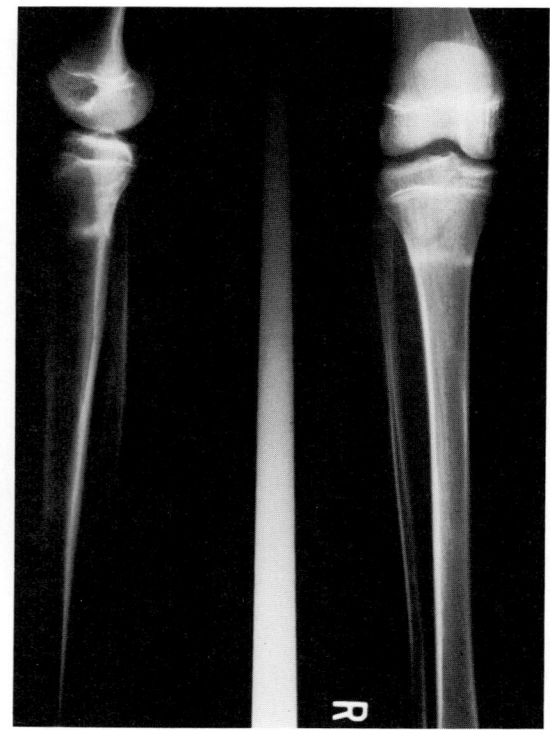

A

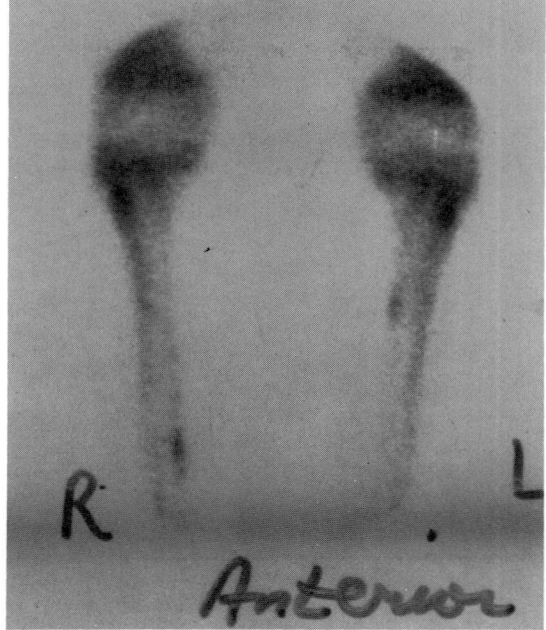

B

FIGURE 31–16. (A) X-rays of the proximal tibia showing location of stress fracture. (B) Bone scan of the tibia showing increased uptake denoting stress reaction.

uncertainty exists.[122, 134] The condition responds to the removal of the athlete from active sports participation (Fig. 31–16). Alternative training to maintain conditioning in the form of stationary cycling, swimming, or running in the pool with a flotation vest is helpful. Symptoms may return if the athlete resumes floor training too soon. Allowing the athlete to continue to participate in the face of isolated bone pain may lead to bone failure, fracture, and possible surgery, resulting in prolonged downtime. Casting may be necessary but should be avoided if possible because the length of time the athlete is immobilized may cause muscle atrophy and thus extend the rehabilitation period beyond the time of fracture healing.

KNEE LIGAMENT INJURIES

Ligament injuries of the knee joint are not as common as those seen in the ankle. The knee ligaments, however, are very important in allowing the basketball and volleyball athletes to perform the necessary running, cutting, decelerating, and jumping maneuvers. Ligamentous integrity provides the stability and confidence players need to perform these activities. The diagnosis and treatment of knee ligament injuries is discussed in detail in Chapters 17, 18, and 19. Here we will concentrate on the treatment of these injuries in the young basketball or volleyball player.

When an athlete presents with a history of a valgus injury, with or without contact, and complains of medial knee pain, a sprain of the *medial collateral ligament* should be suspected. The physical examination must be performed carefully to ensure that other knee structures are not involved. Effusion or swelling of the knee joint may be mild to moderate in an isolated MCL sprain.[58] A tense effusion suggests a more serious injury.

Radiographic examination must be performed on all adolescent knee injuries. Isolated medial collateral sprains will have normal radiographs unless avulsion at the femoral or tibial attachment of the MCL has occurred or there has been an epiphyseal injury. Soft tissue swelling at the medial aspect of the knee on the AP radiograph may be noted. In the skeletally immature athlete, stress radiographs are necessary to rule out an epiphyseal fracture to the distal femur or proximal tibia.

Treatment of isolated MCL injuries is mainly nonoperative. Functional rehabilitation to maintain thigh muscle strength and knee range of motion is instituted early. The athlete has the knee wrapped with a compressive Ace. Ice is applied to the affected area. A hinged knee brace is worn to provide support and stability to the injured knee. Crutches are used until the athlete is comfortable enough to ambulate with full weight on the affected leg. Grade III injuries may require 6 weeks of recovery time before the athlete is able to return to competition. Grades I and II respond quicker and the downtime may be only 1 to 3 weeks. Once at least 90 degrees of comfortable motion is obtained, stationary bicycle riding is started to maintain conditioning.

A neoprene sleeve with hinges is helpful to maintain stability and comfort during the early phase of rehabilitation. Running in a swimming pool with a flotation vest is also instituted. Daily treatments of ice, ultrasound, and high-voltage galvanic stimulation (HVGS) are beneficial for the athlete's comfort. Oral antiinflammatory medications are administered from the time of injury for a period of 2 weeks. Light weights are instituted once a comfortable, full range of motion is established. Resistance training is advanced according to symptoms. Dynamometer testing is performed to document the athlete's progress. The injured leg should regain at least 80 percent of the strength of the normal leg before the athlete can return to court activities.[104]

Free-throw shooting can be resumed when the athlete can ambulate comfortably without crutches. Jump-shooting practice begins once a comfortable range of motion has returned, but the knee should be protected with a hinged brace. Lateral movement, backpedaling, crossover movements, and cutting activities are also done initially with a protective knee brace. The knee brace does not protect the knee from all abnormal knee motions but may give the athlete enough support and protection to increase confidence and activity levels, facilitating return to the court. The athlete may elect to continue with taping of the knee, a knee sleeve, brace, or a combination of both once he or she returns to competition. Clinically, a grade III sprain may still demonstrate a small degree of laxity at 30 degrees of flexion. The athlete will complain of a feeling of looseness, especially with lateral movement and cutting activities, but functionally will still be able to play. The medial collateral ligament heals initially with scar tissue that does not have the normal integrity of the uninjured MCL.[130] This accounts for the noticeable functional laxity.

The *anterior cruciate ligament* (ACL) is the most important static stabilizer for normal knee function on the basketball or volleyball court. This ligament prevents anterior translation of the tibia on the femur during deceleration, prevents anterolateral tibial subluxation with cutting, and stabilizes the knee from hyperextending when landing from a jump.[52]

The ACL may be injured by itself or in combination with the medial collateral ligament or menisci.[33, 63] The mechanism of injury is usually a decelerating cutting movement without contact or hyperextension of knee when landing from a jump such as in rebounding or shooting a lay-up. Contact from another player may or may not be a contributing factor. Many athletes are surprised by the severity of the ligament injury because of the apparently minimal amount of trauma it takes to rupture the anterior cruciate ligament. For a young athlete, this is a serious ligament injury; it is a season-ending injury but should not be a career-ending one.

Sometimes the athlete will not seek medical care after an acute ACL tear. After 2 or 3 weeks the pain may be gone, swelling minimal, and function again possible.[4, 117] The athlete may attempt to play only to experience an episode of instability. The Lachman and pivot-shift tests will be easier to perform in these cases. Instrumented documentation by the use of the KT-1000 or Genucom will confirm the incompetency of the anterior cruciate ligament.

Nonoperative treatment or primary repair of a ruptured anterior cruciate ligament alone does not yield satisfactory results in the young basketball or volleyball player.[15, 51, 86, 107, 133] The age of the patient, the incidence of associated meniscal pathology, and the demands of the sports warrant surgical stabilization. Diagnostic arthroscopy should not replace a good clinical examination. Arthroscopy of the injured knee with definitive repair or reconstructive procedures is the treatment of choice. Extraarticular reconstructions in the form of an iliotibial band tenodesis with arthroscopic meniscal repair or excision is my preference in the athlete with open physes.[3, 76] In the athlete with physes that are nearly closed or closed, the arthroscopically assisted patellar tendon autograft with associated meniscal repair or excision is my preferred treatment, although other surgeons have reported success with other reconstruction techniques.[23, 25, 26, 78, 83, 102, 105, 115] In a basketball or volleyball player, nonoperative treatment will usually lead to repeated episodes of giving way, resulting in further meniscal damage and articular surface wear.[62] Instability that is allowed to continue over many years may ultimately lead to significant degenerative arthritic changes that limit knee joint function.[106]

Avulsion of the anterior cruciate ligament from bone has been classified depending on the displacement of the avulsed fragment. Although the ligamentous tissue does not fail completely because the bone fails instead, it does undergo plastic deformation. Arthroscopic repair with replacement of the bone avulsion to its anatomical position is the treatment of choice. In some instances, the fragment must be returned to its anatomical origin through an open arthrotomy. Closed reduction with casting of the knee in full extension in those avulsions that are minimally displaced may produce a satisfactory result.

Postoperatively, the rehabilitative regimens differ depending on the procedure performed. The postoperative immobilization for those athletes with an extraarticular iliotibial band tenodesis or repair of an avulsed tibial spine may be from 3 to 6 weeks with knee flexed 20 to 30 degrees.[3] Casting may be utilized, but prefabricated hinged postoperative braces are well tolerated by the young patient, are more comfortable than casting, and are easily removed to check wounds. Patients who undergo anterior cruciate ligament reconstruction using the patella tendon autograft are placed in an early motion, aggressive rehabilitation program.[105, 106] The postoperative brace is worn in full extension for a period of 4 weeks. The patient is taken out of the brace for motion therapy and is allowed weight bearing as early as comfort dictates, with crutches for the first 2 weeks and then without crutches. Bathing out of the brace is allowed once skin healing has occurred. Sleeping without the brace is also allowed at 2 weeks postsurgery.

Passive range-of-motion activities on the Biodex machine are started 1 week after surgery and are continued until full range of motion is obtained. At 1 month after surgery, the athlete is allowed out of the brace and is started on light resistive activities with elastic bands. Muscle atrophy occurs rapidly after an ACL injury and is advanced further because of the surgery. Early active motion helps to maintain muscle tone and strength. The remainder of the therapy program consists of regaining full knee motion and developing full muscle strength and endurance, which will ultimately allow the player to return to competition. The time to return for most athletes varies from 6 to 12 months. Strength and stability are continuously checked using the Biodex or Cybex machines and the KT-100 or Genucom throughout the rehabilitative period.

MISCELLANEOUS LOWER EXTREMITY INJURIES

Contusions to the quadriceps muscle occur when a player sustains blunt trauma from another player's knee during defensive or offensive activities. When injured, the quadriceps muscle is usually under contraction and may thus bleed profusely. These contusions may cause significant swelling, pain, and loss of motion. In severe injuries, an organized calcified mass known as *myositis ossificans* may develop.[75] Once the injury occurs, the player is unable to continue and may be out of practice for 2 to 3 weeks, depending on the severity. Treatment consists of immediate compression, ice, and protection of weight bearing with crutches. Deep massage is avoided early on because of the chance of causing further bleeding and aggravating the patient's pain. Active range of motion is limited initially but is allowed to progress according to the athlete's comfort. Injection of corticosteroid medications directly into the injured area is avoided. Oral antiinflammatory medication is given early and continued for 2 weeks. Analgesics are necessary in severe quadriceps contusions.

Full flexion and extension must be achieved before resistive exercises are instituted and before running activities are allowed. HVGS is used along with ultrasound to facilitate muscle recovery. Gentle range of motion in a swimming pool or whirlpool will produce light resistance and help to establish muscle activity.

Protection of the thigh to prevent a contusion from occurring or to protect an already injured muscle may be accomplished with foam pads and Ace wraps or with spandex pants that allow placement of thigh protectors similar to those worn by football players. Thigh protection should be worn at all practices if the player has a history of thigh injuries.

Hamstring and groin muscle injuries also occur but not from direct contact with another player. In these muscles, excessive eccentric contraction overloads the tissue, causing tearing of the muscle fibers.[48, 53, 54] The medial hamstring group is the most common muscle group strained and is usually injured near the ischial tuberosity. In the groin, the adductor magnus or gracilis muscles may also become injured. This is associated with running activities.[82, 110] The player usually did not allow sufficient time for warm-up and flexibility activities before beginning play. The typical muscle strain occurs quite suddenly, with severe pain causing limited lower extremity function. Running and even walking may be difficult. Thigh compression wraps using an Ace wrap are utilized early as well as ice. In severe muscle strains, crutches are necessary to aid in ambulation. HVGS and ultrasound facilitate muscle recovery. Range-of-motion activities are started once pain has decreased. Light resistive activities, either with elastic bands or in the swimming pool, are started as soon as active activity is comfortable. A full range of motion is necessary for cycling or weight machine activities. Approximately 2 to 3 weeks of rehabilitation daily are necessary for the athlete to regain the muscle conditioning of the involved muscle group before returning to sports. The athlete must continue flexibility training, including hamstring and adductor stretching, to prevent recurrence of the injury.

The *semimembranosus tendon insertion* at the posterior medial corner of the tibia may be a site of medial knee pain, usually felt during running and jumping activities.[118] The location of the pain below the joint line must be distinguished from a medial meniscus tear by careful palpation of the semimembranosus insertion with the knee flexed. Semimembranosus insertional tendinitis may present as a primary entity or in association with intraarticular pathology.[118] Conservative treatment of flexibility exercises, antiinflammatory medication, ultrasound, ice massage, and the wearing of a neoprene knee sleeve may help in the resolution of the symptoms. In chronic cases, a bone scan may be helpful in locating the source of the posterior medial knee pain. Surgical intervention is only necessary in those cases refractory to conservative treatment. Arthroscopy of the knee joint in conjunction with exploration of the semimembranosus tendon is very successful in surgically treating this insertional tendinitis.[118]

The *iliotibial band* may also be a source of lateral knee pain where it passes over the lateral femoral condyle. The pain has an insidious onset and is located above the lateral joint line. The onset of the pain coincides with an increase in running activity usually at the start of the practice season.[2, 94, 119, 135] The player's shoes should be inspected for excessive wear and the athlete examined for knee, ankle, and hindfoot malalignment. Orthotics may be required to correct any malalignment problems. Iliotibial band stretching and flexibility activities are necessary as well as ice massage and oral antiinflammatory medications. Neoprene sleeves have been used with success. Injection of the iliotibial band with local anesthetics and soluble corticosteroids may help in treatment. Athletes with iliotibial band syndrome may require surgical removal of the area of irritation if conservative treatment fails.

ANKLE SPRAINS

The sprained ankle is the most common injury that poses a problem to the competing athlete.[7, 123] Ankle sprains limit participation because of the downtime associated with recovery and healing and also have a high recurrence rate if not properly treated. By preventing these injuries, the amount of time away from competition may be lessened and the recurrence rate may be diminished.

The most common mechanism for ankle sprains is one of *plantar flexion* and *inversion* (Fig. 31–17). In this position, the lateral ligaments are placed under maximal tension. The sequence of failure proceeds from the anterior talofibular ligament to the lateral calcaneofibular ligament and then the posterior talofibular ligament. The medial deltoid ligament is the hinge on which the foot rotates as the force is dissipated. With isolated *eversion* of the ankle, a rare sprain of the medial deltoid ligament occurs. *Dorsiflexion* and *eversion* may cause lateral rotation of the fibula to occur and disrupt the anterior inferior tibiofibular ligament and possibly the interosseous membrane. With isolated *external rotation* of the foot and no flexion, an isolated injury to the anterior inferior tibiofibular ligament may occur. With isolated *plantar flexion* of the ankle joint, the anterior syndesmotic ligament may become injured.[7] A careful history may indicate the position of the foot and ankle at the time of injury and thus allow the physician to anticipate which ligaments are most likely to be injured.

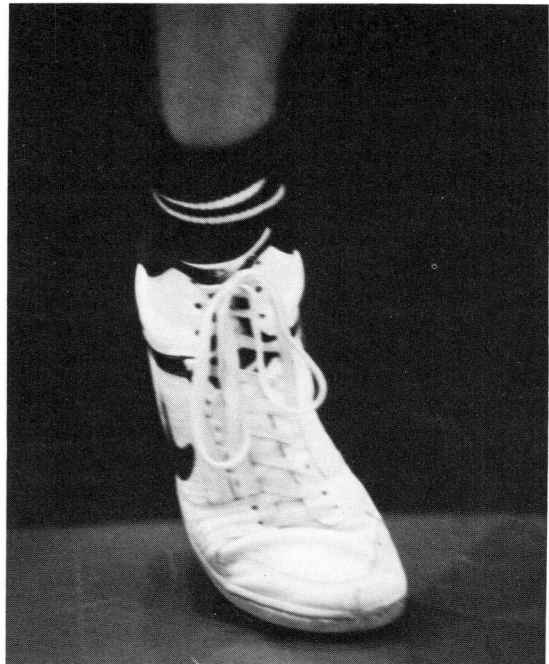

FIGURE 31–17. The position of the ankle for lateral ankle sprain is that of plantar flexion and inversion.

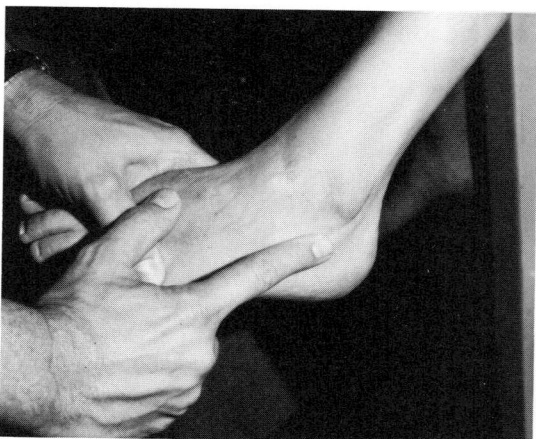

FIGURE 31–18. In ankle sprains, palpation of the lateral ankle ligaments may demonstrate tenderness.

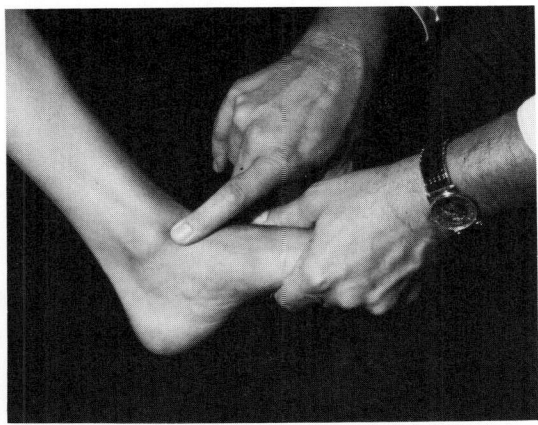

FIGURE 31–19. Palpation of the medial deltoid ligament may reveal tenderness.

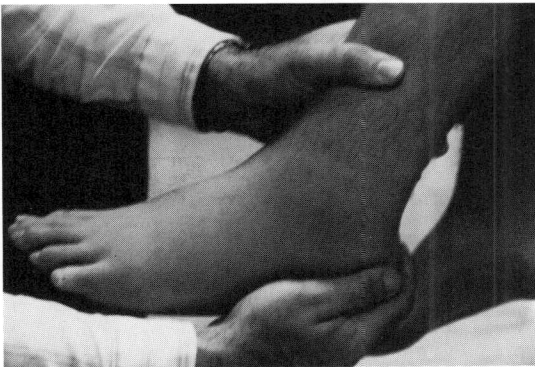

FIGURE 31–21. The anterolateral drawer test signifies anterior talofibular ligament injury.

Inspection of the involved ankle immediately after a sprain may show minimal signs of swelling or ecchymosis (Figs. 31–18 and 31–19). Palpation of the involved ligaments may be painful. The swelling occurs as hemorrhage and edema develop. The amount of edema depends on the severity of the injury. The ecchymosis develops as the hemorrhage dissects up and down the peroneal tendon sheath along the lateral aspect of the lower extremity. The swelling and ecchymosis become more apparent within 24 hours after the injury and may persist for several weeks after the injury.

Swelling of the ankle joint itself may be detected by balloting the anterior aspect of the joint (Fig. 31–20). Swelling, ecchymosis, or tenderness on the medial side of the ankle may reflect deltoid ligament injury. Palpating each ligament for tenderness will help the examiner determine which structures are injured. The anterolateral drawer test is the easiest stability test to perform on the injured ankle.[7, 8] The patient is sitting comfortably on the examining table with the knee flexed over the edge, allowing the lower extremity to hang free. With one hand stabilizing the tibia, the other hand grasps the heel and an anterior force pulls the foot forward (Fig. 31–21). The foot is usually in mild plantar flexion. A positive test subluxes the talus from the ankle mortise in an anteromedial direction. The anterior talofibular ligament has to be disrupted to give a positive test. Inversion of the ankle in mild plantar flexion is performed in order to test the integrity of the lateral calcaneofibular ligament (Fig. 31–22). This test may be painful in the acute case, with resulting peroneal muscle spasm.[7, 8] Subluxation of the talus medially indicates a positive test and suggests disruption of the main stabilizing ligament to the lateral side of the ankle. Injection of a local anesthetic to this area may make the performance of the inversion test more comfortable for the patient. Stress testing devices have been designed to aid in standardizing ankle stress testing for radiographic documentation. Eversion stress testing is performed when a tear of the medial deltoid ligament is suspected (Fig. 31–23).

In performing the stress tests, it is important to grasp the heel and not the forefoot. Movement of the forefoot may give the examiner a false sense of varus instability, as motion occurs at the midtarsal joints instead of the tibiotalar joint. Both ankles must be compared clinically and radiographically when documenting ligamentous laxity. In the adolescent athlete, one must also suspect failure

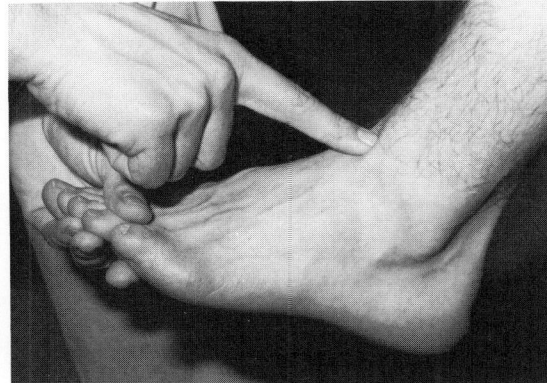

FIGURE 31–20. Balloting of the anterior ankle to demonstrate swelling.

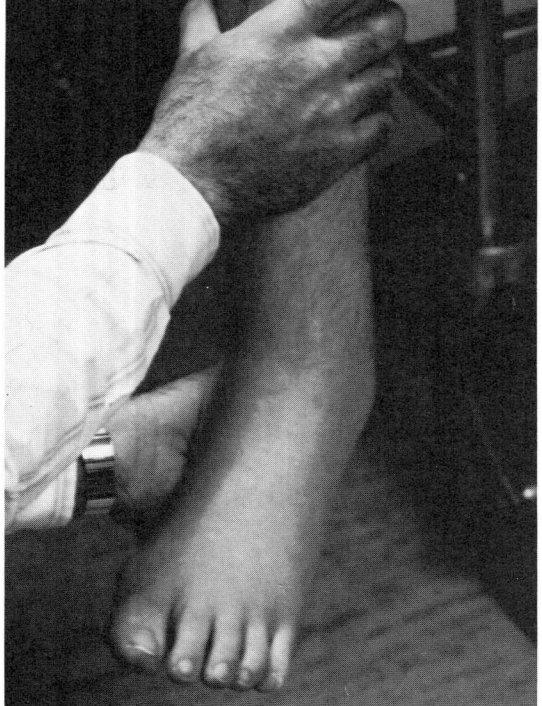

FIGURE 31–22. Inversion stress testing of the ankle evaluates the lateral calcaneolfibular ligament.

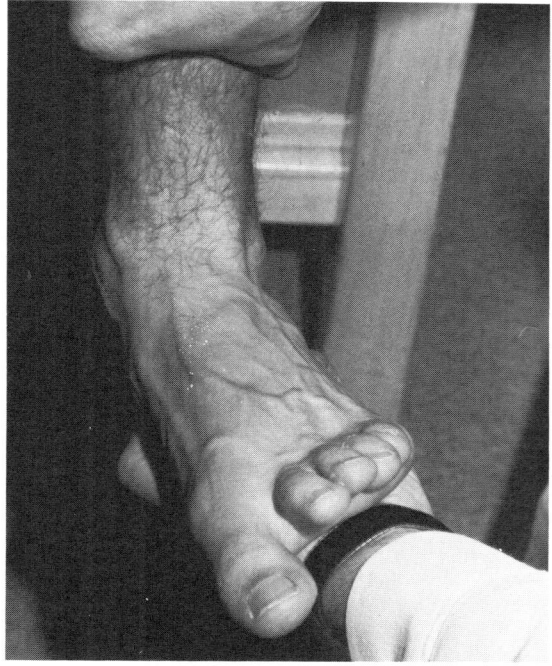

FIGURE 31–23. Eversion stress testing of the ankle to evaluate the medial deltoid ligament.

of the epiphysis to the distal fibula and distal lateral tibia in all ankle sprains. Radiographs are thus necessary in all ankle sprains in this age group.[7, 8]

Three radiographic views are standard: anteroposterior (AP), lateral, and mortise view (Fig. 31–24). Stress radiographs are optional and are performed after the initial films are reviewed and fractures have been ruled out.

Stress radiographs demonstrate abnormal laxity of the lateral ligaments as well as the deltoid ligament medially. Both ankles should be stressed and the amount of instability documented. Stress radiographs may be unreliable, depending on pain and muscle spasm, unless local anesthetic agents are administered.

Arthrography and tenosynoviography have been used to document the degree and severity of ankle sprains but are usually not practical or necessary in the acute injury. Tomograms may also be used if an articular injury of the talar dome is suspected. Bone scans are also used if there are normal radiographs and no physical evidence of lateral or medial ligament injury but persistence of anterior ankle pain. A positive bone scan may indicate increased activity in the area of the syndesmotic ligament, indicating a high ankle sprain from forced dorsiflexion (Fig. 31–25).

Treatment of acute ankle sprains is usually conservative. The principles of rest, ice, compression, and elevation are followed.[97] After evaluation, the patient is placed in a compression wrap and a pneumatic brace (Fig. 31–26). He or she is given crutches but is allowed to bear weight as tolerated. As soon as the patient is bearing full weight on the injured extremity, the crutches are discarded. Frequent follow-up allows the athlete to progress on a functional rehabilitation program. Heat is not used in the early management of an ankle sprain. Galvanic stimulation may be used during treatment sessions under supervision where available. The BAPPS board is used to restore proprioception and elastic bands for resistance training[30] (Fig. 31–27). The stationary bicycle is also instituted early once motion begins to return. The bicycle encourages motion and muscle activity in the lower extremity without loading the ankle joint.

The goals of rehabilitation are to obtain full, pain-free range of motion and improve functional strength. The early phase of rehabilitation may take 1 to 3 weeks, depending

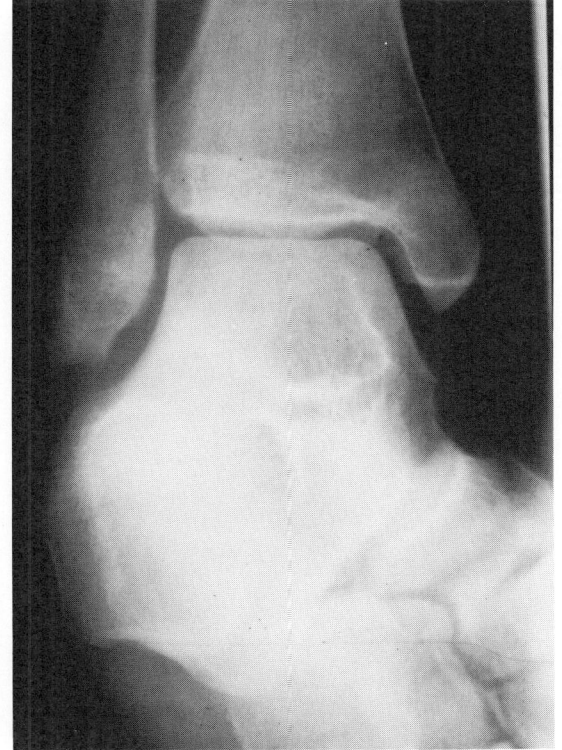
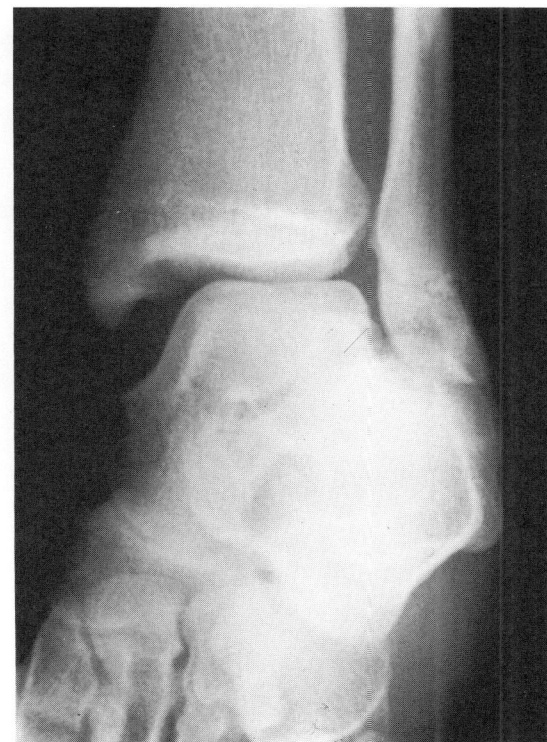
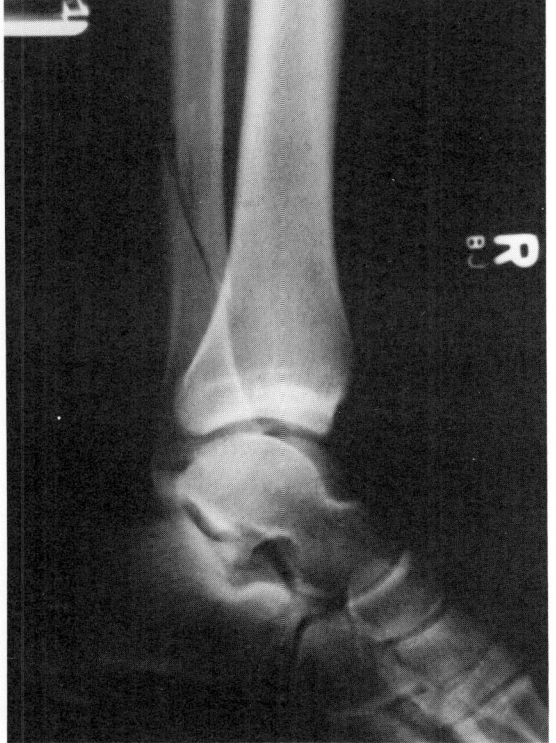

FIGURE 31–24. X-rays of the ankle. (*A*) Normal mortise view. (*B*) Mortise view of the ankle showing widening of the syndesmosis, indicating injury to the syndesmotic and deltoid ligaments. (*C*) Lateral X-ray of the ankle showing fracture of the fibula.

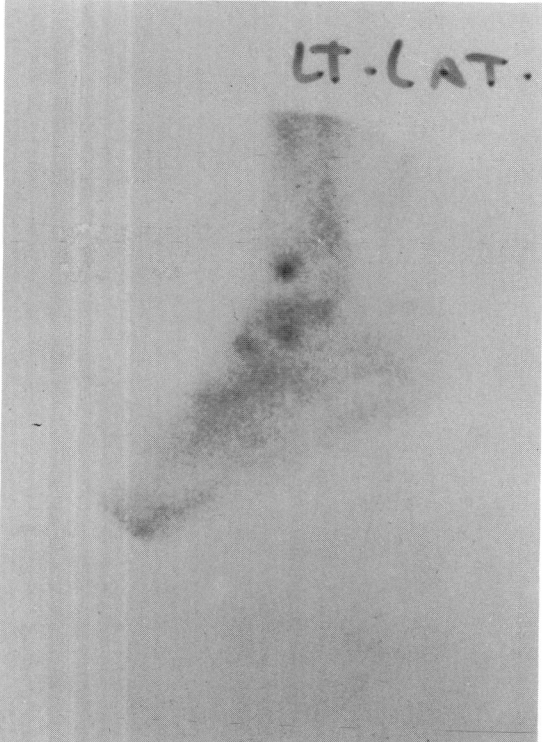

FIGURE 31–25. Bone scan of the ankle showing uptake in the area of the syndesmotic ligament, indicating a high ankle sprain from forced dorsiflexion.

on the severity of the ankle injury. In the advanced stages of treatment, light jogging, figure-of-eight running, and lateral sliding movements similar to defensive drills may be instituted. The athlete is protected with tape on the ankle and the pneumatic brace (Fig. 31–28). This combination of external protection has been shown to be a stable construct that allows early and safe return

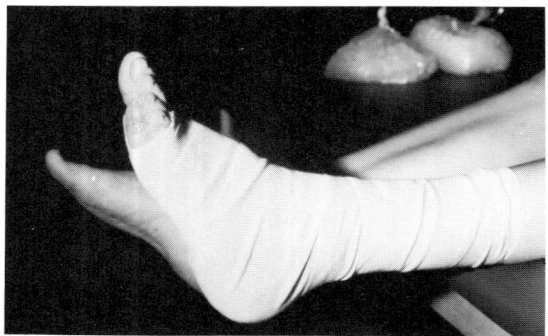

FIGURE 31–26. Initial treatment of an acute ankle sprain is a compressive wrap to the ankle, ice, and elevation.

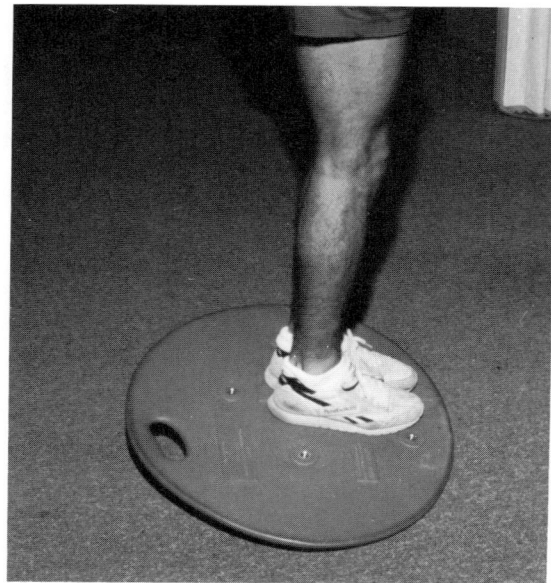

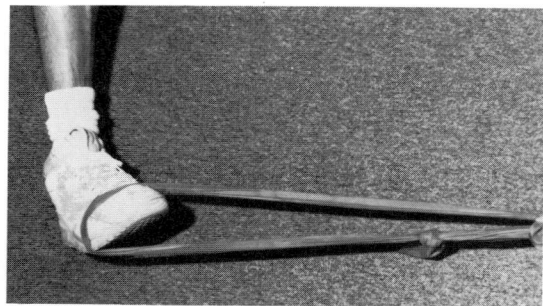

FIGURE 31–27. (A) BAPPS board for ankle motion and proprioception. (B) Theraband for light resistive activities for ankle motion.

to athletic competition.[123] Swelling and soreness may persist for as long as 6 weeks. Treatment and observation as well as protection of the ankle may be necessary for this length of time.

In some isolated cases of nondisplaced epiphyseal fractures of the distal fibula, the pneumatic brace may be used for immobilization in place of casting. Displaced fractures that require closed or open reduction may need extended periods of immobilization to allow time for bone healing. The high ankle sprain may also require immobilization to ensure healing and to help in the reduction of pain. The pneumatic brace may not be effective in these injuries because it does not restrict dorsiflexion.

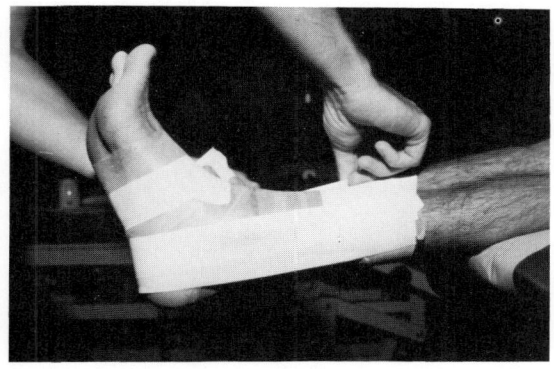 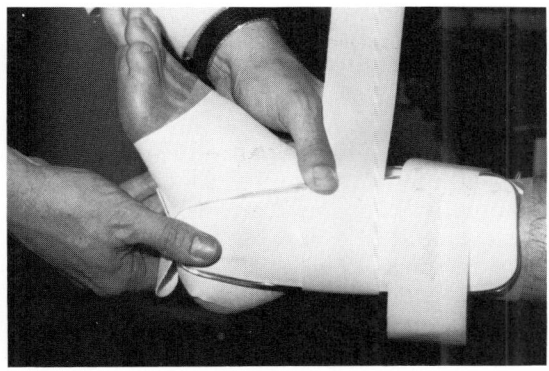

FIGURE 31–28. (A) Taping of the ankle for functional activities combined with (B) pneumatic brace wear is the most stable construct.

Systemic medication in the form of nonsteroidal antiinflammatory medication may also be beneficial. Analgesics may also be necessary early in the course of the injury. Anesthetic, steroid, or enzyme injections are not recommended. Most sprained ankles respond to this regimen of treatment, and return should be expected about the third week and certainly by the sixth week. Using a functional rehabilitation program decreases the

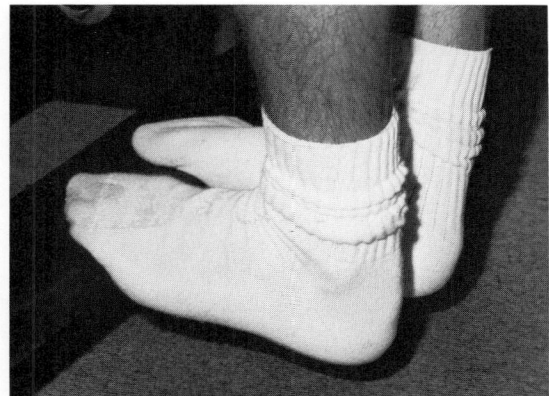

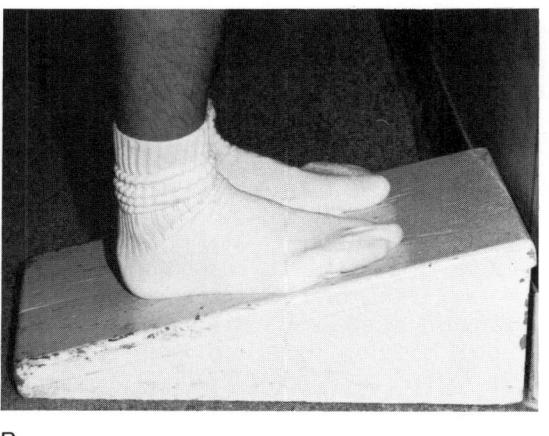

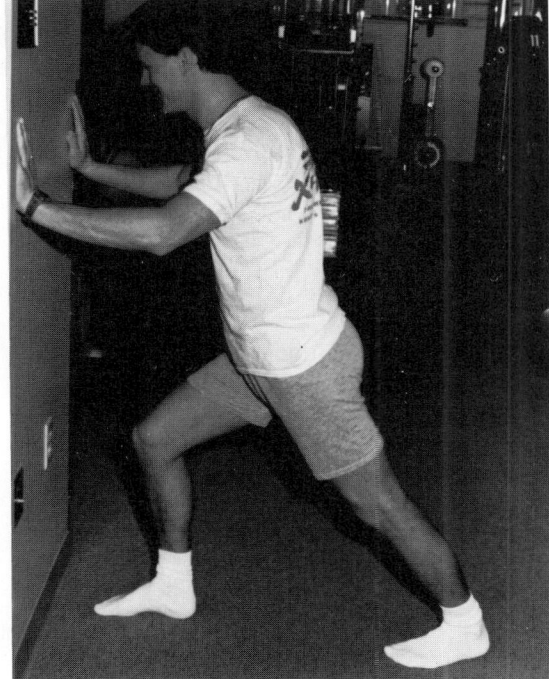

FIGURE 31–29. Heel cord stretching. (A) Heel dips. (B) Incline boards. (C) Leaning against the wall.

amount of conditioning time needed to return the athlete to competition once the sprain has healed. Before returning to full competition, the athlete must achieve full range of motion, functional strength, and no pain. Prophylactic taping of the athlete may be continued for a period of 6 weeks. The pneumatic brace may be worn until the athlete's confidence and functional strength have returned. The use of taping and the pneumatic brace may also help with sensory feedback and decrease the chance of recurrence.

The best treatment of an ankle injury is one of prevention.[143] An ankle exercise routine may be part of the preseason conditioning program as well as prepractice and pregame warm-ups. Heel cord stretching is performed first and may be done in conjunction with stretching of the hamstrings, adductors, and quadricep muscles. Heel cords are stretched by leaning against the wall or by doing heel dips on a step or on various inclined boards (Fig. 31-29). One should never bounce but apply a steady pressure to exert effectively a gradual stretch of the calf muscles. Another way to stretch the calf muscles is to loop a towel around the foot while sitting with the legs straight and actively dorsiflex the foot while pulling with the towel (Fig. 31-30). Rubber tubing is a convenient way to apply a resistive force to the muscle groups of the lower leg to complement the stretching with a strengthening routine (Fig. 31-31). Strengthening of eversion, inversion, dorsiflexion, and plantar flexion may also be performed isometrically or with light weights attached to the forefoot.

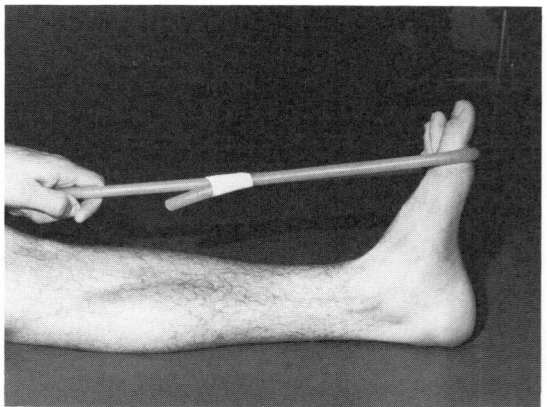

FIGURE 31-31. Rubber tubing may be used for light resistive activities for the muscles of the lower extremity.

Balance may be developed by walking on the heels and on the toes; standing balance may be improved by standing on one leg with the eyes closed. Functional activities that can be included are rope jumping, cutting drills, and figure-of-eight running with progressively smaller circles, both clockwise and counterclockwise. Plyometrics help train muscle activity during jumping and landing.

With strict attention to a preparticipation routine, the athlete may help to reduce the incidence and severity of ankle injuries. Chronic ankle injuries are usually the result of a failed rehabilitation program or an improper diagnosis. Other injuries that may mimic chronic ankle instability are subluxation of the peroneal tendons, osteochondral or chondral defects of the talar dome, tarsal coalition, sinus tarsi syndrome, and stress fracture of the fibula, medial malleolus, or tarsal navicular.[14, 16, 19, 37, 93, 98, 113] (See Chapter 22.)

ACHILLES TENDINITIS

Achilles tendinitis may present as pain and swelling of the tendon approximately 3 to 5 cm above its insertion into the calcaneus.[24, 28, 147] One cause of Achilles inflammation particular to basketball players is irritation from direct contact with the heel counter on "high-top" basketball shoes. Low-cut heel counters usually do not cause this local irritation. A more serious cause of Achilles tendon injury is repeated strains of the tendon with consequent microde-

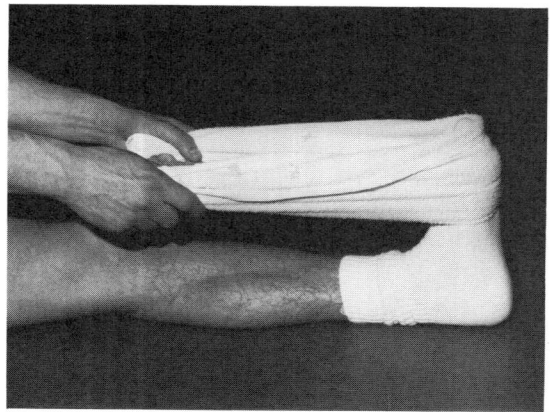

FIGURE 31-30. Heel cord stretching using a towel in the knee extended position.

generation and tearing of the tendon substance.[24, 116] The landing phase of the jump is thought to cause the microfailure of the tendon tissue by eccentrically overloading the tendon. An inflammatory response ensues, thickening the paratendon tissue and resulting in scarring and limited motion. In adolescent basketball and volleyball players, rupture of the Achilles tendon is rare, but partial rupture may occur.

Prevention of Achilles tendon injury is paramount in sports requiring repetitive jumping activities. Heel cord stretching before practice will improve the flexibility of the calf muscles. The athlete should spend sufficient time before practice to ensure the muscles to the lower extremity are warmed up and stretched before engaging in running and jumping activities. This will lessen the incidence of heel cord injuries.

Once an injury occurs, symptoms are usually pain and swelling localized to the tendon itself. Palpation of the tendon substance reproduces the pain. Passive dorsiflexion of the foot or active plantar flexion against resistance may both cause discomfort. The Thompson test for Achilles rupture is usually normal, and no defect in the tendon is palpable.

Radiographs are usually normal but may demonstrate calcification within the tendon substance in chronic cases. Soft tissue swelling of the Achilles may also be noted. Ultrasonography and magnetic resonance imaging (MRI) may give more information concerning the extent of tendon tissue involvement. Both tests may detect tendon tissue calcification, hemorrhage, and partial or complete ruptures.

Rest, ice, compression, and heel cord stretching activities are instituted early. Antiinflammatory medications are helpful and are given for a short period of time, usually 2 weeks. Injections of anesthetics and steroids should be avoided, as this may cause tendon rupture.[74] A heel lift in the form of a heel wedge or heel cup is worn in the shoes to remove the strain from the tendon. Jumping activities are stopped until symptoms resolve. Once the pain and swelling resolve and healing is advanced, jumping activities may be reinstated. Plyometric activities under supervision may be helpful in the advanced stages of rehabilitation of Achilles tendon injuries. Taping the arch of the foot with the foot in equinus may lessen the tension on the Achilles tendon; it should also be instituted during the advanced stages of rehabilitation (Fig. 31–32). When chronic tendon disease becomes refractory to conservative management, surgical intervention may be necessary. The tendon sheath must be explored and the tendon substance must be opened longitudinally to remove the diseased tendon[24, 79, 116] (Fig. 31–33).

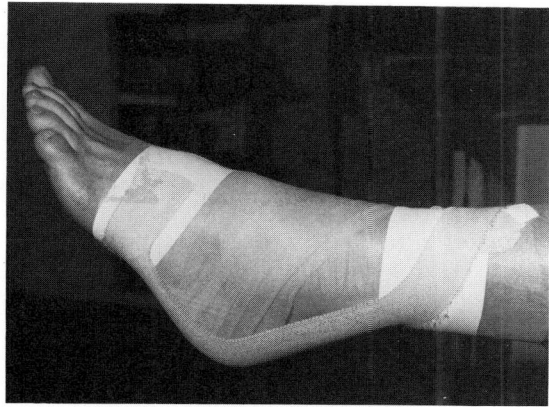

FIGURE 31–32. Taping of the foot and ankle for Achilles tendinitis.

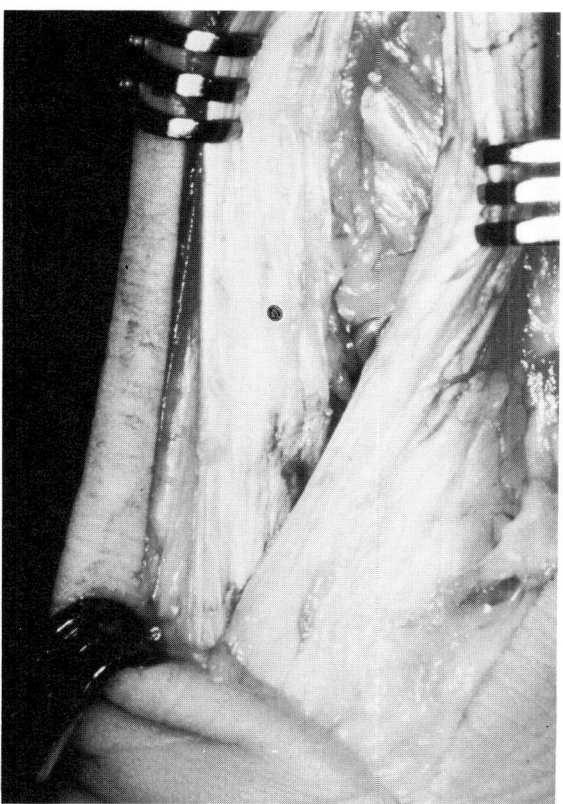

FIGURE 31–33. In refractory cases of gross tendon degeneration, surgical exploration of the Achilles tendon is necessary.

Other conditions of the Achilles complex that may be seen in young athletes include strain of the musculotendinous junction of the medial head of the gastrocnemius, apophysitis of the calcaneus (known as Sever's disease), and retrocalcaneal bursitis. The *calf muscle strain* is treated with rest, ice, compression, protected weight bearing, and stretching activities until symptoms resolve. Light jogging, rope jumping, and figure-of-eight running are instituted as symptoms warrant. Advancement to full activities depends on return of muscle strength, full motion, and no pain.

Sever's calcaneal apophysitis is very painful and limits running and jumping activities. Radiographic examination may reveal sclerosis and fragmentation of the calcaneal apophysis (Fig. 31–34). Treatment is symptomatic and includes a heel lift, taping to limit plantar flexion, stretching, and nonsteroidal antiinflammatories. Ice massage after activities limits the pain and inflammation. The condition is self-limiting and resolves with skeletal maturity.

Retrocalcaneal bursitis presents as lateral heel pain associated with swelling and callous formation at the lateral aspect of the Achilles tendon proximal to its insertion.[20, 21] Palpation of the area of the retrocalcaneal bursa reproduces the pain. Radiographic examination may reveal a prominent posterior calcaneal beak that repeatedly compresses the retrocalcaneal bursa with repeated dorsiflexion of the foot (Fig. 31–35). The swelling and pain cause shoe wear to be difficult because the heel counter crosses this area. Treatment is conservative, including heel lifts, antiinflammatory medication, and ice massage. Local steroid injection into the bursa while carefully avoiding the tendon may be palliative. In extreme cases, surgical removal of the bursa and the calcaneal tuberosity is necessary to resolve the problem.[20]

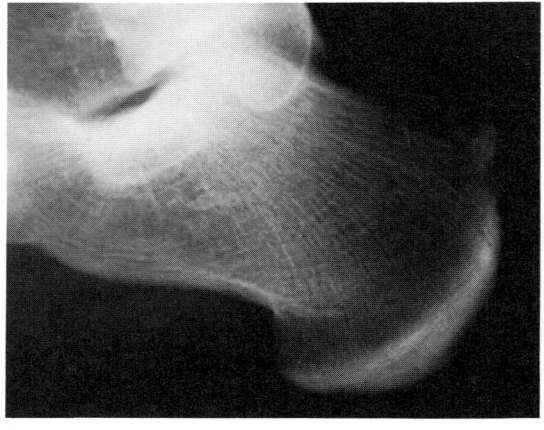

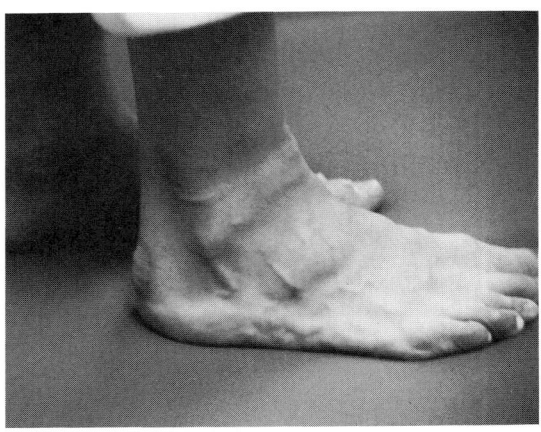

FIGURE 31–35. (*A*) Lateral X ray of the calcaneus demonstrating Haglund disease. (*B*) Pump bumps.

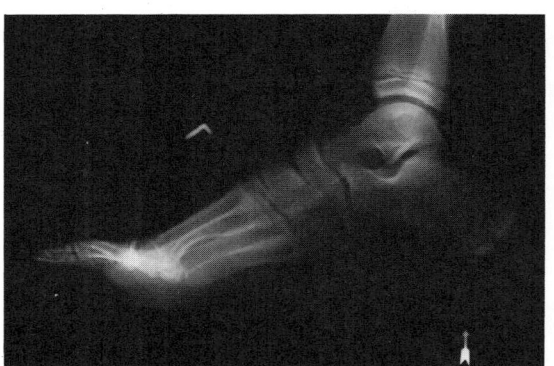

FIGURE 31–34. Lateral X-ray of the calcaneus showing sclerosis and fragmentation of the calcaneal apophysis or Sever's disease.

FOOT INJURIES

The basketball or volleyball athlete is at risk for foot injuries because of the intensity and duration of the activity in these sports. The feet provide the platform from which all running, jumping, landing, and cutting activity must be initiated.[128, 132, 140] Daily maintenance of foot hygiene and treatment of soft tissue injuries are important for keeping these athletes on the court. Choice of footwear and playing surfaces may influence the occurrence of injuries.[38, 44] Other factors contributing to injury include growth, age, and skeletal architecture of the foot as well as lower extremity muscle flexibility and strength.

Besides the Achilles tendon injuries already discussed, insertional tendon injuries are also associated with basketball and volleyball. A painful area of thickening and prominence on the posterosuperior lateral border of the calcaneus is often called a "pump bump" or Haglund syndrome. It is often associated with retrocalcaneal bursitis and may be influenced by shoe wear. The counter of most low-cut basketball or volleyball shoes irritates this area. Radiographs reveal a large calcaneal beak that contributes to the compression of the retrocalcaneal bursa between the calcaneus and the Achilles tendon (Fig. 31–36). Associated Achilles tendon involvement may produce radiopaque calcifications within the tendon.

Shoe wear in general may be painful because of the location of the pump bump. Initial treatment includes a doughnut pad, ice, and oral antiinflammatory medications. A local injection of corticosteroid and local anesthetic medication into the bursa, carefully avoiding the Achilles tendon, may be helpful. Modification of the shoe in order to prevent contact between its counter and the inflamed area is usually helpful. Shoe inserts to avoid overpronation and elevate the heel may help avoid shoe counter contact.

Surgical excision of the bursal tissue and osteotomy of the calcaneal tuberosity with or without exploration of the Achilles tendon may be necessary in those cases that do not respond to conservative treatment.[20, 21] The surgical approach is medial to the Achilles tendon, avoiding the medial neurovascular structures. Performing a proper osteotomy of the calcaneus and smoothing the bony contours of the calcaneus will lead to an excellent resolution of the problem. Postoperative management requires immobilization of the foot in a splint or cast for 3 weeks; then partial weight bearing is begun. Tenderness at the Achilles insertion is experienced for several weeks after active activities begin. A heel lift will limit the stress to the Achilles insertion. Stretching will also help with Achilles tendon rehabilitation. Resistive gastrocnemius activities are instituted after the surgical incision has healed and comfort has returned. Light jogging is started after a full, painless range of motion is obtained. Jumping and cutting are the last activities that are instituted because of the Achilles tendon involvement. This surgery may have a prolonged convalescence and should be scheduled in the off-season to provide sufficient time for rehabilitation and recovery.

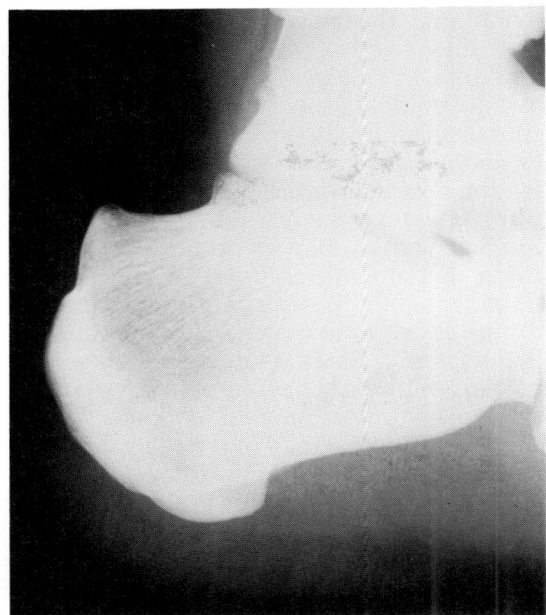

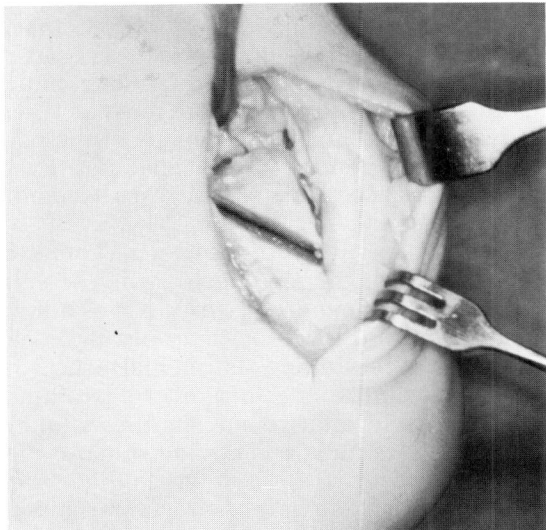

FIGURE 31–36. (A) Lateral X-ray of calcaneus showing Haglund disease. (B) Surgical excision of calcaneal beak.

Posterior tibial tendinitis may present as exertional posterior medial ankle pain. It is usually located posterior to the medial malleolus but may extend proximally to the muscle attachment to the posterior medial tibia and distally to the insertion of the tendon into the tarsal navicular.[20, 21] Tenderness and swelling along the course of the tendon are typical. Excessive pronation is usually evident. Conservative treatment consists of an arch support with a medial heel lift to remove the tension on the posterior tibial tendon during running and jumping. Oral antiinflammatory medication is also helpful. Surgical exploration is indicated in those cases that do not respond to conservative treatment and in which acquired foot deformities are noted. Surgical exploration of the posterior tibial tendon usually reveals partial rupture or attrition of the tendon as it courses behind the medial malleolus.

An *accessory tarsal navicular syndrome* presents as pain at the insertion of the posterior tibialis tendon. This entity is common in the adolescent athlete and may produce pain along the medial aspect of the arch of the foot. Swelling, a noticeable prominence, and excessive pronation may be present. Conservative management consisting of an arch support with a medial heel lift, ice, and antiinflammatory medication is helpful. Injections to this area have a variable response, and surgical exploration with removal of the ossicle may be indicated. Care must be taken to leave intact the main insertion of the posterior tibialis tendon to the navicular. Excision of the accessory ossicle usually eradicates the pain.

The plantar surface of the heel is a common site of pain. *Calcaneal periostitis*, or subcalcaneal pain syndrome, presents as a low-grade pain in the heel with an insidious onset. Tenderness along the medial aspect of the calcaneus in the area of the proximal plantar fascia attachment signifies *plantar fasciitis*. Care must be taken to rule out medial plantar nerve entrapment as the source of the pain. Radiographs are performed to exclude the possibility of a calcaneal neoplasm or cyst. A spur on the plantar aspect of the calcaneus is common in plantar fasciitis. The spur alone does not represent the cause of the pain but is the effect of excessive stress applied to the plantar fascia attachment.[20, 21, 22] The player's shoes and inserts are inspected for abnormal wear patterns. Conservative therapy includes toe flexion exercises, arch stretching, and ice massage. Arch supports are given to those athletes with excessive foot pronation. Athletes with a cavovarus midfoot do not respond to arch support wear. In some instances, an injection of a local anesthetic and a soluble corticosteroid will give temporary relief of the pain. In refractory cases, release of the plantar fascia will resolve the problem.[20, 21] This may be performed under local anesthesia and on an outpatient basis.

Some refractory, atypical cases of heel pain are caused by a *stress fracture of the calcaneus*. Radiographs often appear normal in these cases; bone scan or computerized tomography (CT) may be necessary to make the diagnosis. Taping of the arch, padding of the heel, and arch supports are helpful and are the mainstays of treatment.[148]

Midfoot pain in the running and jumping athlete during competition and at rest may indicate a *stress fracture of the tarsal navicular*.[6, 64, 112, 138, 141] The onset of symptoms may occur over as long as 36 months. Swelling may be minimal. Pain with weighted plantar flexion of the foot during landing and push-off in running is typical. Routine radiographs often do not show this fracture. This injury may result from the precarious blood supply to this bone. Bone scans, tomograms, and CT scans are necessary for evaluating a fracture of the navicular.[13, 50, 112, 138] Treatment is determined by the fracture type. Uncomplicated, nondisplaced fractures should be casted for 6 to 8 weeks while the athlete is non–weight bearing. Surgical intervention is necessary for those fractures that demonstrate delayed healing, avascular fragments, or nonunion. Surgery consists of debridement, cancellous grafting, and screw fixation. The athlete is still immobilized and kept non–weight bearing for at least 6 weeks.

Lateral foot pain involving the fifth metatarsal suggests a stress fracture of the metatarsal known as a *Jones fracture*.[35, 39, 69, 70] This is distinctly different from the tuberosity fracture of the base of the fifth metatarsal.[1, 32, 81, 153] Acute fractures that occur with trauma are treated with immobilization and non–weight bearing for 6 weeks. For fractures that present with several weeks of pain and limited function and demonstrate on radiographs a delayed union or frank nonunion, surgical intervention with intramedullary screw fixation and possibly bone grafting is the treatment of choice[72, 136, 154] (Fig. 31–37).

Another potential area of foot pain is the plantar aspect of the great toe in the area of the sesamoid bones. The tibial sesamoid is more commonly affected.[27, 29, 91, 142] The athlete experiences pain on extension of the toe and weight bearing such as when landing

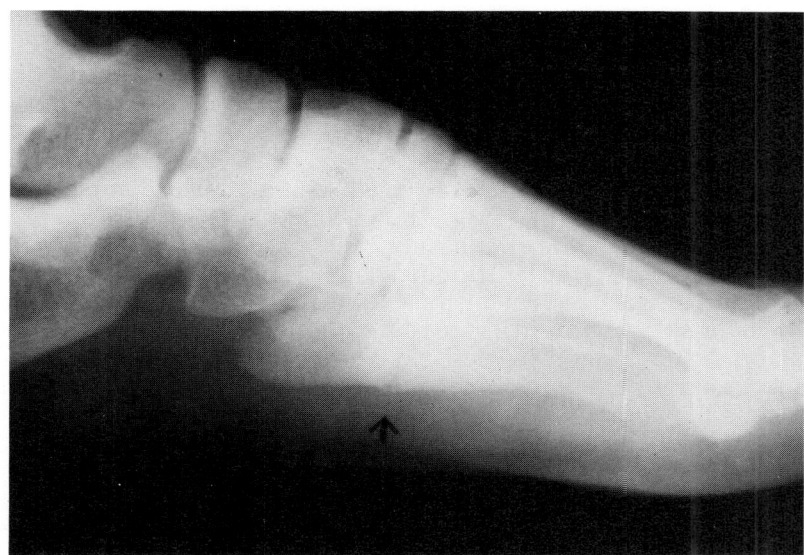

FIGURE 31–37. (A) Lateral X-ray of the foot denoting a Jones fracture. (B) Internal fixation of acute fracture with intramedullary screw.

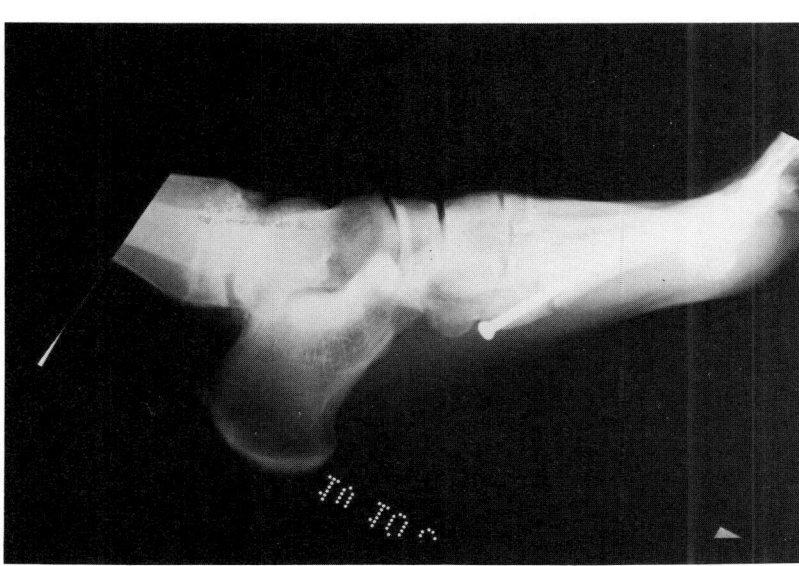

from a jump or running. Palpation of the medial aspect of the first metatarsal joint on the plantar surface of the foot reveals the sesamoid to be quite painful. Radiographs may demonstrate a bipartite sesamoid; a sprinter's view may show incongruity of the articular surface. A bone scan will highlight an acute fracture. Rest, padding, and extension taping are conservative treatments. Surgical treatment is necessary if pain is not controlled by the conservative approach. Although bone grafting has been shown to have success in a number of cases, excision of the painful sesamoid has been my preferred treatment.[120]

Superficial soft tissue injuries to the foot may sometimes severely affect the basketball and volleyball athlete. The medial aspect of the distal phalanx of the great toe, the distal tips of the toes, and the posterior aspect of the heel are the most common sites of *blister* formation. The blisters occur because of friction between the skin and the sock interface caused by movement within the shoe itself. Preventive measures include wearing well-fitted shoes and two pairs of socks, one pair of sweat socks and one of sanitary socks. Conditioning of the plantar aspect of the foot and toes will toughen the skin and aid in preventing further blistering. Treatment includes taping and padding the "hot spots." The blister may be drained at the edge with an 18-gauge needle or an 11-blade scalpel under sterile conditions. The blistered area may be filled with an analgesic ointment or zinc oxide to dry the skin and then covered with a sterile compressive dressing. The occlusive dressings may need to be continued for 3 to 4 days and then skin edges trimmed daily. The common complication of blisters is infection. Areas of skin breakdown must be cared for daily. *Pseudomonas* species and *Staphylococcus aureus* are the common pathogens associated with foot infections.[67, 124, 127]

Continued intermittent pressure on the skin of the foot may cause a thickened, tender area of skin called a *callus* to develop.[67, 71, 80, 127] Bony prominences may produce weight distribution abnormalities on the overlying skin that produce callosities. The callus is avascular and histologically is a keratinized area of the skin produced from the stratum basale.[85] The most common areas are the plantar aspects of the metatarsal heads, with the largest area noted under the first metatarsal head. The treatment should include checking shoe fit and redistribution of weight bearing with orthotic devices made of Plastizote or rubber materials.[57, 92] If the shoe shows signs of wear on the sole as well as the upper body, it should be changed. Pads constructed to provide protection to areas of increased callous formation must be applied directly to the skin. Petroleum jelly is sometimes used to decrease friction that can cause a blister to form in the middle of the callus. Calluses must be trimmed on a regular basis. Daily soaks and the use of a pumice stone to shave the cornified periphery of the callus will help in the management of painful calluses.

Infections of the foot can also inhibit the athlete from competing. Fungal infections result from poor foot skin hygiene. Fungal infections are noted between the toes and may also involve the toenails. The most common skin fungus is tinea corporis, with candidiasis affecting the toenails.[10, 71, 127] Tolnaftate 1 percent will effectively treat the tinea infections of the skin. Miconazole 2 percent cream is quite effective for fungal nail infections. The feet must be inspected daily, cleaned at least three times a day, and dried thoroughly. Foot powders also help to keep the feet dry during athletic activities. Superinfections by *Staphylococcus* species may require hospitalization, debridement, and intravenous antibiotics. Griseofulvin, 500 to 1000 mg daily in divided doses, may be necessary for fulminant cases of foot fungal disease.

Viral infections of the plantar surface of the foot occur under the metatarsal heads or elsewhere. The papovirus is the usual etiological agent.[67, 71, 127] The affected areas are painful to touch and pressure. The areas are irregular in shape; mosaic or cluster patterns are seen. These lesions bleed with surgical debridement. Conservative treatment with salicyclic acid preparations is helpful. Spontaneous regression usually takes place over 4 to 5 months.

Toenails should be carefully manicured to prevent the harboring of fungal agents. An infection due to an ingrown nail is called a *paronychia*. Warm water soaks, nail debridement, and incision and drainage of the infection are necessary in advanced stages. *Subungual hematomas* may occur if shoes do not fit properly or the toenail is too long and is compressed against the end of the shoe. The hematoma, if painful, is drained by puncturing the nail. The athlete should inspect the toenails, the region between the toes, and the plantar aspect of the feet daily for any signs of foot disease. Prevention will limit the severity of the fungal disease, limit infections, and prevent toenail destruction. Daily changes of clean socks, foot powders to prevent excessive perspiration, pads for hot spots, and trimming of calluses are necessary steps for foot protection.

Shoe fit is the most important preventive step in foot care.[44, 92, 145] Basketball shoes have a rubberized sole with patterns that are molded into the sole to help distribute the weight-bearing stresses (Fig. 31–38). The inner lining contains an air cell or foam pad between the sole and the shoe insert. Most basketball shoes come with a removable shoe insert that has a small molded arch support and supplies a surface that decreases the friction at the sock-insert interface. The insert may be removed and a custom-fitted orthotic substituted for an athlete who has problems with calluses, blisters, or other stress-related conditions. The counter of the shoe is padded to protect the Achilles tendon. The high-top basketball shoe is reinforced about the ankle to provide an external support to lessen the severity of ankle sprains. The shoes should be laced from the first to the last hole in a crisscross manner using all the holes available to give the most stable construct.

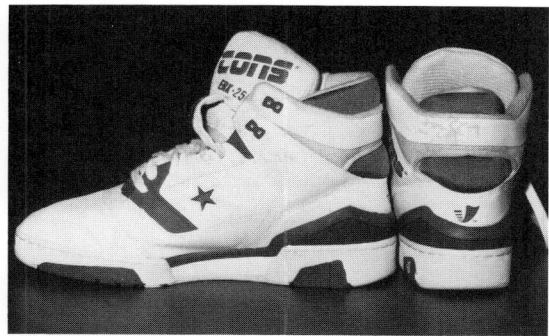

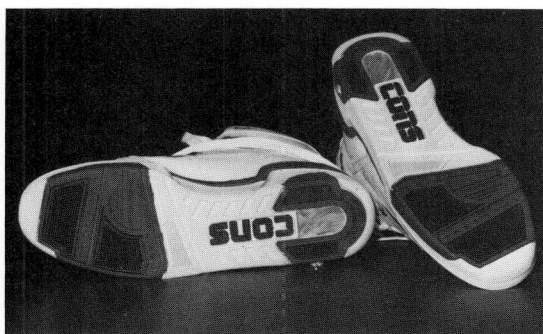

FIGURE 31–38. Basketball shoes showing pattern of the sole for good shoe-surface interface with high heel counter and large tongue for protection of the extensor tendons of the foot.

The tongue of the shoe should fit comfortably over the anterior aspect of the ankle and foot, protecting the extensor tendons that are superficial and subject to compression in this area. The toes should fit comfortably in the toebox, which should have sufficient room to accommodate two pairs of socks without crowding and impinging the toes. The shoes must be replaced if any support structures are damaged, torn, or worn. A shoe in disrepair may lead to an injury that requires the athlete to miss practice or competition.

SUMMARY

Basketball and volleyball are two sports with similar injury patterns. Awareness of situations that can lead to injuries may help in their avoidance and keep the athletes on the court longer. Once an injury is recognized, prompt and careful evaluation, treatment, and rehabilitation will ensure the quick and safe return of the athlete. A knowledge of the type of injuries seen in these two sports will allow the sports medicine specialist to focus on the occurrences of injury patterns and provide prompt and appropriate care.

References

1. Acker, J. H., and Drez, D., Jr.: Nonoperative treatment of stress fractures of the proximal shaft of the fifth metatarsal (Jones fracture). Foot Ankle 7:152–154, 1986.
2. Andrews, J. R.: Overuse syndromes of the lower extremity. Clin. Sports Med. 2:137–148, 1983.
3. Andrews, J. R., and Sanders, R.: A "mini reconstruction" technique in treatment of anterolateral rotatory instability (ALRI). Clin. Orthop. 172:93–96, 1983.
4. Arnold, J. A., Cohen, T. P., Heaton, L. M., et al.: Natural history of anterior cruciate tears. Am. J. Sports Med. 7:305–313, 1979.
5. Beck, J. L., and Wildermuth, B. P.: The female athlete's knee. Clin. Sports Med. 4(2):345–366, 1985.
6. Belkin, S. C.: Stress fractures in athletes. Orthop. Clin. North Am. 11(4):735–742, 1980.
7. Black, H. M.: Operative treatment of ankle sprains—acute and chronic. Am. J. Sports Med. 5:256–257, 1977.
8. Black, H. M.: Roentgenographic considerations in ankle sprains. Am. J. Sports Med. 5:238–240, 1977.
9. Blazina, M. E., Kerlan, R. K., Jobe, F. W., Carter, V. S., and Carlson, G. J.: Jumper's knee. Orthop. Clin. North Am. 4:665–678, 1973.
10. Bordelon, R. L.: Management of disorders of the forefoot and toenails associated with running. Clin. Sports Med. 4:4, 1985.
11. Bowers, K. D., Jr.: Patellar tendon avulsion as a complication of Osgood-Schlatter's disease. Am. J. Sports Med. 9(6):356–359, 1981.
12. Brady, T. A., Cahill, B. R., and Bodnar, L. M.: Weight training–related injuries in the high school athlete. Am. J. Sports Med. 10(1):1–5, 1982.
13. Brill, D. R.: Sports nuclear medicine bone imaging for lower extremity pain in athletes. Clin. Nuc. Med. 8(3):101–106, 1983.
14. Burkus, J. K., Sella, E. J., and Southwick, W. O.: Occult injuries of the talus diagnosed by bone scan and tomography. Foot Ankle 4:6, 1984.
15. Cabaud, H. E., Feagin, J. A., and Rodkey, W. G.: Acute anterior cruciate ligament injury and augmented repair. Experimental studies. Am. J. Sports Med. 8:395–401, 1980.
16. Canale, S. T., and Belding, R. H.: Osteochondral lesions of the talus. J. Bone Joint Surg. 62A:97–192, 1980.
17. Chambers, R. B.: Orthopaedic injuries in athletes (ages 6 to 17). Comparison of injuries occurring in six sports. Am. J. Sports Med. 7(3):195–197, 1979.
18. Chandy, T. A., and Grana, W. A.: Secondary school athletic injury in boys and girls. A three year comparison. Phys. Sports Med. 13(3):106–111, 1985.

19. Chrisman, O. D., and Snook, G. A.: Reconstruction of lateral ligament tears of the ankle. J. Bone Joint Surg. 51A:904–912, 1969.
20. Clancy, W. G., Jr.: Runner's injuries. Part two: evaluation and treatment of specific injuries. Am. J. Sports Med. 8(4):287–289, 1980.
21. Clancy, W. G., Jr.: Symposium: runner's injuries. Am. J. Sports Med. 8:137–138, 1980.
22. Clancy, W. G., Jr.: Tendinitis and plantar fasciitis in runners. Orthopedics 6:217–233, 1983.
23. Clancy, W. G., Jr.: Arthroscopic anterior cruciate ligament reconstruction with patellar tendon. Techniques Orthop. 2:13–22, 1988.
24. Clancy, W. G., Jr., Neidhart, D., and Brand, R. L.: Achilles tendinitis in runners—a report in five cases. Am. J. Sports Med. 4:46–57, 1976.
25. Clancy, W. G., Jr., and Ray, J. M.: Anterior cruciate ligament autografts. In Jackson, D. W., and Drez, D., Jr. (eds.): The Anterior Cruciate Ligament Deficient Knee, New Concepts in Ligament Repair. St. Louis, C. V. Mosby Co., pp. 193–210, 1987.
26. Clancy, W. G., Jr., Ray, J. M., and Zoltan, D.: Acute third degree anterior cruciate ligament injury: a prospective study of conservative nonoperative treatment and operative treatment with repair and patellar tendon augmentation. J. Bone Joint Surg. 70A:1483–1488, 1988.
27. Clanton, T. O., Butler, J. E., and Eggert, A.: Injuries to the metatarsophalangeal joints in athletes. Foot Ankle 7(3):162–176, 1986.
28. Clement, D. B., Taunton, J. E., and Smart, G. W.: Achilles tendinitis and peritendinitis etiology and treatment. Am. J. Sports Med. 12(3):179–184, 1984.
29. Coker, T., Arnold, J., and Weber, D.: Traumatic lesions of the metatarsophalangeal joint of the great toe in athletes. Am. J. Sports Med. 6:326–334, 1978.
30. Cooper, D., and Fair, J.: Ankle rehabilitation using the ankle disk. Phys. Sports Med. 6(6):41, 1978.
31. Cox, J. S.: Patellofemoral problems in runners. Clin. Sports Med. 4(4):699–715, 1985.
32. Dameron, T. B.: Fractures and anatomical variations of the proximal portion of the fifth metatarsal. J. Bone Joint Surg. 57A:788–792, 1975.
33. DeHaven, K. E.: Diagnosis of acute knee injuries with hemarthrosis. Am. J. Sports Med. 8:9–14, 1980.
34. DeHaven, K. E., and Lintner, D. M.: Athletic injuries: comparison by age, sports and gender. Am. J. Sports Med. 14(3):218–224, 1986.
35. DeLee, J. C., Evans, J. P., and Julian, J.: Stress fractures of the fifth metatarsal. Am. J. Sports Med. 11(5):349–353, 1983.
36. Dererrauk, M. D., Parr, G. R., Lachmann, S. M., Page-Thomas, P., and Hazleman, B. L.: The diagnosis of stress fractures in athletes. JAMA 252(4):531–533, 1984.
37. Devas, M. B.: Stress fractures of the fibula. A review of fifty cases in athletes. J. Bone Joint Surg. 30B: 818–829, 1956.
38. Drez, D. J.: Running footwear—examination of the training shoe, the foot and functional orthotic devices. Am. J. Sports Med. 8:140, 1980.
39. Drez, D., Young, D., Johnston, R. D., and Parker, W.: Metatarsal stress fractures. Am. J. Sports Med. 8(2):123–125, 1980.
40. Ferretti, A.: Epidemiology of jumper's knee. Sports Med. 3(4):289–295, 1986.
41. Ferretti, A., Ippolito, E., Mariani, P., and Pudd, M. G.: "Jumper's knee." Am. J. Sports Med. 11(2):58–62, 1983.
42. Fetto, J. F., and Marshall, J. L.: Injury to the anterior cruciate ligament producing the pivot-shift sign. J. Bone Joint Surg. 61A:710–714, 1979.
43. Fornage, B. D., Rifkin, M. D., Touche, D. H., and Segal, P. M.: Sonography of the patellar tendon: preliminary observations. AJR 143(1):179–182, 1984.
44. Frederick, E. C.: Kinematically mediated effects of sport shoe design: a review. J. Sports Sci. 4(3):169–184, 1986.
45. Fritschy, D., and de Gautard, R.: Jumper's knee and ultrasonography. Am. J. Sports Med. 16(6):637–640, 1988.
46. Galway, H. R., and MacIntosh, D. L.: The lateral pivot shift. A symptom and sign of anterior cruciate ligament insufficiency. Clin. Orthop. 147:45–50, 1980.
47. Galway, R. D.: The pivot shift syndrome (abstract). J. Bone Joint Surg. 54B:588, 1972.
48. Garrett, W. E., Jr.: Strains and sprains in athletes. Postgrad. Med. 73(3):200–209, 1983.
49. Garrick, J. G., and Requa, R. K.: Injuries in high school sports. Pediatrics 61:465–469, 1978.
50. Geslien, G. E., Thrall, J. H., Espinosa, J. L., and Older, R. A.: Early detection of stress fractures using ^{99m}Tc-polyphosphate. Radiology 121: 683–687, 1976.
51. Giove, T. P., Sayer, J. H., Kent, B. A., et al.: Nonoperative treatment of the torn anterior cruciate ligament. J. Bone Joint Surg. 65A:184–192, 1983.
52. Gray, J., Taunton, J. E., McKenzie, D. C., Clement, D. B., McConkey, J. P., and Davidson, R. G.: A survey of injuries to the anterior cruciate ligament of the knee in female basketball players. Int. J. Sports Med. 6(6):314–316, 1985.
53. Harvey, J. S., Jr.: Overuse syndromes in young athletes. Pediatr. Clin. North Am. 29(6):1369–1381, 1982.
54. Harvey, J. S., Jr.: Overuse syndromes in young athletes. Clin. Sports Med. 2(3):595–607, 1983.
55. Hecman, J. D., and Alkire, C. C.: Distal patellar pole fractures. A proposed common mechanism of injury. Am. J. Sports Med. 12(6):424–428, 1984.
56. Henry, J. H., Lareau, B., and Neigut, D.: The injury rate in professional basketball. Am. J. Sports Med. 1:16–18, 1982.
57. Hertzman, C. A.: Use of Plastizote in foot disabilities. Am. J. Phys. Med. 52:289, 1973.
58. Holden, P. L., Eggert, A. W., and Butler, J. E.: The nonoperative treatment of grade I and II medial collateral ligament injuries to the knee. Am. J. Sports Med. 11(5):340–344, 1983.
59. Holder, L. E.: Radionuclide bone imaging in the evaluation of bone pain. J. Bone Joint Surg. 64A:1391–1396, 1982.
60. Holder, L. E.: Radionuclide bone imaging in the evaluation of athletic injuries. Diag. Nuc. Med. 2(2):3–8, 1985.
61. Holder, L. E., and Matthews, L. S.: The nuclear physician and sports medicine. In Freeman, L. M., and Weissmann, H. S. (eds.): Nuclear Medicine Annual 1984. New York, Raven Press, pp. 81–140, 1984.
62. Hopkinson, W. J., Mitchell, W. A., and Curl, W. W.: Chondral fractures of the knee. Cause for

63. Hughston, J. C., Andrews, J. R., and Cross, M. J.: Classification of knee ligament instability. Part I. The medial compartment and cruciate ligaments. Part II. The lateral compartment. J. Bone Joint Surg. 58A:159–172, 173–179, 1976.
64. Hunter, L. Y.: Stress fracture of the tarsal navicular. More frequent than we realize? Am. J. Sports Med. 9(4):217–219, 1981.
65. Ismail, A. M., Balakrishman, R., and Rajakamur, M. K.: Rupture of patellar ligament after steroid infiltration. J. Bone Joint Surg. 51B:503–505, 1969.
66. Jackson, D. W., Jennings, L. D., Maywood, R. M., and Berger, P. E.: Magnetic resonance imaging of the knee. Am. J. Sports Med. 16:29–38, 1988.
67. Jahss, M. H.: Disorders of the Foot. Philadelphia, W. B. Saunders Co., 1982.
68. Jakob, R. P., Hassler, H., and Staeubi, H. U.: Observations on rotatory instability of the lateral compartment of the knee. Experimental studies on the functional anatomy and pathomechanism of the knee and the reverse pivot shift sign. Acta Orthop. Scand. 52 (Suppl. 191):1–32, 1981.
69. Jones, K. G.: Results of use of the central one-third of the patellar ligament to compensate for anterior cruciate ligament deficiency. Clin. Orthop. 147:39–44, 1980.
70. Jones, R.: Fracture of the base of the fifth metatarsal by indirect violence. Ann. Surg. 35:697–702, 1902.
71. Kalivas, J.: Treatment of Skin Disorders of the Feet and Nails. AAOS Symposium on the Foot and Ankle. C. V. Mosby Co., 1983.
72. Kavanaugh, J. H., et al.: The Jones fracture revisited. J. Bone Joint Surg. 60A:776–782, 1988.
73. Kelly, D. W., Carter, V. S., Jobe, F. W., and Kerlan, R. K.: Patellar and quadriceps tendon ruptures—jumper's knee. Am. J. Sports Med. 12(5):375–380, 1984.
74. Kennedy, J. C., and Willis, R. B.: The effects of local steroid injections on tendons: a biomechanical and microscopic correlative study. Am. J. Sports Med. 4(1):11–21, 1976.
75. Kirkpatrick, J. S., Koman, L. A., and Rovere, G. D.: The role of ultrasound in the early diagnosis of myositis ossificans. Am. J. Sports Med. 15(2):179–181, 1987.
76. Krackow, K. A., and Brooks, R. L.: Optimization of knee ligament position for lateral extraarticular reconstruction. Am. J. Sports Med. 11:293–302, 1983.
77. Kujala, V. M., Kvist, M., and Osterman, K.: Knee injuries in athletes. Review of exertion injuries and retrospective study of outpatient sports clinic material. Sports Med. 3(6):447–460, 1986.
78. Kurusaka, M., Shinichi, Y., and Andrish, J. T.: A biomechanical comparison of different surgical techniques of graft fixation in anterior cruciate ligament reconstruction. Am. J. Sports Med. 15:225–229, 1987.
79. Kvist, H., and Kvist, M.: The operative treatment of chronic calcaneal paratendonitis. J. Bone Joint Surg. 62B:353–357, 1980.
80. Lapidus, P. W.: Orthopedic skin lesions of the soles and toes, calluses, corns, plantar warts, keratomas, neurovascular growths, onychomas. Clin. Orthop. 45:87, 1966.
81. Lehman, R. C., Torg, J. S., Pavlov, H., and DeLee, J. C.: Fractures of the base of the fifth metatarsal distal to the tuberosity: a review. Foot Ankle 7(4):245–252, 1987.
82. Lehman, W. L., Jr.: Overuse syndromes in runners. Am. Fam. Phys. 29(1)157–161, 1984.
83. Lipscomb, A. B., and Anderson, A. F.: Tears of the anterior cruciate ligament in adolescents. J. Bone Joint Surg. 68A(1):19–28, 1986.
84. Maddox, P. A., and Garth, W. P., Jr.: Tendinitis of the patellar ligaments and quadriceps (jumper's knee) as an initial presentation of hyperparathyroidism. A case report. J. Bone Joint Surg. 68A(2):288–292, 1986.
85. Mann, R. A., and DuVries, H. L.: Intractable plantar keratosis. Orthop. Clin. North Am. 41:67, 1973.
86. Marshall, J. L., Warren, R. F., and Wichiewicz, T. L.: Primary surgical treatment of anterior cruciate ligament lesions. Am. J. Sports Med. 10:103–107, 1982.
87. Martens, M., Wouters, P., Burssens, A., and Miller, J. C.: Patellar tendinitis: pathology and results of treatment. Acta Orthop. Scand. 53:445–450, 1982.
88. Mayba, I. I.: Avulsion fracture of the tibial tubercle apophysis with avulsion of patellar ligament. J. Pediatr. Orthop. 2(3):303–305, 1982.
89. McBryde, A. M., Jr.: Stress fractures in athletes. Am. J. Sports Med. 3:212–217, 1975.
90. McBryde, A. M., Jr.: Stress fractures in runners. Clin. Sports Med. 4(4):737–752, 1985.
91. McBryde, A. M., and Anderson, R. B.: Sesamoid foot problems in the athlete. Clin. Sports Med., 7(1):51–60, 1988.
92. McKenzie, D. C., Clement, D. B., and Taunton, J. E.: Running shoes, orthotics and injuries. Sports Med. 2(5):334–347, 1985.
93. McLennan, J. G.: Treatment of acute and chronic luxations of the peroneal tendons. Am. J. Sports Med. 8:432–436, 1980.
94. McNicol, K., Taunton, J. E., and Clement, D. B.: Iliotibial tract friction syndrome in athletes. Can. J. Appl. Sport Sci. 6(2):76–80, 1981.
95. Micheli, L. J.: Pediatric and adolescent sports injuries: recent trends. Exerc. Sport Sci. Rev. 14:359–374, 1986.
96. Micheli, L. J., and Smith, A. D.: Sports injuries in children. Curr. Probl. Pediatr. 12(9):1–54, 1982.
97. Michlovits, S., Smith, W., and Watkins, M.: Ice and high voltage pulsed stimulation in treatment of acute lateral ankle sprains. J. Orthop. Sports Phys. Therapy 9:301–304, 1988.
98. Miller, J. W.: Dislocation of the peroneal tendons: a new operative approach. Am. J. Orthop. 9:136–137, 1967.
99. Mital, M. A., and Matza, R. A.: Osgood-Schlatter disease: the painful puzzler Phys. Sports Med. 5:60, 1977.
100. Moretz, J. A., III, and Grana, W. A.: High school basketball injuries. Phys. Sports Med. 6(10):92–95, 1978.
101. Moretz, J. A., III, Harlan S. D., Goodrich, J., and Walters, R.: Long term follow up of knee injuries on high school football players. Am. J. Sports Med. 12(4):298–300, 1984.
102. Mott, H. W.: Semitendinosus anatomic recon-

struction for cruciate ligament insufficiency. Clin. Orthop. 172:90–92, 1983.
103. Nanninga, A. J., and Josaputra, H. A.: Tibial tuberosity fractures in adolescents—report of a case and review of the literature. Neth. J. Surg. 39(5):144–146, 1987.
104. Nichollas, J. A., and Marino, M.: The relationship of injuries of the leg, foot and ankle to proximal thigh strength in athletes. Foot Ankle 7(4):218–228, 1987.
105. Noyes, F. R., Butler, D. L., Paulos, L. E., et al.: Intra-articular cruciate reconstruction. I. Perspectives on graft strengths, vascularization, and immediate motion after replacement. Clin. Orthop. 172:71–77, 1983.
106. Noyes, F. R., Matthews, D. S., Mooar, P. A., et al.: The symptomatic anterior cruciate deficient knee. II. The results of rehabilitation, activity modification, and counseling on functional disability. J. Bone Joint Surg. 65A:163–174, 1983.
107. O'Donoghue, D.H.: Surgical treatment of fresh injuries to major ligaments of the knee. J. Bone Joint Surg. 32A:721–738, 1950.
108. Ogden, J. A., McCarthy, S. M., and Jokl, P.: The painful bipartite patella. J. Pediatr. Orthop. 2(3):263–269, 1982.
109. Ogden, J. A., and Southwick, W. O.: Osgood-Schlatter's disease and tibial tuberosity developments. Clin. Orthop. 116:188, 1976.
110. Orava, S., Hulkko, A., and Jormakka, E.: Exertion injuries in female athletes. Br. J. Sports Med. 15(4):229–233, 1981.
111. Orava, S., Osterback, L., and Hurme, M.: Surgical treatment of patellar tendon pain in athletes. Br. J. Sports Med. 20(4):167–169, 1986.
112. Pavlov, H., Torg, J. S., and Freiberger, R. H.: Tarsal navicular stress fractures: radiographic evaluation. Radiology 148:641–645, 1983.
113. Powell, J. H., and Whipple, T. L.: Osteochondritis dissecans of the talus. Foot Ankle 6(6):309–319, 1986.
114. Prichett, J. W.: A statistical study of knee injuries due to football in high school athletes. J. Bone Joint Surg. 64A(2):240–242, 1982.
115. Puddu, G.: Method for reconstruction of ACL using the semitendinosus tendon. Am. J. Sports Med. 8:402–404, 1980.
116. Puddu, G., Ippolito, E., and Postacchini, F.: A classification of Achilles tendon disease. Am. J. Sports Med. 4:145–150, 1976.
117. Ray, J. M.: A proposed natural history of symptomatic anterior cruciate ligament injuries of the knee. Sports Med. 7(4):697–713, 1988.
118. Ray, J. M., Clancy, W. G., Jr., and Lemon, R. A.: Semimembranosus tendinitis: an overlooked cause of medial knee pain. Am. J. Sports Med. 16(4):347–351, 1988.
119. Renne, J. W.: The iliotibial band friction syndrome. J. Bone Joint Surg. 57A:110–111, 1975.
120. Richardson, E. G.: Injuries to the hallucal sesamoids in the athlete. Foot Ankle 7(4):229–244, 1989.
121. Roels, J., Martens, M., and Burssens, A.: Patellar tendinitis (jumper's knee). Am. J. Sports Med. 6:362–368, 1978.
122. Rosenthal, L., Hill, R. O., and Chuang, S.: Observation on the use of ^{99m}Tc-phosphate imaging in peripheral bone trauma. Radiology 119:637–641, 1976.
123. Rovere, G. D., Clarke, T. J., Yates, C. S., and Burley, K.: Retrospective comparison of taping and ankle stabilizers in preventing ankle injuries. Am. J. Sports Med. 16:228–233, 1988.
124. Sammarco, G., and James, S.: Soft tissue conditions in athletes' feet. Clin. Sports Med. 1:149–156, 1982.
125. Savoca, C. J.: Stress fractures. A classification of the earliest radiographic signs. Radiology 100:519–524, 1971.
126. Sinding-Larsen, M. F.: A hitherto unknown affection of the patella in children. Acta Radiol. 1:171, 1922.
127. Singer, K., and Jones, D.: Soft tissue conditions of the ankle and foot. In Nicholas, J. A., and Hershman, E. (eds.): The Lower Extremity and Spine in Sports. St. Louis, C. V. Mosby Co., 1986.
128. Slocum, D. B., and Bowerman, W.: Biomechanics of running. Clin. Orthop. 23:39–45, 1962.
129. Slocum, D. B., James, S. L., and Larson, R. L.: Clinical test for anterolateral rotatory instability of the knee. Clin. Orthop. 118:63–69, 1976.
130. Slocum, D. B., Larson, R. L., and James, S. L.: Late reconstruction of ligamentous injuries of the medial compartment of the knee. Clin. Orthop. 100:23–55, 1974.
131. Stanitski, C. L., McMaster, J. H., and Scranton, P. E.: On the nature of stress fractures. Am. J. Sports Med. 6(6):391–395, 1978.
132. Steingard, P. M.: Foot failures in basketball. Phys. Sports Med. 2(3):64–94, 1974.
133. Strand, T., Engesaeter, L. B., Molster, A. O., et al.: Knee function following suture of fresh tears of the anterior cruciate ligament. Acta Orthop. Scand 55:181–184, 1984.
134. Sullivan, J. A.: Recurring pain in the pediatric athlete. Pediatr. Clin. North Am. 31(5):1097–1112, 1984.
135. Sutker, A. N., Barber, F. A., Jackson, D. W., and Pagliano, J. W.: Iliotibial band syndrome in distance runners. Sports Med. 2(6):447–451, 1985.
136. Torg, J. S., Baldwin, F. C., Zelko, R. R., Pavlov, H., Pefe, T. C., and Das, M.: Fractures of the base of the fifth metatarsal distal to the tuberosity. Classification and guidelines for nonsurgical and surgical management. J. Bone Joint Surg. 66A:209–214, 1984.
137. Torg, J. S., Conrad, W., and Kalen, V.: Clinical diagnosis of anterior cruciate ligament instability in the athlete. Am. J. Sports Med. 4:84–91, 1976.
138. Torg, J. S., Pavlov, H., Cooley, L. H., Bryant, M. H., Arnoczky, S. P., Bergfeld, J., and Hunter, L. Y.: Stress fractures of the tarsal navicular. J. Bone Joint Surg. 64A:700–712, 1982.
139. Torg, J. S., Pavlov, H., and Morris, V. B.: Salter-Harris type III fracture of the medial femoral condyle occurring in the adolescent athlete. J. Bone Joint Surg. 63A(4):586–591, 1981.
140. Torg, J. S., Pavlov, H., and Torg, E.: Overuse injuries in sports: the foot. Clin. Sports Med. 6:2, 1987.
141. Towne, L. C., Blazina, M. E., and Cozen, L. N.: Fatigue fracture of the tarsal navicular. J. Bone Joint Surg. 52A(2):376–378, 1970.
142. Vanshal, M. E., Keene, J. S., Lange, T. A., et al.: Stress fractures of the great toe sesamoids. Am. J. Sports Med. 10:277, 1982.

143. Walsh, W. M., and Blackburn, T.: Prevention of ankle sprains. Am. J. Sports Med. 5:243–245, 1977.
144. Walter, N. E., and Wolf, M. D.: Stress fractures in young athletes. Am. J. Sports Med. 5(4):165–169, 1977.
145. Wickstrom, J., and Williams, R. A.: Shoe corrections and orthopedic foot supports. Clin. Orthop. 70:30, 1970.
146. Wilkins, K.: The uniqueness of the young athlete: musculoskeletal injuries. Am. J. Sports Med. 8(5):377–382, 1980.
147. Williams, J. G. P.: Achilles tendon lesions in sports. Sports Med. 3:114–135, 1986.
148. Wilson, E. S., Jr., and Katz, F. N.: Stress fractures. An analysis of 250 conservative cases. Radiology 92:481–486, 1969.
149. Wirtz, P. D.: High school basketball knee ligament injuries. J. Iowa Med. Soc. 72(3):105–106, 1982.
150. Wong, J. C., and Gregg, J. R.: Knee, ankle, and foot problems in the pre-adolescent and adolescent athlete. Clin. Podiatr. Med. Surg. 3(4):731–745, 1986.
151. Zaricznyj, B., Shattuck, L. J., Mast, T. A., Robertson, R. V., and D'Elia, G.: Sports-related injuries in school-aged children. Am. J. Sports Med. 8(5):318–324, 1980.
152. Zelisko, J. A., Noble, H. B., and Porter, M.: A comparison of men's and women's professional basketball injuries. Am. J. Sports Med. 10(5):297–299, 1982.
153. Zelko, R. R., Torg, J. S., and Rachun, A.: Proximal diaphyseal fractures of the fifth metatarsal—treatment of the fractures and their complications in athletes. Am. J. Sports Med. 7(2):95–101, 1979.
154. Zogby, R. G., and Baker, B. E.: A review of nonoperative treatment of Jones' fracture. Am. J. Sports Med. 15(4):304–307, 1987.

32
RUNNING

WILLIAM G. CLANCY, JR.

Running has often been perceived as a relatively "injury-free" sport for school-age athletes, since most running injuries are of the overuse/overload type. The strength of their youthful tissues and their less intense approach to their sport may be thought to protect children and teenagers in comparison with older runners. This perception is not precisely true. The developmental state of their growth plates makes adolescents uniquely prone to certain injuries unknown in other age groups. Furthermore, there has been an increasing emphasis on higher daily mileage for distance runners, a similar increase in the combination of interval training and overdistance running for short- and middle-distance runners, and an expanding role for endurance running in conditioning programs for athletes in other sports. These factors have combined with the greater number of school-age athletes now participating in organized running sports to increase the number of youngsters presenting to physicians with running-related injuries.[3] This chapter will discuss the injuries themselves; the physiological response of the young body to endurance training is reviewed in Chapter 1.

The loads that the lower extremity sees in running have been reported to range from three times body weight up to eight times body weight. At the time of foot impact, this load must be dissipated. Some of the load is dissipated as sheer; as the foot slides forward, the surface may absorb some load, and the sole of the shoe absorbs some of the reactive force. The lower extremity, however, must absorb most of the ground-reactive force. A significant load is probably absorbed by the bones and the joint surfaces of the ankle, knee, and hip. The muscles of the lower extremity, however, are most important in the dissipation of the resultant ground-reactive force; but muscles are poor third-class lever systems and, as such, must absorb tremendous loads in some instances. It has been reported that the quadriceps muscle may need to generate 22 times body weight at midstance during the running gait. The repetitive forces producing locomotion, in this case running, as well as the ground-reactive force must be within the viscoelastic properties of the lower extremity components or injury will occur. Variations of normal anatomy may lead to stress concentration at certain anatomical locations that may predispose to injury. Patellofemoral stress syndrome, frequently seen in the runner with excessive femoral anteversion, is an example of increased stress concentration due to a variation of normal anatomy. Excessive internal rotation of the hip produces overpronation of the foot at the midstance stage in the running gait. This creates a marked increase of the functional Q angle at the knee, which is felt to produce increased loading of the patellofemoral joint. (The Q *angle* is the angle between a line drawn from the anterior superior iliac spine to the center of the patella and a line drawn from the center of the tibial tubercle to the center of the patella.)

Injuries may also be produced by the fatigue factor. When muscles are fatigued, they lose their ability to dissipate load. Bone, tendon, and articular cartilage are then subjected to increased loading, which may produce microtears in tendon and microfractures in bone. Thus, it would appear that muscle fatigue may play a significant role in muscle strains, tendinitis, avulsion fractures, stress fractures, and joint overload. Anatomical variations, malalignment, and muscle fatigue should be considered the intrinsic factors that play a role in injury production.

Extrinsic factors that may contribute to increased risk of injury are environmental conditions and inappropriate training methods. Among the environmental factors that may predispose to injury are weather conditions, including heat, cold, humidity, and wind. Cold has a significant adverse effect on muscle flexibility and contractibility. Excessive heat may lead to inappropriate fluid and electrolyte loss, which, when combined with high humidity, adversely affects the body's ability to decrease its own temperature and thus affects muscle function.

Another environmental factor that may have an effect on injury production is the running surface. The surface that the foot impacts plays a very important part in how much of the external load will be dissipated. If the surface is somewhat soft and has a low coefficient of friction, such as grass, the foot will sink and slide slightly into the surface. In this case, the body will have to absorb less load in comparison with running on the hard, unyielding concrete or asphalt surface of a sidewalk or road. An additional deleterious factor to be considered when running on roads is the inherent drainage pitch built into them. This drainage pitch forces the runner to compensate his or her body position to maintain balance, producing increased stress concentration. Trochanteric bursitis and iliotibial band syndrome are but two examples of injuries more commonly seen in the downside leg of those who run on roads. In those cases in which the athlete may have a significant variation of normal anatomy, the resultant stress concentration may be greatly increased, producing an overuse or overload type of injury.

Inappropriate training may also predispose to injury. Overdistance training is important to improve performance, but too much overdistance training may lead to muscle fatigue and increase soft tissue loading. Excessive interval training, hill running, or running stadium steps are often associated with overuse injuries. Common sense and good coaching should be able to minimize the potential for injury.

A well-designed shoe may help decrease a runner's injury potential. Continuing attempts are being made in running shoe manufacturing to develop soles that will decrease the impact load the body must absorb.

INJURIES TO THE PELVIS, HIP, AND THIGH

OVERUSE BONY INJURIES

Iliac crest apophysitis is an inflammation of the iliac crest growth plate and probably represents microscopic stress fractures within this growth center. The inciting cause is probably the repetitive pull of the abdominal muscles that insert on the crest. The anterior one half of the iliac crest is by far the more common site of involvement. Iliac apophysitis is usually seen in the 14- to 16-year-old cross-country runner or distance runner. The athlete presents with what he or she calls "hip pain" that was gradual in onset, allowing the athlete to run for 2 or 3 weeks until the pain prevented further training. The pain is generally present only with running. On physical examination, the pain is usually located at the anterolateral pelvic brim, which is painful to palpation and with resisted abduction.

Radiographs are usually negative, but on rare occasions, a partial avulsion of the anterior iliac crest may be seen. Treatment consists of rest from running while substituting some other tolerable aerobic conditioning activity, such as biking or swimming. The usual duration of symptoms before pain-free running can be initiated is 4 to 6 weeks. Recurrence is unusual. Rarely, the posterior iliac crest may be involved, with similar findings.[5]

Osteitis pubis is more frequently seen in the adult but may occasionally be seen in the older teenager who has a very high weekly mileage training program.[2] The athlete usually presents with a prolonged history of bilateral groin (adductor) pain and little, if any, complaints of pubic pain. Palpation of the symphysis pubis, however, should produce a fair amount of pain. Since chronic proximal nontraumatic adductor tendon pain is rare in the runner, particularly the distance runner, one must always consider osteitis pubis. If the radiographs are unrevealing, a bone scan,

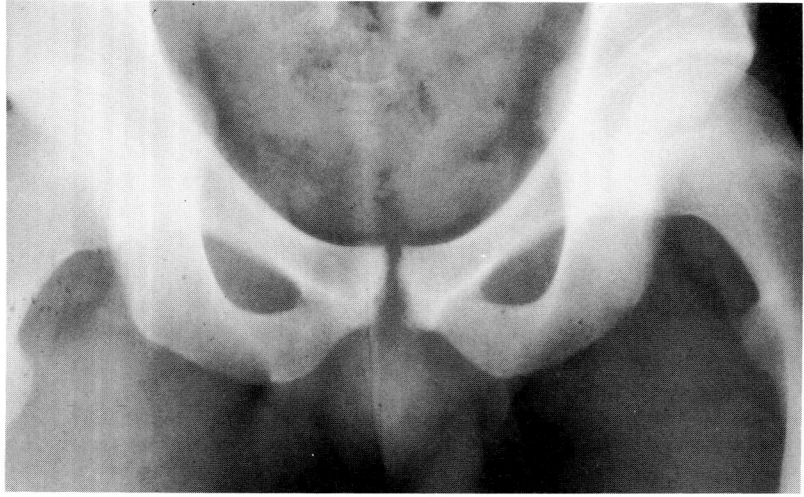
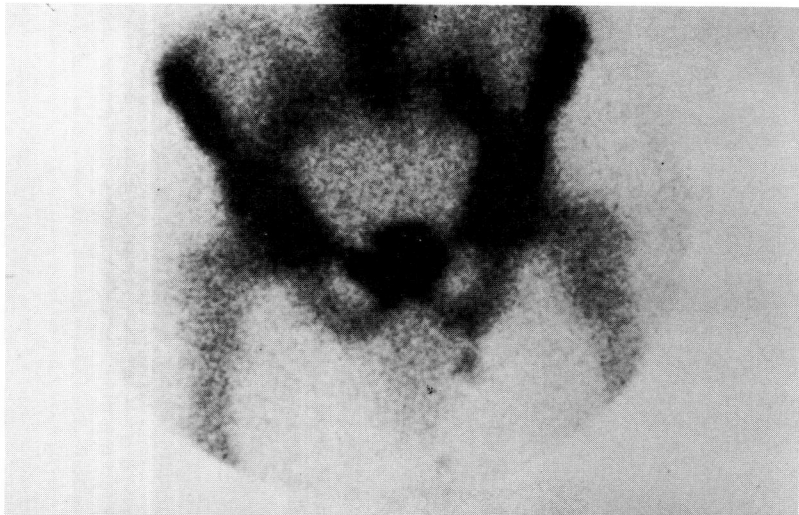

FIGURE 32–1. (*A*) Osteitis pubis may produce radiographic irregularities of the symphysis pubis. (*B*) A bone scan will show increased uptake adjacent to the symphysis.

if positive, confirms the diagnosis (Fig. 32–1). Although the exact pathology is unknown, it is thought that there is a fatigue failure within the ligament at its insertion into the pubic rami at the symphysis. Treatment of this unusual condition requires rest from training, running and bicycling. Nonsteroidal antiinflammatory drugs (NSAIDS) may reduce the pain, which can be severe. Swimming may be allowed after 6 to 12 weeks, according to the patient's response. If there is no improvement after 3 months, an injection of dexamethasone into the pubic symphysis may help.

STRESS FRACTURES

Although very uncommon, stress fractures of the *inferior pubic rami* may be seen in the late teenager and young adult. We have not seen any involving the superior rami. These patients present usually with a prolonged history of pain that may have been present for many weeks to several months.

On physical examination, the maximum area of tenderness should be located at the junction of the inferior ramus with the symphysis. The differential diagnosis would also include chronic adductor strain and osteitis pubis, but radiographic evaluation will elucidate this stress fracture if present. These fractures often take 6 months to heal sufficiently to allow a return to running. Rest from running must be maintained until the patient is asymptomatic to palpation. Any aerobic activities, such as biking or swimming with the legs restricted from kicking, are allowed if they do not produce symptoms.

Stress fractures involving the *femoral neck* have the potential for catastrophic complications and must be carefully evaluated. These fractures are usually seen in long-distance runners who are in their late teens or early adulthood. The early symptoms consist of groin pain with running and progresses to pain with activities of daily living, eventually producing an antalgic gait. Physical examination usually reveals inability to rotate the hip passively internally owing to pain and spasm.

Devas has described two types of fracture patterns that may be seen in those with femoral neck stress fractures.[11] The first type, which is more commonly seen in runners, is the compression type. The fracture appears at the medial aspect of the femoral neck and is most frequently recognized by increased bone density in this area (Fig. 32–2). The second type occurs at the lateral aspect of the femoral neck and is called a distraction or tension fracture.

The compression type of stress fracture tends to be the more stable fracture and, if there is no displacement, may be treated conservatively. The consequences of these fractures are of such great magnitude that this type of stress fracture cannot be taken lightly. The patient should be placed at bedrest until the symptoms subside; then partial weight bearing may be allowed as long as the radiographs show no ominous changes. Stationary bike riding and running in water should be initiated prior to resumption of running.

If the hip symptoms do not resolve with bedrest or if the radiographs demonstrate increased width of the fracture or any signs of displacement, then immediate internal fixation should be considered.[9] Those with the second type of stress fracture, the distraction or tension type of fracture, should be considered for immediate internal fixation, as this type of fracture has a far greater incidence of complications.

If the initial radiographs are negative but the physical examination still reveals signs of hip irritability, then a bone scan is mandatory

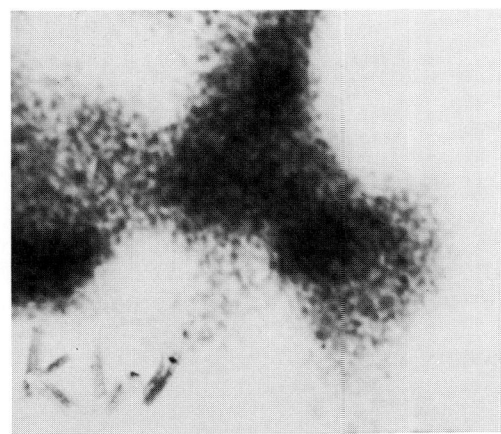

A

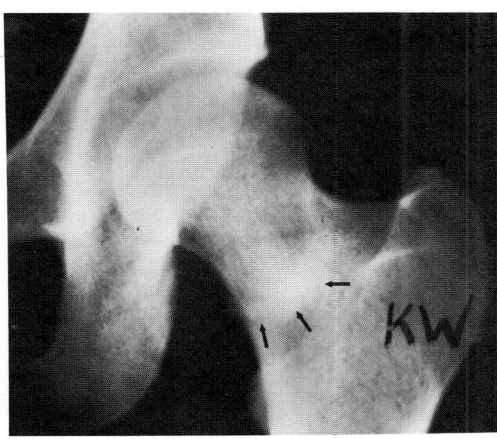

B

FIGURE 32–2. This 17-year-old female cross-country runner presented with groin and thigh pain. Initial radiographs were normal, but a bone scan (*A*) revealed an inferior femoral neck fracture. Radiographs (*B*) taken 1 month later revealed active bone formation.

tory (Fig. 32–2). If the bone scan is positive, then tomograms or a computerized tomography (CT) scan should be obtained to delineate the type of stress fracture. Treatment follows according to the type as described above.

Subtrochanteric stress fractures are rare but, when present, produce vague symptoms of upper thigh or hip pain. The pain is progressive in nature until the runner can no longer tolerate even easy jogging. Radiographs are usually negative in the early stage, but the severity of the symptoms should dictate to the physician that a bone scan is necessary.

Once diagnosed, the patient should be placed on crutches with partial weight bearing. Aerobic activity, such as swimming with both legs supported to prevent kicking, may be allowed if this is not symptomatic. One may progress to running in water when it is tolerated. When the patient's physical examination demonstrates no pain and there are no deleterious signs on the radiographs, a progressive running program is instituted.

In this author's opinion, *proximal femoral shaft stress fractures* are far more common than previously realized. The patient, usually an older teenager or young adult, presents with vague thigh pain without any history of injury. The runner usually states that he or she has a "pulled" thigh muscle even though there was no obvious history of injury. The clinician must be alert to the possibility of a femoral stress fracture whenever a runner presents with such a "muscle pull" without a history of an acute injury. Careful palpation of the bony femoral shaft will elicit marked tenderness at the site of the stress fracture. The radiographs, consisting of an anteroposterior (AP), lateral, and both obliques, may be negative at first, often taking 6 weeks to produce either periosteal or endosteal new bone formation. A bone scan should be performed in the face of negative radiographs.

These fractures heal quite readily if running is stopped. The athlete may be placed on non–weight-bearing endurance exercises, such as running in water or swimming. One may resume training when there is no pain with palpation. The usual amount of time for healing and return to running is 10 to 12 weeks from the date of onset of symptoms. Recurrence is unusual.

AVULSION FRACTURES

Acute avulsion fractures always occur through the apophyses, which are the sites of tendon insertion or origin. They characteristically occur in older adolescents who are approaching the age of apophyseal closure: 11 to 14 years in girls, 12 to 15 years in boys. Clinically, it appears that the apophysis is weaker than the muscle-tendon unit at this age.

Anterior superior iliac spine avulsion fractures occur at the insertion site of the sartorius muscle. The avulsion is the result of excessive contraction of the sartorius muscle. Frequently, this fragment is displaced, but there is seldom a need to anatomically reduce and fix this avulsion unless there is a dramatic amount of displacement. The athlete is placed on crutches until he or she can walk without pain. Stationary bike riding is usually tolerated by the third week. It usually takes 4 to 6 weeks for adequate bony union to allow resumption of running (Fig. 32–3).

The *anterior inferior iliac spine* serves as one of the sites for the rectus femoris muscle attachment. Avulsions of this attachment site are less common than avulsions of the anterior superior iliac spine. The most common mechanism of injury is a fall backward after landing from a jump. There is a maximum contraction of the rectus femoris muscle to maintain balance. Rarely is the apophysis greatly displaced. The athlete usually presents with severe hip pain, which must be differentiated from an acute slipped capital femoral epiphysis, a dislocated hip, or even the rare femoral neck fracture.

Surgical intervention is rarely necessary. This avulsion will heal with bony union in most cases in 6 weeks. Some cases will heal with a strong, fibrous union that seldom leads to problems with sports in the future.

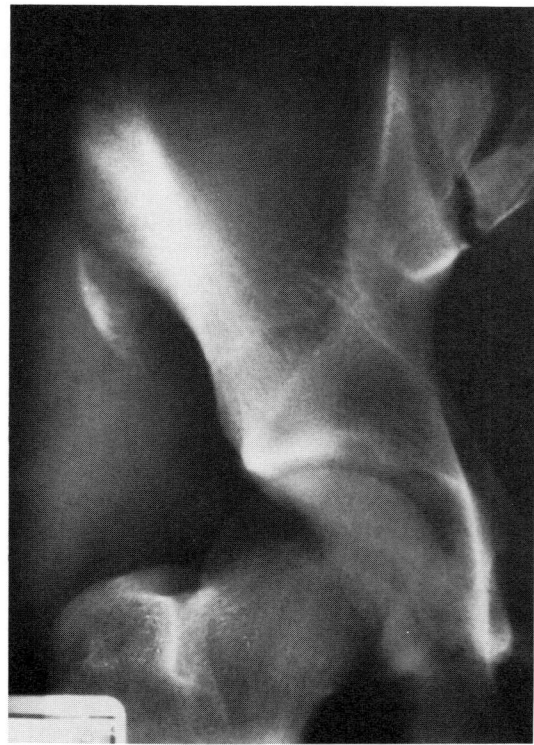

FIGURE 32–3. Avulsion fracture of the anterior superior iliac spine.

The *ischial apophysis* is the main attachment site of the majority of the hamstring musculature. When there is maximum contraction of the quadriceps against unrelaxed and fatigued hamstrings, overload may occur, not at the muscle-tendon junction (the usual site of a muscle strain) but at the growth plate, causing an acute fracture.

In some cases, the growth plate may become significantly displaced and, when so displaced, usually warrants surgical fixation to prevent long-term muscle weakness and/or chronic pain from a pseudoarthrosis or bony prominence on sitting. Usually screw fixation is adequate. Bone healing takes approximately 8 weeks before an aerobic and weight training program can be initiated.

Chronic unrecognized and/or untreated displaced ischial apophyseal avulsion fractures may become quite painful owing to either a massive overgrowth of the apophysis, which is probably a result of fracture hyperemia, or painful micromotion at the fibrous union between the fragment and the pelvis. If this is severely disabling, then surgical intervention may be required. In these cases, there is usually adequate insertion of the hamstrings into the ischium remaining so that simple resection of the fragment may be performed. If there is minimal insertion into the main part of the ischium remaining, internal fixation of the fragment with bone grafting is necessary.

DISORDERS OF THE HIP JOINT

On rare occasions, the athlete may present with hip pain with some loss of hip internal rotation and hip abduction. The differential diagnosis must include slipped capital femoral epiphysis, a femoral neck stress fracture, or a hip joint infection. When the roentgenograms and bone scan are negative, the diagnosis is usually classified as hip joint synovitis. The long-term sequela of this is unknown.

It is of interest that two retrospective studies have shown no correlation between runners and the incidence of late osteoarthritis. Sohn and Micheli's retrospective study of 504 former cross-country runners as compared with a control group of 287 college varsity swimmers found that there was no association between running at moderate levels and the development of osteoarthritis.[21] Puranen et al. found that there was no increase in the incidence of hip osteoarthritis in the older, former elite, Finnish distance runners, who were compared with a similar-aged control nonrunning group.[16]

Slipped capital femoral epiphysis (SCFE) is seldom seen in the school-age runner. However, because it is common in adolescents, the clinician should always keep this in mind in the youngster presenting with groin, thigh, or knee pain. More advanced cases of SCFE will be marked by an external rotation contracture at the hip.

Hip synovitis as a direct result of running is probably an extremely rare entity. There are numerous conditions, as noted previously, that may appear to be located about the hip that, on careful evaluation, are not truly hip joint pain. Iliopsoas tendinitis, chronic adductor tendinitis, and rectus femoris strain are but a few of the potential injuries confused with hip joint synovitis. If true hip joint synovitis is present, one must carefully evaluate for such conditions as femoral neck stress fracture, an intraarticular loose body, slipped capital femoral epiphysis, or Legg-Calvé-Perthes disease.

MUSCLE STRAINS

Muscle strains represent a tear in the muscle-tendon complex and usually occur at the muscle-tendon junction or occasionally at the muscle-tendinous origin from the bone. Although the exact mechanism of failure is still debated, it is theorized that the antagonist muscle or muscle group (usually the stronger muscle) undergoes a very forceful contraction while the affected muscle is still in the contraction phase, stretching the contracted muscle to the point of injury.

Among the thigh muscle groups, the *hamstrings* are most frequently strained, followed by the adductors and quadriceps groups. Approximately half of the injuries seen in the hamstrings appear to occur near the proximal muscle-tendon origin at the pelvis. Pain and tenderness may at first be diffuse but should localize within 24 hours to the proximal muscle mass. Ecchymosis may be noted at the gluteal fold but is more commonly seen in the popliteal fossa several days after the initial injury. The reason the ecchymosis is noted so distally is due to the migration of the extravasated blood by dependent drainage during standing.

Injury to the *adductor* muscles is seen

more commonly in hurdlers, jumpers, and field event athletes than the runner, probably owing to the marked rotational forces produced in these events. The adductor longus muscle appears to be the more common injury site.

The rectus femoris muscle is the most frequent muscle to be injured among the *quadriceps*. Injury to this muscle group is more commonly seen in sprinters and hurdlers.

Treatment of acute muscle strains consists of ice, compression, and elevation for the first 48 hours. The athlete should also be placed on crutches until he or she can ambulate without a limp. Early aggressive stretching should be avoided until the reactive muscle spasm has abated. After 48 hours, moist heat is utilized several times a day, followed by gentle passive stretching and proprioceptive neuromuscular facilitation (PNF). Eccentric muscle strengthening programs are initiated when most of the muscle soreness has abated.

TENDINITIS

In this section, the term *tendinitis* refers to injury to both the tendon and tendon sheath. These injuries are for the most part an overuse/overload fatigue failure within the tendon.

Iliopsoas tendinitis is quite rare but does occur. The patient's symptoms are located deep in the groin, medial and slightly inferior to the femoral head. Deep palpation may produce pain with the hip in external rotation, but the pain disappears with internal rotation. This test should help differentiate this entity from the iliopectineal bursitis or a pectineal muscle strain.

Some patients have a painful, snapping hip that, in reality, is the iliopsoas tendon snapping over the femoral head when the hip rotates from internal to external rotation on hip flexion. Magnetic resonance imaging (MRI) may delineate a significantly enlarged iliopsoas tendon when compared with the opposite side.

Proximal hamstring tendinitis may present with disabling buttock pain. Chronic buttock pain is a problematic but fortunately very uncommon entity seen almost exclusively in distance runners. These athletes complain of deep, vague buttock pain. Palpation reveals that the tenderness is rather consistently located at or near the hamstring tendon insertion into the ischium. The entity must be differentiated from even rarer conditions that have been described to produce buttock pain, such as inferior gluteal artery syndrome, sciatic nerve entrapment, and strains of the short hip external rotators.

Treatment of this tendinitis consists of refraining from the overloading activity and substituting some other nonloading aerobic activity. The athlete is placed on an appropriate flexibility and eccentric strength training program. Antiinflammatory medication is also indicated. When the involved area is no longer tender, a graduated running program is initiated.

BURSITIS

Patients with *trochanteric bursitis* most frequently complain of "hip pain." When asked to point to the area of pain, they delineate their greater trochanteric area as the location of their pain. The entity consists of an inflamed trochanteric bursa and is clinically evident by the fact that their symptoms are present only when the hip moves from full extension to flexion. If the hip is moved only from neutral to flexion, their pain cannot be reproduced. The patients will seldom have the same pain bicycling that they do running, since bicycling does not require as much hip extension.

Clinically, the pain can be reproduced by placing the patient on his or her side with the affected hip upward. The patient then actively moves the lower leg and hip from full extension to 30 degrees of flexion while the examiner places the palm of his or her hand on the greater trochanter. As the hip goes from flexion to extension, the patient should note pain. Frequently, the examiner will feel a pop or snap as the leg goes into flexion. This snap is the iliotibial tract passing over the prominence of the greater trochanter. Some patients demonstrate poor flexibility of the tensor fascia lata and gluteus maximus muscles, producing a tight iliotibial band that can produce significant friction as it passes over the greater trochanter. These patients will frequently have a positive Ober test.[23]

Treatment consists of removing the athlete from running and placing him or her on aerobic activities that prevent the hip from going into extension, such as bicycling or swimming. An iliotibial band stretching program is also initiated. Antiinflammatory medication is recommended for 3 to 4 weeks to help resolve the inflamed bursa. Injection of a soluble steroid is indicated in those who have had a poor response to the initial treatment.

In those rare cases recalcitrant to all treatment, surgical treatment may be indicated. Surgery consists of resection of that portion of the iliotibial band that snaps over the greater trochanter as well as resection of the chronically inflamed bursa.[23]

Ischial bursitis is quite rare but must be distinguished from the more common problem, that being tendinitis of the proximal hamstrings as they insert into the ischium. This entity should resolve quite readily by refraining from prolonged sitting, initiating a flexibility program, and treating the patient with NSAIDS.

KNEE INJURIES

STRESS FRACTURES

Mid- and distal femoral shaft stress fractures are not rare in long-distance runners. The athlete usually complains of vague, poorly localized pain proximal to the knee joint that may be medial or lateral. Not infrequently, this is diagnosed as a quadriceps muscle strain. It is important to note that distal quadriceps muscle strains are quite rare. It has been our principle that vague mid- or distal thigh pain is a stress fracture until proven otherwise (Fig. 32–4).

Radiographs frequently take 6 weeks or longer to demonstrate any periosteal or endosteal changes but should still be obtained. If the initial films are negative, a bone scan should be considered. If there is a stress fracture, the bone scan will delineate it clearly. The athlete is then placed on a nonloading aerobic swimming or biking program as tolerated. It usually takes 6 to 10 weeks from the date that symptoms started before the patient is capable of resuming a running program.

Proximal tibial stress fractures are more common than distal femoral stress fractures and are almost always located on the posterior medial cortex. Often the athlete presents with what appears to be pes anserinus tendinitis or pes bursitis. Both of these entities are rare, and a proximal tibial stress fracture should be the more likely diagnosis.

The average time that asymptomatic running can be resumed varies between 6 and 8 weeks from the onset of symptoms. Usually, the athlete has been training for 2 or 3 weeks with increasing symptoms before running becomes intolerable. Aerobic training can be continued either with an exercise bicycle or running in water. Once the area of the stress fracture is no longer tender, running is begun on a graduated, every-other-day basis for 1 to 2 weeks. If the area becomes symptomatic, running is held for 1 more additional week.

KNEE JOINT PAIN

It is indeed rare for running to produce a knee effusion. If an athlete presents with a true effusion, a complete knee evaluation is mandatory. The common causes of this unusual presentation without any prior history of trauma would include osteochondritis dissecans, loose body, symptomatic patellar subluxation, or a significant articular surface lesion.

All younger adolescent school-age athletes presenting with knee pain must also be evaluated for hip pathology, particularly slipped capital femoral epiphysis.

Anterior knee pain is by far the most common type of knee pain seen in runners; it usually appears to arise from the patellofemoral joint. This syndrome is frequently referred to in the lay literature as "runner's knee." This entity in most cases should be more properly called *patellofemoral stress syndrome*. There are usually only a few findings on clinical evaluation. The most common and almost universal finding is tenderness of the medial facet or undersurface of the patella. Patellofemoral stress syndrome is frequently associated with an increased functional Q angle. The term *functional* Q angle is most important because most physicians evaluate only the static Q angle. A static Q angle consists of the angle formed by drawing a line from the anterior superior iliac spine to the center of the patella and then connecting this point to a line drawn down the center of the patellar tendon to the tibial tubercle.[2] These measurements are frequently made with the patient lying supine and the patella centered and pointing to the ceiling. Unfortunately, if the patient has femoral anteversion or if there is significant foot pronation present, one will not note the marked increase in the functional Q angle. The functional Q angle should be measured while the patient is standing, or if supine, the feet are

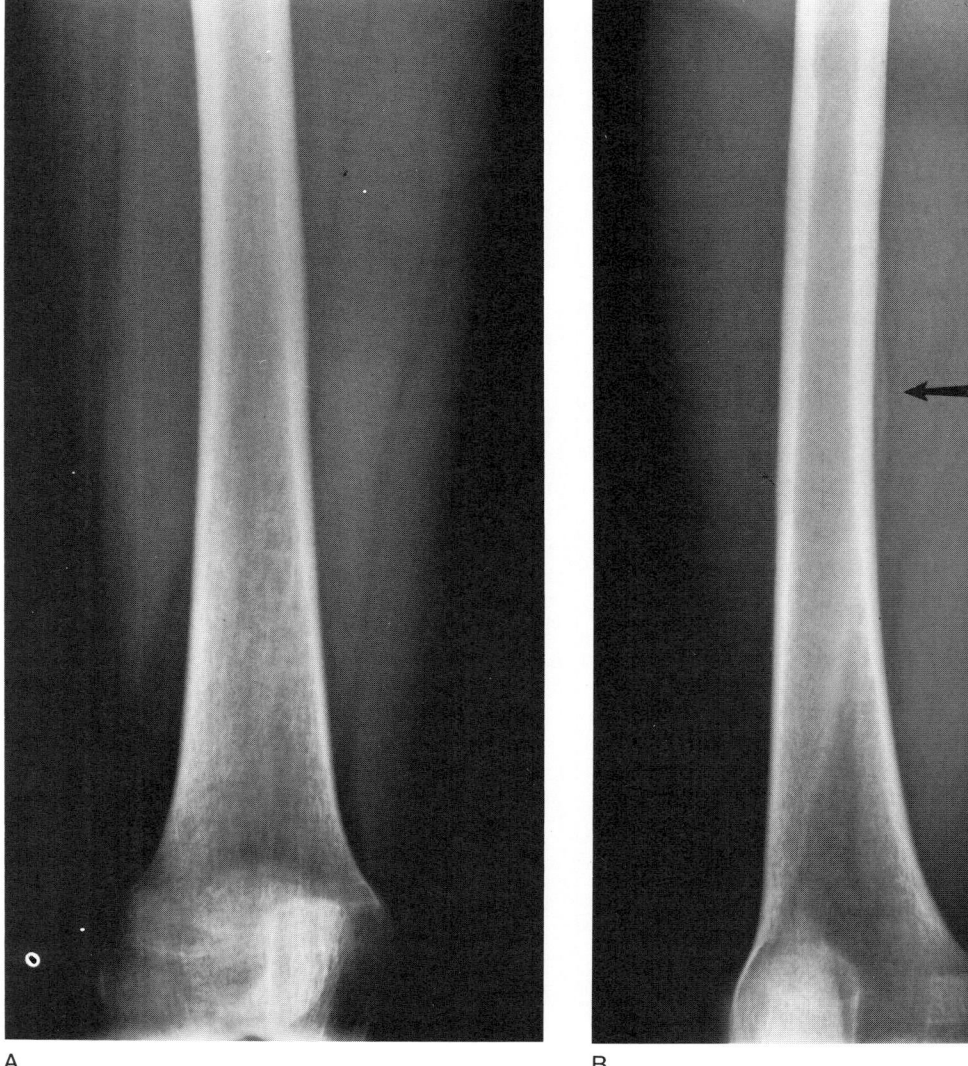

FIGURE 32–4. (A) AP and (B) oblique radiographs of the femur of an 18-year-old female cross-country runner 1 month after the onset of thigh pain. Because the periosteal reaction usually only involves one cortex, it is important to obtain several views.

maximally dorsiflexed with the great toes pointed directly at the patient's nose.

These athletes frequently have little muscle atrophy and rarely benefit from the quadriceps weight training programs that are important in those patients with chondromalacia patella associated with atrophic or disuse quadriceps weakness. Flexibility measurements are important, as we have noted that a number of these patients have marked tightness of their rectus femoris as evidenced when passive knee flexion is performed while the patient is placed prone to maintain the hip in extension (the Ely test).

Treatment is designed to quiet down the patellofemoral symptoms while correcting or alleviating any mechanical malalignment if present. For those with femoral anteversion and/or significant foot pronation, a flexible leather or semirigid orthotic with a $\frac{1}{8}$-inch medial heel wedge is prescribed to be worn in their everyday shoes. When running is resumed, the orthotics are also placed in their running shoes.

There are a number of other causes of anterior knee pain that are dealt with in Chapter 20.

Posterior knee pain, although not common, is not rare. The most common injury is that of a medial or lateral *gastrocnemius muscle strain* at the distal femoral origin site. Although the athlete may complain of just posterior pain, after a careful knee examination with the hip and knee flexed to 90 degrees, the pain will be located either posteromedially or posterolaterally.

Other causes of posteromedial knee pain to be considered are *proximal tibial stress fracture* and *semimembranosus tendinitis*.[17] The causes of posterolateral knee pain include several very rare entities: popliteus tendinitis, biceps tendinitis, bursitis of the biceps bursa over the fibular collateral ligament, and the fabellar syndrome. A tear of the medial or lateral meniscus without a prior history of trauma is very rare in this age group; however, one must consider the possibility of a torn discoid lateral meniscus. Radiographs may help rule out this entity.

Treatment of gastrocnemius strains consists of rest during the acute phase of the injury and the initiation of gentle static stretching exercises. The role of antiinflammatory medication is controversial but clinically seems warranted in those with persistent symptoms. Once there is no tenderness, a weight training program is begun, and a graduated running program is developed for the athlete.

Lateral knee pain in runners is most commonly a manifestation of *iliotibial band syndrome*, although it is occasionally caused by popliteus tendinitis. Iliotibial band syndrome has been considered by many to be a bursitis, but it may be a combination of a bursitis and a tendinitis due to mechanical friction on the iliotibial band by the lateral femoral epicondyle.[18] The iliotibial band may be considered a continuation of the tendinous portions of the tensor fascia lata and the gluteus maximus muscles. As this band or tract passes laterally over the knee joint to insert on the proximal lateral aspect of the tibia, it is fixed to the intermuscular septum at the distal femur by Kaplan's fibers. Kaplan's fibers create a tenodesis effect on the iliotibial tract, producing a taut band over the lateral femoral epicondyle with flexion and extension of the knee. When there is persistent and excessive varus force on the knee, this band becomes even more taut. Since many runners utilize the side of a road for their distance training, the drainage pitch of the road forces the downside knee into excessive varus in order to maintain the body's balance. There appears, in our experience, to be a high correlation between the side with the injury and the side of the road habitually chosen for running. Trochanteric bursitis, essentially the same entity in the proximal lateral thigh, appears to have the same biomechanical and clinical correlations.

On physical examination, the only consistent finding in those with iliotibial band syndrome is tenderness over the lateral femoral epicondyle made worse when the iliotibial band passes over it. The Ober test for a tight iliotibial tract is frequently positive in these patients.

Treatment consists of prohibiting the athlete from running until the area is no longer tender. An iliotibial tract stretching program is begun along with a course of treatment with nonsteroidal antiinflammatory medication. It usually takes a minimum of 6 weeks of rest from running before symptoms or tenderness resolve. In rare cases—that is, when prolonged treatment has failed to resolve the symptoms—the iliotibial tract that passes directly over the lateral femoral epicondyle with flexion and extension is resected along with the underlying bursa.[12]

Popliteus tendinitis, considered by some to be common, has been a very rare cause of lateral knee pain in our experience.[13] Symptoms are produced or aggravated by running down hills. If the symptoms are very mild and clinical evaluation fails to delineate any other cause for the symptoms, the athlete is treated with rest from running but allowed to bicycle and swim. Once there is no tenderness, a running prescription is developed. Antiinflammatory medication and treatment with ultrasound may be beneficial.

Biceps tendinitis is also very uncommon. The athlete complains of vague lateral knee pain that on examination is consistently located at the proximal portion of the fibular head just where the superficial portion of the biceps femoris tendon courses over the most distal portion of the fibular collateral ligament. This entity probably represents a bursitis and not a tendinitis. Injection of Xylocaine into this bursa usually produces immediate relief of pain.

Treatment consists of a course of nonsteroidal antiinflammatory medication or an injection into the bursal area with a soluble short-acting corticosteroid. A complete cessation of running is not necessary.

INJURIES TO THE LOWER LEG AND ANKLE

STRESS FRACTURES

The tibia and fibula are subjected to great repetitive tensile forces during running, and either one may develop a stress fracture. In the author's experience, the *fibular stress fracture* is the most common lower extremity stress fracture in the school-age runner. Persistent soft tissue injury to the muscles around the fibula is rare. Therefore, whenever pain and tenderness have been present around the fibula for 2 weeks or more, a fibular stress fracture is the most likely diagnosis. Unfortunately, it takes approximately 3 weeks for the radiographs to demonstrate any periosteal callus (Fig. 22–30). Frequently, this callus is not demonstrated in the standard anteroposterior and lateral films but is evident only on an oblique film. Thus, it is necessary to order additional oblique films on all suspected stress fractures of the femur, tibia, and fibula. If it is necessary to establish the diagnosis earlier than 3 weeks after the onset of pain, a bone scan should be obtained. A positive bone scan should theoretically be present within 24 hours after the stress fracture becomes clinically evident. Any hot spots noted on the scan that are not related to clinical symptoms are considered by the author as areas of subclinical stress reaction. When an asymptomatic hot spot is noted, the patient is monitored by clinical examination for several weeks, but his or her training is not altered. The only exception would be a hot spot in the femoral neck. Tomograms or a CT scan should be obtained in this case to determine whether or not there was any evidence of an early stress fracture.

The most common location for stress fractures of the fibula in runners is the distal fibula just proximal to the lateral malleolus. Not infrequently, this stress fracture is misdiagnosed as peroneal tendinitis. This is not the site for peroneal tendinitis, which usually occurs between the base of the fifth metatarsal and the distal tip of the fibula. The second most common site for stress fractures is the midfibula, with the proximal fibula the third and least common site.

Treatment of a fibular stress fracture, regardless of the location, consists of refraining from running but allowing normal walking activity. Bicycling, swimming, and running in water are allowed. When there is no tenderness at the fracture site, a graduated running program is begun. The average time to return to running is 6 to 8 weeks from the date of onset of symptoms and does not appear to be related to how long the athlete ran with the stress fracture.

Tibial stress fractures must be distinguished from other causes of lower leg pain in runners including exercise-induced compartment syndrome and the more common "shin splint" syndrome. A careful clinical examination should differentiate these three entities. A tibial stress fracture should have a small focal area of point tenderness, whereas anterior tibial shin splints will produce tenderness over almost the entire length of the tibia but not the anterior muscles themselves. Patients with chronic anterior compartment syndrome will have their greatest amount of tenderness in the adjacent muscles with little or no tenderness of the anterolateral tibial crest. The most common location for tibial stress fractures is the posteromedial cortex of the distal one third of the tibia (Fig. 32–5).

Treatment consists of rest from running, but normal walking activities are allowed without crutches unless the athlete has severe pain. Bicycling, swimming, and running in water are allowed. Running may be resumed on a graduated basis when there is no longer any tenderness of the stress fracture site. The average time back to running is usually between 6 and 8 weeks from the onset of symptoms.

Anterior tibial crest stress fracture is a very rare entity in the school-age athlete but does occur. The patient complains of anterior tibial crest pain that is very well localized. Radiographs could confirm the entity, showing a lucent transverse line at the site of the tenderness. The length of time necessary for healing in this case is difficult to predict and is frequently prolonged. Often the symptoms abate, but the radiographs still demonstrate that complete healing has not taken place. In these cases, a more rigorous treatment program is necessary, and this usually consists of electromagnetic bone stimulation.

MUSCLE STRAINS

Of all the muscle strains that occur in the lower leg, most involve only the gastroc-

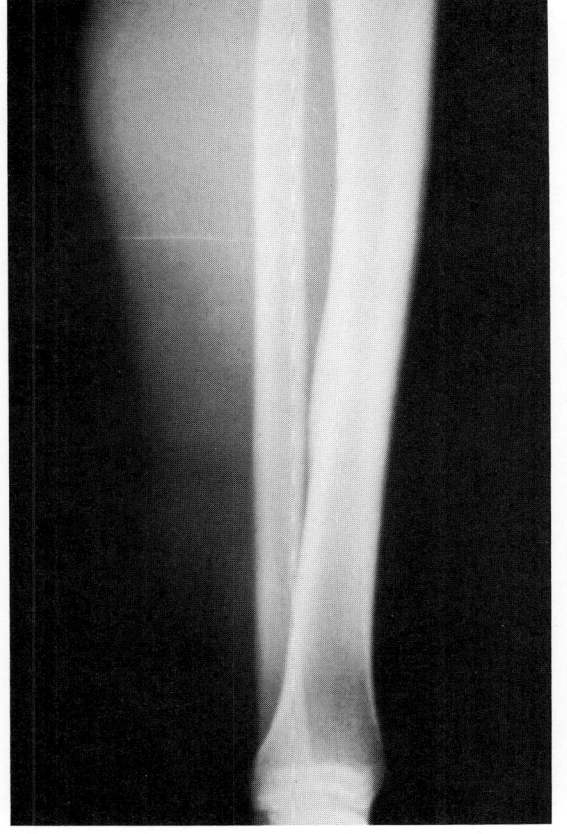
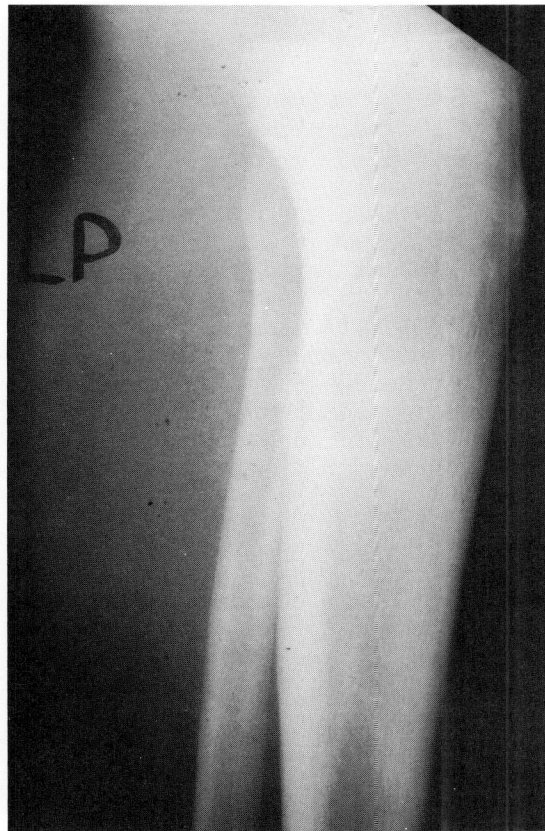
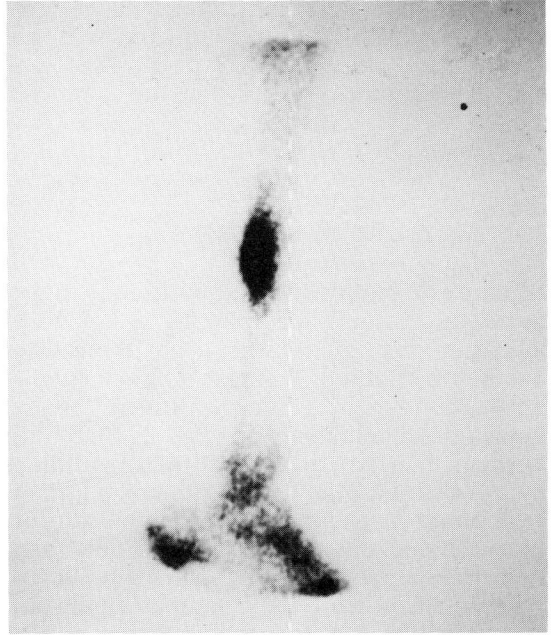

FIGURE 32–5. Midshaft fracture of the tibia seen on (A) radiographs and (B) bone scan. (C) Shows a relatively unusual fracture of the proximal tibial shaft.

nemius and/or soleus. The two sites of injury are the proximal muscle-tendon junction just distal to the origin on the femur and the distal muscle-tendon junction in the posterior proximal calf. The proximal injury has already been discussed. The distal strain is the more common injury and is seen almost exclusively in the sprinter or field event athlete. The athlete usually feels a sharp, stabbing pain or a tearing sensation in his or her calf.

In the past, this entity was thought, at least in some cases, to be a rupture of the plantaris, but it is in reality a tear of the medial head of the gastrocnemius. Rarely is there ever a complete tear and surgery is rarely, if ever, indicated. Cast immobilization, once the accepted mode of treatment, is also unnecessary.

All strains are treated with an early functional rehabilitation program. The functional treatment is progressed according to the athlete's response to the program as described above under thigh strains. This program utilizes ice, compression, and immobilization during the first 48 to 72 hours, followed by the initiation of range-of-motion exercises, both active and active assisted, and a gentle static stretching program. Once these activities are tolerated, a progressive resistance weight program is initiated emphasizing eccentric training. A graduated running program is then begun.

SHIN SPLINTS

Shin splints is a traditional term used to describe any pain located at or about the anterior tibial crest.[7, 10, 19] Over the past few years, a great deal of attention has been paid to anterior tibial pain in the runner, and as a result, anterior tibial pain has been divided into those with tibial stress fractures, those with chronic compartment syndromes, and those with a combined mild muscle strain and shin splints.

Shin splints probably represent a fatigue tear of the collagen fibers that are the bridging connection of the muscle fibers to bone. If a bone scan is performed on those with severe chronic shin splints, a large area of the tibial crest will show increased uptake. This diffuse uptake pattern is quite different from the focal increase in uptake seen in those with tibial stress fractures.

By careful clinical examination, one should be able to differentiate these entities in the majority of cases. If a tibial stress fracture is present, palpation should demonstrate that the maximum area of tenderness is very well localized and that there is no tenderness of the muscle. If a chronic compartment syndrome is present, the maximal area of tenderness will be the muscle itself, particularly near its attachment to the tibia but not immediately adjacent. Those with shin splints will have marked tenderness of a large area medial to the tibial crest with tenderness of the immediately adjacent muscle.

Shin splints are usually seen in the inexperienced younger runner early in his or her training program.[1] Excessive pronation also appears to contribute to the problem in some athletes. If the runner is a well-trained distance runner who has had similar episodes in the past, one must first consider that the athlete has a chronic compartment syndrome.

Treatment depends on the severity of the symptoms and should be initiated only after the more serious potential diagnoses have been eliminated. In those with mild shin splint symptoms, their mileage should be decreased, and if they are running on hard surfaces, they should switch to grass or another soft surface. If they have excessive pronation, a flexible orthotic with a $\frac{1}{8}$-inch medial heel lift is placed in their running shoes. Stretching and eccentric weight training programs are initiated and possibly a course of nonsteroidal antiinflammatory medication. Those with severe symptoms are placed in a nonimpact aerobic activity and held from running until there is no tenderness of the involved area. Treatment is otherwise the same as above.

EXERCISE-INDUCED COMPARTMENT SYNDROMES

There are four muscle compartments in the lower leg; the anterior, the lateral, the deep posterior, and the superficial posterior. The muscles contained in these compartments are surrounded by a thick wall of relatively inelastic fascia. When muscles in the compartment heat up, as they do with running, they expand. The compartments' fascial walls must also expand to compensate for the increased volume. If they cannot, then the intracompartmental pressure greatly increases. In acute traumatic compartment syndromes, this pressure often increases to a level that can cause necrosis of nerves, muscles, and other sensitive tissues. In exercise-induced compartment syndromes, permanent injury is rare; the pressure buildup is usually slow and painful enough that the runner ceases the inciting activity, and the pressure drops before irreversible damage occurs.

The athletes' history is usually quite characteristic. They are experienced runners who have had similar episodes of pain in the past necessitating layoff from running for several weeks. Physical examination reveals that the site of maximum tenderness is the muscle and not the tibial insertion site, which, on occasion, may also exhibit some tenderness. Confirmation also may be obtained by taking intracompartmental pressures after 15 minutes of sustained running. Pressure readings 5 minutes postexercise of over 30 mm of mercury are diagnostic, and those between 20 and 30 mm of mercury are highly suspicious.[8, 10, 14] Treatment consists of stretching and eccentric and concentric weight training of the involved muscle group or of operative release and partial resection of the entire length of the involved fascial covering.

TENDINITIS

The term *tendinitis* is frequently utilized to signify pain in or about a tendon and is thought by many to mean inflammation only of the tendon sheath. Tendinitis in the runner more frequently represents a fatigue microscopic injury to the tendon itself with a secondarily induced inflammation within the surrounding tendon sheath. In some cases though, only the tendon sheath is injured without any involvement of the tendon. It is virtually impossible, however, to differentiate clinically in the acute situation just which entity is present.

Parontendinitis is the term utilized to describe inflammation of only the tendon sheath. In the past, the terms *tenovaginitis*, *tenosynovitis*, and *peritendinitis* were utilized to describe inflammation of the tendon sheath, depending on whether there was a synovial lining (tenosynovitis) or no synovial lining (tenovaginitis).

Tendinosus is a term utilized by Puddu et al. to describe asymptomatic degeneration within the tendon.[15] In those athletes in which spontaneous tendon rupture had occurred without prior symptoms, histological studies clearly demonstrated numerous areas of marked focal degeneration/necrosis without an inflammatory response. Why these areas of focal necrosis did not stimulate an inflammatory response and clinical symptoms is poorly understood.

Parontendinitis with tendinosus is the entity that is found at the time of biopsy on review of most of the reported cases in the literature as well as our own cases of so-called chronic tendinitis. The term *tendinitis* should refer to those instances when both the tendon and the sheath are inflamed. Actual tendon inflammation is seldom seen histologically except in those with gross partial or complete tendon ruptures.

Achilles tendinitis is the most common of all the tendon problems seen in the school-age runner. The athlete in the acute stage presents usually with crepitance over the distal portion of the tendon with motion. Tenderness is quite severe and is usually located two to three finger breadths above the superior edge of the calcaneus. The crepitance usually lasts for 4 to 5 days. Those with chronic Achilles tendinitis rarely have any crepitance present but may have nodularity at these areas, either readily visible or noted on palpation. Gross enlargement of the tendon strongly indicates a partial rupture. Achilles tendinitis must be differentiated from retrocalcaneal bursitis and pre-Achilles bursitis (Table 32–1) (Fig. 32–6).

Treatment of acute Achilles tendinitis consists of complete abstinence from running; however, swimming or bicycling without toe clips may be allowed if there is no pain during or afterward. A $\frac{1}{2}$-inch heel lift is placed in the shoe during daily activity. Heel cord stretching and eccentric strengthening exercises are begun as well as a nonsteroidal anti-inflammatory medication. Steroid injection

TABLE 32–1. Causes of Pain About the Ankle and Foot in Runners

Lateral	Distal fibula stress fracture
	Peroneal tendinitis
Posterior	Achilles tendinitis
	Retrocalcaneal bursitis
Posteromedial	Retrocalcaneal bursitis
	Calcaneal apophysitis
	Achilles tendinitis
Medial	Posterior tibial tendinitis
	Accessory navicular
	Medial malleolus stress fracture
Anteromedial	Navicular stress fracture
Plantar	Plantar fasciitis
	Sesamoid injuries

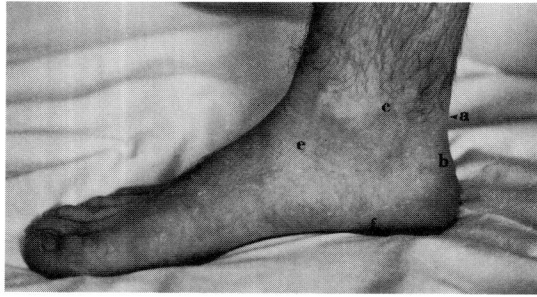

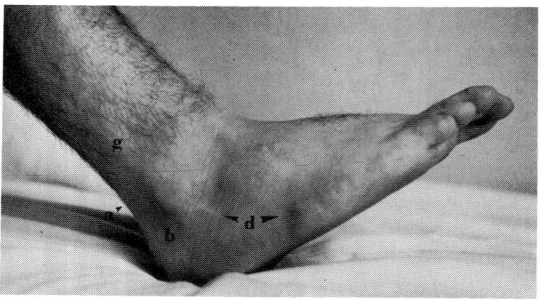

FIGURE 32–6. Sites of tenderness in (*a*) Achilles tendinitis, (*b*) retrocalcaneal bursitis, (*c*) posterior tibial tendinitis, (*d*) peroneal tendinitis, (*e*) accessory navicular pseudoarthrosis, (*f*) plantar fasciitis, and (*g*) fibular stress fracture. (*A*) Medial view. (*B*) Lateral view.

or oral cortisone administration is not indicated. Symptoms of pain with activities and to palpation should abate within 2 to 3 weeks but on occasion may take up to 6 weeks to resolve. Casting or immobilization is rarely indicated.

Those with subacute or chronic symptoms are treated initially as those with acute symptoms; however, it usually requires a minimum of 6 weeks of treatment for the symptoms to subside before painless running can be resumed. When symptoms persist, even with the most rigid treatment program, for greater than 6 months, surgical intervention should be considered. If there is a suggestion of a gross partial rupture, an MRI should be obtained, and if confirmed, surgery should be the treatment of choice. Surgical treatment should never consist of only a decompression of the tendon sheath. Tendon exploration is mandatory both to define any gross in-substance partial rupture and to stimulate an acute healing reaction.[4, 6] It is extremely unlikely, however, that surgery would be necessary for Achilles tendinitis in the school-age runner.

Posterior tibial tendinitis is a far less common entity than Achilles tendinitis and is associated with heavy mileage training and/or significant foot pronation. Pain is almost always located just behind the medial malleolus (Fig. 32–6). Treatment is essentially the same as that for Achilles tendinitis except a flexible leather or semirigid orthotic with a $\frac{1}{8}$-inch medial heel wedge is worn daily during both activities of daily living and on resumption of running. In rare cases, those with what appears to be posterior tibial tendinitis have a stress fracture of the medial malleolus, and this must be kept in mind (Table 32–1).

Peroneal tendinitis is a rare entity whose symptoms are usually present between the insertion of the peroneus brevis at the base of the fifth metatarsal and the inferior tip of the lateral malleolus (Fig. 32–6). Pain in and about the peroneal tendons more proximal to the tip of the fibula is almost always a fibular stress fracture (Table 32–1). Treatment for peroneal tendinitis is essentially the same as utilized for Achilles tendinitis.

INJURIES TO THE FOOT

STRESS FRACTURES

Navicular stress fractures, though uncommon, do occur more frequently than suspected in runners (Table 32–1). Usually, the athlete presents with vague and diffuse midtarsal pain that may also be lateral in nature. As there are very few entities that can produce midtarsal pain, it has been our opinion that this symptom complex should be treated as a navicular stress fracture until proven otherwise. A bone scan will delineate whether a navicular stress fracture is present (Fig. 32–7). If the bone scan is positive, a CT scan should be performed to demonstrate the fracture and for subsequent evaluations of bony union, as the bone scan will remain positive for up to a year even if the bone is healed. The patient should be treated in a short leg, non–weight-bearing cast until union is well established. Failure to recognize a navicular stress fracture may lead to the difficult problem of nonunion.

Metatarsal stress fractures are quite common and may initially present as though the athlete has extensor tenosynovitis. Careful palpation of the entire length of each metatarsal shaft will reveal that the maximum area of

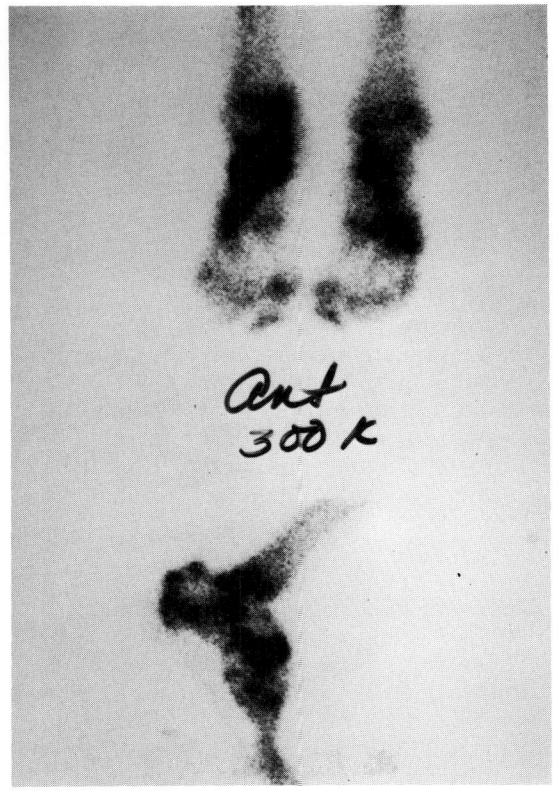 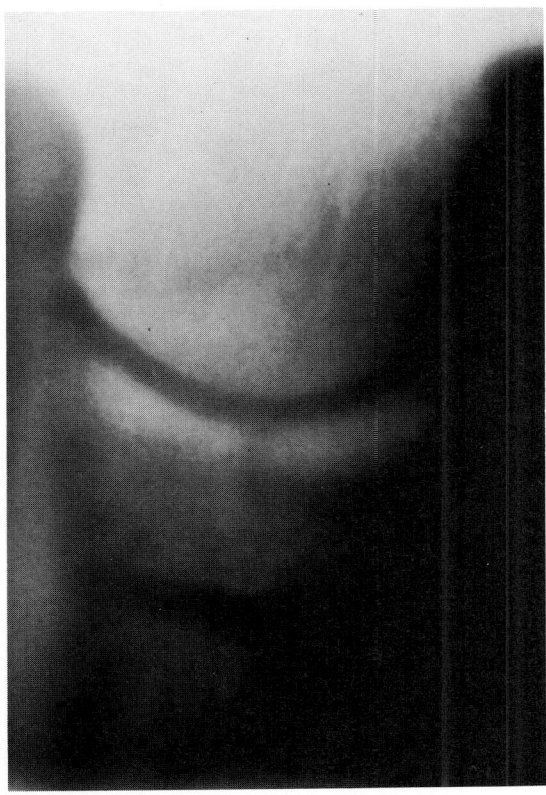

FIGURE 32–7. (*A*) Bone scan of a runner with 3 weeks of vague midfoot pain shows the intense uptake in the navicular typical of a stress fracture. (*B*) Tomogram after 6 weeks of treatment shows the fracture to be healing but not healed.

tenderness will be the shaft of one of the metatarsal bones even though there is also tenderness of the area between the metatarsals suggestive of a Morton's neuroma (Fig. 32–8).

Treatment consists of activity reduction and reduced weight bearing until the athlete can walk without a limp. Aerobic training can be performed on an exercise bicycle or running in water if the appropriate facilities are available. Running is allowed as soon as tolerated. It is the author's experience that it has been virtually impossible, owing to pain, to resume running prior to the sixth week from the date of onset of symptoms.

Sesamoid stress fractures of the great toe, although very uncommon, are still one of the more common causes of pain in or about the first metatarsal phalangeal joint in the school-age runner (Table 32–1). Palpation and compression of the medial or lateral sesamoid should be quite painful if a stress fracture is present. A positive bone scan will differentiate this from chondromalacia of the sesamoid. In reality, some of these stress fractures are probably failure of the fibrous union in a bipartite or tripartite sesamoid, producing a painful pseudoarthrosis. In either case, the initial treatment should be one of aggressive non–weight bearing in a short leg cast for 6 weeks. If conservative treatment fails, then surgical treatment should be considered. If there is a true nonunited stress fracture, then one has the options of surgical removal and early functional weight bearing (the author's preferred treatment) or bone grafting the fracture, which is followed by a non–weight-bearing short leg cast for 6 weeks. Surgical excision of the sesamoid has not been noted to produce any deleterious effects in our patients.[22]

OTHER BONY INJURIES

Calcaneal apophysitis is a stress reaction that probably reflects microstress fractures within the proximal calcaneal growth plate.

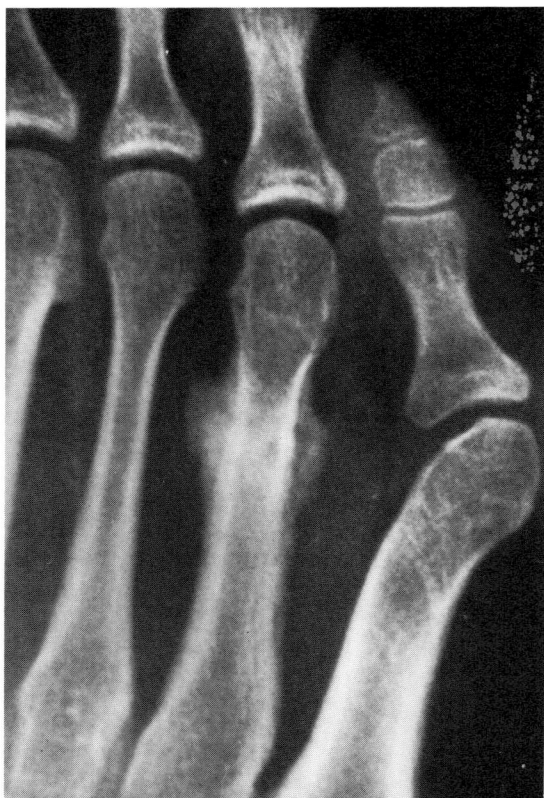

FIGURE 32–8. Radiographic appearance of a stress fracture of the fourth metatarsal.

Since the apophysitis generally closes about age 14 in boys, symptoms present themselves between the ages of 10 and 14. The symptoms are usually low grade in nature and rarely are severe enough to prevent training. This is a self-limited entity that disappears with closure of the growth plate.

Treatment consists of refraining from running if the symptoms are causing the athlete to walk or run with a limp. The athlete is placed on heel cord stretching and eccentric strengthening exercises. A heel lift may be of some benefit, and an orthotic with a $\frac{1}{8}$-inch medial heel lift is utilized if there is excessive foot pronation. This entity must be distinguished from Achilles tendinitis (Table 32–1).

Accessory navicular pseudoarthrosis causes characteristic medial midtarsal pain in runners (Fig. 32–6). Physical examination will reveal tenderness at the site of attachment of the posterior tibial tendon to the navicular (Table 32–1). Careful examination in this entity reveals a very prominent and enlarged medial navicular, which on radiographic evaluation reveals an accessory navicular. A bone scan should be obtained, as it is very rare indeed to develop posterior tibial insertional tendinitis at this location. If the bone scan is positive, it is our belief that it represents a failure of the fibrous union and has produced a painful pseudoarthrosis. One must be very sure that what is viewed on the roentgenograms is truly an accessory navicular and not two parts of a navicular stress fracture.

The treatment consists of short leg cast immobilization and nonsteroidal antiinflammatory medication if the symptoms have not been present for a prolonged time period. If the symptoms have been present for 6 months or longer, conservative treatment is still quite practical; however, surgical excision may be indicated.

PLANTAR FASCIITIS

The plantar fascia, one of the supporting structures of the longitudinal arch, is not truly a tendon, as it does not have a true muscle origin nor a tendon sheath. With each running step, the plantar fascia undergoes tremendous cyclic loading, and in some athletes this will produce a fatigue failure resulting in an inflammatory response and pain—*plantar fasciitis.*

The athlete will notice marked soreness on the inside of the foot near the heel on arising in the morning, necessitating walking on the outside of the foot. The pain will usually diminish during the day but gets worse again with running. Daily running is usually tolerable for about 4 weeks, but the pain increases to the point that training can only be performed every other day. Most athletes do not seek medical care for 4 to 6 weeks after the onset of symptoms, and some wait longer.

Physical examination will reveal marked tenderness of the medial half of the plantar fascia just distal to its insertion onto the calcaneus. There is also usually tenderness of the abductor hallucis at its insertion to the calcaneus. This pain is due to the overuse decompensation of this muscle while attempting to walk with the foot inverted.

Treatment consists of switching aerobic training to cycling, running in water, or swimming until the area is no longer tender, which usually takes a minimum of 6 weeks and, on occasion, up to 6 months. The patient is also placed in an orthotic with a $\frac{1}{8}$-inch medial heel wedge to tilt the foot into inversion, lessening the load on the plantar fascia. Nonsteroidal antiinflammatory medication may be of some benefit. Steroid injections only give temporary relief of symptoms and are not indicated in this condition. If symptoms fail to respond by 6 months, then surgical release offers a very high degree of success in our series of patients. Entrapment of the abductor digiti quinti and/or entrapment of the calcaneal branch of the posterior tibial nerve has been reported to be associated with plantar fasciitis, but this is quite rare in the author's experience.[4, 20]

The above entities must be differentiated from calcaneal periostitis of the medial calcaneal tubercle, which is almost always seen in the middle- and older-age runner. In this entity, there is little or no tenderness of the insertion of the plantar fascia but significant tenderness of the medial calcaneal tubercle.

TENDINITIS

Peroneal tendinitis, as mentioned above, is almost always located in the tendinous area between its insertion on the base of the fifth metatarsal to the inferior tip of the lateral malleolus. Treatment consists of essentially that described for Achilles tendinitis except that an orthotic, flexible leather or semirigid, with a $\frac{1}{8}$-inch lateral heel wedge is worn daily to diminish the eversion loading created by the normal gait pattern.

Extensor digitorum communis tendinitis, though very uncommon, is thought to occur from overcompression on the extensor tendons by too-tight shoelaces. It is believed that the inflammation is limited only to the tendon sheaths and is not a result of microtrauma to the tendon.

Treatment consists of warm soaks and nonsteroidal antiinflammatory medications. This tenosynovitis usually resolves within a few days. If it persists, one needs to rule out a metatarsal stress fracture.

MORTON'S NEUROMA

This entity, although not uncommon in the adult runner, is only occasionally seen in the high school runner. This entity is probably a result of compression of the metatarsal heads on the peripheral nerve proximal to where it branches into the digital nerves. By far the most common site is between the third and fourth metatarsals, perhaps because of their relative hypermobility. Essentially all runners, whether they land heel first, flatfoot, or toe first, strike the ground first with the outside of their foot, then roll into foot flat at midstance. It is this lateral compression with the foot in supination at foot strike that probably leads to the nerve trauma and subsequent fibrosis and nerve enlargement, which then produces a progressive vicious cycle.

A Morton's neuroma must be differentiated from a metatarsal stress fracture. Palpation should reveal that the maximum area of tenderness is in the intermetatarsal space and not the metatarsal shaft. The pain can be reproduced by holding the distal foot in one's hand and then squeezing the metatarsal heads together.

Most cases, if seen early enough, can be best treated by injecting around the affected nerve with dexamethasone, a soluble steroid, and placing a flexible or semirigid orthotic with a metatarsal pad in both the everyday shoe and the running shoe. The athlete should probably be switched to another aerobic training activity until symptoms are improved. If conservative treatment fails, excision of the neuroma is indicated. In most instances, conservative treatment will dissipate the symptoms or reduce them to a tolerable level.

SELECTION OF RUNNING SHOES AND ORTHOTICS

The basic requirements of a good shoe consist of a strong and relatively inflexible heel counter with a good shock-absorbing heel and midsole, a reasonably flexible midsole, and a wide toebox. A semirigid arch pad will accompany any good running shoe. An orthotic, in my opinion, should be utilized in an asymptomatic adolescent or young adult only when there is gross malalignment present. This would include those with obvious femoral anteversion and excessive pronation or those with isolated marked excessive pronation. We recommend a simirigid leather orthotic with a $\frac{1}{8}$-inch medial heel. A rigid orthotic is utilized in those with very unusual bony anatomy.

References

1. Andrish, J. T., Bergfeld, J. A., and Walheim, J.: A prospective study on the management of shin splints. J. Bone Joint Surg. 56A:1697–1700, 1974.
2. Brody, D. M.: Running injuries. CIBA Symp 32, 1980.
3. Clancy, W. G.: Lower extremity injuries in the jogger and distance runner. Phys. Sports Med. 2:46–50, 1974.
4. Clancy, W. G.: Tendinitis and plantar fasciitis in runners. Orthopedics 6:217–233, 1983.
5. Clancy, W. G., and Foltz, A. S.: Iliac apophysitis and stress fractures in adolescent runners. Am. J. Sports Med. 4:214–218, 1976.
6. Clancy, W. G., Neidhart, D., and Brand, R. L.: Achilles tendinitis in runners. Am. J. Sports Med. 4:46–56, 1976.
7. Clement, D. B.: Tibial stress syndrome in athletes. Am. J. Sports Med. 2:82–85, 1974.
8. D'Ambrosia, R. D., Zelis, R. F., and Churnard, R. G.: Interstitial pressure measurements in the anterior and posterior compartments in athletes with shin splints. Am. J. Sports Med. 5:127–131, 1977.
9. DeLee, J. C.: Fractures and dislocations of the hip. In Fractures, Rockwood and Green (eds.). J. B. Lippincott Co., Philadelphia, 1984.
10. Detmer, D. E., Sharpe, K., Sufit, R. L., and Girdleg, F. M.: Chronic compartment syndrome. Am. J. Sports Med. 13:162–170, 1985.
11. Devas, M. D.: Stress fractures of the femoral neck. J. Bone Joint Surg. 47B:728–738, 1965.
12. Martins, M., Libbrecht, P., and Burssens, A.: Surgical treatment of the iliotibial band friction syndrome. Am. J. Sports Med. 17:651–654, 1989.
13. Mayfield, G. W.: Popliteus tendon tenosynovitis. Am. J. Sports Med. 5:31–36, 1977.
14. Mubarak, S. J.: Exertional compartment syndrome. In Prevention and Treatment of Running Injuries, D'Ambrosia and Drez (eds.). Charles B. Slack, Thorofare, NJ, 1982.
15. Puddu, G., Ippolito, E., and Postacchini, F.: A classification of Achilles tendon disease. Am. J. Sports Med. 4:424–425, 1975.
16. Puranen, J., Alahetola, L., and Peltokallio, P.: Running and primary osteoarthritis of the hip. Br. Med. J. 2:424–425, 1975.
17. Ray, J. M., Clancy, W. G., and Lemon, R. A.: Semimembranosus tendinitis: an overlooked cause of medial knee pain. Am. J. Sports Med. 16:347–351, 1988.
18. Renne, J. W.: The iliotibial band friction syndrome. J. Bone Joint Surg. 57A:1110–1111, 1975.
19. Slocum, D. B.: The shin splint syndrome. Am. J. Surg. 114:875–881, 1967.
20. Snider, M. P., Clancy, W. G., and McBeath, A. A.: Plantar fascia release for chronic plantar fasciitis in runners. Am. J. Sports Med. 11:215–219, 1983.
21. Sohn, R. S., and Micheli, L. J.: The effect of running on the pathogenesis of osteoarthritis of the hip and knees. Clin. Orthop. 188:106–109, 1985.
22. Van Hal, M. E., Keene, J. S., Lange, T. A., and Clancy, W. G.: Stress fractures of the great toe. Am. J. Sports Med. 10:122–128, 1982.
23. Zoltan, D. J., Clancy, W. G., and Keene, J. S.: A new operative approach to snapping hip and refractory trochanteric bursitis in athletes. Am. J. Sports Med. 14:201–204, 1986.

33

SOCCER

WILLIAM E. GARRETT, JR.
JOHN LOHNES

Soccer is the fastest-growing team sport among American youth. Exact statistics on participation are difficult to acquire owing to the many municipal and recreational programs and club teams not affiliated with schools or registered with the United States Youth Soccer Federation. However, the total number of participants under age 18 has been estimated between 2 and 5 million.[39] The game is promoted for school-age children because it is relatively safe, requires little in the way of special or expensive equipment, is simple to learn, and does not require unique physical characteristics to excel.

CHARACTERISTICS OF SOCCER AND YOUTH SOCCER PLAYERS

Soccer is a game characterized by noncontinuous running interspersed with high-intensity sprints. Participants can cover up to 10 kilometers during a 90-minute match, with 20 to 30 percent of the time spent sprinting. The game consists of rare stoppages in action and few substitutions; thus, endurance and cardiovascular conditioning are important for players of all ages. The length of matches is usually limited to 60 minutes for youth.

Soccer is unique among team sports in its requirement to use primarily the lower extremities and head to control the ball. With the exception of the goalkeeper, the upper extremities are used only for throwing the ball in bounds. Little protective gear or special equipment is required. Soccer is transitional between a contact and noncontact sport. Injuries may result both directly from collision and indirectly from the tension and torque stresses of running and kicking.

The kick in particular is the primary cause of most soccer injuries, either directly or indirectly. The mechanism of the kicking motion in soccer and American football has been analyzed by Gainor et al.[14] who found that only about 15 percent of the kinetic energy generated is actually imparted to the ball and that the remaining 85 percent is imparted to the carry-through of the leg. Thus, injuries to the kicking leg occur in the deceleration of the leg either by muscular contraction or by collision with another player.

In soccer, a variety of methods are employed to kick the ball, depending on whether the player desires power, control, distance, loft, or some combination of these. The three basic kicks employ the inside, outside, or instep of the foot (Fig. 33–1). The inside kick offers both control and power and is used especially for passing on the ground. It employs use of the hip adductors and foot inverters and stresses the groin and the medial aspect of the knee (Fig. 33–1A and 33–1B). The outside kick uses the hip abductors and external rotators and the foot dorsiflexors to control the ball and direct it short distances laterally (Fig. 33–1C and 33–1D). The instep or straight-ahead kick is used for long volleys or passing shots to direct the ball downfield. It requires forceful contraction of the hip flexors, knee extensors,

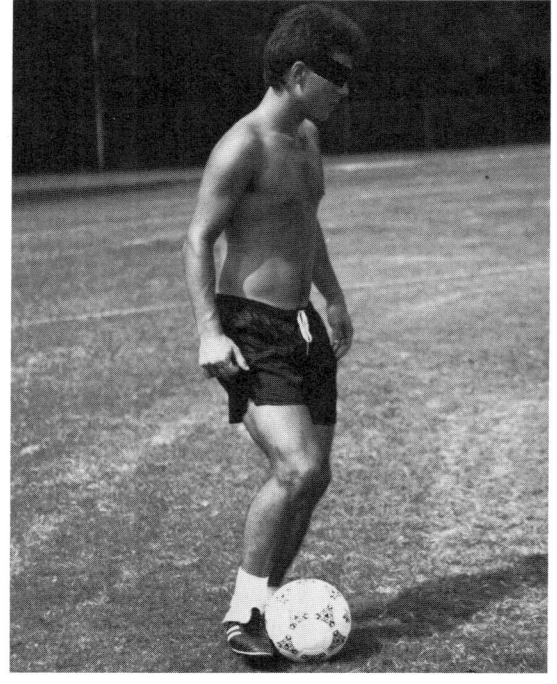
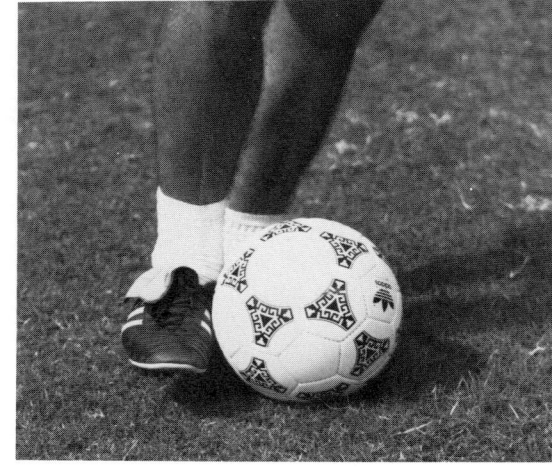
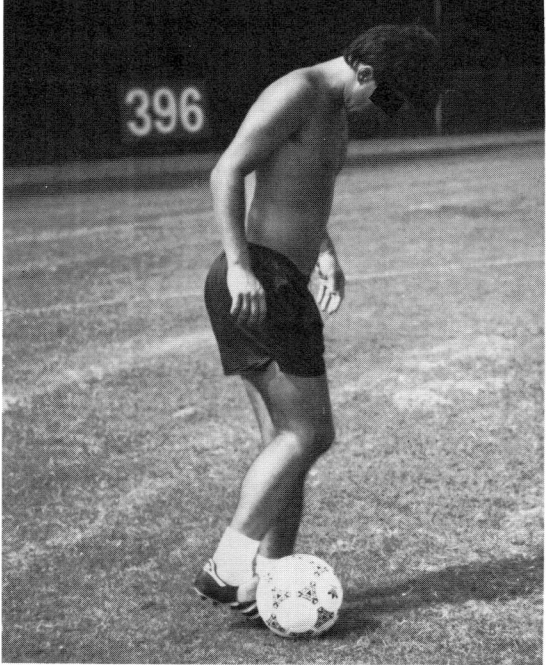
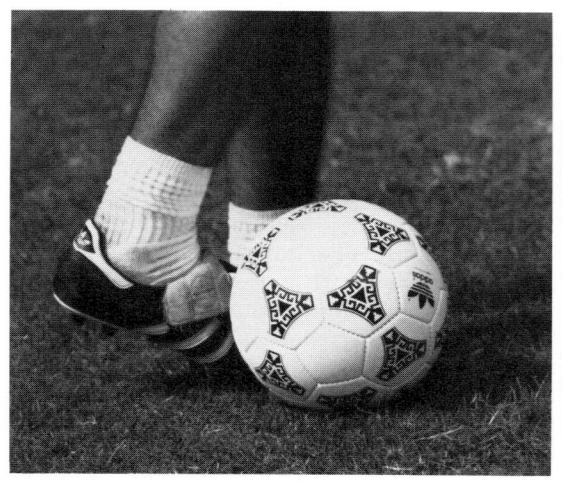

FIGURE 33–1. (*A,B*) The inside kick. (*C,D*) The oustide kick. (*E,F*) The instep kick.

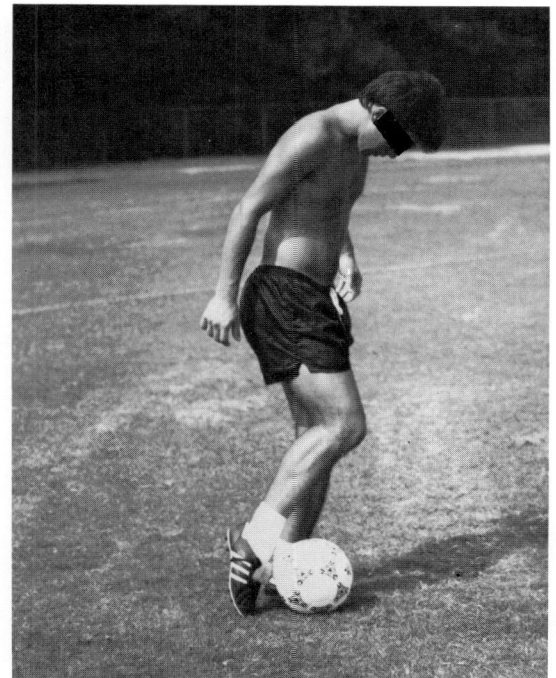
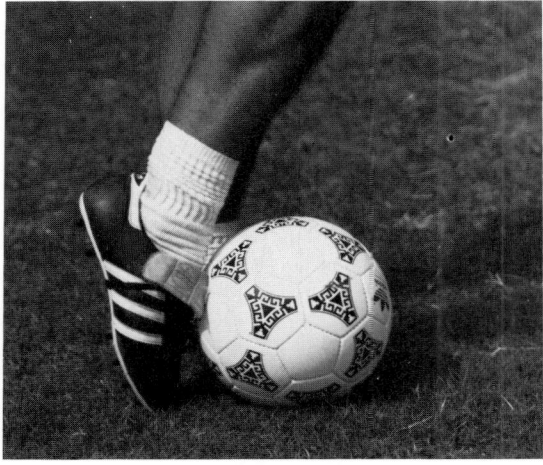

E F

FIGURE 33–1. *Continued*

and ankle dorsiflexors and results in great distance but affords less control (Fig. 33–1E and 33–1F).

Tackling in soccer means removing the ball from the possession of an attacking player. Contact is made with the ball but not with the player. The technique may involve either a blocking or sliding tackle, as illustrated in Figures 33–2 and 33–3.

Heading is an active movement in which the player uses the superior aspect of the forehead to strike the oncoming ball and the rest of the body to impart force and provide direction (Fig. 33–4). It is important to understand that heading is an active, not passive, maneuver and is not painful or injurious when done correctly.

Soccer may be played indoors or outdoors, on natural or artificial turf. The indoor game is played on a smaller field, with fewer players, and is typically faster paced.

Generally, the demands of soccer do not favor any unique morphological attributes such as increased height or weight. Skilled motor coordination, agility, and tactical development are of greater importance. One study of under-16 and under-18 Canadian national teams did demonstrate above-average height and mass, leg strength, and hip flexibility in these elite youth players.[19] However, these differences may have been attributable to selection. Other studies have shown a trend toward taller, heavier, and leaner players, but this may simply reflect the trend in the overall population.[17]

Two studies have investigated the physiological training effects of soccer in children. Berg et al.[4] found no significant changes in cardiorespiratory fitness, peak knee torque, or flexibility in a group of 11-year-old boys following a 12-week soccer conditioning program. However, a study by Mosher et al.[22] did

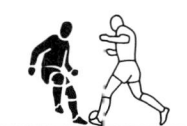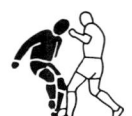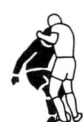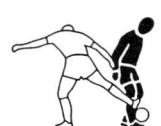

FIGURE 33–2. The blocking tackle.

TABLE 33–1. Summary of Studies of Youth Soccer Injuries

	Nilsson and Roaas[23]	Sullivan et al.[36]	Pritchett[25]	Sadat-Ali and Sankaran-Kutty[28]	Schmidt-Olsen et al.[31]	Hoff and Martin[15] 8-16		Maehlum et al.[20] 12-18		
	Adolescents	7-18	High School	11-20	9-19	Outdoor	Indoor	Total	Boys	Girls
Type of injury (% total)										
Contusion	36%	38%	31%	⎫ 23%	33%	8%	14%	47%	48%	45.5%
Abrasion/laceration	39	—	7	⎭	20	—	—	18	20	14
Sprain	⎫ 20	35	⎫ 38	26	—	16	30	22	19.5	25.5
Strain	⎭	9	⎭	7.5	—	11	17	—	—	—
Fracture	3.5	9	19	29	4	1	6	6	5	6
Location of injury (% total)										
Head/face	10%	15%	9%		5%	22%	8%	17%	20%	12%
Upper extremity	15	17	26			6	20	14	14	14
Pelvis/groin/trunk	7	3	4		4	8	15	7.5	6	10
Lower extremity	68	65	58		81	63	58	61	60	63
Thigh	12			⎫						
Knee	14	12		⎬ 44						
Shin/calf	13			⎬						
Ankle	16	41		⎬						
Foot	13			⎭						

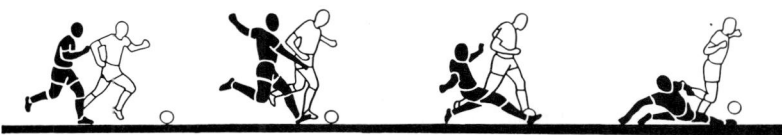

FIGURE 33-3. The sliding tackle.

show significant increases in aerobic fitness in this same age group following a similar 12-week training program.

Other studies of the effects of training in prepubescent children are inconclusive but suggest that some improvement in aerobic fitness can occur with regular training. The interpretation of training-induced physiological changes in prepubescents is difficult owing to the effects of growth and development and the variety of sports and training programs.[3] Considerably more work needs to be done to assess the fitness demands of specific sports on children. For youth soccer participants, however, the emphasis should generally be more on the acquisition of basic skills, agility, and coordination than on improving strength and aerobic capacity.

INCIDENCE OF INJURY

Despite the worldwide popularity of soccer, there have been relatively few studies of the epidemiology of soccer injuries, particularly in youth players. Seven studies of soccer injuries in young soccer players have been published. The results of these series are summarized in Table 33-1.

In general, it has been found in these studies that injuries in youth soccer are uncommon, occurring in only about 5 percent of participants annually. Injuries in soccer occur about one fifth as commonly as in American football. The incidence of injury tends to increase with age, up to 10-fold in high school players. Players under 10 experience injuries only rarely, and these do not usually result in time lost from play. Girls appear twice as likely to be injured as boys in soccer, although the reasons for this have not been identified. Indoor soccer has been found to have a higher rate of injury than outdoor. Youth goalkeepers sustain a disproportionately higher number of injuries than do players in other positions.

TYPES OF INJURIES

Contusions, muscle strains, and ligament sprains account for most of the injuries resulting in time lost from games or practices for all age groups in soccer. In children, contusions and abrasions are the most common injuries, and approximately 75 percent of these are not serious, that is, result in no lost playing time. Most of these injuries involve the lower extremities. Fractures account for about 10 percent of all injuries and most typically involve the upper extremity owing to a fall. Fractures do not appear to be more frequent in youth players despite the decreased strength of growing epiphyseal plates. Serious, permanent injury such as head and spinal cord trauma are fortunately rare, accounting for less than 0.1 percent.

HEAD AND NECK

Despite the absence of protective headgear, soccer injuries to the head, mouth, and face account for only about 10 percent of all injuries in youth. This figure is, however, greater than that for adult players. The reasons for this may be related to lesser skill, greater head-to-body weight ratio, or greater ball-to-body size ratio. As mentioned above, serious concussions, skull fractures, and cervical spine trauma are rare, but lacerations, eye and dental injuries, and facial fractures are not infrequent. Goalkeepers may be more

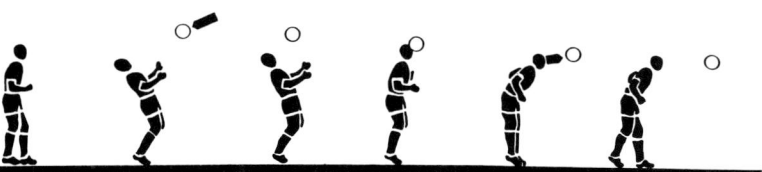

FIGURE 33-4. Heading the ball.

susceptible to head and neck injuries since they are more likely to approach the play headfirst.[13] Head and facial injuries may occur with improper heading or collision with the ground, goalposts, or other players. Hyperflexion-extension injuries to the neck can result when a player is kicked or struck forcefully by the ball. Sane and Ylipaavalniemi[30] reviewed maxillofacial and dental injuries occurring in Finland over a 3-year period in players ages 8 to 47 (mean 25.1). Of 8640 total soccer injuries, 6.4 percent affected the teeth, alveolar processes, or lower or middle third of the facial skeleton. The most common cause of these injuries was direct contact with another player. Players under age 20 were less likely to sustain dental and maxillofacial injuries than older players; only 4.3 percent of these injuries occurred in children under age 15. However, owing to the high cost and potential for permanent impairment from dental injuries in particular, the authors recommend the use of mouthguards.

Burke et al.[5] reported a series of 12 soccerball-induced eye injuries in patients ages 6 to 21. Hyphema and retinal edema were present in all injuries; vitreous hemorrhage, retinal hemorrhage, corneal abrasion, traumatic iritis, angle recession, retinal tear, and traumatic pigmentary retinopathy also occurred, in descending frequency. There were no permanent impairments in any case; nevertheless, Burke recommended the use of protective goggles for youth soccer players. Proper heading technique should also be stressed for beginning players.

Little is known about the chronic effects of repetitive heading. One study observed a higher incidence of electroencephalogram (EEG) changes in a group of soccer players compared with a control group.[38] In this study, the changes were most significant in the younger players (ages 16 to 20). The higher incidence was felt most likely to be due to neuronal changes caused by repeated minor head traumas.

The value of helmets has been observed in American football, hockey, and lacrosse, but no study has evaluated the effectiveness of protective headgear in soccer.

UPPER EXTREMITY

The incidence of upper extremity injuries in youth soccer participants has been reported to average between 15 and 20 percent. This compares with 10 percent in most adult series. Typically, these injuries involve sprains, fractures, or dislocation of the thumb or fingers. Again, goalkeepers are more likely to be injured owing to the specific demands of their position.

Possible reasons for the higher incidence of upper extremity injury observed in young players include more frequent falls, illegal ball contact, decreased technical expertise, and greater fragility of upper extremity epiphyses.[16]

HIP, PELVIS, AND GROIN

Most studies combine injuries to the trunk, back, pelvis, and groin, with incidences ranging generally from 3 to 10 percent for outdoor soccer to as high as 15 percent for indoor youth players. The most common injuries to the hip, pelvis, and groin in soccer are the hip pointer, pelvic avulsion fractures, and groin strains. In children, iliac crest apophysitis, slipped capital femoral epiphysis, and subcapital compression fractures should also be considered.

Hip Pointer

The hip pointer is a contusion to the iliac crest, especially common in goalkeepers and usually caused by a fall on the side. Extreme point tenderness, swelling, and ecchymosis over the iliac crest are diagnostic in cases with a history of a direct blow to the iliac crest. Treatment involves application of ice and compression acutely, followed by an oral nonsteroidal antiinflammatory medicine. Occasionally, the hematoma may be aspirated and the area infiltrated with Xylocaine if pain is severe. Although this injury is often quite painful, the athlete may return to play with protective padding over the iliac crest.

Iliac Crest Apophysitis

Apophysitis of the iliac crest can present like a hip pointer, although the onset is gradual with no clear history of contusion. Pain is aggravated by running. The iliac crest apophysis can be seen radiographically at puberty, appearing first anteriorly and progressing posteriorly with skeletal maturity. Closure usually occurs by age 14 in girls and age 16 in boys but may occur as late as age 18 and 20, respectively. Repetitive, subacute strain of the muscular attachments about the iliac crest during this period of closure results in an inflammatory response. Apophysitis is treated by rest and antiinflammatory medications until pain resolves, followed by a gradual return to activity with emphasis on strengthening the involved muscle group. The player can typically resume soccer after 4 to 6 weeks.

Groin Pain

Chronic groin pain is common in soccer players owing to the repetitive shear stress of the inside kick on the thigh adductors and pubic area. Often there is no acute injury but simply gradually increasing pain during activity, particularly when executing an inside kick or when the leg is stressed in abduction and external rotation. The pain may be felt locally about the groin and pubic area or down the anterior aspect of the thigh. Chronic muscle strains, abdominal wall muscle abnormalities, osteitis pubis, or hernias are all possible causes. A careful physical exam will usually distinguish a hernia from a muscle strain. The adductor longus, adductor brevis, iliopsoas, rectus femoris, and rectus abdominus are most often affected. Recurrent strain of the abdominal wall musculature may lead to a defect at the pubic insertion. While this defect may not result in a palpable hernia, a Bassini-type herniorrhaphy has been found to correct the condition successfully.[34, 41] Osteitis pubis is periostitis of the pubic symphysis and inflammation of the surrounding ligaments. The pubic symphysis does not mature until the third decade, and so youth players are particularly susceptible to this condition. On physical exam, there is usually point tenderness over the pubic symphysis and pain with isolation of the hip adductors. The differentiation of osteitis pubis from adductor strains may be aided by noting characteristic radiologic changes described by Rispoli[26] in which osteolysis and eventual erosion and arthrosis can be observed. A technetium 99 pyrophosphate bone scan may be positive but is not necessarily diagnostic.

Treatment of chronic muscle strains and osteitis pubis both involve rest, antiinflammatory medications, and gradual return to sport, with emphasis on strengthening the abdominal and thigh musculature. Typically, the recovery is long and may take up to 6 months in some cases.

Subcapital Stress Fracture and Slipped Femoral Capital Epiphysis

A young soccer player who complains of vague, aching pain in the hip, groin, thigh, or knee should be examined for possible stress fracture of the femoral head and neck or slipped femoral capital epiphysis. Knee pain in particular is often the primary symptom of hip pathology in children. In preadolescents, the stress fracture is most often a compression type and is evidenced radiographically by a small line of internal callus formation after 2 to 3 weeks. The treatment for this is simply rest until symptoms resolve.

More serious is a slip of the femoral capital epiphysis. This injury occurs most commonly in boys between the ages of 13 and 16 and in girls between the ages of 11 and 14. Classically, the child is prepubescent but obese or of large build. The child will complain of groin or knee pain referred to the anteromedial thigh and knee with weight bearing and may walk with the leg externally rotated. The diagnosis is usually obvious on routine radiographs, and the treatment may involve either surgical stabilization or simply immobilization according to the preference of the orthopedic surgeon.

Avulsion Fractures of the Pelvis and Femur

Pelvic and proximal femoral avulsion fractures occur in both adult and youth soccer and are the result of the extreme stresses placed on the lower extremity musculature during kicking and sudden stops and starts while running. The most common muscles involved are the abdominal external and internal obliques (hip flexion), rectus femoris (hip flexion and knee extension), adductor longus (thigh adduction), iliopsoas (hip flexion), and hamstrings (knee flexion, kick deceleration, and hip extension). In the skeletally immature athlete, the apophyseal attachment of the muscle tendon avulses either completely or partially.

The athlete will experience sudden sharp pain at the time of injury. Pain can be reproduced by isolation of the involved muscle or muscle group. Occasionally, a defect or mass near the muscle origin may be palpable if the avulsion is complete. The diagnosis can be confirmed radiographically. Treatment involves rest, ice, and analgesics initially, followed by a course of antiinflammatory medication. Most of these injuries will improve with conservative treatment only; however, if the avulsed bony fragment is large or considerably displaced, surgical repair may be indicated. The decision to repair is made acutely. Avulsion fractures treated conservatively will usually require 6 to 8 weeks to heal.

LOWER EXTREMITY

Injuries to the lower extremities are easily the most common, accounting for between 58 and 81 percent of all injuries in the published studies (Table 33–1). Ligamentous sprains and muscular strains about the knee, ankle, and foot are the second-most common injuries sustained by youth soccer participants. Again, owing to the comparatively weaker epiphyseal plates, an avulsion fracture involving the ligamentous or tendinous attachments should always be considered when evaluating an apparent sprain or strain.

Contusions

Contusions are the most frequently occurring injury in youth soccer, accounting for approximately 30 to 40 percent of all injuries. Most of these contusions involve the lower extremities, with the anterior thigh, shin, and malleoli of the ankle being particularly vulnerable. Most of these injuries are minor and do not result in lost playing time. However, deep contusions to the thigh and calf muscles can be quite painful and require more extensive treatment and rehabilitation.

A muscle contusion resembles a muscle strain in that it causes disruption of muscle fibers with resultant hemorrhage, edema, and inflammation. Various experimental studies have demonstrated that blunt trauma to the thigh causes rupture of the deep muscles near the bone. Initially, a hematoma forms, followed by an inflammatory response and reorganization of the hematoma as the muscle heals. Myositis ossificans is a possible sequela of muscle contusions and is most common during adolescence.

Muscle contusions are graded from I to III, depending on the severity of the injury and the amount of disability. The treatment of contusions involves ice and compression initially, followed by antiinflammatory medications and gradual stretching and range of motion. Immobilization of the involved extremity may be appropriate for comfort only in grade II or III muscle contusions but is not advisable for long periods and is not necessary for healing to occur. Massage is definitely contraindicated.[2]

Contusions to bony prominences, notably the medial and lateral malleoli of the ankle and the anterior tibia, are extremely common in soccer. These injuries result in a subperiosteal hematoma and may involve a cortical fracture, which becomes visible on follow-up radiographs. Treatment again is largely symptomatic. Protection of the anterior lower extremities and ankles with shin guards is the single-most effective way to reduce the number of contusions. Shin guards should be required equipment for both practices and games.

Thigh Injuries

Contusions to the thigh (charley horse) generally involve the quadriceps and lateral hamstring muscles. Strains, or occasionally rupture, of the rectus femoris, adductor longus, and hamstrings usually occur at the musculotendinous junction. Players sustaining severe muscle contusions should be observed closely for signs of acute compartment syndrome.

Knee Injuries

Knee injuries are probably the most frequent and disabling injuries in soccer. A large-scale study of Swedish soccer injuries over an 8-year period underscores the importance of knee injuries; 35 percent of all injuries involved the knee. Over half of all injuries leading to more than 1 month of disability were injuries to the knee. As in most other sports, the injuries of the knee most common in soccer involve the medial collateral ligaments (MCLs), anterior cruciate ligaments (ACLs), and the menisci. In skeletally immature children with physical findings of ligamentous instability, epiphyseal fractures and avulsions (e.g., of the intercondylar eminence or tibial tubercle) must be ruled out. Injury to the lateral structures of the knee may be more common in soccer than in other sports owing to the greater exposure of the knee to varus stresses. Medial knee injuries in soccer are typically caused by an extreme valgus torque just before a kick and less commonly by a direct blow. Likewise, the mechanism of an ACL injury is usually a sudden deceleration, twisting, and/or hyperextension stress with no contact involved.

Complete rupture of the ACL is an ominous injury for a young soccer player. The natural history of this injury in a young athletic population is one of increasing instability and an inability to accelerate, decelerate, or change directions rapidly. These skills obviously are important in soccer, and one could expect significant alteration in the skill and ability of the player. It is our opinion that young people with ACL injuries should undergo reconstructive surgery of the ACL if they are near or past skeletal maturity. Often players before skeletal maturity will have an avulsion fracture of the intercondylar eminence of the tibia, which includes the tibial attachment site of the ACL. This fracture should be reduced near anatomically and held by either cast or surgical treatment. Occasionally, ACL tears without fracture occur in skeletally immature patients; treatment in this case is controversial. (See Chapter 18.)

Medial collateral ligament injuries are also relatively frequent. Most of these injuries are not complete ruptures but grade I or II injuries. Current practice trends favor treatment of MCL injuries with aggressive rehabilitation and relatively little immobilization when the ACL is intact. (See Chapter 17.)

Meniscus injuries also occur relatively frequently in soccer. Often these injuries are concomitant with injury to knee ligaments. It is now recognized that meniscectomy, particularly in young patients, increases the chance of later arthrosis. There is more emphasis now on meniscus repair; anterior cruciate ligament reconstruction with meniscus repair is favored for young athletes with both injuries.

Chronic overuse injuries about the knee are also common in soccer and include patellar tendinitis, tibial epiphysitis (Osgood-Schlatter disease), patellofemoral pain (chondromalacia patella), symptomatic parapatellar plica, and iliotibial band bursitis.

Ankle Sprains

Ankle sprains are among the most common injuries in soccer players. Chronic ankle instability and pain in adult players are typically the result of multiple, often minor, injuries sustained over many years; therefore, there is great interest in the prevention of ankle injuries during youth. Like other sports, the most common mechanism for ankle sprain is an inversion–plantar flexion stress, injuring the anterior talofibular and calcaneofibular ligaments. The diagnosis and treatment of ankle sprains have been described in Chapter 22.

Controlling the soccer ball typically requires extreme plantar flexion of the foot to increase the ball-to-foot surface area during the dribble and pass. This repetitive loading of the anterior capsule and ligaments often results in a condition known as "footballer's ankle," characterized by chronic pain, swelling, and stiffness in adult players. The development of calcifications and osteophytes about the anterior and posterior talus can be observed radiographically as the condition progresses. Similarly, irritation of an os trigonum is common in soccer because of extreme plantar flexion. This may become symptomatic in early years of sport.

The use of routine taping or ankle orthoses to prevent ankle injuries in children is controversial, although several studies have identified its effectiveness in limiting recurrent sprains.[8, 10, 11] Ankle strengthening and proprioceptive drills to prevent functional instability are extremely important following a severe sprain.[37]

Other Ankle and Foot Injuries

Sprains. In addition to the typical ankle sprain, a variety of other ligaments about the ankle and foot can be injured owing to the specific demands of controlling the soccer ball. On the medial side of the foot are ligaments of the talonavicular, naviculocuneiform, medial tarsometatarsal (Lisfranc), and first metatarsophalangeal joints. On the lateral side are the calcaneocuboid, cuboideonavicular, cuneiocuboid, lateral tarsometatarsal, and second through fifth metatarsophalangeal joints. Sprains of these ligaments are often the result of inversion/plantar flexion stress but may also result from hyperdorsiflexion of the foot.

Turf Toe. A condition known as "turf toe" is the result of repetitive extreme hyperextension of the first metatarsophalangeal joint, resulting in damage to the plantar capsule of this joint and the adjacent sesamoid bones. Playing on hard surfaces in flexible shoes predisposes to this condition, which is characterized by pain on forced extension of the great toe and stiffness. Taping to control hyperextension is helpful symptomatically (Fig. 33–5). (See Chapter 23.)

Tendinitis. Injuries to tendons about the ankle and foot are common and may be caused acutely by a direct blow or by mechanical stress, resulting in strain, avulsion

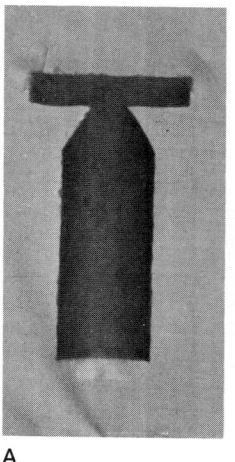 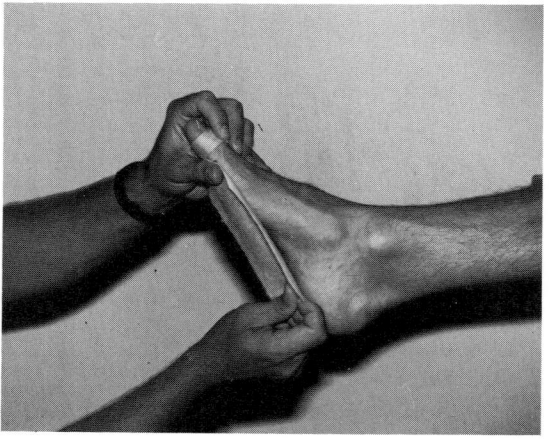 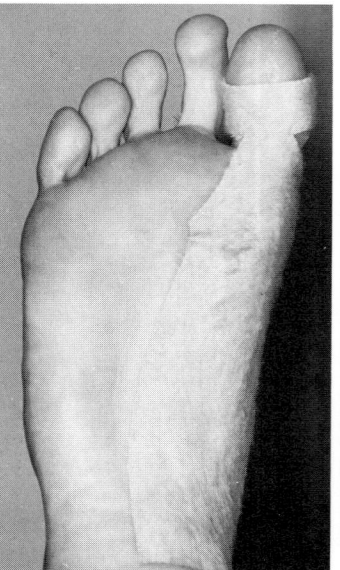

FIGURE 33–5. Taping to limit hyperextension of the great toe. (*A*) Precut moleskin. (*B*) Applying to foot. (*C*) Finished taping.

fracture, or tendinitis or tenosynovitis. The inside kick places particular stress on the posterior tibial tendon, whereas the outside kick stresses the peroneals, extensor hallucis longus, and extensor digitorum communis.

Contusions. Contusions to the toes, either by a direct blow or more often the repetitive trauma of kicking and compression of the toes in the shoe, are familiar to soccer players of all ages. The resulting subungual hematoma can be quite painful and usually results in the eventual loss of the toenail. Acutely, the hematoma should be drained by drilling or burning a hole in the nail to relieve the pressure. If the nail is avulsed, the toe should be taped to protect the nailbed from further injury and keep the nail fold open until a new nail grows in. Particular care should be taken as new toenails develop to avoid an ingrown nail, which is another common problem in soccer players caused not only by the frequent loss of nails but also by the constant compression of the toes in the narrow toebox of the soccer shoe.

TRAINING AND INJURY PREVENTION

PREPARTICIPATION EXAMINATION

Preparticipation sports evaluations for youth soccer should include a thorough history to identify previous injuries, illnesses, and developmental difficulties and a standard screening physical for existing medical and musculoskeletal pathology.[27] In addition to this routine evaluation, some assessment of basic fitness should be performed. It is common wisdom that deficits in strength, flexibility, and endurance predispose to injury, although there have been few studies to verify this in children. There have been no studies to determine fitness norms for youth soccer players and the relation of fitness to soccer injury rates at different developmental ages.

Sapega[42] has emphasized the importance of sport-specific musculoskeletal profiling particularly in the rehabilitation of injuries. Ekstrand and Gillquist[10] identify various "player factors" as contributors to injury in their study of adult soccer players. These included joint instability, muscle tightness, inadequate rehabilitation of old injuries, and lack of training. Muscle strains occurred more commonly in players with relative muscle tightness. Ankle sprains were more frequent in players with sprains or clinical instability. Players sustaining noncontact knee sprains had preexisting reduced strength in the injured leg. Ekstrand has also found adult soccer players to have more muscle tightness than nonsoccer players. Agre and Baxter noted significant preexisting musculoskeletal abnormalities in injuries occurring among a group of male collegiate soccer players.[1]

Based on these few studies, preseason screening is advisable to detect and correct joint instability, muscle tightness, inadequately rehabilitated injuries, and serious lack of conditioning.

WARM-UP AND TRAINING

The importance of warm-up in the prevention of muscle strains has been observed clinically in soccer players[1, 8, 17, 33] and supported experimentally.[29] Warm-up should consist of a 15- to 20-minute period of jogging, controlled passing, and dribbling. Warm-up should be followed by static, contract-relax stretching with emphasis on the lower extremity muscle groups.[18]

Ekstrand[8] noted that a high practice-to-game ratio results in fewer average injuries and concluded that players in better condition are less likely to be injured. For youth players, particularly in the under-12 age groups, the emphasis should be on learning ball control skills and the fundamentals of play rather than on competitive performance. The interval between games should allow 3 to 4 days for recovery.

NUTRITION

Shephard and Leatt[32] have examined the carbohydrate and fluid needs of adult soccer players, noting the substantial depletion of muscle glycogen and fluid volume that occurs during a typical match. A well-balanced diet consisting of 50 percent carbohydrates (preferably complex carbohydrates) should be encouraged. The value of "carbohydrate

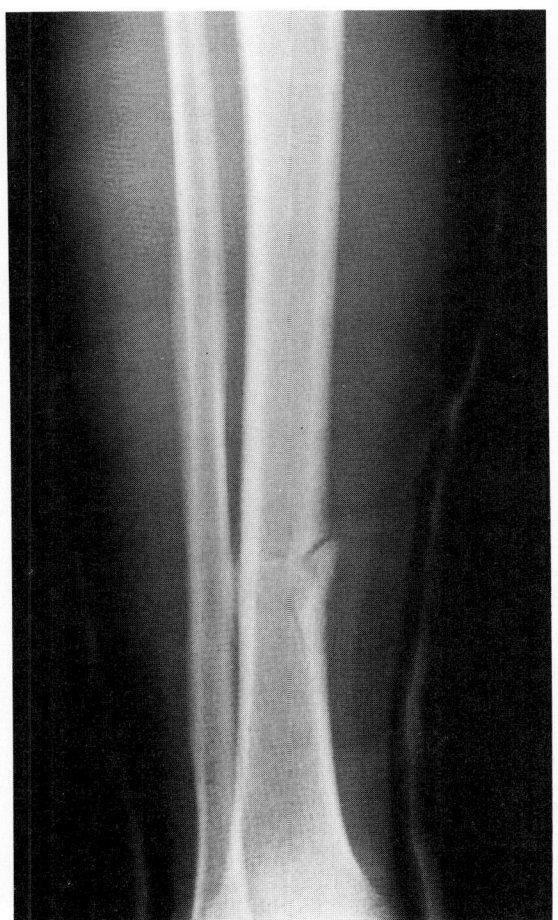
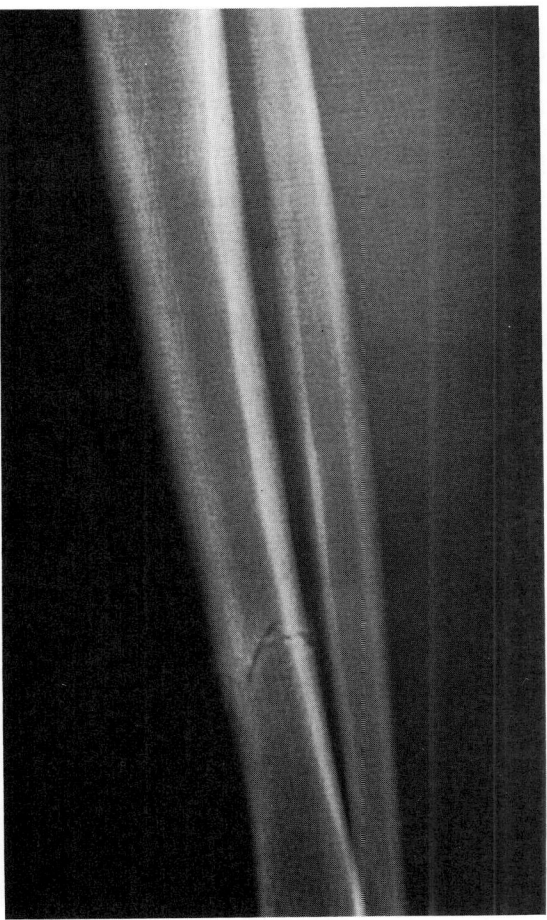

A   B

FIGURE 33-6. Most tibial injuries are contusions and hematomas, although complete fractures periodically occur. This injury occurred in a 17-year-old soccer player.

loading" for soccer is probably minimal and is not necessary for youth players. Increased fluid intake should be encouraged in the hours before a match. At least 3 to 5 ounces of water should be taken every 20 minutes during heavy excercise—more during hot weather. Glucose-polymer fluid preparations can be an aid to replenishing and preserving glycogen stores if given before and during a game. A preparation with lower concentrations and osmolality is preferred (e.g., 7 percent polyglucose: 360 mOsm/liter) in order to enhance absorption.

PROTECTIVE EQUIPMENT AND FIELD MODIFICATIONS

The provision of shin guards has been shown to reduce the incidence of injuries to the lower leg.[10] Shin guards should be required for youth players, in whom contusions to the lower leg and ankle are the most common injuries (Fig. 33–6).

Soccer shoes should be appropriate for the field surface and conditions. Training or "turf" shoes are probably more appropriate footwear for beginning players than are cleated shoes, since they provide greater stability.

The size of the field and goals can be scaled down to the size of the players to reduce the physical demands of the sport. Likewise, smaller ball sizes (sizes 3 and 4) are more easily controlled by young children and may lessen the incidence of head and face injuries.

RULES AND OFFICIATING

An often overlooked measure to prevent injuries involves proper officiating and supervision by coaches and parents. Young players should be instructed in the correct methods of tackling and what constitutes fouls and dangerous plays. The penalties for uncontrolled and dangerous plays should be strictly enforced. The avoidance of poor field conditions and inclement weather is the responsibility of the coach and referee.

REHABILITATION

When injury does occur, supervised, progressive rehabilitation is important in preventing recurrence. When possible, this should be carried out under the supervision of a physician, physical therapist, or trainer, although for most youth players much of the daily supervision will be the responsibility of the coach. Normal endurance and strength with full, painless range of motion is the initial goal of any rehabilitation program, followed by sport-specific functional drills before returning to sport. Owing to the high demands for rapid, coordinated movements in soccer, great emphasis should be placed on coordination and agility exercises. For soccer, these drills can be similar to those used in the warm-up period with modifications to suit the specific injury.

References

1. Agre, J. C., and Baxter, T. L.: Musculoskeletal profile of male collegiate soccer players. Arch. Phys. Med. Rehabil. 68:147–150, 1987.
2. Antao, N. A.: Myositis of the hip in a professional soccer player; a case report. Am. J. Sports Med. 16(1):82–83, 1988.
3. Bar-Or, O.: Trainability of the pre-pubescent child. Phys. Sports Med. 17(5):65–82, 1989.
4. Berg, K. E., LaVoie, J. C., and Latin, R. W.: Physiological training effects of playing youth soccer. Med. Sci. Sports Exerc. 17(6):656–660, 1985.
5. Burke, M. J., Sanitato, J. J., Vinger, P. F., Raymond, L. A., and Kulwin, D. R.: Soccerball-induced eye injuries. JAMA 249:2682–2685, 1983.
6. DeHaven, K. E., and Lintner, D. M.: Athletic injuries: comparison by age, sport, and gender. Am. J. Sports Med. 14(3):218–224, 1986.
7. Ekblom, B.: Applied physiology of soccer. Sports Med. 3:50–60, 1986.
8. Ekstrand, J.: Soccer injuries and their prevention. Linkoping University, Medical Dissertations, no. 130, 1982.
9. Ekstrand, J., and Gillquist, J.: The frequency of muscle tightness and injuries in soccer players. Am. J. Sports Med. 10(2):75–78, 1982.
10. Ekstrand, J., and Gillquist, J.: The avoidability of soccer injuries. Int. J. Sports Med. 4:124–128, 1983.
11. Ekstrand, J., Gillquist, J., and Liljedahl, S.: Prevention of soccer injuries. Am. J. Sports Med. 11(3):116–120, 1983.
12. Ekstrand, J., Gillquist, J., Moller, M., Oberg, B., and Liljedahl, S.: Incidence of soccer injuries and their relation to training and team success. Am. J. Sports Med. 11(2):63–67, 1983.
13. Fields, K. B.: Head injuries in soccer. Phys. Sports Med. 17(1):71–73, 1989.
14. Gainor, B. J., Piotrowski, G., Puhl, J. J., and Allen, W. C.: The kick: biomechanics and collision injury. Am. J. Sports Med. 6(4):185, 1978.
15. Hoff, G. L., and Martin, T. A.: Outdoor and indoor soccer: injuries among youth players. Am. J. Sports Med. 14(3):231–233, 1986.
16. Keller, C. S., Noyes, F. R., and Buncher, C. R.: The medical aspects of soccer injury epidemiology. Am. J. Sports Med. 15(3):230–237, 1987.

17. Kirkendall, D. T.: The applied sport science of soccer. Phys. Sports Med. 13(4):53–59, 1985.
18. Leard, J.: Flexibility and conditioning in the young athlete. In Pediatric and Adolescent Sports Medicine, Micheli, L. J., ed. Little, Brown & Co., Inc., Boston, MA, 1984.
19. Leatt, P., Shephard, R. J., and Plyley, M. J.: Specific muscular development in under-18 soccer players. J. Sports Sci. 5:165, 1987.
20. Maehlum, S., Dahl, E. and Daljord, O. A.: Frequency of injuries in a youth soccer tournament. Phys. Sports Med. 14(7):73–79, 1986.
21. McMaster, W. C., and Walter, M.: Injuries in soccer. Am. J. Sports Med. 6(6):354, 1978.
22. Mosher, R. E., Rhodes, E. C., Wenger, H. A., and Filsinger, B.: Interval training: the effects of a 12-week programme on elite, pre-pubertal male soccer players. J. Sports Med. 25 (1–2):5–9, 1985.
23. Nilsson, S., and Roaas, A.: Soccer injuries in adolescents. Am. J. Sports Med. 14(3):218–224, 1986.
24. Oberg, B., Ekstrand, J., Moller, M., and Gillquist, J.: Muscle strength and flexibility in different positions of soccer players. Int. J. Sports Med. 5(4):213–216, 1984.
25. Pritchett, J.: Cost of high school soccer injuries. Am. J. Sports Med. 9(1):64–66, 1981.
26. Rispoli, F. P.: Sindrome pubica dei calciatori soc emiliana romagnola triveneta ortop. Traumatol. Atti. 8:331, 1963.
27. Rooks, D. S., and Micheli, L. J.: Musculoskeletal assessment and training: the young athlete. Clin. Sports Med. 7(3):641–677, 1988.
28. Sadat-Ali, M., and Sankaran-Kutty, M.: Soccer injuries in Saudi Arabia. Am. J. Sports Med. 15(5):500–502, 1987.
29. Safran, M. R., Garrett, W. E., Jr., Seaber, A. V., Glisson, R. R., and Ribbeck, B. M.: The role of warm-up in muscular injury prevention. Am. J. Sports Med. 16(2):123–129, 1988.
30. Sane, J., and Ylipaavalniemi, P.: Maxillofacial and dental soccer injuries in Finland. Br. J. Oral Maxillofac. Surg. 25:383–390, 1987.
31. Schmidt-Olsen, S., Bunemann, L. K. H., Lade, V., and Brassoe, J. O. K.: Soccer injuries of youth. Br. J. Sports Med. 19:161–164, 1985.
32. Shephard, R. J., and Leatt, P.: Carbohydrate and fluid needs of the soccer player. Sports Med. 4:164–176, 1987.
33. Smodlaka, V. N.: Rehabilitation of injured soccer players. Phys. Sports Med. 7(8):59–67, 1979.
34. Smodlaka, V. N.: Groin pain in soccer players. Phys. Sports Med. 8(8):57–61, 1980.
35. Stanitski, C. L.: Common injuries in preadolescent and adolescent athletes. Sports Med. 7(1):32–41, 1989.
36. Sullivan, J. A., Gross, R. H., Grana, W. A., and Garcia-Moral, C.: Evaluation of injuries in youth soccer. Am. J. Sports Med. 8(5):325–327, 1980.
37. Tropp, H., Askling, C., and Gillquist, J.: Prevention of ankle sprains. Am. J. Sports Med. 13(4):259–261, 1985.
38. Tysvaer, A. T., and Storli, O.: Soccer injuries to the brain. Am. J. Sports Med. 17(4):573–578, 1989.
39. Ward, A.: Soccer: safe kicks for kids. Phys. Sports Med. 15(8):151–156, 1987.
40. Xethalis, J., and Boiardo, R.: Soccer injuries. In The Lower Extremity and Spine in Sports Medicine, Vol. 2, Nicholas, J. A., and Hershman, E. B., eds. C. V. Mosby, St. Louis, MO, 1986.

34
TENNIS

ROBERT NIRSCHL
JANET SOBEL

GOALS OF TENNIS

Physical education in the U.S. school system should leave each graduating pupil with an in-depth ability to play a lifetime sport as well as an understanding of the methods to implement personal physical fitness. Tennis is a wonderful lifetime sport and with appropriate supplemental exercises can be an excellent tool for the achievement of consistent lifelong physical fitness.

Other achievable goals of tennis include the development of highly sophisticated neuromuscular skill patterns and agility. The sport is also an excellent vehicle for social opportunity and teaches discipline, persistence, and self-reliance. For the truly gifted, tennis offers the opportunity of financial rewards. Overall, tennis is a marvelous tool to aid in the transition of youth to adulthood.

THE DEMANDS OF TENNIS

Like many sports, tennis can be a stern taskmaster, and the imposed demands can challenge the individual both emotionally and physically. The coordination patterns of stroking one ball actually require the functions of running, catching, hitting, and throwing. Learning these mechanical skill patterns can be frustrating, and the rigors of competition can challenge the strongest of egos.

Physical demands can result in a variety of deficiencies including acute injury, chronic overuse injury, and musculotendinous imbalance predisposing to injury. The potential for injury is magnified by individual personal physical deficiencies brought to the sport by heredity, disease, or prior injury. Common areas of tennis-imposed muscle-tendon imbalance include the elbow, shoulder, back, and abdomen. Common acute injuries include ankle sprains, patellofemoral and meniscal knee problems, and muscle pulls of the abdomen and legs. Common overuse problems include tendinitis of the shoulder, elbow, patellar tendon, Achilles tendon, and plantar fascia. In growing children, skeletal problems including apophysitis at the medial and posterior elbow, knee, and os calcis are common, and osteochondritis of the elbow capitellum is not uncommon.

FITNESS EVALUATION

As noted, tennis can impose substantial demands that either result in injury or the predisposition to injury through muscle-tendon imbalance. In addition, individual physical deficiency is often brought to the sport. Fitness evaluation is therefore a key ingredient in preventing injury and enhancing tennis performance.

In this regard, we have had an opportunity to play a significant role in the development of the United States Tennis Association (USTA) player development program. It will be of interest to share some early general fitness evaluation data on national-level junior tennis players (ages 16 to 18). The protocol included testing for baseline conditioning, musculoskeletal durability, and performance. This study focused on musculoskeletal durability with reference to individual physical hereditarial variations as well as tennis-imposed muscle-tendon imbalance and actual injury. Overall, of the first group of 80 nationally ranked players who were tested, 70 percent were noted to have shoulder imbalances or injury. Elbow abnormalities, postural problems of the thoracolumbar area, abdominal problems, knee and ankle difficulties, and flexibility deficiencies were also quite common. The high incidence of shoulder problems is consistent with the report of Kibler et al.[1]

The message from these early preliminary data is quite clear: Even in elite, nationally ranked players, significant musculoskeletal deficiencies either resulting in or predisposing to injury were present. It is likely therefore that in all youth, a significant percentage will have problems that should be addressed before injury occurs. Resolution of these problems is undertaken by appropriate individual supplemental exercise programs for strength, endurance, flexibility, aerobic and anaerobic capacity, agility, and skill.

TRAINING TECHNIQUES

The majority of tennis players, whether adult or youth, do not participate in a meaningful, structured tennis training program. The usual approach is merely to play. Adequate stroke mechanics may or may not be taught, and strategy for competitive play is sporadic. This typical approach often results in poor tennis mechanics, poor conditioning, and muscle-tendon imbalance. All these invite injury. If intense play, or a rapid escalation of frequency or duration of play, occurs (two to four times per week, 2- to 3-hour sessions or greater), injury is common. Hard surfaces (cement or asphalt-based) are additionally punishing to the lower extremities. Use of a tennis backboard or a ball machine increases the number of ball impacts per unit of time and also increases potential for overuse to the upper body.

Ideal training programs include the following:

1. Obtain a quality fitness performance exam such as the Level III program outlined in Table 34-1, adopted by the USTA and our institution (Virginia Sports Medicine Institute).

TABLE 34-1. Tennis Fitness Evaluation Protocol

1. History assessment
2. Musculoskeletal durability
    a. Varus-valgus elbow angle
    b. Shoulder slope angle—scapular insufficiency
    c. Spinal postural alignment
    d. Q angle (knees)
    e. Tibial os-calcis alignment
    f. Foot posture
    g. Flexibility—shoulder, back, hip, knee, ankle
    h. Manual strength testing—shoulder, hip groups
    i. Grip strength
    j. Grip (hand) size
3. Performance tests
    a. Upper body anaerobics (medicine-ball toss)
    b. Vertical jump
    c. Reaction time
    d. Hexagon test
    e. Fan run
    f. 20-yard dash
4. Baseline conditioning tests
    a. Submaximal aerobics
    b. Timed sit-ups
    c. Timed push-ups
    d. Sit-reach flexibility
    e. Lean body mass
5. Isokinetic testing
    a. Cybex 340 knee
    b. Cybex 340 shoulder
    c. Cybex 340 testing of clinically indicated areas

2. Obtain and perform supplemental exercises to eliminate deficiencies as identified in the fitness performance exam.
3. Implement equipment changes, counterforce bracing, or orthotics to supplement the deficiencies noted on the fitness performance exam.
4. Start tennis training on a gradual basis for:
    a. Stroke mechanics.
    b. Competitive strategy.
5. Although highly individualized, the following basic schedule for serious youth tennis play is suggested:
    a. Structured tennis program three times per week (2 to 3 hours) with ample rest periods.
    b. Maintenance program of supplemental exercises (1 hour, two times per week) after serious deficiencies have been eliminated by a quality medical rehabilitation program.
    c. Random tennis play per skill level to a frequency and intensity that does not produce overuse injury.
    d. Fitness retesting is recommended every 6 months for competitive

groups to ensure that muscle-tendon imbalance is not occurring secondary to the imposed demands of the sport.

STROKE MECHANICS

As noted, a single tennis stroke encompasses all the attributes of a baseball game (e.g., running, catching, hitting, and throwing). This is accomplished with the use of a 28-inch lever (i.e., the racquet length). Frustration occurs often, as proper body position in relation to the ball requires quickness, speed, and agility. In addition, the process of catching and hitting requires extreme focus on the ball-racquet interface, whereas the act of throwing requires some attention to the proposed target. Neuromuscular confusion is therefore commonplace, especially if attention to the target precedes the focus on the ball-racquet interface.

INJURY-PRODUCING STROKE MECHANICS

In general, quality tennis players place high emphasis on the lower body (e.g., running and body balance). In contrast, inexperienced players place little emphasis on the lower body. Inadequate body position and poor body balance result in arm overload; thus, shoulder tendinitis and tennis elbow of the lateral and medial elbow or apophysitis are commonplace.

PROTECTIVE TENNIS STROKES

Fortunately, good tennis mechanics is also good medicine. The power sources of quality ground strokes are leg power (ground reaction) and forward body balance, with trunk and shoulder rotation (Fig. 34–1). All these physical forces are protective of the arm, elbow, forearm, and wrist. Quality serve and overhead strokes can be punishing to the shoulder and medial elbow, but the quick elevation from backswing cocking to the impact position are more protective than, for example, the throwing motion in baseball.

TENNIS COMPETITIVE STRATEGIES

Tennis is a game of extreme variation. The variations are dependent on physique, skills, fitness, playing environment, and the opponent. Injury-producing strategies result from failure to take into consideration these variations and to adapt appropriately. In general, smooth stroke mechanics, shot selection that adapts to the situation, and consistent play are most helpful for sport success and the prevention of injury. Rapid play, jerky, sudden changes of shot selection, inadequate rest periods, and lack of fluid replacement all contribute to injury.

EQUIPMENT

Equipment encompasses a variety of categories.

PERSONAL EQUIPMENT

Clothing and shoes are intrinsic to sport performance and injury prevention. Light, accommodating wear is always appropriate. In colder climates, proper warm-up clothing is essential. Tennis shoes must adapt to movement in all directions, have an adequate midsole to absorb shock, provide a supportive heel counter, and have an adequate toe-

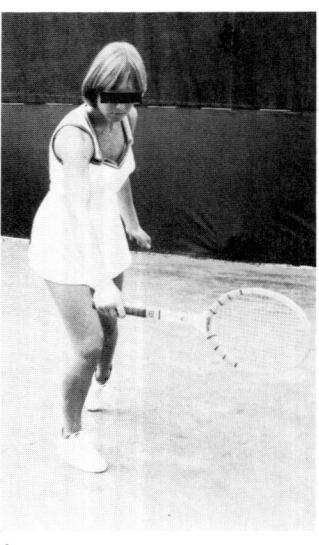
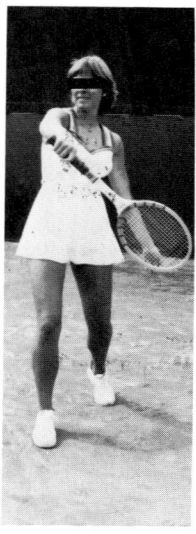

A B

FIGURE 34–1. (A) Quality backhand stroke. Quality tennis strokes utilize the lower body and trunk rotation for the power source. This technique protects the arm. (B) Faulty backhand.

box and flexible forefoot. The insole should be comfortable and offer the opportunity to be replaced by a custom orthotic if necessary.

RACQUETS

The selection of racquets incorporates the concepts of skill and tennis play as well as injury prevention. Powerful players with quality stroke mechanics often choose firm racquets with tight stringing to obtain additional ball control. Less powerful players often choose racquets and softer string tensions that deliver more ball velocity at the expense of control.

The needs of tennis play must be balanced against the needs of injury prevention. Although the data are clinical and anecdotal, it is our recommendation that the following racquet selection be utilized for symptomatic or tennis elbow injured arms:

1. Midsized racquet frame (90 to 110 square inches of hitting zone)
2. Graphite or graphite composite frame (such as graphite plus fiberglass or kevlar); note that the majority of graphite composites racquets contain graphite as the major component
3. Medium to moderate flexibility of the frame
4. Medium to soft string tension
5. Proper handle size (Fig. 34–2)

TENNIS BALLS

Tennis balls may vary considerably (especially solid core balls versus the usual vac-

PROPER GRIP SIZE: TECHNIQUE OF ROBERT P. NIRSCHL, M.D.

Regardless of which grip style you use—eastern, continental, or western—you will still have problems stroking the ball properly unless you have a racquet with the proper grip size for you. If the grip is too big, you'll have trouble holding on to the racquet, especially on very hot days when your hands sweat. Too small a grip, on the other hand, can produce blisters.

For years, sporting good store salesmen and pro-shop assistants have fitted grips mainly on the basis of trial and error, asking you how a particular grip "feels." In some places, the method is a little more "scientific." You hear criteria such as "touching the seventh octagon of the handle" or "the thumb overlaps the third finger."

There is a simpler, more accurate way to check grip size, one that anyone can easily check. It's by means of the palm crease factor.

Look at the palm of your hand. Notice the lateral creases. The bottom crease, running along the middle portion of the hand, is the one you want. If you take a ruler (see drawing) and measure from the tip of your ring finger to a point on the creases between the ring and middle fingers, you should be able to determine the grip you need. If the measurement comes out to say 4⅔ inches, that is the correct grip size for you.

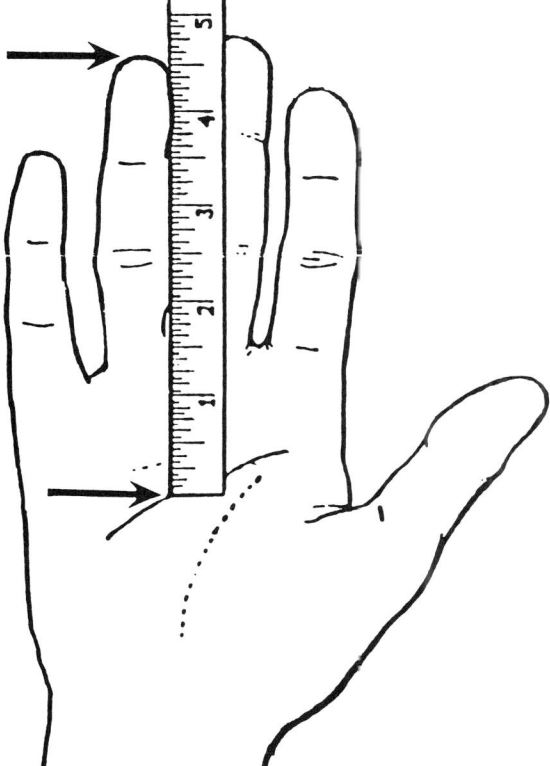

FIGURE 34–2. Nirschl hand measurement technique for proper grip size.

uum ball design). For protection from injury, we recommend the usual vacuum ball. Dead balls or balls that have picked up moisture may cause injury and are to be avoided.

COUNTERFORCE BRACING

The concept of counterforce bracing is to constrain the generation of internal muscle tension forces or prevent tendon migration. Applying a basically nonelastic constraint in appropriate areas has been noted clinically to minimize the symptoms of medial and lateral tennis elbow. Analysis has also revealed biomechanical relevance including decreased angular acceleration and decreased muscle activity in the braced group.[2] At present, counterforce bracing is utilized at the elbow to prevent injury as well as a treatment tool (Fig. 34–3). Overall, it has been clinically noted that a wide brace that controls all muscle groups in a comfortable, balanced manner results in an effective control of pain in symptomatic elbow patients.[3]

Wrist abnormalities of the ulnar-carpal and radial-carpal column are consistently controlled by wrist counterforce braces that allow active finger function.

In the lower extremity, shin splints, posterior tendinitis, and plantar fasciitis are also aided by counterforce bracing.

Metatarsalgia and symptomatic pronated feet are clinically aided by metatarsal pads and firm (not rigid) orthotics.

COMMON INJURIES

A wide variety of injuries occur secondary to tennis activities. As noted, however, many individual hereditarial and prior injury deficiencies are often brought to the sport. The most common problems are as follows:

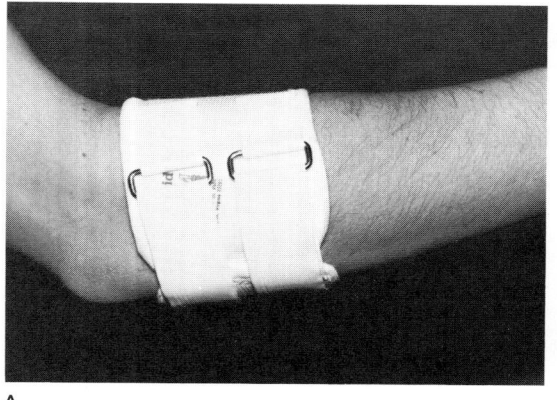
A

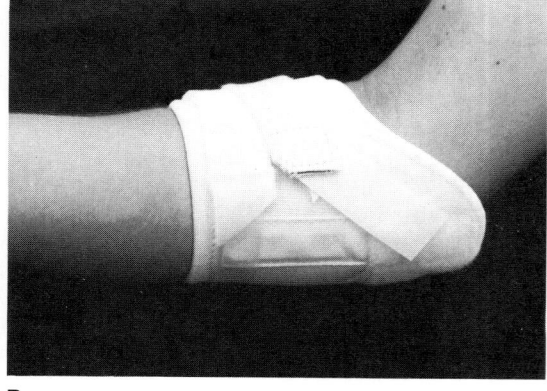
B

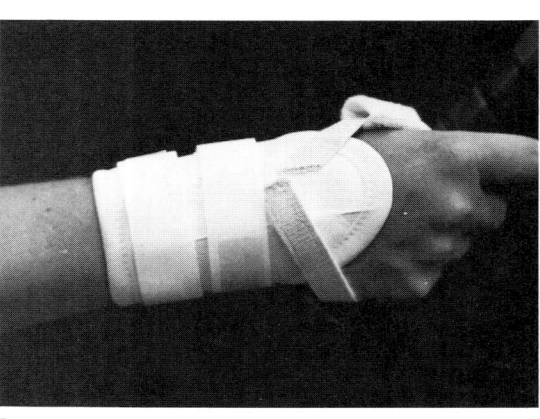
C

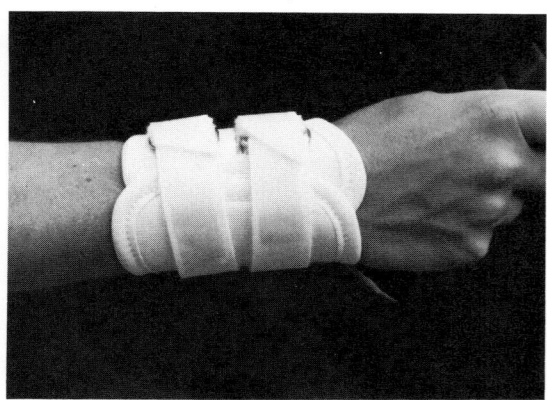
D

FIGURE 34–3. (A) Lateral tennis elbow counterforce brace. (B) Medial tennis elbow counterforce brace. (C) Radial-carpal counterforce wrist brace. (D) Ulnar-carpal counterforce wrist brace.

A. Tendon
   a. Tennis elbow, lateral and medial
   b. Shoulder tendinitis (primarily the supraspinatus aspect of the rotator cuff)
   c. Patellar tendon
   d. Achilles tendon
   e. Plantar fascia
B. Ligament
   a. Wrist, triangular fibrocartilage and ulnar collateral ligament
   b. Ankle sprain (primarily lateral; anterior fibulotalar ligament)
C. Muscle
   a. Lumbar
   b. Calf (medial gastrocnemius)
   c. Abdominal
   d. Thigh (hamstring and adductors)
D. Joint
   a. Shoulder subluxation
   b. Wrist (distal radial-ulnar joint)
   c. Knee (meniscal)
   d. Wrist ganglion
E. Apophysis
   a. Medial elbow (Little League elbow)
   b. Knee, tibial tubercle (Osgood-Schlatter)
   c. Os calcis (Sever)
   d. Vertebral (Scheuermann)
   e. Posterior elbow (olecranon)
F. Bone
   a. Back, lumbar (spondylolysis)
   b. Stress fracture of the tibia
   c. Stress fracture of the metatarsals
G. Neural elements
   a. Ulnar nerve compression at elbow
   b. Lumbar disk

Overall, the injury experience at Virginia Sportsmedicine Institute has been equally divided between upper and lower extremities. As noted, the lower extremity injuries are those typical of running sports. The upper extremity problems are often more challenging and recalcitrant. The major recalcitrant problems in youth include (1) *shoulder tendinitis* and (2) *back and abdominal problems*. Shoulder tendinitis is often associated with scapular weakness and subtle shoulder subluxation. Abdominal muscle pull and lumbar muscle-ligament strain often associated with thoracic kyphosis and lumbar lordosis are also quite common. Lumbar pars interarticularis stress fracture and lumbar disk disease must always be kept in mind, although statistically these maladies are not common. As the individual matures to the later teens, the problems clearly shift to the difficulties of tendon overload. Meniscal and patellofemoral problems of the knee are fairly common in this age group as well.

TYPICAL CLINICAL PRESENTATIONS OF COMMON TENNIS PROBLEMS

The common chronic problems most frustrating to both doctor and patient are the chronic overuse maladies of shoulder tendinitis, medial and lateral tennis elbow, medial and posterior (olecranon) apophysitis, and wrist problems of the radial-carpal and radial-ulnar columns. In the majority of instances, these problems are initiated by tennis play that is frequent, intense, and of long duration (e.g., two to four times per week, 2 to 3 hours per session) or with a sudden increase in activity after a layoff of several months. The usual presentation of symptoms is gradual in onset after an intense session of practice (often in an attempt to change a stroke pattern). Poor stroke mechanics are often associated (e.g., inadequate elevation and poor lower body participation in the serve and overhead and late ground stroke patterns with excessive wrist snap). Young athletes often equate power with success and more likely than not overhit most balls. Constant repetitive overload of this nature not only incites symptoms of pain but also induces muscle imbalances that further exaggerate pain symptoms and spread the area of injury vulnerability.

SHOULDER TENDINITIS

The presenting symptom is pain with the activity of upward acceleration from the backswing cocking position of the serve. The pain is characteristically located over the anterior rotator cuff and bicipital area with referred pain to the deltoid insertion on the proximal one third of the humerus. Posterior pain over the infraspinatus insertion may be noted as well. Although rarely articulated by the patient, close questioning not uncommonly evokes the history of anterior subluxation of the glenohumeral joint. It is important therefore to perform subluxation tests designed to demonstrate anterior shoulder subluxation.

Clinical signs in the typical rotator cuff patient reveal not only the classic areas of tenderness over the supraspinatus attachment point at the greater tuberosity but stretched out and weak scapular muscles (positive rhomboid scapular winging) with tenderness over the levator scapulae attachment to the scapula and weak external rotator and abductor muscles (infraspinatus, supraspinatus, teres minor).

LATERAL TENNIS ELBOW TENDINITIS

The classical presenting symptom is pain just anterior and distal to the lateral epicondyle associated with wrist and finger extensor stress (e.g., drinking from a cup, shaking hands, or hitting tennis backhands). Wrist flexion or triceps-biceps activity cause no pain. Palpation over the extensor brevis origin causes exquisite pain, whereas palpation over the lateral epicondyle causes moderate or no pain. Resisted forearm pronation is usually painful, whereas supination is usually painless.

MEDIAL TENNIS ELBOW TENDINITIS

The presenting symptom is pain at and just distal to the medial epicondyle associated with wrist flexion and forearm pronation stress (e.g., wrist flexor curls, shaving of the face, hitting tennis forehands late, or pronation and wrist snap on first serves). Palpation over the pronator teres and flexor carpi radialis at their attachment point to the medial epicondyle causes exquisite pain.

Associated findings may be a positive Tinel sign at zone 3 of the medial epicondylar groove in the area of the ulnar nerve penetration through the flexor ulnaris arcade. In addition, close examination may reveal evidence of medial collateral ligament insufficiency as manifested by positive valgus instability testing.

MEDIAL EPICONDYLAR APOPHYSITIS (LITTLE LEAGUE ELBOW)

Medial apophysitis is the youth version of medial tennis elbow. Since the pathological changes occur at the medial epicondylar apophysis, however, the pain and palpable tenderness are located directly on the medial epicondyle. Ulnar nerve symptoms are not usual unless an avulsion fracture occurs secondary to more intense trauma. Valgus instability is fairly common, and secondary lateral compartment symptoms can occur in association with capitellar osteochondritis dissecans. Careful review of elbow radiographs is therefore essential.

OLECRANON APOPHYSITIS

Repetitive triceps activity in the tennis serve and overhead can overload the olecranon apophysitis at the level of triceps insertion. This condition is analogous to Osgood-Schlatter disease of the knee. Radiographic changes revealing fragmentation of the apophysis are common. The presenting symptoms are pain at the olecranon with aggressive elbow extension, and signs include palpable tenderness at the distal triceps insertion and olecranon pain with triceps stress testing.

RADIAL COLUMN WRIST PROBLEMS

In adolescents, the most common problems are dorsal ganglion and capsular synovitis (impingement) at the radial-carpal joint. Attritional ligament overload with scapholunate dissociation is rare in adolescents but must be kept in mind. The presenting symptoms of ganglion are a visible and palpable tender mass with mild constraint of wrist flexion and extension. In dorsal capsular impingement, symptoms of pain are similar, but pain is noted more often typically on aggressive dorsiflexion. Palpation reveals capsular thickening, but the cystic mass of the ganglion is not present.

ULNAR COLUMN WRIST PROBLEMS

The most common problem by far is degenerative attrition or tear of the triangular fibrocartilage (TFC) complex. Symptoms of pain distal to the dorsal radial-ulnar joint are commonly noted with relatively intense wrist dorsiflexion and forced supination. Palpable tenderness is located directly over the TFC complex radial to the ulnar styloid and distal to the dorsal radial-ulnar joint. A positive arthrogram confirms the diagnosis, but a partial tear may not be evident by this test.

Less common problems include synovitis of the distal radial-ulnar joint, tendinitis and/or subluxation of the extensor carpi ulnaris tendon, and sprain of the ulnar collateral ligament complex.

Exaggerated wrist positions, wrist roll with tennis spin shots, and a "layed-back wrist" while executing forehand volleys are common etiological factors in the incitement of ulnar column wrist abnormalities.

BASIC TREATMENT APPROACHES

Overall, the basic treatment approach (Table 34–2) for all sport injury has not been altered from our 1973 report[4] and subsequent treatment formulas for adult tennis elbow tendinitis.[3, 5, 6]

TABLE 34–2. Tennis Elbow Rehabilitation Protocol

1. Rest phase—control pain (usually 1 to 2 weeks)
   a. Avoid abusive activities (sports)
   b. Controlled activities of daily living
   c. Use counterforce brace
   d. Modalities of physical therapy (high-voltage electrical stimulation, ice, and heat)
2. Antiinflammatory medication
   a. Aspirin or ibuprofen
   b. Other NSAIDS (less commonly used)
   c. Cortisone (oral or injection) if symptoms of such severity to preclude rehabilitative exercise
3. Start fitness program at the time of rest phase onset
4. Start rehabilitative exercise when activities of daily living are comfortable
   a. Use counterforce brace
   b. Start with 1-pound isotonic program of wrist curls, supination and pronation, and ulnar and radial deviation daily
   c. Proceed to 3 pounds, then alternate isotonic weights with isoflex resistance system (tension cord)
   d. Add hand isometrics and finger extension against rubber band resistance when comfortable with isotonic-isoflex program
   e. End point of isotonic exercises is 5 pounds, 15 repetitions for women, and 8 pounds, 15 repetitions for men; painless anaerobic isoflex sprints, and dynamometer grip strength of dominant arm 10 percent greater than nondominant
   Note: The arm and shoulder muscle groups are often weak in association with tennis elbow; check these muscle groups and if weakness is present, rehabilitation must also include biceps, triceps, rotator cuff, and scapular muscle groups
5. Gradual return to tennis when rehabilitation end point reached; Continue maintenance supplemental exercises three times per week.
   a. Use counterforce brace for 3 months minimum
   b. Check equipment and sports techniques and correct as indicated

NSAIDS = Nonsteroidal antiinflammatory drugs

RELIEF OF INFLAMMATION

The concepts include the mnemonic "PRICEMM"—protection, rest, ice, compression, elevation, medication, and modalities. The relief of pain and inflammation of course does not in any way indicate that a complete healing response has occurred.

PROMOTION OF HEALING

To promote healing requires the stimulation of vascular supply and invasion of mesenchymal (fibroblastic) cells. The ultimate stimulation of mature collagen for tendon and ligament healing and cartilage or bone for joint and skeletal healing completes the healing cycle. In general, rehabilitative exercise programs to gradually develop endurance, strength, and flexibility to promote healing are the key.

PROMOTION OF FITNESS

As rehabilitation of the injured part is initiated, fitness programs for uninjured areas should already be under way. A general fitness program offers many advantages including aiding in the healing process. Psychological support and maintaining or improving previously attained fitness are important goals of any fitness program.

CONTROL OF ABUSE

The goal of sport is to win, not good health. Tennis shares this intended goal with other sports. As such, any opportunity to reduce abusive overloads is welcome. In this context, the following concepts have proved beneficial.
- Proper sport technique
- Control of frequency and duration of activity
- Counterforce bracing
- Appropriate equipment selection
- Proper equipment size

SURGERY

If a quality rehabilitative effort such as outlined above fails, a surgical solution may be indicated. In general, the majority of tennis-related injuries are resolved by a quality rehabilitative program. Those maladies most commonly presenting for surgery in youngsters include:

- Rotator cuff shoulder tendinitis (subluxation)
- Knee abnormalities (patellofemoral and meniscal)
- Elbow (capitellar osteochondritis, medial and lateral tennis elbow)

In young adult groups (20 to 30 years of age), the tendon problems of shoulder and elbow and persistent knee problems are more likely to require surgery. Overall, of course, the variety of surgical problems can encompass body areas from the fingers to the toes.

WHEN TREATMENT FAILS

It is unusual not to be reasonably successful in returning an injured youth back to tennis. Major knee instabilities and recalcitrant lumbar disk syndrome would be more likely to preclude return. Even in these circumstances, surgery can often be restorative. The return to a highly competitive or world level is of course more difficult than recreational competition.

Although we may not be able to return all athletes to a competitive level equal to the preinjury state, it is our experience that the large majority are returned utilizing the principles outlined above.

If treatment is not totally successful, modified tennis activity, such as ground strokes and controlled serving motion, is often an option. Even limited return, although precluding full-scale competition, still offers skill enhancement, fitness potential, and the wide social opportunities of a lifetime sport.

References

1. Kibler, W. B., McQueen, C., and Uhl, T.: Fitness evaluation and findings in competitive junior tennis players. Clin. Sports Med. 7(2):403–416, 1988.
2. Groppel, J., and Nirschl, R. P.: A biomechanical and EMG analysis of the effects of counter-force bracing on the tennis player. Am. J. Sports Med. 14:195–201, 1986.
3. Sobel, J., and Nirschl, R. P.: Conservative treatment of tennis elbow. Phys. Sportsmed. 9:42, June, 1981.
4. Nirschl, R. P.: Tennis elbow. Orthop. Clin. North Am. 4(3):787–801, 1973.
5. Nirschl, R. P.: Prevention and treatment of elbow and shoulder injuries in the tennis player. Clin. Sports Med. 7(2):289–308, 1988.
6. Nirschl, R. P.: Rotator cuff surgery. In Barr, J. (ed.): AAOS Instructional Course Lectures, 38:447–463, 1989.

35

SKIING

THOMAS D. ROSENBERG
JONATHAN L. FRANKLIN
LONNIE E. PAULOS

The popularity of skiing has increased dramatically over the last 20 years. With this increased popularity, more and more children have become involved with this sport, starting at a younger and younger age. Many schools have organized programs ranging from beginning instruction to racing teams. Younger children with better techniques, better equipment, and greater competition have resulted in more high-energy falls and more serious injuries.

Skiing demands aerobic conditioning as well as strength and endurance. A keen sense of balance is necessary as the skier responds to the uneven terrain. This chapter will discuss the training principles to meet these demands as well as prevention techniques to decrease the injury rate. We will discuss the trends in skiing injuries as well as review specific injuries in children related to skiing. Because of the trend toward more serious knee injuries in children while skiing, as well as our own extensive experience in knee injuries, the chapter will emphasize the treatment of knee injuries in children.

INJURY TRENDS IN SKIING

The specific type and frequency of skiing injuries have changed dramatically over the last 20 years. These changes have been influenced by equipment changes (boots, skis, bindings, and poles), changes in skiing techniques, and changes involving machine grooming of the slopes. The earliest reported series of ski injuries noted a very high incidence of ankle injuries and tibia fractures. There was a very high overall injury rate as well. Estimates of the total accident rate have decreased from 7.7 per 1000 skier visits in 1950 to 2.5 per 1000 skier visits in the 1987–1988 season.[1] In 1977, Ellison[9] reported an injury rate for women of 7.9 per 1000 ski days and for men of 4.9 per 1000 ski days. He stated that the number of injuries for children had increased and related this increase to the number of young skiers using poor-quality or ill-fitting equipment.

Perhaps the most thorough evaluation of skiing injuries has been performed by Johnson and his associates at the Sugarbush ski area in Vermont.[21, 22, 23] They performed a comprehensive evaluation of all ski injuries at one ski area between 1972 and 1987. This evaluation evaluated prospectively 5701 ski injuries that came from an estimated group of 1.69 million skier visits. The evaluation included thorough testing of the equipment used by the injured skier. The overall injury rate at the ski area was noted to decline by 50 percent during the 15 year period. The major reduction was seen in lower extremity injuries, especially tibia fractures and ankle sprains, which showed a decrease of 88 and 86 percent, respectively. Spiral fractures of the tibia decreased by 89 percent over the period studied. The only area where the injury rate had increased over the 15-year period was in serious knee injuries where com-

TABLE 35–1. Injury Trends in Past 15 Years

	Trend	Percentage
Overall injury rate	Declined	50
Lower extremity injuries	Declined	60
Injuries below knee	Declined	78
Tibia fractures	Declined	88
Ankle sprains	Declined	86
Knee injuries	Declined	36
Third-degree knee sprains	Increased	172

Source: From Johnson, R. J.; Ettlinger, C. F.; and Shealy, J. E.: Skier injury trends. Presented at the 7th International Symposia on Skiing Trauma and Safety, France, 1989.

plete tears of the anterior cruciate ligament were found to have increased by 172 percent (Table 35–1).

In 1975, Marshall and his associates[27] were the first to emphasize serious knee injuries in skiers. Feagin et al.[15] similarly found a dramatic increase in serious knee injuries, reporting an incidence of 1.2 knee injuries per 1000 skier days, 60 percent of those injuries involved the anterior cruciate ligament. Feagin estimated that over 100,000 anterior cruciate ligaments are injured per year in the United States in skiing alone.

Very few studies have addressed specifically pediatric and adolescent injuries in skiing despite the fact that children appear to be more susceptible to injuries in this sport. In the 1986–1987 season, males less than 10 years old accounted for 5.95 percent of all ski injuries, and females in this age group made up 4.64 percent of all ski injuries. Males in the 11- to 17-year-old group sustained 19.29 percent of all injuries, whereas females in this age group sustained 16.5 percent.[1] Therefore, skiers 17 years old or younger accounted for 46.4 percent of all ski injuries.

Garrick and Requa[17] and Requa and Garrick[33] evaluated a group of over 3500 students involved in five major ski schools in the Seattle area. In this young group of skiers, they reported an injury rate of 9.1 per 1000 skier days. The students 10 years and under had the lowest incidence of injuries, whereas the 11- to 14-year-old age group had the highest overall injury rate. The younger group had a higher rate of fractures, whereas the older group had higher rates of sprains, abrasions, and bruises. The most common injury was injury to the knee, followed by the ankle and upper extremity.

In 1982, Moreland[29] addressed skiing injuries in children and suggested that downhill skiing accounted for the greatest number of injuries to children of all the usual outdoor winter sports. He felt that the incidence of injury in children was somewhat higher than the overall injury rate for all skiers. He stressed several factors accounting for the difference. First, he felt that there was an increased injury rate in beginners, and children make up a high percentage of the beginners. Second, he felt that children would be more prone to reporting their injury to ski patrol or medical personnel. Finally, he felt that there was a higher incidence of lower extremity equipment-related injuries in the younger age group. He concluded that the incidence of injuries in young teenagers was significantly above the rates for all ages and that tibial fractures were a particularly common injury in this age group.

Blitzer et al.[2] in 1984 looked specifically at downhill ski injuries in children at the Sugarbush area in northern Vermont. They found that during the period from 1972 through 1981, 22 percent of injuries occurred in children 16 years of age or younger. The adolescents had the highest injury rate, whereas children under 11 years of age had the same injury rate as adults. Foot and ankle injuries as well as tibia fractures were more common in the younger skiers and gave way to more serious knee injuries in the older age groups. Upper extremity injuries were less common in children than in the adults.

In summary, children are becoming more involved at a younger age in the sport of skiing and appear to have injury rates higher than the overall skiing population, yet there have been few studies addressing injuries specifically in children. Because of the tremendous number of children now skiing and the problems unique to treating children's injuries, this area definitely deserves careful attention.

SPECIFIC INJURIES IN PEDIATRIC AND ADOLESCENT SKIERS

CONTUSIONS AND LACERATIONS

Probably the most common injuries sustained by children while skiing are contusions and lacerations. These are often not severe and are most often not reported to the ski patrol or medical facilities. Lacerations are most often seen on the scalp and face, since those areas are exposed to sharp ski edges and other obstacles. The rest of the body is usually protected by ski clothing, boots, or gloves. With better grooming of ski areas and better warning markings, we see less lacerations and contusions from underbrush or external hazards. Most of these injuries occur from ski edges or skier collisions. With the departure from the traditional safety straps, many of the contusions and lacerations from the skis and ski edges have now been eliminated. With the traditional safety straps, skis stayed close to the falling skier and often resulted in lacerations. Modern ski brakes allow the skier to fall away from the sharp ski edges and yet stop the ski from continuing down the hill. Contusions are treated with rest and icing for the first 24 to 48 hours and then heat, stretching, and gradual mobilization and increase in activities. Lacerations must be thoroughly irrigated, and an assessment is made whether or not suturing is required.

UPPER EXTREMITY INJURIES

Although the overall injury rate has been decreasing over the past 20 years, most of this decrease has been in the lower extremity injuries. With the increased number of skiers, there has been a relative increase in the number of upper extremity injuries.[38] The most common upper extremity injuries are injuries to the shoulder and injuries to the thumb. There have been no reports specifically addressing children's upper extremity injuries, but the most comprehensive reviews of upper extremity injuries in skiing have been by Carr et al.[4] Weaver,[38] and Derkash et al.[8]

Thumb Injuries

Carr et al.[4] reported 40 percent of all upper extremity injuries involved the thumb, with 85 percent of the thumb injuries being to the ulnar collateral ligament of the metacarpal phalangeal joint. The proposed mechanism of injury to the thumb was a forward fall on an outstretched hand still holding the ski pole (Fig. 35–1). The pole would force the thumb into abduction and hyperextension, resulting in a sprain of the ulnar collateral ligament, an injury often called "skier's thumb." The pole manufacturers thought the strap was causing the pole to remain in the hand during these falls and therefore introduced the "new grip" ski poles with molded hand grips on platforms (Fig. 35–2). Carr et

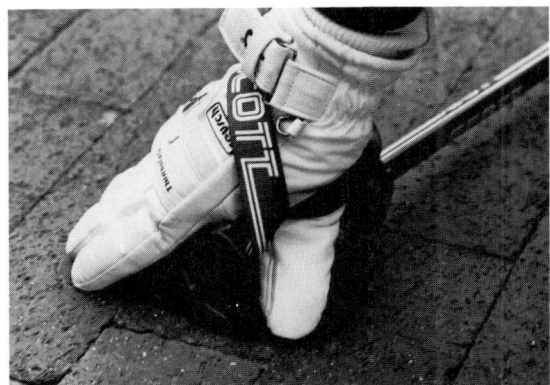

FIGURE 35–1. The proposed mechanism of "skier's thumb."

al.[4] compared the "new grip" ski poles to the traditional straps and found that the "new grip" ski poles did not reduce the thumb or upper extremity injuries. They appeared to hold the pole in the hand during a fall as did the traditional straps and therefore did not reduce injuries to the thumb.

Perhaps the most comprehensive recent review of the "skier's thumb"[18] is the series of Derkash et al.[8] A joint opening of greater than 45 degrees on stress radiographs compared with the opposite side was considered a complete tear of the ulnar collateral ligament requiring surgical intervention. The surgical technique is well described in this article. Again, these authors found that the change in pole design did not decrease the incidence of total ulnar collateral ligament tears. It is important to note that the youngest patient in this series was 16 years old.

Rockwood and his associates[34] address the child's gamekeeper's thumb. They state that the injury can occur in the preadolescent or the adolescent and recommend open repair if the joint opens 45 degrees more than the normal side, similar to the treatment of this injury in an adult (Fig. 35–3A). Complete tears opening less than 45 degrees more than the normal side are treated in a thumb spica cast for 4 weeks. The most common injury in the younger child is a Salter Harris type III fracture of the ulnar corner of the epiphysis of the proximal phalanx (Fig. 35–3B). If the epiphyseal fragment is displaced, open reduction and internal fixation are recommended. One must also be aware of the "pseudo" gamekeeper's thumb in which the ligament is intact but the physis is opening with a Salter Harris type I fracture. A stress X ray may be helpful in this diagnosis (Fig. 35–3C).

676 PART III—SPORT-SPECIFIC SPORTS MEDICINE

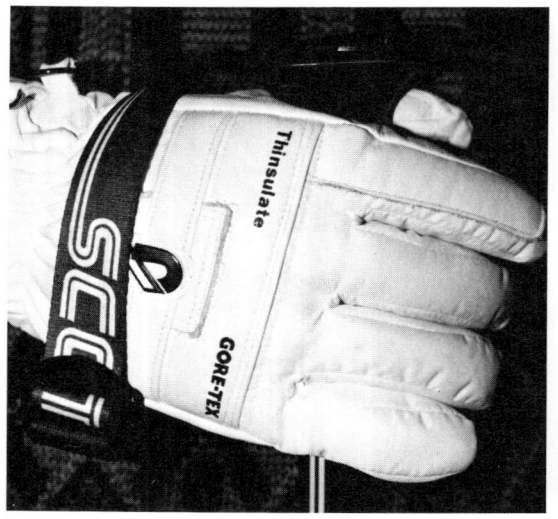 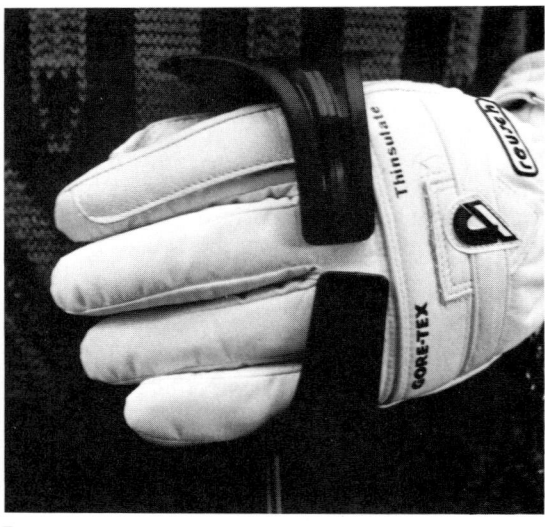

FIGURE 35–2. The "old"-type ski grips, held in place by straps (*A*) are contrasted with the open handles of the "new" type (*B*).

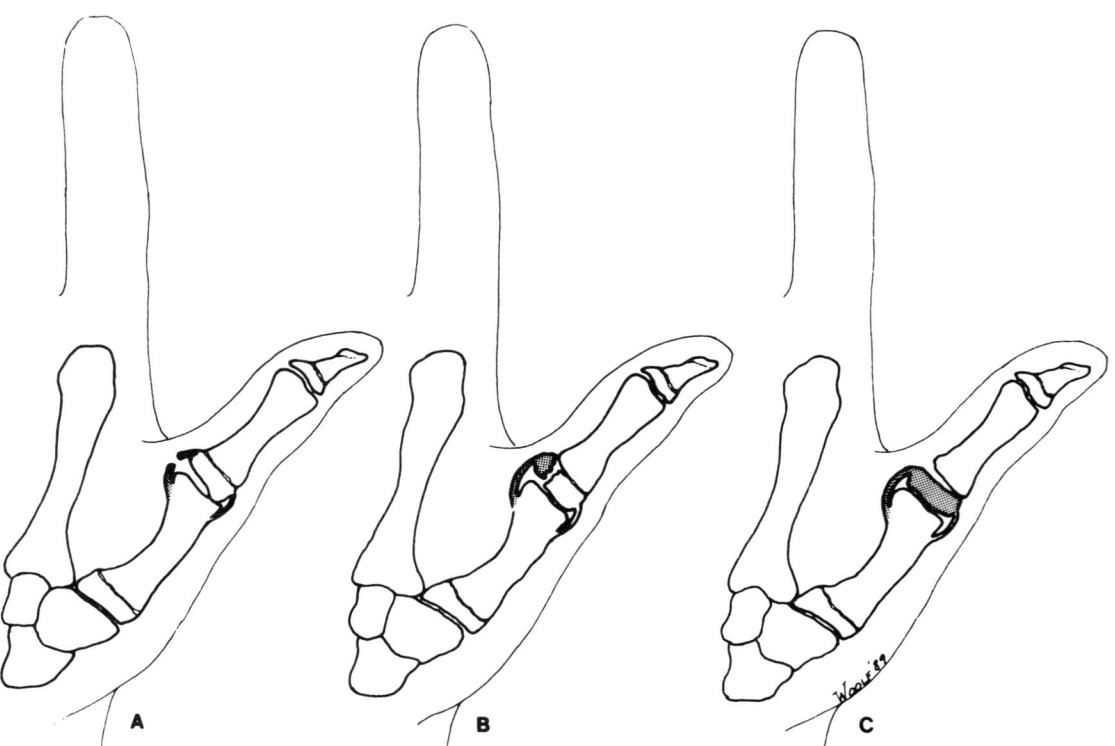

FIGURE 35–3. The child's gamekeeper's thumb. (*A*) True rupture of the ulnar collateral ligament. (*B*) Salter Harris type III fracture with intact ligament attached to epiphyseal fragment. (*C*) Salter Harris type I fracture or "pseudo" gamekeeper's thumb.

Shoulder Injuries

Weaver[38] reviewed 135 consecutive shoulder injuries seen at an Aspen ski clinic during the 1978–1979 ski season. He found anterior dislocation of the shoulder to be the most common ailment, making up 52 percent of the total injuries. Rotator cuff tears were the next most common, accounting for 20 percent of the total injuries, followed by acromioclavicular separations, which made up 18 percent of the injuries. The remaining 10 percent of the injuries were made up of contusions and isolated fractures. Although children's injuries were not specifically addressed, it is interesting to note that the rotator cuff injuries occurred in the older patients, whereas dislocations, especially recurrent dislocations, often occurred in the younger patients.

It has been well established that younger patients have a much higher rate of recurrence after dislocations. Shoulder instability is especially disabling in skiing since the arm is often abducted and externally rotated with pole planting, especially if the pole sticks in the snow as the skier advances forward. This position makes the shoulder vulnerable for an anterior dislocation. Also, skiing often involves falling onto an outstretched arm, again often resulting in recurrent dislocations.

Whenever possible, shoulder dislocation should be carefully documented with radiographs prior to reduction. Proper muscle relaxation is necessary so that the reduction maneuver can be accomplished in a gentle fashion. Once the shoulder is reduced, careful X-ray documentation is mandatory to rule out fractures or persistent dislocations. X-rays should include either an axillary or transscapular view to document reduction (Fig. 35–4). The shoulder is then placed into a sling and swath. Immobilization should be continued for the first 3 weeks with a first-time dislocation to allow adequate healing of the anterior structures. This is especially true in children since recurrent dislocations are the major complication of this injury in children, unlike the shoulder stiffness seen in adults. Once fully rehabilitated, the child may return to skiing, but if recurrence of the dislocation occurs, we would recommend surgical repair before return to skiing for the child. The treatment of clavicular fractures and injuries to the acromioclavicular joint are discussed in Chapter 12. Other shoulder fractures are managed with the techniques described for general trauma.[32, 34]

LOWER EXTREMITY INJURIES

Skiing places a unique challenge on the lower extremity not experienced in any other sport. The ski, binding, and boot create an

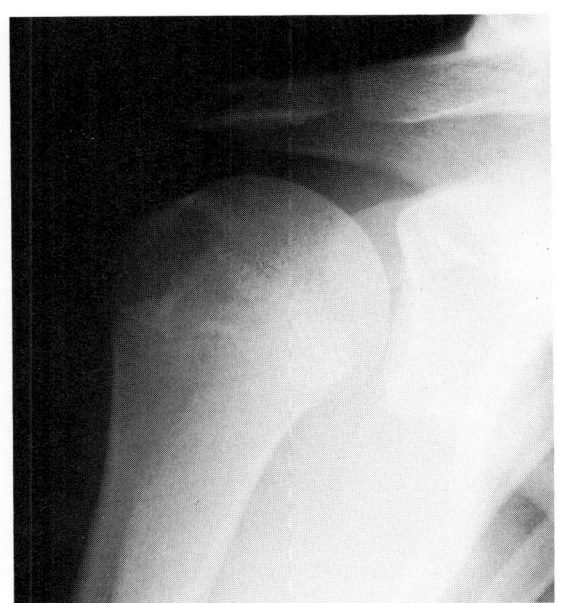 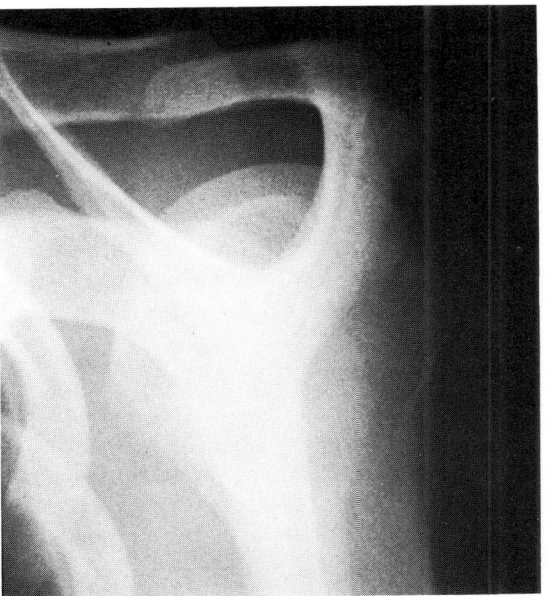

FIGURE 35–4. (*A*) Anteroposterior X ray of shoulder. (*B*) Transscapular lateral view of shoulder.

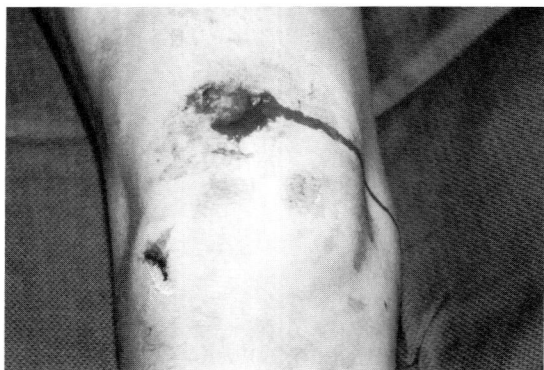

FIGURE 35–5. Knee laceration that communicated with the knee joint and required surgical irrigation and debridement of knee joint.

extension of the normal anatomy of the lower extremity, creating an extremely large lever arm. Forces are transmitted through the lower extremity to the knee. The higher and stiffer boot places most of this stress through the knee joint. Injuries to the knee will be discussed in length in the next section. The other injuries that need to be addressed with the lower extremities are contusions, lacerations, ankle sprains, and fractures.

Contusions and lacerations are treated similarly to the upper extremity injuries. In younger children especially, one should remember that it is difficult to obtain a thorough examination of an injured extremity. Therefore, one should carefully inspect the skin for contusions and lacerations that may be hints at more serious underlying injuries. X rays may be required to confirm that bones are not fractured deep to serious contusions. Lacerations, again, should be thoroughly irrigated and explored. Lacerations around the knee should be very carefully examined to rule out the possibility of penetration of the knee joint, which would require surgical irrigation and drainage (Fig. 35–5).

Ankle Sprains

Ankle sprains are seen much less commonly, now that stiffer and higher boots are available. However, a fair amount of these injuries still occur in younger children, possibly because they tend to wear ill-fitting boots. Since children are growing so fast, the initial fit of the boots is often loose. The sprains are treated in standard fashion, obtaining appropriate X-rays to rule out growth plate injuries and a thorough examination with comparison to the opposite ankle to evaluate ligamentous laxity. Severe ankle sprains may require casting or functional bracing for 3 to 4 weeks as well as a comprehensive rehabilitation program including work on strength, range of motion (ROM), and proprioception training. We have not seen chronic ankle instability produce problems with skiing, since skiing requires only flexion and extension of the ankle. The valgus and varus stresses are prevented by the stiff ski boot. We have therefore not seen the need for ankle ligament reconstruction specifically for skiing.

Fractures

The lower extremity fracture rate has declined over the last 20 years, but tibia fractures and ankle fractures still occur, especially in the younger skiers. Freeman et al.[16] reviewed 734 tibial fractures treated in Aspen, Colorado, from 1968 to 1978 and noted an overall decline in the rate of tibial fractures from 12.9 per 100,000 skier days in 1968 to 2.9 per 100,000 skier days in 1983. The decline was mainly seen in spiral fractures. This group of patients were all adults but may reflect the changing patterns seen in children's fractures also. We have similarly seen a changing pattern in lower leg fractures on the ski slopes. There are less distal tibia and ankle fractures, perhaps owing to the protection of stiffer, better-fitting boots. The decrease in spiral fractures appears to be secondary to side release toe bindings, which eliminate the twisting mechanisms of spiral fractures. However, we see more "boot top" fractures, as the forces are transmitted to the tibia at the top of the stiffer boots.

Peter et al.[31] described the treatment of 91 consecutive fractures of the lower leg using functional bracing. They described excellent results with this method of treatment of these skiing-related fractures. The youngest patient was age 15, and the average age of patients was 34 years. We would refer the reader to the standard fracture textbooks for treatment of lower extremity fractures in children.[32, 34] We would caution the physician caring for children's skiing fractures to be aware of the potential for physeal injuries and have a very high index of suspicion for them. One must carefully palpate the physeal regions. If ligamentous laxity exists around the knee and there is tenderness at the physeal region, a stress X-ray is required to rule out physeal fracture (Fig. 35–6). X-rays are often difficult to interpret in children be-

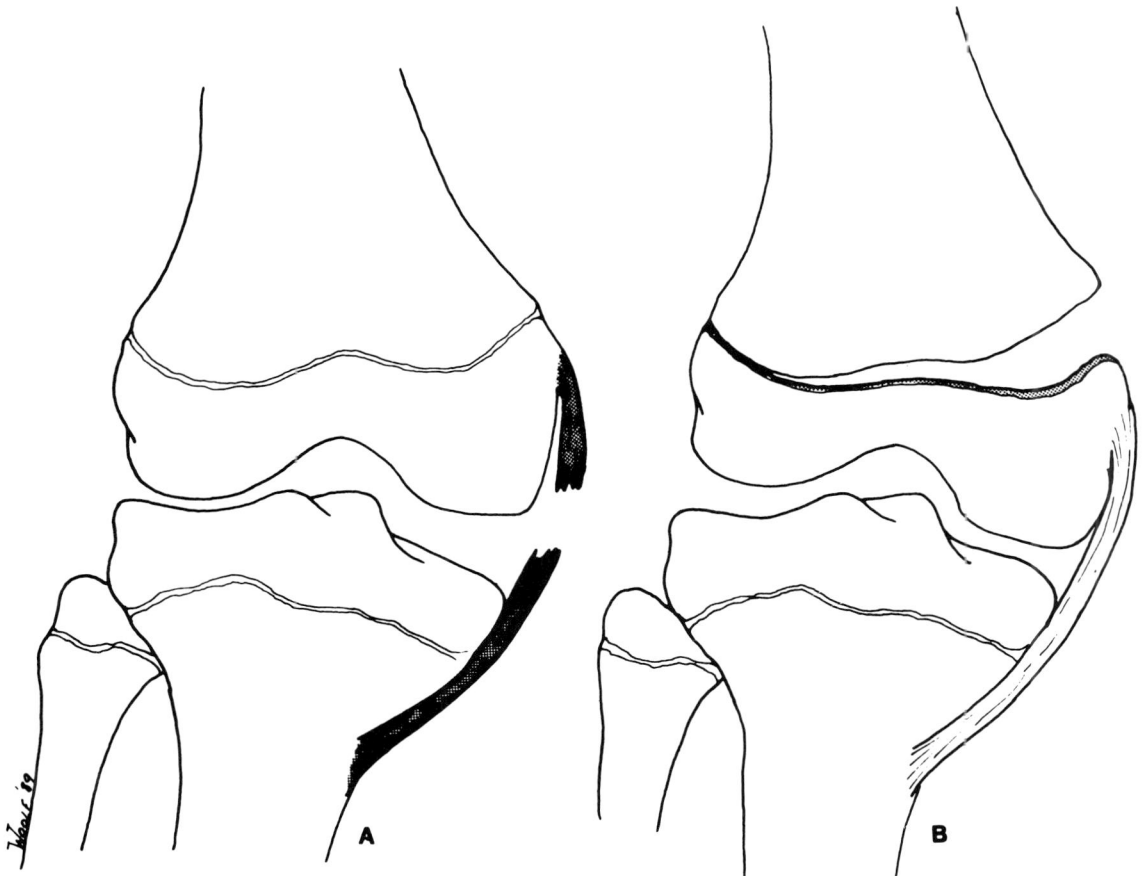

FIGURE 35-6. A stress X-ray can help diagnose a true medial collateral ligament rupture or a Salter-Harris type I fracture. (*A*) Joint opening found with medial collateral ligament rupture. (*B*) Distal femoral physeal opening found with Salter-Harris type I fracture with intact ligament.

cause of the growth plates, and one must remember that the opposite extremity is always available for a comparison view, if necessary.

In our experience, most diaphyseal tibia fractures in adolescents can be treated closed. Initial treatment consists of a long leg cast with the knee slightly flexed to control rotation at the fracture site. Children heal rapidly, especially younger children, and therefore weight bearing can usually begin at 2 to 3 weeks in the long leg cast. A comminuted or markedly displaced fracture requires longer immobilization because of the delayed healing associated with greater soft tissue injury. During the early period of immobilization, frequent radiographic evaluation must be repeated, or the cast can be wedged if any angulation occurs. After 3 to 4 weeks, most "boot top" fractures can be changed to a patellar tendon bearing cast with full weight bearing. Total time of immobilization varies from 6 to 8 weeks to 3 months, depending on the patient's age and the degree of soft tissue trauma.

Even during the immobilization period, an aggressive rehabilitation program is begun. This program includes straight leg raises and isometrics to maintain quadriceps strength. Well-leg cycling and upper extremity strengthening are begun early. Once the immobilization is discontinued, work begins on range of motion at the knee and ankle, cycling, and swimming during the first month. Once full motion is achieved, fracture callus is present on the radiograph, and there is no pain at the fracture site (usually 3 to 4 months postinjury), the skier begins a strengthening program including minisquats, leg press, sports cords, straight-ahead jogging, outdoor cycling, pogo ball, and trampoline. Only after

TABLE 35–2. Tibia Fracture Rehabilitation ("Boot Top" Fracture)

Immobilization (6 to 12 Weeks)
Long leg cast (2 to 4 weeks)
   Straight leg raises, isometrics
Patellar tendon bearing cast (4 to 8 weeks)
   Knee motion
   Weight bearing
   Well-leg cycling, upper extremity strengthening

Early Mobilization (First Month out of Cast)
Ankle and knee motion
Cycling, swimming

Strengthening (Second to Fourth Month out of Cast)
Outdoor cycling, jogging
Minisquats, leg press, sports cords
Pogo ball, trampoline

Return to Skiing (6 to 8 Months Postinjury)
Must have full motion
Must have full strength
Must have radiographic confirmation of healing

---

the child has achieved full strength and range of motion may he or she return to skiing (usually 6 to 8 months) (Table 35–2).

Knee Injuries

As previously described, the overall trend has been for a decrease in injury rate occurring during skiing, yet knee injuries have increased in the past 15 years by a factor of 2.7.[23] Feagin et al.[15] estimated that 100,000 anterior cruciate ligaments are injured per year in skiing. With the high proportion of pediatric and adolescent-age skiers, it is mandatory that physicians treating ski injuries familiarize themselves with the diagnosis and treatment of knee injuries in children.

The anterior cruciate ligament sprain is the most common injury in skiing.[20] The most common mechanism that we see for the anterior cruciate ligament injury is catching a ski tip in heavy snow, producing an external rotation/valgus stress on the knee. This mechanism may partially or completely tear the medial collateral ligament as well. The second common mechanism that we see is forced hyperextension that may occur during deceleration when skiing from a fast, packed surface onto heavy, untracked snow. The anterior cruciate ligament, a normal check to hyperextension, is flattened out against the intercondylar notch and rupture occurs. Another mechanism for rupture is internal rotation of the tibia and extension with or without valgus stress. This most often occurs from catching an outside edge, which draws the ski across the front of the forward-falling skier. McConkey[26] has suggested a new mechanism for anterior cruciate ligament injury seen in expert skiers. In these cases, the skier produces a violent quadriceps contraction to recover from an out-of-control sitting-back posture or to gain control after landing from a jump. The powerful quadriceps contracture exerts an "active" anterior drawer stress on the tibia capable of rupturing the anterior cruciate ligament.

Several different types of anterior cruciate ligament complex injuries occur in children that require different treatment methods. The interstitial tear of the anterior cruciate ligament is less common in children than in adults (Fig. 35–7A). More often, an avulsion without bone occurs at the tibial insertion of this ligament[7] (Fig. 35–7B). Rarely, such avulsions occur near the femoral insertion in older adolescents near skeletal maturity similar to an adult injury. The tibial and femoral avulsions are grouped together since their healing potential and treatment are similar. A third type of injury is the bony tibial eminence avulsion, which occurs in the child for the anatomical reasons stated below (Fig. 35–7C).

There are several factors that make the treatment of children's knee injuries unique. Anatomical considerations make the child's knee injury different from an adult's. The rarity of the midsubstance disruption of the anterior cruciate ligament in the skeletally immature is felt to be related to the insertion of the cruciate. The collagen fibers insert directly into the perichondrium and epiphyseal cartilage of the proximal tibia.[28] This insertion often results in a bony avulsion rather than a ligamentous disruption. The open physis provides a challenge in planning reconstructive procedures without compromising the remaining growth with drill holes. The anterior cruciate ligament attaches just in front of and lateral to the anterior tibial spine. This anatomical location and the relative strength of the ligament also contribute to the occurrence of avulsions of the tibial eminence rather than midsubstance tears with anterior cruciate ligament injuries in children.[7]

Another factor to consider when making treatment decisions regarding children's ligament injuries is the fact that children will have many more years to tolerate the instability than an adult with a similar injury. Several studies have suggested a poor prognosis with anterior cruciate ligament deficiency in

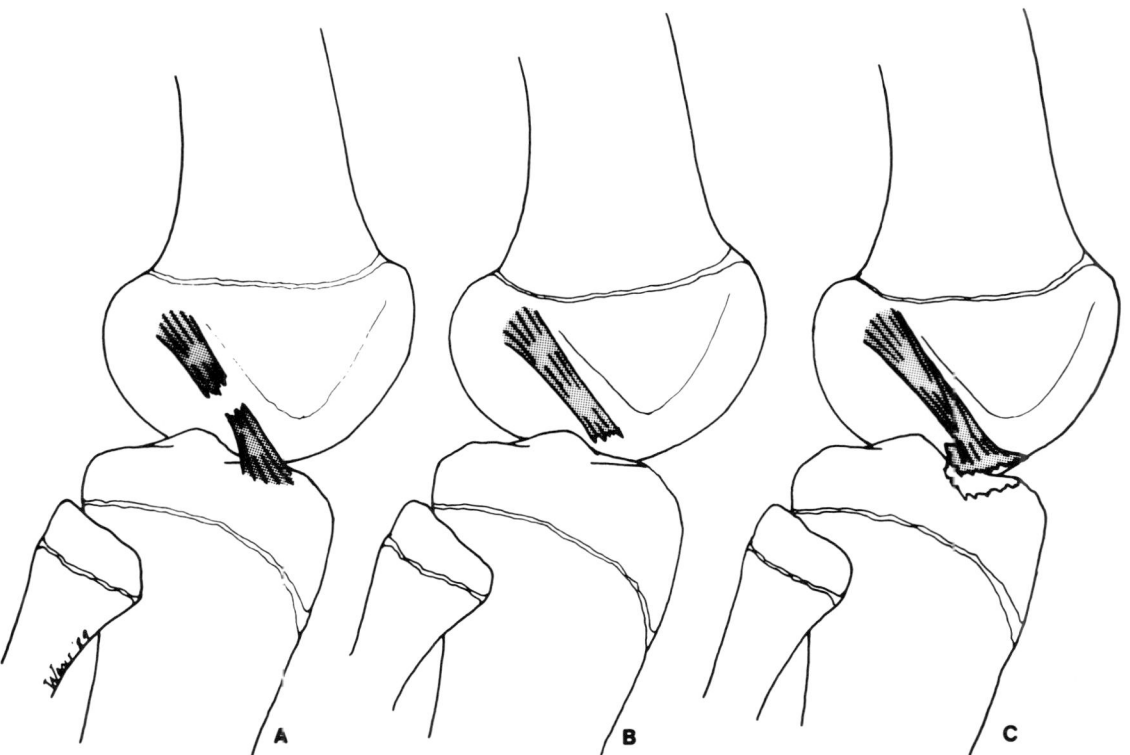

FIGURE 35-7. Type of anterior cruciate ligament complex injuries in the child. (*A*) Midsubstance tear. (*B*) Avulsion near tibial insertion (may also occur rarely near femoral insertion). (*C*) Bony avulsion of tibial eminence.

children.[3, 7] Many extraarticular or bony injuries heal rapidly in children. However, the intraarticular anterior cruciate ligament complex is bathed in synovial fluid, and therefore, as in the adult, the intersubstance tear has little healing potential. Children are also involved in many activities that require an anterior cruciate ligament, whereas adults are often able to modify their activities to accommodate their ligamentous insufficiency. Disruption of the anterior cruciate ligament with or without other associated ligament injuries is becoming more commonly diagnosed in the pediatric and adolescent age group. This may well represent a better awareness and ability to diagnose these injuries, yet there are very few authors that have addressed ligamentous insufficiency in the knees of children.[3, 5, 6, 24]

Before considering treatment options, one must address the question, "Does one need an anterior cruciate ligament for skiing?" It was once thought that skiing does not require an anterior cruciate ligament since the flexed knee position is often maintained during skiing. However, one must thoroughly evaluate associated ligamentous laxity as well as meniscal pathology, either of which would make tolerating this condition more difficult. Considering the current competitiveness of skiing and the jumps that must be executed in downhill racing, a young skier may require an anterior cruciate ligament to face the challenges of skiing safely.[36] When treating a young skier for an anterior cruciate ligament injury, the child's other sports activities must also be considered. A child's play and sports activities often involve running, jumping, and pivoting; these activities must also be considered when choosing a treatment for anterior cruciate ligament injury in a child. For the reasons stated above, we therefore feel that an aggressive approach to the anterior cruciate ligament injury in a child is warranted but that it should be performed in a manner that respects the open physis whenever possible.

For the intersubstance tear, or the disruption at the tibial or femoral insertion, primary repair or immobilization is not likely to

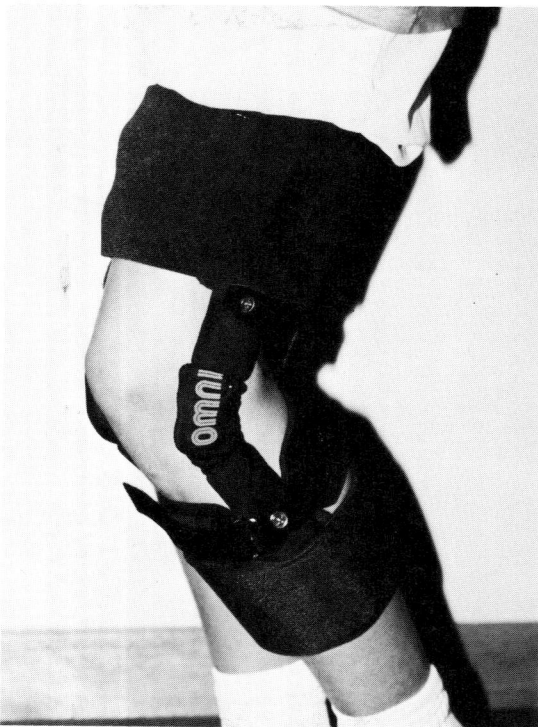

FIGURE 35–8. A functional sports brace may protect the knee prior to surgical reconstruction.

be successful. If the child is within 2 years of skeletal maturity and mechanical symptoms do not exist, then the child can often be protected with a brace for 1 or 2 years (Fig. 35–8) until a standard technique could be used for anterior cruciate ligament reconstruction without affecting the growth plates. It would be mandatory however, that the child is willing to wear a brace and does not experience "giving way" episodes that might cause irreversible damage to the menisci or articular surfaces. Successful bracing can allow a child to return to skiing with no restrictions. A younger child or a child in which bracing is unsuccessful should be treated aggressively with anterior cruciate ligament reconstruction. In these young children, the open physis must be considered when choosing a reconstruction technique.

Lipscomb and Anderson[24] described a surgical reconstruction of the anterior cruciate ligament using the semitendinosus and gracilis tendons through drill holes crossing the physis in 24 children age 12 to 15 years old. This technique utilized tunnels crossing the tibial physis but avoided crossing the femoral physis. Only 1 patient out of 24 in this group showed a significant growth abnormality. They concluded that drilling across the tibial physis and femoral epiphysis did not cause significant growth disturbance.

McCarroll and his associates[25] recently reported the results in 40 patients under age 14 treated for anterior cruciate ligament tears; 10 patients had extraarticular reconstructions, 14 had intraarticular reconstructions, and 16 were treated conservatively. Very few of the conservatively treated patients returned to athletics, whereas all the surgically treated patients returned to athletics. They recommended an aggressive approach to anterior cruciate ligament tears in children under age 14, using the extraarticular approach to children 13 years of age and younger. They observed no growth abnormalities in the surgically treated group.

We feel that the surgeon should avoid violating the physis whenever possible. This becomes important in selecting a graft for reconstruction in a child. The commonly used central one-third patellar tendon graft in adults should not be used in children with open physes: Harvesting the bone block from the tibial tubercle could cause a serious growth abnormality. The hamstring tendons, especially the semitendinosus, are a reasonable choice for an autogenous graft. Again, the surgeon must be careful not to injure the tibial physis during the harvest of this tendon at its distal tibial insertion. An allograft, which requires no sacrifice of autogenous structures, is another option. However, one must consider the possibility of disease transmission with the use of allograft. Although extraarticular reconstruction is another possibility, the authors feel that the chances of success of an isolated extraarticular reconstruction are not good. Also, an extraarticular reconstruction sacrifices an important secondary restraint and may therefore not be a totally benign procedure. If treatment cannot be deferred, such as in the case of a locked meniscus, the authors would cautiously recommend a semitendinosus tendon graft for intraarticular reconstruction. In this difficult situation, one must weigh the risks of growth abnormalities against the likelihood of permanent damage to the menisci and articular surfaces. Another possibility in this difficult situation would be to repair the meniscus and brace the child while meniscal healing occurs, then proceed with anterior cruciate ligament reconstruction at skeletal maturity.

Treatment of tibial eminence fractures has been addressed in recent orthopedic literature.[19, 35] Open reduction has been advocated for displaced fractures of the tibial eminence.[19] Despite healing of the fracture in the normal position, mild degrees of anterior cruciate ligament laxity have been noted to result from its injury. It has been suggested that the anterior cruciate ligament probably stretches before its tibial attachment fractures.[35]

We feel that anatomical reduction of the tibial eminence fracture is essential for an optimum outcome from this injury. There are two treatment options available: closed reduction and casting or open (or arthroscopic) reduction. Extension casting can be a satisfactory method of treatment if anatomical reduction can be confirmed. This often requires tomograms or computerized tomography (CT) scans while in the cast. It is interesting to note that full extension is a position that puts tension on the anterior cruciate ligament and thus might tend to distract the fracture fragment. However, the contour of the intercondylar notch presses against the tibial eminence in full extension and provides a mechanical reduction of the fracture fragment (Fig. 35–9).

If anatomical reduction cannot be achieved with closed techniques, arthroscopic or open techniques are essential. We prefer to use arthroscopic techniques to decrease the morbidity of the procedure. The crater must be thoroughly cleaned of small fragments or early clot formation. The bony fragment on the ligament stump should also be similarly cleaned so that anatomical reduction can be achieved. If the fragment is large enough (greater than 1 cm by 1 cm) and the patient is near skeletal maturity, then an interfragmentary screw can often be placed across the fracture, holding the fragment reduced anatomically. A cannulated system may aid in

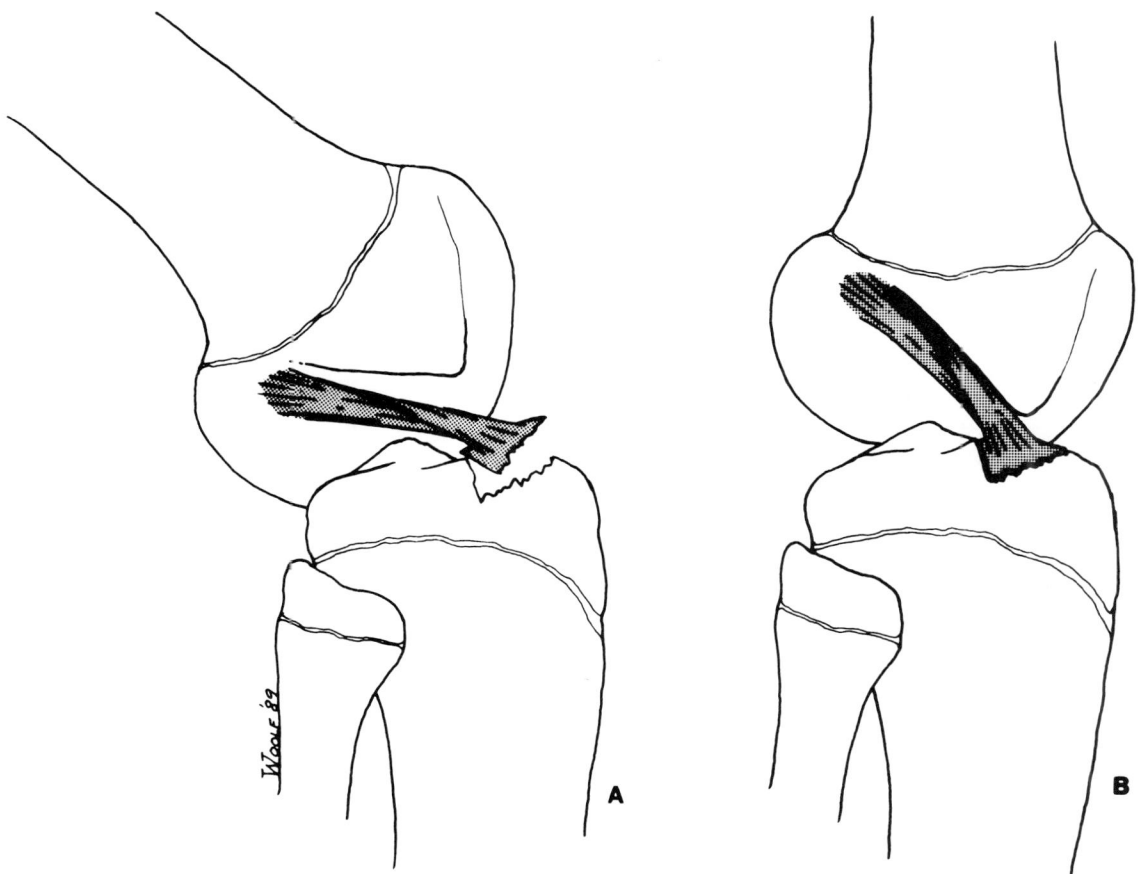

FIGURE 35–9. (*A*) Displaced tibial eminence fracture. (*B*) Full extension reduces the tibial eminence fragment by direct pressure from the adjacent roof of the intercondylar notch.

the reduction and placement of the screw. In cases with smaller fragments or a wide, open physis, a helpful technique is placing sutures into the distal end of the anterior cruciate ligament near its insertion to the bony fragment. These sutures can be placed with an interarticular stitching device. Once these sutures have been placed, small suture channels are drilled through the anterior aspect of the tibia, exiting in the base of the crater. The previously placed sutures are then pulled through these drill holes and tied over a bony bridge on the proximal tibia. These small central drill holes through the physis probably have no effect on later growth.[28] If one wishes to avoid drilling through the physis altogether, the holes can be placed in the epiphysis only and similarly tied over a bony bridge. When pulling these sutures tight, anatomical reduction of the fracture site should be confirmed through direct arthroscopic visualization.

As with an adult patient, a comprehensive rehabilitation program is essential for an optimum result. Depending on the type of graft chosen and the adequacy of fixation, the program may include an initial period of immobilization. With the tibial eminence fractures, this immobilization should occur with the leg near full extension for the added benefit of mechanical reduction at the fracture site. For reconstructive procedures, the knee is often immobilized initially in 45 degrees of flexion to decrease tension on the graft. During this initial 4 weeks, isometric exercises are performed as well as straight leg lifting. Problems with stiffness are rare in children, so the risk of immobilization is not as great as in the adult. Once this initial immobilization is completed, motion is begun. Motion in the 0- to 60-degree range is allowed initially and increased by 10 degrees of flexion each week. Depending on the type of graft and fixation, partial weight bearing is begun approximately at 6 weeks and full weight bearing by 8 weeks. Bicycling, swimming, leg press, and sports cords–type activities start at approximately 3 months and jogging is begun at 6 months (Fig. 35–10). Full return to sports is not attempted until 10 to 12 months following surgery. We recommend a sports brace for the first year or two after returning to sports while maturation and remodeling of the graft are still occurring (Table 35–3).

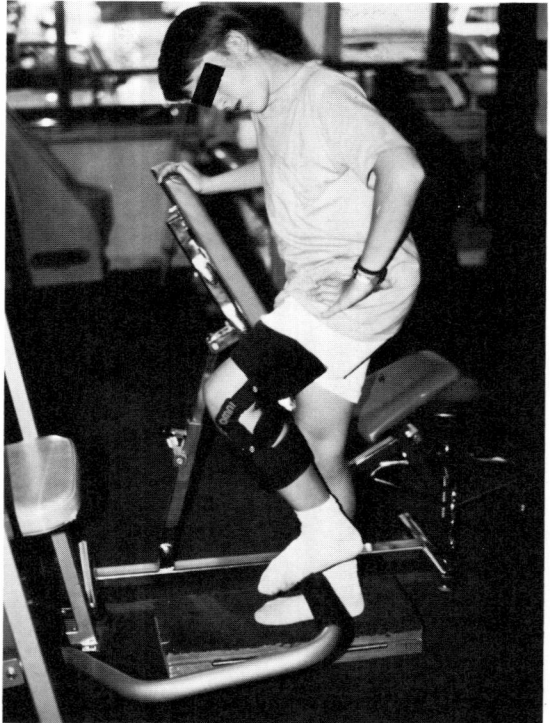
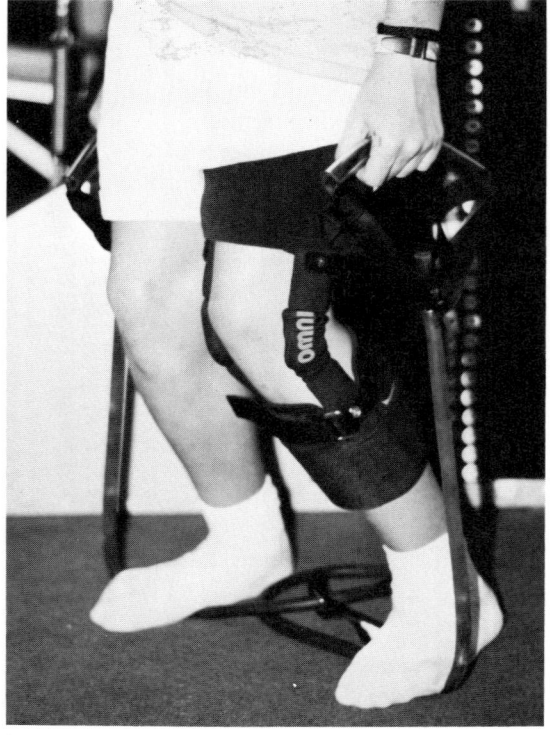

A B

FIGURE 35–10. Postoperative rehabilitation. (*A*) Leg press program. (*B*) Sports cords.

TABLE 35–3. Anterior Cruciate Ligament Rehabilitation for Skiing

Immobilization (0 to 4 Weeks)
Brace locked at 40 degrees for straight leg raising, isometrics
Electrical stimulation optional
Well-leg cycling

Range of Motion (0 to 8 Weeks)
Early passive range of motion (may use prone hamstring curls)
    Begin on first postop week with 0 to 70 degrees, then increase flexion by 10 degrees per week, starting on fourth postop week
Active range of motion
    Begin on first postop week with 0 to 70 degrees, then increase flexion and extension by 10 degrees per week, starting on sixth postop week

Progressive Weight Bearing
Start with 25 percent of weight on the third postop week and increase 25 percent per week (full weight at sixth postop week)

Functional Phase
Swimming and sports cords at fourth postop week
Minisquats, leg press, stationary cycling at eighth postop week
Trampoline, rowing, Nordic Track, outdoor biking (level ground) at twelfth to fourteenth postop week
Pogo ball, balance board at sixteenth postop week
Outdoor biking (hills) at twentieth postop week
Jogging program at 6 months (straight-ahead)

Return to Skiing at 9 to 12 Months While Wearing Sports Brace

---

One must carefully evaluate the associated ligamentous and meniscal injuries at the time of treatment of anterior cruciate ligament injuries. Skiing injuries often involve an external rotation/valgus mechanism, so the medial collateral ligament is often involved. When a grade III disruption of the medial collateral ligament is associated with an anterior cruciate ligament tear, we would not recommend primary repair of the medial collateral ligament. A child's medial collateral ligament is likely to heal at proper tension when treated conservatively. We would recommend anterior cruciate ligament reconstruction if the patient were close to skeletal maturity. In the case of a younger child with anterior cruciate and medial collateral ligament injuries, we would use a collateral brace for 6 weeks to protect the healing medial collateral ligament and then switch to a functional brace for the anterior cruciate ligament.

If the medial collateral ligament injury is an isolated injury, we recommend nonoperative treatment, as described in Chapter 17. With an isolated medial collateral ligament injury, one must always remember that a physeal injury can mimic a ruptured medial collateral ligament by allowing opening at the physis with valgus stress. Stress X rays may be necessary to rule out the physeal injury.

In summary, careful examination with a high index of suspicion should be carried out on any child who presents with a potential injury to the anterior cruciate ligament complex. Hemarthrosis should make one suspicious of injury to this complex. Once the diagnosis is made and all associated injuries are evaluated, we recommend an aggressive approach to the anterior cruciate ligament in the child. This often involves bracing until skeletal maturity is reached, followed by intraarticular reconstruction of the anterior cruciate ligament. Tibial eminence fractures are treated by anatomical reduction of the fracture fragment by closed or open techniques. The choice of graft and reconstruction technique should take into account the open physis and always respect the remaining growth potential.

PREVENTION OF INJURY

As the popularity of skiing increases, there are more and more children and adolescents skiing at younger ages. With this increased enthusiasm, prevention of injury has become a major area of importance. Proper prevention of injury is based on four principles: (1) proper training, (2) proper equipment, (3) skier education, and (4) a search for effective prophylactic bracing techniques.

In order to achieve the proper training, one must have a full understanding of the demands of the sport of skiing. Most of the work in this area has been performed by Steadman and his associates.[37] Steadman states that skiing requires aerobic fitness. A very high oxygen consumption has been documented while skiing as well as a very rapid heart rate. In order to reduce fatigue, therefore, one must have good aerobic conditioning. The highest injury rate has been shown to occur in the afternoon, which suggests fatigue or lack of aerobic fitness.[15, 37] Aerobic conditioning can be achieved with any activity that requires moderate effort for long periods of time. Such training may include bicycling, jogging, rowing, or other similar activities. Strength and endurance are also key elements to prevention of injury.

Strength is especially important in the lower extremities, where appropriate strength and muscle balance are required to maintain a skier's position and balance. Exercises should emphasize quadriceps and hamstring strength since these muscles are important for balance. Strength and endurance, Steadman points out, are best achieved with both concentric training and eccentric training. These can be achieved with leg presses or minisquats utilizing weights or elastic "sports cords" for the quads and leg curls for the hamstrings. It is important to remember to avoid injury to the patellofemoral joint during resistance work. If prior patellofemoral pathology is present, one must modify the training activities to help reduce the patellofemoral forces.

The next element in the prevention of ski injuries is equipment. The best review of the relationship between equipment and injuries is by Ettlinger and Johnson in 1982.[14] The original skis were quite rigid, with the boot being strapped to the ski. The boot was also quite flexible, resulting in many ankle sprains and ankle fractures as well as tibial fractures. The tibia fractures were often of the spiral pattern. In the 1940s and the 1950s, equipment manufacturers began producing release bindings. However, it was not until several years later that there was a change in the pattern of injuries. Much of the change may be related to stiffer, higher boots as well as release bindings. Currently, much of the stress is seen at the knee.

Over the last 5 years, bindings have also been changing dramatically. Manufacturers are now producing bindings that release upward at the toe piece as well as bindings that release in multiple directions besides the traditional side-to-side release. More manufacturers are making children's bindings as sophisticated as adult bindings with ski brakes, low-friction plastic liners for the toe piece, hold-down lugs, more rollers and Teflon pads, increased adjustability, and better materials.[10, 14] Before the last 2 or 3 years, not every manufacturer was offering top-of-the-line adult features in child and junior boots and bindings.[13] Ettlinger stated that children's boots are often fabricated from a softer plastic to allow the boot to flex more easily. The softer materials are usually high in friction, which he points out is a potentially dangerous combination. In addition, children are often growing rapidly and frequently wear hand-me-down equipment from older siblings that is not always the correct size for them. Finally, little equipment is available for a child under 30 pounds, since that is the lower limit for binding settings.[12] Children's equipment should be fitted and adjusted properly. The bindings should be frequently retested and adjusted appropriately for the growing child. Proper equipment and fit are major factors in avoiding injuries in children.

A third factor that may reduce injuries is a sound education program. This education should certainly begin at a young age so that as children are learning to ski, they also learn what precautions help reduce injuries. The National Ski Area Association stresses the importance of the skiers' understanding their responsibilities in order to decrease the risk of injuries.[1] Their skiers' responsibility code stresses skiing under control, knowing not to stop where you might obstruct a trail or not be visible from above, yielding appropriately to other skiers, using devices to help prevent runaway skis, and obeying the posted signs. Proper skier education will likely prevent injuries and is especially important as the popularity of skiing increases and the ski areas become more crowded.

The area of prophylactic bracing to prevent ski injuries is currently under investigation.[30] In our laboratory, we have developed a surrogate knee in order to test various braces under different biomechanical loads. The American Academy of Orthopedic Surgeons Committee for Evaluation of Preventative Knee Braces has listed seven characteristics for an ideal preventative brace:

1. It should supplement stiffness of the knee to injury-producing loads from both contact and noncontact stresses.
2. It should not interfere with normal function.
3. It should not increase risk factors elsewhere in the lower extremity.
4. It should adapt to various anatomical shapes and sizes.
5. It should not be harmful to others.
6. It should be cost-effective and durable.
7. It should have documented efficacy in preventing injuries.

No current brace fulfills all these criteria. We are currently conducting clinical trials of various types of braces for skiing. In the future, there may be braces to help prevent the epidemic of knee injuries that we have recently seen from skiing.

SUMMARY

The popularity of skiing nationwide has increased dramatically over the last 2 decades. There are more and more children and adolescents involved in skiing at younger ages, and subsequently there are increased amounts of serious injuries to children while skiing. The trend in skiing has been a dramatic decrease in the incidence of injury in all areas except for knee injuries over the last 15 years. These knee injuries commonly involve children. Physicians treating ski injuries must become increasingly aware of this specific injury and the treatment of serious knee injuries in children. The child's knee is unique because of several anatomical considerations as well as the activity requirements for children. Because of the demands on a child's knee, we believe in an aggressive program in diagnosis and treating knee injuries in children. All preventative measures possible should be undertaken to help make skiing a safe and enjoyable sport for children and adolescents. Prevention includes proper training, proper equipment, proper education, and perhaps prophylactic bracing in the future.

References

1. Authoritative source at National Ski Areas Association, Springfield, MA, January 1989.
2. Blitzer, C. M., Johnson, R. J., Ettlinger, C. F., and Aggeborn, K.: Downhill skiing injuries in children. Am. J. Sports Med., 12(2):142–147, 1984.
3. Bradley, G. W., Shives, T. C., and Samuelson, K. M.: Ligament injuries in the knees of children. J. Bone Joint Surg., 61A(4):588–591, 1979.
4. Carr, D., Johnson, R. J., and Pope, M. H.: Upper extremity injuries in skiing. Am. J. Sports Med., 9(6):378–383, 1981.
5. Chick, R. R. and Jackson, D. W.: Tears of the anterior cruciate ligament in young athletes. J. Bone Joint Surg., 60A(7):970–973, 1978.
6. Clanton, T. O., DeLee, J. C., Sanders, B., and Neidre, A.: Knee ligament injuries in children. J. Bone Joint Surg., 61A(8):1195–1201, 1979.
7. DeLee, J. C. and Curtis, R.: Anterior cruciate ligament insufficiency in children. Clin. Orthop., 172:112–118, 1983.
8. Derkash, R. S., Matyas, J. R., Weaver, J. K., Oden, R. R., Kirk, R. E., Freeman, J. R., and Cipriano, F. J.: Acute surgical repair of the skiers thumb. Clin. Orthop., 216:29–33, 1987.
9. Ellison, A. E.: Skiing injuries. CIBA Clin. Symp., 29(1):1–40, 1977.
10. Ettlinger, C. F.: Children's bindings. Skiing, pp. 116–117, January 1984.
11. Ettlinger, C. F.: Kids' bindings: what you need to know. Skiing, pp. 121–125, January 1986.
12. Ettlinger, C. F.: Junior bindings: ins and outs. Skiing, pp. 120–129, January 1987.
13. Ettlinger, C. F.: Kids' bindings get better. Skiing, pp. 199–216, December 1987.
14. Ettlinger, C. F. and Johnson, R. J. The state of the art in preventing equipment-related alpine ski injuries. Clin. Sports Med., 1(2):199–207, 1982.
15. Feagin, J. A., Jr., Lambert, K. A., Cunningham, R. R., Anderson, L. M., Reigel, J., King, P. H., and Vangenderen, L.: Consideration of the anterior cruciate ligament injury in skiing. Clin. Orthop., 216:13–18, 1987.
16. Freeman, J. R., Weaver, J. K., Oden, R. R., and Kirk, R. E.: Changing patterns in tibial fractures resulting from skiing. Clin. Orthop., 216:19–23, 1987.
17. Garrick, J. G. and Requa, R. K.: Injury patterns in children and adolescent skiers. Am. J. Sports Med., 7(4):245–248, 1979.
18. Gerber, C. F.: Skier's thumb. Am. J. Sports Med., 9(3):171–181, 1981.
19. Gronkvist, J., Hirsch, G., and Johansson, L.: Fracture of the anterior tibial spine in children. J. Pediatr. Orthop., 4:465–468, 1984.
20. Hogen, J.: The most common ski injury. Snow Country, pp. 62–64, December 1988.
21. Howe, J. and Johnson, R. S.: Knee injuries in skiing. Orthop. Clin. North Am., 16(2):303–314, 1985.
22. Johnson, R. J. and Ettlinger, C. F.: Alpine ski injuries: changes through the years. Clin. Sports Med., 1(2):181–197, 1982.
23. Johnson, R. J., Ettlinger, C. F., and Shealy, J. E.: Skier injury trends. Presented at the 7th International Symposia on Skiing Trauma and Safety, France, 1989.
24. Lipscomb, A. B. and Anderson, A. F.: Tears of the anterior cruciate ligament in adolescents. J. Bone Joint Surg., 68A(1):19–28, 1986.
25. McCarroll, J. R., Rettig, A. C., and Shelbourne, K. D.: Anterior cruciate ligament injuries in the young athlete with open physis. Am. J. Sports Med., 16(1):44–47, 1988.
26. McConkey, J. P.: Anterior cruciate ligament rupture in skiing. Am. J. Sports Med., 14(2):160–164, 1986.
27. Marshall, J. R., Warren, R., and Fleiss, D. J.: Ligamentous injuries of the knee in skiing. Clin. Orthop., 108:196–199, 1975.
28. Matz, S. O. and Jackson, D. W.: Anterior cruciate ligament injury in children. Am. J. Knee Surg., 1(1):59–65, 1988.
29. Moreland, M. S.: Skiing injuries in children. Clin. Sports Med., 1(2):241–251, 1982.
30. Paulos, L. E., Drawbert, J. P., France, E. P., and Rosenberg, T. D.: Lateral knee braces in football: do they prevent injury? Phys. Sports Med., 14(6):119, 1986.
31. Peter, R. E., Rachelin, P., and Fritschy, D.: Skiers' lower leg shaft fracture. Am. J. Sports Med., 16(5):486–491, 1988.
32. Rang, M.: Children's Fractures Ed. 2. J. B. Lippincott Co., Philadelphia, 1982.
33. Requa, R. K. and Garrick, J. G.: Skiing injuries in children and adolescents. Presented at the Second International Conference on Ski Trauma and Skiing Safety, Grenada, Spain, 1978.
34. Rockwood, C. A., Jr., Wilkins, K. E., and King, R. E. (eds.): Fractures in Children, Vol. 3. J. B. Lippincott Co., Philadelphia, 1984.
35. Smith, J. B.: Knee instability after fractures of the

intercondylar eminence of the tibia. J. Pediatr. Orthop., 4:462–464, 1984.
36. Steadman, J. R. and Higgins, R. W.: ACL injuries in the elite skier. In: The Crucial Ligaments, Feagin, J. A., Jr. (ed). Churchill Livingstone, Inc., New York, pp. 471–482, 1988.
37. Steadman, J. R., Swanson, K. R., Atkins, J. W., and Hagerman, G. R.: Training for alpine skiing. Clin. Orthop., 216:34–38, 1987.
38. Weaver, J. K.: Skiing related injuries to the shoulder. Clin. Orthop., 216:24–28, 1987.

INDEX

Note: Page numbers in *italic* refer to illustrations; page numbers followed by t refer to tables.

Abdominal viscera injury, in football, 574
Abduction splint, in physeal fracture, 566
Accessory navicular bone, 384–386, *385*
   in ballet, 496
   in basketball, 624
   in running, 648
   in volleyball, 624
Acetabular dysplasia, 516, *516*
Achilles tendinitis, 379–380, 513
   athletic shoe and, 380
   causes of, 379
   clinical findings in, 379–380
   development of, 513
   in basketball, 620–622, *621*
   in running, 645–646
   in volleyball, 620–622, *621*
   stretch box for, 513, *513*
   treatment for, 380, 513
Achilles tendon, 512–513
Achilles tendon rupture, 513–514
Acromioclavicular joint injury, 197–202
   Alexander view for evaluation of, 197
   classification of, *198*, 198–199
   clinical features in, 197
   differential diagnosis of, 198–199
   dumbbell and, 32
   dysfunction, 466, *466*
   Kenny Howard sling for, *199*
   in football, 565
   overuse of, 205
   padded donut for, *199*
   physical examination in, 197–198
   radiographic examination in, 197–198
   sprain, 73
      in hockey, 597
         prognosis for, 597
         signs and symptoms of, 597
         splint for, *597*
         treatment of, 597
      treatment of, 73t
   treatment of, 199–200
   type III, 200–202
   type IV acromioclavicular separation, 202
   type V acromioclavicular separation, 202
   type VI acromioclavicular separation, 202
Active range-of-motion activity, in therapeutic pool, 77
Acute neck injury, in wrestling, return to competition criteria for, 530t
Addiction
   to anabolic steroid, 55
   to cocaine, 58
Adductor, muscle strain of, 124–125
   hockey, 594–597
Adolescent
   anterior cruciate ligament injury in, 295

   arm development of, 448
   as swimmer, 12–13
   as thrower
      conditioning in, 456–463
      unique challenges for, 447–449
   back pain in
      due to anomalous L5-S1, *152*
      due to central disk protrusion, *152*
   bunion in, 495–496
      spacers for, *496*
   endurance training in, 13–15
      evaluation of, 13
      risks of, 14–15
   kyphosis in, 499
   olecranon process in, 449
   proximal humeral epiphysis in, 448
   strength training of, 36–37
   stress in, 105–106
Aerobic fitness measurement, in endurance training, 8–9
   indirect measures of, 8–9
Age, flexibility and, 46
Air splint, for ankle, *571*
Allograft, for anterior cruciate ligament injury, 304
Amenorrhea
   in ballet, 492–493
   weight and, 492–493
Amnesia, 135
Amphetamine, 59
Anabolic steroid, 52–57
   addiction to, 55
   and cardiovascular disturbances, 55
   blood study of, 55
   cholesterol effects of, 55, 56
   cosmetic uses of, 53
   counseling for, 56
   discontinuance of, 54
   generic names of, 53, 53t
   liver and, 54
   mechanism of action of, 54
   psychological effects of, 52, 55–57
   psychosocial aspects of, 111–112
   reproductive system and, 54
   side effects of, 54
   trade names of, 53, 53t
Ankle
   air splint for, *571*
   anatomy of, *366*
   anterior impingement in, *505*
   brace for, *571*
   flexor hallucis longus and, 507t
   inversion sprain of, 508–510
   lateral ligaments in, *367*
   os trigonum and, 507t
   posterior impingement and, *507*, 507t
   posterior impingement syndrome and, *506*

Ankle (continued)
  posterior pain syndromes and, 507t
  taping of, 571
Ankle avulsion fracture, 378
Ankle fracture, 390–398. See also specific type.
  rehabilitation after, 395
Ankle injury. See also specific type.
  anatomy of, 365–368
  anterior impingement syndrome in, 504–505
  in ballet, 497–498, 504–515
  in basketball, 614–620
  in football, 571–572
  in gymnastics, 426–427
  in hockey, 592–593
  in running, 642–646
    compartment syndrome and, 644–645
    muscle strains and, 642–644
    shin splint and, 644
    stress fractures and, 642
    tendinitis and, 645–646
  in swimming, 442
  in wrestling, 547, 547–549, 548
  lateral ligaments in, 366–368
  ligamentous stability in, 370
  medial ligaments in, 365–367
  posterior impingement syndrome in, 505–507
  pseudomeniscus in, 508
  stress fractures and, 398–400
  tarsal tunnel syndrome and, 508
Ankle-instep flexibility, in ballet, 490, 490
Ankle ligament reconstruction, 511
Ankle pain, chronic, 384–390
Ankle sprain, 370–379, 507, 508–511, 510. See also specific type.
  avulsion fragments in, 378, 378
  classification of, 509, 509t
  in basketball, 614–620, 614–620
  in skiing, 678
  in soccer, 659
  in volleyball, 614–620, 614–620
  medial, 376–378, 377
    deltoid tear in, 376, 377
  persistent pain after, 378–379
  physical treatment modalities for, 72, 72t
  rehabilitation after, 372t, 373
Ankle support, in football, 585–586
Ankle taping, 571–572
Annular ligament, 207
Anorexia nervosa, 112
  in ballet, 494
  in gymnastics, 418
Anterior apprehension maneuver, 167
Anterior capsule attachment, 163
Anterior capsule ligament sprain, shoulder, 466, 466
Anterior cruciate ligament injury, 284–312. See also specific type.
  allograft for, 304
  and safe sport, 296
  arthroscopically assisted techniques in, 304
  arthroscopy in, 300
  associated injuries of, 291–292, 292t
  bilateral, 287
  brace for, 297–298
  contributing factor to, 287
  decision making in, 294–296
  degenerative joint disease and, 294
  dynamometer testing for, 297
  enhancement factor in, 287
  familial occurrence of, 287
  femoral notch dimension variability in, 287
  graft placement in, 303, 303
  in adolescent, 295
  in child, 295, 681
  in football, 568–570
  in preadolescent, 304–305
  interference fit screw fixation in, 303, 304
  intraarticular reconstruction in, 301
  Lachman maneuver in, 289, 289
  lateral collateral ligament disruption in, 291
  lateral meniscus in, 291–292
  mechanism of injury of, 286–287
  medial collateral ligament and, 291
  medial meniscus in, 291–292
  meniscal tear in, 291–292, 292t, 294
  muscle fatigue in, 287–291
  natural history of, 293–294
  nonoperative management of, 296–298
  O'Donoghue's triad in, 291–292
  operative procedure in, 299, 302, 303, 304
  Osgood-Schlatter disease in, 306
  patellar tendon graft in, 301
  patient compliance in, 295
  patient education in, 294–295
  patient history in, 284–286
  patient's perception of severity of, 285
  physical examination in, 287–291
  pivot-shift maneuver in, 289–290, 290
  prosthetic device for, 304
  rehabilitation after, 306–312, 308, 308t, 684–685, 685t
    accelerated protocol for, 307–308
    agility activities for, 309
    basketball, 612–613
    closed-kinetic exercise for, 308
    continuous passive motion for, 309, 309
    full knee extension for, 307
    functional activities for, 309
    in high school seniors, 312
    knee swelling in, 312
    ligament augmentation device for, 307
    overuse injuries in, 312
    patient's attitude in, 312
    prone hangs in, 309, 310, 310
    prosthetic ligament device for, 307
    return to sports and, 310–311
    weight bearing in, 307
  Segond fracture in, 292
  surgical management of, 298–306
    delayed, 298
    immediate, 299
  tibial tubercle apophysitis in, 306
  treatment choices in, 295–296
  vs. medial collateral ligament injury, 275–276
Anterior cruciate ligament rupture, medial collateral ligament tear, 281
Anterior drawer test, for lateral ankle sprain, 371, 371
Anterior glenoid, displaced fracture of, 162
Anterior impingement syndrome, in ankle, 504–505
Anterior shoulder capsule, in wrestling, 533
Anterior shoulder pain syndrome, 465, 465–469
Antiinflammatory agent, for muscle contusion, 127
Apprehension maneuver, 167
Arm, in adolescent, development of, 448
Arm injury, strength training for, 33
Arrhythmia, in preparticipation exam, 93
Arthrography
  in lateral ankle sprain, 372
  in osteochondritis dissecans, 244

Arthroscopic meniscectomy, rehabilitation after, 71, 71t
Arthroscopy, 246
  for ankle pain, 379
  in anterior cruciate ligament injury, 300
  in discoid meniscus, 268
  in meniscal tear, 258, 258t, 264–267, 300, 300t
  of glenohumeral joint, 182–183
  of wrist, 422
Artificial turf, 561
Atlantoaxial instability, in Down syndrome, 99, 137–138
Atopic dermatitis, in wrestling, 555–556
Auricular hematoma, in wrestling, 525, 525–527
Avascular necrosis
  Osgood-Schlatter disease and, 355
  osteochondritis and, 411–412
Avulsion fracture, 121–122. See also specific type.
  in running, 636–637
  in skiing, 683
  in soccer, 657–658
  of anterior cruciate ligament, 295, 612, 683
  of fifth metatarsal, 504

Baby Bennett fracture, 230
Back injury. See also specific type.
  in ballet, 516
  in football, 563
  in gymnastics, 425
  in swimming, 442
  in wrestling, 539
  strength training for, 27–28
Back pain, in adolescent
  anomalous L5-S1 and, 152
  central disk protrusion and, 152
Backstroke, 430, 430–431
Ballet, 484–518
  accessory navicular bone and, 496
  amenorrhea and, 492–493
  ankle in, 497–498
  ankle injury in, 504–515
  ankle-instep flexibility in, 490, 490
  anorexia nervosa in, 494
  body proportions in, 488
  body types in, 487–491
  bulemia and, 494
  discoid lateral meniscus in, 499
  dislocation in, 498
  eating disorder in, 494
  exercise in, 494
  external tibial torsion in, 490
  foot in, 490
  foot injury in, 490–491, 500–504
  forefoot in, 495–496
  full pointe in, 491–492
  hindfoot in, 496–497
  hip in, 499
  hip injury in, 516
  hip turnout in, 488–489
  knee hyperextension in, 489
  knee in, 498–499
  knee injury in, 515–516
  leg alignment in, 489, 489–490
  leg injury in, 514–516
  ligamentous laxity in, 488
  lordosis in, 499
  menarche in, 492–493
  midfoot in, 496
  movements in, 484–486, 486, 487
  natural selection in, 487–491
  nutrition in, 493–494
  Osgood-Schlatter disease and, 498
  osteochondritis dissecans and, 498–499
  patellar malalignment in, 498
  positions in, 484–486, 485
  purging in, 494
  rehabilitation and, 517–518
  scoliosis in, 499
  skeletal growth in, 493
  spine in, 499
  spine injury in, 516–517
  subluxation in, 498
  subtalar joint and, 496–497
  thinness in, 492
  toe in, 491
  training for, 491–494
  upper body strength in, 517
Bar press, narrow grip in, 33
Baseball, 447–483. See also Throwing.
Basketball, 601–627, 602
  accessory tarsal navicular syndrome and, 624
  Achilles tendinitis in, 620–622, 621
  ankle sprain in, 614–620, 614–620
  calcaneal periostitis in, 624
  calcaneus stress fracture in, 624
  foot injury in, 622–627
  groin muscle injury in, 613
  hamstring injury in, 613
  iliotibial band pain in, 614
  injury epidemiology of, 602–603, 603
  Jones fracture in, 624
  knee fracture in, 607–611
  knee injury in, 603–613
  knee ligament injury in, 611–613
  knee pad for, 606
  lower extremity injury in, 613–614
  Osgood-Schlatter disease in, 606–607, 607
  patellar tendinitis in, 603–606
  posterior tibial tendinitis in, 623–624
  quadricep contusion in, 613
  retrocalcaneal bursitis in, 622
  semimembranosus tendon insertion pain and, 613–614
  Sever's calcaneal apophysitis in, 622, 622
  shoe for, 626–627, 627
  tarsal navicular stress fracture in, 624
Bench press, wide-grip, 31
Bennett's fracture, 231, 231
Beta blocker, 61
Bicep curl
  with cam-shaped bar, 34
  with dumbbell, 34
  with straight bar, 33, 34
Biceps tendinitis, 30
Bilateral sacralization, 516
Bipartite patella, 334, 352–353
Bipennate muscle, 118–119, 118–119
Blood doping, 61–62
  risks of, 62
Blood pressure, in endurance training, 5
  and strength training, 25
Blood volume, in endurance training, 5
Body composition
  in endurance training, 5
  in strength training, 26
Body fat, in wrestling, 549
Body size, flexibility and, 46

Bodybuilding, 21
Bone
    in endurance training, 7–8
    in strength training, 26–27
Bony mallet finger, 219
Boutonnière deformity, 224
Boxer's fracture, 229, *229*
Brace. *See also specific type.*
    ankle, 571
    for anterior cruciate ligament injury, 297–298, 568–570, 686
    for medial collateral ligament injury, *277*
    for posterior cruciate ligament injury, 327, *327*, *329*
    in football, 565, *565*, 568–570, 571
Brachial artery, 211
Brachial plexus injury, 141–142
    classification of, 141
    in football, 562
    in wrestling, 530–531
    mechanism of, 141
    pathomechanics of, 141
Brachialis, 211
Breaststroke, *430*, 431
Bronchospasm, exercise-induced, 96–97
Brostrom lateral ankle repair, 511
Bucket handle tear, of intercondylar notch, 261, 261–262
Bulemia, 112
    in ballet, 494
    in gymnastics, 418
Bunion, 495–496
Burner, in football, 562–563, *563*
Burnout, 106–107
    avoidance mechanisms in, 107, 107t
    definition of, 106
Bursitis
    biceps femoris, 641
    in running, 638–639
    ischial, 639
    periscapular, 470
    prepatellar, 350–351, 542–544
    retrocalcaneal, 622
    subacromial, 466
    trachametric, 638
Butterfly stroke, 430, *430*

Cable cross-over, *32*
Caffeine, 60–61
    adverse effects of, 60
    physiological effects of, 60
    urine concentration of, 61, 61t
    withdrawal syndrome, 60–61
Calcaneal apophysitis, 380
    in running, 647–648
Calcaneal periostitis
    in basketball, 624
    in volleyball, 624
Calcaneofibular ligament, 367–368
Calcaneus fracture, 509
Calcaneus stress fracture
    in basketball, 624
    in volleyball, 624
Callus, 500
Capitellum, in osteochondritis dissecans, 476–477
Cardiac output, in endurance training, 4
Cardiovascular examination, in preparticipation examination, 92–94
Carpal fracture-dislocation, 233, 236

Carpal instability, 235–238
Carpus fracture-dislocation, *236*
Cartilage, in endurance training, 7–8
Cephalgia, in strength training, 34–35
Cervical collar, 563
    in football, 585
Cervical cord neuropraxia, 139–141, 563
Cervical disk injury, 139
Cervical instability, 140
Cervical musculature strain, 139
Cervical spine, examination of, *528*
Cervical spine fracture, 137–138
Cervical spine stenosis, Torg's criteria for, *140*
Cervical sprain, 139
Cervical strain, in wrestling, 529–530
Cervical strain syndrome, 28
Cervical vertebral fracture, comminuted, 138
Chest injury, in strength training, 28–29
Child
    acromio-clavicular joint of, 193, 199
    anterior cruciate ligament injury in, 295, *681*
    gamekeeper's thumb in, 675, 676, *676*
    in ballet, 491–492
    in endurance training, 13–15
        risks of, 14–15
    meniscal tear in, 256
        arthroscopy for, 258, 258t
    strength training in, 36–37
Chondral fracture of patella, 351
Chondromalacia of patella, 347
Chrisman-Snook lateral ankle reconstruction, 374–376
Circuit training, 20–21
Clavicle
    anatomy of, 190–191
    function of, 190–191
    insertions of, 191, *191*
    muscular attachments of, 191, *191*
    osteolysis of distal end of, *31*
Clavicle dislocation, in football, 565
Clavicle fracture, 192–197
    classification of, 193, *193*
    clinical features of, 192
    complications of, 196–197
    differential diagnosis of, 193
    harness for, 194
    in hockey
        prognosis in, 599
        shoulder pad for, *599*
        signs and symptoms in, 598
        treatment of, 599
    internal fixation of, 194
    physical examination in, 192–193
    prognosis in, 196
    radiographic examination in, 192–193
    rehabilitation after, 194–195
    sling for, 194
    treatment of, 194–197, *196*, *197*
Clavicle injury, 190–205
Clay shoveler's fracture, 138–139
Cocaine, 58–59
    addiction to, 58
    cardiovascular effects of, 59
    psychological effects of, 58–59
    side effects of, 58–59
Cold compression unit, 70
Collar. *See also specific type.*
    in football, 563, *563*
Collateral ligament injury. *See also specific type.*
    medial. *See* Medial collateral ligament injury.
    of finger metacarpal phalangeal joint, 226

of knee, 272–282
of thumb, 227
Collateral ligament instability, medial, gravity stress test in, 215, *215*
Collateral ligament sprain, medial, *474*, 478
 in football, 570–571
Collateral ligament tear, medial, in anterior cruciate ligament rupture, 281
Commitment, 114
Compartment syndrome, 514–515
Compression fracture, of distal phalanx, 220–221
Compression wrap, for muscle strain, 123
Computerized tomography, of meniscal tear, 257
Concentric contraction, 19
Concussion, 132–136
 and increased intracranial pressure, 135–136
 classification of, 134
 in football, 562
 in wrestling, 523–524
  categories of, 523
  return to competition criteria for, 524
 initial screening examination in, 132–134
 return to competition after, 136t, 136–137
Conduction, 67, 72
Condylar fracture, of finger, 227
Confusion, 135
Congenital C4-C5 fusion, 140, *140*
Congenital cardiovascular disease, in sudden death, 93–94
Connective tissue
 flexibility of, 43
  viscoelastic properties of, 43–44
 in endurance training, 7–8
 in strength training, 26–27
Contact dermatitis, in wrestling, 555–556
Contrast bath, 76–77
 ice immersion in, 77
Contusion
 in skiing, 674–675
 in soccer, 658
 medial, vs. medial collateral ligament injury, 274
Conversion, 72–73
Coracoacromial arch, *181*
Coracoclavicular ligament, *192*
Corn, 500
Counterforce bracing, in tennis, 668, *668*
Crack, 59
Cruciate ligament injury
 anterior. See Anterior cruciate ligament injury.
 posterior. See Posterior cruciate ligament injury.
Cruciate ligament rupture, anterior, 281
Cruciate ligament tear, anterior, 272
Cryotemp, 70, 73, *73*
Cryotherapy, 67–71
 application mode of, 68
 application techniques for, 69–71
 contraindications to, 68
 for medial collateral ligament injury, 276, 277
 for muscle contusion, 127
 for muscle strain, 123
 indications for, 68
 physical principles of, 67–68
 physiological effects of, 68
Cybex dynomometer, isokinetic strengthening, 169

Daily Adjustable Progressive Resistance Exercise, 22, 22t
Dancer's fracture, 502–503

Dancer's tendinitis, 507, 580
Degeneration, in Osgood-Schlatter disease, 355–356
Degenerative joint disease, and anterior cruciate ligament injury, 294
Degenerative spondylolisthesis, 145
Dehydration
 in wrestling, 549–550, 551
 in football, 572–573
Deltoid, strength test of, *529*
Deltoid ligament tear
 in medial ankle sprain, 376
 operative repair of, 377
Demi-pointe, 484
Denial, 109
Dermatitis, in wrestling, 555–556
Dermatological problem, in wrestling, 551–556
Disappointment, 114
 management of, 114–115
Discoid meniscus, 268–269
 arthroscopy of, 268
 classification of, 268
 clinical presentation of, 268
 in ballet, 499
 incidence of, 268
 meniscectomy for, 269
 saucerization for, 269
 treatment of, 269
 Wrisberg ligament type, 268–269
Dislocation. *See also specific type.*
 acromio-clavicular, 197–202
 in ballet, 498
 distal interphalangeal joint, 221
 of elbow, 207–216
 of knee, 328–329
 of metacarpal-phalangeal joint, 224–226
 of patella, 339–347
 of proximal intraphalangeal joint, unstable, 222–224
 of shoulder, 157–189
 sterno-clavicular, 202–205
Distal condylar fracture, treatment of, 228–229
Distal femoral physis fracture, vs. medial collateral ligament injury, 275, 611, 678–679
Distal fibula fracture, 390–391, *391*
 Salter-Harris type I, 390
 Salter-Harris type II, 390, *392*
 Salter-Harris type III, *393*
 treatment of, 391
Distal interphalangeal joint
 dorsal dislocation of, *221*
 thermoplast splint for, *220*
Distal interphalangeal joint injury, 219–222
Distal phalanx
 compression fracture of, *220*, 220–221
 dorsal dislocation of, 221
Distal phalanx fracture, 217, 218, *218*
 intraarticular, *218*
 percutaneous K-wire splinting of, *219*
 thermoplast splint for, *218*
Distal tibia fracture, 391–393
 Salter-Harris type I, 391
 Salter-Harris type II, 391
 Salter-Harris type III, 391–392
 Salter-Harris type IV, 391–392
 signs of, 391
 treatment of, 391
Dorsal dislocation
 of distal phalanx, 221
 of metacarpal phalangeal joint, 224–226, *225*
  complex, 225
 of proximal interphalangeal joint, 222, 223

Dorsal intercalary segmental instability, 235, *237*
Down syndrome
  atlantoaxial instability and, 99, 137–138
  preparticipation exam and, 99
Drug testing, 62–64
  athlete selection for, 62
  confirmation of, 63
  screening test for, 63
  techniques of, 63
  urinary excretion duration in, 63, 63t
  urine manipulation in, 63
Drug use
  enabler in, 111–112
  NCAA-banned, 63, 64, 64t
  psychosocial aspects of, 111–112
  USOC-banned, 63
Dumbbell
  for acromioclavicular joint, *32*
  for pectoralis muscle, *32*
  in bicep curl, *34*
  in decline press, *32*
  in incline press, *32*
Dynamic posterior shift test, in posterior cruciate ligament injury, 322
Dynamic stretching, 44
Dynamometer testing, in anterior cruciate ligament injury, 297

Eating disorder, 112
  in ballet, 494
  in gymnastics, 418
Eccentric contraction, 19
Edema
  in high-volt pulsed galvanic stimulation, 82t
  in medial collateral ligament injury, 273
Effusion, in medial collateral ligament injury, 273
Egyptian foot, 495
Elbow
  anatomy of, 207–210
  arteries of, 209, *209*
  bony architecture of, *208*
  epiphyseal growth plates of, 448, *448*
  ligamentous anatomy of, *210*
  muscles of, 209, *209*
  nerves of, 209, *209*
Elbow dislocation, 207–216
  associated injuries of, 210–211
  classification of, 210
  complications of, 215
  evaluation of, 211
  mechanism of injury of, 210
  medial epidondyle incarceration of, *214*
  nondominant extremity in, 207
  nonoperative treatment of, 212–214
  operative treatment of, 214–215
  pathology of, 210–211
  posterior, *212*
  prognosis of, 216
  vs. lateral condylar fracture, 211
  vs. supracondylar fracture, 211
  vs. transcondylar fracture, 211
Elbow injury. *See also specific type.*
  in swimming, 441–442
    treatment of, 442
  in throwing
    anterior, 471
    flexion contracture in, 477
    flexor-pronator tendinitis in, 477–478, 479

history of, 471
lateral, 471
medial, 476
medial collateral ligament sprain in, 478
medial elbow pain in, 477–481, *478*
medial epicondylar fracture in, 479
physical examination in, 471
posterior, 476
posterior elbow pain in, 481–483
posteromedial impingement in, 478, 481–483
proximal olecranon traction injury in, 480, *481*
ulnar neuritis in, 478, 481
Elbow instability, single axis orthosis and, 214, *214*
Elbow reduction
  puller technique for, *213*
  pusher technique for, *213*
Electrical stimulation, 80–81
  for quadriceps, *83*
  in medial collateral ligament injury, 278
Emergency equipment, 131t
Endurance training, 3–15
  aerobic fitness measurement in, 8–9
    indirect measures of, 8–9
  blood pressure in, 5
  blood volume in, 5
  body composition in, 5
  bone in, 7–8
  cardiac output in, 4
  cartilage in, 7–8
  exercise duration in, 10
  exercise frequency in, 10
  exercise intensity in, 9–10
  factors affecting, 9–10
  fitness level in, 9
  fitness parameters in, 3–6
  heart hypertrophy in, 5
  heart rate in, 4, 4–5, *10*
  in adolescent, 13–15
    evaluation of, 13
    risks of, 14–15
  in child, 13–15
    risks of, 14–15
  in normal individual, 6t
  interval training in, 12
  ligament in, 8
  mitochondria in, 6
  muscle fiber type in, 7
  myoglobin in, 7
  on connective tissue effects of, 7–8
  overtraining in, 12
  oxygen in, 3
  peripheral circulation in, 5–6
  respiratory changes in, 5
  skeletal muscle adaptations to, 6–7
  stroke volume in, 4
  tendon in, 8
  training cessation in, 8
  training program in, 11–13
    competitive period in, 11
    examples of, 12–13
    periods in, 11
    preparatory period in, 11
    transition period in, 11
  training specificity in, 10–11
  ventilary equivalent in, 5
  world-class endurance and, 6t
Energy requirement, in strength training, 26
Epicondylar apophysitis, medial, in tennis, 670
Epicondylar fracture, medial, 479, *479*
Epidural hematoma, 136

Equipment
  for emergency, 131t
  in football, 576–579
  in hockey, 590
  in tennis, 666–668
  in wrestling, 525, 526
Ergogenic aid, 52–65
Evaporation, 67
Exercise. *See also* Rehabilitation.
  duration, in endurance training, 10
  for leg, *458*, 458–459
  for rotator cuff, 460–463, *460–463*
  for trunk, *458*, 458–459
  frequency, in endurance training, 10
  in ballet, 494
  intensity, in endurance training, 9–10
Exercise-induced bronchospasm, 96–97
Exertional headache, 34
Extensor digitorum communis tendinitis, in running, 649
Extensor tendon avulsion, 219–220
External rotation recurvatum test, in posterior cruciate ligament injury, 322
External rotation strengthening, Theraband for, *169*
External tibial torsion, in ballet, 490
Extremity tank, ice immersion, 77
Eye injury, in hockey, 590

Fast-twitch fiber, 119
Fatigue, in running, 632–633
Femoral condyle, in osteochondritis dissecans, *242, 243, 244, 245, 247, 248, 249*
  age distribution in, 242, *242*
  lateral, *243, 246*
  medial, *243, 246*
  site distribution in, 242, *242*
Femoral epiphysis, subclinical slipped, 499
Femoral neck, stress fracture of, 516, 634
Femoral neck fracture, *635*
Femur, *640*
  epiphyseal fracture of, 607
Femur avulsion fracture, in soccer, 657–658
Fibula, 512
  distal fracture of, 390–391
  stress fracture of, 400, *400*, 514, *514*
Fifth metatarsal avulsion fracture, 504
Fifth metatarsal fracture, 502–503, *503*
Finger metacarpal phalangeal joint, in collateral ligament injury, 226
First metatarsophalangeal joint, in football, 572
Fitness evaluation, in tennis, 664–665
  protocols for, 665, 665t
Fitness level, in endurance training, 9
Fitness parameters, in endurance training, 3–6
Flak jacket, in football, *585*, 586
Flexibility
  age and, 46
  body size and, 46
  connective tissue and, 43
    viscoelastic properties in, 43–44
  evaluating, 40–41
  improving, 46–47
  in swimming, 48–49
  injury and, 45–46
  myotactic reflex and, 44
  parameters of, 40–43
  performance effects of, 45
  physiological bases of, 43–44
  program for, 47

sex and, 46
test for, 41–43
  of ankle, 43, *43*
  of calf, 43, *43*
  of hamstrings, 41–42, *42*
  of hip, 41, *41*, *42*
  of hip flexor, 42, *42*
  of hip flexor length, 42
  of knee, *41*
  of quadriceps, 42, *42*
  of shoulder, 41, *41*
  of trunk, *41*, *42*
  of trunk hyperextension, 42
types of, 40
Flexibility training, 40–49
  athletic profile in, 48–49
  in swimming, 49
Flexor hallucis longus, in ankle, 507t
Flexor hallucis longus tendinitis, 505, 507, 508
Flexor-pronator tendinitis, 479, *479*, 670
Fluid replacement, in wrestling, 550, 550t
Fluori-Methane spray, 74
Fluoromethane spray, 70–71
Focal brain injury, 132
Folliculitis, in wrestling, 552–553
Foot, in ballet, 490, 490–491
Foot injury, 365–405, 406–414
  in ballet, 500–504
  in basketball, 622–627
  in football, 571–572
  in running, 646, 646–649, *647, 648*
    stress fractures and, 646–647
  in swimming, 442
  in volleyball, 622–627
  Jones fracture of, *625*
Football, 559–586
  abdominal viscera injury in, 574
  acromioclavicular injury in, 565
  ankle injury in, 571–572
  ankle support in, 585–586
  anterior cruciate ligament injury in, 568–570
  brace in, 565, *565*
  burner in, 562–563, *563*
  cervical collar in, 585
  clavicle dislocation in, 565
  collar in, 563, *563*
  collateral injury in, 570–571
  concussion in, 562
  first metatarsophalangeal joint in, 572
  flak jacket in, *585*, 586
  foot injury in, 571–572
  head injury in, 561–563
  heat illness in, 572–573
    prevention of, 573
  helmet in, 576–579, *577*
    fitting of, 577–579, *578–579*
    maintenance of, 579
  hip injury in, 566–567
  hip pad in, 580, *581*
  historical aspects of, 559
  humerus injury in, 565
  injury epidemiology in, 560–561
  injury prevention in, 560–561
  knee brace in, 568–570, *570*
  knee injury in, 568–571
  lifter in, *566*, 586
  low back pain in, 563–564
  lumbar spine injury in, 563–564
  medial collateral ligament sprain in, 570–571
  mouth guard in, 581

Football (continued)
  muscle contusion in, 567–568
  myositis ossificans in, 567–568
  neck injury in, 561–563
  neck roll in, 585
  neoprene sleeve in, 586, *586*
  orthotic device in, 584, *584*
  padding in, 582–586, *583*
  pelvis injury in, 566–567
  playing surface in, 561
  posterior cruciate injury in, 570
  protective equipment in, 575–586
    fit of, 575
    selection of, 575
  screening in, 560–561
  shoe in, 581–582, *582*
    design of, 561
    fitting of, 581–582
  shoulder harness in, 586
  shoulder injury in, 564–566
  shoulder pad in, 580, *580*
    fitting of, 580
  sideline medical decisions in, 573–576
  socks in, 581
  specialization in, 559
  splinting in, 582–586
    buddy taping in, *582*
  sternoclavicular dislocation in, 565–566
  stress fracture in, 572
  tailbone pad in, 580, 581
  thoracic/rib cage protector in, *585*, 586
  transient quadriplegia in, 563
Forearm injury
  in gymnastics, 424–425
    dowel grips in, 425
  in strength training, 33
Forefoot, in ballet, 495–496
Friedberg's disease, 502, *502*
Full pointe, 484
Fungus infection, in wrestling, 554–555
Furunculosis, 552
  in wrestling, 552–553
Fusiform muscle, 118–119, *118–119*

Gait
  biomechanics of, 368–369, *369*
  stance phase of, 368–369, *369*
  swing phase of, 368–369, *369*
Gamekeeper's thumb, 226, *226*. See also Skier's thumb
  in child, 675, 676, *676*
Gastrocnemius, in muscle strain, 124
Gastrocnemius-soleus complex, in patellar instability, 337
Gel-type cold pack, 69
Gender, and flexibility, 46
Giant set, 22
Glenohumeral joint
  arthroscopy of, 182–183
  bony structures of, 157–158
  capsule of, 158
  ligaments of, 158
  muscle-tendon unit of, 159
Glenohumeral joint dislocation, 598
Glenohumeral joint subluxation, 598
Glenohumeral ligament, inferior, 158
Glenoid, anterior, displaced fracture of, 162
Glenoid margin, osteophyte in, *181*
Godfrey's posterior sag test, in posterior cruciate ligament injury, 320

Gravity stress test, in medial collateral ligament instability, 215, *215*
Great toe metatarsophalangeal joint, 406–412
  anatomy of, *407*
  chronic injuries in, 410–412
  classification of, 408, 408t
  clinical features of, 406
  fracture of, 408–409, *409*
  history of, 407
  physical examination of, 407
  radiographic examination of, 407–408
  sprain of, 409–410
  treatment of, 408
Groin muscle injury
  in basketball, 613
  in hockey, 594–597
  in soccer, 656–658
  in volleyball, 613
Groin pain, in soccer, 657
Growth hormone, 57–58
  and strength training, 27
  side effects of, 57–58
Gymnastics, 413–426
  ankle injury in, 426–427
  anorexia nervosa in, 418
  bulemia in, 418
  eating disorder in, 418
  elbow injury in, 426
  events, 414–416
  forearm injury in, 424–425
    dowel grips in, 425
  historical perspective in, 415
  injury epidemiology in, 419
  knee injury in, 427
  lower extremity injury in, 426–427
  male-female differences in, 416
  men's events in, *416–417*
  nutrition in, 416–417
  shoulder injury in, 426
  spine injury in, 427–428
  upper extremity injury in, 424–425
  women's events in, 418
  wrist injury in, 419–424, *421, 423, 424*
    arthroscopy of, 420–422
    evaluation of, 420–422
    management of, *420*, 420–422
    prevention of, 422–424
    rehabilitation of, 422, *422*

Haglund disease, 623
Hallux rigidus, 408, *408*
Hallux saltans, 508
Hamstring, in eccentric muscle strength training, 125
Hamstring injury
  in basketball, 613
  in running, 637
  in soccer, 658
  in volleyball, 613
  muscle strain and, 124, 125
    physical modalities of, 70
  physical modalities of strain in, 70t
Hand injury, 217–238
  in wrestling, 537
    metacarpophalangeal sprain in, 537, *537*
    proximal interphalangeal sprain in, 537, *537*
Hangman's fracture, 138
Head injury, 130–142
  and increased intracranial pressure, 135–136
  and return to competition, 136–137

classification of, 132, 132t
field decision-making algorithm for, 133t
in football, 561–563
in soccer, 654–656
in wrestling, 523–527
incidence of, 130
logrolling in, *134*
second minor, 135
spine board for, *134*
sports prone to, 130, 131, 131t
transport in, *134*
turning injured athlete in, *134*
Headgear, in wrestling, 525, 526, *526*
Heart hypertrophy, in endurance training, 5
Heart murmur, in preparticipation exam, 93
Heart rate, in endurance training, 4, 4–5
Heat cramp, 573
Heat exhaustion, 573
Heat illness, in football, 572–573
  prevention in, 573
Heat stroke, 573
Heat syncope, 573
Helmet
  in football, 576–579, *577*
    fitting of, 577–579, *578–579*
    maintenance of, 579
  in hockey, 590
Herpes gladiatorum, in wrestling, 553, 553–554, *554*
High-voltage pulsed galvanic stimulation, 80, 81–83
Hill Sachs lesion, 157, 158
Hip, in ballet, 499
Hip adductor strain, in hockey, 594–597
  prognosis in, 596–597
  signs and symptoms in, 594
  spica wrap for, *596*
  treatment of, 594–596, *595–596*
Hip injury
  in ballet, 516
  in football, 566–567
  in running, 633–639
    avulsion fracture of, 636–637
    bursitis in, 638–639
    muscle strain in, 637–638
    overuse bony injuries in, 633
    stress fracture in, 634–636
    tendinitis in, 638
  in soccer, 656–658
Hip joint disorder, in running, 637
Hip pad, in football, 580, 581
Hip pointer,
  in football, 567
  in soccer, 656
Hip synovitis, in running, 637
Hip tendinitis, 516
Hip tendon avulsion, 516
Hip turnout, in ballet, 488–489
Hockey, 590–599
  acromioclavicular sprain in, 597
    prognosis in, 597
    signs and symptoms in, 597
    splint for, *597*
    treatment of, 597
  clavicle fracture in
    prognosis in, 599
    shoulder pad for, *599*
    signs and symptoms in, 598
    treatment of, 599
  epidemiological studies in, 591–592
  eye injury in, 590
  helmet in, 590
  hip adductor strain in, 594–597
    prognosis in, 596–597
    signs and symptoms in, 594
    spica wrap for, *596*
    treatment of, 594–596, *595–596*
  historical aspects of, 590
  injury incidence in, 591
  injury mechanism in, 592, 592t
  injury site in, 592, 592t
  injury types in, 592, 592t
  shoulder dislocation in
    shoulder harness for, *598*
    signs and symptoms in, 598
    treatment in, 598
  shoulder injury in, 597–599
  spinal injury in, 590–591
Hockey ankle, 592–594, *593*
  prognosis in, 593–594
  signs and symptoms in, 592–593
  treatment of, 593, *593*, 594
Humeral head, 157
  Hill Sachs deformity, *161*, *162*
  posterior dislocation of, *178*
    anterior humeral notch in, *179*
Humerus, 207, *208*
Humerus injury, in football, 565
Hydrotherapy
  application techniques of, 76–77
  contraindications to, 76
  indications for, 76
  physical properties of, 76
  physiological effects of, 76
Hyperextension, in wrestling, 527
Hypertension, in preparticipation exam, 92–93

Ice immersion, 70, 73, *73*
  contrast bath, 77
  extremity tank, 77
Ice massage, 69
Ice pack, 69, *69*
Ice pop, *69*
Ice towel, 69
Iliac crest apophysitis
  in running, 633
  in soccer, 656–657
Iliac spine
  avulsion fracture of, anterior superior, 636, *636*
  avulsion of anterior inferior, 122, *122*, 636
  bilateral avulsion of anterior superior, 122, *122*
Iliopsoas insertion avulsion, 122, *122*
Iliopsoas tendinitis, in running, 638
Iliotibial band pain
  in basketball, 614
  in running, 641
  in volleyball, 614
Impetigo, 553
  in wrestling, 553
Impingement syndrome
  of ankle, 504–505
  of shoulder, 469
Inderal, 61
Infection, in Osgood-Schlatter disease, 355
Infrapatellar tendinitis, 515
Infraspinatus fibrosis, 470, *470*
Infraspinatus traction tendinitis, 470, *470*
Injury
  denial of, 109
  determination of, 109

Injury (continued)
　distress in, 109
　flexibility and, 45–46
　lasting deficits from, 110
　personal control and, 110
　problematic adjustment to, 110–111
　vulnerability to, 109
Intercondylar notch
　anterior cruciate ligament, 287
　bucket handle tear of, 261, 261–262
Internal rotation contracture, 470, 470
Internal rotation strengthening, Theraband for, 169
Interval training, in endurance training, 12
Iontophor-PM, 85, 86, 86
Iontophoresis, 80, 84–86
　application methods of, 85–86
　contraindications to, 85
　current generators for, 85
　electrodes in, 85
　indications for, 85
　physical principles of, 85
　physiological effects of, 85
Ischemia, in osteochondritis dissecans, 240
Ischial apophysis avulsion, 122, 122
Ischial apophysis fracture, 637
Ischial bursitis, in running, 639
Isokinetic exercise, 20
Isokinetic strengthening, Cybex dynomometer for, 169
Isometric exercise, 20
Isotonic exercise, 20
Isthmic spondylolisthesis, 145

Jefferson fracture, 138
Jersey finger, 221–222
Jones fracture, 398, 398, 503, 503–504
　in basketball, 624
　in foot, 625
　in volleyball, 624
Jumper's knee, 515

Knee, 240–364. See also Patella.
　effusion, 337
　in ballet, 498–499
　in basketball, 603–614
　in football, 568–571
　in gymnastics, 425
　in hockey, 532
　in running, 639–642
　in skiing, 680–686
　in soccer, 658–659
　in swimming, 440–442
　in tennis, 669
　in volleyball, 603–614
　in wrestling, 541–547
Knee brace, in football, 568–570, 570
Knee joint pain, in running, 639–642
Knee pad, 543, 543
　in basketball, 606
　in volleyball, 606
Knee pain, in swimming, prevention of, 441
Kyphosis, in adolescent, 499

L5 hemisacralization, 516–517
Laceration
　in skiing, 674–675
　in wrestling, 524–525

Lachman maneuver, in anterior cruciate ligament injury, 289, 542
Lateral ankle sprain, 371–376
　anterior drawer test for, 371, 371
　arthrography in, 372
　classification of, 371
　mechanisms of injury of, 371
　radiographic findings in, 372, 372
　surgical treatment of, 374–376, 375, 376
　treatment of, 372–374
Lateral collateral ligament disruption, in anterior cruciate ligament injury, 291
Lateral collateral ligament sprain, of knee, 280, 280
Lateral discoid meniscus, 268
Lateral meniscus, in anterior cruciate ligament injury, 291–292
Lateral patellar glide, in patellar instability, 336
Lateral shoulder pain, 469–470
Lateral tennis elbow tendinitis, 670
Lateral third fracture, of clavicle, 196, 196
Lateral tibial capsular avulsion fracture, in anterior cruciate ligament injury, 292
Latissimus dorsi, in throwing, 455
Laxity, in shoulder tendinitis, 433–434
Leg, exercise for, 458, 458–459
Leg alignment, in ballet, 489, 489–490
Leg injury
　in ballet, 514–516
　in strength training, 29–30
Lifter, in football, 566, 586
Ligament, in endurance training, 8
Ligament injury, of thumb metacarpal phalangeal joint, 226–227
Ligamentous laxity, 165
　in ballet, 488
　in swimming, 431–432
Lisfranc sprain, 504
Little League elbow
　in tennis, 670
　in baseball, 477–478
Liver, anabolic steroid effects on, 54
Long head biceps tendinitis, 465, 465
Lordosis, 517
　in ballet, 499
Low back injury. See also specific type.
　in wrestling, 539, 539–541
　　prevention of, 540
　　treatment of, 540–541, 541t
Low back pain, 144
　in football, 563–564
Lower extremity fracture, in skiing, 678–680
Lower leg injury. See also specific type.
　in basketball, 613–614
　in gymnastics, 426–427
　in running, 642–646
　　compartment syndrome in, 644–645
　　muscle strains in, 642–644
　　shin splint in, 644
　　stress fractures in, 642
　　tendinitis in, 645–646
　in skiing, 677–685, 678
　in soccer, 658–660
　in volleyball, 613–614
　in wrestling, 541–549
Lumbar spine injury, in football, 563–564
Lumbosacral brace
　for spondylolisthesis, 153, 154, 154
　for spondylolysis, 153, 154, 154
Lumbosacral strain, 28

Magnetic resonance imaging
  for achilles tendon, 621
  for meniscal tear, 257
  for osteochondritis dissecans, 244–245
  for patellar tendon, 605
  for shoulder, 161
  for wrist, 421
Maisonneuve fracture, 376, *377*
Malingering athlete
  causes of, 108
  counseling for, 108–109
  fears of, 108
  helpful advice for, 108–109
  need for attention of, 108
  perspective of, 108
Mallet finger, 219–220
Maximum oxygen uptake, different sports compared, 9
Medial collateral ligament
  anatomy of, *273*
  clinical grading of, 274t
  laxity of, *273*
  medial meniscal tear and, 275
Medial collateral ligament injury, 272–282
  adduction exercises for, 278
  anterior cruciate ligament in, 291
  brace in, *277*
  clinical features of, 272
  clinical grading of, 274
  cryotherapy for, 276, *277*
  differential diagnosis of, 274
  edema in, 273
  effusion in, 273
  electrical stimulation in, *278*
  functional rehabilitation program for, 276–279
  immobilization of, 276
  in basketball, 611–612
  in football, 570–571
  in skiing, 685
  in swimming, 442–443
  physical examination in, 272–274
  prognosis in, 279–280
  quadriceps setting in, *278*
  radiographic examination in, 274
  rehabilitation after, 279t
  semitendinosus graft in, 282
  surgical repair of, 280–282
  treatment of, 276–279
  upper body ergometer in, *278*
  vs. anterior cruciate ligament injury, 275–276
  vs. distal femoral physis fracture, 275
  vs. medial contusion, 274
  vs. medial meniscal tear, 275
  vs. patellar subluxation, 275
Medial ligament instability, 378
Medial malleolar stress fracture, 399–400, *400*
Medial meniscal tear, vs. medial collateral ligament injury, 275
Medial meniscus, in anterior cruciate ligament injury, 291–292
Medial patellar glide, patellar instability and, 336
Medial synovitis, in swimming, 443
Medial tennis elbow tendinitis, 670
Medial third clavicle fracture, 195
Menarche
  in ballet, 492–493
  in weight, 493
Meniscal tear, 30, 255–269
  arthroscopy for, 258, 258t, 264–267, 300, 300t
  clinical assessment of, 256–257
  computerized tomography of, 257

diagnostic studies of, 257
discoid, 268–269
excision of, 260, 261–263
excision techniques of, *261*, 261–263, *262*, *263*
history of, 256–257
in anterior cruciate ligament injury, 291–292, 292t, 294
in child, 256
  arthroscopy for, 258, 258t
magnetic resonance imaging in, 257
mechanism of injury of, 256
partial meniscectomy in, 260
physical examination in, 257
rehabilitation in, 264, *264*
stabilization in, 300
total meniscectomy for, 267–268
treatment of, 259–268
types of, 258–259, *259*
vs. lateral collateral ligament sprains, 280
Meniscectomy
  for discoid meniscus, 269
  partial, 260
  total, 267–268
Meniscus
  arthroscopic repair of, 264–267, *265–267*
  development of, 255–256
  discoid. See Discoid meniscus.
  functions of, 255
  hypocellular fibrocartilage in, 255
Metacarpal base fracture, 231–232
Metacarpal fracture, *229*, 229–230, *230*
Metacarpal phalangeal joint, dorsal dislocation of, 224–226, *225*
  complex, 225
Metatarsal stress fracture, *495*, 502
  in running, 646–647
Metatarsalgia, *501*
Metatarsophalangeal joint, great toe, 406–412. See also Great toe metatarsophalangeal joint.
Metatarsophalangeal joint subluxation, *501*
Metoprolol, 61
Microcurrent electrical neuromuscular stimulation, 80, 84
  for pain relief, 84
  for wound healing, 84
Middle phalanx fracture, 227
Middorsal foot pain, 399
Midfoot, in ballet, 496
Mitochondria, in endurance training, 6
Model's foot, 495
Moist hot pack, 75, *75*
Morton's foot, 495
Morton's neuroma, in running, 649
Mouth guard, in football, 581
Multipennate muscle, 118–119, *118–119*
Muscle contusion, 127–128
  antiinflammatory agent for, 127
  cryotherapy for, 127
  in football, 567–568
  mobilization of, 127
  of quadriceps, 127
  pathology of, 127
  prevention of, 128
Muscle fatigue, in anterior cruciate ligament injury, 287–291
Muscle fiber
  composition of, 119
  types of, 119
    in endurance training, 7
Muscle soreness, exercise-induced, 125–126

Muscle strain, 118–129
  body response to, 120–121
  compression wrap for, 123
  cryotherapy for, 123
  grading of, 123
  immobilization of, 123
  in running, 637–638
  mechanism of, 119–120
  of adductor, 124–125
  of gastrocnemius, 124
  of hamstring, 124, 125
  of lumbar paraspinal, 125
  of quadriceps, 124
  of rotator cuff, 125
  pathophysiology of, 119–121
  prevention of, 126–127
  stretching and, 126–127
  treatment of, 123–124
  warm-up and, 126–127
Muscle-tendon unit, anatomy of, 118–119
Myoglobin, in endurance training, 7
Myositis ossificans, 128
  in football, 567–568
Myotactic reflex, and flexibility, 44

Nailbed injury, 217–219
Navicular bone, accessory, 384–386, 385
Navicular bone stress fracture, in running, 646, 647
Navicular stress fracture, in running, 647
Neck exercise program, 532, 532, 533
Neck injury, 130–142
  field decision-making algorithm in, 133t
  in football, 561–563
  in soccer, 654–656
  in turning injured athlete, 134
  in wrestling, 527–533
    on-the-mat assessment of, 527–529
    prevention of, 531–533
    return to competition criteria for, 530
  incidence of, 130
  logrolling in, 134
  spine board in, 134
  sports prone to, 130, 131, 131t
  strength training for, 27–28
  transport in, 134
Neck roll, in football, 585
Neoprene sleeve, in football, 586, 586
Neurogenic pain syndrome, in wrestling, 530–531
  return-to-action criteria for, 531
  treatment of, 530t, 530–531
Neuropraxia, 139–141
Noncompliance, after wrestling injury, 522–523
Nosebleed, in wrestling, 524–525
Nutrition
  and strength training, 35–36
  in ballet, 493–494
  in gymnastics, 416–417
  in soccer, 661–662
  in wrestling, 550–551
    pre-event meal for, 551, 551t

O'Donoghue's triad, in anterior cruciate ligament injury, 291–292
Odontoid fracture, 138

Officiating, in soccer, 662
Olecranon apophysitis, in tennis, 670
Olecranon process, in adolescent, 449
Olympic weight lifting, 21
Orthopedic examination
  90-second screening in, 96, 96t
  preparticipation exam in, 94–95
Orthotics
  for patella pain, 349, 350
  in football, 584, 584
  in running, 649
Os calcis fracture, 509
Os trigonum, 386, 386–387, 505, 506–507
  of ankle, 507t
Osgood-Schlatter disease, 334, 355–359
  and degeneration, 355–356
  and infection, 355
  and patella alta, 359
  and Sever's disease, 357
  and trauma, 356
  avascular necrosis and, 355
  complications in, 359
  differential diagnosis of, 358
  etiology of, 355
  in anterior cruciate ligament injury, 306
  in ballet, 498
  in basketball, 606–607, 607
  in volleyball, 606–607, 607
  of foot, 495–496, 496
  radiographic findings of, 357, 357, 358
  signs and symptoms of, 356–357, 357
  treatment of, 358–359
Osteitis pubis, 634
Osteochondral fracture, Berndt and Harty classification of, 395, 397, 397
Osteochondritis
  avascular necrosis and, 411–412
  in sesamoid, 411–412
Osteochondritis dissecans, 240–252, 334, 351–352, 395, 476
  abnormal ossification in, 241
  arthrography in, 244
  arthroscopy in, 246
  bone grafting and, 247–249
  bone peg fixation and, 247
  clinical features of, 241–246
  drilling for, 248–250, 250
  etiology of, 240–241
  fragment removal in, 247
  genetic predisposition to, 240–241
  history in, 243
  in ballet, 498–499
  in capitellum, 476–477
  in femoral condyle, 242, 243, 244, 245, 247, 248, 249
    age distribution of, 242, 242
    lateral, 243, 246
    medial, 243, 246
    site distribution of, 242, 242
  in talus, 504, 505, 505
  incidence of, 241–242
  ischemia in, 240
  magnetic resonance imaging in, 244
  nonoperative treatment of, 246
  of patella, 351–352, 352
  operative treatment of, 246–252
  physical examination in, 243
  pin fixation in, 247
  radiographic examination of, 243–244
  screw fixation in, 247, 248

trauma and, 241
treatment of, 246–252
in skeletally immature patients, 250–252, 251
in skeletally mature patients, 252
Osteoid osteoma, of tarsal navicular, 505, 506, 506
Osteolysis, of distal end of clavicle, 31, 31, 205
Osteonecrosis, of sesamoid, 501, 501
Overhead throw, 452
Overtraining, 110
in endurance training, 12
Overuse injury, 107–108
of acromioclavicular joint, 205
Overwork, and shoulder tendinitis, 432
Oxygen
in endurance training, 3
uptake stroke volume of, 4

Padding, in football, 582–586, 583
Pain, 110–111
Painful patella syndrome, 515
Parontendinitis, in running, 645
Pars interarticularis, defects of, 146–147
Passive arm adduction, posterior capsule, 169
Patella
articular cartilage of, 332
bipartite, 352–353
in ballet, 498–499
in effusion, 337
osteochondritis dissecans of, 351–352, 352
position of, 335
sleeve fracture of, 609
stress fracture of, 609, 610
supine examination of, 336
turning out below of, 498
Patella alta, 332, 335
Osgood-Schlatter disease and, 359
Patellar pain, 347–350, 515
classification of, 334
history of, 347–348
in swimming, 443
orthotics for, 349
physical examination of, 348–349
rehabilitation of, 349–350
Patella tendinitis, 605
Patella tendon, 604
chronic degenerative change, 605
Patellar dislocation, 275, 334, 339
evaluation of, 339–341
patellar tendon graft and, 328
recurrent, 343
rehabilitation of, 346–347
surgery for, 328
surgical treatment of, 343–346
treatment of, 339–341
Patellar effusion, quadriceps contusion in, 128
Patellar flexion contracture, 257
Patellar fracture, 334, 351
in basketball, 607–611
in volleyball, 607–611
Patellar hyperextension, in ballet, 489
Patellar injury
in ballet, 515–516
in basketball, 603–613
in football, 568–571
in gymnastics, 427
in running, 639–642
in skiing, 678, 680–685
brace for, 682

in soccer, 658–659
in swimming, 442, 442
in volleyball, 603–613
in wrestling, 541–547
by diagnosis, 541–542, 542t
ligament injuries and, 545, 545–547, 546
meniscus injury and, 544, 544–545
on-the-mat assessment of, 541–542
prepatellar bursitis and, 542–544
return to competition criteria for, 542, 542t
rehabilitation after, 684
Patellar instability, 332–347
classification of, 334
effusion in, 337
in gastrocnemius-soleus complex, 337
lateral patellar glide in, 336
medial patellar glide in, 336
physical examination in, 334–337, 335, 335t, 336, 337
quadriceps and, 337
radiographic evaluation of, 338, 338–339, 339
recurrent, 341–342, 343
surgical treatment of, 343–346, 344, 345
rehabilitation of, 342–343, 346t, 346–347
Patellar malalignment, in ballet, 498
Patellar pain, orthotics in, 350
Patellar stress fracture, in running, 639
Patellar subluxation, 275
vs. medial collateral ligament injury, 275
Patellar tendinitis, 334, 359–363
clinical features of, 361, 361
in basketball, 603–606
in volleyball, 603–606
pathogenesis of, 359–360
radiographic evaluation of, 361
treatment of, 361–363, 362, 363
Patellar tendon-bone graft, in posterior cruciate ligament injury, 328
Patellar tendon disorder, 355–363
Patellar tendon graft
in anterior cruciate ligament injury, 301
in knee dislocation, 328
Patellofemoral contact, 332, 333
Patellofemoral joint, biomechanics of, 332–334, 333
Pathologic spondylolisthesis, 145
Patient compliance
in anterior cruciate ligament injury, 295
in wrestling, 522–523
Patient education, in anterior cruciate ligament injury, 294–295
Peasant's foot, 495
Pectoralis
dumbbell for, 32
weighted dip exercise for, 28
Pectoralis major, exercises for, 32
Pectoralis major tendon avulsion, 28
Pelvis avulsion fracture, in soccer, 657–658
Pelvis injury
in football, 566–567
in running, 633–639
avulsion fracture in, 636–637
bursitis in, 638–639
muscle strain in, 637–638
overuse bony injuries in, 633
stress fracture in, 634–636
tendinitis in, 638
in soccer, 656–658
Perimeniscal capillary plexus, 255
Periodization, 23
Periostitis, in ulnar forearm, 34

Peripheral circulation, in endurance training, 5–6
Periscapular bursitis, 470, 470
Peroneal dislocation, 514
Peroneal exercise regimen, 511
Peroneal strength, 511
Peroneal subluxation, 514
Peroneal tendinitis, 380–384, 514
  in running, 646, 649
Peroneal tendon instability, 382–384
Persistence, 115–116
Perspective, 112–113
  guidelines for, 113t
Phalangeal fracture, 227–228
Phenylpropanolamine, 60
Phoresor-PM 700, 85, 86
Physeal fracture, abduction splint for, 566
Physical maturation, and preparticipation exam, 97–99
Physis, premature closure, in triplane fracture, 394
Pitcher
  age limits of, 448
  amateur vs. professional, 455–456, 456t
  conditioning of, 456–463
  training of
    in-season, 457, 457t
    off-season, 457, 457t
Pitching. *See* Throwing.
Pivot-shift maneuver, in anterior cruciate ligament injury, 289–290
Plantar fasciitis, in running, 648–649
Plantar flexion sign, 505
Plyometrics, 21
Postconcussion syndrome, 135
Posterior capsule, in passive arm adduction, 169
Posterior capsule sprain, 470, 470
Posterior cruciate ligament injury, 317–330, 320, 321, 322, 323
  associated injuries of, 323, 323–324
  brace for, 327, 327, 329
  by age, 317
  dynamic posterior shift test in, 322
  external rotation recurvatum test in, 322
  Godfrey's posterior sag test in, 320
  history of, 319
  in football, 570
  incidence of, 317
  intraarticular reconstruction of, 328
  mechanism of injury of, 317–319, 318, 319
  natural history of, 324–325
  nonoperative treatment of, 326–327
  operative management of
    indications for, 327
    technique of, 328–329
  patellar tendon-bone graft in, 328
  physical examination in, 319–323
  posterior drawer test in, 320
  prognosis for, 326
  rehabilitation of, 326, 329
  reverse pivot-shift test in, 322
  Shelbourne's dynamic posterior shift test in, 320
  treatment of, 325–329
Posterior drawer test, for posterior cruciate ligament injury, 320
Posterior impingement syndrome, of ankle, 505–507, 506
Posterior shoulder instability
  acute traumatic posterior dislocation, 177–179
    mechanism of injury of, 177
  anatomical considerations in, 177

  recurrent posterior subluxation in, 179–183, 180, 181
    arthroscopy, 182–183
    surgical treatment of, 182–183
    rehabilitation of, 182, 182t
    surgical procedures for, 183, 183–185, 184
    posterior skin incision in, 183
Posterior shoulder pain, 470–471, 470
Posterior tibial tendinitis, 384, 514
  in basketball, 623–624
  in running, 646
  in volleyball, 623–624
Posteromedial impingement, of elbow, 474, 478, 481
Postinjury adjustment, psychosocial aspects of, 109–111
Postoperative adjustment, psychosocial aspects of, 109–111
Posttraumatic amnesia, 135
Power lifting, 21
Preadolescent, anterior cruciate ligament injury in, 304–305
Preparticipation exam, 88–100
  and sudden death, 93–94
  arrhythmia in, 93
  cardiovascular examination in, 92–94
  disqualifying conditions in, 98, 99–100
  Down syndrome in, 99
  exercise-induced bronchospasm in, 96–97
  format of, 89
  frequency of, 89–90
  heart murmur in, 93
  hypertension in, 92–93
  laboratory tests in, 96
  medical history in, 90, 91, 91
  objectives of, 88–89
  orthopedic examination in, 94–95
  participation recommendations in, 98, 98t
  physical exam in, 90–92, 92
  physical maturation in, 97–99
  timing of, 89–90
Prepatellar bursectomy, 543
Prepatellar bursitis, 334, 350–351
  in wrestling, 543t
  treatment of, 543–544
Profundus avulsion fragment, 221
Profundus tendon avulsion, 221–222
Progressive resistance exercise, 22
Propanolol, 61
Proprioceptive neuromuscular facilitation, 45
Prosthetic device, for anterior cruciate ligament injury, 304
Protective equipment
  in football, 575–586
    fit of, 575
    selection of, 575
  in soccer, 662
Proximal carpometacarpal fracture, 230
Proximal femoral shaft, stress fracture of, 636
Proximal fifth metacarpal fracture, 230
Proximal hamstring tendinitis, in running, 638
Proximal humeral epiphysiolysis, 471
Proximal humeral epiphysis, in adolescent, 448
Proximal interphalangeal joint injury, 222–224
  and dislocation, unstable, 222–224
  and dorsal dislocation, 222, 223, 223
  and volar dislocation, 224, 224
  traveling fellow for, 223
Proximal medial olecranonectomy, 482
Proximal olecranon epiphysiolysis, 480, 480, 481

Proximal olecranon traction injury, 480, 481
Proximal phalanx fracture, 227–228, 228
Proximal radioulnar, 207
Proximal tibia, development of, 356, 356
Pseudo-hallux rigidus, 508
Pseudomeniscus, of ankle, 508
Pubic ramus, inferior, stress fracture in, 634
Purging, in ballet, 494

Q angle, 335, 632, 639
Quadriceps
  electrical stimulation of, 33
  knee effusion in, 128
  muscle contusion of, 127
    in basketball, 613
    in volleyball, 613
  muscle strain of, 124
  patellar instability and, 337
Quitting, 115–116

Rabbit tibialis anterior muscle strain
  histological appearance at 7 days of, 121
  histological appearance at 24 hours of, 121
  histological appearance at 48 hours of, 121
  immediate histological appearance of, 120
Racquet, in tennis, 667
  grip size of, 667, 667
Radial collateral, 207
Radial collateral ligament injury, 227
Radial column wrist problem, in tennis, 670
Radial head dislocation, 210
Radiocapitellar, 207
Radius, 207
Recurvatum, excessive, 498
Rehabilitation
  following anterior stabilization, 176t
  in anterior shoulder instability, 176–177
  in arthroscopic meniscectomy, 71, 71t
  in ballet, 517–518
  in clavicle fracture, 194–195
  in knee injury, 684
  in meniscal tear, 264, 264
  in patella pain, 349–350
  in patellar instability, 342–343, 346t, 346–347
  in patellofemoral pain, 349–350
  in posterior cruciate ligament injury, 326, 329
  in posterior shoulder instability, 182, 182t
  in rotator cuff, 467–468t, 467–469
  in soccer, 662
  in tennis elbow, 671, 671t
  in tibia fracture, 680, 680t
  of ankle fracture, 395
  of ankle sprain, 372t, 373
  of anterior cruciate ligament, 685t
  of anterior cruciate ligament injury, 306–312, 308, 308t, 684–685
    accelerated protocol for, 307–308
    agility activities in, 309
    closed-kinetic exercise in, 308
    continuous passive motion in, 309, 309
    full knee extension in, 307
    functional activities in, 309
    knee swelling and, 312
    ligament augmentation device in, 307
    of high school seniors, 312
    of overuse injuries, 312
    patient's attitude in, 312
    prone hangs in, 309, 310, 310
    prosthetic ligament device in, 307
    return to sports and, 310–311
    weight bearing and, 307
  of posterior shoulder instability, 182t
  of shoulder, anterior dislocation in, 169t
  strength training and, 34–35
  ultrasound and, 78–80
    application techniques of, 79–80
    contraindications to, 78–79
    indications for, 78–79
    physical principles of, 78
    physiological effects of, 78
Repetition, 21
Resistance training, 19. *See also* Strength training.
  program for, 22–23
Retrocalcaneal bursitis
  in basketball, 622
  in volleyball, 622
Retrograde amnesia, 135
Reverse pivot-shift test, in posterior cruciate ligament injury, 322
Rhomboid strain, 470, 470
Rib cage injury, in wrestling, 538, 538
Rotator cuff
  exercise for, 460–463, 460–463
  muscle strain in, 125
  rehabilitation of, 467–468t, 467–469
  throwing and, 456
Rotator cuff dysfunction syndrome, 466, 466
Rotator cuff tear, 469
Running, 632–649
  accessory navicular pseudoarthrosis in, 648
  Achilles tendinitis in, 645–646
  ankle injury in, 642–646
    compartment syndrome in, 644–645
    muscle strains in, 642–644
    shin splint in, 644
    stress fractures in, 642
    tendinitis in, 645–646
  bursitis in, 638–639
  calcaneal apophysitis in, 647–648
  extensor digitorum communis tendinitis in, 649
  fatigue in, 632–633
  foot injury in, 646, 646–649, 647, 648
    stress fractures in, 646–647
  hip injury in, 633–639
    avulsion fracture in, 636–637
    bursitis in, 638–639
    muscle strain in, 637–638
    overuse bony injuries in, 633
    stress fracture in, 634–636
    tendinitis in, 638
  hip joint disorder in, 637
  hip synovitis in, 637
  iliac crest apophysitis in, 633
  iliopsoas tendinitis in, 638
  in chanteric bursitis, 638
  injury risk in, 632–633
  ischial bursitis in, 639
  knee injury in, 639–642
  knee joint pain in, 639–642
  knee stress fracture in, 639
  lower extremity load in, 632
  lower leg injury in, 642–646
    compartment syndrome in, 644–645

Running (continued)
    muscle strains in, 642–644
    shin splint in, 644
    stress fractures in, 642
    tendinitis in, 645–646
    metatarsal stress fracture in, 646–647
    Morton's neuroma in, 649
    muscle strain in, 637–638
    navicular stress fracture in, 646, 647, *647*
    orthotics in, 649
    pain causes in, 645t
    parontendinitis in, 645
    pelvis injury in, 633–639
        avulsion fracture in, 636–637
        bursitis in, 638–639
        muscle strain in, 637–638
        overuse bony injuries in, 633
        stress fracture in, 634–636
        tendinitis in, 638
    peroneal tendinitis in, 646, 649
    plantar fasciitis in, 648–649
    posterior tibial tendinitis in, 646
    proximal hamstring tendinitis in, 638
    running surface for, 633
    sesamoid stress fracture in, 647
    shoe for, 649
    slipped capital femoral epiphysis in, 637
    tendinitis in, 638, 649
    tendinosus in, 645
    thigh injury in, 633–639
        avulsion fracture in, 636–637
        bursitis in, 638–639
        muscle strain in, 637–638
        overuse bony injuries in, 633
        stress fracture in, 634–636
        tendinitis in, 638
Running program, 456, 456t
Russian stimulation, 80, 83–84

Saucerization, of discoid meniscus, 269
Scaphoid fracture, 233, *235*
    displaced, 233, 235
    nondisplaced, 233
Scapularis, in throwing, 455
Scheuermann's disease, 499
Scoliosis
    idiopathic, 499
    in ballet, 499
Segond fracture, *292*
    in anterior cruciate ligament injury, 292
Semimembranosus tendon insertion pain
    in basketball, 613–614
    in volleyball, 613–614
Semitendinosus graft, in medial collateral ligament injury, 282
Sesamoid
    in osteochondritis, 411–412
    in osteonecrosis, 501, *501*
    symptomatic partite, 410
Sesamoid fracture, 500
Sesamoid stress fracture, 410, 411, 412
    in running, 647
Sesamoiditis, 410–411, 500
Set, in weightlifting, 21
Sever's calcaneal apophysitis, 380–381
    in basketball, 622, *622*
    in volleyball, 622, *622*

Sever's disease, 380, 381, *381*
    and Osgood-Schlatter disease, 357
    risk factors of, 380
    treatment of, 380
Shelbourne's dynamic posterior shift test, in posterior cruciate ligament injury, 320
Shin splint, 514–515
Shoe
    in Achilles tendinitis, 380
    in basketball, 626–627, *627*
    in football, 581–582, *582*
        fitting of, 581–582
    in running, 649
    in volleyball, 626–627, *627*
Shoulder, 192
    bony structures of, 157–158
    capsule of, 158
    circle concept of, 158
    double sheet reduction of, *163*
    epiphyseal plate of, 475, *475*
    functional anatomy of, 431–432
    in swimming, 431–441
    ligaments of, 158
    manual flexibility program for, 472–474, *472–474*
    muscle-tendon unit of, 159
    prone reduction of, *163*
    rehabilitation of, 169t
Shoulder dislocation, 30
    anterior
        acute, treatment of, 168–169
        recurrent, 165
        treatment of, 168–177
    in hockey
        shoulder harness in, *598*
        signs and symptoms of, 598
        treatment of, 598
Shoulder harness, in football, 586
Shoulder impingement syndrome, 469
Shoulder injury. *See also* specific type.
    in football, 564–566
    in gymnastics, 426
    in hockey, 597–599
    in skiing, 677, *677*
    in strength training, 30–33
    in throwing, 463–471
        acromioclavicular dysfunction in, 466
        anterior capsule ligament sprain in, 466
        anterior shoulder pain syndrome in, 465–469
        history of, 463
        infraspinatus fibrosis in, 470
        infraspinatus traction tendinitis in, 470
        internal rotation contracture in, 470
        lateral shoulder pain in, 469–470
        long head biceps tendinitis in, 465
        periscapular bursitis in, 470
        physical examination in, 463–464
        posterior capsule sprain in, 470
        posterior shoulder pain in, 470
        proximal humeral epiphysiolysis in, 471
        rhomboid strain in, 470
        rotator cuff dysfunction syndromes in, 466
        shoulder impingement syndrome in, 469
        shoulder instability in, 464–465
        sternoclavicular sprain in, 465
    in wrestling, 533–537
        physical examination in, 534–536, *535, 536*
        return to competition criteria for, 537t
Shoulder instability, 157–188, 434
    anatomical considerations in, 157–159

anterior, 162–177
  acute tramuatic dislocation of, 162–164
  anterior subluxation
    rehabilitation in, 176t
    surgical treatment of, 174–176, *174, 175, 176*
    treatment of, 170, *170*
  harness, 565, 598
  classification of, 159t, 159–160
  complications of, 187–188
  degree of, 160
  direction of, 160
  etiology of, 159
  frequency of, 159
  H-plasty in, *187*
  in baseball, 464–465
  in football, 564–565
  in hockey, 597–598
  in skiing, 677
  in swimming, 433–434
  in wrestling, 533–536
  posterior. See *Posterior shoulder instability*.
  radiographic evaluation of, 160–161
  recurrent, 165
  subluxation in, 165–168
  surgical techniques for, 172–174, *173*
  treatment of, 170
  rehabilitation after, 176–177
  stretching exercise in, *168*
  supine stress test for, *167*
  surgical treatment of, 171–177, 187–188
  T-plasty capsular shift in, *187*
  treatment selection in, 170–171
  West Point axillary radiograph of, 160–161, *160–161*
Shoulder multidirectional instability
  sulcus sign in, 185
  surgical treatment of, 186–187, *187*
  treatment of, 185
Shoulder pad, in football, 580, *580*
  fitting of, 580
Shoulder pain syndrome
  anterior, *465*, 465–469
  posterior, *470*, 470–471
Shoulder pointer, 73
  treatment of, 73t
Shoulder tendinitis
  anterior instability in
    prevention of, 441
    treatment of, 441
  causal factors in, 433
  clinical features of, 436
  hypovascularity of, 433
  in tennis, 669–670
  in training, 437
  laxity in, 433–434
  overwork and, 432
  physical examination in, *434*, 434–436, *435, 436*
  posterior instability in
    prevention of, 441
    treatment of, 441
  prevention of, 436–439
  strengthening of, 437, *437, 438*
  stretching of, 437–438, *438*
  stroke mechanics of, 433, 438–439
  subacromial loading and, 432–433, *433*
  treatment of, 439–441
Sidearm throw, 455
Simian foot, 495

Sinding-Larsen-Johansson syndrome, 334, 359, 360, *360*, 603
Sinus tarsi syndrome, 512
Skeletal growth, in ballet, 493
Skeletal muscle
  in endurance training, 6–7
  in strength training, 25
Skier's thumb, 675, *675*, 676
Skiing, 673–687
  ankle sprain in, 678
  contusion in, 674–675
  injury prevention in, 685–686
  injury trends in, 673–674, *674*
  knee injury in, *678*, 680–685
    brace for, *682*
  laceration in, 674–675
  lower extremity fracture in, 678–680
  lower extremity injury in, 677–685, *678*
  shoulder injury in, 677, *677*
  thumb injury in, 675, *675*, 676, *676*
  upper extremity injury in, 675–677
Skin disease, in wrestling, 551–556
Slipped capital femoral epiphysis
  in running, 637
  in soccer, 657
Slow-twitch fiber, 119
Soccer, 651–662
  ankle sprain in, 659
  blocking tackle in, *653*
  contusion in, 658
  femur avulsion fracture in, 657–658
  groin injury in, 656–658
  groin pain in, 657
  head injury in, 654–656
  heading ball in, *654*
  hip injury in, 656–658
  hip pointer in, 656
  iliac crest apophysitis in, 656–657
  injury incidence in, 654, 655
  injury prevention in, 660–662
  injury types in, 654, 655t
  kick types in, 651–662, *652–653*
  knee injury in, 658–659
  lower extremity injury in, 658–660
  neck injury in, 654–656
  nutrition and, 661–662
  officiating in, 662
  pelvis avulsion fracture in, 657–658
  pelvis injury in, 656–658
  player characteristics in, 651–654
  preparticipation examination in, 660–661
  protective equipment in, 662
  rehabilitation in, 662
  sliding tackle in, 654
  slipped femoral capital epiphysis in, 657
  subcapital stress fracture in, 657
  tendinitis in, 659
  thigh injury in, 658
  tibial contusion in, *661*
  training in, 660–662
  turf toe in, 659
    taping in, *660*
  upper extremity injury in, 656
Socks, in football, 581
Soft tissue injury, 139
Spinal injury
  in ballet, 516–517
  in gymnastics, 427–428
  in hockey, 590–591

Spinal stenosis, 140
Spine
  congenital anomalies in, 516
  in ballet, 499
Spinous process avulsion, 138–139
Spinous process tip, avulsion in, *139*
Splayfoot, 495
Splinting, in football, 582–586
  buddy taping in, *582*
Spondylolisthesis, 28, 144–155
  classification of, 145, 145t
  clinical findings of, 148–153
  etiology of, 146–148
  grade I, *150*
  history of, 145–146, 148–149
  in ballet, 517
  in football, 563–564
  in swimming, 443
  in wrestling, 540
  incidence of, 144, 148
  lumbosacral brace in, 153, 154, *154*
  physical examination in, 149–150
  radiographic findings in, 150–153
  surgical treatment of, 155
  terms in, 145–146
  treatment of, 153–155
Spondylolysis, 28, 144–155, 517, *517*
  active spine extension in, *149*
  classification of, 145, 145t
  clinical findings of, 148–153
  etiology of, 146–148
  history of, 145–146, 148–149
  incidence of, 144, 148
  L4, *150, 151*
  L5, *150*
  lumbosacral brace in, 153, 154, *154*
  passive spine extension in, *149*
  physical examination in, 149–150
  radiographic findings in, 150–153
  surgical treatment of, 155
  terms in, 145–146
  treatment of, 153–155
Sports, classification of, 99, 99t
Sports medicine
  psychosocial aspects of, 105–116
  psychosocial-emotional issues of, 112–116
Staphylococcal infection, in wrestling, 552–553
Static stretching, 44–45
Stationary bicycle, seat adjustment in, *30*
Sternoclavicular dislocation, in football, 565–566
Sternoclavicular injury, 202–205, 465
  classification of, 203
  computed tomography scan in, *203*
  differential diagnosis in, 203
  physical examination in, 202–203
  radiographic examination in, 202–203
  treatment of, 203–205, *204*
Sternoclavicular ligament, 190
Steroid. See Anabolic steroid.
Stimulant, 58–61
Stinger, in wrestling, 530–531. See also Brachial plexus injury; Burner.
  return-to-action criteria of, 531
  treatment of, 530t, 530–531
Strap, *569*
Strength training, 19–37
  arm injury in, 33
  back injury in, 27–28
  body composition in, 26
  bone in, 26–27
  cardiovascular effects of, 24–25
  cephalgia in, 34–35
  chest injury in, 28–29
  concepts of, 19–21
  connective tissue in, 26–27
  definition of, 19
  energy requirement of, 26
  flexibility in, 34
  for shoulder injury, 30–33
  forearm injury in, 33
  growth hormone in, 27
  hormonal effects in, 27
  in adolescent, 36–37
  in child, 36–37
  injuries in, 27–34
  leg injury in, 29–30
  modalities of, 19
  neck injury in, 27–28
  neural effects of, 23–24
  nutrition and, 35–36
  physiological effects of, 23–27
  psychological effects of, 26
  rehabilitation and, 34–35
  skeletal muscle in, 25
  strength effect of, 26
  testosterone in, 27
  wrist injury in, 33
Streptococcal infection, in wrestling, 553
Stress, in adolescent, 105–106
Stress fracture. *See also specific type.*
  in football, 572
  navicular, 399, 624, 646
  of ankle, 398–400
  of femoral neck, 516, 634, 657
  of femur, 639–640
  of fibula, 400, 514, *514*, 642
  of inferior pubic ramus, 634
  of knee, 610, 639
  of medial malleolus, 399–400
  of metatarsal, 502, 646
  of patella, *609*–610
  of proximal femoral shaft, 636
  of pubis, 634
  of sesamoid, *410*, 411, *411*, 412, 647
  of tibia, 514–515, *610*
  subtrochanteric, 635
Stretch box, for Achilles tendinitis, 513, *513*
Stretching
  muscle strain and, 126–127
  shoulder tendinitis and, 437–438, *438*
  technique for, 44–45
Stroke volume
  in endurance training, 4
  oxygen uptake, 4
Subacromial loading, in shoulder tendinitis, 432–433, *433*
Subdural hemorrhage, 136
Subluxation of patella
  evaluation of, 339–341
  in ballet, 498
  recurrent, 343
  rehabilitation of, 346–347
  surgical treatment of, 343–346
  treatment of, 339–341
Subluxing cuboid, 504
Subscapularis tendon, 158
Subtalar joint, 497, *497*
Subtrochanteric stress fracture, 635

Sudden death
  causes of, 95, 95t
  congenital cardiovascular disease in, 93–94
  preparticipation exam and, 93–94
  screening study usefulness in, 95, 95t
Sulcus sign, 168
  of shoulder multidirectional instability, 185
Superset, 22
Supine stress test, for shoulder instability, 167
Suprascapular nerve palsy, 167
Supraspinatus, selective strengthening of, 169
Swimmer, adolescent, 12–13
Swimmer's shoulder
  icing in, 439
  prevention of, 436, 436t
  treatment of, 439, 439t
Swimming, 427–443
  ankle injury in, 442
  back injury in, 442–443
  elbow injury in, 439–440
    treatment of, 440
  flexibility in, 47–48
  flexibility training in, 49
  foot injury in, 442
    treatment of, 442
  freestyle, 428, 428
  knee injury in, 440, 440
  knee pain prevention in, 442
  medial collateral ligament injury in, 440–441
  medial synovitis in, 441
  patellofemoral pain in, 441
  shoulder in, 429–439
  strokes in, 427–429
  training in, 429
Symptomatic partite sesamoid, 410
Syndesmotic complex, 368, 368
Synthetic turf, 561

Tailbone pad, in football, 580, 581
Talocalcaneal coalition, 390
Talocalcaneal ligament, 368
Talofibular joint, 365, 366
Talofibular ligament
  anterior, 367, 370, 371
  in ballet, 508–509
  in basketball, 616, 618
  in hockey, 592
  posterior, 368
Talus
  neck of, 497, 497
  osteochondritis dissecans of, 504, 505, 505
Talus fracture, 512, 512
Talus transchondral fracture, 395–398, 396
  diagnosis of, 395
  mechanism of injury of, 395
Tarsal coalition, 388, 388–390
  conservative treatment of, 390
  incidence of, 388
  physical examination of, 389
  radiographic examination of, 389–390
  surgical treatment of, 390
  symptoms of, 388
Tarsal navicular, osteoid osteoma in, 505, 506, 506
Tarsal navicular stress fracture, 399, 399
  in basketball, 624
  in volleyball, 624
Tarsal tunnel syndrome, in ankle, 508

Tear-drop fracture, 138
Tendinitis, 379–384. See also specific type.
  in running, 638, 649
  in soccer, 659
Tendinosus, in running, 645
Tendinous lesion, 120
Tendon, in endurance training, 8
Tendon insertion, 118
Tennis, 664–672
  common injuries of, 668–669
  competitive strategies of, 666
  counterforce bracing in, 668, 668
  demands of, 664
  equipment in, 666–668
  fitness evaluation in, 664–665
    protocols for, 665, 665t
  goals of, 664
  injury treatment in, 671–672
  Little League elbow in, 670
  medial epicondylar apophysitis in, 670
  olecranon apophysitis in, 670
  racquet in, 667
    grip size of, 667, 667
  radial column wrist problem in, 670
  shoulder tendinitis in, 669–670
  stroke mechanics in, 666, 666
    injury-producing, 666
    protective, 666, 666
  training in, 665–666
  ulnar column wrist problem in, 670–671
Tennis elbow, rehabilitation of, 671, 671t
Testosterone, in strength training, 27
Theobromine, 60
Theophylline, 60
Theraband
  in external rotation strengthening, 169
  in internal rotation strengthening, 169
Therapeutic pool, 77
  active range-of-motion activity in, 77
Thermoconductivity, 67
Thermotherapy, 71–75
  application techniques of, 75
  contraindications to, 74–75
  indications for, 74–75
  physical principles of, 72–74
  physiological effects of, 74
  ultrasound in, 75
Thigh, ultrasound in, 79
Thigh injury
  in running, 633–639
    avulsion fracture in, 636–637
    bursitis in, 638–639
    muscle strain in, 637–638
    overuse bony injuries in, 633
    stress fracture in, 634–636
    tendinitis in, 638
  in soccer, 658
Thigh pad, 581
Thompson peroneal tendon stabilization, 383, 383
Thoracic/rib cage protector, in football, 585, 586
Three-quarter throw, 452–455
Throwing, 447–452. See also specific type.
  acceleration in, 451
  coaching in, 455
  cocking in, 449, 450
  deliveries in, 452–455
  elbow injury in
    anterior, 471
    flexion contracture in, 477

Throwing (continued)
    flexor-pronator tendinitis in, 477–478, 479
    history in, 471
    lateral, 471
    medial, 476
    medial collateral ligament sprain in, 478
    medial elbow pain in, 477–481, 478
    medial epicondylar fracture in, 479
    physical examination in, 471
    posterior, 476
    posterior elbow pain in, 481–483
    posteromedial impingement in, 478, 481–483
    proximal olecranon traction injury in, 480, 481
    ulnar neuritis in, 478, 481
  follow-through in, 451–452
  in adolescent
    conditioning for, 456–463
    pain in, 447–449
  internal rotation in, 464
  latissimus dorsi in, 455
  rotator cuff muscle in, 456
  scapularis in, 455
  shoulder abduction in, 453–454
  shoulder injury in, 463–471
    acromioclavicular dysfunction in, 466
    anterior capsule ligament sprain in, 466
    anterior shoulder pain syndrome in, 465–469
    history in, 463
    infraspinatus fibrosis in, 470
    infraspinatus traction tendinitis in, 470
    internal rotation contracture in, 470
    lateral shoulder pain in, 469–470
    long head biceps tendinitis in, 465
    periscapular bursitis in, 470
    physical examination in, 463–464
    posterior capsule sprain in, 470
    posterior shoulder pain in, 470
    proximal humeral epiphysiolysis in, 471
    rhomboid strain in, 470
    rotator cuff dysfunction syndromes in, 466
    shoulder impingement syndrome in, 469
    shoulder instability in, 464–465
    sternoclavicular sprain in, 465
  windup in, 449, 450
Thumb injury, in skiing, 675, 675, 676, 676
Thumb metacarpal fracture, 231, 231–232
  base fracture patterns of, 231, 231
Thumb metacarpal phalangeal joint, ligament injury in, 226–227
Thumb to forearm sign, 165
Tibia
  midshaft fracture in, 643
  stress fracture in, 610
Tibia fracture, rehabilitation of, 680, 680t
Tibial apophysis, avulsion injuries in, 357
Tibial eminence, hypoplastic, 287
Tibial eminence fracture, 683
Tibial epiphyseal fracture, 608
Tibial stress fracture, 514–515
Tibial tendinitis, posterior. See Posterior tibial tendinitis.
Tibial tubercle apophysitis, in anterior cruciate ligament injury, 306
Tibiofibular joint, 365, 366
Tibiotalar joint, 365, 366
Tillaux fracture, 393, 393–394
Toe, in ballet, 491
Training
  in ballet, 491–494

  in shoulder tendinitis, 437
  in swimming, 431
  in tennis, 665–666
  of pitcher
    in-season, 457
    off-season, 457
Training cessation, in endurance training, 8
Training program, in endurance training, 11–13
  competitive period in, 11
  examples of, 12–13
  periods in, 11
  preparatory period in, 11
  transition period in, 11
Transcutaneous nerve stimulation, 80, 84
  indications for, 80
Transient quadriplegia, in football, 563
Trauma
  in Osgood-Schlatter disease, 356
  in osteochondritis dissecans, 241
Traumatic spondylolisthesis, 145
Triangular fibrocartilage complex, 233
Tricep tendon rupture, 33
Trigonal process fracture, 512
Triplane fracture, 394, 394
  anatomical reduction of, 394
  physis premature closure of, 394
Trochanteric bursitis, in running, 638
Trochlear-olecranon, 207
Trunk, exercise for, 458, 458–459
Trunk injury, in wrestling, 538–541
Tuft injury, 217, 218, 219
Turf toe, 410
  in football, 572
  in soccer, 659
    taping in, 660

Ulna, 207, 208
Ulnar collateral ligament injury, 226, 226–227
Ulnar column wrist problem, in tennis, 670–671
Ulnar forearm, periostitis, in, 34
Ulnar nerve, 211
Ulnar neuritis, 474, 478, 481
Ultrasound
  and patellar tendinitis, 603–605
  in rehabilitation, 78–80
    application techniques of, 79–80
    contraindications to, 78–79
    indications for, 78–79
    physical principles of, 78
    physiological effects of, 78
  of thigh, 79
  thermotherapy and, 75
Unconsciousness, 135
  algorithm for, 131, 133
  disaster plan for, 131
  equipment for, 131, 131t
  management of, 131–132
  moving patient in, 131–132, 134
  training for, 131
Underhand throw, 455
Unipennate muscle, 118–119, 118–119
Upper body strength, in ballet, 517
Upper extremity injury. See also specific type.
  in gymnastics, 424–425
  in skiing, 675–677
  in soccer, 656
  in wrestling, 533–537

Vapocoolant spray, 70–71
Variable-resistance exercise, 20
Ventilary equivalent, in endurance training, 5
Viral infection, in wrestling, 553–554
Volar dislocation, 224
  of proximal interphalangeal joint, 224
Volar intercalary segmental instability, 235
Volleyball, 601–627, *602*
  accessory tarsal navicular syndrome in, 624
  Achilles tendinitis in, 620–622, *621*
  ankle sprain in, 614–620, *614–620*
  calcaneal periostitis in, 624
  calcaneus stress fracture in, 624
  foot injury in, 622–627
  groin muscle injury in, 613
  hamstring injury in, 613
  iliotibial band pain in, 614
  injury epidemiology of, 602–603, *603*
  Jones fracture in, 624
  knee fracture in, 607–611
  knee injury in, 603–613
  knee ligament injury in, 611–613
  knee pad in, *606*
  lower extremity injury in, 613–614
  Osgood-Schlatter disease in, 606–607, *607*
  patellar tendinitis in, 603–606
  posterior tibial tendinitis in, 623–624
  quadriceps contusion in, 613
  retrocalcaneal bursitis in, 622
  semimembranosus tendon insertion pain in, 613–614
  Sever's calcaneal apophysitis in, 622, *622*
  shoe for, 626–627, *627*
  tarsal navicular stress fracture in, 624

Warm-up, muscle strain and, 126–127
Weight
  in amenorrhea, 492–493
  in menarche, 493
Weight lifter's shoulder, 30, *31*
Weight loss methods, in wrestling, 549–550
Weight training, 21
Weighted dip exercise, pectoralis muscle in, *28*
Whirlpool, 72, 75, 76
Working weight, adjustment guidelines in, 23
Wrestling, 520–556
  acute neck injury in, return to competition criteria of, 530t
  ankle injury in, *547*, 547–549, *548*
  anterior shoulder capsule in, *533*
  atopic dermatitis in, 555–556
  auricular hematoma in, *525*, 525–527
  banned holds in, 520–521, *521*
  body fat in, 549
  cervical strain in, 529–530
  concussion in, 523–524, 524t
    categories of, 523
    return to competition criteria for, 524
  contact dermatitis in, 555–556
  dehydration in, 549–550, 551
  dermatitis in, 555–556
  dermatological problem in, 551–556
  fluid replacement in, 550, 550t
  folliculitis in, 552–553
  fungus infection in, 554–555
  furunculosis in, 552–553
  hand injury in, 537
    metacarpophalangeal sprain in, 537, *537*
    proximal interphalangeal sprain in, 537, *537*
  head injury in, 523–527
  headgear in, 525, 526, *526*
  herpes gladiatorum in, 553–554
  high injury rate in, 520
  historical aspects of, 520
  hyperextension in, *527*
  impetigo in, 553
  injuries by region in, 522t
  knee injury in, 541–547
    by diagnosis, 541–542, 542t
    ligament injuries in, *545*, 545–547, *546*
    meniscus injury in, *544*, 544–545
    on-the-mat assessment in, 541–542
    prepatellar bursitis in, 542–544
    return to competition criteria for, 542, 542t
  laceration in, 524–525
  low back injury in, *539*, 539–541
    prevention of, 540
    treatment of, 540–541, 541t
  lower extremity injury of, 541–549
  mastoid dressing in, 527, *527*
  match injury in, 522
  neck injury in, 527–533
    on-the-mat assessment in, 527–529
    prevention of, 531–533
    return to competition criteria for, 530
  neurogenic pain syndrome in, 530–531
    return-to-action criteria for, 531
    treatment of, 530t, 530–531
  noncompliance in, 522–523
  nosebleed in, 524–525
  nutrition and, 550–551
    pre-event meal for, 551, 551t
  permanent neurological loss in, *531*
  potentially dangerous hold in, *521*, 521–522, *522*
  practice injury in, 522
  prepatellar bursitis in, 543t
  return to competition criteria for, 524t
  rib cage injury in, 538, *538*
  shoulder injury in, 533–537
    physical examination in, 534–536, *535*, *536*
    return to competition criteria for, 537t
  staphylococcal infection in, 552–553
  stinger in, 530–531
    return-to-action criteria for, 531
    treatment of, 530t, 530–531
  streptococcal infection in, 553
  tournament injury in, 522
  trunk injury in, 538–541
  upper extremity injury in, 533–537
  viral infection in, 553–554
  weight loss methods in, 549–550
Wrist
  arthroscopy for, 422
  Terry Thomas sign in, *237*
Wrist injury, 217–238, 232–238
  evaluation of, 232–233
  in gymnastics, 419–424, *421*, *423*, *424*
    arthroscopy for, 420–422
    evaluation of, 420–422
    management of, *420*, 420–422
    prevention of, 422–424
    rehabilitation of, 422, *422*
  strength training in, 33
  Thermoplast splint in, *232*
  transscaphoid perilunate fracture dislocation in, *236*
Wrist pain, evaluation of, 233, *233*

p. 91 – Good lux questions for pre-exam forum.